PRINCIPLES OF CEREBROVASCULAR DISEASE

PRINCIPLES OF CEREBROVASCULAR DISEASE

Harold P. Adams, Jr., MD
Professor of Neurology
Division of Cerebrovascular Diseases
Carver College of Medicine
University of Iowa
Iowa City, Iowa

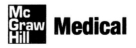

New York   Chicago   San Francisco   Lisbon   London   Madrid   Mexico City   Milan
New Delhi   San Juan   Seoul   Singapore   Sydney   Toronto

Principles of Cerebrovascular Disease

1 2 3 4 5 6 7 8 9 0   CCW CCW   0 9 8 7 6

ISBN-13: 978-0-07-141653-5
ISBN-10: 0-07-141653-6

This book was set in Garamond by TechBooks.
The editors were Anne Sydor, Karen G. Edmonson, and Lester A. Sheinis.
The production supervisor was Catherine H. Saggese.
Project management was provided by TechBooks.
The cover designer was Cathleen Elliott.
The cover image was provided by Scott Camazine/Photo Researchers, Inc.
The indexer was Suneethi Raaja.
Courier Westford was printer and binder.

This book is printed on acid-free paper.

Library of Congress Cataloging-in-Publication Data

Adams, Harold P., 1944-
    Principles of cerebrovascular disease / Harold Adams.
        p. ; cm.
    Includes index.
    ISBN 0-07-141653-6 (alk. paper)
        1. Cerebrovascular disease. I. Title.
        [DNLM: 1. Cerebrovascular Accident. 2. Cerebrovascular Disorders. WL 355 A214p 2006]

RC388.5.A33 2006
616.8'1—dc22
                                                        2006043633

This book is dedicated to my family, particularly my wife, Leah.
They have supported me in my professional activities.
They have always been there when I needed them.

This book also is dedicated to my colleagues, particularly at
the University of Iowa, and my patients who have taught me
and advised me over the last 30 years.

CONTENTS

PREFACE

Cerebrovascular disease is a leading cause of death and human suffering around the world. Despite advances in prevention and treatment, far too many people suffer severe neurological injuries that result in changes to their lives and to those of their loved ones. The effects of stroke on patients' families and to society are huge. The economic consequences of stroke in both health care–related costs and lost productivity are massive. Thus, actions to forestall stroke or limit the subsequent neurological damage following stroke must be expanded. These efforts include continued advances in the knowledge of the basic science underpinnings for the diagnosis and treatment of stroke. These efforts also include translational and clinical research, which already is resulting in dramatic changes in patient care. These advances need to be complemented by increased public and professional understanding about stroke. This book is aimed at providing information about clinical findings, diagnostic studies, and treatment of persons with cerebrovascular disease, including therapies to prevent or treat stroke. While some information about the anatomy and pathophysiology of stroke is included, this is not a neuroscience text. Rather, the book is oriented toward providing clinical insights that might be useful to practicing physicians, residents, and students.

This book is organized to run parallel with the course of evaluation and treatment of a hypothetical patient with cerebrovascular disease. It includes chapters about both ischemic stroke and hemorrhagic stroke that are intermixed throughout the volume. Whenever possible, I included figures and tables to convey information.

The first chapters generally relate to the epidemiology of stroke, identification of persons who are highest risk for stroke, and the risk factors for stroke that can be modified or treated. The third chapter describes the organization of stroke treatment resources (public education, emergency medical services, hospitals, and physicians) that could improve patient care, especially in an acute setting. Chapters describing transient ischemic attacks, ocular manifestations of cerebrovascular disease, ischemic stroke, and hemorrhagic stroke follow. Chapter 8 reviews the usually ordered diagnostic studies including brain, vascular, and cardiac imaging and other tests performed in the evaluation of a patient with stroke. Chapters 9 through 16 then describe the gamut of diseases that may produce either ischemic or hemorrhagic stroke. Also included are chapters describing the causes of stroke in children and young adults and venous thrombosis, pituitary apoplexy, and spinal cord vascular disease. The subsequent chapters describe interventions to prevent and treat ischemic and hemorrhagic stroke. The evidence for the safety and utility of specific medical and surgical therapies is described. In the case of medications, I included some information about the pharmacology of the agents. Complications of stroke and their prevention and treatment are included in this section. The book closes with a review of rehabilitation after stroke and measures to help an individual to return to society.

This is a single-author text and, thus, my perceptions about the utility of specific interventions are expressed. However, I tried to be dispassionate in approach to my evaluation of the data and provide any recommendations about treatment using the rules of evidence. Thus, both therapies that have been shown to be effective and those that are not established as useful are discussed. Some therapies that hold promise but for which there are limited data also are reviewed. The limitations of current knowledge about management and areas where continued research is needed also are discussed. Because new information about stroke is appearing rapidly, I tried to make this book as up-to-date as possible. While I recognize that a book that has a strong emphasis on management may become dated, I hope that this book will provide a foundation for the interpretation of the results of future clinical trials.

ACKNOWLEDGMENTS

The task of writing a book is a considerable undertaking and I have a large number of people to thank. Their contributions to this book are huge and I would not have been able to complete this book without their help.

I thank Dr. Sydney Schochet, Department of Pathology, University of West Virginia; the late Dr. Daniel Jacobson, Department of Neurology, Marshfield Clinic; Dr. Duke Samson, Department of Neurosurgery, University of Texas Southwestern School of Medicine; Dr. Patrick Hitchon, Department of Neurosurgery, University of Iowa; Dr. Enrique Leira, Department of Neurology, University of Iowa; Dr. Patricia Davis, Department of Neurology, University of Iowa; Dr. John Chaloupka, Department of Radiology, University of Iowa; and Mr. Edwin Miller, Department of Surgery, University of Iowa, for providing some of the pictures that are used in this book.

I thank Dr. Kevin Faber and Dr. Matthew Jensen for proofreading this book. Their comments and corrections were very helpful. I thank Karla Grimsman, RN, for her help in organizing the figures and other assistance in development of the book. I also thank Kimberly Aggson, Beth Stecher, and Jessica Fritz for their secretarial support. They helped me with the huge tasks of preparing text, indexing, and completing the bibliographies. Any mistakes in this book are my fault, not theirs.

PRINCIPLES OF CEREBROVASCULAR DISEASE

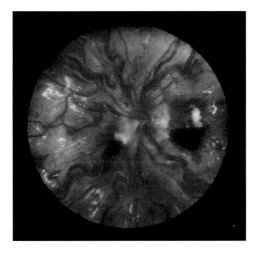

Figure 5-2. Subhyloid (preretinal hemorrhage) found in left eye of an elderly woman with an occlusion of the central retinal vein. Similar findings can be seen with subarachnoid hemorrhage. (*Courtesy of Daniel Jacobson, M.D., Marshfield Clinic, Marshfield, WI.*)

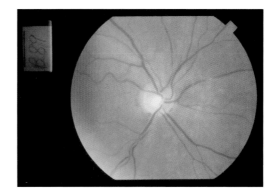

Figure 5-3. Ophthalmoscopic examination of the right eye shows a fibrin-platelet embolus in a branch retinal artery in a patient with amaurosis fugax. (*Courtesy of Daniel Jacobson, M.D., Marshfield Clinic, Marshfield, WI.*)

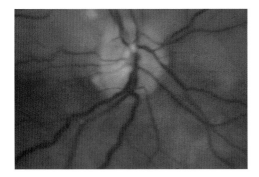

Figure 5-4. Ophthalmoscopic examination of the right eye shows calcific emboli in the proximal segment of the superior branch of the central retinal artery. (*Courtesy of Daniel Jacobson, M.D., Marshfield Clinic, Marshfield, WI.*)

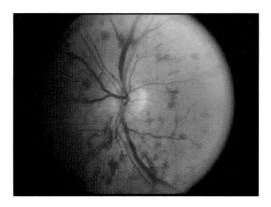

Figure 5-5. Venous stasis retinopathy visualized in the left eye of an elderly man with severe atherosclerotic disease of the internal and external carotid arteries. Note the presence of hemorrhages and the dilated veins. (*Courtesy of Daniel Jacobson, M.D., Marshfield Clinic, Marshfield, WI.*)

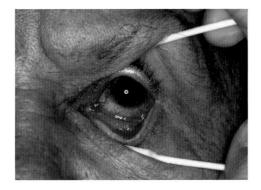

Figure 5-6. Direct visualization of the eye of a patient with severe venous stasis retinopathy shows a large poorly reactive pupil, a cataract, and dilated conjunctival veins. (*Courtesy of Daniel Jacobson, M.D., Marshfield Clinic, Marshfield, WI.*)

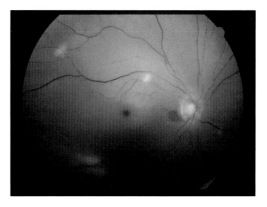

Figure 5-7. Ophthalmoscopic examination of the right eye in a patient with a central retinal artery occlusion shows a cherry red foveal spot, boxcar arteriolar flow, and attenuated arteries. (*Courtesy of Daniel Jacobson, M.D, Marshfield Clinic, Marshfield, WI.*)

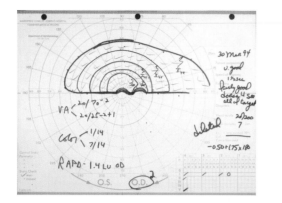

Figure 5-8. Altitudinal loss of the inferior visual field is demonstrated from a branch retinal artery infarction. (*Courtesy of Daniel Jacobson, M.D., Marshfield Clinic, Marshfield, WI.*)

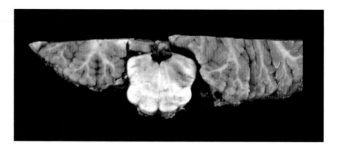

Figure 6-33. Cross section of the medulla and inferior cerebellum shows an infarction in the left dorsolateral medulla. The findings are consistent with occlusion of small branches of the vertebral artery producing the clinical findings of the dorsolateral medullary syndrome of Wallenberg. (*Courtesy of S.S. Schochet, M.D. Department of Pathology, University of West Virginia, Morgantown, WV*)

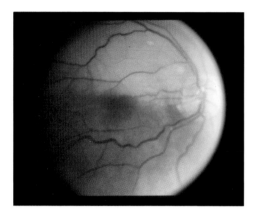

Figure 5-9. Ophthalmoscopic examination of the right eye in a patient with an occlusion with the superior branch of the central retinal artery shows a whitish appearing retina in the superior portion of the eye. (*Courtesy of Daniel Jacobson, M.D., Marshfield Clinic, Marshfield, WI.*)

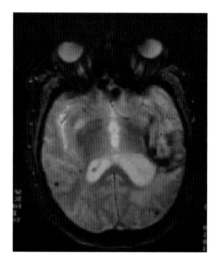

Figure 8-22. Gradient echo MRI shows small area of hemorrhage. Findings are consistent with amyloid angiopathy with small hemorrhage.

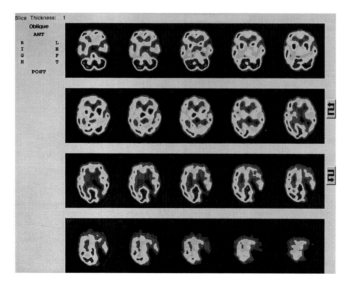

Figure 8-27. A single photon emission CT study (SPECT) reveals an area of hypoperfusion in a patient with a left parietal infarction.

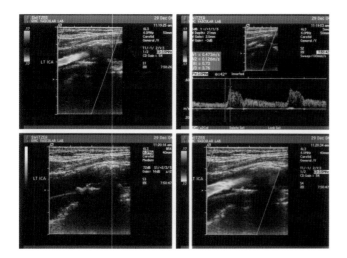

Figure 8-37. Carotid duplex study shows mild to moderate stenosis of the origin of left internal carotid artery.

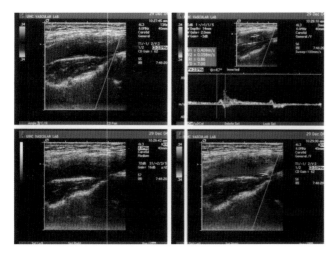

Figure 8-39. Normal carotid duplex study.

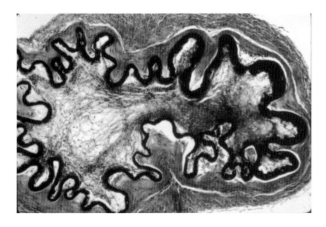

Figure 10-7 Cross section of the middle cerebral artery from a patient with moyamoya disease is stained with elastin stain. Thickening of the elastin-stained components of the arterial wall is seen. (*Courtesy of S.S. Schochet, M.D., Department of Pathology, University of West Virginia, Morgantown, WV*)

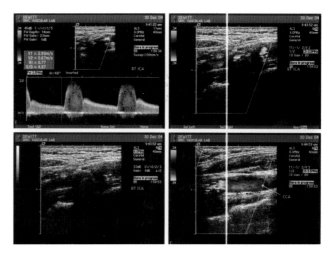

Figure 8-38. Carotid duplex study demonstrates moderate stenosis of the internal carotid artery.

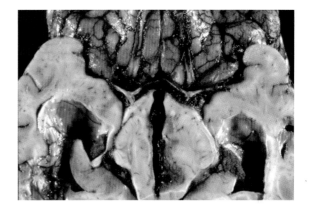

Figure 10-6. Basal view of the brain from a patient dying of moyamoya disease shows the reduction in the caliber of the anterior cerebral and middle cerebral arteries. In addition, small vessels can be seen bilaterally in the Sylvian cisterns. (*Courtesy of S.S. Schochet, M.D., Department of Pathology, University of West Virginia, Morgantown, WV*)

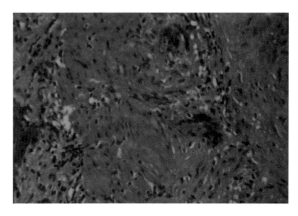

Figure 11-5. A biopsy from the superficial temporal artery in a patient with giant cell arteritis shows marked inflammatory changes, obliteration of the vascular lumen, and giant cells. (*Courtesy of S.S. Schoche, M.D., Department of Pathology, University of West Virginia.*)

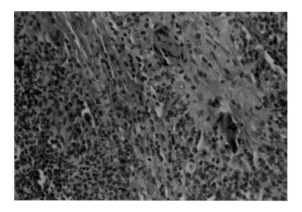

Figure 11-6. An orbital tissue specimen reveals marked inflammatory changes found with a necrotizing vasculitis. The pathological findins are supportive of the diagnosis of Wegener disease. (*Courtesy of S.S. Schochett, M.D., Department of Pathology, University of West Virginia.*)

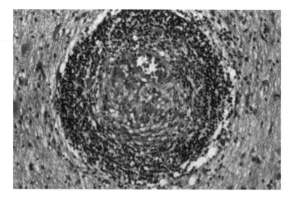

Figure 11-7. Results of brain biopsy demonstrates marked perivascular inflammatory changes consistent with vasculitis. Note that the lumen of the vessel is almost completely obliterated. (*Courtesy of S.S. Schochett, M.D., Department of Pathology, University of West Virginia.*)

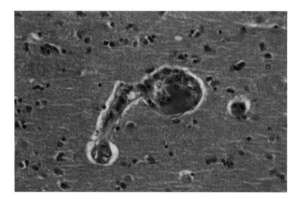

Figure 14-2. Microscopic specimen shows arteriolar occlusions in a patient dying of TTP. (*Courtesy of S.S. Schochet, M.D., Department of Pathology, University of West Virginia, Morgantown, WV*)

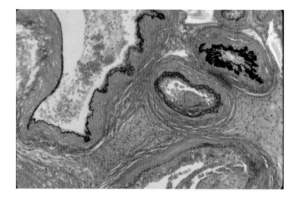

Figure 15-11. Elastic stained surgical specimen demonstrates both arterial and venous structures. The findings are consistent with an arteriovenous malformation. (*Courtesy of S.S. Schochet, M.D., Department of Pathology, University of West Virginia, Morgantown WV*)

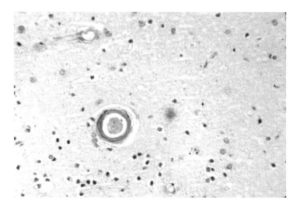

Figure 16-7. Surgical specimen of the brain stained with Congo red shows perivascular amyloid deposits. The findings are those of cerebral amyloid angiopathy. (*Courtesy of S.S. Schochet, M.D., Department of Pathology, University of West Virginia, Morgantown, WV*)

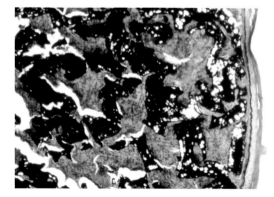

Figure 23-9. Elastic stained surgical specimen of an arteriovenous malformation that was treated previously with embolization shows the polymerization material within the lumen of the vessels. (*Courtesy of S.S. Schochet, M.D., Department of Pathology, University of West Virginia, Morgantown, WV*)

CHAPTER 1

Classification of Stroke, Commonly Used Terms in Cerebrovascular Disease, and the Pathophysiology of Stroke

All physicians, regardless of their practice, encounter patients with cerebrovascular disease. Because strokes are common, serious neurological diseases, physicians are faced with decisions about emergency treatment of these conditions. Because of the widespread prevalence of cerebrovascular disease, physicians are required to make recommendations for the prevention of stroke.

And because cerebrovascular diseases are a leading cause of long-term disability, physicians are responsible for organizing care of chronically ill patients who have had strokes. In order to provide an update on the management of these patients, this book focuses on the principles for the diagnosis and treatment of vascular diseases of the central nervous system.

▶ CEREBROVASCULAR ACCIDENT

Many physicians and other health care providers use the term *cerebrovascular accident* (CVA) to denote stroke. This usage is inappropriate because there is nothing accidental about stroke. The term CVA also implies that nothing can be done to prevent stroke or to limit its neurological consequences, which in turn can lead to a sense of nihilism in stroke care. However, strokes can be prevented. Strokes are due to vascular diseases of the brain, which can be treated. Acute strokes can be treated and patients' neurological outcomes can be improved. The term CVA should be abandoned.

▶ CLASSIFICATION OF STROKE

In this book, the terms *cerebrovascular disease* and *stroke* include hemorrhagic and ischemic vascular

diseases that affect any location of the central nervous system. Several different systems are used to classify these strokes. Cerebrovascular disease is most commonly separated into events that are secondary to bleeding or ischemia, the location of the brain or spinal cord that is affected, the involved vascular territory, the presumed cause, the clinical course, or the time course (Table 1-1). In addition, cerebrovascular disease also includes vascular events that affect eyes or ears. Most strokes are due to occlusion or rupture of an artery or arteriole. Less commonly, stroke can be secondary to venous disease.

Ischemic Stroke

Ischemic stroke secondary to arterial occlusion accounts for approximately 80 percent of all cerebrovascular events. Most cases of arterial occlusion are secondary to *thromboembolism*. The term *cerebral thrombosis* encom-

▶ **TABLE 1-1.** CLASSIFICATION OF
CEREBROVASCULAR DISEASES

General classification
  Ischemic cerebrovascular disease
    Ischemic stroke (arterial thromboembolic stroke)
    Cerebral infarction
    Cerebral thrombosis
    Cerebral embolism
  Hemorrhagic cerebrovascular disease
    Hemorrhagic stroke
    Traumatic intracranial hemorrhage
    Spontaneous intracranial hemorrhage
  Venous thrombosis
  Spinal cord hemorrhage or infarction
  Pituitary apoplexy

passes those cases of occlusion that are secondary to de novo formation of a clot in an artery. In *cerebral embolism*, the thrombus develops in the heart or a proximal extracranial or intracranial artery and subsequently migrates to a distal artery resulting in an occlusion. Occasionally, embolism can be secondary to nonthrombotic material, such as fat or atherosclerotic debris.

Hemorrhagic Stroke

Bleeding in the brain, spinal cord, or adjacent structures accounts for the cases of *hemorrhagic stroke*.

▶ VASCULAR CLASSIFICATION

Knowledge of the vascular anatomy of the central nervous system is crucial for understanding the myriad variations of cerebrovascular disease and for making educated decisions about evaluation and treatment of affected patients. Categorization of vascular events often is based on the involved vascular territory—*carotid* or *vertebrobasilar* circulation. This differentiation is particularly important when deciding about local interventions (surgery or endovascular procedure). The location of an ischemic stroke often is denoted by the name of the occluded artery, for example, the middle cerebral artery (Table 1-2). In addition, recognition of the involved vessel is crucial for the diagnosis and management of patients with hemorrhagic stroke. For example, the location of an aneurysm influences decisions about surgical treatment.

Aorta

Thromboembolic events to the brain can arise from the left atrium, the left ventricle, the ascending aorta, or the *arch of the aorta* (Fig. 1-1). Atherosclerotic disease of the aorta is an increasingly recognized cause of embolic

events to the brain. The descending aorta gives rise to intercostal branches that serve as the parents of radicular arteries, which in turn send branches to the *anterior* and *posterior spinal arteries* that perfuse the spinal cord. The largest of these collateral vessels, named the *artery of Adamkiewicz*, usually arises from the lower segment of the thoracic aorta. In addition, the cervical portion of

▶ **TABLE 1-2.** ARTERIAL VASCULAR
ANATOMY OF THE BRAIN

Arch of the aorta
  Brachiocephalic (innominate) artery
    Right common carotid artery
      Right internal carotid artery
      Right external carotid artery
    Right subclavian artery
      Right vertebral artery
  Left common carotid artery
    Left internal carotid artery
    Left external carotid artery
  Left subclavian artery
    Left vertebral artery
Carotid (anterior) circulation - internal carotid artery
  Ophthalmic artery
  Anterior choroidal artery
  Posterior communicating (posterior cerebral) artery
  Anterior cerebral artery
    Recurrent artery of Huebner
    Anterior communicating artery
    Orbito-frontal artery
    Fronto-polar artery
    Calloso-marginal artery
    Pericallosal artery
  Middle cerebral artery
    Lenticulostriate arteries
    Anterior, middle, and posterior temporal arteries
    Prefrontal artery
    Precentral artery
    Central artery
    Superior and inferior parietal arteries
    Angular artery
Vertebrobasilar (posterior) circulation
  Vertebral artery
    Posterior inferior cerebellar artery
    Anterior spinal artery
  Basilar artery
    Anterior inferior cerebellar artery
    Internal auditory (labyrinthine) artery
    Penetrating (pontine) arteries
    Superior cerebellar artery
    Posterior cerebral artery
      Interpeduncular-thalamic artery
      Posterior choroidal artery
      Thalamo-perforating artery
      Thalamo-geniculate artery
      Anterior and posterior temporal arteries
      Parieto-occipital artery
      Calcarine artery

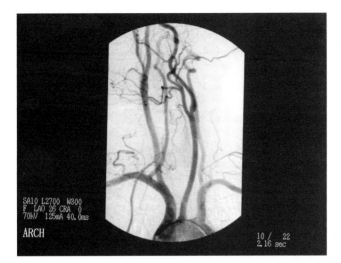

Figure 1-1. Anteroposterior view of a normal arch aortogram demonstrates the major branches of the aorta including the brachiocephalic, left common carotid, and left subclavian arteries. Both vertebral arteries and the bifurcations of the carotid arteries are also shown.

the spinal cord receives collateral branches from the vertebral arteries and the anterior spinal artery receives blood supply from the distal portions of the vertebral arteries. At this location, the anterior spinal artery can perfuse the medial portion of the caudal medulla and its occlusion can lead to bilateral pyramidal infarctions. The venous drainage of the spinal cord is largely via a dorsal plexus of vessels. Vascular malformations, most commonly located dorsal to the cord, can be a cause of hemorrhagic or ischemic lesions of the spinal cord.

Vertebrobasilar Circulation

The *vertebral* and *basilar arteries* supply the brain stem, cerebellum, and the posterior portions of the cerebral hemispheres. The two vertebral arteries arise from the subclavian arteries. In most persons, the *left subclavian artery* is a branch of the arch of the aorta and the *right subclavian artery* is a branch of the *brachiocephalic (innominate) artery*. Occlusive disease of the subclavian artery proximal to the origin of the vertebral artery can give rise to the *subclavian steal syndrome*, in which blood ascends via one vertebral artery and then diverts down the other vessel to perfuse the arm—a circumstance that results in blood being shunted from the cerebral circulation. The vertebral arteries ascend to the head through the transverse foramina located in the lateral processes of the sixth through the second cervical vertebrae. The arteries then perforate the dura to enter the cranial vault via the foramen magnum. The two vertebral arteries unite to form the basilar artery at approximately the pontomedullary junction. The major branches

of the vertebral arteries are the anterior spinal artery, short penetrating arteries that perfuse the dorsolateral medulla, and the *posterior inferior cerebellar artery* (PICA). This vessel sends penetrating branches to the dorsolateral medulla and provides blood to the inferior and lateral aspects of the cerebellum. Branches of the vertebral artery can be involved in vascular malformations located in the posterior fossa and the origin of PICA can be the site of a saccular aneurysm.

The basilar artery sits in the pre-pontine and interpeduncular cisterns in front of the brain stem. The artery divides into its terminal branches, the *posterior cerebral arteries*, at the mesencephalic-diencephalic junction (Fig. 1-2). Several short penetrating arteries rising from the basilar artery enter the anterior and medial portions of the pons and midbrain. Besides the posterior cerebral arteries, the other major branches include the *anterior inferior cerebellar arteries* (AICA) and the *superior cerebellar arteries*. The superior cerebellar artery perfuses rostral cerebellum and the dorsolateral aspects of the midbrain. The dorsolateral pons and the medial and anterior aspects of the cerebellum receive blood via AICA. The *internal auditory artery (labyrinthine artery)* provides blood to the inner ear. This vessel can arise either directly from the basilar artery or as a branch of the AICA. The perfusion beds of the cerebellum can vary considerably between individuals. In some circumstances, one or more of the cerebellar arteries can be hypoplastic or absent and the vascular beds can differ between the left and right cerebellar hemispheres. Venous drainage from the brain stem and cerebellum is

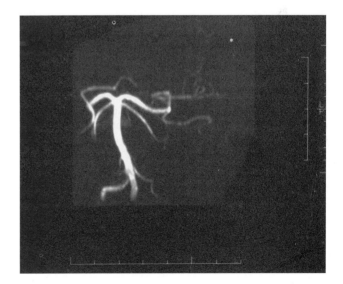

Figure 1-2. Anteroposterior view of a magnetic resonance angiogram of the posterior circulation shows the distal segments of the vertebral arteries, the origin of the posterior inferior cerebellar arteries, the superior cerebellar arteries, and the posterior cerebral arteries.

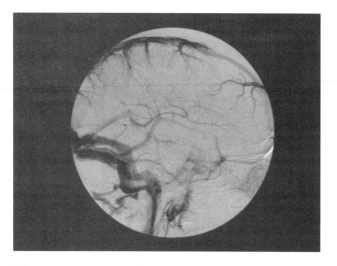

Figure 1-3. Lateral view of the venous phase of the right carotid arteriogram shows both the deep and superficial venous systems draining the cerebral hemisphere.

via small vessels that empty into the *basal vein of Rosenthal*, the *great vein of Galen*, or the *transverse* or *sigmoid sinuses* (Fig. 1-3, Table 1-3).

The diencephalon receives blood from multiple small penetrating arteries that arise from the basilar artery, the proximal portion of the posterior cerebral arteries, or the *posterior communicating artery*. Anatomists have given several names to these arteries, and the resultant confusion has complicated our understanding of these vessels and their vascular territories. In this book, *interpeduncular-thalamic artery*, *posterior choroidal artery*, *thalamoperforating artery*, and *thalamogeniculate artery* are used when describing the small arteries that perfuse the thalamus and adjacent diencephalic structures. The posterior cerebral artery also can receive blood from the internal carotid artery via the posterior communicating artery. In approximately

▶ **TABLE 1-3.** VENOUS DRAINAGE OF THE BRAIN

Cavernous sinus
Venous drainage of the cerebral cortex
    Superior sagittal sinus
      Cortical veins
      Veins of Trolard and Labbé
    Inferior sagittal sinus
Venous drainage of deep hemispheric structures
    Internal cerebral vein
    Basal vein of Rosenthal
    Great vein of Galen
Straight sinus
Transverse sinus
Sigmoid sinus
Internal jugular vein

20 percent of persons, one posterior cerebral artery is a direct branch of the internal carotid artery and the proximal portion of the artery corresponds to the posterior communicating artery. This variation is sometimes described as an embryonic origin of the posterior cerebral artery. The basilar bifurcation and the origin of the posterior communicating artery from the internal carotid artery are frequent sites for saccular aneurysms. The cortical branches of the posterior cerebral artery perfuse the occipital lobe, the medial and inferior portions of the temporal lobe, and the superior and medial aspects of the parietal lobe. The *calcarine artery*, which supplies the primary visual cortex, is a branch of the posterior cerebral artery.

Carotid Circulation

In most persons, the *left common carotid artery* is a direct branch of the aorta, arising proximal to the left subclavian artery, and the *right common carotid artery* is a branch of the brachiocephalic artery (see Fig. 1-1). Both common carotid arteries ascend in the anterior aspect of the neck just lateral to the trachea and medial to the *internal jugular vein*. The common carotid artery bifurcates into *internal* and *external carotid arteries* at approximately the angle of the jaw (Fig. 1-4). The external carotid artery perfuses the soft tissues of the face, the scalp, and the meninges. The external carotid artery is an important collateral channel (usually via orbital and meningeal branches) for maintaining blood flow in a patient with an occlusion of the internal carotid artery.

The internal carotid artery supplies the ipsilateral eye and most of the ipsilateral cerebral hemisphere (Fig. 1-5(a) to 5(c)). Deep penetrating branches of the internal carotid artery provide blood to the basal ganglia, internal capsule, and deep hemispheric white matter. Cortical branches perfuse the insula, the frontal lobe, the superior aspect of the temporal lobe, and the anterior, lateral, and inferior portions of the parietal lobe. The extracranial (cervical) portion of the internal carotid artery ascends just lateral to the vertebral bodies. This portion of the artery is the most common site for atherosclerosis or arterial dissection. The internal carotid artery enters the cranial vault via the carotid canal (this segment is called the petrous portion). The artery then moves anteriorly and medially in an S-shaped curve to lie in the *cavernous sinus* (cavernous portion). Atherosclerotic disease can involve this portion of the artery. Injury to the cavernous portion of the carotid artery can lead to a carotid cavernous fistula. Aneurysms also can arise from the cavernous portion of the internal carotid artery. Branches to the pituitary gland arise from the internal carotid artery as it penetrates the dura to enter the subarachnoid space. The portions of both anterior cerebral arteries are connected via the *anterior communicating artery*. Approximately one-third of intracranial saccular aneurysms arise in the region of the anterior communicating artery.

The middle cerebral artery moves laterally from the internal carotid artery to enter the Sylvian cistern and Sylvian fissure. Thereafter it moves posteriorly and superiorly, giving rise to several cortical branches that supply the lateral and inferior portions of the frontal lobe, the insula, the inferior and anterior portions of the parietal lobe, and the superior portion of the temporal lobe (see Fig. 1-5(a) and Fig. 5(b)). These vessels, which are located along the pial surface of the hemisphere, are aligned from anterior to posterior to form a series of wedges that extend from the cortical surface to deep, adjacent portions of the lobar white matter. These branches are named *prefrontal, precentral, central, superior parietal, inferior parietal, angular,* and *anterior, middle,* and *posterior temporal* arteries. Aneurysms arising from the proximal portion of the middle cerebral artery are most commonly located in the Sylvian fissure. Several deep penetrating branches of the middle cerebral artery *(lenticulostriate arteries)* supply the putamen, the head of the caudate nucleus, and the anterior limb of the internal capsule.

Venous Anatomy of the Hemispheres

The cavernous sinus consists of a plexus of smaller veins that drain blood from eyes, nose, and face (see Table 1-3). There are prominent collateral channels between the two cavernous sinuses. These collateral veins pass around the region of the pituitary. Venous drainage of the cerebral hemispheres is via cortical and deep channels. In general, flow is in an anterior to posterior direction. The cortical veins generally drain into the *superior sagittal sinus, inferior sagittal sinus,* and *transverse sinus*; the largest cortical veins are named the *vein of Labbe* and the *vein of Trolard* (see Fig. 1-3). The former vessel usually drains inferiorly, while the latter vein empties into the superior sagittal sinus. The deep hemispheric structures are drained via the *thalamostriate vein* and *septal vein*. At the foramen of Munro, these two veins merge to form the *internal cerebral vein*, which moves posterior along the medial aspect of the thalamus. The internal cerebral vein joins the basal vein of Rosenthal to form the great vein of Galen at the mesencephalic—diencephalic junction. The great vein of Galen and the inferior sagittal sinus unite to create the *straight sinus*. At the torcula, the straight sinus joins the superior sagittal sinus to form the transverse sinuses. The left and right transverse sinuses often are asymmetrical in caliber and the majority of venous blood may travel via one of the sinuses. The transverse sinuses move laterally and anteriorly along the tentorium and the petrous portion of the temporal bone. From this point

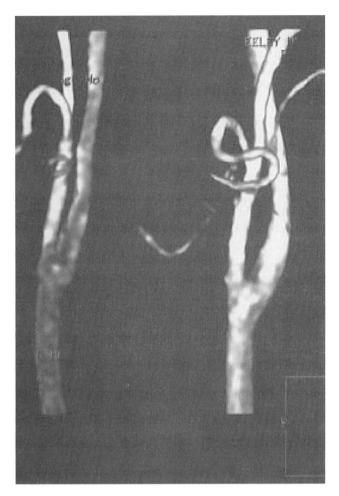

Figure 1-4. Magnetic resonance angiograms of both internal and external carotid arteries show the normal appearance of the bifurcations. The first branches of the external carotid arteries are seen.

ophthalmic artery, which supplies the eye, is the first major intracranial branch. Other important branches of the internal carotid artery are the posterior communicating artery, *anterior choroidal artery, anterior cerebral artery,* and *middle cerebral artery* (see Fig. 1-5(a) and 1-5(b)). The middle cerebral artery is the terminal branch. The anterior choroidal artery perfuses the optic tract, the posterior limb of the internal capsule, adjacent portions of the basal ganglia and thalamus, and the lobar white matter.

The anterior cerebral artery moves anteriorly and medially to a parasagittal location along the medial aspect of the frontal lobe (see Fig. 1-5(a) and 1-5(b)). A deep penetrating branch, the *recurrent artery of Huebner* perfuses the inferior and anterior portion of the head of the caudate nucleus. Cortical branches supply the medial and anterior aspects of the frontal lobe. The major cortical branches are named the *orbito-frontal, fronto-polar, calloso-marginal,* and *pericallosal* arteries. The proximal

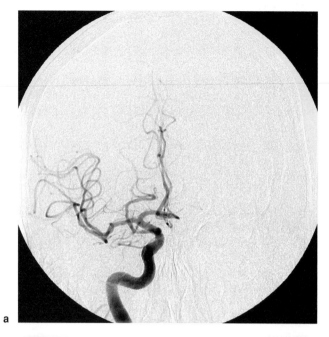

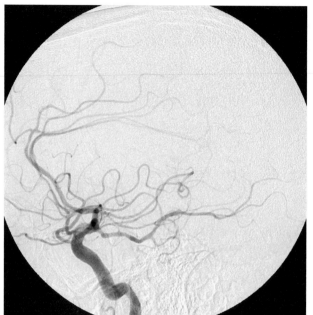

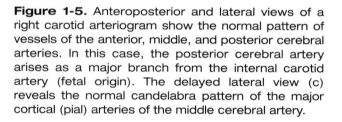

Figure 1-5. Anteroposterior and lateral views of a right carotid arteriogram show the normal pattern of vessels of the anterior, middle, and posterior cerebral arteries. In this case, the posterior cerebral artery arises as a major branch from the internal carotid artery (fetal origin). The delayed lateral view (c) reveals the normal candelabra pattern of the major cortical (pial) arteries of the middle cerebral artery.

onward, the sinus is known as the *sigmoid sinus*. The sigmoid sinus exits the skull via the jugular foramen; from this point onward, the vessel is known as the *internal jugular vein*.

Penetrating Arteries

Several short penetrating arteries perfusing the brain stem and the deep structures of the cerebral hemispheres are end vessels (see Table 1-2). Occlusions of these vessels produce relatively small (<1.5-cm diameter) strokes (*lacunar infarction*) and fairly stereotyped neurological syndromes (*lacunar syndromes*). These

short penetrating arteries are vulnerable to the effects of hypertension, and thus, *hypertensive hemorrhage* occurs primarily in the areas of the brain perfused by these vessels. Larger deep hemispheric infarctions are secondary to thromboembolic occlusion of larger cerebral arteries; the most common is occlusion of the middle cerebral artery that causes a stroke in the distribution of several lenticulostriate arteries (*striatocapsular infarction*).

Collaterals

A broad spectrum of neurological impairments can occur with occlusion of major arteries. For example,

▶ **TABLE 1-4.** COLLATERAL CIRCULATIONS

External carotid artery/internal carotid artery
Circle of Willis
Pial collaterals—terminal branches of cerebral
hemispheres
    Middle cerebral artery
    Anterior cerebral artery
    Posterior cerebral artery
Pial collaterals—terminal branches of the cerebellum
    Posterior inferior cerebellar artery
    Anterior inferior cerebellar artery
    Superior cerebellar artery

one patient may die from a multilobar infarction secondary to an internal carotid artery occlusion while another person may be asymptomatic. The discrepancies partially result from the anatomic presence of collateral vessels of adequate caliber (Table 1-4). Three major systems of collaterals can protect the brain from an arterial occlusion: branches of the external carotid artery, the circle of Willis, and the pial arteries. First, anastomoses between branches of the external carotid artery and branches of the internal carotid artery can maintain adequate brain perfusion in a patient with an occlusion of the internal carotid artery (Fig. 1-6). Muscular branches in the neck can connect with vessels

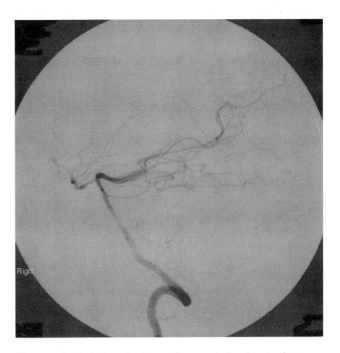

Figure 1-7. Lateral view of a vertebral arteriogram demonstrates flow in the middle cerebral artery via collateral flow through the posterior communicating artery.

in the posterior circulation. The *circle of Willis* constitutes the second major collateral system (Figs. 1-7 and 1-8). The integrity of the circle of Willis differs between persons; in particular, the anterior communicating artery or one or both of the posterior communicating arteries can be atretic. Depending upon the presence of these collateral arteries, the vascular bed of the internal carotid artery can be isolated. In these circumstances, an infarction also can affect the territories of both the anterior and middle cerebral arteries. In some patients, the proximal segment of the anterior cerebral artery may be hypoplastic and the distal anterior cerebral artery receives blood from the contralateral anterior cerebral artery via the anterior communicating artery. The third collateral circulation for the cerebral hemisphere is based on the pial cortical branches of the anterior, middle, and posterior cerebral arteries. A similar pial collateral circulation for the cerebellar hemisphere involves distal branches of the superior cerebellar artery, AICA, and PICA. Because the distal branches of the pial arteries interdigitate, it is possible for blood to be diverted from cortical branches of a patent artery distally to an occlusion of another pial artery. On the other hand, these cortical branches represent the distal arterial territories of the major intracranial vessels. Because perfusion pressure is lowest in these terminal regions, the areas of the brain supplied by these terminal vessels are affected with hypotensive ischemia, leading to *watershed (borderzone)* infarctions.

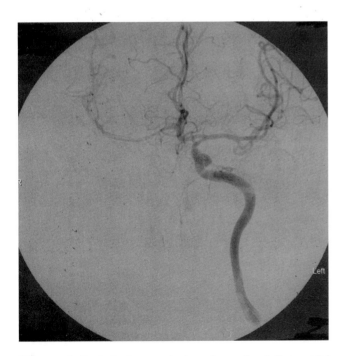

Figure 1-6. Anterior–posterior view of a left carotid arteriogram demonstrates flow in the right middle cerebral artery via collateral flow through the anterior communicating artery. The patient had an occlusion of the right internal carotid artery.

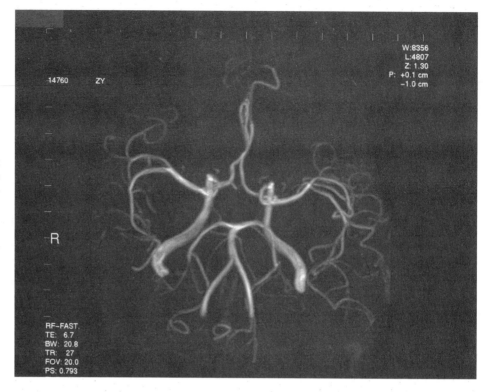

Figure 1-8. Submental vertex view of a magnetic resonance angiogram demonstrates the distal segments of the vertebral arteries, the basilar artery, and the posterior cerebral arteries. Also shown are the origins of the superior cerebellar arteries. In addition, the study visualizes both internal carotid arteries and the anterior and middle cerebral arteries. This view provides important information about the anatomy of the circle of the Willis.

▶ CLASSIFICATION BY THE TYPE AND DURATION OF SYMPTOMS

Ischemic cerebrovascular events are categorized by the presence and the duration of neurological symptoms. While the subcategories are sometimes considered as different diseases, in reality, these ischemic events should be considered as part of a continuum from asymptomatic disease to a fatal stroke (Table 1-5).

Clinically Silent Stroke

In some cases, the neurological symptoms might be so subtle that neither the patient nor observers are aware

▶ **TABLE 1-5.** TIME-RELATED CLASSIFICATION OF ISCHEMIC CEREBROVASCULAR DISEASE

Asymptomatic arterial disease
  Asymptomatic bruit
  Asymptomatic stenosis
Clinically silent stroke
Transient ischemic attack
  Amaurosis fugax
Cerebral infarction with transient symptoms
Minor stroke
Acute ischemic stroke
  Hyperacute stroke (brain attack)
  Stroke-in-evolution (progressing stroke)
Completed stroke
Vascular dementia (multi-infarction dementia)

that a stroke has occurred. Brain imaging subsequently leads to discovery of the vascular brain injury—a *clinically silent stroke.*[1,2] Most of these lesions, which often are discovered during the evaluation following another stroke or unrelated neurological complaints, are located in the deep structures of the cerebral hemispheres. Clinically silent infarctions are most common among patients with other evidence of vascular disease.[2] Similarly, asymptomatic arterial disease might be detected by physical examination or by vascular imaging. The most common situation is an *asymptomatic bruit* or *stenosis* of the internal carotid artery.

Transient Ischemic Attack

A *transient ischemic attack* (TIA) is diagnosed when a patient has focal neurological symptoms that completely resolve and are ascribed to vascular disease.[3] A TIA should not be considered as different from ischemic stroke. Rather, it is the mildest form of ischemic cerebrovascular disease that forms a continuum to include life-threatening cerebral infarction.[4] A TIA represents a thromboembolic event that abates because of lysis of the clot or because collateral flow permits adequate reperfusion to the brain. While a TIA does not leave any neurological residuals, it is a warning that the patient's vascular disease has changed and that the risk of impending stroke is considerable.[3,5] For these reasons, a patient should be managed urgently, instituting effective stroke prophylaxis. Unfortunately, the diagnosis of TIA is difficult and not all transient episodes of neurological dysfunction are due to ischemia. While the definition of TIA includes duration of up to 24 h, most events last only a few minutes.[6] Physicians should not wait 24 h to exclude the diagnosis of TIA so as to initiate treatment of patients with ischemic stroke. When a patient has neurological signs persisting for more than 1 h, the prudent course is to diagnose acute ischemic stroke rather than TIA. Most patients with neurological signs that resolve after 1 h will subsequently have a stroke detected by brain imaging.[7,8] In these cases, the term *cerebral infarction with transient symptoms* (CITS) is often used.

Minor Ischemic Stroke

In the past, diagnoses such as *reversible ischemic neurological deficit* (RIND) or *partially reversible ischemic neurological deficit* (PRIND) were made when a patient's symptoms lasted for prolonged periods (even>24 h) or when a patient's impairments largely resolved. These terms probably are not very useful and their use has been abandoned in favor of the diagnosis of a *minor ischemic stroke* because in fact affected patients have had strokes that largely resolved.[9] More recently, the term *acute recovered cerebral ischemia* (ACRI) has been used to distinguish those patients whose strokes have largely resolved within a few hours and who appear to have a very high risk for another, more serious stroke.[10] The reason to substitute this term for minor ischemic stroke is not obvious. The diagnosis of minor ischemic stroke is important because it not only implies that the underlying vascular pathology is unstable but that the collateral circulation and other compensatory mechanisms may not be sufficient to completely ease the consequences of recurrent thromboembolism. There is evidence that the risk of a major stroke is higher among patients with a minor stroke than among persons with TIA. Because the ophthalmic artery is the first major branch of the internal carotid artery, ischemia of the eye also portends an increased risk of ischemic stroke in the ipsilateral cerebral hemisphere. A painless, brief episode of monocular visual loss *(amaurosis fugax)* is the result of transient thromboembolic occlusion of the ophthalmic artery or its retinal branches.

Brain Attack

Advances in treatment are prompting a change in the approach to management of patients with acute ischemic or hemorrhagic cerebrovascular disease. Because of the time-linked changes in the brain and vasculature, the interval from onset of symptoms to treatment is crucial. During the first few hours following onset, the patient has the potential for either neurological improvement or worsening. In an effort to highlight the importance of urgent treatment, public-awareness programs are using the term *brain attack* to describe stroke.[11] The aim is to make the public respond to stroke with the same alacrity as for a heart attack.[12,13] Patients seen within the first few hours following an arterial occlusion can be diagnosed as having an *acute (hyperacute) ischemic stroke.*[14] In general, the time limit for acute ischemic stroke is 12–24 h, while the hyperacute designation would include a shorter time limit of 3–6 h. This is the time limit for treatment with interventions such as thrombolytic agents.

Stroke-in-Evolution

Some patients have neurological worsening during the first hours following stroke. These patients are thought to have a *stroke-in-evolution (progressing stroke)* secondary to early recurrent embolization, progression of thrombosis, or perfusion failure secondary to inadequate collateral flow.[15,16] However, these patients must be differentiated from patients whose neurological status declines secondary to medical or neurological complications of the stroke or other medical illnesses. Patients with stroke-in-evolution represent a group that demands urgent care because their outcomes are poorer than those whose neurological status remains stable.

Cerebral Infarction

Patients with mild-to-severe neurological impairments that persist for more than 24 h are considered to have had a *completed stroke (cerebral infarction)*. Strokes range in size from small lesions that produce mild, focal neurological impairments to multilobar infarctions that can cause severe neurological deficits or death (Table 1-6).[17] The priorities in therapy reflect the size and location of the brain lesion and the type and severity of neurological deficits. Still, patients who survive an ischemic stroke have a high risk of recurrent cerebrovascular events.

Vascular Dementia

While a single stroke produces focal neurological deficits that correspond with the location of the brain injury, multiple recurrent strokes can lead to dysfunction causing cognitive decline *(vascular dementia)*.[18,19] Patients with a history of either ischemic or hemorrhagic cerebrovascular disease have an enhanced risk of dementia. Vascular disease is second to degenerative disease (Alzheimer disease) as a cause of dementia; it accounts for approximately one-third of the cases of dementia.[18] Approximately one-fourth of survivors of stroke will subsequently develop dementia.[20,21] In addition, stroke is recognized as a contributing factor in the development of symptomatic Alzheimer disease.[22]

▶ **TABLE 1.6.** OXFORDSHIRE CLASSIFICATION OF STROKE SYNDROMES

Lacunar infarction
  Contralateral motor or sensory impairments
    Alone or in combination
    Usually affect face, upper extremity, and lower extremity
  Dysarthria
  Cognitive, behavioral, or visual impairments are mild or absent
Partial anterior cerebral infarction
  Prominent cognitive or behavioral impairments
    Differ in dominant or nondominant hemisphere
  Contralateral motor and sensory impairments
    Face, upper extremity, and lower extremity not equally affected
  Contralateral visual field impairment
Total anterior cerebral infarction
  Normal to slightly depressed consciousness
  Prominent cognitive or behavioral impairments
    Differ in dominant or nondominant hemisphere
  Contralateral motor and sensory impairments
    Usually affect face, upper extremity, and lower extremity
  Contralateral visual field impairment
  Ipsilateral conjugate eye deviation
  Dysarthria
Posterior circulation infarction
  Normal consciousness to coma
  Unilateral (contralateral) or bilateral motor impairments
  Contralateral sensory impairments (can be dissociated)
  Disturbances in ocular motility
  Ipsilateral cranial nerve palsies
  Dysarthria
  Ipsilateral cerebellar signs

Adapted from Bamford et al.[17]

Differentiating vascular dementia from Alzheimer disease can be difficult. A number of clinical and imaging findings are used to help distinguish these causes of cognitive decline. A widely used clinical scale is that developed by Hachinski et al.,[23] which includes a number of historical and physical findings. While cases of vascular dementia often are ascribed to multiple small infarctions deep in the cerebral hemisphere (*multi-infarction dementia*), the development of new brain imaging technologies has allowed for the detection of extensive white matter changes in a sizable number of patients with cognitive impairments (Table 1-7). The imaging changes, which are primarily periventricular in location, are known as *leukoaraiosis* and often are ascribed to disease of small arterioles.[19] These white matter changes are associated with an increased probability of dementia.[24] Still, evidence correlating the imaging findings with other types vascular disease seems to be circumstantial. The cause-and-effect relationship between microvascular disease and leukoaraiosis has

▶ **TABLE 1-7.** HACHINSKI SCALE TO DIFFERENTIATE VASCULAR (MULTI-INFARCTION) DEMENTIA FROM DEGENERATIVE (ALZHEIMER DISEASE) DEMENTIA

Abrupt onset of neurological symptoms	2 points
History of focal neurological symptoms	2 points
History of focal neurological signs	2 points
History of stroke	2 points
Fluctuating course of symptoms	2 points
Stepwise neurological deterioration	1 point
Nocturnal confusion	1 point
Relative preservation of personality	1 point
Depression	1 point
Prominent somatic complaints	1 point
Pseudobulbar affect	1 point
History of hypertension	1 point
Evidence of atherosclerosis	1 point

7 or more points suggests vascular dementia and 4 or fewer points suggests degenerative dementia.
Adapted from Hachinski et al.[23]

not been established. However, the imaging findings have prompted an increase in the diagnosis of *Binswanger disease* as a variety of vascular dementia.[25] This diagnosis remains difficult and controversial.

▶ SPECTRUM OF CEREBROVASCULAR DISEASES (STROKE AS A SYMPTOM)

Besides having a variety of clinical findings based on the location and size of the ischemic stroke, the cause of an arterial occlusion (stroke subtype) also affects the patient's symptoms and signs.[26] It also influences decisions about management. The differential diagnosis for the cause of ischemic stroke is extensive and uncommon etiologies should be considered when a patient presents with atypical symptoms.

▶ **TABLE 1-8.** GENERAL CATEGORIES CAUSES OF ISCHEMIC STROKE

Hypotension and perfusion failure
  Watershed (borderzone) infarction
Thromboembolism
  Atherosclerosis
    Extracranial large artery disease
    Intracranial large artery disease
    Small (penetrating artery) disease
  Cardioembolism
  Nonatherosclerotic vasculopathies
    Infectious vasculitic
    Noninfectious, inflammatory vasculitic
    Noninflammatory vasculopathies
  Hypercoagulable (prothrombotic) disorders
  Other causes of embolism

▶ **TABLE 1-9.** CATEGORIZATION OF SUBTYPES OF ISCHEMIC STROKE

Large artery atherosclerosis
    Clinical findings of cortical or multilobar hemispheric infarction or findings of major brain stem or cerebellar infarction
    Brain imaging findings compatible with cortical or multilobar hemispheric infarction or findings of major brain stem
      or cerebellar infarction
    Demonstration of high-grade stenosis or occlusion of appropriate artery by vascular imaging
      (Probable—absence of another equally plausible explanation for stroke)
Cardioembolism
    Clinical findings of cortical or multilobar hemispheric infarction or findings of major brain stem or cerebellar infarction
    Brain imaging findings compatible with cortical or multilobar hemispheric infarction or findings of major brain stem or
      cerebellar infarction
    Demonstration of high-risk cardiac lesion by cardiac evaluation or demonstration of a lower (or undetermined) risk
      cardiac lesion during evaluation and absence of any other etiology
      (Probable—absence of another equally plausible explanation for stroke)
Small artery occlusion
    Clinical findings of a traditional lacunar syndrome
    Brain imaging findings of small (<1.5-cm diameter) subcortical hemispheric or brain stem infarction
      (Probable—absence of high-grade stenosis or occlusion of relevant major intracranial or extracranial artery and absence
        of high-risk cardiac lesion)
Stroke of other etiology
    Broad spectrum of clinical findings
    Brain imaging shows infarction
    Evaluation demonstrates a nonatherosclerotic vasculopathy or prothrombotic state
      (Probable—absence of other cause of stroke)
Stroke of undetermined etiology
    Broad spectrum of clinical findings
    Brain imaging shows infarction
    Evaluation not performed
    Evaluation negative for cause of stroke
    Evaluation demonstrates two or more causes that are equally plausible

Large Artery Atherosclerosis

Atherosclerosis is the leading arterial disease that promotes thromboembolism (Tables 1-8 and 1-9). Thrombosis of a large extracranial or intracranial artery usually is secondary to an atherosclerotic plaque or stenosis *(large artery atherosclerosis)* (Fig. 1-9). The thrombosis can lead to occlusion or artery-to-artery embolism.

Small Artery Occlusive Disease

Persons with risk factors for large artery atherosclerosis also have a high likelihood of developing occlusion of a small penetrating artery that leads to a lacunar infarction *(small artery disease.)*

Hypoperfusion

Profound declines in blood pressure can aggravate the effects of impaired flow distal to a stenosis. Global *hypotension,* such as that which occurs during cardiovascular operations, also can lead to brain ischemia. The most vulnerable areas of the cerebral hemispheres for hypotensive injury are at the end of the perfusion beds of the major intracranial arteries. The resultant infarctions are often described as having a watershed pattern of ischemic stroke.

Cardioembolic Stroke

Approximately one-fourth of ischemic strokes are secondary to emboli that arise in the heart *(cardioembolism)* (Fig. 1-10).

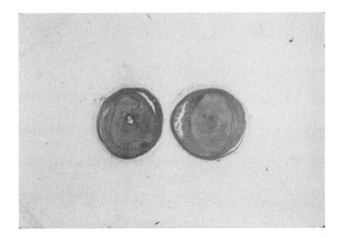

Figure 1-9. Cross section of a basilar artery demonstrates thrombotic occlusion of the artery superimposed on an atherosclerotic plaque. (*Courtesy of S.S. Schochet, M.D., Department of Pathology, University of West Virginia.*)

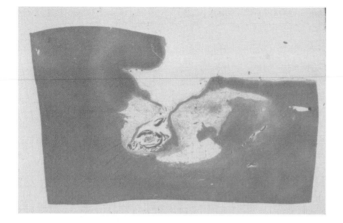

Figure 1-10. Microscopic specimen obtained from a patient dying of a cerebellar infarction. Findings include a loss of neurons and edema and are consistent with a recent ischemic injury.

Other Causes of Ischemic Stroke

Smaller numbers of patients will have arterial occlusions secondary to *nonatherosclerotic vasculopathies* but these diseases are especially important among children and young adults. *Prothrombotic (hypercoagulable) disorders*, which are either inherited or acquired, are relatively uncommon causes of ischemic stroke. Still, screening for these disorders is important if the patient or family has a history of recurrent venous or arterial thrombotic events. In most cases, the cause of stroke cannot be established with certainty based on the clinical evaluation. Ancillary diagnostic studies, such as cardiac and vascular imaging or screening for hematological disorders, are required. The cause of stroke might not be established in many patients. In some cases, no likely cause can be found despite an extensive evaluation. Finally, in some circumstances, more than one potential cause for the stroke is found and the physician is uncertain as to which of the etiologies is most likely.

Hemorrhagic Stroke

Approximately 20 percent of strokes are secondary to bleeding into or adjacent to the brain or spinal cord (hemorrhagic stroke). Craniocerebral trauma, including relatively mild head injuries, is a leading cause of bleeding that occurs in the brain, subarachnoid space, subdural space, or epidural space (Table 1-10). In general, patients with *traumatic intracranial hemorrhage* are not considered to have hemorrhagic stroke because the presence of associated injuries and differing pathogenesis, prognosis, and treatment of the brain illness. In some instances, differentiating a traumatic brain hemorrhage from a hemorrhagic stroke can be difficult. The typical situation for this scenario is when a comatose patient, for whom no history is available, is found to

have intracranial bleeding. Cases of *spontaneous* (nontraumatic) *intracranial hemorrhage* constitute the population of persons with hemorrhagic stroke. Hemorrhagic strokes are categorized into subgroups depending upon the primary anatomic location of the bleeding. A localized clot in the brain, subdural space, or epidural space is called a *hematoma*.

Intracerebral Hemorrhage

The primary location of *intracerebral hemorrhage* is the brain parenchyma. While the cerebral hemispheres are the usual locations for hemorrhages, bleeding also occurs in the cerebellum or brain stem. The hemorrhages are often denoted by the primary location of the bleeding: *putaminal (basal ganglia) hemorrhage, thalamic hemorrhage, lobar hemorrhage, pontine hemorrhage,* or *cerebellar hemorrhage.*

Intraventricular Hemorrhage

In cases of *intraventricular hemorrhage*, the bleeding is found primarily in the fourth, third, and the lateral ventricles. An intraventricular hemorrhage can arise within the ventricle or more commonly as an extension of bleeding elsewhere in the brain.

Subarachnoid Hemorrhage

In patients with *subarachnoid hemorrhage*, the bleeding is found primarily in the basal cisterns and sulci. Primary subarachnoid hemorrhage accounts for approximately one-third of cases of hemorrhagic stroke. Differentiation of subarachnoid from intracerebral hemorrhage is important because clinical presentations differ; patients with subarachnoid hemorrhage may have headache without other neurological signs. In fact, the

▶ **TABLE 1-10.** CLASSIFICATION OF HEMORRHAGIC STROKE

Anatomic location of bleeding
  Intracerebral (intraparenchymal) hemorrhage
    Putamen
    Thalamus
    Brain stem
    Cerebellar
    Lobe
  Intraventricular hemorrhage
  Subarachnoid hemorrhage
  Subdural or epidural hemorrhage
Categories of hemorrhagic stroke
  Hypertensive hemorrhage
  Aneurysmal hemorrhage
  Vascular malformation
  Bleeding diathesis
  Amyloid angiopathy

absence of focal neurological deficits is a distinct feature of subarachnoid hemorrhage.

Subdural Hematoma

A *subdural hematoma* is located external to the arachnoid but internal to the dura mater. Although trauma is the primary cause of subdural bleeding, occasionally hemorrhage in this location is secondary to a hemorrhagic stroke, particularly bleeding from a ruptured aneurysm. Spontaneous subdural bleeding also can complicate hemodialysis or the use of anticoagulants.

Epidural Hematoma

An *epidural hematoma* is located within the skull but external to the dura mater. Almost all cases of epidural hematomas are secondary to trauma. In many cases, patients will have hemorrhage involving several intracranial structures. A relatively common scenario is an intracerebral hemorrhage with intraventricular or subarachnoid extension of the blood.

Spinal Cord Hemorrhage

Most cases of bleeding involving the spinal cord will be secondary to closed or penetrating trauma. However, cases of *spinal cord hemorrhage*, with most events being extra-axial and causing cord compression, can occur.

Patients with hemorrhagic stroke usually have their vascular events attributed to an underlying cause. The most common cause of intracerebral hemorrhage is hypertension and is known as *hypertensive hemorrhage*. A ruptured aneurysm is the leading cause of spontaneous subarachnoid hemorrhage (*aneurysmal subarachnoid hemorrhage*). Other leading causes of hemorrhagic stroke include *vascular malformations, amyloid angiopathy*, and *bleeding diatheses* (see Table 1-10). Medications also are among the most common causes of bleeding disorders that promote hemorrhagic stroke.

Venous Thrombosis

Cerebrovascular events due to venous occlusions are much less common that those secondary to arterial events. The clinical findings of *venous thrombosis* are markedly different from other forms of stroke. Because of the nonapoplectic nature of the presentation and the relatively low frequency of the illness, venous thrombosis often is not recognized clinically.

Pituitary Apoplexy

Pituitary apoplexy is diagnosed when a patient has either a hemorrhagic or ischemic vascular event that primarily affects the pituitary gland. These vascular events have a clinical profile that differs from other forms of stroke and often complicates a pituitary tumor.

▶ PATHOPHYSIOLOGY OF STROKE

The pathophysiology of either ischemic or hemorrhagic stroke is complex. A number of time-linked metabolic and cellular events follow the onset of the brain injury.

Hemorrhagic Stroke

In hemorrhagic stroke, a blood vessel ruptures and leads to bleeding into the brain or spinal cord and adjacent structures results. With subarachnoid hemorrhage, the bleeding occurs primarily in the subarachnoid space and localized clots can occur as a result of the trabeculations of tissue between the pia and arachnoid layers of the meninges. More disseminated extension of blood also might occur. With intraparenchymal hemorrhage, the bleeding spreads along planes of white matter leaving areas of intact neural tissue surrounding the hematoma.[27] Tissue in the area of the hematoma demonstrates neuronal injury, edema, and an inflammatory reaction. The bleeding can progress for several hours with expansion of the hematoma.[28,29] Expansion of the hematoma can be the result of continued bleeding from the original site or disruption of adjacent vessels.[27] The hemorrhage damages adjacent brain tissue and provokes the development of vasogenic and cytotoxic edema. Part of the neurological injury probably is the result of hypoperfusion and ischemia in adjacent areas of the brain. Neuronal death in hemorrhage probably is the result of both apoptotic and necrotic events.[27] The edema may in part be due to the accumulation of proteins within the clot as well as disruption of the blood-brain barrier secondary to ischemia.

Ischemic Stroke

The scientific understanding of the pathophysiology of infarction in the central nervous system continues to change dramatically. Ischemia can result from any mechanism that reduces blood flow to the brain and deprives the central nervous system of the needed oxygen and glucose. It also allows for the retention of metabolic waste products that are neurotoxic. Several mechanisms of infarction have been described. Air bubbles, pieces of atherosclerotic debris, fat globules, amniotic fluid, or tumor cells also rarely occlude blood vessels. More commonly, blood vessels are occluded by thrombi that develop in situ or from pieces of clot that migrate to the brain—a process known as *embolization*. Occasionally, ischemia can result from the inability of the blood to provide adequate levels of oxygen to the central nervous system; such events are very rare but could be the mechanism of brain injury due to carbon monoxide poisoning, profound anemia, or severe hypoxia.

Cerebral Blood Flow

Normally cerebral blood flow is approximately 50–55 mL/100 g/min. Autoregulation maintains this flow despite a wide range of arterial blood pressures.[30,31] Autoregulation is lost in the acute brain ischemia and blood flow becomes pressure-dependent. Blood flow is also influenced by cerebral perfusion pressure, which in turn is directly affected by intracranial pressure. A decline in cerebral perfusion pressure by a reduction in mean arterial pressure or an increase in intracranial pressure can potentiate ischemia. These concerns have lead to caution about rapid lowering of arterial blood pressure in patients with stroke, especially if the patient also has signs of increased intracranial pressure. As cerebral blood flow is reduced, electrical activity of the relevant area of the brain changes and these changes are associated with clinical abnormalities. As blood flow drops to approximately 20–30 mL/100 g/min, cellular metabolic abnormalities are detected.[32] At lower levels, cellular apoptotic or metabolic changes begin to lead to cell death.

Hypoperfusion-induced ischemia of the central nervous system usually occurs in the setting of orthostatic hypotension, cardiac arrest, shock, or surgery, in which blood supply is globally reduced. Presumably, the natural autoregulatory mechanisms are not sufficiently effective to maintain adequate perfusion to the brain. The most common neurological symptoms of such ischemia are syncope or anoxic encephalopathy. Ischemia can occur at the end of perfusion beds that are most vulnerable to general reductions in flow. This phenomenon is the presumed mechanism for watershed or borderzone infarctions.[33] However, less severe episodes of hypoperfusion can cause focal ischemia presumably on the basis of an underlying arterial stenosis. In this circumstance, local arterial thrombosis might aggravate the effects of hypoperfusion. In addition, some neural tissues, for example, the medial temporal lobe, might be more vulnerable to the effects of a hypotensive event.

Arterial Occlusion

Most infarctions are secondary to an acute arterial occlusion. This occlusion initiates a very complex process that involves intravascular, endothelial, neuronal, glia, and inflammatory phenomena.[32,34–36] Ischemic neural tissue can either die or survive depending upon the ability of the body or physicians to intervene to protect the tissue. Time truly is critical. The time course for either death or survival of ischemic neural tissue probably is measured in minutes to hours.[37,38]

Ischemic Penumbra

Some neural tissue may be irreversibly injured while adjacent cells might be salvaged if interventions are prescribed quickly. The theory of the ischemic penumbra is a foundation behind the current approach to the management of patients with acute infarctions of the central nervous system.[30,31,34,35,37,39] This phenomenon has been demonstrated in both experimental models and humans.[40–42] Following the arterial occlusion, a core of tissue might rapidly die because of lack of perfusion and cell dysfunction.[43–45] This tissue might not be saved by any medical or surgical intervention. However, surrounding areas of the brain might have borderline blood flow. These cells may be dysfunctional but have the potential for recovery. Neither apoptosis nor irreversible cellular necrotic events have occurred. The rationale for screening with diffusion and perfusion mismatch on magnetic resonance imaging is based on the concept of the potential viability of the ischemic penumbra. The diffusion defects reflect the area of irreversible injury, while the area of hypoperfusion could represent the penumbra. Rapid restoration of blood flow to this region or the administration of agents that might halt some of the cellular or metabolic consequences of acute ischemia might save the injured area. Clinical studies evaluating the utility of interventions, such as thrombolytic agents, have already demonstrated reversibility of ischemic damage and potential salvage of the penumbral region.[39,44,46]

Cellular Consequences of Ischemia

The understanding of the cellular, metabolic, and inflammatory changes that lead to infarction continues to expand[36] (Fig. 1-11). With hypoxia, the cell's ability to maintain active metabolism of glucose and creation of adenosine triphosphate fails.[35,47] This metabolic failure leads to a dysfunction of energy-dependent pumps that regulate the flow of ions into and out of the cell, resulting in both cellular depolarization and intracellular edema. Presumably, some measures, such as hypothermia, which could lower brain metabolic activity could be protective of ischemic neurons.

Ischemia also leads to increases of extracellular concentrations of excitatory amino acids.[48] The accumulation of excitatory amino acids, in particular glutamate, promotes the influx of calcium into ischemic neurons.[49] Glutamate-sensitive receptors are found in neural tissue; the ionotropic receptors are *n*-methyl-*d*-aspartate (NMDA), α-amino-3-hydroxy-5-methyl-4-isoxazole propionic acid (AMPA), and kainate receptors. The

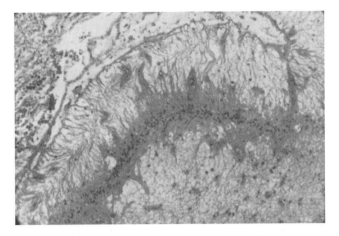

Figure 1-11. Embolus in a pial artery of the brain with adjacent cortical infarction is found on this autopsy specimen. (*Courtesy of S.S. Schochet, M.D., Department of Pathology, University of West Virginia.*)

metabotropic receptor (mGluR) has eight different subunits.[36] Several agents with putative effects on inhibiting the glutamate-sensitive ionotropic receptors have been evaluated.[50] For example, glycine and zinc are important factors for the activation of the NMDA receptor while magnesium has inhibitory effects. In addition, agents that block the influx of calcium might have neuroprotective effects.

Increases in intracellular calcium is associated with a number of metabolic effects that lead to changes in activity of proteins and genes. Some of the up-regulated genes, such as those that increase the activity of heat shock proteins and chaperones, might help protect the cell.[36] Other proteins such as phospholipases, proteases, and nucleases cause further injury to intracellular elements including the nucleus and mitochondria.[35,47] High concentration of intracellular calcium in combination with metabolic acidosis stimulates the release of reactive oxygen and nitrogen species (free radicals).[51] These reactive species probably are produced by injured mitochondria within neurons, glia, and inflammatory cells. Among the reactive agents are nitric oxide and peroxynitrite. Nitric oxide is produced from *l*-arginine via the action of nitric oxide synthase (NOS), the inducible form of which is activated by stimulation of the NMDA receptor. These reactive species interact with macromolecules and may activate apoptosis and inflammation.[36,50] Free radical antagonists or inhibitors of NOS might be useful in limiting neuronal injury secondary to the release of reactive oxygen and nitrogen species. The endothelial form of NOS might be helpful in the setting of stroke because it promotes dilation of blood vessels. The HMG-coA reductase inhibitors (statins), which are cholesterol-lowering agents, also might be useful in

stroke because of their effects on stimulating the endothelial form of NOS.[36]

An influx of inflammatory cells into the ischemic area occurs during reperfusion.[52] This inflammatory reaction might have both positive and negative effects. The presence of white blood cells and macrophages can help with repair and recovery. On the other hand, these cells can produce reactive oxygen and nitrogen species or toxic proteases that may augment brain ischemia.[36] Strategies such as preventing infiltration of white blood cells, halting activation of microglia, or limiting the production of toxins and reactive species by the white blood cells might lessen the neurological injury caused by ischemia.[53,54]

Apoptosis

Apoptosis, which involves fragmentation of DNA, also may contribute to cell death in stroke.[47,49,55] Caspases, proenzymes that promote cleavage of DNA, are central to the process of apoptosis. Several capsases can be released through mitochondrial injury or may be activated extrinsic to the mitochrondria.[36] Studies of interventions that limit or reverse the effects of apoptosis will occur in the years ahead.

Additional new information about the cellular and metabolic consequences is likely. This information will spawn the study of promising interventions to protect ischemic tissue.

REFERENCES

1. Davis PH, Clarke WR, Bendixen BH, Adams HP, Jr., Woolson RF, Culebras A. Silent cerebral infarction in patients enrolled in the TOAST Study. *Neurology* 1996; 46:942–948.
2. Giele JLP, Witkamp TD, Mali WPTM, Van Der Graaf Y, for the SMART Study Group. Silent brain infarcts in patients with manifest vascular disease. *Stroke* 2004;35:742–746.
3. Johnston SC. Transient ischemic attack. *N Engl J Med* 2002;347:1687–1692.
4. Koudstaal PJ, van Gijn J, Frenken CW, et al. TIA, RIND, minor stroke: a continuum, or different subgroups? Dutch TIA Study Group. *J Neurol Neurosurg Psychiatry* 1992; 55:95–97.
5. Kleindorfer D, Panagos P, Pancioli A, et al. Incidence and short-term prognosis of transient Ischemic attack in a population-based study. *Stroke* 2005;36:720–724.
6. Albers GW, Caplan LR, Easton JD, et al. Transient ischemic attack—proposal for a new definition. *N Engl J Med* 2002; 347:1713–1716.
7. Bogousslavsky J, Regli F. Cerebral infarct in apparent transient ischemic attacks. *Neurology* 1985;35:1501–1503.
8. Evans GW, Howard G, Murros KE, Rose LA, Toole JF. Cerebral infarction verified by cranial computed tomography and prognosis for survival following transient ischemic attack. *Stroke* 1991;22:431–436.

9. Caplan LR. Are terms such as completed stroke or RIND of continued usefulness. *Stroke* 1983;14:431–433.

10. Johnston SC, Gress DR, Browner WS, Sidney S. Short-term prognosis after emergency department diagnosis of TIA. *JAMA* 2000;284:2901–2906.

11. Hill MD, Hachinski V. Stroke treatment: time is brain. *Lancet* 1998;352(suppl 3):SIII10–SIII14.

12. Fuster V. Epidemic of cardiovascular disease and stroke: The three main challenges. Presented at the 71st scientific sessions of the American Heart Association. Dallas, Texas. *Circulation* 1999;99:1132–1137.

13. Fuster V, Smaha L. AHA's new strategic impact goal designed to curb epidemic of cardiovascular disease and stroke. *Circulation* 1999;99:2360

14. Adams HP, Jr. Treating ischemic stroke as an emergency. *Arch Neurol* 1998;55:457–461.

15. Toni D, Fiorelli M, Gentile M, et al. Progressing neurological deficit secondary to acute ischemic stroke. A study on predictability, pathogenesis, and prognosis. *Arch Neurol* 1995;52:670–675.

16. Yamamoto H, Bogousslavsky J, Van Melle G. Different predictors of neurological worsening in different causes of stroke. *Arch Neurol* 1998;55:481–486.

17. Bamford J, Sandercock P, Dennis M, Burn J, Warlow C: Classification and natural history of clinically identifiable subtypes of cerebral infarction. Lancet, 1991;337:1521–1526.

18. Bowler JV, Hachinski V. Criteria for vascular dementia: replacing dogma with data. *Arch Neurol* 2000;57: 170–171.

19. Roman GC, Tatemichi TK, Erkinjuntti T, et al. Vascular dementia: diagnostic criteria for research studies. Report of the NINDS-AIREN International Workshop. *Neurology* 1993;43:250–260.

20. Kokmen E, Whisnant JP, O'Fallon WM, Chu CP, Beard CM. Dementia after ischemic stroke: a population-based study in Rochester, Minnesota (1960–1984). *Neurology* 1996; 46:154–159.

21. Censori B, Manara O, Agostinis C, et al. Dementia after first stroke. *Stroke* 1996;27:1205–1210.

22. Honig LS, Tang M-X, Albert S, et al. Stroke and the risk of Alzheimer disease. *Arch Neurol* 2003;60:1707–1712.

23. Hachinski VC, Iliff LD, Zilhka E, et al. Cerebral blood flow in dementia. *Arch Neurol* 1975;32:632–637.

24. Prins ND, van Dijk EJ, den Heijer T, et al. Cerebral white matter lesions and the risk of dementia. *Arch Neurol* 2004; 61:1531–1534.

25. Roman GC. From UBOs to Binswanger's disease. Impact of magnetic resonance imaging on vascular dementia research. *Stroke* 1996;27:1269–1273.

26. Adams HP, Jr., Bendixen BH, Kappelle LJ, et al. Classification of subtype of acute ischemic stroke. Definitions for use in a multicenter clinical trial. TOAST. Trial of Org 10172 in Acute Stroke Treatment. *Stroke* 1993; 24:35–41.

27. Qureshi AI, Tuhrim S, Broderick JP. Spontaneous intracerebral hemorrhage. *N Engl J Med* 2001;344:1450–1460.

28. Brott T, Broderick J, Kothari R, et al. Early hemorrhage growth in patients with intracerebral hemorrhage. *Stroke* 1997;28:1–5.

29. Kazui S, Hiroaki N, Yamamoto H, Sawada T, Yamaguchi T. Enlargement of spontaneous intracerebral hemorrhage. *Stroke* 1996;27:1783–1787.

30. Hakim AM. The cerebral ischemic penumbra. *Can J Neurol Sci* 1987;14:557–559.

31. Heiss WD, Graf R. The ischemic penumbra. *Curr Opin Neurol* 1994;7:11–19.

32. Pulsinelli W. Pathophysiology of acute ischaemic stroke. Lancet 1992;339:533–536.

33. Leblanc R, Yamamoto YL, Tyler JL, Diksic M, Hakim A. Borderzone ischemia. *Ann Neurol* 1987;22:707–713.

34. Ginsberg MD. Adventures in the pathophysiology of brain ischemia: penumbra, gene expression, neuroprotection. The 2002 Thomas Willis Lecture. *Stroke* 2003;33:214–223.

35. Lee JM, Zipfel GJ, Choi DW. The changing landscape of ischaemic brain injury mechanisms. *Nature* 1999;399:A7–14.

36. Yenari MA. Pathophysiology of acute ischemic stroke. *Cleve Clin J Med* 2004;71(suppl 1):S25–S27.

37. Ginsberg MD, Pulsinelli WA. The ischemic penumbra, injury thresholds, and the therapeutic window for acute stroke. *Ann Neurol* 1994;36:553–554.

38. Pulsinelli WA, Jacewicz M, Levy DE, Petito CK, Plum F. Ischemic brain injury and the therapeutic window. *Ann N Y Acad Sci* 1997;835:187–193.

39. Davis SM, Donnan GA. Advances in penumbra imaging with MR. *Cerebrovasc Dis* 2004;17(suppl 3):23–27.

40. Karonen JO, Ostergaard L, Liu Y, et al. Combined diffusionand perfusion MRI with correlation to single-photon emission CT in acute ischemic stroke. Ischemic penumbra predicts infarct growth. *Stroke* 1999;30:1583–1590.

41. Heiss W-D. Imaging the ischemic penumbra and treatment effects by PET. *Keio J Med* 2001;50:249–256.

42. Heiss W-D. Best measure of ischemic penumbra: positron emission tomography. *Stroke* 2003;34:2534–2535.

43. Kaufmann AM, Firlik AD, Fukui MB, Wechsler LR, Jungries CA, Yonas H. Ischemic care and penumbra in human stroke. *Stroke* 1999;30:93–99.

44. Karonen JO, Ostergaard L, Vainio P, et al. Diffusion and perfusion MR imaging in acute ischemic stroke: a comparison to SPECT. *Comput Methods Programs Biomed* 2001;66:125–128.

45. Liu Y, Karonen JO, Vanninen RL, Nuutinen J, Perkio J, Vainio PA. Detecting the subregion proceeding to infarction in hypoperfused cerebral tissue: a study with diffusion and perfusion weighted MRI. *Neuroradiology* 2003;45:345–351.

46. Heiss WD, Grond M, Thiel A, et al. Tissue at risk of infarction rescued by early reperfusion: a positron emission tomography study in systemic recombinant tissue plasminogen activator thrombolysis of acute stroke. *J Cereb Blood Flow Metab* 1998;18:1298–1307.

47. Morgenstern LB, Pettigrew LC. Brain protection–human data and potential new therapies. *New Horizons* 1997;5:397–405.

48. Castillo J, Davalos A, Noya M. Progression of ischaemic stroke and excitotoxic aminoacids. *Lancet* 1997;349:79–83.

49. Dirnagl U, Iadecola C, Moskowitz MA. Pathobiology of ischaemic stroke: an integrated view. *Trends Neurosci* 1999;22:391–397.

50. Zheng Z, Lee JE, Yenari MA. Molecular mechanisms and potential targets for treatment. *Curr Mol Med* 2003; 3:361–372.

51. Zivin JA. Factors determining the therapeutic window for stroke. *Neurology* 1998;50:599–603.

52. Chamorro A. Role of inflammation in stroke and atherothrombosis. *Cerebrovasc Dis* 2004;17(suppl 3):1–5.

53. Han HS, Yenari MA. Cellular targets of brain inflammation in stroke. *Curr Opin Investig Drugs* 2003;4:522–529.

54. Barone FC, Feuerstein GZ. Inflammatory mediators and stroke: new opportunities for novel therapeutics. *J Cereb Blood Flow Metab* 1999;19:819–834.

55. Pulera MR, Adams LM, Liu H, et al. Apoptosis in a neonatal rat model of cerebral hypoxia-ischemia. *Stroke* 1998;29:2622–2630.

CHAPTER 2

Epidemiology of Stroke

The importance of stroke will grow dramatically in the twenty-first century. With the exception of acquired immune deficiency syndrome, the worldwide scourge of infectious diseases is declining. As the result of the combination of public health measures, improvements in medical care, and economic advances, life expectancy is expected to increase for people throughout the world. With advancing age, diseases such as atherosclerosis will become endemic around the world. In the United States,

life expectancy has grown for men and women of all ethnic groups. Increases in the average age of populations and changes in lifestyle in developing countries portend increases in the rates of common diseases of affluence that already affect persons in industrialized countries. Thus, the emphasis of health care in the twenty-first century will move to the management of common, noncommunicable diseases that lead to death or disability, including heart disease, cancer, dementia, and stroke.

▶ GLOBAL IMPACT OF CEREBROVASCULAR DISEASE

While the worldwide importance of stroke will increase during the next century, it already is a leading cause of death and disability (Fig. 2-1). The World Health Organization estimates that worldwide a stroke occurs every 5 s—a figure that translates to approximately 25,000 persons having a stroke every day (Table 2-1). Approximately 5 million people per year die of cerebrovascular disease.[1,2] Although the frequency of stroke has declined in North America, Japan, Australia, and western Europe during the last 30 years, probably as the result of improved management of common risk factors that lead to cerebrovascular disease, the frequency of stroke has been increasing rapidly in eastern Europe and parts of East Asia.[3–7] Stroke is the primary cause of death in China and other countries in eastern Asia.[8]

The effects of stroke on society, including the costs of health care, are considerable. Management of stroke and its consequences accounts for a large portion of health care budgets; for example, approximately 3 percent of the medical care costs in the Netherlands are attributed to care of patients with

cerebrovascular diseases.[9] An Australian-population-based study found that the total lifetime costs for ischemic strokes were greater than those for hemorrhagic strokes, largely because of the higher prevalence of infarction.[10] However, the same study demonstrated that the per-patient economic costs were greatest for hemorrhages and least for lacunar infarctions. Similar high health care costs occur throughout the world. Although expenses vary between countries, they are high regardless of the type of health care insurance system.[11]

In the United States, approximately 750,000 Americans have a stroke or recurrent stroke every year.[12,13] On average, someone in the United States has a stroke every 45 s. The American Heart Association estimates that approximately 930,000 hospitalizations in the United States are secondary to stroke.[12] The differences in numbers reflect the necessity of some patients to be hospitalized more than once for the treatment of stroke or its consequences (see Table 2-1). Annually, approximately 165,000 people in the United States die as a direct consequence of stroke and another 140,000 deaths are indirectly attributed to cerebrovascular disease.[12] Approximately 12 percent of patients with

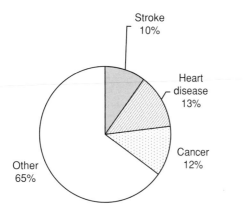

Figure 2-1. World Health Organization estimates on mortality around the world. Stroke (solid segment) accounts for 5.5 million deaths, approximately 10 percent of all deaths. For comparison, heart disease (striped segment) (7.2 million deaths/10 percent) and cancer (speckled segment) (7.1 million deaths/12 percent) are shown.

ischemic stroke and 38 percent of patients with hemorrhagic stroke are dead within 30 days of the vascular event.[12] Although the incidence of stroke in the United States declined during the last 30 years, the decline has slowed and future increases in stroke are anticipated. The advanced life expectancy of Americans in general and, in particular, patients with heart disease (a group at very high risk for stroke) forecasts an explosion in the future incidence of cerebrovascular disease. For example, Elkins and Johnston[14] estimate that the number of deaths from stroke will double in the next 30 years and that increases in stroke-related mortality will outpace overall population growth. Despite the increased ability to detect minor hemorrhagic strokes with the use of brain imaging, the decline in intracranial bleeding parallels the decline in ischemic stroke.[6,15,16] This decline has occurred despite the increasing use of antithrombotic medications, which have an inherent bleeding risk, to prevent cerebral infarction and other ischemic events. The drop in the frequency of intracranial hemorrhage probably reflects improved treatment of arterial hypertension. Unlike other forms of stroke, the incidence of subarachnoid hemorrhage has not changed; it remains at approximately 6.9–19 per 100,000.[15,17,18]

Vascular diseases of the nervous system have other societal implications as well. In the United States, there are an estimated 4.8 million stroke survivors and similar high prevalence rates are reported from other parts of the world.[12] While some patients completely recover, stroke remains a common cause of disability and human suffering. Cerebrovascular disease (recurrent stroke/vascular dementia) is an important cause of cognitive decline. In addition, the neurological effects of stroke can compound the consequences of degenerative neurological diseases, such as Alzheimer disease. As a result, the mental, behavioral, and physical sequelae of stroke are among the leading reasons for long-term institutionalized care. A disabling stroke also affects the patient's family and community. Family members need to assume caregiver responsibilities and other roles or duties that have been those of the patient. An adult child might need to take up the role of caregiver of an elderly parent because the other parent is infirm or might not be living. The community often needs to provide medical services, including nursing home care, when a patient does not have a family caregiver or when the severity of neurological impairments prohibits the family from providing sufficient care.

Stroke is an economically expensive illness.[19] The fiscal costs of preventive or acute management, rehabilitation, and long-term institutionalized care are considerable (Table 2-2). While some preventive measures are

▶ **TABLE 2-1.** STROKE AS A PUBLIC HEALTH PROBLEM

Incidence	
Worldwide	9,000,000 cases
United States	750,000 cases
Annual mortality	
Worldwide	5,000,000 deaths
United States	
Direct cause	165,000 deaths
Indirect cause	140,000 deaths
30-day mortality—United States	
Hemorrhage	38%
Infarction	12%
Stroke survivors—United States	4,800,000 people

Adapted from American Heart Association.[12]

▶ **TABLE 2-2.** ECONOMIC COSTS OF STROKE

Direct
  Prevention
    Physicians' fees
    Medications
    Surgical procedures
    Behavioral interventions
  Acute treatment
    Emergency medical services
    Hospitalization
      Diagnostic studies
      Medications
      Surgical procedures
    Physicians' fees
  Rehabilitation
  Long-term care
Indirect
  Loss of productivity of patient and family
  Social security or disability payments

relatively inexpensive (i.e., stopping smoking or use of aspirin), some medications to treat risk factors for atherosclerosis or to prevent thromboembolism are expensive. Prescription of some of these medications to large populations of at-risk persons could result in huge increases in health care costs. For example, treating all Americans with hypercholesterolemia with one of the new cholesterol-lowering medications would be very costly. In addition, the expenses of surgical or endovascular procedures that are prescribed in stroke prophylaxis can surpass $15,000 per patient. The costs of acute hospitalization and treatment are also great, especially for management of patients with intracranial hemorrhage (see Table 2-2). Inpatient hospital costs for the acute treatment of stroke account for approximately 70 percent of the medical expenses in the first year after stroke.[12] Expenses relate to general hospital care (50 percent), medical treatments (21 percent), and diagnostic tests (19 percent). The per-patient costs of acute treatment of a patient with a ruptured intracranial aneurysm can exceed $100,000 and the lifetime costs exceed $200,000.[20] Many stroke survivors require a prolonged period of rehabilitation, often in an inpatient setting. The current costs of long-term nursing home care in the United States often are in excess of $4000 per month. Besides the expense of direct health care for treating stroke, the indirect economic consequences from lost productivity by the patient and caregivers expand the financial impact of stroke. The community may need to provide social or disability payments to support the patient and family. Such a situation is most likely to occur when stroke affects a young adult. Already, the fiscal costs of stroke in the American population are estimated to be approximately $30–$50 billion per year.[12,20]

The indirect social and economic costs of stroke during the twentieth century are reflected in world history. During the last century, Woodrow Wilson, Vladimir Lenin, Franklin D. Roosevelt, Winston Churchill, and Josef Stalin had strokes that were fatal or resulted in cognitive or physical disability while they were leading world powers. One can speculate whether these strokes altered history during and after World War I and World War II, the Russian Revolution, or the cold war. The economic and human consequences of these leaders' strokes might be beyond calculation. One can hypothesize whether the advances in stroke care that have occurred during the last 50 years could have prevented these leaders' strokes or limited their neurological consequences.

▶ EPIDEMIOLOGY OF CEREBROVASCULAR DISEASE

While a stroke can affect any person, a number of epidemiological factors denote those people who have the

▶ **TABLE 2-3.** EPIDEMILOGICAL FACTORS FOR INCREASED RISK FOR STROKE

Age	Increases with each decade of life
Sex	Men > women
Ethnicity	African Americans > whites
	Hispanic Americans > whites (younger ages)
	Asian Americans = whites
Geography	East Asia > rest of the world
	Eastern Europe > Western Europe
	Europe > United States or Canada
	Developing countries > industrialized countries
Social status	Poor > wealthy
	Lower social class > upper social class
	Uneducated > educated
Family	Family history of premature stroke > absence
	Parents with stroke > absence
	Vascular disease in young relatives > older relatives
Environment	Cold weather > temperate weather
	Winter > spring, fall, or summer
	Monday > other days
	Weekend > weekdays
	Morning > other times of day

highest risk for cerebrovascular disease (Table 2-3). Not only do the overall rates of stroke vary among subgroups of the population, the types and causes of stroke are influenced by factors such as the patient's age, gender, ethnicity, geographical location, social or economic status, environmental factors, and family history. Some factors that portend an increased risk of stroke cannot be controlled or modified. Other factors might be indirectly related to an increased stroke risk, such as the influence of personal behavior or lifestyle. A scale that adds the contribution of both treatable risk factors and epidemiological findings is given in Table 2-4. This scale can be used to predict the risk of stroke among asymptomatic adults.

Age

Advancing age is the single most important forecaster of a high risk for stroke. Although a majority of stroke deaths are among elderly patients, stroke is a leading cause of death among all age groups and cerebrovascular disease is among the top 10 causes of mortality in children. Not surprisingly, survival after stroke is influenced by the patient's age. Higher mortality rates among the elderly might reflect the presence of severe concomitant diseases. Other factors such as the plasticity of the nervous system or the patient's stamina also affect age-related prognosis, including survival.

▶ **TABLE 2-4.** FRAMINGHAM SCALE FOR
CALCULATING RISK OF STROKE

| | | Systolic Blood Pressure (mm Hg) | |
Points	Age	Untreated	Treated
Men			
0	≤56	97–105	97–105
1	57–59	106–115	106–112
2	60–62	116–125	113–117
3	63–65	126–135	118–123
4	66–68	136–14	124–129
5	69–71	146–155	130–135
6	72–75	156–165	136–142
7	76–78	166–175	143–150
8	79–81	176–185	151–161
9	82–84	186–195	162–178
10	>84	>195	>178
Women			
0	<56	<95	<95
1	57–59	95–106	95–106
2	60–62	107–118	107–113
3	63–64	119–130	114–119
4	65–67	131–143	120–125
5	68–70	144–155	126–131
6	71–73	156–167	132–139
7	74–76	168–180	140–148
8	77–78	181–192	149–160
9	79–81	193–204	161–204
10	>81	≥205	≥205

Add points for age and relevant systolic blood pressure reading.
Also add points for the following:
　For men—add 2 points for diabetes mellitus; add 3 points for
　current smoker; add 4 points for cardiovascular disease; add
　4 points for atrial fibrillation; add 5 points for left ventricular
　hypertrophy.
　For women—add 3 points for diabetes mellitus; add 3 points for
　current smoker; add 2 points for cardiovascular disease; add 6
　points for atrial fibrillation; add 4 points for left ventricular hyper-
　trophy.
Estimated 10-year risk of stroke:
　10 points—men 10%; women 6%
　15 points—men 20%; women 16%
　20 points—men 37%; Women 37%
　25 points—men 63%; women 71%
Adapted from Goldstein et al.[12]

The likelihood of stroke increases rapidly after the age of 55 (Fig. 2-2). For both men and women of all ethnic groups, the chances of stroke approximately double for each decade of life after 55. Data from an epidemiological study in Cincinnati, OH, demonstrate that the risk of hemorrhagic stroke is seven times higher among persons older than 70 than it is in younger persons.[21] The relationship between stroke and advancing age is a leading reason for the predicted explosion in the frequency of stroke during the next 50 years. The high frequency of stroke among women in developed countries likely reflects their long life expectancy.

Because stroke is the most common cause of acute neurological symptoms among persons older than 55, it

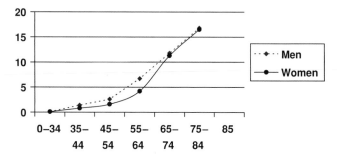

Figure 2-2. The incidence of stroke among white American men (solid line) and women (dashed line). Adapted from American Heart Association.[12]

is a primary diagnostic consideration. On the other hand, the lower frequency of cerebrovascular disease among younger persons often requires exclusion of other disease prior to a diagnosis of stroke. The patient's age impacts on the rates of complications.[22–24] For example, elderly persons are likely to have severe comorbid diseases such as dementia, Parkinson disease, heart disease, arthritis, or diabetes mellitus that increase the risk of complications or influence acute general management.[25,26] In addition, the patient's age affects decisions about medical or surgical therapies to prevent stroke and decisions about acute stroke management. For example, the risk of major bleeding complications following intravenous administration of thrombolytic agents is higher among persons older than 75 than among younger patients.

While there is a strong age relationship with the overall frequency of stroke, differences in the types and causes of cerebrovascular disease are found among different age groups (Fig. 2-3). The proportion of strokes that are secondary to ischemia is high among persons older than 55 (Fig. 2-4). This relationship largely explains the finding that 80 percent of strokes are of ischemic origin. Hemorrhages account for the majority of cerebrovascular events among children and young adults. Still, approximately 3–5 percent of ischemic strokes occur in persons younger than 45.[27]

Stroke is a leading cause of death in children.[28] The incidence of ischemic stroke in children is approximately 0.58–2.6 per 100,000.[29,30] The incidence of hemorrhagic stroke is estimated to be 1.5 per 100,000 children.[30] The causes of stroke in children and young adults appear more diverse than among older persons[31–33] (see Chapter 17). Congenital vascular anomalies or inherited disorders of coagulation that lead to bleeding, such as hemophilia, are important causes of hemorrhagic stroke in childhood.[28] Other inherited diseases leading to arterial disease also are important causes of stroke in childhood.[34] Congenital cardiac diseases, including cyanotic heart disease, and nonatherosclerotic vasculopathies, such as moyamoya, are potential causes of ischemic stroke in children and young

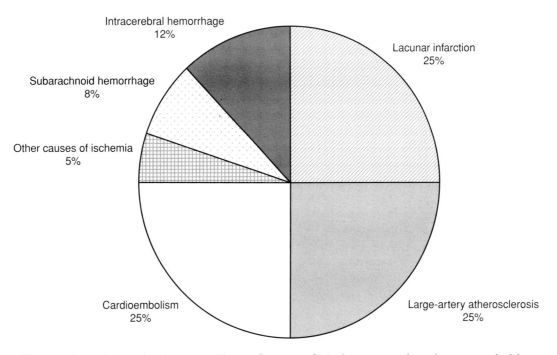

Figure 2-3. Approximate proportions of cases of stroke among Americans aged older than 55.

adults, but generally are not considered as a cause of stroke in the elderly.

Saccular aneurysms are an important cause of intracranial hemorrhage in young and middle-aged adults. Although aneurysmal subarachnoid hemorrhage

does affect older persons, the average age for affected persons is 55.[35] Other leading causes of hemorrhagic stroke in young adults include bleeding diatheses, drug abuse, trauma, and vascular malformations. Although young adults with risk factors such as hypertension,

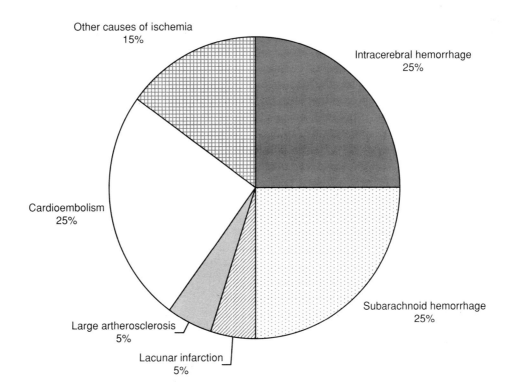

Figure 2-4. Approximate proportions of causes of stroke among Americans aged 15–45.

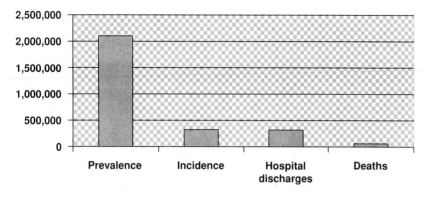

Figure 2-5. Impact of stroke among men in the United States. Adapted from the American Heart Association.[12]

diabetes mellitus, and smoking can have accelerated atherosclerosis as the cause of ischemic stroke, nonatherosclerotic vasculopathies, heart diseases, and prothrombotic disorders are etiologies of stroke in this age group.[36,37] In addition, ischemic and hemorrhagic stroke, including venous thrombosis, are recognized as important complications of pregnancy[38,39] (see Chapter 17).

Atherosclerosis generally evolves slowly over a person's lifetime; thus, it is not surprising that it is the leading arterial cause of ischemic stroke among persons older than 55 (see Chapters 4 and 9). For many years, controversy has existed about the relationship between some of the traditional risk factors for atherosclerosis and the occurrence of ischemic stroke. Some of this controversy may be attributed to the relatively advanced age of many persons who have stroke. Persons who live into the ninth and tenth decades often lack some of the traditional risk factors, such as tobacco use, which might cause heart disease or cancer, leading to death at a younger age. The absence of some of these factors may be a partial explanation for these persons' longevity. While these persons with very advanced age probably have stroke secondary to atherosclerosis, the development of arterial pathology probably relates more to their age than to the presence or absence of traditional risk factors, such as hypercholesterolemia. In addition, premature mortality from coronary artery disease among patients with multiple risk factors may explain the lack of a similar relationship to ischemic stroke. Coronary artery disease that leads to structural cardiac abnormalities and atrial fibrillation is an indirect atherosclerotic cause of stroke. In addition, the patient's age can affect decisions about medical or surgical treatment of atherosclerotic cerebrovascular disease. Still, no medical intervention or modification of behavior is likely to reverse the effects of advancing age on increasing the risk of stroke.

Gender

Stroke is a leading cause of death and disability among both men and women (Figs. 2-5 and 2-6). Thus, stroke is an important health problem for both sexes. Approximately 327,000 men and 373,000 women have a stroke in the United States each year.[12] Nearly 2,700,000 American women and 2,100,000 American men have had a stroke in the past. Stroke kills more women than men (100,000 vs 63,000) annually.[12] In the United States, approximately one in six women will die of stroke. This risk is compared to that which occurs with carcinoma of the breast, an illness that kills 1 in 25 women. In nearly all age groups, the rates of stroke are higher among men than among women. One exception is the slightly higher frequency of stroke among women aged 15–30, which is attributed to the potential for cerebrovascular complications of pregnancy or the puerperium[40] (see Chapter 17). Pregnancy-related cerebrovascular events happen at a particularly high rate in developing countries.

In most countries, the life expectancy of women is several years longer than that of men. As a result, the strong influence of advancing age on stroke risk accounts for the higher aggregate rate of stroke in women (Figs. 2-7 and 2-8). While women account for approximately 60 percent of the deaths from stroke, a majority of women who die from stroke are older than 80. Still, age-specific mortality figures are similar among men and women. During the last 30 years, the decline

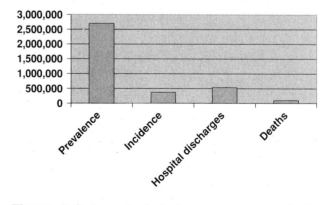

Figure 2-6. Impact of stroke among women in the United States. Adapted from the American Heart Association.[12]

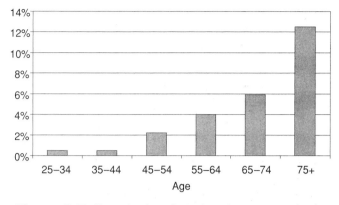

Figure 2-7. Prevalence of stroke among men in the United States as influenced by age. Adapted from the American Heart Association.[12]

in stroke incidence and mortality has been steeper among women than among men.[41] No major differences in recovery following stroke are noted between men and women. However, because many women are elderly and live alone, the likelihood that a woman surviving a stroke will be able to return home is less than that of her male counterpart.

The prognosis following a transient ischemic attack (TIA) is also influenced by the patient's sex. In general, women have a lower risk of a major vascular event (ischemic stroke, myocardial infarction, or vascular death) following a TIA than do men. The relatively benign prognosis following TIA among women might be reflected by a perceived lack of favorable treatment responses to some stroke-prevention therapies. Because the prognosis is better in women, a treatment effect of any prophylactic intervention will be hard to demonstrate due to the lack of serious adverse events including stroke. For example, when aspirin was first found to be effective in stroke prophylaxis, the benefit was limited to men. However, subsequent studies, including large meta-analyses that included larger numbers of women, have shown that men and women respond equally to antiplatelet aggregating agents.[42] Similar differences in responses between men and women were shown following carotid endarterectomy for treatment of severe, asymptomatic narrowing of the internal carotid artery.[43]

Women account for approximately 60 percent of cases of aneurysmal subarachnoid hemorrhage.[35] The main locations for ruptured aneurysms differ between women and men. Aneurysms of the middle cerebral artery are more common among women, while they are more commonly located on the anterior communicating artery in men. The average age of women with ruptured aneurysms is higher than that found in men. Women have an increased rate of serious complications and their prognosis is generally poor. The responses to treatment of subarachnoid hemorrhage also seem to differ between men and women.

Because the population of women older than 80 is much greater than that of men, the frequency of hemorrhagic stroke secondary to amyloid angiopathy is higher in women. On the other hand, there is some evidence for the protective effect of estrogens in forestalling Alzheimer disease in elderly women and, by implication, this hormone also might slow down the angiopathy that leads to intracerebral hemorrhage.

Pregnancy-related hemorrhagic stroke is an important cause of maternal mortality and morbidity; among the causes are ruptured aneurysms, ruptured vascular malformations, and venous thrombosis[44] (see Chapter 17). In particular, pregnancy is a leading contributing factor to the development of cerebral venous thrombosis (see Chapter 18). After the introduction of oral contraceptives, a strong relationship between their use and the risk of stroke was suggested; however, this correlation is less strong with the lower dose preparations that are prescribed currently[45] (see Chapter 17). The evidence for a potential relationship between the use of oral contraceptives and stroke appears to be strongest for the chances of aneurysmal subarachnoid hemorrhage.

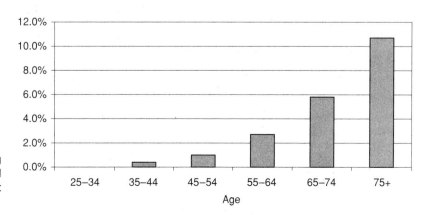

Figure 2-8. Prevalence of stroke among women in the United States as influenced by age. Adapted from the American Heart Association.[12]

Some strokes in young adults are attributed to migraine. Because of the high prevalence of migraine among young women, strokes in this group of patients are often attributed to migraine. The complex interactions between migraine and stroke are described in Chapter 17.

The higher frequency of alcohol and drug abuse among young men compared to young women may explain the higher rates of hemorrhagic and ischemic stroke. The high rate of serious trauma among young men leads to stroke secondary to extracranial or intracranial arterial injury. In addition, traumatic intracranial bleeding is common among young men. Some unusual causes of ischemic stroke such as Fabry–Anderson disease are X-linked. Because hemophilia is inherited in an X-linked recessive pattern, secondary hemorrhagic stroke is restricted to boys.

Accelerated atherosclerosis occurs at a younger age among men than among women; this difference probably is the major reason for the increased frequency of ischemic stroke among men in most age groups. In general, the rate of symptomatic atherosclerosis rises rapidly after the age of 40–50 in men and 50–60 in women. There have been potential explanations for the slower rate of atherosclerosis among women, with the protective effect of estrogens being the most widely cited reason. In general, the causes of ischemic stroke among postmenopausal women are similar to those found in men. The influence of postmenopausal use of estrogen or progesterone replacement therapy on the risk of stroke is controversial. The most recent evidence suggests that the combination of estrogen and progesterone might increase the likelihood of ischemic stroke.[46] Recent data also suggest that postmenopausal use of estrogen alone may be correlated with an increase in the risk of stroke. However, there is no evidence that postmenopausal use of estrogens and progesterone affects the course of atherosclerosis.

In general, men and women respond similarly to medical and surgical therapies to prevent or treat stroke. Measures to control risk factors for atherosclerosis can be prescribed with equal efficacy to men and women. The efficacy of antithrombotic medications in preventing ischemic events is similar in men and women. However, one should be aware of potential teratogenic effects of medications, such as warfarin, when prescribing these agents to women who may become pregnant. Carotid endarterectomy may be recommended for treatment of symptomatic men or women who have high-grade stenosis of the internal carotid artery. The effectiveness of this operation in asymptomatic women is not as apparent as in asymptomatic men. Endovascular procedures also can be recommended for both men and women. Measures for emergent evaluation and treatment of patients with suspected stroke are used in men and women. Thrombolytic therapy can be recommended for treatment of male and female patients with acute ischemic stroke. Treatment of hemorrhagic stroke also appears to not be affected by the patient's gender. Both male and female patients seem to respond equally to rehabilitation measures.

Geography and Ethnicity

Both hemorrhagic and ischemic stroke affect persons in all ethnic groups in all parts of the world.[47–49] Although cerebrovascular disease is a worldwide scourge, rates vary greatly among countries and regions. Some of the disparity may be secondary to differences in diet or lifestyle. Diets in eastern Asia differ markedly from those consumed in Mediterranean countries. The prevalence of smoking varies considerably in different countries. In addition, variations in health care and public health resources, reporting of the causes of death, and cultural norms can be reflected in the diverse stroke rates. Ethnic differences in the rates of stroke have been reported from multicultural societies. In general, rates of ischemic and hemorrhagic stroke are higher in eastern Europe than in western Europe, North America, or Australia.[5,50] Case fatality rates for intracranial hemorrhage are higher in eastern than in western Europe.[50] In addition, the frequency of stroke is increasing in eastern Europe possibly as a result of the poor state of health care in some of these countries, including the lack of modern medications, small numbers of stroke specialists and stroke programs, and the nonavailability of modern technology. The rate of stroke in the United Kingdom is higher than that in most other countries in western Europe; this high incidence is not explained. Recently, a differentiation of rates of stroke in Britain was noted with higher rates in the northern parts of the country than in the south.[51] Differences in diet may explain some of the variations between stroke rates in European countries. For example, the Mediterranean diet that emphasizes fish, vegetable oils, fruits, and vegetables has been associated with low rates of atherosclerotic disease. Similarly, a lower risk of heart disease and presumably stroke could accompany the drinking of red wine.

The incidence of stroke, in particular hemorrhage, is especially high in eastern Asia, an area of the world in which stroke is the leading cause of death. A recent report from China demonstrated that approximately 27 percent of strokes were secondary to hemorrhage.[52] The relative proportion of hemorrhagic stroke in eastern Asia is higher than that in other parts of the world. Presumably, this difference reflects the high rate of hypertension in Asian populations, which may be related to the high salt content of the diet or a genetic predisposition. The importance of hypertension is supported by the relatively high rate of lacunar infarction among Asians with ischemic stroke. A J-shaped relationship exists between blood cholesterol concentrations and the incidence and types of stroke. While hypercholesterolemia is associated with an increased chance of ischemic stroke secondary to advanced atherosclerosis, the incidence of brain hemorrhage is high among patients with low serum cholesterol values. Because Asian populations have relatively low cholesterol levels, this observation also may explain the prominence of hemorrhagic stroke. The shift from a low-fat, high-sodium diet based on fish proteins to a diet higher in animal proteins and fats is occurring in parts of Asia. The new, more western diet might result in future changes in the frequency and types of stroke in eastern Asia. Zhang et al.[52] have reported that the majority of strokes in China are the result of brain infarction. In addition, the risk of stroke, recurrent stroke, or death among Chinese is secondary to both intracranial and extracranial atherosclerosis.[53] Kubo et al.[7] report that the frequency of hemorrhagic stroke in Japan declined more rapidly than that of ischemic stroke. This difference in declines means that the relative proportions of the subtypes of stroke in eastern Asia may soon correspond to those found in western cultures.

Epidemiological data from Latin America, South and Southeast Asia, Africa, and most parts of the Middle East do not provide definitive estimates about the rates of stroke in these geographic regions. However, one can safely assume that strokes are an important public health problem, which will grow in the future. A survey from South America demonstrates that the rates and types of stroke are similar to those found in North America.[54] However, most of these data are from Argentina and Chile, which have an ethnic profile similar to that found in Europe and North America. Additional data from Central America and other parts of South America are needed. The geographic location of the patient does influence decisions about diagnosis and treatment. Some causes of stroke, for example, infectious diseases, are restricted to specific parts of the world. An example is stroke as a consequence of cysticercosis in persons living in Central America and Mexico. In addition, geographic location also is associated with the patient's ethnicity. Differences in the types and causes of stroke between European and Asian populations reflect the diverse nature of cerebrovascular disease. For example, the highest rates of moyamoya in the world are found in East Asian populations. Moyamoya disease, diagnosed in East Asia, appears to be an inherited disease, while moyamoya syndrome, diagnosed elsewhere in the world, probably is acquired. Because the ancestors of Native Americans appear to have migrated to North and South America from eastern Asia, they might share

some genetic risks with persons living in eastern Asia. These potential genetic similarities might impact on the causes of stroke. Clustering of Takayasu disease is seen in northeastern Asia and Mexico.

The incidence of and mortality from stroke in the United States and Canada are lower than that in most other parts of the world. Although the two countries have differing systems of health care, both report relatively dramatic declines in stroke during the last 30 years. The causes for the lower rates are debated but probably reflect professional and public health efforts to control risk factors for stroke, especially hypertension and smoking. Geographic variations in stroke also are noted within the United States. A recent report from the Centers for Disease Control and Prevention found that age-adjusted incidence for stroke ranged from 33 per 100,000 in New Hampshire to 83.8 per 100,000 in South Carolina.[13] The so-called Stroke Belt is described as an area in the United States that extends from Virginia to Texas.[13,55] These states have high rates of stroke with the greatest incidence found in the Carolinas. A notable exception is Florida, which has had a large immigration of persons from other parts of the United States. Potential explanations include high rates of hypertension and tobacco use, dietary differences, and ethnicity. Declines in stroke rates are noted in most parts of the United States, including the Stroke Belt.[56] In general, the area of the Stroke Belt seems to be shrinking possibly due to migration, changes in lifestyle, and the blending of regional cultures.[57,58] However, some recent increases in the rates of stroke are reported from western states. While rates in these states are relatively low, the immigration of older persons to Arizona and other Sunbelt states may explain some of this increase.

While most of the reports on ethnic influences in stroke are from the United States, similar findings have been described in Canada and the United Kingdom. In New Zealand, the rates of stroke are higher among persons of Maori or Pacific Island ancestry than those of European background.[59] The differences in rates in most countries cannot be explained by factors such as age, sex, or social class and, as a result, some ethnic relationship may be presumed.

In the United States, stroke is a particularly important health problem for African Americans[13,60] (Figs. 2-9 and 2-10). The burden of stroke in African Americans is one of the most serious public health problems that American medicine is facing.[61] Every year, approximately 110,000 African Americans have a stroke.[12] Increased risks are present for both hemorrhagic and ischemic stroke. In comparison to whites, the incidence of stroke is increased by a factor of 2 among both African-American men and women.[12] This racial disparity is most marked among younger persons. Among

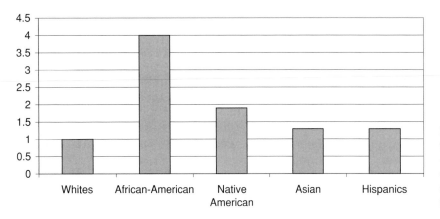

Figure 2-9. Relative risk of death from stroke mortality among young (age 35–44) Americans as affected by ethnicity. The other ethnic groups are compared to whites (rate = 1). Adapted from the American Heart Association.[12]

persons younger than 45, the risk of ischemic stroke is up to four times higher in African Americans than in whites (see Fig. 2-9).[62] The frequency of hemorrhagic strokes is two to four times higher in African Americans than in other ethnic groups.[63–66] In addition to a higher number of strokes, the vascular events themselves appear to be more severe among African Americans. Part of this difference may be reflected by a relatively lower rate of TIA in African Americans. Mortality from stroke in all age groups is approximately twice as high in African Americans as in whites and among persons under the age of 45; the relative risk for mortality is approximately 4.[63] Likewise, African-American children have a higher risk for stroke-related deaths than do children of other ethnic groups.[28] Despite an overall trend for a decline in stroke mortality within the United States, deaths from stroke have not dropped among African Americans.[67] Even further, the risk of recurrent stroke appears higher among African Americans than in other ethnic groups.[68] Thus, the high frequency of stroke with all its consequences among African Americans represents a critically important public health problem for the United States. The impact of all aspects of stroke care must emphasize interventions aimed at this minority group.

The causes of stroke are also affected by ethnicity. For example, sickle-cell disease, which is restricted largely to persons of African or Middle Eastern ancestry, is an important cause of hemorrhagic or ischemic stroke in children and young adults.[69] The prevalence of risk factors that predispose to stroke, in particular hypertension and obesity, is more common among African Americans.[70,71] Atherosclerosis is common in the African-American population, but the locations of advanced lesions differ from those reported among persons of European ancestry. While severe stenosis of the extracranial portion of the internal carotid artery is common in whites, intracranial atherosclerosis is more frequently found in African Americans.

Under the age of 65, the rate of stroke is higher among Hispanic Americans than among persons of European ancestry. However, at older ages, the rates of stroke are similar. The increased frequency of stroke may be explained partially by the high prevalence of diabetes mellitus in the Hispanic-American population. In addition, the risk of hemorrhagic stroke is increased modestly among Hispanic Americans.[63] The rates of stroke among younger Native Americans and whites are similar. However, over the age of 65, Native Americans have the lowest rate of stroke of any ethnic group in the

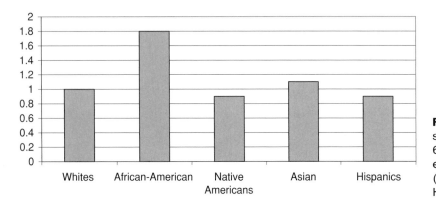

Figure 2-10. Relative risk of death from stroke mortality among Americans aged 65–74 as affected by ethnicity. The other ethnic groups are compared to white (rate = 1). Adapted from the American Heart Association.[12]

United States. The frequency of stroke among Asian Americans does not differ markedly from that found among non-Hispanic white Americans. The rate of stroke among Asian Americans is lower than that reported in eastern Asia. The types of stroke among Asian Americans also differ from those reported in Asia. Severe atherosclerotic lesions in Asian Americans are primarily intracranial in location.

The ethnicity of the patient does influence decisions in the diagnosis and treatment of cerebrovascular disease. Further research on ethnic influences on cerebrovascular disease will grow in importance.

Social and Economic Status

Reports from around the world demonstrate a trend for a higher rate of ischemic and hemorrhagic stroke among persons from lower socioeconomic classes than among more affluent and educated populations[72] (see Table 2-3). The high rate of stroke in the poor may be explained by several factors. Many poor or uneducated people have limited knowledge about health and limited access to health information, including the importance of the control of risk factors. The prevalence of heart disease, diabetes mellitus, obesity, alcohol and drug abuse, and smoking is relatively high among lower socioeconomic groups. In addition, access to health care can be limited and patients might not be able to afford expensive medications. Diets differ between affluent and poorer populations because of the costs of healthy food. The metabolic syndrome, which is linked to obesity, may be especially prominent among lower socioeconomic groups in the United States. While some of the differences between socioeconomic classes in the United States might reflect the costs of health care, similar trends are found in countries with national health insurance schemes. Thus, personal financial factors that might reduce the availability of professional care do not appear to be the major determinant for the high stroke rate among poor.

Work-related stresses associated with jobs that have high demands and low rewards are reported as potential factors leading to vascular disease and stroke. These stresses seem to be greatest among persons who have limited ability to change their occupational duties. Thus, they seem to be less of a problem among professionals than other groups. Occupational relationships may be partially related to development of hypertension or associated with alcohol, tobacco, and drug abuse.

The likelihood of stroke is increased among persons with psychiatric or behavioral disorders. Both depression and anger appear to be risk factors.[73] In addition to being a factor that contributes to cerebrovascular disease, these psychiatric disorders may affect all aspects of care including efforts to recover

from a stroke. Married persons have a lower risk of stroke than do single persons of the same age. Besides being associated with a high chance of cerebrovascular events, living alone also affects the likelihood of a person rapidly reaching medical attention for stroke. In addition, a single person is less likely to be able to return home after stroke because there may be no one to serve as a caregiver in the house. In particular, elderly women, many of whom are widows, often are unable to return home following a stroke.

Family History of Vascular Disease

Both hemorrhagic and ischemic stroke can result from inherited diseases that are described in subsequent chapters, in particular Chapters 12, 14, 16, and 17. Intracranial aneurysms and vascular malformations occur in familial clusters and both can be components of multisystem genetic diseases, such as polycystic kidney disease or hereditary hemorrhagic telangiectasia. Moyamoya disease, which appears to be an inherited vasculopathy especially prominent in eastern Asia, can present with subarachnoid hemorrhage in young adults. In comparison to the general population, a patient with a family history of subarachnoid hemorrhage has approximately a three to five times increased risk of aneurysmal rupture. Siblings of patients with ruptured aneurysms have approximately a 4 percent percent risk of subarachnoid hemorrhage. Inherited disorders of coagulation, such as hemophilia, also may induce hemorrhagic stroke. Brain hemorrhage is an important complication of sickle-cell disease.

Ischemic stroke can result from several inherited prothrombotic diseases. A family history of deep vein thrombosis, pulmonary embolism, premature stroke or myocardial infarction, or spontaneous abortions provides evidence for an inherited prothrombotic disorder. In addition, familial disorders, such as diseases of lipid or amino acid metabolism, can accelerate development of atherosclerosis. Some of these are secondary to polygenetic disorders, while others can be ascribed to specific genetic diseases, such as the X-linked Fabry–Anderson disease. This rare disease is a recognized cause of atherosclerosis in young men. Both diabetes mellitus and migraine, which can lead to ischemic stroke, also seem to cluster in families. In addition, the list of inherited disorders that lead to vasculopathy and stroke is growing. The most prominent inherited vasculopathy is cerebral autosomal dominant arteriopathy with subcortical ischemic leukoencephalopathy (CADASIL), which is a cause of recurrent stroke and vascular dementia in young adults.

However, because of the high prevalence of cerebrovascular disease in the general population, many patients report that one or more relatives have had a stroke. Depending upon the age of the patient and the age of his/her affected relatives, this history may or may not be helpful. Strokes that occur in elderly relatives probably are not as significant as those events that affect younger persons (<60 years). Events in young adults might portend an inherited predisposition to stroke. Some of the familial relationship to stroke may be secondary to common environmental factors such as diet, the use of alcohol or tobacco, physical inactivity, a lack of knowledge about health care, or limited access to medical services. Vascular events in multiple family members appear to be more ominous than when a single relative has had a myocardial infarction or stroke. When a stroke occurs in a monozygotic twin, the risk of stroke in the other twin is increased by a factor of 5. Maternal or paternal history of stroke appears to be associated with a higher risk of vascular events in a child. The relative risk increases by approximately 2-4 when the father has had a stroke and by 1.4 if the mother has had stroke. Tentschert et al.[74] found that a sex-specific relationship exists between a maternal history of stroke and the prevalence of hypertension and left ventricular hypertrophy in women with ischemic cerebrovascular disease. In general, the risk of stroke is greater when parents have strokes than when such events occur in siblings or other relatives.

Environmental Factors

The incidence of both hemorrhagic and ischemic stroke has been associated with changes in weather, season of the year, day of the week, or time of the day.[75] The significance of some of these relationships should be explored. An increased frequency of stroke, in particular intracranial hemorrhage, is correlated with cold weather and winter months. Strokes are also more frequent on Mondays than other days of the week. Among young adults, a peak in subarachnoid hemorrhage and ischemic stroke occurs on weekends, and this finding is speculated to be associated with excessive consumption of alcohol. Subarachnoid hemorrhage is most frequent in the early morning hours. Ischemic stroke also peaks during the first hours after awakening in the morning. This time relationship might be secondary to hypertension or changes in coagulation factors that appear early in the morning. An increased frequency of stroke has also been correlated with environmental factors such as air pollution.[76,77]

▶ PROGNOSIS OF ISCHEMIC OR HEMORRHAGIC STROKE

A number of issues need to be addressed when considering the prognosis of patients with cerebrovascular disease.

▶ **TABLE 2-5.** PREDICTORS OF INCREASED RISK OF ISCHEMIC STROKE OR RECURRENT ISCHEMIC STROKE

Asymptomatic bruit or stenosis
Symptomatic atherosclerotic disease
   Coronary artery disease
   Peripheral artery disease
Atrial fibrillation
Amaurosis fugax
Transient ischemic attack
Ischemic stroke

Patients with hemorrhagic and ischemic stroke have a high risk of death or disability from the event itself. In addition, patients with symptomatic cerebrovascular disease have a high potential for recurrent neurological events. Patients with stroke secondary to atherosclerosis are also at risk for other vascular events, including myocardial infarction or vascular death. Besides stroke and myocardial infarction, other causes of vascular death include pulmonary embolism, rupture of an aortic aneurysm, or peripheral arterial disease. Several factors affect a patient's prognosis. Persons with asymptomatic cerebrovascular disease have a more favorable course than those who have had recent neurological events (Table 2-5). Because a patient with a TIA does not have residual neurological impairments, the primary prognostic issue is the potential for a disabling stroke.[78] The transient neurological symptoms reflect a change in the underlying vascular disease. Patients with hemorrhagic stroke have a higher risk of early death (<1 month) than do persons with ischemic stroke. Among patients with either type of stroke, age, severity of neurological impairments, size of the stroke on brain imaging, and presence of concomitant diseases predict outcomes. In addition, the cause of stroke affects acute prognosis and the likelihood of recurrent events.

Asymptomatic Cerebrovascular Disease

Compared to healthy, age-matched persons, patients with an asymptomatic carotid bruit or atherosclerotic stenosis have an increased risk for stroke, myocardial infarction, and vascular death. Myocardial infarction is the leading cause of death among this group of persons. The yearly risk of clinically overt stroke is estimated as 1–3 percent.[43,79] The risk is higher among persons with more severe narrowing (80–90 percent stenosis) and those who have progression of the plaque detected by sequential noninvasive studies.[79–81] Persons with active tobacco use, hypercholesterolemia, or hypertension have a greater risk of rapid progression of asymptomatic plaques. A sizable percentage of patients who have subsequent stroke will have warning symptoms of TIA. The chances of stroke are as high in the vascular territory of the contralateral internal carotid artery or the posterior circulation as that found ipsilateral to the stenotic lesion. These features add difficulty to any decision about treatment. The relatively low rates of ischemic stroke ipsilateral to the stenotic lesion mean that data demonstrating efficacy of any local intervention (surgery or endovascular therapy) are difficult to achieve.

An unruptured saccular aneurysm can be detected in several situations. It may be found on brain or vascular imaging performed to assess another condition. An unruptured aneurysm can produce ischemic or mass-related symptoms. Nearly 25 percent of patients with subarachnoid hemorrhage have more than one aneurysm. Only one of the aneurysms would have ruptured and the others remain asymptomatic. The annual rate of aneurysmal rupture is relatively low among asymptomatic persons but it is greater among persons who have had a prior subarachnoid hemorrhage.[82] Several factors predict the likelihood of aneurysmal rupture. Patients with prior subarachnoid hemorrhage have an increased risk of bleeding. Persons with hypertension and those who smoke or abuse alcohol have a higher risk of aneurysmal rupture. While the location of the aneurysm does not affect the risk of bleeding, the size of the aneurysm does; the greatest risk is among patients with aneurysms greater than 6 mm in diameter.

Prognosis Following TIA

Approximately 10 percent of patients with ischemic stroke report premonitory symptoms (TIA). A TIA is an important omen for impending stroke (see Chapter 5). Besides marking the patient as having a high risk for stroke, a TIA also predicts a high likelihood of myocardial infarction or vascular death. Overall, the chances of a stroke are approximately 20 percent within 5 years of a TIA.[83] The risk of stroke following a TIA appears to be front-loaded. In one study that assessed the frequency of events among persons seen in an emergency department for evaluation of TIA, the risk of stroke was found to be approximately 10 percent during the first 3 months, with 5 percent risk within 48 h[84]. Lovett et al.[85] recently reported that the risk of stroke following a first-ever TIA was 8.6 percent within 7 days and 12.0 percent within 30 days. Multiple events (crescendo TIA) appear to be more ominous than a single event (Table 2-6). The definition of crescendo TIA includes several events that occur in a cluster within a few hours or days, including at least three events within 24–48 h. Because the risk of stroke appears to be especially high, crescendo TIA should be considered a neurological emergency and aggressive investigation and treatment are necessary.

▶ **TABLE 2-6.** FACTORS THAT PREDICT HIGHEST RISK OF STROKE FOLLOWING TIAs

Interval since last event
Multiple events (crescendo TIA)
Events that are prolonged (>1 h)
Events that occur upon awakening in the morning
Events that are associated with major impairments

Although any patient who has a TIA is at risk for stroke, some happen to have a heightened risk. A minor stroke or hemispheric TIA is accompanied by a higher risk than an episode of amaurosis fugax. TIAs associated with severe neurological impairments (such as weakness of one-half of the body) or prolonged deficits (generally >1 h in duration) are more ominous than those associated with brief or minor events.[84] Events lasting more than 1 h usually occur among patients with severe extracranial atherosclerotic disease or cardiac lesions. An event that is present upon awakening in the morning is also associated with a high risk for ischemic stroke. A high-grade stenosis of the internal carotid artery has a high risk for stroke.[86] The presence of extensive vascular disease, such as contralateral internal carotid artery occlusion or intracranial disease, also portends a high chance for stroke. Persons with a symptomatic occlusion of the internal carotid artery and who have borderline reduced perfusion in the ipsilateral cerebral hemisphere have an approximately 20–25 percent rate of stroke within 2 years.[87] Patients with a history of diabetes mellitus or congestive heart failure have a high risk of vascular death following a TIA.[88,89]

Recurrent Ischemic Stroke

Patients who have had one stroke also have a high risk for another event. These patients appear to have a higher likelihood of another stroke than do patients with TIA. Presumably, the risk of recurrence is highest in the first days following the first stroke. Recent clinical trials provide important evidence about the chances of another cerebrovascular event within the first days following ischemic stroke.[90–92] Overall, the likelihood of recurrent stroke is approximately 1.5 percent within 1 week, 2–3 percent within 2 weeks, and 2–5 percent within 4 weeks. Most recurrent strokes are in the same vascular territory as that of the original stroke. Some of the recurrent strokes are preceded by a TIA. The probability of recurrent stroke is increased among African Americans, Hispanic Americans, or persons with elevated blood pressure, congestive heart failure, or valvular heart disease. The subtype of ischemic stroke generally does not affect the likelihood of new cerebrovascular events.

Concerns persist that recurrent embolism is high among persons with cardiac diseases. For example, the presence of an intra-atrial thrombus might portend a high likelihood of early stroke. A similar scenario might occur among persons with intra-arterial thrombi. Not surprisingly, the prognosis of a second stroke is poorer than that following a single event. The poor prognosis of recurrent stroke often is due to cognitive deficits; multiple recurrent strokes can lead to vascular dementia.

Prognosis Following Ischemic Stroke

Outcomes following ischemic stroke are discussed in terms of mortality and unfavorable outcomes (Table 2-7). The group of unfavorable outcomes includes those patients who survive stroke but have severe residual neurological impairments that result in disability, serious handicap, or institutionalized care. Approximately one-fourth of stroke survivors are cared for on a long-term basis in a nursing home.[12] Survival with severe motor or cognitive deficits that result in long-term care is considered by many persons to be an outcome worse than death. The leading causes of long-term disability include visual loss, cognitive or language impairments, motor or sensory deficits, and poor balance. In addition, a secondary depression can cause major disability. By 3 months following ischemic stroke, approximately 30–40

▶ **TABLE 2-7.** PREDICTORS OF POOR OUTCOMES FOLLOWING ACUTE ISCHEMIC STROKE

Neurological status
  Decreased level of consciousness
  Major focal neurological impairments
    (High score on NIHSS)
  Stroke due to large artery occlusion
    Internal carotid artery
    Proximal middle cerebral artery
    Basilar artery
  Recurrent strokes
Cause of stroke
  Large artery atherosclerosis
  Cardioembolism
Epidemiological features
  Advanced age
  African Americans
Comorbid diseases
  Diabetes mellitus or hyperglycemia
  Heart disease—congestive heart failure
  Lung disease
Baseline brain imaging findings
  Multilobar infarction
  Dense artery sign
  Shift of midline structures (mass effect)
  Hemorrhagic transformation

percent of patients have made a complete recovery or have minimal residual impairments.[12] By 1 year, approximately 65 percent of stroke survivors are independent. The rate of recovery is highest among younger persons and those with lacunar or brain stem infarctions. Still, most young adults describe stroke as a negative event that changes their lives.[93]

Approximately 10–20 percent of patients die within 1 month of stroke.[12,94] In general, mortality directly secondary to the brain disease occurs within 1 week (Table 2-8). These deaths are the result of the brain injury itself, brain edema with increased intracranial pressure and herniation, secondary intracranial hemorrhage, or recurrent stroke (see Chapter 24). Medical complications of stroke including infections, cardiac events, or venous thromboembolic events are the leading causes of death in the subsequent 2–3 weeks. A similar-sized percentage of affected persons will die during the subsequent months. Approximately 30 percent of the patients with stroke will be dead by 1 year, and by 5 years, more than one-half of patients will die.[95] Approximately 50 percent of persons aged 65 or less at the time of stroke will be dead within 8 years of their cerebrovascular event.[12] Both acute and long-term mortality rates are higher among the old than younger persons.[26] Most late (>30 days following stroke) deaths are due to cardiovascular disease, pulmonary infections, or complications of the original stroke. Cancer and recurrent stroke are other potential causes of late deaths. When compared to similarly aged healthy persons, the increase in mortality among patients with ischemic cerebrovascular disease persists up to 20 years following stroke. Overall, the risk of death among persons who survive stroke is approximately 2–2.5 times that of similarly aged healthy persons.

Several factors influence the prognosis of persons with ischemic stroke[96] (see Table 2-7). Unfavorable

▶ **TABLE 2-8.** CAUSES OF DEATH FOLLOWING ISCHEMIC STROKE

Deaths occurring within 1 week of stroke
  Neurological effects of acute stroke
  Brain edema (increased intracranial pressure, herniation)
  Hemorrhagic transformation of stroke
Deaths occurring during 1 week–1 month of stroke
  Pneumonia
  Urinary tract infection/sepsis
  Pulmonary embolism
  Cardiorespiratory failure
Deaths occurring after 1 month of stroke
  Myocardial infarction
  Sudden or vascular death
  Recurrent stroke
  Infection (pneumonia, urinary tract infection)
  Comorbid diseases

outcomes are more common among elderly persons (especially >85 years) and those with severe comorbid diseases including diabetes mellitus, heart disease, lung disease, or preexisting dementia. The presence of hyperglycemia following stroke forecasts an unfavorable outcome regardless of other clinical features[97,98] (Chapter 21). The adverse effects of hyperglycemia may be secondary to lactic acidosis from anaerobic glycolysis, which occurs with the combination of hypoxia and elevated glucose levels. In addition, hyperglycemia might be a marker of a stress response to a very severe stroke. Other comorbid diseases, such as emphysema or coronary artery disease, may affect decisions for acute management, predispose to serious medical complications, or limit the patient's ability to undergo rehabilitation. Because they have a higher likelihood of having a severe event, African Americans have a poorer prognosis than do other ethnic groups. Overall, when adjusting for age and other comorbid diseases, the prognoses of men and women appear to be similar.

The most important forecaster of outcome is the severity of the patient's neurological impairments, which in turn reflects the location and size of the stroke. Patients with large cortical or subcortical infarctions have a high chance of residual neurological deficits that lead to disability, although these strokes probably will not prove fatal. Patients with isolated or mild neurological impairments usually recover completely or have nondisabling residual complaints. The extent of the neurological deficits influences decisions about management of the acute stroke itself. In addition, patients with severe deficits are also at high risk for medical or neurological complications. Coma, the most important clinical predictor of an unfavorable outcome, is rarely detected during the first 24 h following cerebral infarction.

Patients with multilobar infarctions secondary to occlusion of a major extracranial or intracranial artery have extensive deficits. These patients are prone to development of malignant brain edema that may be fatal, and they are likewise vulnerable to bleeding complications of thrombolytic therapy. The National Institutes of Health Stroke Scale (NIHSS) is commonly used to quantify the severity of the stroke (Table 2-9). Scores range from 0 to 42 points. The NIHSS score predicts outcome.[99–101] The baseline NIHSS score predicts response to

▶ **TABLE 2-9.** NATIONAL INSTITUTES OF HEALTH STROKE SCALE

Item	Range of Scores
Level of consciousness 0—alert, 1—drowsy, 2—stupor, 3—coma	0–3 points
Responses to two questions 0—knows age and month, 1—answers one correctly, 2—cannot answer either question	0–2 points
Responses to two commands 0—follows two commands, 1—follows one command, 2—cannot follow either command	0–2 points
Lateral eye movements (best gaze) 0—normal eye movements, 1—partial gaze paresis, 2—forced gaze palsy	0–2 points
Visual fields 0—no visual loss, 1—partial hemianopia, 2—complete hemianopia, 3—bilateral visual loss	0–3 points
Facial weakness 0—no facial weakness, 1—minor unilateral facial weakness, 2—partial unilateral facial weakness, 3—complete paralysis of one or both sides of face	0–3 points
Upper extremity weakness (both right and left scored) 0—normal movement, 1—drift of limb, 2—some effort against gravity, 3—no effort against gravity, 4—no movement	0–4 points (up to 8)
Lower extremity weakness (both right and left scored) 0—normal movement, 1—drift of limb, 2—some effort against gravity, 3—no effort against gravity, 4—no movement	0–4 points (up to 8)
Limb ataxia (cannot be tested in presence of paresis) 0—no limb ataxia, 1—present in one limb, 2—present in two limbs	0–2 points
Sensory 0—no sensory loss, 1—mild-to-moderate sensory loss, 2—severe-to-total sensory loss	0–2 points
Language 0—normal language, 1—mild-to-moderate aphasia, 2—severe aphasia, 3—mute	0–3 points
Articulation 0—normal, 1—mild-to-moderate dysarthria, 2—severe dysarthria	0–2 points
Extinction or inattention 0—absent, 1—visual or sensory inattention or extinction, 2—profound hemiattention	0–2 points

Adapted from Brott et al.[128]

treatment with thrombolytic agents.[102] Patients with occlusion of the basilar artery and secondary pontine infarction leading to coma or locked-in syndrome have a particularly poor prognosis. Patients with large (>3 cm in diameter) cerebellar infarctions have an increased risk of death due to mass effects, which can lead to hydrocephalus or brain stem compression.

The results of brain imaging provide prognostic information. A large, multilobar infarction with effacement of the cortical sulci, obliteration of the insular cortex, and the appearance of a subcortical hypodensity can be found following an occlusion of the middle cerebral artery.[103] These changes are most commonly found among patients with severe neurological impairments. The correlation between the score on the NIHSS and the volume of the infarction is strong.[104] In subsequent hours, imaging findings of a shift of midline structures and the development of a large area of hypodensity are correlated with an unfavorable outcome. Detection of the dense artery sign (thrombus in the middle cerebral artery) also forecasts a high chance of poor outcome. Besides predicting a high probability of brain edema, these imaging changes forecast an increased risk for major intracranial bleeding from interventions such as thrombolytic therapy.

Prognosis Following Hemorrhagic Stroke

In comparison to patients with ischemic stroke, the prognosis of patients with intracranial bleeding is much more guarded. Approximately 35 percent of patients with hemorrhagic stroke will die within 30 days of the event.[12,105–107] In a Japanese population study, Kubo et al.[7] reported that the mortality following intracerebral hemorrhage was 61 percent. The 30-day mortality rate among children exceeds 20 percent, making intracranial hemorrhage a leading cause of death in childhood.[30] Approximately 10–25 percent of patients die within 24 h of the ictus and many patients are not able to reach medical attention.[106,108] Intracranial hemorrhage is often detected as part of a medical examiner evaluation of a person found dead (Table 2-10). Hemorrhagic stroke is second to cardiac ischemia and arrhythmias as a cause of sudden death.[15] Some early deaths following brain hemorrhage probably are secondary to respiratory arrest or acute cardiovascular complications, including malignant arrhythmias. While mortality is high among persons with hemorrhagic stroke, the prognosis for neurological recovery among survivors can be relatively good. Because blood often dissects along the course of nerve fibers, the area of brain destruction may be relatively limited and recovery might be better than that anticipated at the time of the initial examination.

▶ **TABLE 2-10.** CAUSES OF DEATH IN ACUTE HEMORRHAGIC STROKE

Within 24 h
  Acute brain injury
  Cardiovascular complications
  Acute pulmonary edema
24 h–1 week
  Increased intracranial pressure
    Brain edema
    Mass of hematoma
    Hydrocephalus
  Complications of medical treatment
  Complications of surgical treatment
Greater than 1 week
  Medical complications
    Pneumonia and other infections
    Pulmonary embolism
Ruptured aneurysms
  Recurrent hemorrhage
  Vasospasm and ischemic stroke

Several factors predict outcomes following hemorrhagic stroke (Table 2-11). Elderly persons have poorer outcomes than do younger patients.[109] The patient's sex and ethnicity does not affect prognosis. Severe comorbid diseases, such as heart disease or diabetes mellitus, have an adverse impact on outcomes.[110] The etiology of the hemorrhage affects both acute and long-term prognoses. Hemorrhages secondary to a coagulopathy, including antithrombotic or thrombolytic treatment, are often associated with severe or prolonged bleeding and a poor prognosis. Patients with lobar hemorrhages sec-

▶ **TABLE 2-11.** PREDICTORS OF POOR OUTCOME FOLLOWING HEMORRHAGIC STROKE

Clinical
  Decreased level of consciousness
  Major focal neurological impairments
Cause
  Bleeding diathesis
  Amyloid angiopathy
  Ruptured aneurysm
Epidemiological features
  Advanced age
Comorbid diseases
  Hyponatremia
Baseline brain imaging findings
  Deep hemispheric hematoma
  Brain stem hematoma
  Hematoma > 2.5 cm in diameter
  Intraventricular hemorrhage
  Extensive subarachnoid hemorrhage
  Acute hydrocephalus

ondary to amyloid angiopathy have a relatively high risk for recurrent bleeding and a generally poor prognosis. Advanced age and the presence of Alzheimer disease also influence the poor prognosis of patients with hemorrhagic stroke secondary to amyloid angiopathy. The annual risk for recurrent bleeding from a ruptured arteriovenous malformation is approximately 2 percent. The risk is not particularly high during the first days following the initial hemorrhage. In some instances, the hemorrhage may obliterate a small vascular malformation. Because many patients with ruptured vascular malformations are children and young adults, their prognosis is better. There may be an increased risk for recurrent hemorrhage from arteriovenous malformations during the third trimester of pregnancy or labor. Patients with nonaneurysmal subarachnoid hemorrhage, particularly those with blood restricted to the perimesencephalic cistern, have a good prognosis and low rates of complications.

The size and location of the hematoma also affect prognosis. Generally, patients with bleeding in the cortical white matter adjacent to the cortex, especially those with hemorrhages in the frontal and occipital poles, have a better prognosis than do those with bleeding into deep hemispheric structures, the brain stem, or the cerebellum.[111,112] Patients with large deep hemorrhages (>2.5 cm in diameter) usually have poor outcomes. Prior to the advent of brain imaging, intraventricular extension of the bleeding was considered to be uniformly fatal because it was detected only by autopsy. Now intraventricular blood is detected in approximately 15 percent of cases of hemorrhagic stroke. While the finding of intraventricular hemorrhage remains an unfavorable prognostic sign, it does not forecast fatality. Intraventricular hemorrhage can cause acute hydrocephalus secondary to obstruction of the cerebrospinal fluid pathways. Hydrocephalus also is associated with mass effects of the hematoma, and thus its presence is correlated with more severe hemorrhages.[113] Large cerebellar hemorrhage (>2.5 cm in diameter) can cause acute hydrocephalus and secondary brain stem compression.[114] Since the development of brain imaging, small intraparenchymal hemorrhages, most commonly in the basal ganglia and brain stem, have been increasingly recognized. The prognosis of this group of patients is relatively good. Their course is often similar to that noted among persons with small subcortical infarctions.

The size and location of the hemorrhage also are correlated with the severity of the neurological impairments. The most important prognostic sign is the patient's level of consciousness[109,115,116] (see Table 2-11). Depression in consciousness, including coma, is common among patients with hemorrhagic stroke. Coma is most common among patients with large brain stem or basal ganglia hematomas. Patients with fever or tachycardia also have a poor prognosis following intracranial hemorrhage.[117,118]

Prognosis Following Aneurysmal Subarachnoid Hemorrhage

Patients with ruptured intracranial saccular aneurysm have a very guarded prognosis. Patients die or are disabled as a consequence of the initial hemorrhage, recurrent aneurysmal rupture, vasospasm with secondary ischemic stroke, or complications of medical or surgical interventions.[119] Approximately 80 percent of deaths happen within 1 week of the aneurysmal rupture. Recurrent aneurysmal rupture occurs primarily within the first 10 days. Overall, the risk is approximately 20 percent, but within the first 24 h the chances of a second hemorrhage are approximately 4 percent.[108] Vasospasm leading to ischemic stroke also peaks within the first 7–10 days. Because most of the serious consequences of subarachnoid hemorrhage occur within the first 2 weeks of the initial ictus, the interval from aneurysmal rupture greatly influences prognosis.

Despite the relatively young age of the affected patients, the 30-day mortality is approximately 50 percent (see Table 2-10). Approximately 10 percent of the deaths occur within 24 h of the aneurysmal rupture. Approximately 50 percent of survivors will have major neurological impairments. The patient's age does affect prognosis; patients older than 65 have poorer outcomes than do younger persons.[120] The presence of severe comorbid diseases, such as heart disease, also adversely affects prognosis. While women generally are older than men, their prognosis is poorer even when adjusting for age.[35] Women have a higher risk for recurrent hemorrhage and vasospasm than do men. No ethnic relationships are found for either mortality or unfavorable outcomes. The patient's neurological status is a strong forecaster; mortality is approximately 15 percent among alert patients and it is approximately 75 percent among comatose patients. Seriously ill patients have a high rate of medical and neurological complications. The presence of focal signs, such as hemiparesis, does not affect outcomes.

Several rating scales have been used to quantify the neurological impairments following subarachnoid hemorrhage. The most widely used are the Hunt–Hess Scale and the World Federation of Neurological Surgeons Scale[121] (Table 2-12). The latter scale is based on the features in the Glasgow Coma Scale (Table 2-13). While the Glasgow Coma Scale was originally developed for evaluation of the seriousness of brain injury following trauma, the ratings seem to work well when predicting outcomes following brain hemorrhage.

▶ **TABLE 2-12.** WORLD FEDERATION OF NEUROLOGICAL SURGEONS' RATING SCALE

Grade	Glasgow Score	Focal Signs
I	15	Absent
II	13–14	Absent
III	13–14	Present
IV	7–12	Present/absent
V	3–6	Present/absent

Adapted from Ogungbo.[129]

▶ **TABLE 2-14.** MODIFIED RANKIN SCALE

Score	Impairments
0	No symptoms at all
1	No disability despite symptoms
2	Slight disability but does not require assistance
3	Moderate disability but can walk
4	Moderately severe disability
5	Severe disability and often bedridden
6	Dead

Adapted from Bamford et al.[130]

Approximately 20–30 percent of patients have one or more severe headaches in the days and weeks prior to the major subarachnoid hemorrhage. These symptoms often are ascribed to a minor rupture of the aneurysm (warning or sentinel leak). Patients with warning symptoms have a much poorer prognosis than do patients with a single hemorrhage; the overall mortality approximately doubles.

The location of the aneurysm influences outcomes. Aneurysms of the anterior communicating artery and the posterior circulation are associated with poorer prognoses than are aneurysms of the internal carotid artery or the middle cerebral artery. The size of the aneurysm also affects prognosis. Patients with giant

aneurysms (>25 mm) have a much higher mortality than those with smaller aneurysms. Patients with hyponatremia have a poor prognosis.

Several imaging findings affect prognosis. Persons with normal CT scans and those with small, thin collections of subarachnoid blood generally do very well[122] (see Table 2-11). They have a low risk for vasospasm and the primary concern focuses on prevention of recurrent aneurysmal rupture. Patients with diffuse or localized thick collections of blood have a high risk for vasospasm.[123] The presence of extensive subarachnoid blood, hydrocephalus, intracerebral hemorrhage, or intraventricular hemorrhage is associated with poor neurological signs and poor outcomes. These CT changes do not forecast vasospasm or ischemic stroke.

▶ ASSESSING OUTCOMES OF STROKE

Because the spectrum of outcomes following stroke is broad and because nonfatal events are often considered as unfavorable, several scales have been developed to rate disability or societal impairments that limit the return to prestroke activities. These scales evaluate different components of the neurological status than do the acute stroke scales, which focus on discrete neurological impairments. The Glasgow Outcome Scale, used

▶ **TABLE 2-13.** GLASGOW COMA SCALE

Best eye-opening response
- 4   Eyes open spontaneously, not necessarily aware of environment
- 3   Eyes open to speech, not necessarily in response to command
- 2   Eyes open in response to painful stimulus
- 1   No eye opening in response to painful stimulus

Best motor response
- 6   Follows simple commands, can have paresis or hemiplegia
- 5   Responds to painful stimulus by attempting to remove source of pain
- 4   Withdraws to painful stimulus
- 3   Develops abnormal flexor (decorticate) posturing in response to painful stimulus
- 2   Develops abnormal extensor (decerebrate) posturing in response to painful stimulus
- 1   No motor response to painful stimulus

Best verbal response
- 5   Patient oriented to time, place, and person
- 4   Patient confused but responds to conversation
- 3   Language is intelligible and no sustained sentence
- 2   Has incomprehensible sounds, moans, and groans—no words
- 1   No verbal response

Adapted from Teasdale et al.[124]

▶ **TABLE 2-15.** BARTHEL INDEX

	Dependent	Partial	Independent
Feeding	0	5	10
Chair/bed transfers	0	5/10	15
Grooming	0	0	5
Toilet transfers	0	5	10
Bathing	0	0	5
Walking	0	5/10	15
Stairs	0	5	10
Dressing	0	5	10
Bowel control	0	5	10
Bladder control	0	5	10

Adapted from Mahoney and Barthel.[126]

initially to evaluate survivors of severe head injuries, has applicability to stroke, especially subarachnoid hemorrhage.[124] The modified Rankin Scale examines the patient's overall performance[125] (Table 2-14). It is the most widely used stroke-outcome-rating instrument. It has high interrater agreement and it is employed extensively in acute stroke treatment trials. The Barthel index consists of several questions designed to examine the patient's ability to perform activities of daily living[126] (Table 2-15). The Barthel index rates disability but it is heavily influenced by motor impairments. Other scales, which have not been used as widely, measure quality of life and other global outcomes.

REFERENCES

1. Bogousslavsky J, Aarli J, Kimura J. Stroke and neurology: a plea from the WFN. *Lancet* 2003;2:212–213.
2. Bogousslavsky J, Aarli J, Kimura J, for the Board of Trustees WFoN. Stroke: time for a global campaign? *Cerebrovasc Dis* 2003;16:111–113.
3. Thorvaldsen P, Asplund K, Kuulasmaa K, Rajakangas AM, Schroll M. Stroke incidence, case fatality, and mortality in the WHO MONICA project. World Health Organization monitoring trends and determinants in cardiovascular disease. *Stroke* 1995;26:361–367.
4. Stegmayr B, Asplund K, Kuulasmaa K, Rajakangas AM, Thorvaldsen P, Tuomilehto J. Stroke incidence and mortality correlated to stroke risk factors in the WHO MONICA project. An ecological study of 18 populations. *Stroke* 1997;28:1367–1374.
5. Asplund K. Stroke in Europe. Widening gap between East and West. *Cerebrovasc Dis* 1996;6:3–6.
6. Broderick J, Brott T, Tomsick T, Leach A. Lobar hemorrhage in the elderly. The undiminishing importance of hypertension. *Stroke* 1993;24:49–51.
7. Kubo M, Kiyohara Y, Kato I, et al. Trends in the incidence, mortality, and survival rate of cardiovascular disease in a Japanese community. The Hisayama Study. *Stroke* 2003;34:2349–2354.
8. Jackson MR, Chang AS, Robles HA, et al. Determination of 60 percent or greater carotid stenosis: a prospective comparison of magnetic resonance angiography and duplex ultrasound with conventional angiography. *Ann Vasc Surg* 1998;12:236–243.
9. Evers SM, Engel GL, Ament AJ. Cost of stroke in The Netherlands from a societal perspective. *Stroke* 1997;28:1375–1381.
10. Dewey HM, Thrift AG, Mihalopoulos C, et al. Lifetime cost of stroke subtypes in Australia. Findings from the North East Melbourne Stroke Incidence Study (NEMESIS). *Stroke* 2003;34:2502–2507.
11. Levy E, Gabriel S, Dinet J. The comparative medical costs of atherothrombotic disease in European countries. *Pharmacoeconomics* 2003;21:651–659.
12. American Heart Association. Heart disease and stroke statistics—2005 update. 2005. (This is a widely distributed document that is not published in a journal. I do not know how to add more. If you believe it needs to be treated by a book, would add Dallas, Texas: American Heart Association as the location and publisher).
13. Williams JE, Ayala CS, Croft JB, et al. State-specific mortality from stroke and distribution of place of death–United States, 1999. *JAMA* 2002;288:309–310.
14. Elkins JS, Johnston SC. Thirty-year projections for deaths from ischemic stroke in the United States. *Stroke* 2003;34:2109–2112.
15. Phillips LH, II, Whisnant JP, O'Fallon WM. The unchanging pattern of subarachnoid hemorrhage in a community. *Neurology* 1980;30:1034–1040.
16. Broderick JP, Brott T, Tomsick T, Huster G, Miller R. The risk of subarachnoid and intracerebral hemorrhages in blacks as compared with whites. *N Engl J Med* 1992;326:733–736.
17. Ostbye T, Levy AR, Mayo NE. Hospitalization and case-fatality rates for subarachnoid hemorrhage in Canada from 1982 through 1991. The Canadian Collaborative Study Group of Stroke Hospitalizations. *Stroke* 1997;28:793–798.
18. Menghini VV, Brown RDJ, Sicks JD, O'Fallon WM, Wiebers DO. Incidence and prevalence of intracranial aneurysms and hemorrhage in Olmsted County, Minnesota, 1965 to 1995. *Neurology* 1998;51:405–411.
19. Martinez-Vila E, Irimia P. The cost of stroke. *Cerebrovasc Dis* 2004;17(suppl 1):124–129.
20. Taylor TN, Davis PH, Torner JC, Holmes J, Meyer JW, Jacobson MF. Lifetime cost of stroke in the United States. *Stroke* 1996;27:1459–1466.
21. Brott T, Thalinger K, Hertzberg V. Hypertension as a risk factor for spontaneous intracerebral hemorrhage. *Stroke* 1986;17:1078–1083.
22. Al Rajeh S. Stroke in the elderly aged 75 years and above. *Cerebrovasc Dis* 1994;4:402–406.
23. Mayo NE, Neville D, Kirkland S, et al. Hospitalization and case-fatality rates for stroke in Canada from 1982 through 1991. The Canadian Collaborative Study Group of Stroke Hospitalizations. *Stroke* 1996;27:1215–1220.
24. Tanne D, Yaari S, Goldbourt U. Risk profile and prediction of long-term ischemic stroke mortality: a 21-year follow-up in the Israeli Ischemic Heart Disease (IIHD) project. *Circulation* 1998;98:1365–1371.
25. Kalra L. Does age affect benefits of stroke unit rehabilitation? *Stroke* 1994;25:346–351.
26. Marini C, Baldassarre M, Russo T, et al. Burden of first-ever ischemic stroke in the oldest old: evidence from a population-based study. *Neurology* 2004;62:77–81.
27. Adams HP, Jr., Butler MJ, Biller J, Toffol GJ. Nonhemorrhagic cerebral infarction in young adults. *Arch Neurol* 1986;43:793–796.
28. Fullerton HJ, Chetkovich DM, Wu YW, Smith WS, Johnston SC. Deaths form stroke in US children, 1979 to 1998. *Neurology* 2002;59:34–39.
29. Earley CJ, Kittner SJ, Feeser BR, et al. Stroke in children and sickle-cell disease: Baltimore–Washington Cooperative Young Stroke Study. *Neurology* 1998;51:169–176.
30. Broderick J, Talbot GT, Prenger E, Leach A, Brott T. Stroke in children within a major metropolitan area: the

surprising importance of intracerebral hemorrhage. *J Child Neurol* 1993;8:250–255.

31. Ganesan V, McShane MA, Liesner R, Cookson J, Hann I, Kirkham FJ. Inherited prothrombotic states and ischaemic stroke in childhood. *J Neurol Neurosurg Psychiatry* 1998;65:508–511.

32. Garcia JH, Pantoni L. Strokes in childhood. *Semin Pediatr Neurol* 1995;2:180–191.

33. Kittner SJ. Stroke in the young. Coming of age. *Neurology* 2002;59:6–7.

34. Pavlakis SG, Kingsley PB, Bialer MG. Stroke in children: genetic and metabolic issues. *J Child Neurol* 2003;15:308–315.

35. Kongable GL, Lazino G, Germanson TP. Gender-related differences in aneurysmal subarachnoid hemorrhage. *J Neurosurg* 1996;84:43–48.

36. Williams LS, Garg BP, Cohen M, Fleck JD, Biller J. Subtypes of ischemic stroke in children and young adults. *Neurology* 1997;49:1541–1545.

37. Adams HP, Jr., Kappelle LJ, Biller J, Gordon DL, Love BB. Ischemic stroke in young adults. *Arch Neurol* 1995;52:491–495.

38. Lanska DJ, Kryscio RJ. Risk factors for peripartum and postpartum stroke and intracranialvenous thrombosis. *Stroke* 2000;31:1274–1282.

39. Lanska DJ, Kryscio RJ. Stroke and intracranial venous thrombosis during pregnancy and puerperium. *Neurology* 1998;51:1622–1628.

40. Hershey LA. Gender differences in cerebrovascular disease. *Neurology* 1993;3:1–4.

41. Falkeborn M, Persson I, Terent A, Bergstrom R, Lithell H, Naessen T. Long-term trends in incidence of and mortality from acute myocardial infarction and stroke in women: analyses of total first events and of deaths in the Uppsala Health Care Region, Sweden. *Epidemiology* 1996;7:67–74.

42. Antithrombotic Trialists' Collaboration. Collaborative meta-analysis of randomised trials of antiplatelet therapy for prevention of death, myocardial infarction, and stroke in high risk patients. *BMJ* 2002;324:71–86.

43. Executive Committee for the Asymptomatic Carotid Atherosclerosis Study. Endarterectomy for asymptomatic carotid artery stenosis. *JAMA* 1995;273:1421–1428.

44. Kittner SJ, Stern BJ, Feeser BR, et al. Pregnancy and the risk of stroke. *N Engl J Med* 1996;335:768–774.

45. Schwartz SM, Petitti DB, Siscovick DS, et al. Stroke and use of low-dose oral contraceptives in young women: a pooled analysis of two US studies. *Stroke* 1998;29:2277–2284.

46. Writing Group for the Women's Health Initiative Investigators. Risks and benefits of estrogen plus progestin in healthy postmenopausal women. Principal results from the Women's Health Initiative Randomized Controlled Trial. *JAMA* 2002;288:321–333.

47. Poungvarin N. Stroke in the developing world. *Lancet* 1998;352(suppl 3):SIII19–SIII22.

48. Sudlow CL, Warlow CP. Comparing stroke incidence worldwide: what makes studies comparable? *Stroke* 1996;27:550–558.

49. Sudlow CL, Warlow CP. Comparable studies of the incidence of stroke and its pathological types: results from an international collaboration. International Stroke Incidence Collaboration. *Stroke* 1997;28:491–499.

50. Truelen T. Piechowski-Jozwiak B, Bonita R, et al. Stroke incidence and prevalence in Europe. A review of the available data. *Eur J Neurol,* 2006;13:581–598.

51. Morris RW, Whincup PH, Emberson JR, Lampe FC, Walker M, Shaper AG. North–South gradients in Britain for stroke and CHD. Are they explained by the same factors? *Stroke* 2003;34:2604–2611.

52. Zhang LF, Yang J, Hong Z, et al. Proportion of different subtypes of stroke in China. *Stroke* 2003;34:2091–2096.

53. Wong KS, Li H. Long-term mortality and recurrent stroke risk among Chinese stroke patients with predominant intracranial atherosclerosis. *Stroke* 2003;34:2361–2366.

54. Saposnik G, Del Brutto OH, for the Iberoamerican Society of Cerebrovascular Diseases. Stroke in South America. A systematic review of incidence, prevalence, and stroke subtypes. *Stroke* 2003;34:2103–2107.

55. Lanska DJ, Peterson PM. Geographic variation in reporting of stroke deaths to underlying or contributing causes in the United States. *Stroke* 1995;26:1999–2003.

56. Lanska DJ, Peterson PM. Geographic variation in the decline of stroke mortality in the United States. *Stroke* 1995;26:1159–1165.

57. Casper ML, Wing S, Anda RF, Knowles M, Pollard RA. The shifting stroke belt. Changes in the geographic pattern of stroke mortality in the United States, 1962 to 1988. *Stroke* 1995;26:755–760.

58. Howard G, Evans GW, Pearce K, et al. Is the stroke belt disappearing? An analysis of racial, temporal, and age effects. *Stroke* 1995;26:1153–1158.

59. McNaughton H, Weatherall M, McPherson K, Taylor W, Harwood M. The comparability of resource utilisation for Europeans and non-Europeans following stroke in New Zealand. *NZ Med J* 2002;115:101–103.

60. Gorelick PB. Cerebrovascular disease in African Americans. *Stroke* 1998;29:2656–2664.

61. Kissela B, Schneider A, Kleindorfer D, et al. Stroke in a biracial population. The excess burden of stroke among blacks. *Stroke* 2004;35:426–431.

62. Kittner SJ, McCarter RJ, Sherwin RW, et al. Black–white differences in stroke risk among young adults. *Stroke* 1993 (12 Suppl):I13–I15.

63. Morgenstern LB, Spears WD, Goff DCJ, Grotta JC, Nichaman MZ. African Americans and women have the highest stroke mortality in Texas. *Stroke* 1997;28:15–18.

64. Qureshi AI, Suri MA, Safdar K, Ottenlips JR, Janssen RS, Frankel MR. Intracerebral hemorrhage in blacks. Risk factors, subtypes, and outcome. *Stroke* 1997;28:961–964.

65. Qureshi A, Giles W, Croft J. Racial differences in the incidence of intracerebral hemorrhage: effects of blood pressure and education. *Neurology* 1999;52:1617–1621.

66. Gebel JM, Broderick JP. Intracerebral hemorrhage. *Neurol Clin* 2000;18:419–438.

67. Gillum RF. Stroke mortality in blacks. Disturbing trends. *Stroke* 1999;30:1711–1715.

68. Sheinart KF, Tuhrim S, Horowitz DR, et al. Stroke recurrence is more frequent in blacks and Hispanics. *Neuroepidemiology* 1998;17:188–198.

69. Prengler M, Pavlakis SG, Prohovnik I, Adams RJ. Sickle cell disease: the neurological complications. *Ann Neurol* 2002;51:543–552.

70. Sacco RL, Kargman DE, Zamanillo MC. Race-ethnic differences in stroke risk factors among hospitalized patients with cerebral infarction: the Northern Manhattan Stroke Study. *Neurology* 1995;45:659–663.

71. Worrall BB, Johnston KC, Kongable G, Hung E, Richardson D, Gorelick PB. Stroke risk factor profiles in African American women: an interim report from the African-American antiplatelet stroke prevention study. *Stroke* 2002;33:913–919.

72. Cox AM, McKevitt C, Rudd AG, Wolfe CD: Socioeconomic status and stroke Lancet Neurology, 2006;5:181–188.

73. Williams JE, Nieto J, Sanford CP, Couper DJ, Tyroler HA. The association between trait anger and incident stroke risk: the Atherosclerosis Risk in Communities (ARIC) study. *Stroke* 2002;33:13–19.

74. Tentschert S, Greisenegger S, Wimmer R, Lang W, Lalouschek W. Association of parental history of stroke with clinical parameters in patients with ischemic stroke or transient ischemic stroke. *Stroke* 2003;34:2114–2119.

75. Field TS, Hill MD. Weather, chinook, and stroke occurrence. *Stroke* 2002;33:1751–1758.

76. Low RB, Bielory L, Qureshi Al, et al. The relation of stroke admissions to recent weather, airborne allergans, air pollution, seasons, upper respiratory infections, and asthma incidence, September 11, 2001, and day of the week. *Stroke*, 2006;37:951–957.

77. Maheswaran R, Elliott P. Stroke mortality associated with living near main roads in England and Wales. A geographical study. *Stroke* 2003;34:2776–2780.

78. Johnston SC. Transient ischemic attack. *N Engl J Med* 2002;347:1687–1692.

79. Norris JW. Risk of cerebral infarction, myocardial infarction and vascular death in patients with asymptomatic carotid disease, transient ischemic attack and stroke. *Cerebrovasc Dis* 1992;2(suppl):2–5.

80. Mackey AE, Abrahamowicz M, Langlois Y, et al. Outcome of asymptomatic patients with carotid disease. Asymptomatic Cervical Bruit Study Group. *Neurology* 1997;48:896–903.

81. Bogousslavsky J, Despland PA, Regli F. Asymptomatic tight stenosis of the internal carotid artery: long-term prognosis. *Neurology* 1986;36:861–863.

82. Wiebers DO, Piepgras DG, Brown RD, Jr., et al. Unruptured aneurysms. *J Neurosurg* 2002;96:50–51.

83. Giles MF, Rothwell PM. Prediction and prevention of stroke after transient ischemic attack in the short and long term. *Expert Rev Neurother*, 2006;6:381–395.

84. Johnston SC, Gress DR, Browner WS, Sidney S. Short-term prognosis after emergency department diagnosis of TIA. *JAMA* 2000;284:2901–2906.

85. Lovett JK, Dennis MS, Sandercock PA, Bamford J, Warlow CP, Rothwell PM. Very early risk of stroke after a first transient ischemic attack. *Stroke* 2003;34:e138–e140.86. North American Symptomatic Carotid Endarterectomy Trial Collaborators. Beneficial effect of carotid endarterectomy in symptomatic patients with high-grade carotid stenosis. *N Engl J Med* 1991;325:445–453.

87. Grubb RL, Jr., Derdeyn CP, Fritsch SM, et al. Importance of hemodynamic factors in the prognosis of symptomatic carotid occlusion. *JAMA* 1998;280:1055–1060.

88. Evans BA, Sicks JD, Whisnant JP. Factors affecting survival and occurrence of stroke in patients with transient ischemic attacks. *Mayo Clin Proc* 1994;69:416–421.

89. Bruno A, Jeffries L, Lakind E, Qualls C. Predictors of cerebral infarction following transient ischemic attack. *J Stroke Cerebrovasc Dis* 1993;3:23–28.

90. International Stroke Trial Collaborative Group. The International Stroke Trial (IST): a randomised trial of aspirin, subcutaneous heparin, both, or neither among 19435 patients with acute ischaemic stroke. *Lancet* 1997; 349:1569–1581.

91. CAST (Chinese Acute Stroke Trial) Collaborative Group. CAST: randomised placebo-controlled trial of early aspirin use in 20,000 patients with acute ischaemic stroke. *Lancet* 1997;349:1641–1649.

92. The Publications Committee for the Trial of ORG 10172 in Acute Stroke Treatment (TOAST) Investigators. Low molecular weight heparinoid, ORG 10172 (danaparoid), and outcome after acute ischemic stroke: a randomized controlled trial. *JAMA* 1998;279:1265–1272.

93. Kappelle LJ, Adams HP, Jr., Heffner ML, Torner JC, Gomez F, Biller J. Prognosis of young adults with ischemic stroke. A long-term follow-up study assessing recurrent vascular events and functional outcome in the Iowa Registry of Stroke in Young Adults. *Stroke* 1994;25:1360–1365.

94. Kiyohara Y, Kubo M, Kato I, et al. Ten-year prognosis of stroke and risk factors for death in a Japanese community. The Hisayama Study. *Stroke* 2003;34:2343–2347.

95. Vernino S, Brown RD, Sejvar JJ, Sicks JD, Petty GW, O'Fallon WM. Cause-specific mortality after first cerebral infarction. A population-based study. *Stroke* 2003;34:1828–1832.

96. Appelros P, Nydevik I, Viitanen M. Poor outcome after first-ever stroke: predictors for death, dependency, and recurrent stroke within first year. *Stroke* 2003;34:122–126.

97. Bruno A, Biller J, Adams HP, Jr., et al. Acute blood glucose level and outcome from ischemic stroke. Trial of Org 10172 in Acute Stroke Treatment (TOAST) Investigators. *Neurology* 1999;52:280–284.

98. Bruno A, Levine SR, Frankel M, et al. Admission glucose level and clinical outcomes in the NINDS rt-PA Stroke Trial. *Neurology* 2002;59:669–674.

99. Adams HP, Jr., Davis PH, Leira EC, et al. Baseline NIH Stroke Scale score strongly predicts outcome after stroke. *Neurology* 1999;53:126–131.

100. Appelros P, Terént A. Characteristics of the National Institute of Health Stroke Scale: results from a population-based stroke cohort at baseline and after one year. *Cerebrovasc Dis* 2004;17:21–27.

101. Weimar C, König IR, Kraywinkel K, Ziegler A, Diener HC, on behalf of the German Stroke Study Collaboration. Age and National Institutes of Health Stroke Scale score within 6 hours after onset are accurate predictors of outcome after cerebral ischemia. Development and external validation of prognostic models. *Stroke* 2004;35:158–162.

102. The NINDS t-PA Stroke Study Group. Generalized efficacy of t-PA for acute stroke. Subgroup analysis of the NINDS t-PA Stroke Trial. *Stroke* 1997;28:2119–2125.

103. von Kummer R, Nolte PN, Schnittger H, Thron A, Ringelstein EB. Detectability of cerebral hemisphere ischaemic infarcts by CT within 6 h of stroke. *Neuroradiology* 1996;38:31–33.

104. Brott T, Marler JR, Olinger CP, et al. Measurements of acute cerebral infarction: lesion size by computed tomography. *Stroke* 1989;20:871–875.

105. Drury I, Whisnant JP, Garraway WM. Primary intracerebral hemorrhage: impact of CT on incidence. *Neurology* 1984;34:653–657.

106. Broderick JP. Natural history of primary intracerebral hemorrhage. In: Whisnant JP, ed. *Population-Based Clinical Epidemiology of Stroke.* Oxford, England: Butterworth Heinemann; 1993.

107. Tatu L, Moulin T, El Mohamad R, Vuillier F, Rumbach L, Czorny A. Primary intracerebral hemorrhages in the Besancon Stroke Registry. Initial clinical and CT findings, early course and 30-day outcome in 350 patients. *Eur Neurol* 2000;43:209–214.

108. Schievink WI, Wijdicks EFM, Parisi JE. Sudden death from aneurysmal subarachnoid hemorrhage. *Neurology* 1995;45:871–874.

109. Franke CL, van Swieten JC, Algra A. Prognostic factors in patients with intracerebral haematoma. *J Neurol Neurosurg Psychiatry* 1992;55:653–657.

110. Wong K. Risk factors for early death in acute ischemic stroke and intracerebral hemorrhage: a prospective hospital-based study in Asia. Asian Acute Stroke Advisory Panel. *Stroke* 1999;30:2326–2330.

111. Schievink WI, Wijdicks EFM, Piepgras DG. The poor prognosis of ruptured intracranial aneurysms of the posterior circulation. *J Neurosurg* 1995;82:791–795.

112. Baptista MV, vanMelle G, Bogousslavsky J. Prediction of in-hospital mortality after first-ever stroke: the Lausanne Stroke Registry. *J Neurol Sci* 1999;166:107–114.

113. Wijdicks EF, St Louis E. Clinical profiles predictive of outcome in pontine hemorrhage. *Neurology* 1997;49: 1342–1346.

114. Wijdicks EF, St Louis EK, Atkinson JD, Li H. Clinician's biases toward surgery in cerebellar hematomas: an analysis of decision-making in 94 patients. *Cerebrovasc Dis* 2000;10:93–96.

115. Juvela S. Risk factors for impaired outcome after spontaneous intracerebral hemorrhage. *Arch Neurol* 1995;52: 1193–1200.

116. Rosenow F, Hojer C, Meyer-Lohmann C, et al. Spontaneous intracerebral hemorrhage. Prognostic factors in 896 cases. *Acta Neurol Scand* 1997;96:174–182.

117. Wijdicks EFM, Vermuelen M, Hijdra A. Hyponatremia and cerebral infarction in patients with ruptured intracranial aneurysms: is fluid restriction harmful? *Ann Neurol* 1985;17:137–140.

118. Wijdicks EFM, Vermuelen M, Ten Haaf JA. Volume depletion and natriuresis inpatients with ruptured intracranial aneurysm. *Ann Neurol* 1985;18:211–216.

119. Torner JC, Kassell NF, Wallace RB. Preoperative prognostic factors for rebleeding and survival in aneurysm patients receiving fibrinolytic therapy: report of the Cooperative Aneurysm Study. *Neurosurgery* 1981;9:506–513.

120. Lanzino G, Kassell NF, Germanson TP, et al. Age and outcome after aneurysmal subarachnoid hemorrhage: why do older patients fare worse? *J Neurosurg* 1996;85:410–418.

121. Hunt WE, Hess RM. Surgical risk as related to time of intervention in the repair of intracranial aneurysms. *J Neurosurg* 1968;28:14–20.

122. Adams HP, Jr., Kassell NF, Torner JC. Usefulness of computed tomography in predicting outcome after aneurysmal subarachnoid hemorrhage. *Neurology* 1985;35:1263–1267.

123. Fisher CM, Kistler JP, Davis JM. Relation of cerebral vasospasm to subarachnoid hemorrhage visualized by computerized tomographic scanning. *Neurosurgery* 1980;6:1–9.

124. Teasdale GM, Pettigrew LE, Wilson JT, Murray G, Jennett B. Analyzing outcome of treatment of severe head injury: a review and update on advancing the use of the Glasgow Outcome Scale. *J Neurotrauma* 1998;15:587–597.

125. Bamford J, Sandercock P, Dennis M, et al. A prospective study of acute cerebrovascular disease in the community: the Oxfordshire Community Stroke Project 1981–1986—1. Methodology, demography and incident rates of first-ever stroke. *J Neurol Neurosurg Psychiatry* 1988;51:1373–1380.

126. Mahoney FI, Barthel DW. Functional evaluation: the Barthel index. *Md State Med J* 1965;14:61–65.

127. Goldstein LA, Adams R, Alberts MJ et al. Primary prevention of ischemic stroke. A guideline from the American Heart Association/American Stroke Association. *Stroke,* 2006;37:1583–1633.

128. Brott T, Adams HP Jr, Olinger CP. Developing measurements of acute cerebral infarction. I. A reliable, valid, and brief clinical examination scale. *Stroke,* 1989;20:864–870.

129. Ogungbo B. The World Federation of Neurological Surgeons scale for subarachnoid hemorrhage. *Surg Neurol,* 2003;59:236–237.

130. Bamford J, Sandercock PA, Warlow CP, Slattery J Interobserver agreement for assessment of handicap in stroke patients. *Stroke,* 1989;20:828.

CHAPTER 3

Organizing Stroke Management Resources

▶ USING THE RULES OF EVIDENCE AND GUIDELINES

For too long, physicians were dependent upon opinions of experts, teachers, or their personal experience when making decisions about the management of stroke. This tradition, for the better, is now being abandoned. The public, third party payers, and the medical community demand that therapies of proven utility be prescribed and interventions that have little utility be avoided. In an attempt to improve management, medical community has adopted ways to assess and rate the quality of data supporting the use or nonuse of specific treatments. Similar standards (levels of evidence) are used to examine the utility of diagnostic studies. These standards are now being used widely and the employed methodology is widely known. Physicians should have a working knowledge about the information that supports their decisions for management of stroke.

Guidelines

Guidelines are used to provide advice on ways to improve patient care.[1] Panels of experts, which critically review the available information, usually write the guidelines. They examine the data using the rules of evidence, which are based on the strength and origin of the data. Information collected by prospectively performed, scientifically rigorous clinical trials is rated as the strongest and most valid (Tables 3-1 and 3-2). Data from smaller clinical trials, nonrandomized comparison studies, studies involving historical controls, or anecdotal experiences (case reports or small series) are given less emphasis. Depending upon the level of the data, the guidelines give recommendations of varying strength. If data strongly support an intervention, a high (Grade A) recommendation is given to administer the therapy. Depending upon the circumstances, the guidelines also provide comments about specific indications or contraindications for an intervention and details about the administration of the medication including ancillary care. If available data do not support a potential benefit of a specific therapy, the panel should advise that the intervention not be given. The panel also can give recommendations for components of a particular treatment based on consensus rather than scientific data as many parts of patient care are based on traditional practice. An obvious situation is the recommendation to protect the airway with endotracheal intubation in a patient with a decreased level of consciousness. Surely, a clinical trial would be ill-advised to address this particular question. In addition, data from clinical trials testing interventions in other clinical settings may be applicable to the management of patients with cerebrovascular disease. For example, data about the use of specific anticonvulsants are used when recommending treatment of seizures following stroke.

During the last decade, several stroke-related guidelines have been published.[2–8] Not surprisingly, these guidelines emphasize different components of management. In addition, the available data might be interpreted in slightly different ways by the panels that advised the guidelines. Consequently, some discrepancies exist. While minor conflicts in advice exist between the various statements, the general recommendations are similar. The differences should be viewed as strengths because they allow clinicians to seek opinions from several sources. The contents of the above-cited guidelines are used extensively in the management sections of this book. However, one should recognize the limitations of guidelines because clinical trials cannot test every

▶ **TABLE 3-1.** STRENGTH OF SUPPORTING DATA TREATMENT GUIDELINES

Level	Features of Data
I	Data from large, well-designed clinical trials
	Data should not be vulnerable to false positive/negative results
	More than one trial with similar results
	Meta-analyses of trials provide subgroup information
II	Data from smaller clinical trials
	Some risk for false positive/negative results
III	Data from nonrandomized prospective studies
IV	Data from uncontrolled prospective studies
	Often compared to historical controls
V	Data from small series or case reports

Adapted from Guyatt et al.[82]

permutation of the diverse spectrum of either ischemic or hemorrhagic cerebrovascular diseases. Some diseases that lead to stroke are uncommon and thus no clinical trial can be performed to test therapies for these conditions. The wide spectrum of patients with stroke and the diversity of presentations mean that clinical research usually involves broad categories. Thus, some recommendations might not apply to every individual patient. Clinicians will need to adapt the available information to their patients and make the best decision possible.

▶ METHODOLOGY OF CLINICAL TRIALS IN STROKE

Physicians should be aware of the results of ongoing clinical research. The results of several clinical trials become available annually and these new data have the potential to change practice dramatically. With the advent of mass electronic communication, new data become available long before a guideline can be updated. Physicians need to judge the validity of any newly available information about diagnosis and treatment of patients with cerebrovascular disease. Unfortunately, some very promising

▶ **TABLE 3-2.** STRENGTH OF RECOMMENDATIONS TREATMENT GUIDELINES

Strength	Features
A	Supported by Level I data
	Large randomized controlled trial(s)
B	Supported by Level II data
	Smaller randomized controlled trial(s)
C	Supported by Levels III, IV or V data
	Nonrandomized controlled studies
	Historical control studies
	Small series or case reports

Adapted from Guyatt et al.[82]

advances are not sustained when evaluated in subsequent trials. Thus, clinicians should evaluate the quality of the research.

Criteria for a modern clinical trial include measures to avoid bias in recruitment (randomization) and rating of responses (blinding) as well as an adequate cohort (number) of patients (sample size calculation) in order to avoid a chance misinterpretation of results (type I or type II error) (Table 3-3). In addition, a well-designed

▶ **TABLE 3-3.** CRITERIA TO ASSESS CLINICAL TRIALS FOR EFFICACY

Strong rationale to test the intervention
  Experimental evidence
  Clinical studies—normal volunteers, patients
    Determination of dose
    Determination of treatment regimen
    Estimate of potential risks and benefits
Hypotheses—primary, secondary, and null
  Sample size calculations
Study population to be recruited
  Inclusion criteria
  Exclusion criteria
  Informed consent or surrogate consent
Randomization to avoid bias in treatment assignment
  Stratification by site or clinical variables
  Randomization scheme
Ancillary care
  During and following acute treatment
  Treatment of concomitant illnesses
  Medical and surgical interventions
  Rehabilitation
Assessment of responses to treatment
  Timing of assessments
    Acute treatment period
    Duration of follow-up
    End of study assessment
  Types of assessments
    Clinical
    Laboratory and imaging
  Clinical assessments using standardized instruments
    Measurements of impairments
    Measurements of disability or handicap
    Measurements of new events
    Deaths and causes of death
Quality control measures
  Standardized protocol and operations manual
  Education of investigators and other study personnel
  Certification of investigators in rating instruments
  Monitoring of data at sites and centrally
  Adjudication of major outcome events
Detailed statistical plans including interim analyses
Monitoring of participants' safety
  Study specific safety monitoring including external board
Attention to regulatory requirements
  Governmental
  Institutional review boards

trial should include measures to assure the quality of the data, such as standardization of clinical and laboratory assessments, comparisons with source documents, and data editing. It is not possible to mask treatment allocation in some trials, such as one testing a surgical therapy. In such a situation, the trial can include an independent panel to adjudicate results. These methodologies are used widely in clinical trials in cerebrovascular disease and results from studies that do not meet these stringent criteria should be viewed with caution.

▶ ORGANIZATION OF STROKE RESOURCES

Management of patients with stroke is predicated on early treatment. The goal is to evaluate and treat patients as rapidly as possible.[9,10] A number of obstacles to emergency care can be identified.[11,12] Each of these roadblocks must be overcome in order to increase the number of patients who receive acute therapy.

Management of patients with cerebrovascular disease is complex. Successful treatment of the stroke-prone patient involves primary prevention, treatment of the acute neurological illness, prevention or control of complications, rehabilitation to maximize recovery, and initiation of therapies to prevent recurrent stroke. Successful treatment involves collaboration of physicians from several specialties (Table 3-4). Successful treatment also entails participation of nonphysician health care professionals (Table 3-5). Most importantly, successful treatment requires active involvement of the patients and their family and community. With the advent of interventions that improve outcomes, all aspects of treatment should be coordinated in an expeditious manner.[13–17] Stroke now is being treated appropriately as a life-threatening or changing disease.

▶ TABLE 3-4. PHYSICIANS STROKE MANAGEMENT

Neurology
    Vascular neurology
    Interventional neurology
    Intensive care
Neurosurgery
Neuroradiology
Primary care specialists
Emergency medicine
Intensive care specialists
Physical medicine and rehabilitation
Vascular surgery
Cardiology
Cardiovascular surgery
Hematology
Psychiatry

▶ TABLE 3-5. NONPHYSICIAN HEALTH CARE PROVIDERS—STROKE

Nurses
    Stroke unit
    Other acute care units
Rehabilitation specialists
    Physical therapy
    Occupational therapy
    Speech pathology
    Vocational rehabilitation
    Cognitive rehabilitation—neuropsychology
Social services—discharge planner
Chaplain
Dietician
Pharmacy
Laboratory personnel
    Radiology
    Pathology

▶ PUBLIC RESPONSE

Patients with impaired consciousness, seizures, major impairments, or brain hemorrhage are most likely to reach attention quickly.[18] On the other hand, persons with mild strokes or gradually evolving signs usually do not arrive in time for emergent stroke care.[19,20] In particular, mildly affected patients do not arrive within the 3-h time window required for the safe and effective intravenous administration of r-tPA. Approximately one-fifth of patients wake up in the morning with their symptoms; in these circumstances, the time of onset is unknown. Still, a sizable percentage of patients with stroke present upon awakening might be treated successfully if they arrive at an emergency department within a few hours of first detection.[21] Patients who call emergency medical services and are transported by ambulance arrive in an emergency department sooner than those who first contact their primary care physician. Also, strokes that occur in a public place, such as a store, are more likely to prompt activation of emergency medical services that are those events that occur at home.[22,23] Persons who live alone often do not receive medical attention for several hours after the event.

Brain Attack

Because of the similarities between acute myocardial infarction (heart attack) and stroke (brain attack), much of the public message for stroke care imitates that employed for acute heart disease.[24–28] The likenesses between these two types of vascular disease are several (Table 3-6). Both acute diseases are associated with serious complications. Stroke is a major complication of heart disease and heart disease often complicates stroke. Acute cardiac events are important complications of

▶ **TABLE 3-6.** SIMILARITIES AND DIFFERENCES BETWEEN HEART ATTACK AND BRAIN ATTACK

Similarities
    Leading causes of death
    Usually due to an acute arterial occlusion
    Might be treated with reperfusion therapy
    Time is critical for successful treatment
    Stroke complicated by cardiac problems
    Myocardial infarction complicated by stroke
    Care improved by treatment in specialized unit
    Patients often ignore symptoms
Differences
    Pain is the primary symptom of heart attack but
        Most patients with stroke do not have pain
    Stroke produces a variety of symptoms
        Reflect area of brain injury
    Stroke can cause decreased alertness or inattention
        Patient unable to seek help
        Patient not thinking clearly
    Stroke due to a variety of conditions including hemorrhage

neurological lesions, particularly hemorrhagic stroke. Both myocardial infarction and ischemic stroke are secondary to arterial thromboembolic occlusions and can be treated successfully with thrombolytic agents. The sense of urgency shown to acute heart disease should also be given to stroke.

Educating the public about the symptoms of stroke is challenging because most strokes are not associated with prominent headache or pain. Since most persons recognize pain as important, its absence might convey another meeting. In addition, the diverse nature of stroke symptoms, reflecting the locations of the brain affected by the vascular events, muddles the message even more.[29] Most individuals do not know the symptoms of stroke and the level of knowledge is lowest among the elderly, the very group at highest risk[30–32] (Table 3-7).

▶ **TABLE 3-7.** PUBLIC EDUCATION FOR STROKE "BRAIN ATTACK"

Seek medical attention immediately
    Dial 911—emergency number
    Go to an emergency department
Time course of symptoms of acute stroke
    Sudden onset
    Can be present upon awakening
Nature of symptoms of acute stroke
    Loss of consciousness
    Paralysis, weakness, numbness, or clumsiness
    Usually one side of body
    Loss of vision or part of vision in one or both eyes
    Difficulty understanding others or speaking
    Slurred speech
    Intense dizziness (vertigo)
    Unusually severe headache

Younger persons, those who have had a prior stroke or TIA, or those who have had multiple health problems, are more likely to be aware of the symptoms of stroke. In addition, because stroke affects the brain, the patient's thinking or consciousness might be impaired. The person might not be aware of the seriousness of the brain illness. As a result, an observer often must recognize that a person is having a stroke. Thus, educational efforts should involve relatives, friends, neighbors, and the general public as well as the patient. Elderly persons living alone should participate in community programs that involve visitors or neighbors (such as a postal employee or a person delivering meals) to check on them at regular intervals. While this system might not permit urgent stroke care, access to treatment may still be improved.

The public does not need to be educated about all the permutations of stroke. Rather, they should be informed of the most important and frequent symptoms; this information can be presented in a very straightforward manner (see Table 3-8). The message should emphasize the sudden nature of stroke and that the focal symptoms reflect the loss of function of one part of the brain. Also any educational program should respect the cultural norms of the community. For example, the term *brain attack* means epilepsy in some Spanish-speaking communities. In addition, the public should be informed about the correct response to a new neurological event; they should seek medical attention immediately. The public should also be aware that effective therapies that improve outcomes are available but that successful treatment is directly correlated with the interval from the onset of stroke symptoms. The message should emphasize that the sudden onset of

▶ **TABLE 3-8.** SUMMARY OF STATEMENTS OF INTERNATIONAL STROKE ADVOCACY GROUPS

Primary and secondary prevention are cost-effective
    Control risk factors for atherosclerosis
    Medical or surgical interventions for highest risk persons
Development of local, regional, and national stroke programs (services)
    Out-of-hospital and hospital services
    Acute stroke care units
    Rehabilitation services and return to society
    Special issues—geography, density of population, culture
Management of acute stroke
    Importance of skilled professionals including physicians
    Use of evidence-based therapies
Rehabilitation
Importance of quality of life of stroke survivors and caregivers
    Patient education
    Advocacy groups
    Activities of daily living
    Community care and support

focal neurological signs is a marker of a serious brain illness. In this situation, the most likely alternative diagnosis to ischemic stroke is hemorrhagic stroke and vice versa. Both can be treated. While other neurological diseases can mimic stroke, the number of alternatives is relatively small and conditions such as seizures or profound hypoglycemia are serious illnesses in themselves that mandate treatment. A transient event (TIA) should be viewed as a warning sign of impending stroke and rapid initiation of medical treatment may prevent a major brain injury. Thus, a TIA is of equal importance to an acute stroke and patients should be informed to seek medical attention even if the neurological symptoms begin to abate. In one series of 100 patients seen for a possible acute stroke, vascular events were diagnosed in 87.[33] With aggressive educational efforts, community knowledge about the warning signs and risk factors for stroke can improve.[32,34] This experience suggests that patients seeking medical attention for suspected stroke will likely have a cerebrovascular lesion.

911

Patients with a possible stroke should call emergency medical services (dialing 911 in most parts of the United States) or go directly to an emergency department. Transportation by private vehicle is slower than via an ambulance and the patient should not drive to the hospital. The patient should not delay treatment by seeking the advice of friends or relatives. If a person having a stroke calls a friend, the correct response is to advise seeking medical attention immediately. A patient or relative should not call a physician's office because this response often delays treatment.[35] In one study, the median time from onset of stroke until clinical assessment was 84 min if the patient first called 911 but was 270 min if the patient first called a physician's office.[36] Devices that can be activated during an emergency are available in some nursing homes or retirement communities. Most importantly, patients should not stay at home hoping that the symptoms will resolve. Patients must know that therapies of proven usefulness are available if they seek medical attention quickly.[37]

► LOCAL AND REGIONAL ORGANIZATION OF STROKE RESOURCES

In an effort to speed treatment, communities should organize health care resources to speed transportation, evaluation, and initiation of treatment. Such programs are being developed around the world.[24,27,28,38,39] While most of the effort is aimed at increasing the number of patients with ischemic stroke who can be treated with r-tPA, much of emergent management is equally applicable to persons

► **TABLE 3-9.** COORDINATED INSTITUTIONAL STROKE CARE

Acute stroke care team—treatment largely in emergency department
   Services, including brain imaging, available 24 h/day, 7 days/week
   Personnel summoned on an emergency (call) basis
   Neurologist—vascular neurologist (usually directs team)
   Neurosurgeon
   Emergency medicine/primary care physicians
   Radiology—interventional neuroradiology
   Nurses
   Laboratory personnel—radiology and pathology
   Pharmacy
   Acute stroke care protocols
Acute stroke care unit
   Geographically defined facility
   Monitoring capability
   Nurses
   Physicians—usually vascular neurologist
   Stroke treatment care maps and protocols
   Coordinated evaluation and treatment
   Rehabilitation
Stroke rehabilitation team
   Physician rehabilitation specialists
   Other rehabilitation specialists
   Social services and discharge planning

with intracranial hemorrhage. In recent years, advocacy groups have authored important statements aimed at improving stroke care (Table 3-9). Fortunately, governmental and public interest groups have begun to implement these programs. In particular, several initiatives are underway in the United States and Operation Stroke is one such model in this direction. The Operation Stroke is being sponsored by the American Stroke Association.[34] Much of the regional and local organization of stroke care resources is modeled after programs used to treat patients with major traumatic injuries. In the future, regional hospital-based stroke centers may be created. Stroke care could be organized such that all patients are triaged to one or two units within a metropolitan area.[39] Such a regional approach can be very successful. For example, Katzan et al.[34] found that a majority of patients could reach a hospital within 6 h of onset of stroke. Interested parties such as stroke advocacy organizations, local government, public health agencies, emergency medical services, hospitals, and physicians should develop a regional plan that will work for their communities. Among the thornier issues is the referral of patients to designated hospitals. Many institutions do not have the facilities or physician expertise to provide the required level of care.[40,41] Institutions that do not have modern stroke care resources should be bypassed en route to a regional stroke center. The components of coordinated acute stroke care (see Table 3-9) are a benchmark that can be used to assess medical centers. In addition, insurance companies, health maintenance organizations, governmental health plans, and other third party payers should avoid placing obstacles to the reimbursement for rapid treatment of stroke. Patients should be taken to the closest *appropriate* care facility to receive emergent care. Both the public and health care providers should demand inclusion of emergent stroke care, regardless of the location, in insurance plans.

▶ EMERGENCY MEDICAL SERVICES

The regional acute stroke care program should include instructions for all components of emergency medical services, including responding to calls from the public, emergent (in-the-field) treatment, and urgent transportation to the closest appropriate hospital that can manage patients with stroke. The dispatcher at the emergency telephone center must first recognize the features of stroke and the importance of the call. Training dispatchers about the clinical findings of stroke is critically important. In one study, dispatchers recognized the symptoms of stroke in only 52 percent of cases.[42] In particular, they must learn the critical time-linked relationship between stroke and its successful treatment. Receptionists at physicians' offices or telephone operators (paging services) at hospitals also need to be aware of the importance of stroke-related calls. These persons should either directly call the emergency medical services or advise the caller to dial 911. They also should inform the appropriate physicians of the call. The emergency medical services dispatcher should send an ambulance to the site on a high-priority basis.[25,43] The approach should be the same as that used when a patient is thought to have a myocardial infarction.

Emergency Assessment

The activities of the paramedics are critical. Programs are available to educate paramedics about the nuances of stroke and the importance of emergent treatment.[44,45] The paramedics should evaluate the patient quickly. Besides providing initial life support and examining the vital signs, the paramedics also can do a relatively brief neurological assessment. Stroke-rating scales, which can be used easily by paramedics, have been developed to expedite the examination of the patient[45] (Table 3-10). Paramedics already are adept at performing the Glasgow Coma Scale, which provides important prognostic information for stroke (see Table 2.13). Although this scale was developed for the emergent assessment of patients with craniocerebral trauma, it can be used to assess patients with decreased levels of consciousness.[46] Because most patients with ischemic stroke will be alert, the score on the Glasgow Coma Scale likely will be normal. However,

▶ **TABLE 3-10.** LOS ANGELES PREHOSPITAL STROKE SCALE

Screening Criteria	Yes	No	?
Age >45			
No seizure/epilepsy			
Symptoms <24 h			
Not in wheelchair/bedridden			
Blood glucose >60/ <400			

Examination	Normal	Right	Left
Facial smile		Droop____	Droop____
Grip		Weak____	Weak____
		None____	None____
Arm strength		Drift____	Drift____
		Falls____	Falls____
Has only unilateral weakness	Yes____	No____	

Adapted from Kidwell et al.[45]

low scores might be seen in case of basilar artery thrombosis or massive intracerebral hemorrhage.

Emergency History

Often, the history of the event is not obtainable from a patient with decreased consciousness or cognitive or language impairments. As a result, relatives or other observers are the usual sources of information. The paramedics should ask them about the time of onset, course, and nature of symptoms. The paramedics also should inquire about recent medical illnesses and the use of any medications, such as anticoagulants. This information can be transmitted to physicians and hospital personnel before arrival in the emergency department. This step is crucial because some of the observers (shopkeepers, neighbors, etc.) probably will not be going to the hospital. The patient will be transported to the hospital by ambulance and family members will likely come by private vehicle. As a result, the relatives will arrive at the emergency department some time (minutes or hours) after the patient—this lag is important when physicians are making decisions about emergent care.

Emergency Treatment

In the future, emergency stroke treatment might even begin in the field. Although emergency medical services personnel currently cannot administer any stroke-specific therapy, development of effective neuroprotective medications, which could be administered safely to patients with either hemorrhagic or ischemic stroke, could improve initial care. An agent, such as magnesium, might be given while the patient is being transported for additional treatment, such as thrombolytic agents.[47] Such early interventions, which are currently under intense investigation, might increase the time window for subsequent definitive treatment by limiting the brain injury. In addition to immediate life support and stabilizing the patient's cardiovascular status, paramedics also can check the blood glucose concentration and administer thiamine and glucose if hypoglycemia is present.

Air Transportation

In cities and suburban areas, land ambulances and mobile critical care units are used to transport most patients with stroke. However, emergency land transportation can be potentially time-consuming if a patient lives in a rural location. Distances are considerable and medical resources (hospitals and personnel with expertise in stroke) are limited. Emergency air transportation (helicopter or fixed wing aircraft) is an option.[48–50] However, such services are often located only in larger cities and logistics in arranging such transportation can be time-consuming. The time saved by air transportation might be marginal when a patient is within 100 miles (160 km) of a stroke center. Other variables, such as weather conditions, also can limit the availability of emergency air transportation.

Telemedicine

Telemedicine is a potential and emerging option if a patient is first evaluated in a small hospital that has brain imaging available.[51–53] This strategy brings the expertise to the patient rather than vice versa. The patient is evaluated and imaged locally. A radiologist or stroke specialist at a tertiary hospital can interpret the brain imaging that is transmitted electronically. A neurologist could assess the patient via television because most of the neurological examination can be visualized easily. The neurologist and the local physician could make decisions jointly about emergent stroke care that could be given at the community hospital prior to transportation to a larger medical center. Already, such programs are underway in the United States and other countries. The evaluation of patients with suspected stroke, including the performance of the NIH Stroke Scale, is done reliably using telemedicine technology.[54] Such strategies can increase the number of patients who can be treated with r-tPA.[55] In addition, and equally important, such consultation can help a local physician in deciding when to withhold acute stroke therapies. Technical advances in electronic telecommunication likely will increase the feasibility of telemedicine. An alternative is telephone consultation. While telephone consultation does not permit direct observation of the patient, it does allow the physician in a small hospital to gain advice from a stroke specialist.

► EMERGENCY DEPARTMENT

Professional and stroke advocacy organizations are working with governmental groups to develop a method to designate acute stroke treatment centers.[56] These centers would be modeled on programs used to treat patients with severe trauma. Such institutions would serve as the hub for local or regional stroke programs. Patients would be transported preferentially to these hospitals. The stroke treatment center would have the professional and support services to provide early care of patients with stroke (see Table 3-9). In most instances, initial and critical treatment of stroke occurs primarily in an emergency department. However, in some instances, patients subsequently require emergent endovascular or surgical treatment given in other areas of the hospital. The acute stroke treatment center should have close relationships with acute inpatient care services and a rehabilitation program so that coordinated patient management can be facilitated.

Time Goals for Treatment

Specific time goals for components of emergency evaluation and treatment have been developed.[39,57,58] The time begins the moment the patient arrives in the hospital. These time goals are difficult to achieve unless there is a concerted effort to speed evaluation and treatment.[34] A coordinated acute stroke care team, which can be activated prior to or upon arrival of the patient, expedites treatment.[13,59] If the ambulance personnel call the hospital in advance of the patient's arrival, such a team can be assembled to meet the patient. Physician members of the team usually include neurologists, primary care physicians, or emergency medicine physicians. With the approved steps of increased education and certification of neurologists who have special expertise in cerebrovascular disease (vascular neurologists), these individuals will lead the acute stroke care team. Because of the importance of surgical management of intracranial hemorrhage, a neurosurgeon should be readily available. In the future, the acute stroke care team might include a neurologist, neurosurgeon, or neuroradiologist who has expertise in the endovascular treatment of stroke.

Code Stroke

In addition, the emergency department should have a well-defined plan for the emergency management of patients with stroke. Unfortunately, many hospitals have not implemented such policies. For example, Burgin et al.[60] found that the guidelines for emergency stroke care often are not followed in smaller community hospitals. However, with aggressive educational and quality improvement efforts, the management of patients with stroke can be improved. Katzan et al.[61] found that

▶ **TABLE 3-11.** FEATURES OF STROKE UNITS

Observation of the patient
  Clinical evaluation (history and physical examination)
  Diagnostic tests
    General laboratory
    Brain, vascular, and cardiac imaging
  General care needs
    Vital signs and neurological monitoring
    Nutrition, hydration, and swallowing
    Assessment of impairments and functions
Early management
  Management of fluids and food—intravenous fluids
  Treatment of swallowing problems
  Monitoring and treatment of complications such as
   hypoxia, hypoglycemia, fever, or infection
  Early mobilization
  Positioning and handling of bedridden patients
  Skin care
  Avoid use of bladder catheters
Rehabilitation
  Multidisciplinary team
  Patient education
  Early assessment of discharge needs
  Discharge planning

Adapted from Langhorne and Dennis, Lancet 2004;13:834.

educational programs improved compliance with the guidelines for administration of r-tPA and a reduction in the rate of hemorrhagic complications resulted.

Physician Activities

Physicians are responsible for emergent assessment of the patient (history and physical examination) and for ordering resuscitative measures. The key components of the clinical assessments are listed in Table 3-11. The physician develops a differential diagnosis based on the available clinical findings and orders the emergency diagnostic tests. The availability of preprinted orders would expedite this task. The severity of the stroke is quantified by the use of the NIH Stroke Scale (see Table 2.9). The physician also makes decisions about emergency treatment of the stroke.

Nursing Activities

Nurses perform regular assessments of the patient's vital signs and neurological status. The nurses also administer emergency medications.

Emergency Diagnostic Studies

The laboratory and radiology personnel perform the required ancillary tests on an urgent basis and a pharmacist prepares the necessary medications to be administered. Most guidelines list a limited number of diag-

nostic studies that should be available on an emergency basis[58] (see Table 8.1). The recommendations focus on resources that can be performed at most moderate-to-large hospitals across the United States. The goal is to use tests that can be performed quickly and that provide key information to guide the medical or surgical management of the stroke. While CT currently is listed as the recommended brain imaging study, advances in MRI technology and knowledge suggests that, in the future, this test might replace CT as the initial imaging procedure of choice.[58] In addition, the results of the diagnostic tests are helpful in management to prevent or control medical or neurological complications. Treatment usually is initiated in the emergency department and the patient is subsequently admitted to the hospital.

▶ ACUTE HOSPITALIZATION

While decisions about admission to the hospital are made on a case-by-case basis, most patients with acute stroke should be hospitalized[58,62] (see Chapter 24). An exception might be a patient with severe preexisting disease, such as advanced dementia, who might receive only palliative care and who could be transferred directly to a skilled nursing facility following a stroke. Overall, the interval from onset of stroke is a crucial factor about recommending admission. Patients who have had a mild ischemic stroke or TIA and who did not seek medical attention until several days following the event usually can be evaluated and treated as an outpatient. Patients with a recent TIA or resolving ischemic stroke should be admitted. Johnston et al.[63] demonstrated the ominous nature of such events. Most patients with intracranial hemorrhage are admitted because of potentially life-threatening complications of the disease. In particular, alert patients with minimal symptoms from subarachnoid hemorrhage should be admitted because of the high risk for early recurrent bleeding. The presence of serious comorbid diseases also affects decisions about hospitalization; the most common are cardiovascular disease, diabetes mellitus, or lung disease. Concomitant neurological diseases also affect decisions about hospitalization. Depending upon the type and cause of stroke, the severity of neurological impairments, and the types of treatment, most patients are admitted to a stroke unit or an intensive care unit (ICU). In some cases, the patient will be admitted to an inpatient unit following emergency surgery or endovascular therapy.

Follow-up management of the stroke itself is an important component of acute treatment after admission (Table 3-12). Several components of management commence simultaneously during the first few days after

▶ **TABLE 3-12.** COMPONENTS OF MANAGEMENT DURING HOSPITALIZATION FOR STROKE

Medical or surgical management of acute brain injury
 Continue interventions started in emergency department
 Surgical/endovascular management of vascular lesion
Prevent or control acute or subacute neurological complications
Prevent or control acute or subacute medical complications
Evaluate for cause of stroke
Institute medical or surgical therapies to prevent recurrent stroke
Rehabilitation and plans for discharge and posthospital care

stroke. In addition, the patient should be evaluated for the cause of stroke, neurological and medical complications, or the presence of severe comorbid diseases. Patients should be assessed frequently for changes in neurological or medical status. Determination of the likely cause of stroke affects the selection of medical or surgical measures to prevent recurrent events. Rehabilitation and restorative interventions are also started in the hospital.

▶ **STROKE UNITS**

Because stroke is a potentially life-threatening disease and because patients have a high risk for serious complications during the first days following stroke, patients usually are admitted to a monitored bed for observation and treatment. Patients with severe strokes often are admitted to an ICU.[27,64-66] The indications for admission to an ICU include the need for ventilatory assistance, aggressive management of increased intracranial pressure, arterial hypertension or cardiovascular complications, and close observation following surgical or endovascular treatment. Patients with severe intracranial hemorrhage, including those with ruptured aneurysms, usually are treated initially in an ICU. Most patients with ischemic stroke, including those treated with r-tPA, and persons with recent TIA can be admitted to a non-ICU monitored bed for close observation and treatment.

During recent years, stroke care units have been developed to expedite treatment.[67,68] The components of a stroke unit vary between institutions; however, a focus should be on early treatment in an acute care setting[69] (see Tables 3-9 and 3-11). In Germany, a system of intensive care stroke units is being developed. The units emphasize the first 3–4 days of care.[69] The units have as a goal reducing long-term health care costs by decreasing morbidity and improving outcomes through aggressive acute management, including the use of thrombolytic agents, neuroprotective therapies, therapies to treat complications, and rehabilitation.

In some institutions, a stroke unit might emphasize longer-term care or rehabilitation.[70] A stroke unit usually involves a geographically defined facility that includes monitoring equipment and that is staffed by a group of skilled nurses, who have a special interest in treating patients with neurological disease. Several studies demonstrate the utility of stroke care units in improving outcomes following stroke.[71-76] Launois et al.[77] demonstrated that stroke units are very cost-effective. The units improve care by preventing complications, expediting evaluation, facilitating rehabilitation, and starting measures to prevent recurrent neurological events. These benefits can persist up to 10 years following stroke.[78]

Stroke Team

Some institutions have implemented a *stroke team* that primarily consists of rehabilitation specialists seeing patients on several nursing units. However, this strategy lacks some critical components of specialized medical and nursing care. A geographically defined facility that includes all components of stroke care is optimal (see Table 3-11). One study comparing a stroke unit to a stroke team approach showed the superiority of the stroke unit.[79] The number of beds in a stroke unit depends upon the level of activity but a minimal number probably is four. The hospital administration and the physicians should agree to the plan to have a stroke bed available (open) for admission at all times. This step helps assure the prompt admission of patients and is important when interacting with physicians at other institutions. The physicians should have a plan to arrange for a new "open" bed whenever the emergency bed is filled by a new admission. A way to facilitate the efficacy of the unit may be the institution of a policy that most patients will be moved to another acute care bed or a rehabilitation bed after the first 24–72 h. In some larger hospitals, a stroke unit could be incorporated in the administrative structure of the inpatient neurology service.

The location of the stroke unit should allow for easy access to both rehabilitation facilities and diagnostic laboratories. The unit should permit for easy direct observation by nurses and a central monitoring facility.[80] The unit should have technical resources to permit monitoring of cardiac rate and rhythm, blood pressure, level of oxygenation, and respiratory rate. The blood pressure could be monitored via the use of noninvasive devices or intra-arterial lines. This equipment is often needed if aggressive lowering of the arterial blood pressure is needed. Some stroke units or neurological ICU have other capabilities including ventilators and endotracheal intubation. However, because most patients with stroke do not need this aggressive treatment, patients requiring intubation and ventilatory assistance often are transferred to an independent medical or surgical ICU.

A *stroke service* (stroke team) includes physicians, nurses, and other personnel who have special interest and expertise in treating patients with stroke. The membership of this group can overlap with that listed in the acute stroke care team. In particular, the physicians are likely to be members of both groups. However, additional physicians including ICU specialists might also be members. A physician, usually a vascular neurologist, directs both the stroke team and the stroke unit. The physicians are responsible for the overall management of the patient, including medical assessments and writing orders for all aspects of care.[59] Nurses have frequent interactions with patients and are responsible for administering medications and other direct patient care activities. Nurses also work with rehabilitation specialists to start mobilization and to perform range-of-motion exercises. The nurses also help educate the patient and family about stroke, prognosis, acute treatment, rehabilitation, and long-term treatment. The nurses are also important in coordinating discharge planning. An independent discharge planner might assume this latter activity. Rehabilitation specialists include physical therapists, occupational therapists, speech pathologists, vocational counselors, and neuropsychologists. These professionals work closely with the nurses and physicians. Depending upon the institution, a physician specializing in rehabilitation might direct the rehabilitation activities. A social worker can advise the patient, family, and physician about governmental programs and health insurance coverage that affect long-term treatment decisions. The social worker can help the patient apply for disability.

▶ CENTERS OF EXCELLENCE IN STROKE

Centers of excellence are being developed for management of patients with other diseases including heart disease.[81] A similar approach makes a great deal of sense for management of cerebrovascular disease.[15] Resources to speed diagnosis and treatment can be concentrated at the locations where physicians and surgeons with special expertise are available.[39] For example, the sophisticated endovascular and neurosurgical techniques to treat patients with intracranial vascular disease can be housed at one institution. Such specialization will result in improved patient care. It might also avoid duplication of costly services and technologies.

▶ REHABILITATION

Planning for rehabilitation begins as soon as the patient's medical condition permits (see Chapter 25).

The goal of rehabilitation is to assist the patient recover as much as possible and as quickly as possible from his/her cerebrovascular event. Some patients with acute cerebrovascular disease, such as those with a TIA or ischemic stroke that was treated successfully with r-tPA, might not need rehabilitation because their neurological status has recovered. Other patients are not candidates for rehabilitation because of the severity of their neurological impairments or because of serious preexisting comorbid medical diseases. For example, patients with depressed consciousness or severe cognitive impairments will not be able to participate in a rehabilitation plan.

Physicians with expertise in neurological rehabilitation may be consulted. In addition, rehabilitation professionals include physical therapists, speech pathologists, occupational therapists, neuropsychologists, and vocational counselors. Planning should include the types of rehabilitation activities and their intensity. While the first assessments and treatments begin during acute hospitalization, a key component of initial management involves planning for subsequent treatment. Options include inpatient rehabilitation either in a freestanding institution or a unit attached to the hospital, outpatient treatment either at home or through clinic visits, or rehabilitation in a skilled nursing facility. These plans need to be finalized prior to discharge from the acute care setting.

▶ DISCHARGE PLANNING AND RETURN TO SOCIETY

The planning for the patient's ultimate return to society begins in concert with the planning for rehabilitation (see Chapter 25). Although stroke is a leading cause of death, most patients survive—although many with residual, often severe, neurological impairments. Some patients will go to an intensive inpatient rehabilitation program following their acute care. Other patients will be able to return to their homes with minimal or no assistance. Some patients will be able to return to their home with a family member serving as caregiver or may use community-provided services. A minority requires long-term institutionalized care. The physician treating the patient in the acute care hospital can predict the likely location for the patient based on a number of clinical variables including the patient's neurological impairments, coexisting neurological and medical problems, epidemiological factors, the social situation, community resources, and economic considerations (Table 3-13). Many institutions have professional discharge planners (either a social worker or nurse) to assist the physician in making the necessary arrangements for the patient to return home.

▶ **TABLE 3-13.** FACTORS AFFECTING PLANS FOR DISCHARGE FROM HOSPITAL FOLLOWING STROKE

Neurological impairments
    Severity and type of impairments
    Plans for rehabilitation
Preexisting neurological diseases
    Dementia
    Movement disorder
    Neuromuscular disease
Comorbid medical diseases
    Heart disease
    Lung disease
    Diabetes mellitus
Epidemiological variables
    Age
    Gender
    Required medications
    Alcohol or drug abuse
Social situation
    Occupation
    Marital status
    Availability of family or friend as caregiver
    Health status of spouse or caregiver
    Children or other dependents in household
    Locations/availability of extended family members
    Previous living environment
Community
    Size of community
    Community resources for home care
Economic considerations
    Governmental programs
    Private insurance programs

REFERENCES

1. Demaerschalk BM. Evidence-based clinical practice education in cerebrovascular disease. *Stroke* 2004;35:392–396.
2. Sacco RL, Adams R, Albers G et al. Guidelines for prevention of stroke in patients with ischemic stroke or transient ischemic attack. A statement for healthcare professionals from the American Heart Association/American Stroke Association Council on Stroke. *Circulation*; 2006;113:409–449.
3. Adams HP, Jr., Brott TG, Furlan AJ, et al. Guidelines for thrombolytic therapy for acute stroke: A supplement to the guidelines for the management of patients with acute ischemic stroke. *Stroke* 1996;27:1711–1718.
4. Mayberg MR, Batjer HH, Dacey R, et al. Guidelines for the management of aneurysmal subarachnoid hemorrhage. A statement for healthcare professionals from a special writing group of the Stroke Council, American Heart Association. *Stroke* 1994;25:2315–2328.
5. Broderick JP, Adams HP, Jr., Barsan W, et al. Guidelines for the management of spontaneous intracerebral hemorrhage: A statement for healthcare professionals from a special writing group of the Stroke Council, American Heart Association. *Stroke* 1999;30:905–915.
6. Goldstein LB, Adams R, Alberts MJ et al. Primary prevention of ischemic stroke. A guideline from the American Heart Association/American Stroke Association Stroke Council. *Circulation*, 2006;113:873–923.
7. Albers GW, Amarenco P, Easton JD, Sacco RL, Teal P. Antithrombotic and thrombolytic therapy for ischemic stroke. *Chest* 2001;119:300S–320S.
8. Norris JW, Buchan A, Cote R, et al. Canadian guidelines for intravenous thrombolytic treatment in acute stroke. A consensus statement of the Canadian Stroke Consortium. *Can J Neurol Sci* 1998;25:257–259.
9. Hill MD, Hachinski V. Stroke treatment: Time is brain. *Lancet* 1998;352(suppl 3):SIII10–SIII14.
10. Diez-Tejedor E, Fuentes B. Acute care in stroke: The importance of early intervention to achieve better brain protection. *Cerebrovasc Dis* 2004;17(suppl 1):130–137.
11. Fogelholm R, Murros K, Rissanen A, Ilmavirta M. Factors delaying hospital admission after acute stroke. *Stroke* 1996;27:398–400.
12. Smith MA, Doliszny KM, Shahar E, McGovern PG, Arnett DK, Luepker RV. Delayed hospital arrival for acute stroke: The Minnesota Stroke Survey. *Ann Intern Med* 1998;129:190–196.
13. Alberts MJ, Chaturvedi S, Graham G, et al. Acute stroke teams: Results of a national survey. National Acute Stroke Team Group. *Stroke* 1998;29:2318–2320.
14. Alberts MJ, Hademenos G, Latchaw RE, et al. Recommendations for the establishment of primary stroke centers. *JAMA* 2001;283:3102–3109.
15. Adams RE, Acker J, Alberts M, et al. Recommendations for improving the quality of care through stroke centers and systems: An examination of stroke center identification options. Multidisciplinary consensus recommendations from the Advisory Working Group on Stroke Center Identification Options of the American Stroke Association. *Stroke* 2002;33:1–7.
16. Moser DK, Kimble LP, Alberts MJ et al. Reducing delay in seeking treatment by patients with acute coronary syndrome and stroke. A scientific statement from the American Heart Association Council on Cardiovascular Nursing and Stroke Council. *Circulation*, 2006;114:168–182.
17. Kennedy J, Buchan AM. Acute neurovascular syndromes: Hurry up, please, it's time! *Stroke* 2004;35:360–362.
18. Yu RF, San Jose MC, Manzanilla BM, Oris MY, Gan R. Sources and reasons for delays in the care of acute stroke patients. *J Neurol Sci* 2002;199:49–54.
19. Kothari R, Jauch E, Broderick J, et al. Acute stroke: Delays to presentation and emergency department evaluation. *Ann Emerg Med* 1999;33:3–8.
20. Kothari R, Sauerbeck L, Jauch E. Patients' awareness of stroke signs, symptoms, and risk factors. *Stroke* 1997;28:1871–1875.
21. Serena J, Davalos A, Segura T, MOstacero E, Castillo J. Stroke on awakening: Looking for a more rational management. *Cerebrovasc Dis* 2003;16:128–133.
22. Streifler JY, Davidovitch S, Sendovski U. Factors associated with the time of presentation of acute stroke patients in an Israeli community hospital. *Neuroepidemiology* 1998;17:161–166.
23. Wester P, Radberg J, Lundgren B, Peltonen M. Factors associated with delayed admission to hospital and in-hospital

delays in acute stroke and TIA: A prospective, multicenter study. Seek- Medical-Attention-in-Time Study Group. *Stroke* 1999;30:40–48.

24. Brown MM. Brain attack: A new approach to stroke. *Clin Med* 2002;2:60–65.

25. Adams HP, Jr. Treating ischemic stroke as an emergency. *Arch Neurol* 1998;55:457–461.

26. Heros RC, Camarata PJ, Latchaw RE. Brain attack. Introduction. *Neurosurg Clin N Am* 1997;8:135–144.

27. Brainin M, Olsen TS, Chamorro A, et al. Organization of stroke care: Education, referral, emergency management and imaging, stroke units and rehabilitation. *Cerebrovasc Dis* 2004;17(suppl 2):1–14.

28. Rymer MM, Thrutchley DE. Organizing regional stroke networks to increase acute stroke intervention. *Neurol Res,* 2005;27(suppl 1)S9–S16.

29. Yoon SS, Byles J. Perceptions of stroke in the general public and patients with stroke: A qualitative study. *BMJ* 2002; 324:1065

30. Montaner J, Vidal C, Molina C, Alvarex-Sabín J. Selecting the target and the message for a stroke public education campaign: A local survey conducted by neurologists. *Eur J Epidemiol* 2001;17:581–586.

31. Pancioli AM, Broderick J, Kothari R, et al. Public perception of stroke warning signs and knowledge of potential risk factors. *JAMA* 1998;279:1288–1292.

32. Schneider AT, Pancioli AM, Khoury JC, et al. Trends in community knowledge of the warning signs and risk factors for stroke. *JAMA* 2003;289:343–346.

33. Zweifler RM, Drinkard R, Cunningham S, Brody ML, Rothrock JF. Implementation of a stroke code system in Mobile, Alabama. Diagnostic and therapeutic yield. *Stroke* 1997;28:981–983.

34. Katzan IL, Graber TM, Furlan AJ, et al. Cuyahoga County Operation Stroke speed of emergency department evaluation and compliance with National Institutes of Neurological Disorders and Stroke time targets. *Stroke* 2003;34:799–800.

35. Salisbury HR, Banks BJ, Footitt DR, Winner SJ, Reynolds DJ. Delay in presentation of patients with acute stroke to hospital in Oxford. *QJM* 1998;91:635–640.

36. Barsan WG, Brott TG, Broderick JP, Haley EC, Levy DE, Marler JR. Time of hospital presentation in patients with acute stroke. *Arch Intern Med* 1993;153:2558–2561.

37. Famularo G, Polchi S, Panegrossi A. Thrombolysis enters the race: A new era for acute ischaemic stroke?. *Eur J Emerg Med* 1998;5:249–252.

38. Gil Nunez AC, Vivancos Mora J. Organization of medical care in acute stroke: Importance of a good network. *Cerebrovasc Dis* 2004;17(suppl 1):113–123.

39. Kennedy J, Ma C, Buchan AM. Organization of regional and local stroke resources: Methods to expedite acute management of stroke. *Curr Neurol Neurosci Rep* 2004; 4:13–18.

40. Ruland S, Gorelick PB, Schneck M, Kim D, Moore CG, Leurgans S. Acute stroke care in Illinois: A statewide assessment of diagnostic and treatment capabilities. *Stroke* 2002;33:1334–1340.

41. Goldstein LB, Hey LA, Laney R. North Carolina stroke prevention and treatment facilities survey: Statewide availability of programs and services. *Stroke* 2000;31:66–70.

42. Kothari R, Barsan W, Brott T, Broderick J, Ashbrock S. Frequency and accuracy of prehospital diagnosis of acute stroke. *Stroke* 1995;26:937–941.

43. Broderick JP. Logistics in acute stroke management. *Drugs* 1997;54(suppl 3):109–116.

44. Kothari R, Hall K, Brott T, Broderick J. Early stroke recognition: Developing an out-of-hospital NIH Stroke Scale. *Acad Emerg Med* 1997;4:986–990.

45. Kidwell CS, Starkman S, Eckstein M, Weems K, Saver JL. Identifying stroke in the field. Prospective validation of the Los Angeles Prehospital Stroke Screen (LAPSS). *Stroke* 2000;31:71–76.

46. Teasdale GM, Pettigrew LE, Wilson JT, Murray G, Jennett B. Analyzing outcome of treatment of severe head injury: A review and update on advancing the use of the Glasgow Outcome Scale. *J Neurotrauma* 1998;15: 587–597.

47. Muir KW. Magnesium in stroke treatment. *Postgrad Med J* 2002;78:641–645.

48. Conroy MB, Rodriguez SU, Kimmel SE, Kasner SE. Helicopter transfer offers a potential benefit to patients with acute stroke. *Stroke* 1999;30:2580–2584.

49. Silbergleit R, Scott PA, Lowell MJ. Cost-effectiveness of helicopter transport of stroke patients for thrombolysis. *Acad Emerg Med* 2003;10:966–972.

50. Thomas SH, Kociszewski C, Schwamm L, Wedel S. The evolving role of helicopter emergency medical services in the transfer of stroke patients to specialized centers. *Prehosp Emerg Care* 2002;6:210–214.

51. Audebert HJ, Kukla C, Vatankhah B, et al. Comparison of tissue plasminogen activator administration management between telestroke network hospitals and academic medical centers. *Stroke,* 2006:37:1822–1827.

52. Handschu R, Littmann R, Reulbach U, et al. Telemedicine in emergency evaluation of acute stroke. Interrater agreement in remote video examination with a novel multimedia system. *Stroke* 2003;34:2842–2846.

53. Wiborg A, Widder B, for the TESS Study Group. Teleneurology to improve stroke care in rural areas. The Telemedicine in Stroke in Swabia (TESS) Project. *Stroke* 2003;34:2951–2957.

54. Wang S, Lee SB, Pardue C, et al. Remote evaluation of acute ischemic stroke: Reliability of national institutes of health stroke scale via telestroke. *Stroke* 2003;34:e188–e192.

55. LaMonte MP, Bahouth MN, Hu P, et al. Telemedicine for acute stroke: Triumphs and pitfalls. *Stroke* 2003;34: 725–728.

56. Alberts MJ, Latchaw RE, Selman WR, et al. Recommendations for comprehensive stroke centers. A consensus statement from the Brain Attack Coalition. *Stroke,* 2005;36:1597–1616.

57. Gropen TI, Gagliano PJ, Blake CA, et al. Quality improvement in acute stroke. The New York State Stroke Center Designation Project. *Neurology,* 2006;67:88–93.

58. Adams HP, Adams RJ, Brott T, et al. Guidelines for the early management of patients with ischemic stroke. A scientific statement from the stroke council of the American Stroke Association. *Stroke* 2003;34:1056–1083.

59. California Acute Stroke Pilot Registry Investigators. The impact of standardized stroke orders on adherence to best practices. *Neurology,* 2005;65:360–365.

60. Burgin WS, Staub L, Chan W, et al. Acute stroke care in non-urgan emergency departments. *Neurology* 2001;57: 2006–2012.

61. Katzan IL, Hammer MD, Furlan AJ, Hixson ED, Nadzam DM. Quality improvement and tissue-type plasminogen activator for acute ischemic stroke: A Cleveland update. *Stroke* 2003;34:799–800.

62. The European Ad Hoc Consensus Group. Optimizing intensive care in stroke. A European perspective. *Cerebrovasc Dis* 1997;7:113–128.

63. Johnston SC, Gress DR, Browner WS, Sidney S. Short-term prognosis after emergency department diagnosis of TIA. *JAMA* 2000;284:2901–2906.

64. Hund E, Grau A, Hacke W. Neurocritical care for acute ischemic stroke. *Neurosurg Clin N Am* 1997;8:271–282.

65. Mitsias P. Ischemic stroke management in the critical care unit: The first 24 hours. *J Stroke Cerebrovasc Dis* 1999;8: 151–159.

66. Qureshi AI, Tuhrim S, Broderick JP. Spontaneous intracerebral hemorrhage. *N Engl J Med* 2001;344:1450–1460.

67. Indredavik B. Stroke units—the Norwegian experience. *Cerebrovasc Dis* 2003;48:21–22.

68. van Gijn J, Dennis MS. Issues and answers in stroke care. *Lancet* 1998;352(suppl 3):SIII23–SIII27.

69. Treib J, Grauer MT, Woessner R, Morgenthaler M. Treatment of stroke on an intensive stroke unit: A novel concept. *Intensive Care Med* 2000;26(11):1598–1611.

70. Indredavik B, Bakke F, Slordahl SA, Rokseth R, Haheim LL. Treatment in a combined acute and rehabilitation stroke unit. *Stroke* 1999;30:917–923.

71. Stroke Unit Trialists Collaboration. How do stroke units improve patient outcomes? A collaborative systematic review of the randomized trials. *Stroke* 1997;28:2139–2144.

72. Stroke Unit Trialists' Collaboration. Collaborative systematic review of the randomised trials of organised inpatient (stroke unit) care after stroke. *BMJ* 1997;314:1151–1159.

73. Ronning OM, Guldvog B. Stroke unit versus general medical wards, II: Neurological deficits and activities of daily living. A quasi-randomized controlled trial. *Stroke* 1998;29: 586–590.

74. Ronning OM, Guldvog B. Stroke units versus general medical wards, I: Twelve- and eighteen-month survival. A randomized, controlled trial. *Stroke* 1998;29:58–62.

75. Langhorne P, Williams BO, Gilchrist W, Howie K. Do stroke units save lives? *Lancet* 1993;342:395–398.

76. Jorgensen HS, Nakayama H, Raaschou HO, Larsen K, Hubbe P, Olsen TS. The effect of a stroke unit: Reductions in mortality, discharge rate to nursing home, length of hospital stay, and cost. A community-based study. *Stroke* 1995;26:1178–1182.

77. Launois R, Giroud M, Mégnigbêto AC, et al. Estimating the cost-effectiveness of stroke units in France compared with conventional care. *Stroke* 2004;35:770–775.

78. Indredavik B, Bakke F, Slordahl SA, Rokseth R, Haheim LL. Stroke unit treatment. 10-year follow-up. *Stroke* 1999; 30:1524–1527.

79. Evans A, Harraf F, Donaldson N, Kalra L. Randomized controlled study of stroke unit care versus stroke team care in different stroke subtypes. *Stroke* 2002;33:449–455.

80. Dayno JM, Mansbach HH. Acute stroke units. *J Stroke Cerebrovasc Dis* 1999;8:160–170.

81. Willerson JT. Centers of excellence. *Circulation* 2003;107: 1471–1472.

82. Guyatt GH, Cook DJ, Sackett DL, Eckman M, Pauker S: Guides for recommendation for antithrombotic agents. *Chest* 1998;114:441S–444S.

CHAPTER 4

Modifiable Risk Factors for Stroke: Diagnosis and Management

▶ GENERAL COMMENTS

Several conditions, which can be controlled or treated, and which are usually associated with an accelerated course of atherosclerosis, predict an increased risk of stroke (Table 4-1). While most of the risk factors for stroke are associated primarily with the risk of ischemic events secondary to thromboembolism, some are also correlated with an increased risk of hemorrhagic stroke. Some additional factors are linked with a heightened likelihood of intracranial bleeding. Most of these conditions can be modified, treated, or controlled by changes in lifestyle or medical interventions. In addition, these conditions are very prevalent in the American population. They are found among men and women of all ethnic groups and of all ages, and they compound the effects of age, gender, family history, and ethnicity in denoting persons who have a high risk for either hemorrhagic or ischemic stroke (Table 4-2). These findings, which are correlated with the premature development of advanced atherosclerosis, are associated with an increased chance of myocardial infarction and ischemic stroke. Furthermore, when detected during adolescence, these findings are also associated with accelerated atherosclerosis in young adulthood, including severe disease of the carotid arteries.[1–3]

While effective management of these factors is associated with a modest but real reduction in the risk of stroke for an asymptomatic individual patient, the aggregate effect of control of these conditions on the public's health is very large. In addition, management of these conditions may be as effective as antithrombotic medications or surgical interventions in reducing the risk of ischemic stroke.[4,5] Advances in treatment of hypercholesterolemia and hypertension have the potential for producing dramatic declines in the chances of stroke. Some of these advances reflect new strategies in therapies to protect the vascular endothelium and to stabilize atherosclerotic plaques in patients with ischemic cerebrovascular disease.[6] Unfortunately, management of these conditions in patients who have had either a transient ischemic attack (TIA) or a stroke is not particularly successful.[7] Many patients have difficulty complying with the required changes in behavior or the use of medications. The patient's health or social situation can compound issues with compliance. Additional efforts including public and individual educational programs are required if these risk-modifying treatments are to meet their full potential.

An open discussion with the patient should include a review of the risk factors and the best strategies for their successful control. Physicians and other medical personnel must support patients in their efforts to affect change in personal behavior. An aggressive approach involving behavioral and pharmacological interventions aimed at treatment of hyperglycemia, hypertension, and hyperlipidemia, when combined with efforts to prevent thromboembolism, can achieve a reduction in the risk of cardiovascular events.[8] Such an approach will be required for improved management of patients with cerebrovascular disease.

▶ ARTERIAL HYPERTENSION

Arterial hypertension is the leading modifiable risk factor for both hemorrhagic and ischemic stroke.[9,10] It is calculated to be a contributing factor for approximately

▶ **TABLE 4-1.** COMMON MODIFIABLE RISK FACTORS FOR STROKE

Both ischemic and hemorrhagic stroke
    Arterial hypertension
    Smoking/tobacco use
    Alcohol abuse
    Drug abuse
    Use of oral contraceptives
Ischemic stroke
    Diabetes mellitus and increased insulin resistance
    Hypercholesterolemia
    Hyperhomocysteinemia
    Obesity
    Physical inactivity
    Sleep apnea and snoring
Hemorrhagic stroke
    Hypocholesterolemia
    Anticoagulants, antiplatelet agents, and thrombolytic
      agents

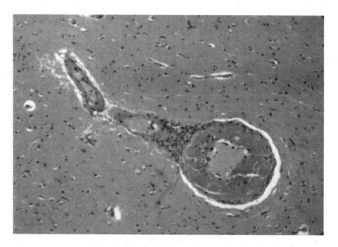

Figure 4-1. Pathological evidence of lipohyalinosis is seen in a penetrating artery of the brain of a patient with chronic hypertension. (*Courtesy of S.S. Schochet, M.D., Department of Pathology, University of West Virginia, Morgantown, WV*)

70 percent of cerebrovascular events. Besides being an independent cause of death and renal failure, arterial hypertension is also associated with accelerated atherosclerosis, hypertensive heart disease, and hypertensive cerebrovascular disease.[11] The primary effects of hypertension result in changes in the vascular endothelium. Elevated blood pressure increases smooth muscle lipoxygenase activity, inflammation, oxidation of low-density lipoprotein (LDL) cholesterol, and formation of superoxide radicals.[12] Simply put, these changes promote the development of atherosclerosis. Additionally, elevated blood pressure leads to increased vascular turbulence that independently promotes atherosclerosis in medium and large caliber arteries, particularly at vascular bifurcations. Furthermore, chronic arterial hypertension promotes development of lipohyalinosis or atherosclerosis in smaller penetrating brain arteries, which in turn leads to lacunar infarction or hypertensive brain hemorrhage[13] (Fig. 4-1). The relationship between hypertension and lacunar infarction is so strong that the diagnosis is called into question when a normotensive patient has a lacunar

syndrome.[14] Similarly, the absence of a strong history of hypertension generally precludes the diagnosis of hypertensive hemorrhage. Hypertensive hemorrhage is generally attributed to rupture of Charcot–Bouchard aneurysms that are found on vessels that perfuse the deep structures of the cerebral hemispheres and brain stem. Besides being a cause of primary brain hemorrhage, arterial hypertension can also lead to rupture of cerebral arteries or vascular abnormalities, including aneurysms and vascular malformations. This scenario may occur acutely in situations such as eclampsia, sympathomimetic drug use, pheochromocytoma, or acute renal dysfunction. Hypertension also indirectly leads to ischemic stroke via heart disease (most commonly coronary artery disease and ischemic cardiomyopathy) by serving as a source of thromboembolism.

Epidemiology

Approximately 50 million Americans (one in four adults) have arterial hypertension, as defined by a systolic blood pressure of greater than or equal to 140 mm Hg or diastolic blood pressure of greater than or equal to 90 mm Hg[15] (Table 4-3). A diastolic blood pressure of 80–90 mm Hg is considered to be borderline elevated. Arterial hypertension is present in 60–70 percent of persons older than 60, although in many cases, it may be in the form of isolated systolic hypertension[16] (Fig. 4-2). Its prevalence increases rapidly above the age of 60. Isolated systolic hypertension is associated with an increased likelihood of stroke among older persons, whereas an elevated diastolic blood pressure denotes a heightened risk for stroke. This relationship is particularly strong among younger persons.

▶ **TABLE 4-2.** PREVALENCE AND ASSOCIATED INCREASE IN RELATIVE RISK—COMMON RISK FACTORS FOR STROKE

Factor	Prevalence (%)	Relative risk
Arterial hypertension	25–40	3–5 times
Total cholesterol >240 mg/dL	40	2–3 times
Current smoker	25	1.5 times
Inactivity	25–50	2.7 times
Obesity	18–22	1.8–2.4 times
Alcohol abuse	2–5	1.6 times

Adapted from Goldstein et al.[10]

▶ **TABLE 4-3.** PREVALENCE OF COMMON MODIFIABLE RISK FACTORS FOR STROKE IN THE UNITED STATES

Arterial hypertension	50 million people
Diabetes mellitus	16 million people
Impaired fasting glucose (not diabetic)	14 million people
Metabolic syndrome	47 million people
Obesity	130 million people
Total cholesterol >200 mg/dL	104 million people
Total cholesterol >240 mg/dL	41 million people
Smoking	48 million people
Chewing tobacco	5 million people

Adapted from American Heart Association.[15]

▶ **TABLE 4-4.** PREVALENCE OF ARTERIAL HYPERTENSION AMONG ETHNIC GROUPS IN THE UNITED STATES

	Men (%)	Women (%)
Non-Hispanic whites	25.2	20.5
African Americans	36.7	36.6
Mexican Americans	24.2	22.4
Asian/Pacific Islanders	9.7	8.4
Native Americans	26.8	27.5

Adapted from American Heart Association.[15]

Rates of hypertension vary among several subgroups in the population. Arterial hypertension is particularly common among African Americans.[17] Approximately 40 percent of African Americans have hypertension. The prevalence of hypertension among African Americans is the highest of any population in the world[15] (Table 4-4; Fig. 4-3). Elevated blood pressures are more common among persons living in the southeastern United States and those in lower socioeconomic groups. It is also more common among women taking oral contraceptives and persons who are obese or inactive.[15] An elevated blood pressure is also common among diabetic patients, especially those who have nephropathy. The high rates of hemorrhagic stroke and lacunar infarction in eastern Asia likely reflect the high prevalence of hypertension, which may be attributed partially to the high daily salt consumption. Reduction of the salt content in the diet and in processed foods might reduce the frequency of cardiovascular events.[18]

Approximately 30 percent of persons with arterial hypertension are not aware of their elevated blood pressure.[15] Since arterial hypertension usually is asymptomatic, it is unrecognized in most affected persons. Even more, a sizable proportion of treated patients have not achieved adequate control of their blood pressure. Approximately only 25 percent of Americans with hypertension have adequate treatment and in Britain the proportion of persons with effective control is under 10 percent. Management of hypertension is often erratic

with numerous switches in medications primarily due to side effects.[19] Efforts to improve blood pressure control greatly reduce the risk of stroke. The current target is a diastolic blood pressure of 70–80 mm Hg and a systolic blood pressure of less than 130 mm Hg. Lowering the diastolic blood pressure by only 5 mm Hg reduces the incidence of stroke by approximately 42 percent and its mortality by nearly 30 percent. Among persons above the age of 65, a 30 percent decline in the incidence of stroke can accompany an 11-mm-Hg drop in systolic blood pressure. The desired level of blood pressure for most persons is under 120/80 mm Hg.[9,10,20] However, lowering blood pressure should be performed with caution. Some patients with severe intracranial or extracranial arterial disease might need higher values of blood pressure to maintain adequate cerebral perfusion through stenotic vessels. Postural syncope or presyncope are the usual symptoms of cerebral hypoperfusion. Patients often complain of increased symptoms of light-headedness or wooziness with standing or other postural changes. Focal neurological symptoms, in particular posterior circulation TIA, also can occur with orthostatic hypotension in a patient whose blood pressure has been lowered excessively or too rapidly.

Treatment

In general, the greatest reductions in the risk of stroke are achieved with vigorous control of blood pressure.[9] Numerous options are available for lowering blood

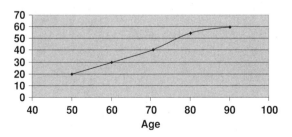

Figure 4-2. Estimated prevalence of hypertension among Americans as adjusted by age. (*Adapted from American Heart Association.[15]*)

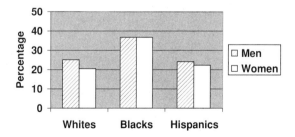

Figure 4-3. Estimated prevalence of hypertension among different adult ethnic groups in the United States. Rates in men are shown in hatched bars and in women in clear bars. (*Adapted from American Heart Association.[15]*)

► **TABLE 4-5.** OPTIONS FOR MANAGING
ARTERIAL HYPERTENSION

Lifestyle changes
   Weight reduction
   Increased exercise
   Diet
      Low sodium
      Calorie reduction
Medications
   Diuretics
   Beta-blockers
   α-1-adrenergic blockers
   Calcium channel blockers
   ACE inhibitors
   Clonidine
   Hydralazine
   Methyldopa
   Minoxidil

pressure, including changes in lifestyle and medications (Table 4-5). Management of arterial hypertension must be individualized.[9,10,21] Diets that emphasize weight loss or sodium restriction are often prescribed.[22] Exercise also provides benefits, including lowering blood pressure, better glucose control in diabetes, and weight reduction. Medications that cause vasoconstriction or elevate blood pressure should be avoided when treating common illnesses, such as an upper respiratory tract infection. Most patients with arterial hypertension will require antihypertensive medications and, in many cases, multiple medications are needed to achieve the desired blood pressure. Treatment should be prescribed on a case-by-case basis.[21] Beta-blockers and diuretics are the usual initially prescribed medications. In particular, diuretics are often prescribed as the first therapy to African Americans and persons older than 65 because of strong evidence of efficacy in these populations. Beta-blockers, on the other hand, improve efficacy in many persons of European heritage. Many studies continue to demonstrate the efficacy of these older medications.[23] In a study comparing a thiazide diuretic, lisinopril, or amlodipine, the frequency of major cardiovascular events was lowest among patients receiving the diuretic.[24] Beta-blockers are often prescribed for lowering blood pressure among patients who also have coronary artery disease. Now, there is evidence of efficacy of this class of antihypertensives beyond simply lowering blood pressure. For example, the addition of metoprolol to a lipid-lowering regimen can slow down the evolution of atherosclerosis among patients with elevated lipids.[25] Yet, not all evidence is positive, as one trial of beta-blockers did not demonstrate a benefit in reducing the risk of ischemic stroke among patients with TIA.[26] Based on a meta-analysis, Wink[27] concluded that beta-blockers were effective in reducing cardiovascular mortality or

morbidity only when the medications were combined with a diuretic. Recently, the Blood Pressure Lowering Treatment Trialists' Collaboration listed the effects of different blood-pressure-lowering regimens on major cardiovascular events.[28] While this group did not find major differences in the responses to different medications, they concluded that the reduction of risk in major vascular events, including stroke, was correlated directly with the degree of blood pressure reduction. Another international trial found that the combination of verapamil and trandolapril was as effective as the combination of atenolol and hydrochlorothiazide in preventing vascular events among persons with hypertension and known coronary artery disease.[29]

Potential endothelial protective properties have been reported with the calcium-channel-blocking agents, the angiotensin converting enzyme (ACE) inhibitors, and angiotensin receptor blockers, and theoretically, these agents might be particularly efficacious in reducing the number of ischemic events among persons with severe arterial disease. There is some evidence that the calcium-channel-blocking medications are effective in lowering the risk of major vascular events, including stroke, in high-risk persons.[30,31] However, Opie[32] reported that the utility of calcium channel blockers in preventing stroke was marginal. Black et al.[33] reported that the frequencies of major cardiovascular events were approximately the same among patients receiving verapamil, as they were among patients treated with either atenolol or hydrochlorothiazide. Although no significant differences were noted among the three treatment groups, the hazard ratio for cerebrovascular events was slightly higher among the patients treated with verapamil. Further, Pahor et al.[34] concluded that patients treated with calcium-channel-blocking drugs were at higher risk for major vascular events than were patients given other antihypertensive agents.

The data demonstrating success of the ACE inhibitors and the angiotensin receptor blockers with high tissue affinity in preventing major vascular appear stronger than that found with other antihypertensive agents. These medications preserve endothelial function and lead to vasodilation.[6,9,10,35,36] Some of these agents slow down the conversion of angiotensin I to angiotensin II and lower the release of endothelin I.[37] Angiotensin II is a potent vasoconstrictor that can induce hypertension and might stimulate the progression of atherosclerosis.[12,38] These medications also promote prostacyclin production and increase the release of nitrous oxide, both of which cause vasodilation.[39] Due to these effects, the ACE inhibitors and angiotensin receptor blockers might help stabilize large atherosclerotic plaques.[6] They also appear to improve the microcirculation in the heart and could also affect the cerebral microcirculation.[40]

Several studies demonstrate the utility of newer ACE inhibitors and angiotensin receptor blockers in preventing ischemic vascular events, including stroke.[31] Niskanen et al.[41] found that captopril was superior to the combination of a beta-blocker and a diuretic among hypertensive diabetic patients. The addition of ramipril to other therapies was effective in lowering the risk of stroke among high-risk persons, including those with diabetes mellitus.[42,43] A subgroup analysis in the same study also found that the administration of ramipril reduced the frequency of cognitive impairments, presumably secondary to ischemia, among high-risk hypertensive patients.[44] Another trial found that the combination of perindopril and indapamide reduced the risk of recurrent stroke among patients with prior TIA or stroke.[45–47] This particular trial enrolled a large number of participants from Asia. The combination was effective among patients with either hemorrhagic or ischemic stroke and normotensive patients also had a positive response. Benefit was present regardless of the patient's age, sex, ethnicity, or the presence of diabetes mellitus.[4,48,49] They also found that the regimen was effective in treating patients with all subtypes of stroke.[50] The same investigators found that perindopril reduced the likelihood of disability from vascular disease.[51] Another trial compared the utility of losartan, an angiotensin receptor blocker, with atenolol in the treatment of hypertension among persons with left ventricular hypertrophy.[52,53] In comparison to atenolol, losartan reduced the risk of fatal or nonfatal stroke by approximately 25 percent. In the trial, both groups had similar baseline and end-of-treatment blood pressure levels. Therefore, there was no confounding effect of blood pressure reduction. In a companion study in the same group, losartan was superior to atenolol by preventing stroke independent of blood pressure reduction among patients without clinically evident vascular disease.[54] These trials suggest that ACE inhibitors or angiotensin receptor blockers could become the primary medications to treat hypertensive patients with cerebrovascular disease. However, it is not yet clear whether all the ACE inhibitors have the same therapeutic effects.[55]

The management of hypertension is a cornerstone of the strategy to prevent stroke.[9,10,56] While some of the medications are expensive, the long-term costs of not treating hypertension are even higher.[57] Antihypertensive treatment also is cost-effective in preventing death, disability, and human suffering. Treatment with any commonly prescribed antihypertensive regimen reduces the chances of ischemic vascular events. Furthermore, the degree of reduction is proportional to the degree of lowering in blood pressure.[28] At present, the most prudent approach is to prescribe one medication that has been shown to be effective in reducing cardiovascular and cerebrovascular events. One of the advantages is their utility in preventing recurrent events among patients with hemorrhagic cerebrovascular disease. At present,

treatment of hypertension is the primary public health strategy to prevent hemorrhagic stroke. The results of the previously described recent trials imply that these medications may also be effective as stroke prophylactic therapies for treatment of nonhypertensive patients. While this finding has major public health implications, most physicians and patients likely will be slow to implement therapies to lower blood pressure among nonhypertensive persons. The expense of the medications must be weighed against the decreased risk of stroke. Additional research demonstrating the utility of these medications in forestalling stroke in hypertensive patients is needed to bolster this treatment approach. Nonpharmacological methods, such as lifestyle changes, might be the most cost-effective approach.

▶ DIABETES MELLITUS AND INCREASED INSULIN RESISTANCE

Diabetes mellitus accounts directly for approximately 200,000 deaths annually in the United States. More people die from diabetes mellitus than from either acquired immune deficiency syndrome or carcinoma of the breast. Diabetes mellitus is also a leading risk factor for vascular disease and this relationship compounds the importance of this disease. Both type I (insulin-dependent) and type II (noninsulin-dependent) diabetes mellitus are associated with an increased risk of accelerated atherosclerosis, including coronary artery disease, small artery disease, and stroke.[58] The frequency of both hypertension and hyperlipidemia is increased among diabetic persons. Hyperglycemia is associated with endothelial cell dysfunction, increased levels of fibrinogen, and increased platelet aggregation, which in turn promotes thrombosis.[58] Endothelial dysfunction may be due to oxidized LDLs, hyperglycemia, hyperinsulinemia, oxidative stress, or increased concentrations of free fatty acids.[58] Hyperglycemia also augments inflammation of the arterial wall and promotes the growth of atherosclerotic plaques. Diabetic neuropathy also can lead to autonomic disturbances and hypotension. Patients with diabetes mellitus have an increased risk of coronary artery disease and thus, indirectly, have an increased risk of cardioembolic stroke. Ho et al.[59] found that diabetic women without a history of vascular disease had a risk of fatal stroke similar to that of persons with a history of previous stroke. They concluded that diabetes was an especially important risk factor for stroke. In addition, persons with diabetes mellitus have an increased likelihood of death or severe disability following stroke.[60]

Insulin Resistance

Insulin resistance is strongly associated with the subsequent development of diabetes mellitus. In insulin resistance, skeletal muscle and fat have impaired uptake and utilization of glucose. In turn, the liver compensates by increasing glucose production.[61] Pancreatic beta cells increase insulin production, until at some point this compensation fails and glucose intolerance or diabetes mellitus develops. Some of the proatherosclerotic effects of diabetes mellitus are associated with insulin resistance.[62–64] Insulin resistance is associated with increased release of triglycerides and abnormal endothelial function.[61,65] It may also be associated with abnormalities in coagulation and inflammation that predispose to ischemic events.[62] Abnormalities in insulin resistance, which may be found in nondiabetic patients, are correlated with advanced atherosclerosis, coronary artery disease, and ischemic events[64,66–69] (Fig. 4-4). However, it should be mentioned that not all data show these relationships. For example, Adachi et al.[70] found no interaction between insulin resistance and stroke in a Japanese population.

Surprisingly, diabetic patients may have a lower incidence of hemorrhagic stroke than that of the general population, although data are conflicting. In particular, the frequency of aneurysmal subarachnoid hemorrhage is low among diabetic patients. The cause of any potential inverse relationship between diabetes mellitus and intracranial bleeding is unclear or unknown.

Epidemiology

Increases in the incidence and prevalence of diabetes mellitus are occurring around the world and dramatic rises are expected in developing countries during the next several decades. Similar increases are also occurring in the United States. Approximately 10,600,000 Americans (5,700,000 women) have physician-diagnosed diabetes mellitus.[15] Annually, nearly 800,000 new cases of type II diabetes mellitus are diagnosed. In addition, an estimated 5,600,000 Americans have undiagnosed diabetes mellitus, based on a fasting blood glucose concentration of greater than 125 mg/dL. Approximately 14 million Americans have impaired fasting blood glucose, defined as a value greater than 110 mg/dL. The prevalence of diabetes mellitus has increased from 4.9 to 6.5 percent during the last decade of

the twentieth century, likely as a reflection of the rapid increase in obesity. The increase in prevalence has occurred among men and women of all age groups, all ethnic groups, in urban regions, and all socioeconomic groups across the United States. The prevalence of diabetes is greatest in Mississippi and lowest in Alaska. In the United States, the prevalence of diabetes mellitus or impaired fasting blood glucose is greater among African Americans and Mexican Americans than among non-Hispanic whites[15] (Table 4-6). Diabetes mellitus is a particularly important risk factor for vascular disease among Mexican Americans.[71] Alarmingly, the frequency of type II diabetes mellitus is increasing rapidly among children and adolescents in the United States. This explosion in diabetes mellitus is attributed to obesity and physical inactivity.

Other situations also are associated with an increased risk of diabetes mellitus. Gestational hyperglycemia is a potential complication of pregnancy. In addition, elevated blood glucose levels can complicate the use of corticosteroids to treat autoimmune disease.

Metabolic Syndrome

The metabolic syndrome (syndrome X) is recognized as a risk factor for diabetes mellitus and atherosclerotic vascular disease.[71–74] The metabolic syndrome is diagnosed when a patient has at least three of the following characteristics: (1) waist circumference greater than 40 in. in men or greater than 35 in. in women, (2) a serum triglyceride level greater than or equal to 150 mg/dL, (3) high-density lipoprotein (HDL) cholesterol lesser than 40 mg/dL in men or lesser than 50 mg/dL in women, (4) blood pressure greater than or equal to 130/85 mm Hg, or (5) fasting blood glucose level greater than or equal to

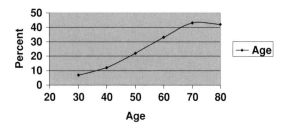

Figure 4-4. Estimated prevalence of insulin resistance among Americans as adjusted by age. (*Adapted from American Heart Association.*[15])

▶ **TABLE 4-6.** PREVALENCE OF DIABETES MELLITUS AND ABNORMAL FASTING BLOOD GLUCOSE VALUES AMONG ETHNIC GROUPS IN THE UNITED STATES

	Men (%)	Women (%)
Non-Hispanic whites		
Diagnosed diabetes mellitus	5.4	4.7
Undiagnosed diabetes mellitus	3.0	2.1
Abnormal fasting glucose	9.4	4.8
African Americans		
Diagnosed diabetes mellitus	7.6	9.5
Undiagnosed diabetes mellitus	2.8	4.7
Abnormal fasting glucose	8.0	6.8
Mexican Americans		
Diagnosed diabetes mellitus	8.1	11.4
Undiagnosed diabetes mellitus	5.8	3.9
Abnormal fasting glucose	12.1	6.7

Adapted from American Heart Association.[15]

▶ **TABLE 4-7.** COMPONENTS OF SYNDROME X (METABOLIC SYNDROME)

Truncal obesity
  Waist circumference >40 in.—men
  Waist circumference >35 in.—women
Hypertension
  Blood pressure >130/85
Glucose intolerance—insulin resistance
  Fasting blood glucose >110 mg/dL
Hyperlipidemia
  Triglycerides >150 mg/dL
  HDL cholesterol <40 mg/dL—men
  HDL cholesterol <50 mg/dL—women

▶ **TABLE 4-8.** MEASURES TO TREAT HYPERGLYCEMIA AND INSULIN RESISTANCE

Lifestyle changes
  Diet
  Weight reduction
  Increase exercise
Medications
  Insulin
  Oral agents

110 mg/dL.[75] There also appears to be a relationship with elevations of apolipoprotein B (100) (Table 4-7).[76] It is also strongly associated with the development of cardiovascular disease.[73] Elevated plasma triglycerides, a high ratio of triglycerides to HDL cholesterol, and high insulin concentrations can predict which obese patients are at highest risk for insulin resistance.[77] While most of the focus has been directed at premature coronary artery disease, a comparable risk for accelerated cerebrovascular atherosclerosis likely exists.

By these criteria, nearly 47 million Americans (23.7 percent of the population) likely have metabolic syndrome[15] (Fig. 4-5). The prevalence appears highest among Mexican Americans.[72] An increase in weight also predicts development of the metabolic syndrome.[78] At present, management focuses on weight loss through diet and exercise. Future public health efforts will need to focus on patients with metabolic syndrome. Saydah et al.[79] emphasized that control of risk factors for vascular disease, including weight, arterial blood pressure, and hypercholesterolemia, is generally poor among diabetic patients. In recent years, the Atkins diet has become a popular way to reduce weight, although it does involve consumption of large amounts of meat and saturated fat. Surprisingly, however, it may reduce LDL cholesterol and triglycerides as well as leading to weight

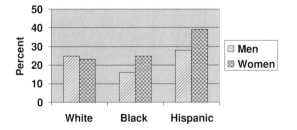

Figure 4-5. Estimated prevalence of metabolic syndrome among different adult ethnic groups in the United States. Rates in men are shown in hatched bars and women in clear bars. (*Adapted from American Heart Association.*[15])

loss. Therefore, it may be especially important for diabetic patients. Vigorously performed trials are needed to properly evaluate the efficacy and safety of this diet.

Treatment

The utility of vigorous control of hyperglycemia in preventing stroke is not evident[56] (Table 4-8). However, effective management of diabetes likely improves the overall health of the patient and indirectly lessens the likelihood of stroke. In some patients, diabetes mellitus will be controlled with changes in diet and lifestyle. In others, oral agents or insulin are often required to lower the blood glucose levels to normoglycemic values. In addition to lowering levels of blood glucose, medications that lower insulin resistance may lessen the risk of ischemic stroke by lowering blood pressure and increasing the level of HDL cholesterol.[9,62] The thiazolidinediones in particular may be useful in reducing insulin resistance as well as preventing stroke and other cardiovascular events.[61,63,80] These medications increase the levels of glucose transporters 1 and 4, lower the levels of free fatty acids, enhance insulin signals, reduce the level of tumor necrosis factor alpha (TNF α), and remodel adipose tissue.[81] These actions increase uptake and utilization of glucose in peripheral organs and decrease hepatic gluconeogenesis, thereby lessening insulin resistance.[81] Kernan et al.[82] found that pioglitazone increased insulin sensitivity and reduced concentrations of C-reactive protein (CRP) among patients with a recent TIA or stroke. While these results are promising, the utility of these medications is not yet established. In addition, some data suggest that their use may be associated with an increased risk of congestive heart failure and ventricular dysfunction. Clearly, more research is needed to evaluate the safety and efficacy of this class of oral agents.

▶ HYPERCHOLESTEROLEMIA

A mature atherosclerotic plaque consists of a large lipid core covered by a thin intraluminal cap. Passage of LDL cholesterol through the surface of the plaque accelerates growth of the lipid core. The presence of HDL cholesterol reduces the oxidation of LDL cholesterol and limits intramural lipid deposition. Decreasing serum concentrations of total and LDL cholesterol reduces intraplaque concentrations of lipids. Because of the pivotal role of cholesterol in atherosclerosis, elevations of the total cholesterol are associated with an increased risk of ischemic stroke. Unstable plaques are the likely substrate for acute occlusions secondary to atherosclerosis. Prevention of plaque rupture is becoming a leading component of medical management.[6]

In the past, the impact of hypercholesterolemia on increasing the risk of stroke was not clear. Some of this uncertainty was secondary to the advanced age of many persons with stroke, a potential inverse association of elevated blood cholesterol levels and hemorrhagic stroke, and the large number of nonatherosclerotic causes of ischemic stroke. However, the association of ischemic stroke secondary to atherosclerosis with hypercholesterolemia has been demonstrated, particularly among persons younger than 65. The prevalence of coronary artery disease and atherosclerosis of major intracranial or extracranial arteries increases with rising levels of serum cholesterol. An increased risk of atherosclerosis is directly associated with increases in levels of total cholesterol, LDL cholesterol, and triglycerides. Conversely, increased levels of HDL cholesterol are associated with a lower risk of ischemic disease. Thus, the risk of stroke is lowest among persons with the highest levels of HDL cholesterol. The risk of stroke is estimated to increase by a factor of 1.8 for persons with a total cholesterol of 240–279 mg/dL (mmol/L) and by 2.6 when the value is greater than 280 mg/dL (mmol/L). The desired levels of total, LDL, and HDL cholesterol are less than 200 mg/dL (<5.20 mmol/L), less than 130 mg/dL (<3.36 mmol/L), and greater than 35 mg/dL (0.9 mmol/L), respectively.

Epidemiology

More than 104 million Americans are estimated to have a total cholesterol level higher than 200 mg/dL.[15] More than 41 million Americans have a total cholesterol level greater than 240 mg/dL. Hypercholesterolemia is found in men and women of all ethnic groups but rates are higher in women than in men[15] (Table 4-9; Fig. 4-6). While elevated cholesterol is diagnosed primarily in adults, approximately 10 percent of teenage Americans have total cholesterol values greater than 200 mg/dL (>5.20 mmol/L). Identification of hypercholesterolemia and measures to lower the levels of cholesterol should begin early in life. The goal of modern management is to reduce both total and LDL cholesterol and increase HDL cholesterol levels.[9] Among patients with ischemic cerebrovascular disease, the aim is to lower LDL cholesterol

▶ **TABLE 4-9.** PREVALENCE OF HYPERCHOLESTEROLEMIA IN ETHNIC GROUPS IN THE UNITED STATES

	Men (%)	Women (%)
Non-Hispanic whites aged 20–74		
Total level >200 mg/dL	52	49
Total level >240 mg/dL	18	20
LDL level >130 mg/dL	49.6	43.7
LDL level >130 mg/dL	20.4	16
HDL level <40 mg/dL	40.5	14.5
African Americans aged 20–74		
Total level >200 mg/dL	45	46
Total level >240 mg/dL	15	18
LDL level >130 mg/dL	46.3	41.6
LDL level >160 mg/dL	19.3	18.8
HDL level <40 mg/dL	24.3	13
Mexican Americans aged 20–74		
Total level >200 mg/dL	53	48
Total level >240 mg/dL	18	17
LDL level >130 mg/dL	43.6	41.6
LDL level >160 mg/dL	16.9	14
HDL level <40 mg/dL	40.1	18.4

Adapted from American Heart Association.[15]

to approximately 100 mg–130 mg/dL and to increase HDL cholesterol concentrations to greater than 50 mg/dL.[83] The goal is to reduce LDL cholesterol to below 100 mg/dL for patients with coronary artery disease, peripheral vascular disease, abdominal aortic aneurysm, diabetes mellitus, or ischemic stroke.[84] Hypercholesterolemia is an important risk factor for death, including vascular death, among persons having chronic hemodialysis.[85]

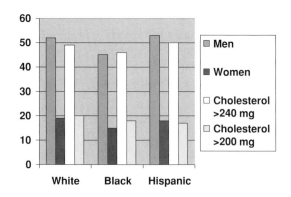

Figure 4-6. Estimated prevalence of hypercholesterolism among different adult ethnic groups in the United States. Rates with a level of total cholesterol greater than 200 mg/dL are shown for men (hatched bar) and women (clear bar). Rates with a level of total cholesterol greater than 240 mg/dL are shown for men (stropped bar) and women (light bar). (*Adapted from American Heart Association.[15]*)

Treatment

Treatment of hypercholesterolemia starts with dietary and lifestyle changes, including increased exercise. Unfortunately, less than 50 percent of eligible patients with hypercholesterolemia are being treated and most are not receiving any lipid-lowering medications.[15] A diet high in vegetables, fruits, whole grains, fiber, and low-fat dairy products is recommended.[86] The major sources of saturated fat in the American diet are red meat, whole milk, butter, and eggs and the consumption of these foods should be limited. In addition, the preparation of food is especially important. Patients should avoid foods that are fried, especially deep fried foods. Consumption of foods such as pizza, Chinese food, French fries, and hamburgers should be limited because these "fast foods" are very high in calories and fat. Regular aerobic exercise can reduce LDL and increase HDL levels. While the exercise must be commensurate with the patient's health, virtually all persons can engage in some physical activity. Vigorous activity is not necessary. For example, patients with painful neuromuscular conditions can have exercise by walking or swimming in a warm pool.

If exercise and diet are not successful, a number of cholesterol-lowering medications are available (Table 4-10). Several of the older medications are no longer prescribed widely. Several reasons may account for their nonuse, including inconvenience of administration, prevalence of side effects, and relatively poor efficacy. Since their introduction, the HMG Co-A reductase inhibitors (statins) have become the primary treatment of hypercholesterolemia.[6,9] These medications can achieve a 20–40 percent reduction in total cholesterol. Secondary increases in HDL cholesterol are somewhat less impressive. In addition, several trials demonstrate their efficacy in lowering the risk of ischemic events, including stroke, among high-risk patients.[87–91] In a randomized trial that enrolled approximately 20,500 patients with coronary artery disease, the Heart Protection Study Group[92] found that the simvastatin reduced the risk of fatal or nonfatal

▶ **TABLE 4-10.** CHOLESTEROL-LOWERING INTERVENTIONS

Lifestyle
  Diet
    Lowered saturated fat and cholesterol
      Daily cholesterol intake <300 mg
      Daily fat <30% of calories
      Saturated fat <10% of calories
    Increased dietary fiber
      Daily dietary fiber intake >25 g
  Weight loss
  Increase exercise
Medications
  Statins
  Ezetimibe
  Niacin

stroke from 5.7 to 4.3 percent (nearly a 25 percent relative risk reduction). These medications may be prescribed to patients with only modest increases in total cholesterol. For example, Sever et al.[93] recently reported that atorvastatin could dramatically prevent both myocardial infarction and stroke among patients with hypertension and average or below average levels of total cholesterol.[24] These medications were also used to reduce vascular events among persons with diabetes mellitus or who had a renal transplantation.[94,95] Comparable responses are found among persons of all age groups.[90] Aggressive lowering of serum cholesterol concentrations is associated with more success in slowing down the progression of atherosclerosis than that of less-intensive treatment regimens.[96] Overall, treatment of hypercholesterolemia conveys a 20–30 percent reduction similar to that achieved with the use of antiplatelet aggregating agents.

The effects of lowering the risk of ischemic events are greater than those expected by simply lowering cholesterol concentrations, implying additional mechanisms for the utility of the statins (Table 4-11). For one, the statins improve endothelial function and reduce platelet

▶ **TABLE 4-11.** PREVENTION OF STROKE CLINICAL TRIALS OF HMG CO-A REDUCTASE INHIBITORS

Trial	Medication	Treatment (Strokes/Patients)	Control (Strokes/Patients)
WOSCOPS	Pravastatin	46/3302	51/3292
SSSS	Simvastatin	75/2221	102/2223
CARE	Pravastatin	54/2081	78/2078
LIPID	Pravastatin	171/4512	198/4502
ACAPS	Lovastatin	0/460	2/459
KAPS	Pravastatin	2/224	4/223

WOSCOPS = West of Scotland Coronary Prevention Study, SSSS = Scandinavian Simvastatin Survival Study, CARE = Cholesterol and recurrent events, LIPID = Long-term intervention with pravastatin in ischemic disease, ACAPS = Asymptomatic Carotid Artery Progression Study, KAPS = Kuopio Atherosclerosis Prevention Study.

activity.[65] They reduce smooth muscle cell proliferation in the artery, limit inflammation, and reduce cytokine levels—effects that appear to stabilize the atherosclerotic plaque and improve vasomotor control.[97–102] In addition, there is now evidence that these medications may cause regression of atherosclerotic lesions. Smilde et al.[103] found that aggressive lowering of LDL-cholesterol levels with atorvastatin led to regression of carotid artery intima-media thickness in patients with hypercholesterolemia. It appears that the statins may also have neuroprotective properties[104] and positive effects in lessening injury in the ischemic penumbra.

Some obstacles that prevent the widespread use of the statins remain. While they have demonstrated efficacy in lowering cholesterol and reducing ischemic events, their use can be complicated by myopathy or hepatic dysfunction.[105,106] Patients should be monitored for these symptoms and laboratory tests may be performed to screen for toxicity. These medications are relatively expensive, although they are easy to use. Efforts to maintain compliance with the treatment regimen are important because many patients will halt their use of these very important medications.[107] The use of these medications likely will grow in the future. Statins should be prescribed to most patients with ischemic stroke, especially if they have heart disease or elevated serum cholesterol levels.[5]

Combinations of the different classes of cholesterol-lowering medications also may be used with a reasonable degree of efficacy and safety.[108] Ezetimibe, a medication that limits absorption of cholesterol at the brush border of the small intestine, was introduced for treatment of persons with hypercholesterolemia.[108–110] This medication may augment the effects of the statins or be used as a monotherapy for lowering cholesterol if a patient cannot tolerate the statin medications. Gagne et al.[111] reported that the combination of ezetimibe and a statin was tolerated well and that its addition resulted in a substantial additional decline in LDL cholesterol. Niacin has been used to treat hyperlipidemia. It does increase HDL-cholesterol levels and reduces both LDL cholesterol and triglycerides.[112] Niacin can cause flushing and other bothersome symptoms. In addition, niacin may affect glucose concentrations and insulin sensitivity, which also could limit its utility.[112] Recently, Nissen et al.[113] found that recombinant ApoA-Milano/phospholipid complex can lead to regression of atherosclerotic plaques in the coronary arteries. While this observation is exciting, additional research is needed to establish the role of this intervention in the treatment of patients with hypercholesterolemia.

An increase in the chances of hemorrhagic stroke has been associated with very low serum total cholesterol concentrations.[114,115] A diet low in saturated fats and high in fish-based proteins also is correlated with an increased risk of intracranial bleeding. However, the relationship between hypocholesterolemia and hemorrhagic stroke is murky. For example, the use of statins seems not to increase the risk of hemorrhage.[116] The relationship between low levels of cholesterol and brain hemorrhage might be a marker for another process, such as excessive alcohol use rather than a direct cause of intracranial bleeding. Additional information is needed about the potential interactions of low cholesterol levels and intracranial hemorrhage.

Lipoprotein (a)

Elevated concentrations of lipoprotein (a) appear to be associated with a two to three times relative increase in the risk of stroke. This highly thrombogenic and atherogenic protein is structurally similar to LDL cholesterol that interacts with the plasminogen receptor. Ethnic minorities in the United States appear to have higher blood levels of lipoprotein (a) than do whites. Additional research is needed on the role of lipoprotein (a) in accelerating the course of atherosclerosis and in predisposing to ischemic stroke. At present, the current strategy is to treat patients with elevated levels of lipoprotein (a) in a manner that is similar to that recommended for patients with elevated LDL-cholesterol concentrations.

▶ OBESITY AND OTHER DIETARY FACTORS

The prevalence of obesity is increasing dramatically in North America, largely as the result of increased daily calorie consumption and a decline in physical activity. Approximately 130 million Americans are either overweight or obese.[15] The rates of obesity are similar in all ethnic groups. In the United States, the prevalence of obesity and diabetes mellitus is highest among persons living in the southeastern states. Approximately 4 million American children, aged 6–11, and 5 million American teenagers are overweight.[15] These numbers have been increasing rapidly. The increase in the prevalence of obesity among children and teenagers is of particular concern.[117] Weiss et al.[118] found that obese children and adolescents with intra-abdominal fat and intracellular lipid accumulation in muscle cells predict the development of severe peripheral insulin resistance. McLaughlin et al.[77] identified genetic markers that appear to predict which obese patients will develop insulin resistance and possibly diabetes. Obesity increases the risk of arterial hypertension, type II diabetes mellitus, hypercholesterolemia, and ischemic heart disease.[117] Overall, obesity is associated with an increase in the relative risk of stroke by a factor of 1.5–2. Obesity is one of the key components of the metabolic syndrome (syndrome X), an important forecaster of insulin resistance and vascular disease; it is a syndrome predicted by rapid weight gain.[74,78] Elevated plasma concentrations of leptin, important components of the body's weight mechanism, are associated with an increased risk of hemorrhagic stroke. Weight reduction is an important component of any strategy to reduce the risk of vascular disease, including stroke.[5] However, weight loss is difficult to achieve and sustain, and many patients show little progress with these efforts.

The risk of vascular disease, including stroke, is reduced among persons with diets high in fiber, potassium, vitamin C, fruits, and vegetables. It has been[86,119] found that high dietary intake of vitamin C and, in smokers, vitamin E reduces the risk of stroke. Daily intake of five or more servings of fruits and vegetables reduces the risk of stroke by nearly 30 percent as compared to those persons who eat little of these foods. In general, the risk of stroke is reduced by approximately 6 percent per each serving of fruits or vegetables. Sauvaget et al.[120] reported that high consumption of green or yellow vegetables and fruits is associated with a reduced risk of both hemorrhagic and ischemic stroke. In a Danish study, Johnsen et al.[121] found that increased intake of fruits reduced the risk of ischemic stroke. It is unclear if these foods directly reduce stroke risk or if they replace other components of the diet that would increase the likelihood of vascular disease. Similarly, patients who eat fruits and vegetables may have other lifestyles, including physical activity and abstinence from tobacco, which lower the risk of stroke. On the other hand, Steffen et al.[122] found that increased consumption of whole grains, fruits, and vegetables was associated with a reduction in heart disease but not stroke. He et al.[123] recently reported that regular consumption of small amounts of fish (1–3 servings per month) lowers the risk of stroke. Surprisingly, among obese persons, consumption of dairy products may reduce the risk of insulin resistance and vascular disease.[124] Although in other studies high dietary consumption of fats is associated with an increased risk of obesity and other factors, including hypertension, diabetes, hypercholesterolemia, and heart disease.[125] Supplemental administration of vitamin E has not reduced mortality, cardiovascular events, or stroke.[126] A British trial that tested vitamin E, vitamin C, and beta-carotene did not demonstrate a reduction in the frequency of vascular events with the use of these antioxidant vitamins.[127] A low serum concentration of magnesium is associated with stroke among patients with advanced atherosclerosis, and supplementation of the mineral to reduce stroke risk has been proposed.[128]

▶ PHYSICAL INACTIVITY

The lack of physical exercise is a well-known risk factor for coronary artery disease and it is associated with obesity,

diabetes mellitus, and hypertension. Overall, physical inactivity increases the risk of heart disease or stroke by a ratio of 2.7 among both men and women.[15] It is also correlated with low serum levels of HDL cholesterol. Increased physical exercise lowers insulin resistance and platelet aggregation. Approximately 30 percent of adult Americans exercise regularly with the highest rates reported among young people, non-Hispanic whites, men, higher socioeconomic groups, and in the West part of the United States. However, large segments of the population, including teenagers, report no regular physical activity during their leisure time. In addition, many secondary school students are not participating in physical exercise or education programs at school. Experimental models demonstrate that increased physical activity can lower stroke risk by reducing brain injury during an ischemic event and by increasing blood flow, presumably by increasing endothelial nitric oxide synthase activity.[129] Conversely, a lack of physical exercise is associated with an increased use of tobacco and increased frequency of obesity.[15]

Gillum et al.[130] found a strong relationship between a low level of exercise and a high risk for stroke. The reduction in stroke risk with exercise may be greater than the reduction in the risk for heart disease. Lee et al.[131] recently reported that moderate or greater exercise reduces the risk of both ischemic and hemorrhagic stroke, with a goal of approximately 30 min of moderate-intensity exercise five to six times weekly. However, many patients with neuromuscular impairments might not be able to perform some of these activities. In addition, older patients cannot perform vigorous exercise. Still, moderate exercise is helpful and should be recommended to most patients with cerebrovascular disease.[5] A study that enrolled healthy female nurses demonstrated that moderate activity, such as walking, is associated with a decline in the risk of stroke.

It should be noted that both hemorrhagic and ischemic stroke have been attributed to vigorous physical activity. Arterial dissection leading to ischemic stroke has been described as a complication of a number of sports including biking and skiing. In general, these vascular events occur during falls or if the individual hyper-rotates or extends the neck, leading to traction of the artery against a bony prominence. While arterial dissection is an important cause of stroke in young adults, the potential for this complication should not be a reason to avoid physical exercise. Hemorrhagic stroke also has been described as a complication of vigorous exercise. In particular, rupture of a saccular aneurysm is described in association with athletic activity, manual labor, heavy lifting, and coitus.[132–134] Still, the risk of intracranial hemorrhage is relatively low and the potential for bleeding should not be a reason to avoid physical exercise.

► HYPERHOMOCYSTEINEMIA

Homocysteine is an amino acid metabolite of methionine metabolism that is methylated in the presence of folate, pyridoxine, and vitamin B-12. High concentrations of homocysteine appear to potentiate the atherogenic effects of risk factors, such as smoking and hypertension. In addition, the amino acid can injure the endothelium and alter coagulability.[135] Epidemiological studies suggest that high concentrations of homocysteine are associated with an increased risk of stroke.[125,136] An elevated plasma homocysteine level is an independent predictor of coronary artery disease among persons with type II diabetes mellitus.[137] Slightly elevated levels of homocysteine are associated with an increased risk of atherosclerotic stroke.[12] Some of the interactions between homocysteine and atherosclerosis may be related to other factors, including diet.[138] Kelly et al.[139] recently proposed that low levels of pyridoxine and inflammation might partially explain some of the relationships between hyperhomocysteinemia and vascular events. Still, there is uncertainty about the importance of elevated homocysteine concentrations and premature atherosclerosis.[138]

Epidemiology

Approximately 5–10 percent of the population has an elevated plasma level of homocysteine. Concentrations of the amino acid increase with advancing age, renal disease, diabetes mellitus, hypothyroidism, smoking, and malignancy. Levels are higher in men than in women. The risk of stroke is increased among persons with a homocysteine level greater than 15.4 μmol/L. The effects of homocysteine appear to be most pronounced among young adults and, in this population, elevations of the amino acid are recognized as an independent predictor of stroke. Screening for homocysteine levels should probably be restricted to those patients who are young or who have relatives who have had vascular events at a young age (<50 years old).

Treatment

The process of macromolecule hypomethylation mediates the toxic effects of homocysteine.[140] Supplementation of the diet with folic acid (1–2 mg/day), pyridoxine (10–50 mg/day), and vitamin B-12 (500 μg/day) reduces the level of homocysteine. In particular, folic acid appears to be effective.[6] Consumption of folate, either in the diet or as a supplement, appears to reduce the risk of ischemic stroke in men.[141] In the mid-1990s, the U.S. Food and Drug Administration approved the addition of folate to grain products in an effort to reduce the frequency of congenital spinal deformities. As a result, homocysteine levels in the population have dropped. However, a correlation between this homocysteine level

and a reduction in ischemic cerebrovascular events has yet to be demonstrated. Ongoing clinical trials are testing the utility of vitamin supplements in reducing the risk of stroke among high-risk persons.[142] Large carefully designed clinical trials tested the utility of the administration of high doses of folic acid, pyridoxine, and vitamin B-12 when given to patients with recent cerebral infarction.[143,144] Modest reductions in the level of homocysteine with this regimen had no effect on vascular outcomes within 2 years. Therefore, it is unclear if additional vitamin supplementation will provide any added benefit in reducing the risk of stroke.

► SMOKING/TOBACCO USE

Smoking is a leading cause of death around the world.[145] Approximately 400,000 Americans die annually from smoking-related diseases.[15] Educational campaigns by governments and public health groups throughout the world emphasize the importance of not smoking and quitting. Despite these educational programs and a number of governmental restrictions on smoking, the use of tobacco remains widespread. In some parts of the world, the prevalence of tobacco use is increasing dramatically.

Epidemiology

Death from any cause is approximately twice as high among young adults who smoke than that among nonsmokers.[146] Tobacco use is a powerful factor for the development of accelerated atherosclerosis, coronary artery disease, and stroke.[125] Smoking is implicated in approximately one-half of the cases of stroke. The effects of smoking on increasing the chance of stroke are greatest among young adults. This risk is dose dependent; the longer and greater the use of cigarettes, the greater the likelihood of stroke. Although cigarette smoking is most commonly incriminated, those who smoke cigars and pipes or chew tobacco also have an increased risk of vascular disease. Additionally, passive exposure to smoke entails some added stroke risk. The relative increase in risk (1.8) is nearly the same for passive smoke exposure as for active smokers. Otsuka et al.[147] found that passive exposure to cigarette smoke acutely impairs coronary flow velocity reserve in healthy nonsmokers, presumably on the basis of endothelial dysfunction. You et al.[148] found that the spouses of smokers had twice the risk of stroke compared to spouses of nonsmokers. While smoking is an important risk factor for ischemic stroke, the use of tobacco also greatly increases the risk of hemorrhagic stroke among men and women.[149] Kurth et al.[150] reported that the risk of subarachnoid hemorrhage and other types of intracranial bleeding in women was directly related to tobacco use and the amount of smoking.[151,152] Passive and active smoking is associated with an increased risk of bleeding.[152] Subarachnoid hemorrhage occurs at younger ages among persons who smoke than among nonsmokers.[151] The combination of smoking and hypertension appears particularly ominous; the relative risk of subarachnoid hemorrhage increases by approximately 15 in hypertensive smokers.[151] A history of recent smoking increases the likelihood of symptomatic vasospasm after subarachnoid hemorrhage.

Nearly all young adults with ischemic stroke secondary to large artery atherosclerosis are smokers. Smoking also has numerous negative cellular effects, including inducing structural changes in the arterial wall, increasing immune responses, and decreasing endothelial function, which lead to accelerated atherosclerosis.[147] In addition, smoking affects platelet aggregation, increases serum fibrinogen concentrations, increases LDL cholesterol, and decreases HDL cholesterol in the blood. Smoking induces progression of atherosclerotic lesions of the carotid artery, coronary arteries, and the aorta. The development of the moyamoya syndrome in young women also has been associated with the combination of oral contraceptive use and smoking. Smoking may compound the prothrombotic effects or oral contraceptives, thereby increasing stroke risk among young women even in the absence of moyamoya syndrome.

Buerger Disease

Buerger disease (thromboangiitis obliterans), which is marked by ischemia and necrosis of the digits and is strongly associated with tobacco abuse, is a rarely diagnosed cause of stroke.

Epidemiological Aspects of Smoking

In the United States, the overall prevalence of smoking declined by approximately 40 percent among persons older than 18 during the last one-third of the twentieth century. Unfortunately, that decline has stopped (Fig. 4-7). While number of adults that smoke continues to fall, more young people are smoking than in the past. This trend portends future increases in tobacco use despite current efforts with the antismoking campaigns aimed at children and adolescents. Presently, approximately 48 million Americans smoke regularly.[15] Additionally, approximately 5 million Americans use chewing tobacco. Throughout the world, tobacco use is on the rise, particularly in Asian and developing countries. The constraints on tobacco advertisements, high taxes on the product, and educational campaigns are less successful than hoped. The efforts to avoid smoking must be aimed at teenagers because approximately 80 percent of those who use tobacco begin prior to the age of 18, with the most common ages being between 14 and 15.

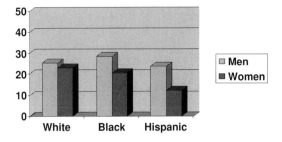

Figure 4-7. Estimated prevalence of active smoking among different adult ethnic groups in the United States. Rates in men are shown in hatched bars and women in clear bars.

Nearly 38 percent of male teenagers and 29 percent of female teenagers in the United States currently smoke, a habit that is most common among young white men from lower socioeconomic families.[15] Regardless of age or sex, smoking is much more common among white Americans than among either African Americans or Mexican Americans. However, as many as 40 percent of Native Americans smoke and, overall, the highest rates of smoking are among persons who live below the poverty level.[15] The use of chewing tobacco is greatest in rural areas and the southern states.

Management

Smoking cessation is very cost effective, the expense of the product is avoided, and the likelihood of medical complications is less.[5,9,10,56,125] The effects of stopping smoking on a patient's health are dramatic. Within 2–5 years of halting the use of tobacco, a person's risk of stroke returns to that found among nonsmokers. Young persons should be encouraged to never start smoking or to stop before becoming addicted. Thus, educational programs aimed at teenagers and young adults remain crucial. A smoke-free environment in public places, such as restaurants, hotels, airports, public transportation, and the workplace, should be encouraged. Still, physicians must recognize the difficulty in quitting. Approximately 80 percent of smokers wish to quit and many have attempted stopping at least once but most resume their habit. The average number of attempts to stop smoking is 4 or 5. Those who are least likely to quit are men, patients with no disability, blue-collar workers, and persons living alone.[153] Obese patients and those with high dependence on nicotine may not achieve smoking cessation even with the use of nasal spray or transdermal nicotine replacement therapy.[154]

Most patients will not be successful without assistance. Pharmacological support and counseling increase the likelihood of success.[153] The use of bupropion and nicotine replacement medications is safe and effective. These medications should be prescribed to patients who have had a stroke and wish to stop smoking.

▶ ALCOHOL ABUSE

The relationship between alcohol use and stroke is complicated. Mild-to-moderate consumption of alcohol appears to lower the risk of myocardial infarction and ischemic stroke, presumably because of alcohol's effects on increasing HDL cholesterol and slowing down the progression of atherosclerosis.[125,155] These beneficial effects are particularly prominent among middle-aged adults.[156] Mild-to-moderate consumption is defined as weekly consumption of less than 100 g of alcohol. A modest decline in the risk of ischemic stroke occurs with drinking one alcoholic beverage per week. This benefit appears to be present among men and women of all ages and ethnic groups, although the benefit seems greatest among persons aged 60–69.[156] The reduction in risk of ischemic vascular events appears to be greater among persons consuming wine than either beer or distilled liquors.[156] Still, drinking a glass of wine daily should not be considered an antidote to eating an unhealthy, high-fat diet. Conversely, Ding et al.[157] recently reported that low-to-moderate alcohol intake was not associated with a reduction in the risk of cerebral infarction. Thus, additional research on the presumed protective effects of alcohol clearly is needed. Alcoholic beverages also are high in calories, which could increase the likelihood of obesity and play a negative role in controlling weight. Goude et al.[158] found that alcohol consumption increases insulin-mediated glucose uptake.

On the other hand, alcohol abuse increases the risk of ischemic stroke.[155] Djousse et al.[156] found that daily consumption of greater than 12 g of alcohol per day increases the risk of stroke by a factor of 2.4 among men. Changes in viscosity as well as fibrinolytic and coagulation factors may promote arterial thrombosis. In addition, alcohol may increase blood pressure, triglyceride levels, and serum glucose concentrations, and may increase the incidence of cardiac arrhythmias. These acute effects, which may in part be ascribed to the diuretic effects of the alcohol, may also explain some of the cases of ischemic stroke in young adults that are seen on weekends and holidays. Thus, binges of alcohol consumption may be as dangerous as chronic abuse. In addition, chronic alcohol abuse may cause a dilated cardiomyopathy, a possible source of cardioembolic events. In addition to the factors described above, abuse of alcohol is often associated with other behavior, including tobacco or drug use that are themselves associated with an increased risk of stroke. In both men and women, a strong correlation also exists between the level of alcohol consumption and the hemorrhagic stroke.[114,159,160] While there appears to be little interaction with modest alcohol consumption and brain hemorrhage, the association between bleeding and alcohol abuse is stronger.[161–163] The relationship is strongest

among persons who are using large amounts of alcohol. A pattern of an increased frequency of subarachnoid hemorrhage on the weekends is ascribed to heavy consumption of alcohol. Finally, heavy alcohol consumption is associated with an increased likelihood of brain atrophy found by imaging studies.[157]

The potential benefits of alcohol on lowering the risk of ischemic vascular disease, including stroke, are not so convincing that physicians should advise nonusers to consume alcoholic beverages.[9,10] Alcohol should not be considered a medication to prevent atherosclerosis or stroke. There are potential adverse health effects from even modest alcohol consumption, which must be considered before any advice about consumption is provided. In fact, current evidence supports the contention that heavy alcohol use (either chronic alcohol abuse or bouts of heavy consumption) does increase the chances of either hemorrhagic or ischemic stroke. Persons who are abusing alcohol should be encouraged to stop.[56] Alcoholism is an illness difficult to treat, and both the physician and the patient need to avail themselves of educational services, support groups, and medications in order to achieve the necessary changes in behavior. More details about alcohol abuse as a cause of stroke in young persons are found in Chapter 17.

▶ DRUG ABUSE

Abuse of drugs, particularly stimulants, causes both hemorrhagic or ischemic stroke.[164,165] The potential relationship between drug abuse and stroke is most overt among young adults and appears stronger for intracranial bleeding than for thromboembolism (see Chapter 17). Cocaine, amphetamines, and other vasoactive agents of abuse may cause abrupt and marked increases in blood pressure and vasoconstriction. The hypertensive surge following drug use may cause rupture of an aneurysm or vascular malformation. Cocaine and amphetamines have also been implicated as a putative cause of vasospasm, which leads to ischemic stroke. Intravenous injection of drugs, such as cocaine or heroin, can also be complicated by infective endocarditis, which in turn leads to septic embolic events of the brain.

▶ USE OF ORAL CONTRACEPTIVES OR POSTMENOPAUSAL USE OF ESTROGENS

The interactions between the use of estrogen and progesterone compounds, and the risk of vascular disease are exceedingly complex. There is evidence that women have a slower evolution of atherosclerotic disease than that of men. Estrogen and other female hormones may affect cholesterol metabolism or other factors that alter the course of atherogenesis.

Oral Contraceptives

Following the introduction of oral contraceptives approximately 40 years ago, a series of reports described a potential interaction between their use and an increased risk of stroke. The mechanisms for this increase are not described, but assumptions included changes in coagulation factors or blood viscosity. The association with oral contraceptive use is strongest for subarachnoid hemorrhage, but the reasons for the increased risk for bleeding are not known.[166] The risk of aneurysmal rupture appears to be associated with the dosage of oral contraceptives and it appears to be relatively small if low doses of estrogen are used.[166,167] Women older than 35 years and those with other risk factors for stroke, including hypertension or smoking, appear to be at the highest risk for cerebrovascular events. In general, this group of women should be encouraged to use alternative forms of birth control. While a small number of strokes in young women may be ascribed to the use of oral contraceptives, other causes of ischemic or hemorrhagic stroke should be sought. Most women who have stroke while taking oral contraceptives ultimately will have another etiology found. Rather than the primary cause of stroke, oral contraceptives should be viewed as a contributing factor. The potential role of oral contraceptive use as a cause of stroke in young women is described in more detail in Chapter 17.

Postmenopausal Use of Estrogens

The most recent evidence suggests that prolonged postmenopausal use of the combination of estrogen and progesterone is associated with a small but real increase in the risk of vascular events.[168,169] Although the actual numbers of events were quite small (212 events among 16,608 women), the Women's Health Initiative reported that combination hormone replacement therapy increased the relative risk of stroke by approximately 40 percent. The increased risk of ischemic stroke was present in all subgroups of postmenopausal women.[169,170] A subsequent report found that postmenopausal estrogen monotherapy was associated with a small but statistically significant increase in risk of stroke. Another study also was unable to demonstrate a benefit from estrogen replacement therapy for preventing vascular events following ischemic stroke.[171] Thus it appears that postmenopausal hormone replacement is not protective and that these medications should not be prescribed in an effort to lower stroke risk. Shearman et al.[172] speculated that estrogen receptor variation may explain some of the conflicting data about the interactions between supplemental estrogen use and the susceptibility to vascular events.

▶ MIGRAINE

Migraine affects approximately 20 percent of American women and 10 percent of American men. Due to its widespread prevalence and because focal neurological symptoms often occur with migraine, a potential cause-and-effect relationship between migraine and stroke has been implicated. In addition, many patients with stroke, particularly those with intracranial hemorrhage, have severe headache that may mimic the symptoms of migraine. Undoubtedly, some cases of migrainous stroke do occur. The usual scenario is a case of recurrent migraine with focal neurological symptoms but with one attack that results in persistent impairments following a usual event. In addition, some cases of migraine may be symptomatic of an underlying cerebrovascular disease, such as an arteriovenous malformation that will subsequently cause hemorrhagic stroke. However, the potential risk of stroke among persons with migraine appears to be relatively low. More details about the relationships between migraine and stroke are described in Chapter 17.

▶ SLEEP DISORDERS AND PULMONARY DISEASE

A potential relationship exists between excessive snoring or sleep apnea and stroke.[172] In general, the risk of stroke is correlated with the severity of snoring. The relationship between sleep apnea and stroke is complicated by the presence of other risk factors. Many affected individuals are also obese or have other serious illnesses, including hypertension or diabetes mellitus, which are themselves major risk factors for stroke. While disorders of sleep appear to be an important marker of a high-risk population, evidence that treatment of sleep apnea will lessen the risk of stroke is not yet available. In addition, sleep disorders are relatively common, following stroke, and may be the result of partial airway obstruction from bulbar dysfunction or due to disturbances in central mechanisms of sleep regulation. Persons with impaired pulmonary function (emphysema and chronic obstructive lung disease) have a modestly increased risk of stroke. However, this relationship is confounded by tobacco use.

▶ USE OF ANTITHROMBOTIC AGENTS

Intracranial hemorrhage is recognized as the leading potentially life-threatening complication of the use of antithrombotic agents, antiplatelet aggregating agents, and thrombolytic medications. Hemorrhagic stroke is the most feared complication of the use of these medications when they are used in either primary or secondary prevention of ischemic disease. In general, intracranial bleeding associated with use of these medications is more extensive and associated with a poorer prognosis than hemorrhagic stroke due to other causes, such as hypertension. The risk of bleeding must be compared to the impressive efficacy of these medications in preventing ischemic stroke. These medications are the mainstay in medical management of patients with cerebrovascular disease and are described in more detail in Chapter 19.

▶ INFLAMMATION AND INFECTION

Atherosclerosis is an arteriopathy that progresses over a lifetime. Many of the previously described modifiable risk factors for stroke are in reality conditions that promote atherosclerosis.[6,102,174,175] Recognition of the important contribution of inflammation to the evolution of atherosclerosis is prompting new strategies to halt or even reverse the arterial disease.[12,176] Inflammation may compound some of the traditional risk factors that promote the growth of atheromatous lesions. Inflammatory responses to the accumulation of LDL cholesterol within the arterial wall may be critical in the initial stages of growth of an atherosclerotic plaque.[12] Some of the potential positive effects of antioxidants on atherosclerosis may be mediated via their anti-inflammatory actions.

In addition to facilitating the deposition of atherosclerotic plaques, various components of the inflammatory response may also affect an established lesion. The migration of T-lymphocytes, mast cells, and macrophages into plaques is pivotal for progression of the atherosclerotic lesion. Increased concentrations of interleukins (ILs) 1, 2, 4, and 6, IFN γ, TNF α, ICAM-1 and -2, and VCAM-1 are associated with an unstable atherosclerotic plaque that is prone to rupture.[6] On the other hand, IL-10 may have some plaque protection properties. Elevations of CRP, D-dimer, and fibrinogen are markers of an increased risk of cardiovascular events after stroke.[177,178] Recently, Asanuma et al.[179] and Roman et al.[180] reported that atherosclerosis occurs prematurely among persons with systemic lupus erythematosus. Affected patients are younger than those with traditional risk factors for accelerated atherosclerosis, and systemic lupus erythematosus appears to be an independent forecaster of advanced atherosclerosis. This association adds further credence to the concept that inflammation plays a role in the arterial changes of atherosclerosis.

In addition, infections may directly or indirectly stimulate progression of atherosclerosis. Grau et al.[181] correlated the presence of periodontal disease as a risk factor for ischemic stroke. Presumably, the relationship is secondary to an infectious or inflammatory reaction. *Chlamydia pneumoniae*, *Helicobacter pylori*, herpes, and cytomegalovirus are among the potential offending organisms.[12,176,182] Prager et al.[183] reported a high rate of infection with chlamydia in atherosclerotic plaques removed at carotid endarterectomy. Increased blood levels of high-sensitivity CRP are associated with an increased risk of hypertension and vascular events including stroke.[102] It has been found that elevated levels of CRP increased the risk of new vascular events following stroke by a factor of 4.[177,184–186] This acute phase reactant protein is produced in the liver and can increase up to 100 times. Elevated levels can indicate chronic low levels of inflammation. An elevation in high-sensitivity CRP may compound the effects of hypercholesterolemia and other risk factors for the development of premature atherosclerosis. Some of the benefit from the statins may be secondary to their anti-inflammatory effects.[102,184] In addition, it is hypothesized that some of the efficacy of aspirin in preventing arterial thromboembolism may be via its anti-inflammatory effects. Other anti-inflammatory agents or even antibiotics may be useful in stabilizing atherosclerotic plaques and preventing arterial thrombosis. To date, no clinical trial has been able to establish any therapeutic efficacy of antibiotics in slowing down the course of atherosclerosis.[176] Brassard et al.[187] did not find any relationship between stroke risk and the use of antibiotics, such as fluoroquinolones, macrolides, tetracyclines, or cephalosporins, but some data suggest a possible association with penicillin.

▶ CORONARY ARTERY DISEASE

Many patients with ischemic cerebrovascular disease also have evidence of coronary artery disease. The coronary artery disease is usually overt. Many stroke patients have a history of angina pectoris, myocardial infarction, endovascular treatment of coronary artery disease, or previous coronary artery bypass surgery. Many of the risk factors described in this chapter portend an increased likelihood of advanced atherosclerosis in the cerebral and coronary arteries. The presence of atherosclerotic disease of the intracranial or extracranial vasculature also forecasts an increased risk of coronary artery disease (see Chapter 5). Because myocardial infarction and sudden cardiac death are among the leading causes of mortality following TIA or cerebral infarction, management of the concomitant heart disease is a crucial component of treatment. Thus, the evaluation and treatment of coronary artery disease should accompany management of risk factors that predispose to stroke.[188]

REFERENCES

1. Li S, Chen W, Srinivasan SR, et al. Childhood cardiovascular risk factors and carotid vascular changes in adulthood. The Bogalusa Heart Study. *JAMA* 2003;290:2271–2276.

2. Raitakari OT, Juonala M, Kähönen M, et al. Cardiovascular risk factors in childhood and carotid artery intima-media thickness in adulthood. The cardiovascular risk in Young Finns Study. *JAMA* 2003;290:2277–2283.

3. Kieltyka L, Urbina EM, Tang R, Bond MG, Srinivasan SR, Berenson GS. Framingham risk score is related to carotid artery intima-media thickness in both white and black young adults: the Bogalusa Heart Study. *Atherosclerosis* 2003;170:125–130.

4. Gorelick PB. Stroke prevention therapy beyond antithrombotics. Unifying mechanisms in ischemic stroke pathogenesis and implications for therapy. *Stroke* 2002;33:862–875.

5. Leys D, Deplanque D, Mounier-Vehier C, Mackowiak-Cordoliani MA, Lucas C, Bordet R. Stroke prevention: management of modifiable vascular risk factors. *J Neurol* 2002;249:507–517.

6. Forrester JS. Prevention of plaque rupture: a new paradigm of therapy. *Ann Intern Med* 2002;137:823–833.

7. Mouradian MS, Majumdar SR, Senthilselvan A, Khan K, Shuaib A. How well are hypertension, hyperlipidemia, diabetes, and smoking managed after a stroke or transient ischemic attack? *Stroke* 2002;33:1656–1659.

8. Gaede P, Vedel P, Larsen N, Jensen GV, Parving HH, Pedersen O. Multifactorial intervention and cardiovascular disease in patients with type 2 diabetes. *N Engl J Med* 2003;348:383–393.

9. Sacco RL, Adams R, Albers G, et al. Guidelines for prevention of stroke in patients with ischemic stroke or transient ischemic attack. A statement for healthcare professionals from the American Heart Association/American Stroke Association Council on Stroke. *Stroke* 2006;37:577–617

10. Goldstein LB, Adams R, Alberts MJ, et al. Primary prevention of ischemic stroke. A guideline from the American Heart Associatin/American Stroke Association Stroke Council. *Stroke* 2066;37:1583–1633

11. Alexander RW. Hypertension and the pathogenesis of atherosclerosis. *Hypertension* 1995;25:155–161.

12. Ross R. Atherosclerosis—an inflammatory disease. *N Engl J Med* 1999;340:115–126.

13. Mast H, Thompson JL, Lee SH, Mohr JP, Sacco RL. Hypertension and diabetes mellitus as determinants of multiple lacunar infarcts. *Stroke* 1995;26:30–33.

14. Ferro JM, Crespo M, Ferro H. Role of vascular risk factors in lacunar and unexplained stokes in young adults: a case-control study. *Cerebrovasc Dis* 1995;5:188–193.

15. American Heart Association. Heart disease and stroke statistics—2004, Dallas TX, American Heart Association.

16. Nawrot T, Den Hond E, Thijs L, Staessen JA. Isolated systolic hypertension and the risk of vascular disease. *Curr Hypertens Rep* 2003;5:372–379.

17. Burt VL, Whelton P, Roccella EJ, et al. Prevalence of hypertension in the U.S. adult population. *Hypertension* 1995;25:305–313.

18. Murray CJ, Lauer JA, Hutubessy R, et al. Effectiveness and costs of interventions to lower systolic blood pressure and cholesterol: a global and regional analysis on reduction of cardiovascular-disease risk. *Lancet* 2003;361:717–725.

19. Ambrosioni E, Leonetti G, Pessina AC, Rappelli A, Trimarco B, Zanchetti A. Patterns of hypertension management in Italy: results of a pharmocoepidemiological survey on antihypertensive therapy. Scientific Committee of the Italian Pharmacoepidemiological Survey on Antyhypertensive Therapy. *J Hypertens* 2000; 18:1691–1699.

20. Droste DW, Ritter MA, Dittrich R, et al. Areteral hypertension and ischaemic stroke. *Acta Neurol Scand* 2003;107:241–251.

21. Naidech AM, Weisberg LA. Treatment of chronic hypertension for the prevention of stroke. *South Med J* 2003;96:359–362.

22. He FJ, MacGregor GA. How far should salt intake be reduced? *Hypertension* 2003;42:1093–1099.

23. Hansson L, Lindholm LH, Ekbom T, et al. Randomised trial of old and new antihypertensive drugs in elderly patients: cardiovascular mortality and morbidity the Swedish trial in old patients with hypertension-2 study. *Lancet* 1999;354:1751–1756.

24. The ALLHAT Officers and Coordinators for the ALLHAT Collaborative Research Group. Major outcomes in moderately hypercholesterolemic, hypertensive patients randomized to Pravastatin vs usual care. The Antihypertensive and Lipid-Lowering Treatment to Prevent Heart Attack Trial (ALLHAT-LLT). *JAMA* 2002;288:2998–3007.

25. Wiklund O, Hulthe J, Wikstrand J, Schmidt C, Olofsson S, Bondjers G. Effect of controlled release/extended release metoprolol on carotid intima-media thickness in patients with hypercholesterolemia: a 3-year randomized study. *Stroke* 2002;33:572–577.

26. The Dutch TIA Study Group. The Dutch TIA Trial: protective effects of low-dose aspirin and atenolol in patients with transient ischemic attacks or nondisabling stroke. *Stroke* 1988;19:512–517.

27. Wink K. Are beta-blockers efficacious as first-line therapy for hypertension in the elderly? *Curr Hypertens Rep* 2003;5:221–224.

28. Blood Pressure Lowering Treatment Trialists' Collaboration. Effects of different blood-pressure-lowering regimens on major cardiovascular events: results of prospectively-designed overviews of randomised trials. *Lancet* 2003;362:1527–1535.

29. Pepine CJ, Handberg EM, Cooper-DeHoff RM, et al. A calcium antagonist vs a non-calcium antagonist hypertension treatment strategy for patients with coronary artery disease. The International Verapamil-Trandolapril Study (INVEST): a randomized controlled trial. *JAMA* 2003;290:2805–2816.

30. Hansson L, Hedner T, Lund-Johansen P, et al. Randomised trial of effects of calcium antagonists compared with diuretics and beta-blockers on cardiovascular morbidity and mortality in hypertension: the Nordic Diltiazem (NORDIL) study. *Lancet* 2000;356:359–365.

31. Neal B, MacMahon S, Chapman N, Blood Pressure Lowering Treatment Trialists' Collaboration. Effects of ACE inhibitors, calcium antagonists, and other blood-pressure-lowering drugs: results of prospectively designed overviews of randomised trials. Blood Pressure Lowering Treatment Trialists' Collaboration. *Lancet* 2000; 356:1955–1964.

32. Opie LH. Calcium channel blockers in hypertension: reappraisal after new trials and major meta-analyses. *Am J Hypertens* 2001;14:1074–1081.

33. Black HR, Elliott WJ, Grandits G, et al. Principal results of the Controlled Onset Verapamil Investigation of Cardiovascular End Points (CONVINCE) trial. *JAMA* 2003;289: 2073–2082.

34. Pahor M, Psaty BM, Alderman MH, et al. Health outcomes associated with calcium antagonists compared with other first-line antihypertensive therapies: a meta-analysis of randomised controlled trials. *Lancet* 2000;356:1949–1954.

35. Lazar HL, Bao Y, Rivers S, Colton T, Bernard SA. High tissue affinity angiotensin-converting enzyme inhibitors improve endothelial function and reduce infarct size. *Ann Thorac Surg* 2001;72:548–553.

36. Taddei S, Virdis A, Ghiadoni L, Mattei P, Salvetti A. Effects of angiotensin converting enzyme inhibition on endothelium-dependent vasodilatation in essential hypertensive patients. *J Hypertens* 1998;16:447–456.

37. Enseleit F, Hurlimann D, Luscher TF. Vascular protective effects of angiotensin converting enzyme inhibitors and their relation to clinical events. *J Cardiovasc Pharmacol* 2001;37:S21–S30.

38. Iadecola C, Gorelick PB. Hypertension, angiotensin, and stroke: beyond blood pressure. *Stroke* 2004;35:348–350.

39. Arnold M, Nedeltchev K, Sturzenegger M, et al. Thrombolysis in patients with acute stroke caused by cervical artery dissection: analysis of 9 patients and review of the literature. *Arch Neurol* 2002;59:549–553.

40. Schwartzkopff B, Brehm M, Mundhenke M, Stauer B. Repair of coronary arterioles after treatment with perindopril in hypertensive heart disease. *Hypertension* 2000;36: 220–225.

41. Niskanen L, Hedner T, Hansson L, Lanke J, Niklason A, The CAPPP Study Group. Reduced cardiovascular morbidity and mortality in hypertensive diabetic patients on first-line therapy with an ACE inhibitor compared with a diuretic/beta-blocker-based treatment regimen: a subanalysis of the Captopril Prevention Project. *Diabetes Care* 2001;24:2091–2096.

42. The Heart Outcomes Prevention Evaluation Study Investigators. Effects of angiotensin-converting-enzyme inhibitor, Ramipril, on cardiovascular events in high-risk patients. *N Engl J Med* 2000;342:145–153.

43. Yusuf S, Sleight P, Pogue J, Bosch J, Davies R, Dagenais G. Effects of an angiotensin-converting-enzyme inhibitor, ramipril, on cardiovascular events in high-risk patients. The Heart Outcomes Prevention Evaluation Study Investigators. *N Engl J Med* 2000;342:145–153.

44. Bosch J, Yusuf S, Pogue J, et al. Use of ramipril in preventing stroke: double blind randomised trial. *BMJ* 2002;324:699–702.

45. PROGRESS Collaborative Group. Randomised trial of a perindopril-based blood-pressure lowering regimen among 6,105 individuals with previous stroke or transient ischaemic attack. *Lancet* 2001;358:1033–1041.

46. MacMahon S, Rodgers A, Neal B, Woodward M, Chalmers J, on behalf of the PROGRESS Collaborative Group. The lowering of blood pressure after stroke. *Lancet* 2002;358: 1994–1995.

47. Staessen JA, Wang J. Blood-pressure lowering for the secondary prevention of stroke. *Lancet* 2001;358:1026–1027.

48. Chalmers J. Trials on blood pressure-lowering and secondary stroke prevention. *Am J Cardiol* 2003;91:3G–8G.

49. Ratnasabapathy Y, Lawes CM, Anderson CS. The Perindopril Protection Against Recurrent Stroke Study (PROGRESS): clinical implications for older patients with cerebrovascular disease. *Drugs Aging* 2003;20:241–251.

50. Chapman N, Huxley R, Anderson C, et al. Effects of perindopril-based blood pressure-lowering regimen on the risk of recurrent stroke according to stroke subtype and medical history. The PROGRESS Trial. *Stroke* 2004; 35:116–21.

51. Perindopril Protection Against Recurrent Stroke Study (PROGRESS) Collaborative Group. Effects of a perindopril-based blood pressure-lowering regimen on disability and dependency in 6105 patients with cerebrovascular disease. A randomized controlled trial. *Stroke* 2003;34: 2333–2338.

52. Lindholm LH, Ibsen H, Beevers G, et al. Cardiovascular morbidity and mortality in patients with diabetes in the Losartan Intervention For Endpoint reduction in hypertension study (LIFE): a randomized trial against atenolol. *Lancet* 2002;359:1004–1010.

53. Dahlöf B, Devereux RB, Kjeldsen SE, et al. Cardiovascular morbidity and mortality in the Lasartan Intervention For Endpoint reduction in hypertension study (LIFE): a randomised trial against atenolol. *Lancet* 2002;359:995–1003.

54. Devereux RB, Dahlof B, Kjeldsen SE, et al. Effects of losartan or atenolol in hypertensive patients without clinically evident vascular disease: a substudy of the LIFE randomized trial. *Ann Intern Med* 2003;139:169–177.

55. Furberg CD, Pitt B. Are all angiotensin-converting enzyme inhibitors interchangeable? *J Am Coll Cardiol* 2001;37: 1456–1460.

56. Leys D, Kwiecinski H, Bogousslavsky J, et al. Prevention. *Cerebrovasc Dis* 2004;17(suppl 2):15–29.

57. Swales JD. The costs of not treating hypertension. *Blood Press* 1999;8:198–199.

58. Hurst RT, Lee RW. Increased incidence of coronary atherosclerosis in Type 2 diabetes mellitus: mechanisms and management. *Ann Intern Med* 2003;139:824–834.

59. Ho JE, Paultre F, Mosca L. Is diabetes mellitus a cardiovascular disease risk equivalent for fatal stroke in women? Data from the Women's Pooling Project. *Stroke* 2003;34:2812–2816.

60. Di Bonito P, Di Fraia L, Di Gennaro L, et al. Impact of known and unknown diabetes on in-hospital mortality from ischemic stroke. *Nutr Metab Cardiovasc Dis* 2003; 13:148–153.

61. Laakso M. Insulin resistance and its impact on the approach to therapy of type 2 diabetes. *Int J Clin Pract* 2001;suppl(117):8–12.

62. Sakkinen PA, Wahl P, Cushman M, Lewis MR, Tracy RP. Clustering of procoagulation, inflammation, and fibrinolysis variables with metabolic factors in insulin resistance syndrome. *Am J Epidemiol* 2000;152:897–907.

63. Kernan WN, Inzucchi SE, Viscoli CM, Brass LM, Bravata DM, Horwitz RI. Insulin resistance and risk for stroke. *Neurology* 2002;59:809–815.

64. Facchini FS, Hua N, Abbasi F, Reaven GM. Insulin resistance as a predictor of age-related diseases. *J Clin Endocrinol Metab* 2001;86:3574–3578.

65. Dumont AS, Hyndman ME, Dumont RJ, et al. Improvement of endothelial function in insulin-resistant carotid arteries treated with pravastatin. *J Neurosurg* 2001;95:466–471.

66. Riina HA, Spetzler RF. Unruptured aneurysms. *J Neurosurg* 2002;96:61–62.

67. Pihlajamaki J, Austin M, Edwards K, Laakso M. A major gene effect on fasting insulin and insulin sensitivity in familial combined hyperlipidemia. *Diabetes* 2001;50:2396–2401.

68. Kareinen A, Viitanen L, Halonen P, Lehto S, Laakso M. Cardiovascular risk factors associated with insulin resistance cluster in families with early-onset coronary heart disease. *Arterioscler Thromb Vasc Biol* 2001;21:1346–1352.

69. Kuusisto J, Lempiainen P, Mykkanen L, Laakso M. Insulin resistance syndrome predicts coronary heart disease events in elderly type 2 diabetic men. *Diabetes Care* 2001;24:1629–1633.

70. Adachi H, Hirai Y, Tsuruta M, Fujiura Y, Imaizuml T. Is insulin resistance or diabetes mellitus associated with stroke? An 18-year follow-up study. *Diabetes Res Clin Pract Suppl* 2001;51:215–223.

71. Meigs J. Epidemiology of the metabolic syndrome. *Am J Manag Care* 2002;8:S283–S292.

72. Reaven G. Metabolic syndrome: pathophysiology and implications for management of cardiovascular disease [Clinical Update]. *Circulation* 2002;106:286–288.

73. Grundy SM. Obesity, metabolic syndrome, and coronary atherosclerosis. *Circulation* 2002;105:2696–2698.

74. Ovbiagela B, Saver JL, Lynn MJ, et al. Impact of metabolic syndrome on prognosis of symptomatic intracranial atherostenosis. *Neurology* 2006;66:1344–1349.

75. Reusch J. Current concepts in insulin resistance, type 2 diabetes mellitus, and the metabolic syndrome. *Am J Cardiol* 2002;90:19G–26G.

76. Relimpio F, Losada F, Pumar A, Mangas MA, Morales F, Astorga R. Relationships of apolipoprotein B(100) with the metabolic syndrome in Type 2 diabetes mellitus. *Diabetes Res Clin Pract* 2002;57:199–207.

77. McLaughlin T, Abbasi F, Cheal K, Chu J, Lamendola C, Reaven G. Use of metabolic markers to identify overweight individuals who are insulin resistant. *Ann Intern Med* 2003;139:802–809.

78. Bosello O, Zamboni M. Visceral obesity and metabolic syndrome. *Obes Rev* 2000;1:47–56.

79. Saydah SH, Fradkin J, Cowie CC. Poor control of risk factors for vascular disease among adults with previously diagnosed diabetes. *JAMA* 2004;291:335–342.

80. Hevener AL, Reichart D, Janez A, Olefsky J. Thiazolidinedione treatment prevents free fatty acid-induced insulin resistance in male wistar rats. *Diabetes* 2001;50:2316–2322.

81. Smith U. Pioglitazone: mechanism of action. *Int J Clin Pract* 2001;suppl(117):13–18.

82. Kernan WN, Inzucchi SE, Iscoli CM, et al. Pioglitazone improves insulin sensitivity among nondiabetic patients with a recent transient ischemic attack or ischemic stroke. *Stroke* 2003;34:1431–1436.

83. Prosser LA, Stinnett AA, Goldman PA, et al. Cost-effectiveness of cholesterol-lowering therapies according to selected patient characteristics. *Ann Intern Med* 2000;132:769–778.

84. Ansell BJ. Cholesterol, stroke risk, and stroke prevention. *Curr Atheroscler Rep* 2000;2:92–96.

85. Liu Y, Coresh J, Eustace JA, et al. Association between cholesterol level and mortality in dialysis patients. Role of inflammation and malnutrition. *JAMA* 2004;291:451–459.

86. Hu FB, Willett WC. Optimal diets for prevention of coronary heart disease. *JAMA* 2002;288:2569–2578.

87. Crouse JR, Byington RP, Furberg CD. HMG-CoA reductase inhibitor therapy and stroke risk reduction: an analysis of clinical trials data. *Atherosclerosis* 1998;138:11–24.

88. Hebert PR, Gaziano JM, Chan KS, Hennekens CH. Cholesterol lowering with statin drugs, risk of stroke, and total mortality. An overview of randomized trials. *JAMA* 1997;278:313–321.

89. Schwartz GG, Olsson AG, Ezekowitz M, et al. Effects of atorvastatin on early recurrent ischemic events in acute coronary syndromes: the MIRACL study: a randomized controlled trial. *JAMA* 2001;285:1711–1718.

90. Collins R, Armitage J. High-risk elderly patients PROSPER from cholesterol-lowering therapy. *Lancet* 2002;360:618–619.

91. Amarenco P, Lavallee P, Touboul PJ. Statins and stroke prevention. *Cerebrovasc Dis* 2004;17(suppl 1):81–88.

92. Heart Protection Study Collaborative Group. MRC/BHF Heart Protection Study of cholesterol lowering with simvastatin in 20,536 high-risk individuals: a randomized placebo-controlled trial. *Lancet* 2002;360:7–22.

93. Sever PS, Dahlof B, Poulter NR, et al. Prevention of coronary and stroke events with atorvastatin in hypertensive patients who have average or lower-than-average cholesterol concentrations, in the Anglo-Scandinavian Cardiac Outcomes Trial-Lipid Lowering Arm (ASCOT-LLA): a multicentre randomised controlled trial. *Lancet* 2003;361:1149–1158.

94. Holdaas H, Fellstrom B, Jardine AG, et al. Effect of fluvastatin on cardiac outcomes in renal transplant recipients: a multicentre, randomised, placebo-controlled trial. *Lancet* 2003;361:2024–2031.

95. Heart Protection Study Collaborative Group. MRC/BHF Heart Protection Study on cholesterol-lowering with simvastatin in 5963 people with diabetes: a randomised placebo-controlled trial. *Lancet* 2003;361:2005–2016.

96. Nissen SE, Tuzcu EM, Schoenhagen P, et al. Effect of intensive compares with moderate lipid-lowering therapy on progression of coronary atherosclerosis. A randomized controlled trial. *JAMA* 2004;291:1071–1080.

97. Sterzer P, Meintzschel F, Lanfermann H, Steinmetz H, Sitzer M. Pravastatin improves cerebral vasomotor reactivity in patients with subcortical small-vessel disease. *Stroke* 2001;32:2817–2820.

98. Corsini A, Pazzucconi F, Arnaboldi L, et al. Direct effects of statins on the vascular wall. *J Cardiovasc Pharmacol* 1998;31:773–778.

99. Cucchiara B, Kasner SE. Use of statins in CNS disorders. *J Neurol Sci* 2001;187:81–89.

100. Van de WA, Caillard CA. Statins and the stroke-cholesterol paradox. *Neth J Med* 2002;60:4–9.

101. Werner N, Nickenig G, Laufs U. Pleiotropic effects of HMB-CoA reductase inhibitors. *Basic Res Cardiol* 2002; 97:105–116.

102. Ridker PM. Inflammatory biomarkers, statins, and the risk of stroke: cracking a clinical conundrum. *Circulation* 2002;105:2583–2585.

103. Smilde TJ, van Wissen S, Wollersheim H, Kastelein JJP, Stalenhoef AFH. Effects of aggressive versus conventional lipid lowering on atherosclerosis progression in familial hypercholesterolaemia (ASAP): a prospective, randomised, double-blind trial. *Lancet* 2001;357:577–581.

104. Vaughan CJ, Delanty N. Neuroprotective properties of statins in cerebral ischemia and stroke. *Stroke* 1999;30: 1969–1973.

105. Pasternak RC, Smith SC, Bairey-Merz CN, Grundy SM, Cleeman JI, Lenfant C. ACC/AHA/NHLBI clinical advisory on the use and safety of statins. *Stroke* 2002;33:2337–2341.

106. Davidson MH. Safety profiles for the HMG-CoA reductase inhibitors: treatment and trust. *Drugs* 2001;61:197–206.

107. Benner JS, Glynn RJ, Mogun H, Neumann PJ, Weinstein MC, Avorn J. Long-term persistence in use of statin therapy in elderly patients. *JAMA* 2002;288:455–461.

108. Davidson MH. Combination therapy for dyslipidemia: safety and regulatory considerations. *Am J Cardiol* 2002; 90:50K–60K.

109. Davidson MH, McGarry T, Bettis R, Melani L, Lipka LJ, LeBeaut AP. Ezetimibe coadministered with simvastatin in patients with primary hypercholesterolemia. *J Am Coll Cardiol* 2002;40:2125–2134.

110. Leitersdorf E. Selective cholesterol absorption inhibition: a novel strategy in lipid-lowering management. *Int J Clin Pract* 2002;56:116–119.

111. Gagne C, Bays HE, Weiss SR, et al. Efficacy and safety of *ezetimibe* added to ongoing statin therapy for treatment of patients with primary hypercholesterolemia. *Am J Cardiol* 2002;90:1084–1091.

112. Miller M. Niacin as a component of combination therapy for dyslipidemia. *Mayo Clin Proc* 2003;78:735–742.

113. Nissen SE, Tsunoda T, Tuzcu EM, et al. Effect of recombinant ApoA-I Milano on coronary atherosclerosis in patients with acute coronary syndromes. A randomized controlled trial. *JAMA* 2003;290:2292–2300.

114. Leppala JM, Virtamo J, Fogelholm R, Albanes D, Heinonen OP. Different risk factors for different stroke subtypes: association of blood pressure, cholesterol, and antioxidants. *Stroke* 1999;30:2535–2540.

115. Segal AZ, Chiu RI, Eggleston-Sexton PM, Beiser A, Greenberg SM. Low cholesterol as a risk factor for primary intracerebral hemorrhage: a case-control study. *Neuroepidemiology* 1999;18:185–193.

116. White H, Simes RJ, Anderson NE, et al. Pravastatin therapy and the risk of stroke. *N Engl J Med* 2000;343:317–326.

117. Lawlor DA, Martin RM, Gunnell D, et al. Association of body mass index measured in childhood, adolescence, and young adulthood with risk of ischemic heart disease and stroke. Findings from 3 historical cohort studies. *Am J Clin Nutr* 2006;83:767–773

118. Weiss R, Dufour S, Taksali SE, et al. Prediabetes in obese youth: a syndrome of impaired glucose tolerance, severe insulin resistance, and altered myocellular and abdominal fat partitioning. *Lancet* 2003;362:951–957.

119. Voko Z, Hollander M, Hofman A, Koudstaal PJ, Breteler MMB. Dietary antioxidants and the risk of ischemic stroke: the Rotterdam Study. *Neurology* 2003;61:1273–1275.

120. Sauvaget C, Nagano J, Allen N, Kodama K. Vegetable and fruit intake and stroke mortality in the Hiroshima/Nagasaki life span study. *Stroke* 2003;34:2355–2360.

121. Johnsen SP, Overvad K, Stripp C, Tjonneland A, Husted SE, Sorensen HT. Intake of fruit and vegetables and the risk of ischemic stroke in a cohort of Danish men and women. *Am J Clin Nutr* 2003;78:57–64.

122. Steffen LM, Jacobs DR, Jr., Stevens J, Shahar E, Carithers T, Folsom AR. Associations of whole-grain, refined-grain, and fruit and vegetable consumption with risks of all-cause mortality and incident coronary artery disease and ischemic stroke: the Atherosclerosis Risk in Communities (ARIC) Study. *Am J Clin Nutr* 2003;78:383–390.

123. He K, Rimm EB, Merchant A, et al. Fish consumption and risk of stroke in men. *JAMA* 2002;288:3130–3136.

124. Pereira MA, Jacobs DR, Jr., Van Horn L, Slattery ML, Kartashov AI, Ludwig DS. Dairy consumption, obesity, and the insulin resistance syndrome in young adults: the CARDIA Study. *JAMA* 2002;287:2081–2089.

125. Boden-Albala B, Sacco RL. Lifestyle factors and stroke risk: exercise, alcohol, diet, obesity, smoking, drug use, and stress. *Curr Atheroscler Rep* 2000;2:160–166.

126. Vivekananthan KP, Penn MS, Sapp SK, Hsu A, Topol EJ. Use of antioxidant vitamins for the prevention of cardiovascular disease: meta-analysis of randomised trials. *Lancet* 2003;361:2017–2023.

127. Heart Protection Study Collaborative Group. MRC/BHF Heart Protection Study of antioxidant vitamin supplementation in 20,536 high-risk individuals: a randomised placebo-controlled trial. *Lancet* 2002;360:23–33.

128. Amighi J, Sabeti S, Schlager O, et al. Low serum magnesium predicts neurological events in patients with advanced atherosclerosis. *Stroke* 2004;35:22–27.

129. Endres M, Gertz K, Lindauer U, et al. Mechanisms of stroke protection by physical activity. *Ann Neurol* 2003; 54:582–590.

130. Gillum RF, Mussolino ME, Ingram DD. Physical activity and stroke incidence in women and men. The NHANES I Epidemiologic Follow-up Study. *Am J Epidemiol* 1996; 143:860–869.

131. Lee CD, Folsom AR, Blair SN. Physical activity and stroke risk. A meta-analysis. *Stroke* 2003;34:2475–2481.

132. Vermeer SE, Rinkel GJ, Algra A. Circadian fluctuations in onset of subarachnoid hemorrhage. New data on aneurysmal and perimesencephalic hemorrhage and a systematic review. *Stroke* 1997;28:805–808.

133. Lammie GA, Lindley R, Keir S, Wiggam MI. Stress-related primary intracerebral hemorrhage: autopsy clues to underlying mechanism. *Stroke* 2000;31:1426–1428.

134. Nencini P, Basile AM, Sarti C, Inzitari D. Cerebral hemorrhage following a roller coaster ride. *JAMA* 2000;284: 832–833.

135. Faraci FM, Lentz SR. Hyperhomocysteinemia, oxidative stress, and cerebral vascular dysfunction. *Stroke* 2004; 35:345–347.

136. Tanne D, Sela BA. Neurological implications of hyperhomocysteinemia in patients with atherothrombotic disease. *Ital Heart J* 2003;4:577–579.

137. Soinio M, Marniemi J, Laakso M, Lehto S, Rönnemaa T. Elevated plasma homocysteine level is an independent predictor of coronary heart disease events in patients with Type 2 diabetes mellitus. *Ann Intern Med* 2004; 140:94–100.

138. Falk E, Zhou J, Moller J. Homocysteine and atherothrombosis. *Lipids* 2001;36:S3–S11.

139. Kelly PJ, Kistler JP, Shih VE, et al. Inflammation, homocysteine, and vitamin B6 status after ischemic stroke. *Stroke* 2004;35:12–5.

140. Ingrosso D, Cimmino A, Perna AF, et al. Folate treatment and unbalanced methylation and changes of allelic expression induced by hyperhomocysteinaemia in patients with uraemia. *Lancet* 2003;361:1693–1699.

141. He K, Merchant A, Rimm EB, et al. Folate, vitamin B_6 and B_{12} intakes in relation to risk of stroke among men. *Stroke* 2004;35:169–174.

142. The VITATOPS Trial Study Group. The VITATOPS (Vitamins to Prevent Stroke) Trial: rationale and design of an international, large, simple, randomised trial of homocysteine-lowering multivitamin therapy in patients with recent transient ischaemic attack or stroke. *Cerebrovasc Dis* 2002;13:120–126.

143. Loon E, Yusuf S, Arnold MJ, et al. Homocysteine lowering with folic acid and B vitamins in vascular disease. *N Engl J Med* 2006;354:1567–1577.

144. Toole JF, Malinow MR, Chambless LE, et al. Lowering homocysteine in patients with ischemic stroke to prevent recurrent stroke, myocardial infarction, and death. The Vitamin Intervention for Stroke Prevention (VISP) randomized controlled trial. *JAMA* 2004;291:565–575.

145. Ezzati M, Lopez AD. Estimates of global mortality attributable to smoking in 2000. *Lancet* 2003;362:847–852.

146. Vessey M, Painter R, Yeates D. Mortality in relation to oral contraceptive use cigarette smoking. *Lancet* 2003;362:185–191.

147. Otsuka R, Watanabe H, Hirata K, et al. Acute effects of passive smoking on the coronary circulation in healthy young adults. *JAMA* 2001;286:436–441.

148. You RX, Thrift AG, McNeil JJ, Davis SM, Donnan GA. Ischemic stroke risk and passive exposure to spouses' cigarette smoking. Melbourne Stroke Risk Factor Study (MERFS) Group. *Am J Public Health* 1999;89:572–575.

149. Thrift AG, McNeil JJ, Forbes A, Donnan GA. Risk of primary intracerebral haemorrhage associated with aspirin and non-steroidal anti-inflammatory drugs: case-control study. *BMJ* 1999;318:759–764.

150. Kurth T, Kase CS, Berger K, Schaeffner ES, Buring JE, Gaziano JM. Smoking and the risk of hemorrhagic stroke in men. *Stroke* 2003;34:1151–1155.

151. Weir BK, Kongable GL, Kassell NF, Schultz JR, Truskowski LL, Sigrest A. Cigarette smoking as a cause of aneurysmal subarachnoid hemorrhage and risk for vasospasm: a report of the Cooperative Aneurysm Study. *J Neurosurg* 1998;89:405–411.

152. Anderson CS, Feigin V, Bennett D, et al. Active and passive smoking and the risk of subarachnoid hemorrhage. An international population-based case-control study. *Stroke* 2004;35:633–637.

153. Bolin K, Lindgren B, Willers S. The cost utility of bupropion in smoking cessation health programs. Simulation model results for Sweden. *Chest* 2006;129:651–660.

154. Lerman C, Kaufmann V, Rukstalis M, et al. Individualizing nicotine replacement therapy for the treatment of tobacco dependence. A randomized trial. *Ann Intern Med* 2004;140:426–433.

155. Reynolds K, Lewis LB, Nolen JDL, Kinney GL, Sathya B, He J. Alcohol consumption and risk of stroke. A Meta-analysis. *JAMA* 2003;289:579–588.

156. Djousse L, Ellison RC, Beiser A, Scaramucci A, D'Agostino RB, Wolf PA. Alcohol consumption and risk of ischemic stroke: the Framingham Study. *Stroke* 2002;33:907–912.

157. Ding J, Eigenbrodt ML, Mosley TH, Jr., et al. Alcohol intake and cerebral abnormalities on magnetic resonance imaging on a community-based population of middle-aged adults. The Atherosclerosis Risk in Communities (ARIC) Study. *Stroke* 2004;35:16–21.

158. Goude D, Fagerberg B, Hulthe J, AIR Study Group. Alcohol consumption, the metabolic syndrome and insulin resistance in 58-year-old clinically healthy men (AIR study). *Clin Sci* 2002;102:345–352.

159. Juvela R, Hillborn M, Palomaki H. Risk factors for spontaneous intracerebral hemorrhage. *Stroke* 1995;26:1558–1564.

160. Leppala JM, Paunio M, Virtamo J, et al. Alcohol consumption and stroke incidence in male smokers. *Circulation* 1999;100:1209–1214.

161. Klatsky A, Armstrong M, Friedman G, Sidney S. Alcohol drinking and risk of hemorrhagic stroke. *Neuroepidemiology* 2002;21:115–122.

162. Thrift A, Donnan G, McNeil J. Heavy drinking, but not moderate or intermediate drinking, increases the risk of intracerebral hemorrhage. *Epidemiology* 1999;10:307–312.

163. Berger K, Ajani UA, Kase CS, et al. Light-to-moderate alcohol consumption and the risk of stroke among U.S. male physicians. *N Engl J Med* 1999;341:1557–1564.

164. Petitti DB, Sidney S, Quesenberry C, Bernstein A. Stroke and cocaine or amphetamine use. *Epidemiology* 1998;9:596–600.

165. Neiman J, Haapaniemi H, Hillbom M. Neurological complications of drug abuse: pathophysiological mechanism. *Eur J Neurol* 2000;7:595–606.

166. Schwartz SM, Petitti DB, Siscovick DS, et al. Stroke and use of low-dose oral contraceptives in young women: a pooled analysis of two US studies. *Stroke* 1998;29:2277–2284.

167. Johnston SC, Colford JMJ, Gress DR. Oral contraceptives and the risk of subarachnoid hemorrhage: a meta-analysis. *Neurology* 1998;51:411–418.

168. Writing Group for the Women's Health Initiative Investigators. Risks and benefits of estrogen plus progestin in healthy postmenopausal women. Principal results from the Women's Health Initiative Randomized Controlled Trial. *JAMA* 2002;288:321–333.

169. Wassertheil-Smoller S, Hendrix SL, Limacher M, et al. Effect of estrogen plus progestin on stroke in post-menopausal women. The Women's Health Initiative: a randomized trial. *JAMA* 2003;289:2673–2684.

170. Yaffe K. Hormone therapy and the brain. Déjà vu all over again? *JAMA* 2003;289:2717–2718.

171. Viscoli CM, Brass LM, Kernan WN, Sarrel PM, Suissa S, Horwitz RI. A clinical trial of estrogen-replacement therapy after ischemic stroke. *N Engl J Med* 2001;345:1243–1249.

172. Shearman AM, Cupples LA, Demissie S, et al. Association between estrogen receptor □ gene variation and cardio-vascular disease. *JAMA* 2003;290:2263–2270.

173. Brown DL. Sleep disorders and stroke. *Semin Neurol* 2006;26:117–122.

174. Fuster V, Badimon JJ, Chesebro JH. Atherothrombosis: mechanisms and clinical therapeutic approaches. *Vasc Med* 1998;3:231–239.

175. Malek AM, Alper SL, Izumo S. Hemodynamic shear stress and its role in atherosclerosis. *JAMA* 1999;282:2035–2042.

176. Ridker PM. On evolutionary biology, inflammation, infection, and the causes of atherosclerosis. *Circulation* 2002;105:2–4.

177. Di Napoli M, Papa F, for the Villa Pini Stroke Data Bank Investigators. Inflammation, hemostatic markers, and antithrombotic agents in relation to long-term risk of new cardiovascular events in first-ever ischemic stroke patients. *Stroke* 2002;33:1763–1771.

178. Albert M, Ridker PM. The role of C-reactive protein in cardiovascular disease risk. *Curr Cardiol Rep* 2002;1:99–104.

179. Asanuma Y, Oeser A, Shintani AK, et al. Premature coro-nary-artery atherosclerosis in systemic lupus erythemato-sus. *N Engl J Med* 2003;349:2407–2415.

180. Roman MJ, Shanker B-A, Davis A, et al. Prevalence and correlates of accelerated atherosclerosis in systemic lupus erythematosus. *N Engl J Med* 2003;349:2399–2406.

181. Grau AJ, Becher H, Ziegler CM, et al. Periodontal disease as a risk factor for ischemic stroke. *Stroke* 2004;35:496–501.

182. Kalayoglu MV, Libby P, Byrne GI. Chlamydia pneumo-niae as an emerging risk factor in cardiovascular disease. *JAMA* 2002;288:2724–2731.

183. Prager M, Turel Z, Speidl W, et al. Chlamydia pneumo-niae in carotid artery atherosclerosis: a comparison of its presence in atherosclerotic plaque, healthy vessels, and circulating leukocytes from the same individuals. *Stroke* 2002;33:2756–2761.

184. Libby P, Ridker PM, Maseri A. Inflammation and athero-sclerosis. *Circulation* 2002;105:1135–1143.

185. Ridker PM, Stampfer M, Rifai N. Novel risk factors for sys-temic atherosclerosis: a comparison of C-reactive protein, fibrinogen, homocysteine, lipoprotein(a), and standard cholesterol screening as predictors of peripheral arterial disease. *JAMA* 2002;285:2481–2485.

186. Sesso HD, Buring JE, Rifai N, Blake GJ, Gaziano JM, Ridker PM. C-reactive protein and the risk of developing hypertension. *JAMA* 2003;290:2945–2951.

187. Brassard P, Bourgault C, Brophy J, Kezouh A, Suissa S. Antibiotics in primary prevention of stroke in the elderly. *Stroke* 2003;34:e163–e167.

188. Adams RJ, Chimowitz MI, Alpert JS, et al. Coronary risk evaluation in patients with transient ischemic attack and ischemic stroke: a scientific statement of healthcare profes-sionals from the Stroke Council and the Council on Clinical Cardiology of the American Heart Association/American Stroke Association. *Circulation* 2003;108:1278–1290.

CHAPTER 5

Asymptomatic Carotid Artery Disease, Transient Ischemic Attacks, and Ocular Manifestations of Cerebrovascular Disease

▶ ASYMPTOMATIC CAROTID BRUIT OR STENOSIS

A cervical bruit is usually secondary to an arterial stenosis causing turbulence in the circulating blood. Because the carotid artery is relatively superficial in the neck, an examining physician can often hear a sound that represents the bruit. The presence of a cervical bruit usually is a marker for generalized atherosclerosis and portends an increased risk for myocardial infarction, ischemic stroke, and vascular death.[1,2] Detection of a cervical bruit is relatively common by auscultating the neck of an elderly patient. Approximately 5 percent of persons older than 65 have a bruit and the prevalence of this finding increases rapidly with advancing age.[3] Carotid bruits are more commonly found among persons with symptomatic coronary artery disease and peripheral vascular disease. A bruit also may be auscultated over an asymptomatic carotid artery in a patient who had a TIA or stroke occurring in the contralateral carotid or the vertebrobasilar circulation.

Clinical Findings

The usual location of a carotid bruit is just anterior to the sternocleidomastoid muscle and inferior to the angle of the mandible. Cervical bruits also can be heard in the supraclavicular area, the posterior aspect of the neck, or diffusely over the neck. Occasionally, cervical bruits radiate over the ipsilateral mastoid process, the temple, or the orbit.[4] The quality, pitch, tone, and duration of the bruit help discriminate those sounds secondary to arterial stenosis from sounds due to other causes. A high-pitched, pistol-shot, systolic sound often is secondary to an arterial stenosis. Other causes of cervical bruits usually produce low-pitched sounds that extend through both systole and diastole.

Most patients usually are not aware of the sound; however, some complain of hearing the sound in their head or in one ear hearing a low-pitched swishing sound (*pulsatile tinnitus*). The sound often is drowned out by ambient noise and thus it is most obvious to patients when they are in a quiet environment. Some patients note that the sound is synchronous with the pulse or that the sound diminishes if they put pressure on the carotid artery. Pulsatile tinnitus often is augmented with exercise, increased blood pressure, or a lateral recumbent position on the affected side. Thus, patients often complain that the sound is most bothersome when they are trying to go to sleep.

Differential Diagnosis

While a cervical bruit is most commonly associated with atherosclerotic stenosis of the internal carotid artery, other conditions can induce turbulence in the arteries or adjacent jugular veins (Table 5-1). Excessive pressure on a pliable carotid artery with the stethoscope can produce a temporary bruit in a child or a young adult. A focal

▶ **TABLE 5-1.** DIFFERENTIAL DIAGNOSIS OF A CERVICAL BRUIT

Atherosclerotic disease
   Stenosis of the internal carotid artery
   Stenosis of the external carotid artery
   Stenosis of the common carotid artery
   Stenosis of the subclavian artery
   Augmentation bruit
Other diseases of the cervical arteries
   Takayasu disease
   Fibromuscular dysplasia
   Arterial dissection
   Compression of the artery
   Arterial kink or loop
Transmitted cardiac murmur
Venous hum
High-flow states
   Cerebral arteriovenous malformation
   Dural arteriovenous malformation
   Carotid-cavernous fistula
   Vascular fistula in the arm (hemodialysis)
   Severe anemia
   Hyperthyroidism

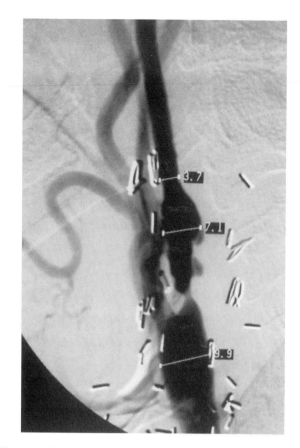

Figure 5-1. Angiogram stenosis origin ICA. Lateral view of a left carotid arteriogram demonstrates stenosis with an ulcerated plaque at the origin of the left internal carotid artery. The measurements are the estimates of the degree of narrowing, including an area of posteristenolie dilation. Chips from a prior contralateral carotid endarterectomy are also seen.

cervical bruit has a sensitivity and specificity of approximately 60 percent in predicting an underlying stenosis of more than 50 percent.[5,6] However, a bruit occurs only if there is sufficient flow to cause turbulence and sound. Thus, a patient with a very high-grade stenosis or occlusion of the internal carotid artery might not have a cervical bruit because the flow in the artery is minimal or nonexistent. In addition, bruits may also be secondary to atherosclerotic stenosis of the external carotid artery, common carotid artery, or subclavian artery. A cranial bruit also may result from stenosis of the intracavernous segment of the internal carotid artery. An augmentation bruit can be heard over the neck contralateral to an occlusion of the internal carotid artery.[4] In this situation, increased flow through the contralateral carotid artery, which is a primary source of collateral blood supply, produces turbulence that leads to confusion about which artery has the most serious disease. A loud continuous bruit that is present in both systole and diastole, especially in a child or young adult, should prompt consideration of a high-flow cerebral arteriovenous malformation or other high-flow states including severe anemia and hyperthyroidism. Dural arteriovenous fistulas at times produce pulsatile tinnitus and a cranial bruit.

Diagnostic Studies

The presence of an asymptomatic carotid bruit usually prompts evaluation of the relevant vessel with carotid duplex ultrasonography, computed tomographic angiography, magnetic resonance angiography, or conventional arteriography (see Chapter 8) (Fig. 5-1). The goal is to determine the presence and extent of local arterial disease. However, the physician should keep alternative diagnoses in mind. The absence of arterial pathology should prompt an assessment for an alternative explanation of the bruit, particularly intracranial pathology.

Asymptomatic Narrowing of the Internal Carotid Artery

Severe narrowing of the internal carotid artery not associated with either a bruit or other clinical findings may be detected during routine vascular evaluation. Asymptomatic narrowing of the internal carotid artery is detected in nearly 6 percent of healthy persons older than 75.[3] The arterial abnormality is most commonly found among elderly men. The asymptomatic stenosis may or may not be associated with the presence of a bruit. The usual scenarios for the detection of an asymptomatic stenosis include routine vascular imaging during a health fair or clinic visit, screening prior to a cardiovascular or another operation, or discovery during evaluation for contralateral carotid or vertebrobasilar symptoms.

Prognosis

The risk of stroke among patients with an asymptomatic bruit or stenosis of the internal carotid artery is much lower than that found among patients with recent ischemic symptoms. This correlation is not surprising because the underlying vascular atherosclerotic plaque has not become sufficiently unstable to induce thrombosis or embolism. The interaction between plaque instability or ulceration and symptomatology has been demonstrated by pathological examination of arterial specimens obtained by carotid endarterectomy. The rate of histologically identified intraplaque hemorrhage or ulceration among asymptomatic patients is much lower than that found among persons with recent ischemic symptoms. Still, a sizable percentage of patients with asymptomatic carotid stenosis have clinically covert ischemic lesions found on brain imaging studies. Thus, the prognosis of persons with asymptomatic stenoses of the internal carotid artery is not entirely benign. They have a higher risk of ischemic events than their peers. A reasonable estimate of the chance of an ipsilateral ischemic stroke is approximately 2 percent per year.[7,8] Some patients will have warning symptoms (TIA) prior to the stroke.[9] Additionally, carotid stenosis forecasts ischemic stroke in other vascular territories and predicts myocardial infarction and vascular death. However, the presence of an asymptomatic carotid bruit or stenosis does not portend a high stroke risk among patients having major operations, including cardiovascular procedures.[10,11] Thus, the presence of a stenosis is not a contraindication to surgery and prophylactic carotid endarterectomy is not necessary in this setting.

Treatment

Treatment options begin with aggressive management of risk factors. Halting smoking and controlling hypercholesterolemia and hypertension may slow the progression of the arterial narrowing. Most patients are treated with antiplatelet aggregating agents. Carotid endarterectomy or carotid angioplasty with stenting is often recommended when the arterial narrowing exceeds 60 percent.[7] (see Chapter 20). At present, carotid endarterectomy is the usual operative procedure to prevent stroke. The relative utility of carotid angioplasty and stenting has not yet been established in comparison to carotid endarterectomy (see Chapter 20).

▶ TRANSIENT ISCHEMIC ATTACK

Many patients, particularly elderly persons, complain of a brief, transient episode of neurological dysfunction and the diagnosis of TIA often is considered.[12,13] While not all episodes of transient neurological dysfunction represent a TIA, these events are relatively common. Brown et al.[14] estimated that the incidence of TIA in the carotid circulation was 38/100,000 and the frequency of TIA in the vertebrobasilar circulation was 14/100,000. However, this report is from the largely white population of Olmstead County, MN, and rates may differ in other ethnic groups and other parts of the world. These events occur in men and women of all ages, although most persons are older than 60.

While some reports list TIA as a risk factor for stroke, it should not be considered a separate entity or risk factor.[15] Rather, a TIA is secondary to thromboembolic occlusion of a blood vessel supplying the brain. In this event, the arterial occlusion resolves as the embolus is lysed or the collateral circulation improves sufficiently to resolve the patient's symptoms. Thus, a TIA could be considered as an ischemic stroke that spontaneously resolves. Therefore, a TIA represents the mildest form of symptomatic ischemic cerebrovascular disease.[16] Its greatest importance is that it denotes a change of the underlying vascular disease to a state yielding a high risk for stroke. While TIA is associated most commonly with atherosclerotic cerebrovascular disease, these events can also be secondary to other diseases including cardioembolism or thromboembolism arising from nonatherosclerotic vasculopathies.

Prognosis

In general, TIA is most strongly correlated with atherosclerotic disease of major intracranial or extracranial vessels. Because the TIA reflects instability of the underlying arterial pathology, the risk of a serious stroke is much higher among persons with warning symptoms than among persons with an asymptomatic arterial stenosis. While the overall risk of stroke within 5 years is estimated at 20 percent, this risk is front-loaded. Approximately 10 percent of strokes occur within 3 months of a TIA and nearly one-half of those events happen within 48 h.[13,17] Recently, Lovett et al.[18] found that the 7-day and 30-day risks of stroke following a first TIA were 8.6 and 12.0 percent, respectively. In addition, a TIA portends an increased risk of myocardial infarction or vascular death. The potentially ominous nature of TIA suggests that patients must seek immediate medical attention and that the health-care system should respond with alacrity.

However, not all transient vascular events have the same prognosis. Patients with *amaurosis fugax* have a better prognosis than those with focal hemispheric symptoms. Severe neurological impairments (such as a hemiparesis) or events lasting longer than 1 h appear to be more ominous than episodes that are brief (under 10 min) or associated with minor symptoms. A TIA that is present upon awakening in the morning or is associated with severe stenosis of the extracranial internal carotid artery also is accompanied with a high risk of stroke. Several events occurring in a short interval, typically defined as three or more events within a 24-h period (*crescendo TIA*), is particularly worrisome.[19,20] A TIA that is sufficiently severe to prompt a patient to visit an emergency room also appears to be especially dangerous. These events portend considerable instability in the underlying arterial disease.

Differential Diagnosis

The symptoms usually clear by the time a patient reaches medical attention and the diagnosis of TIA is inferred from the history obtained from the patient or observers.[21] The differential diagnosis is broader than for stroke.[22] Several other conditions mimic TIA and approximately one-third of patients with these conditions are misdiagnosed[21,23,24] (Table 5-2). Likewise, patients with TIA may be misdiagnosed with a mimicking condition. The symptoms of transient ischemia in the vertebrobasilar circulation are somewhat more nondescript and difficulties in accurate diagnosis are more likely to occur among patients with these events. In particular, lightheadedness, changes in clarity of thinking, sudden collapse, or loss of consciousness often are ascribed to TIA. The nuances that often help to differentiate TIA from other common causes of transient neurological symptoms are listed in Tables 5-3 and 5-4.

▶ **TABLE 5-2.** DIFFERENTIAL DIAGNOSIS OF TRANSIENT ISCHEMIC ATTACKS

Migraine
  Complex migraine with focal neurological symptoms
  Migraine equivalents (migraine without headache)
Transient global amnesia
Partial simple or generalized seizures
  Postictal impairments (Todd's paralysis)
Mass lesions that produce "transient" symptoms
  Subdural hematoma
  Brain tumor (most commonly glioma)
  Arteriovenous malformation
Metabolic disorders
  Hypoglycemia
  Hyponatremia
Primary labyrinthine diseases
  Meniere disease
  Benign positional vertigo
Syncope or presyncope
  Cardiac arrhythmias
  Orthostatic hypotension
  Side effects from medications
Conversion reaction

▶ **TABLE 5-3.** CLINICAL FEATURES OF TRANSIENT ISCHEMIC ATTACKS

Attacks are discrete with a defined onset and resolution
  Sudden onset of symptoms
  Symptoms are maximal at onset
  Symptoms should not spread from one body part to another
  Symptoms resolve slowly
  Attacks usually are not provoked
Duration of attacks is usually 5–20 min in duration
  Rarely attacks can last up to 1 h
Symptoms reflect dysfunction of one part of the brain
  Single vascular territory
  Loss of neurological function (negative symptoms)
    Weakness, heaviness, heaviness, or clumsiness
      Hand and one side of face
      One side of body
    Visual loss in one or both eyes
    Slurred speech
    Trouble understanding or producing language
Approximately 25% of events are associated with headaches
Involuntary movements are uncommon
Loss of consciousness or confusion is uncommon
Wooziness, dizziness, or lightheadedness usually is not a TIA

Clinical Findings

The definition of TIA is relatively clear. It is a discrete vascular event that causes dysfunction of one part of the brain. The diagnosis of TIA should be questioned if the patient or observers are unable to describe an onset and resolution of the event. A course of waxing and waning or gradual worsening over days to weeks is atypical; such symptoms are more suggestive of an intracranial mass, such as a subdural hematoma or tumor, rather than TIA.

While the description of TIA includes an extended time period (≤24 h), this time window is excessively broad. Most events last only a few minutes and a better time frame for a TIA should be less than 25 min.[25] In general, events lasting longer than 1 h are minor strokes.[12,13] On the other hand, very brief or fleeting events also likely are not due to thromboembolism. An episode that lasts a few seconds probably is not a TIA.

A TIA usually is also not provoked by positional changes or activities as often feared by elderly patients who presents with posturally related symptoms. Rarely, a TIA in the posterior circulation can be triggered by turning, flexion, or extension of the neck if the artery is compressed by a bony structure. In addition, the presence of a severe stenosis of the internal carotid artery or an intracranial vessel may be associated with a flow-related, limb-shaking TIA.[26] In this situation, a sudden

▶ **TABLE 5-4.** CLINICAL ASPECTS OF LEADING ALTERNATIVE DIAGNOSES TO TIA

Migraine
    Onset of neurological symptoms usually precede headache
    March of symptoms from one body part to another
        Visual—marching from periphery to center
            marching from right-to-left (vice versa)
            Sensory—paresthesias more than numbness
            Sensory symptoms more prominent than motor
    Visual symptoms usually are binocular
    Visual symptoms usually are positive (not loss of function)
        Scintillating scotoma, sparkles, or shimmering
        Fortification spectra or lightening bolts
        Can be followed by graying or loss of vision
    Migraine equivalents (above symptoms without headache)
    Headache usually is prominent (chief complaint)
        Unilateral, intense, and throbbing in quality
        Usually lasts longer than neurological symptoms
        Associated nausea, vomiting, photophobia, and phonophobia
Seizures
    Loss or alteration of consciousness usually is prominent
    May have aura (focal neurological symptoms) at onset
    March of symptoms from one body part to another
    Positive symptoms rather than loss of function
        Sensory—paresthesias more than numbness
        Motor—involuntary movements, jerking, or posturing
    Incontinence, tongue-biting, or sore muscles
    Residual weakness (Todd's paralysis) or mental status changes
    Can have residual headache
Brain tumor or subdural hematoma
    Symptoms usually are slowly evolving or worsening
    Symptoms usually not sudden onset but can wax and wane
    Symptoms accumulate over time
    Confusion or behavioral symptoms
    Headaches gradually increasing and not associated with events
Hypoglycemia
    Occurs primarily in diabetic patients taking insulin
    Symptoms usually are not sudden onset but gradually evolve
    Confusion and decreased alertness may be subtle
    Can have focal neurological impairments
Syncope
    Occur spontaneously or provoked by activity such as standing
    Sudden onset of symptoms
    Binocular visual blurring
    Dizziness, lightheadedness, or wooziness is prominent
    Brief loss of consciousness or collapse
    Focal weakness or numbness is uncommon
    Seizure activity not found
    Can be associated with chest pain or palpitations

drop in blood pressure such as that occurring when standing upright might induce hypoperfusion distal to the stenosis. While vertigo is a symptom of ischemia in the vertebrobasilar circulation, its occurrence as a solitary symptom usually is secondary to nonvascular diseases. Attacks of vertigo provoked by positional charges usually are not due to TIA. The development of vertigo with bending, head turning, or rolling over in bed is usually seen with primary labyrinthine diseases (benign positional vertigo).

In general, the neurological symptoms of TIA are of maximum severity at onset. A migration or a march of symptoms from one body part to another over several minutes is atypical. The presence of such a march suggests migraine or seizures as the likely diagnosis. Still, a patient may not be aware of all the neurological findings at symptom onset and thus might give a history suggesting a march. While the onset of neurological symptoms is sudden with TIA, their resolution may be gradual with devolution of findings over several minutes.

The symptoms of TIA are included in Table 5-3. Symptoms correspond to dysfunction of an area of the brain perfused by one artery.[27] Neurological symptoms that suggest impaired function of multiple brain areas or the entire brain simultaneously, such as giddiness, lightheadedness, dizziness, wooziness, confusion, or loss of consciousness, usually are not due to TIA, particularly if the symptoms are provoked by postural changes. Such symptoms usually reflect syncope or presyncope.[28] Very few patients collapse or lose consciousness during a TIA. Such events, including drop attacks, probably are secondary to seizures or hypoperfusion (syncope). Positive symptoms, such as bright visual phenomena or involuntary movements, usually occur with migraine or seizures rather than TIA (see Table 5-4). One exception is the limb-shaking TIA, which is relatively rare.

Nearly 25 percent of patients have headache, particularly with TIA in the vertebrobasilar circulation.[29] A TIA in the carotid circulation may be associated with a unilateral eye pain or headache ipsilateral to the affected hemisphere; an event in the vertebrobasilar circulation can have occipital or nuchal pain. Still, headache usually is not the chief complaint but if it is, the likelihood increases that migraine is the cause of the transient neurological symptoms. Nausea, vomiting, photophobia, and phonophobia usually do not occur with TIA.

Transient changes in cognition, memory, or thinking usually are not secondary to TIA. In such circumstances, a seizure is more likely. In addition, patients older than 60 may have isolated events of amnesia that can persist for several hours (*transient global amnesia*). During one of the episodes, the patient appears confused and repetitively attempts to become oriented to time and other recent events. Other neurological signs, such as language disturbances or visual loss, are absent. This condition, which may be secondary to a metabolic or vasospastic event causing hippocampal dysfunction, should not be diagnosed as a TIA. In general, the prognosis of persons with transient global amnesia is excellent. Rarely patients may have one or more recurrent episodes, but this does not appear to be associated with a high risk for ischemic stroke.

Carotid TIA

The symptoms of TIA in the carotid circulation generally differ from those that occur with ischemia in the vertebrobasilar circulation[27] (Table 5-5). Some symptoms, such as dysarthria or unilateral limb weakness, may occur with transient ischemia in either circulation. In such circumstances, the history of other symptoms such as aphasia, vertigo, or visual loss may help distinguish the symptomatic circulation. The simultaneous occurrence of vertigo, ataxia, bilateral motor or sensory symptoms, and dysarthria are suggestive of an event in the posterior circulation. Visual loss in a pattern of homonymous hemianopia may occur with ischemia in either the anterior or posterior circulation. The physician should differentiate this symptom from amaurosis fugax, although such a distinction can be difficult. Patients should be asked to distinguish visual loss on one side (the right field, for example) from that occurring in one eye. Many patients will not be able to do so. In general, a homonymous visual loss occurs simultaneously with other neurological symptoms, while amaurosis fugax is most often an isolated symptom. One of the sources of confusion about the involved vascular territory may be due to anatomic variations in the origin of

▶ **TABLE 5-5.** SYMPTOMS OF TIA IN THE CAROTID AND VERTEBROBASILAR CIRCULATIONS

Carotid circulation
  Ipsilateral amaurosis fugax (transient monocular
    blindness)
  Contralateral weakness, numbness, or clumsiness
    Face and arm usually affected more than leg
  Contralateral homonymous hemianopia
  Aphasia (with dominant hemisphere ischemia)
  Dysarthria
Vertebrobasilar circulation
  Binocular visual loss (blurring)
  Vertigo
  Weakness, numbness, clumsiness, or incoordination
    Unilateral (contralateral) weakness, numbness
    Unilateral (ipsilateral) incoordination, limb ataxia
    Bilateral
    Crossed (ipsilateral face and contralateral limbs)
  Gait ataxia
  Diplopia
  Dysarthria

the posterior cerebral artery; in 20 percent of cases, the artery is a branch of the internal carotid artery.

Symptoms in the carotid circulation involve ischemia in the ipsilateral eye or cerebral hemisphere. Although patients may have both retinal and hemispheric symptoms, these events usually do not occur simultaneously. Patients with either retinal or neurological symptoms should be quizzed about the occurrence of other symptoms. In particular, patients often ignore transient monocular visual symptoms that do not lead to complete monocular blindness. The symptoms of retinal ischemia are discussed later in this chapter. The most common neurological symptoms are contralateral weakness or numbness of the hand, arm, or lower face. Rather than presenting with complete paralysis, patients often describe the hand as being heavy, clumsy, or not working correctly. Physicians should not exhaustively attempt to differentiate the symptoms of weakness (presumably motor loss) from numbness (presumably sensory loss) because patients often have great difficulty distinguishing between these transient symptoms.[21] In addition, such differentiation does not add much precision to the diagnosis. Most patients have simultaneous hand and facial symptoms. The diagnosis of TIA may be difficult when a patient has transient symptoms restricted to the hand because a peripheral nerve or radicular lesion may cause intermittent limb dysfunction. Involvement of a portion of the hand or individual digits is rarely due to TIA. Pain or paresthesias (needles and pins) usually do not occur with TIA. Facial symptoms are described as numbness (such as that occurring with local anesthesia for a dental procedure) by the patient, although observers often notice sagging or drooping of one side of the face or an asymmetry in the smile. Observers are often confused; they might say the normal side is "drawn up" when in fact the abnormal side is sagging. The facial symptoms generally involve the cheek and the mouth, although buccal or tongue symptoms can happen. The tongue symptoms usually are unilateral and ipsilateral to other facial symptoms. While paresthesias restricted to the lips (corner of the mouth), tongue, and hand (*cheiro-oral syndrome*) may occur with TIA, migraine is an important alternative diagnosis. In general, numbness or weakness of the lower limb alone or in conjunction with the upper limb is relatively infrequent. However, if the patient has an event while walking or standing, a gait disturbance including dragging of the leg may be reported. Rarely, a transient dystonic movement, posturing, or shaking of the limb may occur but these symptoms usually are restricted to the upper limb.

A language disturbance may occur with ischemia in the dominant hemisphere, but since patients are often alone during the attack, this symptom is not reported as frequently as numbness or weakness. Observers often report the language disturbance because they recognize that the patient is not speaking clearly or making sense.

Commonly, detection of the language problem occurs during a telephone conversation. The language problem may be described as confusion, nonsensical speech, or trouble finding words. A transient episode of aphasia (primarily a language deficit) should be differentiated from dysarthria (abnormal articulation but with normal language). A listener usually describes the latter as slurred or indistinct speech. Patients use the correct words but their articulation is abnormal. In some cases, the dysarthria is so severe that the speech is not comprehensible. Sometimes the speech abnormality can be associated with motor impairments and the pattern of motor signs can help distinguish dysarthria or aphasia. For example, a speech disturbance reflecting dysfunction of the nondominant (right) hemisphere usually is dysarthria. Presumably, a TIA in the nondominant hemisphere could have symptoms of neglect, but the subtle nature of these signs indicates that most patients and observers do not recognize them.

Vertebrobasilar TIA

The symptoms of TIA in the vertebrobasilar circulation are secondary to dysfunction of the brainstem, ear, cerebellum, diencephalon, or medial and posterior aspects of the cerebral hemispheres (see Table 5-5). Because some symptoms of posterior circulation TIA overlap with those of global ischemia or presyncope, diagnosing the events can be difficult. In addition, the diversity of symptoms in the posterior circulation may lead to misdiagnoses. While some patients have isolated symptoms, most will have a combination of complaints reflecting multiple areas of brain and brainstem/cerebellar dysfunction. Vertigo (not dizziness or lightheadedness) and binocular visual symptoms (blurring or loss of vision) are the two most common symptoms.[22,30] True vertigo (spinning or whirling) should be differentiated from wooziness or a sense of imbalance. Simultaneously, many patients describe nonspecific fuzziness or blurring of vision. Unfortunately, neither vertigo nor blurred vision, when occurring alone, is particularly specific for a vertebrobasilar TIA. Isolated vertigo is more likely to be due to a primary labyrinthine disease than due to transient ischemia.[22] If the visual disturbance is defined with more precision, the diagnosis of occipital ischemia may be included. Loss of vision (blackening) in part of the visual field would be more suggestive of ischemia than a distortion of visual clarity or positive visual phenomena such as sparkles, shimmers, or jagged bright lines. Patients with complaints of transient vertigo or binocular visual loss should be queried closely for other neurological symptoms because the presence of these symptoms strengthens the likelihood of TIA.

Motor or sensory symptoms occurring with vertebrobasilar TIA often are complicated or confusing to the clinician. The symptoms may be unilateral, crossed, or bilateral. Separating a transient episode of unilateral weakness secondary to vertebrobasilar ischemia from that secondary to carotid ischemia may be particularly difficult. A transient attack with right-sided weakness or sensory loss followed by a transient episode of symptoms on the left (*alternating hemiparesis*) much more likely represents pontine ischemia secondary to basilar artery disease than nearly simultaneous attacks in both carotid circulations. The presence of vertigo, imbalance, binocular visual dysfunction, severe dysarthria, or diplopia provides support for the diagnosis of vertebrobasilar TIA as the cause of a transient episode of hemiparesis. Circumoral numbness or tingling that involves the tongue, buccal mucosa, and both sides of the face may develop with transient ischemia in the brainstem but not with carotid circulation events. A sense of imbalance (ataxia) is relatively common and it should be differentiated from vertigo. Observers may report clumsiness or incoordination of the limbs, or a staggering gait, that at times leads to a fall. While bilateral ischemia of the basis pontis can lead to quadriparesis and collapse (*drop attack*), these events are uncommon.[31]

The *subclavian steal syndrome*, a rare but possible cause of vertebrobasilar ischemia, usually occurs with a severe stenosis or occlusion of the proximal portion of the left subclavian artery.[32–34] While angiographic evidence of subclavian steal in which, for example, blood rises in the right vertebral artery and is diverted down the left vertebral artery to perfuse the left arm can be found, the associated clinical syndrome is relatively rare. The typical scenario is symptoms of vertebrobasilar TIA provoked by vigorous exercise of the arm, most commonly the left.

Examination

Most TIA resolve before a physician sees the patient and usually the neurological examination is normal. Still, the physical examination provides clues that support the diagnosis of TIA and likely cause. For example, evaluation of the ear may provide evidence of a nonvascular cause of vertigo. The presence of persisting neurological impairments may mean that the patient has had a stroke or that a nonvascular cause of the symptoms is present. If the patient is seen during a TIA, the neurological deficits should match the symptoms. The general examination also may provide evidence for a nonvascular cause of the patient's symptoms. The vital signs provide information about the patient's overall health and the presence of risk factors, such as hypertension. Asymmetry of the blood pressure or strength of the pulses between the two arms suggests possible severe stenosis or occlusion of a subclavian artery. The presence of an irregular pulse, cardiac murmur, or cardiomegaly provides important evidence for TIA or cardiogenic syncope as the cause of the neurological symptoms. The presence of a cervical bruit, especially ipsilateral to the symptomatic internal carotid artery, also provides supportive evidence for the diagnosis of TIA. However, auscultation of a bruit should not automatically lead to the diagnosis of TIA particularly if the patient had atypical symptoms.

Diagnostic Studies

The goals of the evaluation are to confirm TIA as the cause of the patient's symptoms, to help determine the symptomatic vascular territory, and to establish the most likely etiology of the TIA. In general, brain imaging studies are done to exclude an intracranial mass or a stroke. An electroencephalogram may help exclude seizures. Vascular and cardiac imaging and hematological, coagulation, biochemistry, and immunological studies are done to screen for other etiologies that mimic TIA. The components of the evaluation are described in more detail in Chapter 8.

Treatment

The management of patients with TIA involves management of risk factors, antithrombotic medications, and local therapies, including surgery or endovascular interventions. The prescription of the HMG-CoA reductase inhibitors (statins) and newer antihypertensive agents (particularly the angiotensin converting enzyme inhibitors or angiotensin receptor blockers) are efficacious in reducing the chances of stroke among high-risk patients (see Chapter 4). Antithrombotic agents are usually prescribed (see Chapter 19). Some patients require treatment with carotid endarterectomy, while others require reconstructive operations or endovascular procedures (see Chapter 20).

► OCULAR MANIFESTATIONS OF CEREBROVASCULAR DISEASE

Abnormal ocular findings (symptoms or signs) are found in a sizable percentage of patients with hemorrhagic or ischemic cerebrovascular disease (Table 5-6). In some cases, ocular findings may be the primary manifestation of vascular disease. The most common symptom is the transient monocular loss of vision (amaurosis fugax). The symptoms may include blurring, graying, or blackening of vision in the part or all of the visual field in the eye. It is distinctly unusual for both eyes to be affected simultaneously, given the embolic nature of these events. Permanent monocular visual loss that occurs suddenly is usually due to vascular disease and can be due to central retinal artery occlusion, branch retinal artery occlusion, or anterior ischemic optic neuropathy. The latter is due to an infarction of the optic nerve.

Abnormalities of perfusion to the eye may be used to evaluate the extent of extracranial and proximal

► **TABLE 5-6.** OCULAR MANIFESTATIONS OF CEREBROVASCULAR DISEASE

Hemorrhagic stroke
  Conjunctival or extraocular hemorrhages
  Intraocular hemorrhages (subhyloid)
  Papilledema
  Hypertensive retinopathy
Amaurosis fugax
Retinal changes for underlying disease
  Hypertensive retinopathy
  Diabetic retinopathy
  Retinal intra-arterial embolus
    Fibrin-platelet
    Cholesterol embolus (Hollenhorst plaque)
  Roth spot
Acute partial or total monocular visual loss
  Anterior ischemic optic neuropathy
  Central retinal artery occlusion
  Branch retinal artery occlusion
  Retinal pallor
  Optic disk atrophy
Venous stasis retinopathy
Chronic ocular ischemia
  Retinal microaneurysms
  Retinal hemorrhages
  Optic disk edema
  Chemosis and conjunctival hyperemia
  Glaucoma
  Corneal edema
  Rubeosis iridis
Cavernous sinus thrombosis

intracranial atherosclerotic disease because the ophthalmic artery is the first major branch of the internal carotid artery. This relationship was the basis of some of the first clinical tools to evaluate patients with extracranial atherosclerosis. In the past, ophthalmologists performed *central retinal artery pressure* measurements using tonometry during direct visualization of the ocular fundus. A difference in pressure between the two eyes pointed to severe disease of the internal carotid artery on the side ipsilateral to the lower reading, suggesting compromised flow to the eye ipsilateral to a severe stenosis. *Directional Doppler* evaluation was used to determine the direction of the flow of the supraorbital artery, a branch of the ophthalmic artery. In normal individuals, the flow is toward the face but with severe disease of the internal carotid artery the flow reverses and moves intracranially. Neither of these tests is specific or sensitive and they have been abandoned in favor of better noninvasive diagnostic tests. However, examination of the eye may provide supportive evidence of underlying vascular disease. Chronic hypertension may lead to a retinopathy with arterial narrowing, retinal hemorrhages, and cotton-wool spots. Diabetic retinopathy or changes consistent with a vasculitis may also be detected. Fluorescein angiography can be used to detect disturbances of retinal blood flow. Detection of a postganglionic Horner syndrome can point to a dissection of the internal carotid artery as the cause of a hemispheric stroke.

► OCULAR CHANGES IN HEMORRHAGIC STROKE

Approximately 20–25 percent of patients with hemorrhagic stroke have concomitant ocular hemorrhages.[35] These are found most commonly following severe (coma producing) subarachnoid hemorrhage. Most commonly, the blood is found within the eye—*subhyloid hemorrhages*[36] (Fig. 5-2). The presence of intraocular bleeding is an important clue for an intracranial hemorrhage as a cause of nontraumatic coma. A reasonable rule of thumb is to assume that intracranial hemorrhage is the underlying cause of coma in any patient who also has an intraocular hemorrhage. Subconjunctival hemorrhages also can occur with intracranial bleeding.[37] In addition, the ophthalmoscopic examination may reveal optic disk edema (papilledema) or retinal hemorrhages associated with hypertensive disease or increased intracranial pressure. These findings may suggest a major intracranial hemorrhage or venous thrombosis. The presence of hypertensive changes in the retina may point toward chronic

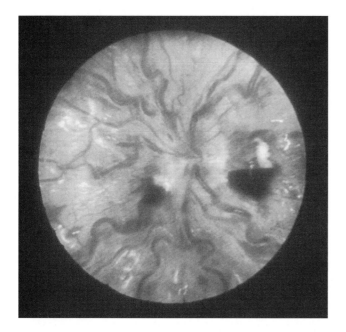

Figure 5-2. Subhyloid (preretinal hemorrhage) found in left eye of an elderly woman with an occlusion of the central retinal vein. Similar findings can be seen with subarachnoid hemorrhage. (*Courtesy of Daniel Jacobson, M.D., Marshfield Clinic, Marshfield, WI.*)

hypertension as the cause of an intracerebral hemorrhage. Additionally, a carotid-cavernous fistula can produce proptosis, chemosis, and a cranial bruit.[38] Vascular malformations or aneurysms also can produce oculomotor palsies or visual field deficits.[38]

► OCULAR CHANGES IN ISCHEMIC DISEASE

Amaurosis Fugax

Amaurosis fugax is the most specific symptom of transient ischemia in the carotid circulation.[39,40] The usual cause is embolization to the central retinal artery or its branches. Ocular symptoms generally are not due to hemodynamic events.[41] The occurrence of amaurosis fugax is a strong piece of evidence of severe atherosclerotic disease of the ipsilateral internal carotid artery.[41] While the classic description of amaurosis fugax is that of a descending curtain covering part of the visual field, which reflects the vascular supply to the eye that respects the horizon, most patients will describe painless blurring, fuzziness, or graying of vision in one eye. Complete loss of the vision can occur. Some patients with ischemia attributed to hypoperfusion will note a gradual loss of vision from the periphery with preservation of central vision.[42] Very rarely, positive visual phenomena including sparkles, shimmers, or bright spots are reported. In addition, some patients with very poor perfusion of the eye report the loss of vision (gray out) provoked by sudden exposure to bright light.[43,44] This event presumably is due to a sudden increase in metabolic demands that overwhelms the vascular reserve. It usually is seen among patients with occlusion or severe narrowing of the internal carotid artery or ophthalmic artery. Attacks of amaurosis fugax are usually shorter than TIA; most lasting a few seconds or minutes. In general, retinal ischemic symptoms correlate strongly with the presence of severe atherosclerotic disease of the ipsilateral internal carotid artery.[45]

Most patients are not seen during an attack. However, examination of the retina during an attack may demonstrate a fibrin-platelet embolus within a retinal artery (Fig. 5-3). These intra-arterial lesions, pale white in appearance, are rarely seen because they lyse before the patient can be examined. A cholesterol embolus (Hollenhorst plaque) is found more frequently because these emboli persist for some time[46,47] (Fig. 5-4). Cholesterol emboli are highly refractile and found at the bifurcation of the retinal arteries. The usual source of these emboli, which represent pieces of atherosclerotic debris, is an ulcerated plaque of the internal carotid artery or the aorta. At times, a Hollenhorst plaque may be found during examination of a patient who denies any visual symptoms.[48,49] The presence of retinal emboli is associated with risk factors for atherosclerosis and an increased

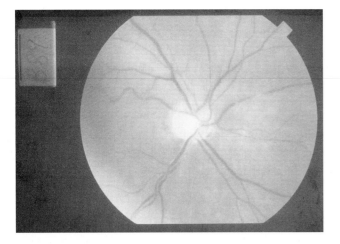

Figure 5-3. Ophthalmoscopic examination of the right eye shows a fibrin-platelet embolus in a branch retinal artery in a patient with amaurosis fugax. (*Courtesy of Daniel Jacobson, M.D., Marshfield Clinic, Marshfield, WI.*)

risk of stroke-related death.[50] A branch retinal artery infarction with a segmental area of pallor of the fundus may be seen.

However, not all transient episodes of visual dysfunction are due to ischemia. *Retinal (ocular) migraine* is an important diagnostic consideration for the cause of transient monocular visual loss in a young person. The symptoms presumably are due to vasospasm. Unlike episodes of amaurosis fugax, these attacks can be accompanied by photopsia and other positive phenomena. Central vision is not lost. In addition, most attacks are associated with headache. Occasionally, retinal migraine may be induced by exercise.

Persistent Ocular Ischemia

An occlusion or severe stenosis of the extracranial internal carotid artery may lead to gradually evolving but *persistent ocular ischemia* due to hypoperfusion. Initially, patients may have transient visual loss that evolves over a few minutes and then persists for several minutes to hours. Occasionally, vision may be lost from the periphery to the center of the field. Postural changes or bright lights may induce the transient symptoms. As the ischemia progresses, changes occur in the anterior segment of the eye (see Table 5-6). Aching pain in the orbit and temple develops. Subsequently, increased intraocular pressure (*neovascular glaucoma*) or a cataract may appear.[51]

Venous Stasis Retinopathy

Venous stasis retinopathy is secondary to persistently low retinal artery pressure that results in sluggish perfusion to the eye.[52,53] The slow arterial flow leads to stagnation in the venous circulation. Findings include microaneurysms, peripheral small retinal hemorrhages, segmental narrowing and dilation of the retinal veins, and swelling of the optic disk (Figs. 5-5 and 5-6). The changes appear similar to those found with diabetic retinopathy.

Retinal Artery Occlusions

Occlusion of the central retinal artery causes sudden, painless, complete loss of vision in one eye[53] (Fig. 5-7). The occlusion usually is due to local arterial thrombosis, embolism from the heart or a proximal atherosclerotic plaque, arteritis, or rarely migraine. The patient has blindness in the eye and an amaurotic pupil (afferent

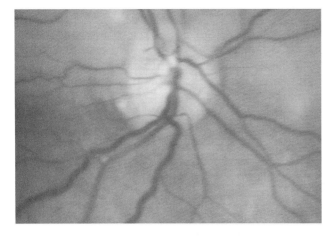

Figure 5-4. Ophthalmoscopic examination of the right eye shows calcific emboli in the proximal segment of the superior branch of the central retinal artery. (*Courtesy of Daniel Jacobson, M.D., Marshfield Clinic, Marshfield, WI.*)

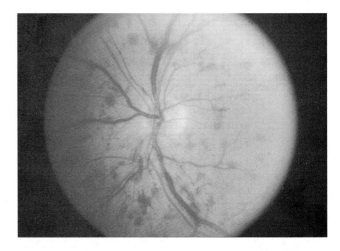

Figure 5-5. Venous stasis retinopathy visualized in the left eye of an elderly man with severe atherosclerotic disease of the internal and external carotid arteries. Note the presence of hemorrhages and the dilated veins. (*Courtesy of Daniel Jacobson, M.D., Marshfield Clinic, Marshfield, WI.*)

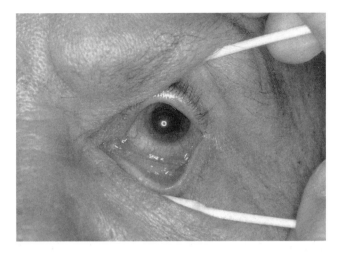

Figure 5-6. Direct visualization of the eye of a patient with severe venous stasis retinopathy shows a large poorly reactive pupil, a cataract, and dilated conjunctival veins. (*Courtesy of Daniel Jacobson, M.D., Marshfield Clinic, Marshfield, WI.*)

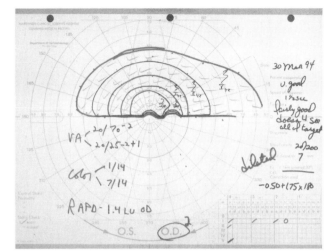

Figure 5-8. Altitudinal loss of the inferior visual field is demonstrated from a branch retinal artery infarction. (*Courtesy of Daniel Jacobson, M.D., Marshfield Clinic, Marshfield, WI.*)

pupillary defect). Intraocular pressure often is reduced. On visualization of the fundus, boxcar segmental narrowing of the arteries, pallor of the retina, and a cherry-red macula are seen. Emboli can also be visualized and eventually optic atrophy develops. Treatment options include ocular massage, anterior chamber paracentesis, and thrombolytic therapy.[54]

A *branch retinal artery occlusion* usually is secondary to embolism (Figs. 5-8 and 5-9). The patient typically presents with sudden onset of a persistent loss of vision in one part of the visual field. Usually the defect is quadrantic, although the visual loss can involve either

the superior or inferior hemifields. An embolus often is found on ophthalmoscopic examination. An area of retinal pallor corresponding to the occluded branch may be visualized.

Anterior Ischemic Optic Neuropathy

Infarction of the optic nerve is an important cause of sudden visual loss among persons older than 60. *Anterior ischemic optic neuropathy* usually is due to arteritic

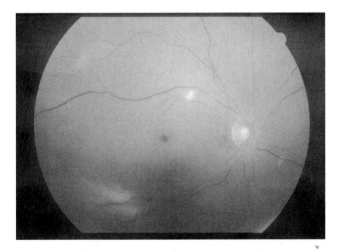

Figure 5-7. Ophthalmoscopic examination of the right eye in a patient with a central retinal artery occlusion shows a cherry red foveal spot, boxcar arteriolar flow, and attenuated arteries. (*Courtesy of Daniel Jacobson, M.D, Marshfield Clinic, Marshfield, WI.*)

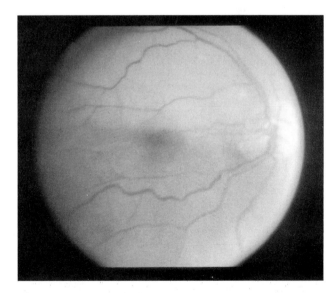

Figure 5-9. Ophthalmoscopic examination of the right eye in a patient with an occlusion with the superior branch of the central retinal artery shows a whitish appearing retina in the superior portion of the eye. (*Courtesy of Daniel Jacobson, M.D., Marshfield Clinic, Marshfield, WI.*)

involvement of the posterior ciliary artery among persons with *giant cell (temporal) arteritis.* Occasionally, the arterial occlusion can be secondary to embolism or diabetic small artery disease.[55] The usual course is the sudden onset of complete visual loss in one eye. Patients with ischemic optic neuropathy usually have a history of headaches, polymyalgia rheumatica, or jaw claudication, and often are markers of underlying giant cell arteritis. On examination, the patient has an afferent pupillary defect and markedly decreased visual acuity. The optic disk is pale and swollen (see Chapter 12).

REFERENCES

1. Ingall TJ, Homer D, Whisnant JP, Baker HLJ, O'Fallon WM. Predictive value of carotid bruit for carotid atherosclerosis. *Arch Neurol* 1989;46:418–422.

2. Norris JW. Risk of cerebral infarction, myocardial infarction and vascular death in patients with asymptomatic carotid disease, transient ischemic attack and stroke. *Cerebrovasc Dis* 1992;2(suppl):2–5.

3. Josse MO, Touboul PJ, Mas JL, Laplane D, Bousser MG. Prevalence of asymptomatic internal carotid artery stenosis. *Neuroepidemiology* 1987;6:150–152.

4. Chambers BR, Norris JW. Clinical significance of asymptomatic neck bruits. *Neurology* 1985;35:742–745.

5. Sauve JS, Thorpe KE, Sackett DL, et al. Can bruits distinguish high-grade from moderate symptomatic carotid stenosis? The North American Symptomatic Carotid Endarterectomy Trial. *Ann Intern Med* 1994;120:633–637.

6. Sauve JS, Laupacis A, Ostbye T, Feagan B, Sackett DL. Does this patient have a clinically important carotid bruit? *JAMA* 1993;270:2843–2845.

7. Executive Committee for the Asymptomatic Carotid Atherosclerosis Study. Endarterectomy for asymptomatic carotid artery stenosis. *JAMA* 1995;273:1421–1428.

8. Olin JW, Fonseca C, Childs MB, Piedmonte MR, Hertzer NR, Young JR. The natural history of asymptomatic moderate internal carotid artery stenosis by duplex ultrasound. *Vasc Med* 1998;3:101–108.

9. Bogousslavsky J, Despland PA, Regli F. Asymptomatic tight stenosis of the internal carotid aartery: Long-term prognosis. *Neurology* 1986;36:861–863.

10. Hart RG, Easton JD. Management of cervical bruits and carotid stenosis in preoperative patients. *Stroke* 1983;14: 290–297.

11. Ropper AH, Wechsler LR, Wilson LS. Carotid bruit and the risk of stroke in elective surgery. *N Engl J Med* 1982;307: 1388–1390.

12. Johnston SC. Clinical practice. Transient ischemic attack. *N Engl J Med* 2002;347:1687–1692.

13. Johnston SC. Transient ischemic attack. *N Engl J Med* 2002; 347:1687–1692.

14. Brown RD, Jr., Petty GW, O'Fallon WM, Wiebers DO, Whisnant JP. Incidence of transient ischemic attack in Rochester, Minnesota, 1985–1989. *Stroke* 1998;29:2109–2113.

15. Albers GW, Caplan LR, Easton JD, et al. Transient ischemic attack—proprosal for a new definition. *N Engl J Med* 2002; 347:1713–1716.

16. Koudstaal PJ, van Gijn J, Frenken CW, et al. TIA, RIND, minor stroke: A continuum, or different subgroups? Dutch TIA Study Group. *J Neurol Neurosurg Psychiatry* 1992;55: 95–97.

17. Johnston SC, Gress DR, Browner WS, Sidney S. Short-term prognosis after emergency department diagnosis of TIA. *JAMA* 2000;284:2901–2906.

18. Lovett JK, Dennis MS, Sandercock PA, Bamford J, Warlow CP, Rothwell PM. Very early risk of stroke after a first transient ischemic attack. *Stroke* 2003;34:e138–e140.

19. Crespo M, Melo TP, Oliveira V, Ferro JM. Clustering transient ischemic attacks. *Cerebrovasc Dis* 1993;3:213–220.

20. Rothrock JF, Lyden PD, Yee J, Wiederholt WC. 'Crescendo' transient ischemic attacks: Clinical and angiographic correlations. *Neurology* 1988;38:198–201.

21. Price TR, Gotshall RA, Poskanzer DC, et al. Cooperative study of hospital frequency and character of transient ischemic attacks. VI. Patients examined during an attack. *JAMA* 1977;238:2512–2515.

22. Hotson JR, Baloh RW. Acute vestibular syndrome. *N Engl J Med* 1998;339:680–685.

23. Ferro JM, Falcao I, Rodrigues G, et al. Diagnosis of transient ischemic attack by the nonneurologist. A validation study. *Stroke* 1996;27:2225–2229.

24. Kraaijeveld CL, van Gijn J, Schouten HJ, Staal A. Interobserver agreement for the diagnosis of transient ischemic attacks. *Stroke* 1984;15:723–725.

25. Kimura K, Minematsu K, Yasaka M, Wada K, Yamaguchi T. The duration of symptoms in transient ischemic attack. *Neurology* 1999;52:976–980.

26. Leira EC, Ajax T, Adams HP, Jr. Limb-shaking carotid transient ischemic attacks successfully treated with modification of the antihypertensive regimen. *Arch Neurol* 1997;54: 904–905.

27. Futty DE, Conneally M, Dyken ML, et al. Cooperative study of hospital frequency and character of transient ischemic attacks. V. Symptom analysis. *JAMA* 1977;238: 2386–2390.

28. Koudstaal PJ, Algra A, Pop GA, Kappelle LJ, van Latum JC, van Gijn J. Risk of cardiac events in atypical transient ischaemic attack or minor stroke. The Dutch TIA Study Group. *Lancet* 1992;340:630–633.

29. Koudstaal PJ, van Gijn J, Kappelle LJ. Headache in transient or permanent cerebral ischemia. Dutch TIA Study Group. *Stroke* 1991;22:754–759.

30. Gomez CR, Cruz-Flores S, Malkoff MD, Sauer CM, Burch CM. Isolated vertigo as a manifestation of vertebrobasilar ischemia. *Neurology* 1996;47:94–97.

31. Brust JCM, Plank CR, Healton EB, Sanchez GF. The pathology of drop attacks. A case report. *Neurology* 1979;29: 786–790.

32. Fields WS, Lemak NA. Joint Study of Extracranial Arterial Occlusion. VII. Subclavian steal—a review of 168 cases. *JAMA* 1972;222:1139–1143.

33. Hennerici M, Klemm C, Rautenberg W. The subclavian steal phenomenon: A common vascular disorder with rare neurologic deficits. *Neurology* 1988;38:669–673.

34. Zelenock GB, Cronenwett JL, Graham LM, et al. Brachiocephalic arterial occlusions and stenoses. Manifestations and management of complex lesions. *Arch Surg* 1985;120:370–376.

35. Keane JR. Retinal hemorrhages. Its significance in 100 patients with acute encephalopathy of unknown cause. *Arch Neurol* 1979;36:691–694.

36. Choudhari KA, Pherwani AA, Gray WJ. Terson's syndrome as the sole presentation of aneurysmal rupture. *Br J Neurosurg* 2003;17:355–357.

37. Gondim FA, Leacock RO. Subconjunctival hemorrhages secondary to hypersympathetic state after a small diencephalic hemorrhage. *Arch Neurol* 2004;60:1803–1804.

38. Biousse V, Mendicino ME, Simon DJ, Newman NJ. The ophthalmology of intracranial vascular abnormalities. *Am J Ophthalmol* 1998;125:527–544.

39. Adams HP, Jr., Putman SF, Corbett JJ, Sires BP, Thompson HS. Amaurosis fugax: The results of arteriography in 59 patients. *Stroke* 1983;14:742–744.

40. Burde RM. Amaurosis fugax. *J Clin Neuro-Ophthalmol* 1989;9:185–189.

41. Anderson DC, Kappelle LJ, Eliasziw M, Babikian VL, Pearce LA, Barnett HJM. Occurance of hemispheric and retinal ischemia in atrial fibrillation compared with carotid stenosis. *Stroke* 2002;33:1963–1968.

42. Bruno A, Corbett JJ, Biller J, Adams HP, Jr., Qualls C. Transient monocular visual loss patterns and associated vascular abnormalities. *Stroke* 1990;21:34–39.

43. Wiebers DO, Swanson JW, Cascino TL, Whisnant JP. Bilateral loss of vision in bright light. *Stroke* 1989;20:554–558.

44. Furlan AJ, Whisnant JP, Kearns TP. Unilateral visual loss in bright light. An unusual symptom of carotid artery occlusive disease. *Arch Neurol* 1979;36:675–676.

45. Lawrence PF, Oderich GS. Ophthalmologic findings as predictors of carotid artery disease. *Vasc Endovascular Surg* 2002;36:415–424.

46. Hollenhorst RW. The ocular manifestations of internal carotid artery thrombosis. *Med Clin N Am* 1960;44: 897–908.

47. Klein R, Klein BE, Jensen SC, Moss SE, Meuer SM. Retinal emboli and stroke: The Beaver Dam Eye Study. *Arch Ophthalmol* 1999;117:1063–1068.

48. Bruno A, Russell PW, Jones WL, Austin JK, Weinstein ES, Steel SR. Concomitants of asymptomatic retinal cholesterol emboli. *Stroke* 1992;23:900–902.

49. Bruno A, Jones WL, Austin JK, Carter S, Qualls C. Vascular outcome in men with asymptomatic retinal cholesterol emboli. *Ann Intern Med* 1995;122:249–253.

50. Klein R, Klein BE, Moss SE, Meuer SM. Retinal emboli and cardiovascular disease: The Beaver Dam Eye Study. *Arch Ophthalmol* 2003;121:1446–1451.

51. Biousse V, Touboul PJ, d'Anglejan-Chatillon J, Levy C, Schaison M, Bousser MG. Ophthalmologic manifestations of internal carotid artery dissection. *Am J Ophthalmol* 1998;126:565–577.

52. Klijn CJM, Kappelle LJ, van Schooneveld MJ, et al. Venous stasis retinopathy in symptomatic carotid artery occlusion: Prevalence, cause, and outcome. *Stroke* 2002;33:695–701.

53. Biousse V. Carotid disease and the eye. *Curr Opin Ophthalmol* 1997;8:16–26.

54. Rumelt S, Brown GC. Update on treatment of retinal arterial occlusions. *Curr Opin Ophthalmol* 2003;14:139–141.

55. Fry CL, Carter JE, Kanter MC, Tegeler CH, Tuley MR. Anterior ischemic optic neuropathy is not associated with carotid artery atherosclerosis. *Stroke* 1993;24:539–542.

CHAPTER 6

Clinical Manifestations of Ischemic Stroke

The diagnosis of ischemic stroke is based on the patient's history and the results of the physical and neurological examinations. Diagnostic studies, including brain imaging, should be considered as tools that support the clinical diagnosis. Because many of the findings on examination can occur with other neurological conditions, including hemorrhagic stroke, the history of the illness becomes key (Table 6-1). In addition, the history and pattern of the impairments should reflect involvement of one part or one vascular territory of the brain. Because arterial perfusion is fairly stereotyped, clinical findings generally are relatively similar among patients. The deficits usually represent damage to an area of brain perfused by one intracranial artery (Fig. 6-1). In general, the alternative diagnoses included in Table 6-1 are excluded by the time course, the pattern of neurological impairments, and the presence of headache, nausea, vomiting, or decreased consciousness. Several clinical features outlined in Table 6-2 point to an ischemic stroke as the cause of the patient's neurological deficits.

▶ DIFFERENTIAL DIAGNOSIS OF ISCHEMIC STROKE

The list of alternative diagnoses to ischemic stroke is relatively limited (see Table 6-1). Although 5–15 percent of patients suspected as having ischemic stroke subsequently are diagnosed with another neurological illness, most of these disorders also are potentially serious.[1,2] The mimics are as important as stroke itself. Hemorrhagic stroke is the most important alternative diagnosis because both conditions present with prominent focal neurological impairments of sudden onset. The clinical features by history and examination that point to hemorrhagic stroke are given in Table 6-3. Because management of hemorrhagic stroke differs markedly from that prescribed to patients with ischemic stroke, differentiating the two disorders is the foremost step in emergent evaluation.[3] In general, headache and depression of consciousness are more severe among patients with a hemorrhage. In addition, nausea and vomiting occurring together with other neurological signs that point to a hemispheric stroke also portend an intracranial hemorrhage. Still, some patients with minor hemorrhages might not have altered consciousness, headache, nausea, or vomiting, and these patients may be misdiagnosed as having an infarction unless brain imaging is done. Thus differentiation of ischemic stroke from hemorrhagic stroke based only on clinical features is difficult.[4,5]

The time course (tempo) of other illnesses in the differential diagnosis usually differs from that of ischemic stroke, and thus the history is key. Some conditions, including brain tumors, have a slower course than vascular disease. Central nervous system infections, which produce focal neurological signs, such as brain abscess or encephalitis often have prodromal symptoms and course that evolves over several days. Hypoglycemia is another important and easily treated alternative diagnosis.[6] Confusion or a disturbance in cognition or consciousness may provide a hint that hypoglycemia is the etiology of focal neurological signs in a diabetic patient.

▶ **TABLE 6-1.** DIFFERENTIAL DIAGNOSIS OF ACUTE ISCHEMIC STROKE

Hemorrhagic stroke
Craniocerebral trauma
Subdural hematoma
Brain tumor (primary or metastatic)
Venous thrombosis
Encephalitis
Hypoglycemia
Seizures with postictal neurological impairments

▶ GENERAL FEATURES OF ISCHEMIC STROKE

Because a majority of ischemic strokes are secondary to an acute embolic occlusion of an artery, the events are usually of sudden onset. While patients can have warning symptoms (transient ischemic attack, TIA), many patients have a stroke as their first neurological symptom. The

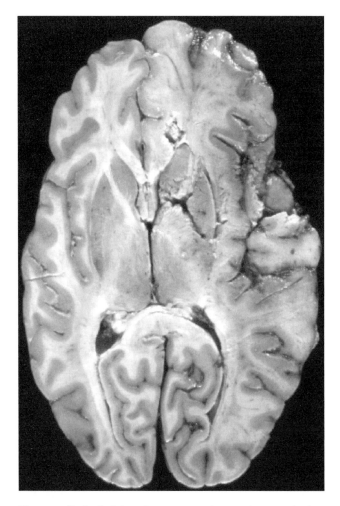

Figure 6-1. Axial autopsy specimen demonstrates infarction of the right frontal lobe, insular cortex, and basal ganglia. The findings are compatible with an occlusion of the proximal portion of the middle cerebral artery. (*Courtesy of S.S. Schochet, M.D., Department of Pathology, University of West Virginia, Morgantown, WV*)

▶ **TABLE 6-2.** CLINICAL FEATURES OF ISCHEMIC STROKE

Time course
  Sudden onset (usually at maximal severity at onset)
  May evolve or gradually worsen (usually <24 h)
  May have waxing or waning of signs during first few hours
Time of onset
  May occur at any time—usually without provocation
  Approximately one-fifth of cases occur during sleep
    Time of onset not obvious in such cases
Consciousness usually is preserved
  Coma may occur with basilar artery occlusion
  Large hemispheric strokes—grogginess or drowsiness
Focal neurological deficits are prominent
  Generally reflect injury to one area of the brain
  Signs reflecting multiple areas of injury are uncommon
Focal neurological deficits reflect vascular territory of one artery
Associated neurological symptoms
  Seizures in approximately 5% of cases
  Headache in approximately 20% of cases
  Nausea and vomiting can occur with brain stem strokes

neurological deficits usually are maximal almost immediately. Other patients may have a gradual or stepwise worsening, or a waxing and waning of their signs. In general, a course of neurological deterioration is usually complete within the first 24 h of stroke. The progression has been ascribed to failure of collateral blood flow, early recurrent embolism, progression of the thrombus, or the metabolic consequences of the ischemic lesion. Approximately one-third of patients have a stroke during sleep, with impairments present upon awakening. In these circumstances, details are lacking about the onset of the event. Still, patients with stroke upon awakening are not different from those persons who have strokes during the day in regard to age, sex, ethnicity, or the presence of risk factors. Thus, these strokes likely are akin to those that happen during waking hours.

▶ **TABLE 6-3.** FEATURES THAT POINT TO HEMORRHAGE IN A PATIENT WITH SUSPECTED ISCHEMIC STROKE

Depression in consciousness can appear early
  Drowsy, stupor, or coma
  Delirium or agitation
Focal neurological signs do not fit one vascular territory
Headache is often severe
Nausea and vomiting—particularly if other signs point to an ischemic stroke in cerebral hemisphere
Nuchal rigidity
Unstable vital signs
  Respiratory abnormalities
  Fever
  Cardiac arrhythmias
  Marked arterial hypertension

Consciousness is preserved in most patients (see Table 6-2). However, patients with multilobar infarctions may be stunned or drowsy immediately following the event. Subsequently, brain edema and increased intracranial pressure may develop, and thereafter patient's level of consciousness may decline. While most infarctions in the brain stem do not cause coma, patients with basilar artery occlusion may present with a sudden decline in consciousness.[7] Approximately 5 percent of patients have one or more seizures in association with the stroke.[8,9] Seizures are usually associated with cortical infarctions secondary to embolism. If the patient's seizure becomes generalized, the level of consciousness may become depressed. Rarely, status epilepticus may occur.

Nearly 20 percent of patients complain of headache.[10–12] However, the headache generally is not the chief complaint. Headaches are more common with events that occur in the posterior circulation and with larger thromboembolic strokes. Headache is distinctly uncommon with lacunar infarctions. Headache, face pain, ear pain, or neck pain can be prominent among patients with arterial dissections and their presence should prompt recognition of the cause of stroke.[13,14] Nausea and vomiting are uncommon with ischemic strokes in the cerebral hemispheres but may be prominent with lesions in the brain stem or cerebellum (Fig. 6-2) Hiccups or unilateral hearing loss also can occur with ischemic events in the posterior circulation.

The spectrum of focal neurological complaints is broad and reflects the location of the brain injury and the size of the occluded artery. Depending upon the size and location of the infarction, most patients have some combination of motor, sensory, visual, and cognitive impairments.

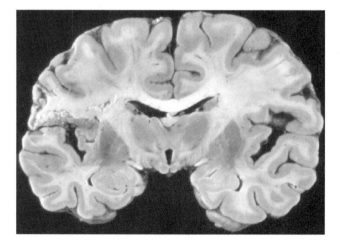

Figure 6-2. Coronal autopsy section of the cerebral hemispheres demonstrates a restricted area of infarction in the right insula and the inferior gyrus of the frontal lobe. The findings are consistent with an embolic occlusion of a branch of the middle cerebral artery. (*Courtesy of S.S. Schochet, M.D., Department of Pathology, University of West Virginia, Morgantown, WV*)

▶ EXAMINATION OF A PATIENT WITH AN ISCHEMIC STROKE

The examination permits detection of signs that are crucial for localizing the stroke and the size of the ischemic lesion. This information influences prognosis, diagnosis of the most likely cause, and decisions about acute treatment of stroke, rehabilitation, and measures to prevent recurrent ischemic stroke. In general, infarctions are differentiated by their anatomic location—left (usually dominant) or right (nondominant) hemisphere or the brain stem and cerebellum. In addition, hemispheric infarctions are subdivided into large (multilobar), branch cortical or small, subcortical strokes. Watershed (border zone) infarctions most commonly occur at the junctions of the terminal branches of the middle, anterior, and posterior cerebral arteries but may also occur at the terminal junctions of the arteries perfusing the cerebellum.

Localization of the stroke is based upon the pattern of the neurological impairments. The presence of decreased consciousness, cranial nerve palsies, nystagmus, limb or gait ataxia, bilateral or crossed motor or sensory signs, or severe dysarthria and dysphagia points to an infarction in the brain stem with or without cerebellar involvement. Infarctions restricted to the cerebellum cause vertigo and truncal, gait, or limb ataxia. Cognitive or behavioral impairments (including aphasia), visual field defects, or unilateral motor signs are usually secondary to infarctions of the cerebral hemisphere. The behavioral and cognitive signs will reflect the affected hemisphere (dominant or nondominant) (Table 6-4). These features have been used in determining the subtypes in the Oxfordshire classification of strokes into *total anterior cerebral infarction* (TACI), *partial anterior cerebral infarction* (PACI), *lacunar anterior cerebral infarction* (LACI), or *posterior circulation infarction* (POCI).[15] This differentiation is of value for predicting outcome after stroke, for establishing the most likely cause, and for making decisions about acute treatment.

Multilobar infarction (TACI), which affects both cortical and subcortical structures, is usually secondary to occlusion of the internal carotid artery or the proximal portion of the middle cerebral artery (see Fig. 6-1). The most common cause is thrombosis of an atherosclerotic internal carotid artery often with secondary embolism intracranially (artery-to-artery embolism). Alternatively, cardioembolism may be the etiology of this type of stroke. Patients with TACI generally have a poor prognosis with a high probability of either death or disability. Deaths are usually due to brain edema and increased intracranial pressure. Patients with cortical infarction secondary to occlusion of a branch artery (PACI) have an intermediate prognosis (Figs. 6-2 and 6-3). These strokes are usually due to embolism (cardioembolism or artery-to-artery embolism). While these patients have a relatively low risk of mortality, they often

▶ **TABLE 6-4.** CLINICAL FEATURES OF SUBTYPES OF ISCHEMIC STROKE

Feature	Multilobar (TACI)	Branch Cortical (PACI)	Subcortical (LACI)	Posterior Circulation (POCI)
Consciousness	Alert to drowsy	Alert	Alert	Alert to coma
Behavioral or cognitive signs	Prominent	Prominent	Uncommon	Absent
Visual field defect	Present Contralateral	Present Contralateral	Uncommon	Absent
Oculorotatory Abnormality	Present Conjugate gaze palsy	Uncommon	Absent	Prominent Varied
Cranial nerve palsy	Absent	Absent	Absent	Present Ipsilateral
Dysarthria	Present	Uncommon	Present	Prominent
Motor defects	Prominent Contralateral	Present Contralateral	Prominent Contralateral	Prominent Contralateral Bilateral Crossed
Sensory defects	Prominent Contralateral	Present Contralateral	Prominent Contralateral	Prominent Contralateral Bilateral Dissociated Crossed
Motor and sensory Defects	Equal Pattern	Equal Pattern	Unequal Pattern	Unequal Pattern
Ataxia	Absent	Absent	Absent	Present Ipsilateral

TACI = total anterior cerebral infarction, PACI = partial anterior cerebral infarction, LACI = lacunar anterior cerebral infarction, POCI = posterior circulation infarction.
Adapted in part from Bamford et al.[15]

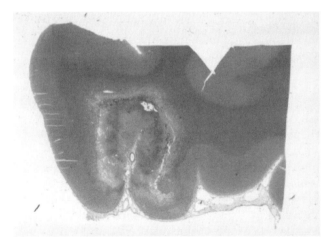

Figure 6-3. Small area of infarction restricted to the cortex due to embolic occlusion of a pial artery. (*Courtesy of S.S. Schochet, M.D., Department of Pathology, University of West Virginia, Morgantown, WV*)

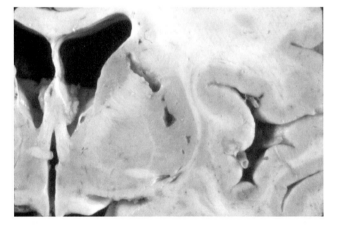

Figure 6-4. Coronal autopsy specimen shows multiple small infarctions in the left putamen, internal capsule, and the head of the caudate nucleus. The findings are compatible with the diagnosis of several lacunar infarctions involving occlusions of the lenticulostriate arteries. (*Courtesy of S.S. Schochet, M.D., Department of Pathology, University of West Virginia, Morgantown, WV*)

have major behavioral, cognitive, and language seque-lae. Infarctions restricted to hemispheric subcortical nuclear or white matter structures (LACI) have rather stereotyped clinical presentations (lacunar syndromes). These strokes are usually secondary to occlusion of small penetrating arteries, although some lacunar syn-dromes may result from embolic occlusions of one or more penetrating arteries (Fig. 6-4). These latter infarc-tions are often larger than lacunes on computed tomog-raphy (CT), although the signs are similar. In general, patients with LACI have a favorable prognosis with a low risk for mortality. However, recurrent lacunar strokes may lead to dementia (multi-infarction dementia). The clinical spectrum of strokes in the posterior circulation (POCI) is varied. Prognosis largely depends upon the site and extent of the ischemic lesion and the underlying cause. Occlusion of the basilar artery often leads to death, whereas chances of mortality are low with a minor brain stem lacunar stroke. Posterior circulation strokes may be secondary to thromboembolic occlusions of major, long, circumferential, or penetrating arteries.

▶ CLINICAL MANIFESTATIONS OF ISCHEMIC STROKES IN THE CEREBRAL HEMISPHERES

Occlusion of the Internal Carotid Artery

The consequences of an occlusion of the internal carotid artery vary (Fig. 6-5). Some patients will have no neuro-logical symptoms, while others may have a multilobar infarction that can be fatal. The severity of the stroke is influenced by the presence of collateral channels and the adequacy of blood flow via the ipsilateral external carotid artery, the circle of Willis from the contralateral internal

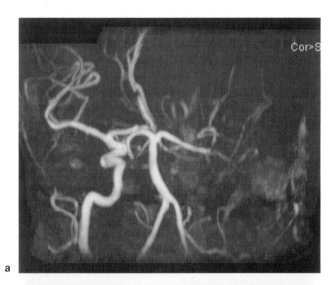

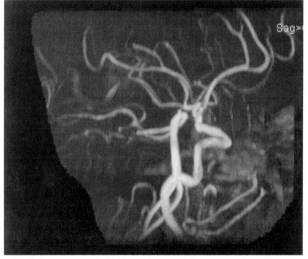

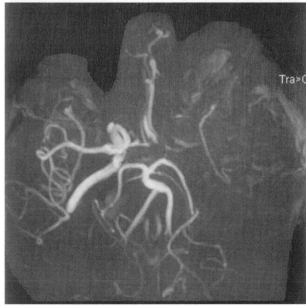

Figure 6-5. (a) Anteroposterior, (b) lateral, and (c) basal views of a magnetic resonance angiography demonstrate an occlusion of the left internal carotid artery.

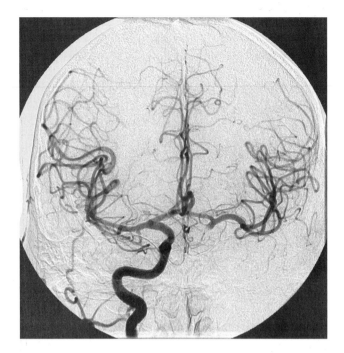

Figure 6-6. Anteroposterior view of a right internal carotid arteriogram demonstrates collateral flow to the left hemisphere via the anterior communicating artery in a patient with an occlusion of left internal carotid artery.

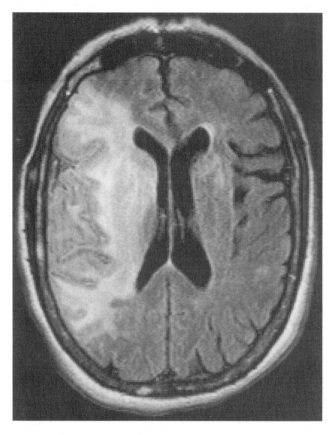

Figure 6-7. Fluid attenuation inversion recovery (FLAIR) sequence magnetic resonance imaging demonstrates a very large infarction of the right hemisphere. The findings are consistent with either an occlusion of the internal carotid artery or the proximal segment of the middle cerebral artery.

carotid artery or posterior circulation, and distal pial vessels from the anterior or posterior cerebral arteries (Fig. 6-6). In general, infarctions secondary to occlusion of the internal carotid artery involve subcortical structures of the cerebral hemisphere (internal capsule, putamen, and caudate nucleus) as well as the frontal, temporal, and parietal lobes (Fig. 6-7). The vascular territories of both the middle and anterior cerebral arteries are often affected. Patients with major infarction secondary to occlusion of the internal carotid artery are often seriously ill and have clinical findings of both cortical and deep hemispheric injury (Table 6-5; Fig. 6-8). An ipsilateral Horner syndrome may be found with dissection of the internal carotid artery. The carotid pulse can be diminished. Because of the extent of the ischemic injury, the prognosis of most patients with symptomatic occlusions of the internal carotid artery is often quite poor.

Occlusion of the Proximal Portion of the Middle Cerebral Artery

Artery-to-artery embolism (a thrombus arising at the carotid bifurcation and migrating distally) or cardioembolism are the primary causes of occlusions of the first (proximal) portion of the middle cerebral artery (Fig. 6-9).[16–18] Atherosclerotic stenosis of the proximal portion of the middle cerebral artery also may lead to thrombotic occlusion of the artery. In general, the clinical findings of patients with occlusion of

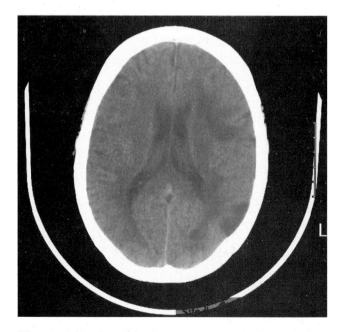

Figure 6-8. CT of the brain shows a multiloar infarction of the right hemisphere.

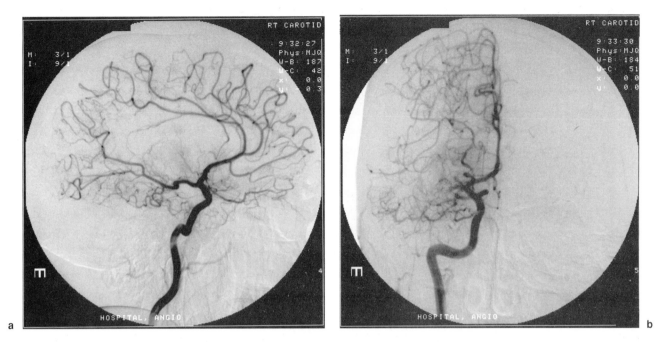

a   b

Figure 6-9. Views of a right carotid arteriogram demonstrate the absence of filling of the middle cerebral artery. Both the anterior and posterior cerebral arteries are well visualized. The most likely explanation for this pattern would be a thromboembolic occlusion of the proximal segment of the middle cerebral artery.

the middle cerebral artery mimic those of patients with occlusion of the internal carotid artery (see Table 6-5; Figs. 6-10 and 6-11). However, some subtle differences may be detected (Fig. 6-12). For example, the lower limb may not be as severely affected as the upper limb or face.

▶ **TABLE 6-5.** FINDINGS OF ACUTE INFARCTION OCCLUSION OF INTERNAL CAROTID ARTERY

Consciousness
    Usually drowsy or inattentive initially
    Subsequently can develop stupor or coma (secondary brain edema)
Cognitive or behavioral impairments
    Global aphasia (dominant hemisphere)
    Apraxia of nonparalyzed limbs (dominant hemisphere)
    Neglect, anosognosia, or asomatognosia (nondominant hemisphere)
    Visuospatial or topographic disorientation (nondominant hemisphere)
    Aprosody of language (nondominant hemisphere)
Dysarthria
Contralateral homonymous hemianopia
Conjugate gaze preference (away from paresis and toward lesion)
Contralateral hemiparesis (involving face, upper limb, and lower limb)
Contralateral hemisensory loss (involving face, upper limb, and lower limb)
With some lesions may have ipsilateral Horner syndrome

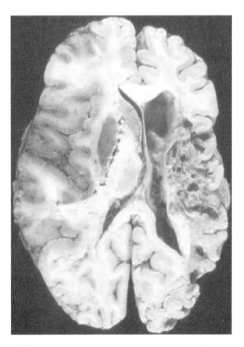

Figure 6-10. Axial autopsy section of both cerebral hemispheres demonstrates an old infarction of the left hemisphere and a more recent infarction involving the right hemisphere. The left ventricle is dilated and the area of infarction on the left consists of multiple cystic areas. The right hemisphere is swollen, areas of hemorrhage are found, and the right lateral ventricle is compressed. (*Courtesy of S.S. Schochet, M.D., Department of Pathology, University of West Virginia, Morgantown, WV*)

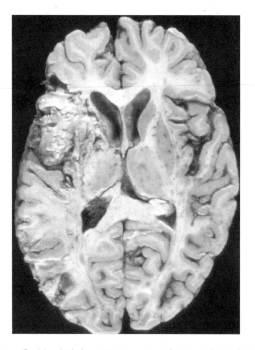

Figure 6-11. Axial autopsy specimen shows cystic changes in the left right caudate, putamen, internal capsule, insula, and frontal lobe. The findings are compatible with an old infarction in the territory of the middle cerebral artery with occlusion of the proximal segment of the vessel. (*Courtesy of S.S. Schochet, M.D. Department of Pathology, University of West Virginia, Morgantown, WV*)

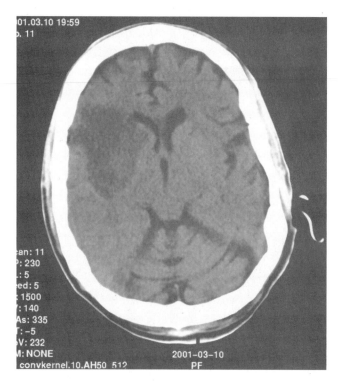

Figure 6-12. Unenhanced CT scan reveals a large infarction of the insula, basal ganglia, and frontal lobe of the right hemisphere. These imaging findings are consistent with an occlusion of proximal portion of the middle cerebral artery.

Striatocapsular Infarction

Some patients with embolic occlusions of the proximal portion of the middle cerebral artery will not develop major cortical infarctions. Pial collateral flow from the terminal branches of the anterior and posterior cerebral arteries will preserve the viability of most of lateral cortical portion of the hemisphere. Instead, the infarction is restricted to deep hemispheric structures (head of caudate, anterior limb of internal capsule, and putamen) that are perfused by the lenticulostriate branches of the middle cerebral artery (striatocapsular infarction)[19–21] (Figs. 6-13 and 6-14). Table 6-6 outlines the impairments that are found with these infarctions. In general, motor deficits predominate but striatocapsular infarctions of the dominant hemisphere produce an atypical aphasia with mildly impaired fluency and repetition but normal comprehension. Nondominant hemisphere lesions may produce behavioral signs including neglect.

Occlusion at the Bifurcation at the Middle Cerebral Artery

In the Sylvian fissure, the middle cerebral artery divides into two major branches. Emboli may reach this bifurcation and occlude one or both vessels. These clots are

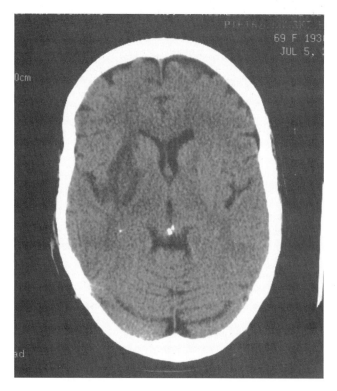

Figure 6-13. Unenhanced CT scan of the brain shows a large striatocapsular infarction in the distribution of the lenticulostriate branches of the middle cerebral artery.

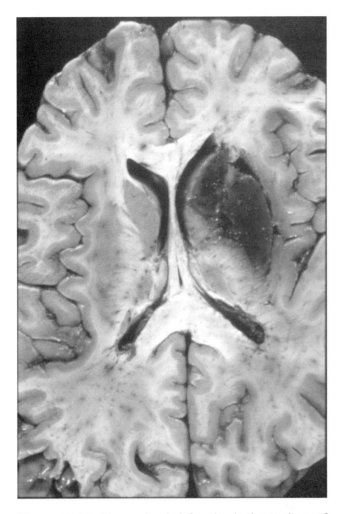

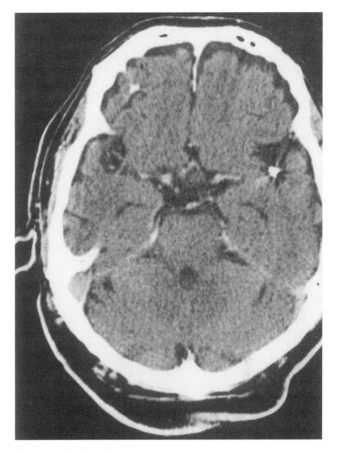

Figure 6-15. CT study demonstrates a dot sign secondary to an embolism in the left middle cerebral artery.

Figure 6-14. Hemorrhagic infarction in the territory of the left lenticulostriate arteries is found on this sagittal autopsy specimen. The findings are consistent with a striatocapsular infarction secondary to occlusion of the proximal portion of the middle cerebral artery. (*Courtesy of S.S. Schochet, M.D., Department of Pathology, University of West Virginia, Morgantown, WV*)

▶ **TABLE 6-6.** FINDINGS OF STRIATOCAPSULAR INFARCTION

Contralateral hemiparesis (involving face, upper limb, and
  lower limb)
Contralateral sensory loss (involving face, upper limb, and
  lower limb)
  Usually less prominent than motor findings
Dysarthria
Hemichorea
Cognitive or behavioral impairments
  Apathy
  Atypical aphasia (dominant hemisphere)
  Hemisensory neglect (nondominant hemisphere)

---

often visualized on brain imaging (*dense artery sign or dot sign*) (Fig. 6-15). Because these clots are distal to the origin of the lenticulostriate arteries, the deep structures of the hemisphere are usually spared. The infarction usually affects the insula and parts of the frontal, temporal, and parietal lobes. The lateral surface of the cerebral cortex is the primary area of ischemia. Patterns of infarction vary considerably. In general, the neurological impairments of a major hemispheric stroke will mimic the findings following occlusion of the internal carotid artery. However, some differences may be detected. Motor and sensory impairments will primarily affect the face and upper limb. The lower limb is usually minimally affected or not involved.

Rarely, pial collateral channels will be sufficiently robust to allow for preservation of most of the hemispheric cortex, and the ischemic injury is restricted to the insular region (*isolated insular infarction*) (Figs. 6-16 and 6-17). Patients with isolated insular infarction have contralateral paresis of the face and hand. Sensory loss usually is not detected. Conduction aphasia may be present if the stroke occurs in the dominant hemisphere. Vertigo, nausea, and contralateral limb ataxia have also

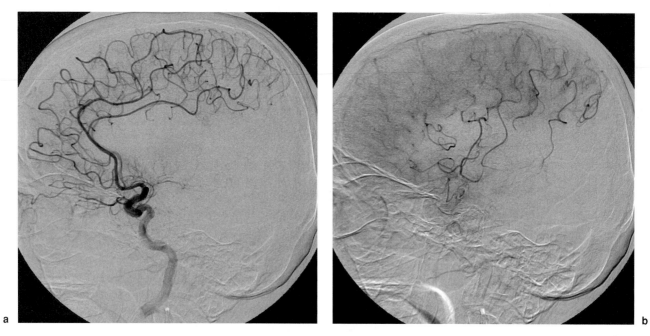

Figure 6-16. Two views of a right carotid arteriogram show (a) an occlusion of proximal segment of the middle cerebral artery and (b) retrograde flow into branch cortical (pial) vessels via collateral channels arising from the anterior cerebral artery.

been described. Cardiac disturbances also may complicate infarction, particularly in the right hemisphere.

Occlusion of Cortical Branches of the Middle Cerebral Artery

Most infarctions in the distribution of the cortical (pial) branches of the middle cerebral artery are secondary to embolism.[22–25] The clinical findings differ depending upon the number of occluded branches and the location of the occlusion. A distal occlusion of one branch may lead to a very restricted neurological impairment, while more proximal or multiple arterial lesions will produce more extensive deficits. Some clots will partially lyse and move distally, and these smaller emboli may occlude one or two pial vessels.[26] As a result, patients may have two or more infarctions, reflecting individual branch occlusions interspersed with relatively preserved areas of the brain (Fig. 6-18). This scenario is a potential explanation for the finding of global aphasia without hemiparesis. In this situation the lesions are in anterior and posterior language areas, while the primary motor cortex is preserved. Because the superficial (cortical/pial) arteries are branches of the two major divisions of the middle cerebral arteries, their vascular territories are generally divided into an anterior/superior grouping that supplies primarily the frontal lobe and a posterior/inferior grouping that perfuses primarily the parietal lobe and superior portion of the temporal lobe (Fig. 6-19). The neurological findings of an anterior/superior division infarction differ from those seen with the more posterior/inferior

lesions (Table 6-7). Depending upon the location in the dominant hemisphere, branch infarctions will cause language disturbances ranging from fluent or nonfluent aphasia to mutism. Fluent aphasias are usually found with posterior/inferior infarctions, while a paucity of spontaneous speech may be found with frontal lobe lesions. Disturbances in emotion or behavioralso may occur with frontal lobe infarctions. Infarctions in the posterior/inferior

▶ **TABLE 6-7.** FINDINGS OF BRANCH CORTICAL INFARCTIONS OF MIDDLE CEREBRAL ARTERY

Anterosuperior
  Contralateral hemiparesis (primarily involving face and
  upper limb)
    May be monoparesis
  Contralateral sensory loss (primarily involving face and
  upper limb)
  Conjugate gaze preference (away from paresis and
  toward lesion)
  Cognitive and behavioral impairments
    Mutism or nonfluent aphasia (dominant hemisphere)
    Neglect (nondominant hemisphere)
Posteroinferior
Contralateral sensory or motor signs less than with
  anterosuperior
Contralateral homonymous hemianopia
Cognitive and behavioral impairments
    Fluent aphasia (dominant hemisphere)
    Gerstmann syndrome (dominant hemisphere)
    Neglect, anosognosia, and asomatognosia
    (nondominant hemisphere)

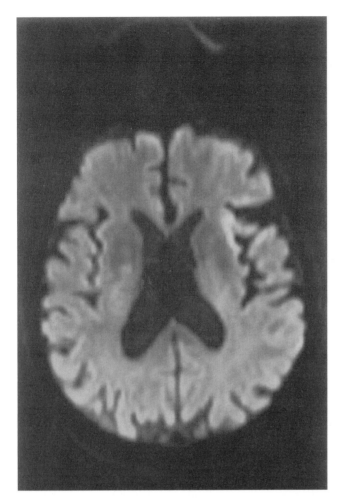

Figure 6-17. Diffusion weighted imaging (DWI) sequence magnetic resonance imaging shows an infarction isolated to the insular cortex in the left hemisphere.

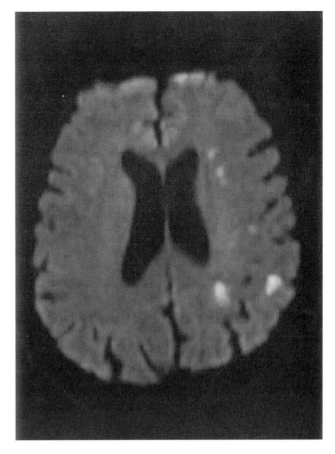

Figure 6-18. Multiple areas of infarction in the left hemisphere are found on an unenhanced CT scan of the brain. The locations of the infarctions are compatible with embolic occlusions of branch pial arteries.

branches of the middle cerebral artery also can cause left–right disorientation, alexia, acalculia, and agraphia. In general, motor and sensory impairments are more prominent with infarctions in the anterior/superior branches. Motor impairments are secondary to infarction of the primary or supplemental motor areas.

Border Zone Infarctions

Border zone (*watershed*) infarctions are usually found at the junctions of the terminal branches of the middle, anterior, and posterior cerebral arteries. Profound hypotension, such as that occurring with major cardiovascular operations, may cause border zone infarctions in both cerebral hemispheres. Border zone infarctions affecting one hemisphere are usually secondary to microemboli combined with hypoperfusion, often resulting from severely stenotic disease of proximal intracranial or extracranial arteries.[27–29] Imaging of the brain demonstrates a series of lesions just lateral to the

▶ **TABLE 6-8.** CLINICAL FINDINGS OF UNILATERAL OR BILATERAL BORDER ZONE INFARCTIONS

Anterior infarctions
   Motor impairments, sensory loss, nonfluent aphasia, and behavioral signs
Posterior infarctions
   Visual field defects, sensory loss, and fluent aphasia
Unilateral—contralateral paresis involving shoulder more than face or hand
   Bilateral—man-in-the-barrel syndrome
   Bilateral—weakness of tongue and limbs with sparing of face
Sensory loss can mimic motor impairments
Cognitive and behavioral impairments
   Unilateral—transcortical motor or sensory aphasia (dominant hemisphere)
   Unilateral—mutism, apathy, and abulia (dominant hemisphere)
   Unilateral—anosognosia (nondominant hemisphere)
   Bilateral—abulia, mutism, and akinetic mutism
Cortical blindness with bilateral strokes

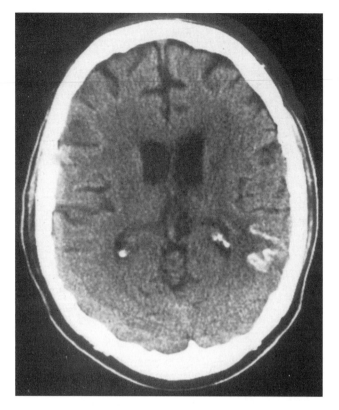

Figure 6-19. CT scan with contrast enhancement demonstrates a small subacute left parietal infarction consistent with an embolic occlusion to a branch of the middle cerebral artery.

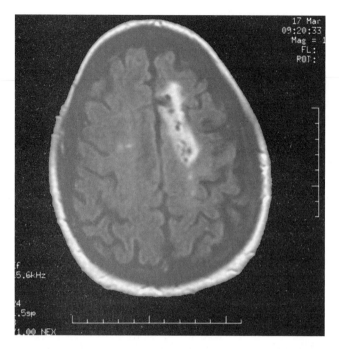

Figure 6-20. Area of hyperintensity in the left cerebral hemisphere is noted on fluid attenuation inversion recovery (FLAIR) magnetic resonance imaging. The pattern of the lesion is consistent with a watershed (border zone) infarction.

parasagittal portions of the hemisphere extending from front to back (Fig. 6-20). The clinical features of unilateral or bilateral border zone infarctions are summarized in Table 6-8. The so-called *man-in-the-barrel syndrome* is found with bilateral border zone infarctions.[30] Clinically, the examination demonstrates paralysis of both shoulders with relative preservation of strength in the lower extremities and the hands. Lesions of the dominant hemisphere produce transcortical aphasia. An infarction in the border zone region of the frontal lobe causes a nonfluent aphasia with preserved repetition. An infarction in the more common posterior (parietal lobe) location produces a fluent aphasia with preserved repetition and echolalia. Dominant hemisphere or bilateral lesions may also produce apathy, abulia, mutism, or akinetic mutism. Severe bilateral border zone infarctions may even produce dementia (anterior lesions) or cortical blindness (posterior lesions).

Other Infarctions in the Territory of the Middle Cerebral Artery

Occlusion of individual penetrating branches of the middle cerebral artery may produce lacunar infarctions that primarily occur in the caudate nucleus, anterior limb of the

internal capsule, or basal ganglia. The lacunar syndromes are described subsequently in this chapter. The most common syndrome is that of pure motor hemiparesis. Large infarctions involving the corona radiata (centrum semiovale) may produce signs that mimic those of a multilobar infarction secondary to occlusion of the middle cerebral artery or internal carotid artery (Fig. 6-21).[31,32] Small infarctions in the same territory may produce isolated motor or sensory impairments that mimic a lacunar infarction.[33] Bilateral infarctions in the territory of the middle cerebral arteries may produce dementia, visual loss, bilateral motor or sensory impairments, and pseudobulbar palsy.

Occlusion of the Anterior Choroidal Artery

The anterior choroidal artery may be occluded secondary to emboli arising from the heart or proximal arteries, or to thrombi that develop in the vessel. This artery perfuses the optic tract, posterior limb of the internal capsule, dorsolateral portion of the thalamus, the posteromedial aspect of the globus pallidus, and inferior portions of the centrum semiovale[34] (Fig. 6-22). The signs of a stroke can range from an isolated hemiparesis to more extensive neurological impairments[35,36] (Table 6-9). Among the more common lacunar syndromes are pure motor hemiparesis, purse sensory stroke, or the combination of homolateral ataxia and

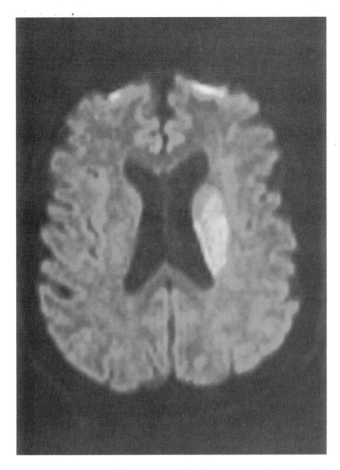

Figure 6-21. Diffusion weighted imaging (DWI) sequence magnetic resonance imaging shows an infarction in centrum semiovale in the left hemisphere.

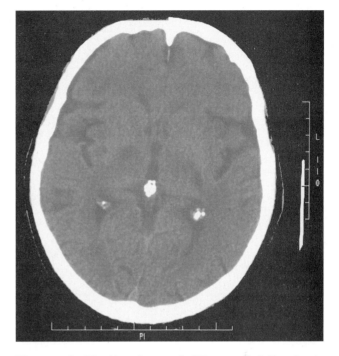

Figure 6-22. Unenhanced CT scan of the brain demonstrates lacunar infarctions in both cerebral hemispheres. The infarction in the left hemisphere is in posterior limb of the internal carotid artery and in the distribution of the anterior choroidal artery. The infarction in the right hemisphere is located in the genu of the internal capsule.

hemiparesis. The motor and sensory findings generally predominate. The behavioral, cognitive, and visual impairments are subtle and atypical. While visual impairments are uncommon, the field defects are often incongruous. One of the potential visual field abnormalities is a homonymous sectoranopia (a segmental area of visual loss that can cross the horizon), reflecting ischemia in the lateral geniculate nucleus.

▶ **TABLE 6-9.** FINDINGS OF INFARCTION OF ANTERIOR CHOROIDAL ARTERY

Contralateral hemiparesis (involving face, upper limb, and lower limb)
Contralateral hemisensory loss (involving face, upper limb, and lower limb)
   Motor and sensory findings can occur concurrently or in isolation
Contralateral homonymous hemianopia
Cognitive and behavioral impairments
   Atypical aphasia, apraxia, or amnesia (dominant hemisphere)
   Contralateral neglect (nondominant hemisphere)

Occlusion of the Anterior Cerebral Artery

Infarctions in the distribution of the anterior cerebral artery are relatively uncommon. Among the leading causes of ischemia is vasospasm following rupture of an anterior communicating artery. In this situation, arterial narrowing may affect one or both anterior cerebral arteries. Less commonly, local atherosclerotic disease develops in the proximal segment of the anterior cerebral artery. Embolization to the anterior cerebral artery is relatively uncommon. The anterior cerebral artery provides blood to the anterior, medial, and inferior aspects of the frontal lobe as well as to the medial and anterior aspects of the parietal lobe, the corpus callosum, a portion of the caudate nucleus, the anterior portion of the thalamus, and part of the anterior limb of the internal capsule. The deep hemispheric structures are largely supplied by the recurrent artery of Huebner (anterior lenticulostriate), which arises from the proximal segment of the artery. An occlusion restricted to the recurrent artery of Huebner causes a lacunar syndrome that might mimic a striatocapsular infarction, producing hemiparesis, limb ataxia, and dysarthria (Figs. 6-23 to 6-25).[37–39]

   The neurological abnormalities with proximal occlusion of the anterior cerebral artery are outlined in

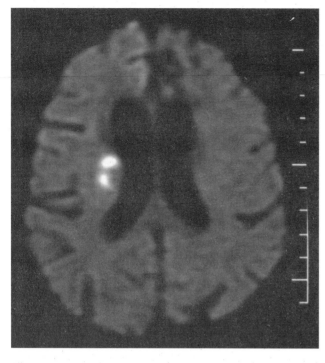

Figure 6-23. Diffusion weighted imaging (DWI) imaging study shows an infarction in the centrum semiovale on the right.

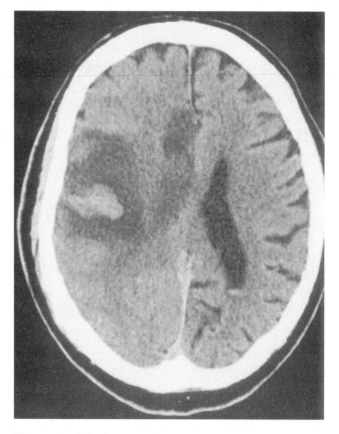

Figure 6-24. Axial CT study demonstrates two areas of infarction. A large infarction with secondary hemorrhage is seen in area of the right middle cerebral artery. A parasagittal lesion consistent with an infarction in area of the right anterior cerebral artery is also present.

► **TABLE 6-10.** FINDINGS OF INFARCTION OF ANTERIOR CEREBRAL ARTERY

Unilateral infarction
  Contralateral hemiparesis (involving primarily the lower limb)
  Contralateral hemisensory loss (involving primarily the lower limb)
  Ipsilateral limb apraxia
  Impairment of bowel and bladder control
  Cognitive and behavioral impairments
    Transcortical motor aphasia (dominant hemisphere)
    Contralateral neglect (nondominant hemisphere)
    Abulia or apathy (either hemisphere)
    Euphoria or disinhibition (either hemisphere)
    Impaired executive function (either hemisphere)
Bilateral infarctions
  Bilateral hemiparesis (involving primarily the lower limbs)
    Motor signs may mimic a paraparesis
  Bilateral hemisensory loss (involving primarily the lower limbs)
    Sensory signs may mimic a spinal sensory level
  Impairment of bowel and bladder control
  Cognitive and behavioral impairments
    Severe abulia or apathy
    Akinetic mutism
    Disturbances in effect

Table 6-10.[40] Cognitive and behavioral abnormalities are prominent, especially when bilateral infarctions occur. Infarctions in the corpus callosum, secondary to occlusion of distal branches, can produce a disconnection syndrome of apraxia, agraphia, and alien hand.[41] With major strokes secondary to occlusion of the internal carotid artery, the signs of anterior cerebral artery infarction develop in addition to those reflecting occlusion of the middle cerebral artery.

Occlusion of the Posterior Cerebral Artery

The posterior cerebral arteries usually are the terminal branches of the basilar artery. While localized atherosclerosis may develop in the proximal portion of the posterior cerebral artery, most occlusions are secondary to cardioembolism or artery-to-artery embolism. Occlusions may affect one or both vessels. The posterior cerebral artery perfuses the medial and inferior portions of the temporal lobe, the parasagittal aspects of the parietal lobe, the occipital lobe, thalamus, and rostral brain

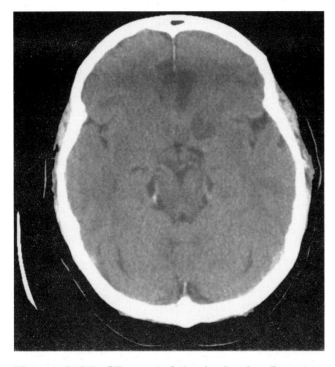

Figure 6-25. CT scan of the brain visualizes two areas of infarction in the distribution of the right anterior cerebral artery. One lesion is located parasagittally and represents ischemia in the area of frontal branches, and the second (deeper) lesion is the territory of the recurrent artery of Huebner.

▶ **TABLE 6-11.** FINDINGS OF UNILATERAL OR BILATERAL INFARCTIONS OF POSTERIOR CEREBRAL ARTERIES

Distal occlusion of posterior cerebral artery
    Contralateral homonymous hemianopia (quadrantanopia)
        With or without macular sparing
    Cognitive and behavioral impairments
        Visual hallucinations or metamorphopsia
        Alexia without agraphia (dominant hemisphere)
        Transcortical sensory aphasia (dominant hemisphere)
        Hemiachromatopsia (dominant hemisphere)
        Amnesia (dominant or nondominant hemisphere)
        Visual hemineglect (nondominant hemisphere)
Proximal occlusion of posterior cerebral artery
    Visual impairments as listed above
    Cognitive and behavioral impairments as listed above
    Contralateral hemiparesis (involving face, upper limb, and lower limb)
    Contralateral hemisensory loss (involving face, upper limb, and lower limb)
Bilateral occlusions of the posterior cerebral arteries
    Bilateral visual loss
    Cortical blindness
    Anton syndrome
    Balint syndrome
    Prosopagnosia
    Amnesia

stem. While distal occlusions of the posterior cerebral artery may produce primarily visual impairments, more proximal occlusions also cause motor and sensory loss[42–44] (Table 6-11). The visual loss is usually a congruous homonymous hemianopia with or without macular sparing (Figs. 6-26 to 6-28). A superior homonymous quadrantanopia results from an infarction restricted to the infracalcarine portions of the occipital lobe. A similar relationship to an inferior homonymous hemianopia can occur with a small infarction restricted to the occipital lobe above the calcarine fissure. Achromatopsia can occur with infarction in the lingual and fusiform gyri. Alexia without agraphia complicates a dominant occipital lobe infarction that extends into the splenium of the corpus callosum. Visual hallucinations, visual perseverations, and visual distortions also occur. Complex behavioral impairments, including amnesia or disturbances in the sleep–wake cycle, also can be prominent. Bilateral occlusions produce marked visual-behavioral deficits, including *Balint syndrome, Anton syndrome*, and *prosopagnosia*.[45] Marked hand–eye incoordination (optic ataxia), inability to see the full visual field at one time (asimultanagnosia), and inability to fixate the eyes on an object (apraxia of gaze) are found in Balint syndrome. In Anton syndrome, the patient has cortical blindness but the patient denies the visual loss. Prosopagnosia is marked by the inability to differentiate subcategories of visual phenomena and most markedly involves the inability to recognize persons by their facial appearance. In addition, patients may have nausea, vomiting, and headache.

Top-of-the-Basilar Occlusion and Thalamic Infarctions

Occlusion of the distal basilar artery (the so-called top-of-the-basilar syndrome) can lead to unilateral or bilateral infarctions in the territory of the posterior cerebral arteries. In addition, the midbrain and thalamus are also infarcted. The top-of-the-basilar syndrome presents with the combination of visual field impairments, oculorotatory disturbances (especially impaired vertical gaze), memory loss, and altered consciousness that may wax and wane[46] (Table 6-12). Motor and sensory impairments may also be detected.

The proximal segment of the posterior cerebral artery and the distal portion (bifurcation) of the basilar artery are the origin of several small penetrating arteries that perfuse the thalamus and the midbrain. Isolated infarctions in the thalamus or rostral brain stem may result from thrombosis of or embolism to the parent arteries. Local small-artery disease also occurs. Anatomists have given different names to these small vessels. In this book, these arteries are called the thalamogeniculate

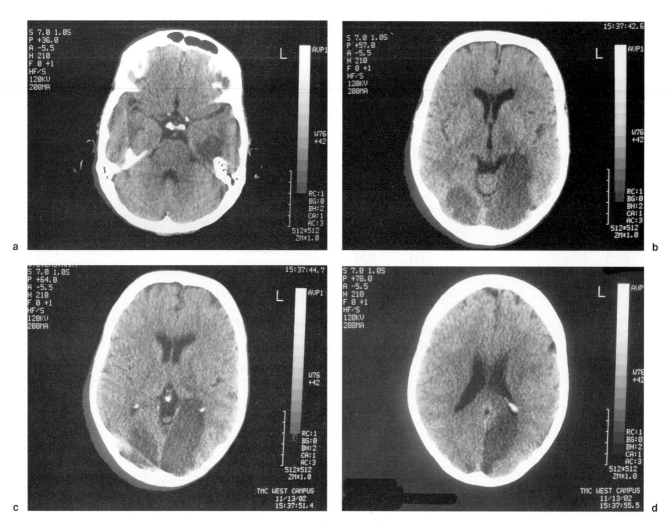

Figure 6-26. Series of CT images of the brain demonstrate bilateral posterior cerebral artery infarctions in a patient with an occlusion of the top of the basilar artery. The infarctions involve both cortical and thalamic structures.

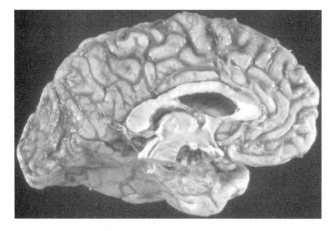

Figure 6-27. Midsagittal view of the left cerebral hemisphere shows an infarction in the occipital lobe, and medial and inferior aspect of the temporal lobe secondary to an occlusion of the posterior cerebral artery. (*Courtesy of S.S. Schochet, M.D., Department of Pathology, University of West Virginia, Morgantown, WV*)

▶ **TABLE 6-12.** TOP-OF-THE-BASILAR SYNDROME

Disturbance in consciousness
   Periodic alterations
   Hypersomnolence
Cognitive and behavioral impairments
   Amnesia
   Akinetic mutism
Ipsilateral oculomotor nerve palsy
   Bilateral superior rectus muscle weakness or ptosis
      Involvement of oculomotor nucleus
   Impaired vertical (up more than down) gaze
Contralateral hemiparesis (involving face, upper limb, and lower limb)
Contralateral hemisensory loss (involving face, upper limb, and lower limb)
Ipsilateral or contralateral limb ataxia
Ipsilateral or contralateral flapping (wing-beating) tremor

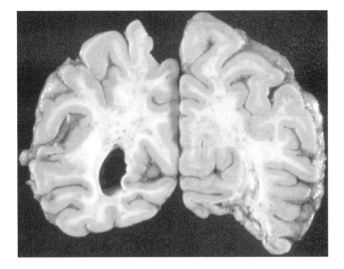

Figure 6-28. Area of infarction in the inferior portion of the temporal lobe is noted in this coronal autopsy specimen. The findings are consistent with the diagnosis of infarction in the territory of the posterior cerebral artery. (*Courtesy of S.S. Schochet, M.D. Department of Pathology, University of West Virginia, Morgantown, WV*)

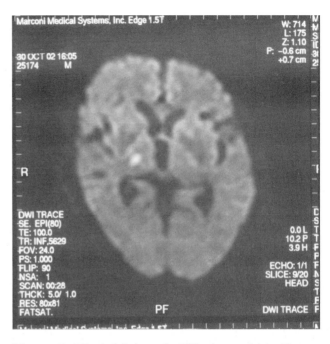

Figure 6-30. Axial view of a Diffusion weighted imaging (DWI) MRI study shows a right thalamic infarction in the distribution of the thalamogeniculate artery.

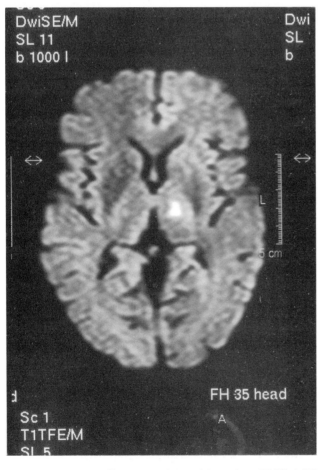

Figure 6-29. Diffusion-weighted imaging (DWI) MRI magnetic resonance imaging study shows an infarction in the anterior portion of the left thalamus.

and posterior choroidal arteries, which arise from the posterior cerebral artery, the tuberothalamic artery, which usually arises from the posterior communicating artery, and the interpeduncular-thalamic artery, which usually arises from the basilar bifurcation or the very proximal portion of the posterior cerebral artery (Figs. 6-26 to 6-28). Infarctions in the territories of these arteries produce distinct clinical syndromes[47,48] (Table 6-13; Figs. 6-29 to 6-31). Patients may have isolated motor or sensory impairments (lacunar syndromes), behavioral disturbances, or hypersomnolence.[49–53] Bilateral thalamic infarctions, which occur most commonly with occlusion of the interpeduncular-thalamic artery, produce profound behavioral impairments.[54,55] Recently, three additional patterns of thalamic infarction have been described. The locations of the causative lesions are in anteromedian, central, and posterolateral aspects of the thalamus. Less-common manifestations of thalamic infarction include thalamic ataxia, which involve impairments in sensation and coordination due to a lesion affecting the ventrolateral, ventroposterolateral, and ventroposteromedial nuclei. Affected patients may have imbalance with falling (astasia-abasia) to the direction opposite to the lesion.[56,57] Thalamic astasia occurs with lesions in the superoposterolateral aspect of the thalamus, in which falling in the direction contralateral to the stroke is observed. Motor and coordination testing is usually normal, although some patients may have mild sensory loss.

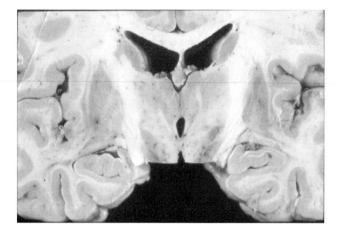

Figure 6-31. Coronal autopsy specimen visualizes an infarction involving the subthalamic nucleus and the globus pallidus on the left. (*Courtesy of S.S. Schochet, M.D., Department of Pathology, University of West Virginia, Morgantown, WV*)

▶ CLINICAL MANIFESTATIONS OF ISCHEMIC STROKES IN BRAIN STEM AND CEREBELLUM

Occlusion of the Vertebral Artery or Posteroinferior Cerebellar Artery

Atherosclerosis and arterial dissection are the most common causes of occlusion of the distal vertebral artery.[58] Less commonly, an embolus from the heart or proximal vertebral artery may lead to obstruction of the distal vertebral artery or the origin of the posteroinferior cerebellar artery (PICA). Penetrating arteries arising from the vertebral artery perfuse the dorsolateral portions of the medulla. Less commonly, these vessels arise from PICA, which also sends vessels to the inferior and medial portions of the cerebellum. As a result infarctions may involve the cerebellum and/or dorsolateral medulla (*lateral medullary syndrome of Wallenberg*) (Figs. 6-32 and 6-33; Table 6-14). Patients may have sensory loss, disturbed ocular motility, Horner syndrome, palatal paralysis, and vocal cord paralysis without the limb or gait ataxia if the infarction is restricted to the medulla.[59–61] Kim[58,62] recently evaluated the clinical findings of 130 patients with lateral medullary infarctions. Sensory abnormalities were found in nearly all patients. In some cases, the sensory loss was isolated to the limbs or body, whereas in others the face was solely involved. Rarely, infarctions were associated with sensory loss in the contralateral or bilateral trigeminal distributions. Other common symptoms or signs included dizziness, Horner syndrome, hoarseness, dysphagia, gait or limb ataxia, headache, and diplopia. If the lesion extends in a rostral direction, diplopia, gaze palsies, facial palsy, and a skew

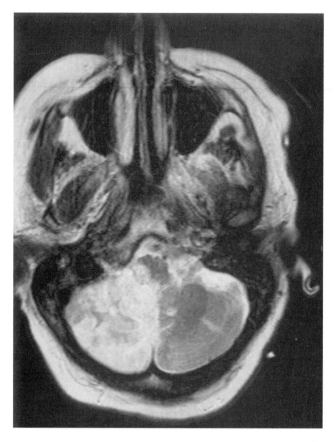

Figure 6-32. Axial T-2-weighted magnetic resonance imaging reveals a large infarction of right side of the cerebellum and darsolateral aspect of the medulla.

deviation may be found. Isolated cerebellar infarction secondary to occlusion of the vertebral or PICA leads to gait ataxia, ipsilateral limb incoordination, and nystagmus without the other signs found with medullary involvement.[63] On occasion, loss of vibratory or position sense may result from involvement of the posterior columns of

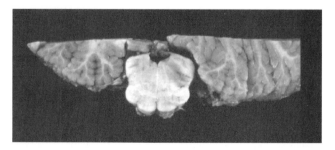

Figure 6-33. Cross section of the medulla and inferior cerebellum shows an infarction in the left dorsolateral medulla. The findings are consistent with occlusion of small branches of the vertebral artery producing the clinical findings of the dorsolateral medullary syndrome of Wallenberg. (*Courtesy of S.S. Schochet, M.D. Department of Pathology, University of West Virginia, Morgantown, WV*)

▶ **TABLE 6-13.** FINDINGS OF THALAMIC INFARCTIONS

Thalamogeniculate artery—inferolateral thalamus
  Contralateral hemisensory loss (involving face, upper limb, and lower limb)
  Thalamic pain syndrome
  Contralateral incoordination or ataxia of the limbs
  Contralateral dystonic posturing or involuntary movements
Interpeduncular-thalamic artery—paramedian thalamus
Unilateral
  Decreased consciousness with disturbed sleep–wake cycle
  Disorientation
  Amnesia
  Impaired vertical gaze
  Dystonia or tremor
  Atypical aphasia (dominant hemisphere)
  Hemispatial neglect (nondominant hemisphere)
Bilateral
  Coma
  Loss of sleep–wake cycle
  Amnesia
  Aphasia
  Neglect
  Vertical gaze palsy
Posterior choroidal artery—pulvinar and lateral geniculate
  Contralateral hemiparesis (involving face, upper limb, and lower limb)
  Contralateral hemisensory loss (involving face, upper limb, and lower limb)
  Homonymous sector or quadrantic visual field defect
Tuberothalamic (polar) artery—ventroanterior thalamus
  Abulia
  Amnesia
  Aphasia (dominant hemisphere)
  Contralateral hemiparesis (involving face, upper limb, and lower limb)
  Contralateral hemisensory loss (involving face, upper limb, and lower limb)
Anteromedian infarction—anterior and paramedian thalamus
  Decreased executive function
  Amnesia
  Transcortical motor pattern of aphasia (dominant hemisphere)
  Vertical gaze paresis
  Decreased consciousness
Central infarction—central thalamus
  Decreased executive function
  Transcortical motor pattern of aphasia (dominant hemisphere)
  Contralateral hemisensory loss
  Contralateral ataxia
Posterolateral infarction—inferolateral and posterior thalamus
  Transcortical motor pattern of aphasia (dominant hemisphere)
  Contralateral hemisensory loss
  Contralateral ataxia

Adapted in part from Schmahmann.[48]

▶ **TABLE 6-14.** FINDINGS OF INFARCTIONS OF THE MEDULLA

Lateral medullary infarction (Wallenberg syndrome)
  Ipsilateral facial pain and numbness
    Dissociated sensory loss to pain and temperature
  Contralateral hemisensory loss (upper limb, trunk, and lower limb)
    Dissociated sensory loss to pain and temperature
  Ipsilateral palatal and vocal cord paralysis
  Hiccups
  Ipsilateral limb ataxia, dysmetria, dyssynergia, and dysdiadokinesia
  Gait ataxia with ipsilateral lateropulsion
  Ipsilateral Horner syndrome
  Skew deviation
  Ipsilateral horizontal, gaze-evoked nystagmus
  Ipsilateral tonic deviation of the eyes
Medial medullary infarction
  Ipsilateral tongue paralysis
  Contralateral hemiparesis (upper limb and lower limb)
  No facial weakness
  Contralateral hemisensory loss (upper limb, trunk, and lower limb)
    Dissociated sensory loss to proprioception and fine touch
  Gaze-evoked nystagmus
Bilateral medial medullary infarction
  Quadriparesis (appears similar to locked-in syndrome)
  Bilateral paralysis of tongue
  Bilateral sensory loss (upper limb, trunk, and lower limb)
    Dissociated sensory loss to proprioception and fine touch

the rostral portion of the cervical cord or from the crossing axons that constitute the internal arcuate fibers.

Medial medullary infarction may be secondary to occlusion of the distal vertebral artery or its final major branch, the anterior spinal artery. Infarctions, which may be either unilateral or bilateral, are relatively uncommon[62,64–66] (see Table 6-14 and fig. 6-34). Bilateral medial medullary infarction mimics the findings with midline pontine infarction (the locked-in syndrome.) In this variation of the locked-in syndrome, the facial and extraocular muscles are spared, while the limbs and tongue are paralyzed. The majority of the corticospinal fibers pass from the pyramid (located in the anterior and medial portion of the medulla) through the pyramidal decussation to the contralateral dorsolateral portion of the spinal cord.[67] Fibers that innervate the upper and lower extremities cross at different levels, and thus it is possible for a unilateral medial medullary infarction to cause paresis of the ipsilateral upper limb and contralateral lower limb. Infarction in the territory of the anterior spinal artery affecting the lower medulla or rostral spinal cord can produce abnormal respiratory function, including Ondine curse, in which the patient loses automatic breathing.[68]

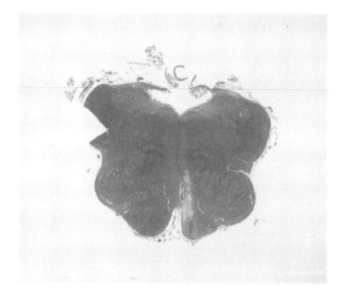

Figure 6-34. Cross section of the medulla shows the findings of a remote infarction. The infarction has affected the left pyramid and the ventral portion of the left medial lemniscus. The findings of a medial medullary syndrome would be found. (*Courtesy of S.S. Schochet, M.D., Department of Pathology, University of West Virginia, Morgantown, WV*)

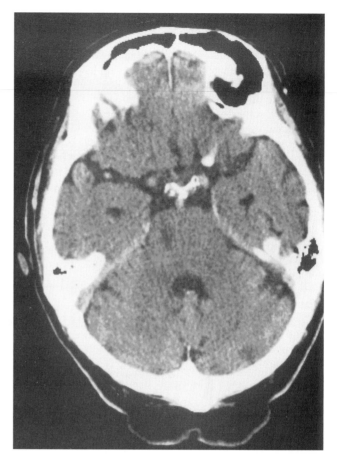

Figure 6-35. Axial CT study demonstrates a small right pontine infarction.

Occlusion of the Basilar Artery, Anteroinferior Cerebellar Artery, or Penetrating Branches of the Basilar Artery

Thrombotic occlusion of the basilar artery most commonly occurs with atherosclerotic disease; resultant occlusions are usually in the midportion of the artery.[69] Other causes include dolichoectasia of the basilar artery, dissection of the artery, and embolism from either the heart or the proximal atherosclerotic disease. Depending on whether the basilar artery, its penetrating branches, or the anteroinferior cerebellar artery (AICA) are occluded, infarction can involve the pontine base and tegmentum, a small area of pontine tegmentum, or the medial aspects of the cerebellum.[70,71] Because the internal auditory (labyrinthine) (figs. 6-35 and 6-36) artery is a branch of AICA or the basilar artery, infarction of the inner ear leading to unilateral or bilateral hearing loss may occur.[72] Intrinsic disease of the small penetrating arteries also may cause infarction that produces discrete brain stem or lacunar syndromes, including pure motor hemiparesis, pure sensory stroke, ataxia-hemiparesis, dysarthria-clumsy hand syndrome, and sensorimotor stroke. An isolated internuclear ophthalmoplegia also can be found with a small brain stem infarction.

The focal neurological impairments in pontine infarction are complex and often involve motor, sensory, and oculomotor signs[69,73] (Table 6-15). Other findings include ataxia, vertigo, nausea, tinnitus, hearing loss, and headache. The motor and sensory impairments may be unilateral, bilateral, or crossed. The sensory loss may be dissociated with isolated pain and temperature or proprioception and touch loss depending upon the location of the stroke. The *locked-in syndrome* may occur with major pontine infarctions.[70,74–76] Affected patients have facial diplegia, impaired horizontal gaze, and quadriplegia with preserved vertical eye movements (Fig. 6-35). Most patients with infarctions involving the basis pontis have dysarthria and dysphagia, and some can have anarthria or mutism. Abnormal horizontal eye movements, ocular bobbing, skew deviation, and small unreactive pupils may be found. Different patterns of motor and oculomotor disturbances that occur with small tegmental infarctions have also been described (Fig. 6-37). The *Millard–Gubler syndrome* is diagnosed when a patient has paresis of the contralateral upper and lower limbs and ipsilateral facial weakness. Ipsilateral conjugate gaze paresis, ipsilateral facial weakness, and contralateral paresis of the upper and lower limbs are found in the *Foville syndrome*. The presence of ipsilateral abducens palsy and a contralateral hemiparesis occurs in the *Landry*

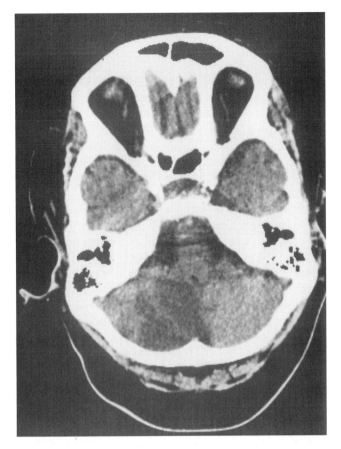

Figure 6-36. Axial CT study demonstrates a major infarction of the pons with involvement of the ipsilateral cerebellar hemisphere in a patient with locked-in syndrome.

syndrome. The *Raymond-Cestan syndrome* includes ipsilateral conjugate gaze palsy and contralateral motor and sensory impairments. Infarction in the territory of AICA involves the dorsolateral pons and the cerebellum (see Table 6-15).

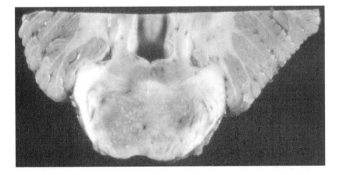

Figure 6-37. Cross section of the pons shows an infarction in the right basis pontis. This finding is consistent with an occlusion of a penetrating artery arising from the basilar artery. (Courtesy of S.S. Schochet, M.D., Department of Pathology, University of West Virginia, Morgantown, WV.)

▶ **TABLE 6-15.** FINDINGS OF INFARCTION OF THE PONS

Unilateral or partial tegmental infarction
  Ipsilateral facial palsy
  Ipsilateral facial sensory loss
  Contralateral hemiparesis (involving upper limb and
    lower limb)
  Contralateral hemisensory loss (involving upper limb
    and lower limb)
    Dissociated sensory loss to proprioception and fine
      touch or pain and temperature
  Ipsilateral abducens palsy
  Ipsilateral conjugate gaze palsy
  Internuclear ophthalmoplegia
  One and one-half syndrome
Dorsolateral (anteroinferior cerebellar artery occlusion)
 infarction
  Ipsilateral facial palsy
  Ipsilateral facial sensory loss
  Ipsilateral deafness
  Ipsilateral Horner syndrome
  Ipsilateral limb ataxia, dyssynergia, dysmetria, and
    dysdiadokinesia
  Contralateral hemisensory loss (involving upper limb
    and lower limb)
    Dissociated sensory loss to pain and temperature
Locked-in syndrome
  Quadriparesis
  Bilateral facial palsies
  Lingual and pharyngeal paresis
  Anarthria
  Bilateral horizontal gaze palsy
  Retained vertical gaze
  Retained consciousness
Massive pontine infarction
  Coma
  Quadriparesis
  Bilateral facial palsies
  Lingual and pharyngeal paresis
  Anarthria
  Bilateral horizontal gaze palsy
  Ocular bobbing
  Small, unreactive pupils (pinpoint pupils)
  Skew deviation

Occlusion of the Superior Cerebellar Artery or Mesencephalic Infarctions

Penetrating branches of the distal portion of the basilar artery perfuse the midbrain.[77,78] In addition, the superior cerebellar artery (SCA) also supplies the dorsolateral midbrain and the superior and medial portion of the cerebellum. Cerebellar infarctions can be from large-artery or small-artery occlusions. {Kim & Kim 2005 ID: 12326} Many of the clinical findings of rostral midbrain infarction comprise the top-of-the-basilar syndrome.[77] In addition, midbrain infarctions produce motor and sensory loss, disturbed ocular motility, visual hallucinations, and altered consciousness.[79] Anteriomedial infarctions are associated with ataxia, oculorotatory impairments, and sensory loss in the hand and face. {Kim & Kim 2005 ID: 12326} Anterolateral infarctions produce hemiparesis and ataxia. {Kim & Kim 2005 ID: 12326} Small infarctions can cause isolated oculomotor nerve or trochlear nerve palsies. A series of discrete vascular syndromes of the midbrain have been described.[80] A contralateral hemiparesis and ipsilateral oculomotor nerve palsy constitute the *Weber syndrome*. Ipsilateral oculomotor nerve palsy and contralateral tremor, chorea, or athetosis are found in the *Benedikt syndrome*. *Claude syndrome* includes ipsilateral oculomotor nerve palsy and contralateral limb ataxia. Other oculomotor disturbances include unilateral and bilateral ptosis, vertical gaze palsy, upbeat nystagmus, skew deviation, and convergence-retraction nystagmus. The findings of stroke in the territory of the SCA include ipsilateral limb ataxia, ipsilateral Horner syndrome, ipsilateral trochlear nerve palsy, and contralateral hemisensory loss of pain and temperature.

Cerebellar Infarction

Infarctions of the cerebellum may occur alone or in conjunction with brain stem ischemia.[81–86] Most infarctions are secondary to embolic events. Larger cerebellar infarctions are usually due to occlusion of the SCA, AICA, or PICA (Figs. 6-38 to 6-39). Because of the anatomic variations in these arteries, secondary cerebellar infarctions can vary considerably among patients. Larger cerebellar infarctions also cause headache, nausea, vomiting, vertigo, and gait incoordination. The limb ataxia is usually ipsilateral to the infarction (Table 6-16). Mass-producing cerebellar infarctions may compress the brain stem and fourth ventricle, leading to decreased consciousness, facial palsy or sensory loss, oculorotatory palsies, or hemiparesis. While these findings are usually not present within the first hours after cerebellar infarction, they may appear during the first 24–48 h following the event. Subsequently, pupillary abnormalities, ocular bobbing, respiratory disturbances, and cardiac arrhythmias may also occur. Lacunar infarctions of the cerebellum may present with isolated signs. In addition, infarctions restricted

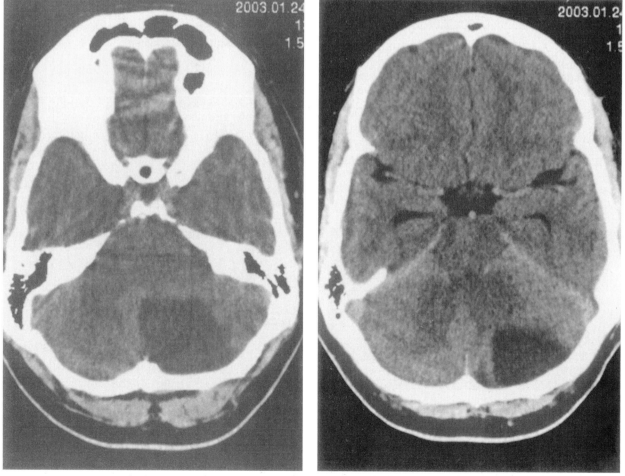

Figure 6-38. Axial CT study shows a cerebellar infarction in the territory of the left PICA.

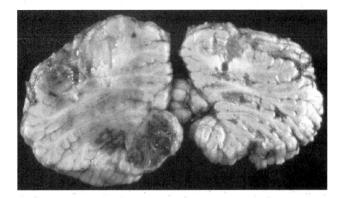

Figure 6-39. Coronal autopsy specimen of both cerebellar hemispheres demonstrates bilateral infarctions. A large lesion of the superior portion of the right hemisphere is compatible with a remote infarction in the territory of the SCA. The large hemorrhagic lesion in the inferior portion of the right hemisphere is consistent with a recent occlusion of the PICA. The smaller cystic lesions in the left hemisphere are secondary to remote lacunar infarctions. (*Courtesy of S.S. Schochet, M.D., Department of Pathology, University of West Virginia, Morgantown, WV*)

to the inferior portion of the cerebellum may mimic an acute vestibular syndrome. Patients may have intense vertigo, vomiting, and imbalance but with no or subtle unilateral limb incoordination.

► LACUNAR INFARCTIONS AND LACUNAR SYNDROMES

Small infarctions secondary to occlusion of small penetrating arteries may be found in the brain stem, cerebellum, or deep hemispheric structures among persons

▶ **TABLE 6-16.** FINDINGS OF CEREBELLAR INFARCTION

Truncal and gait ataxia
Ipsilateral limb ataxia, dyssynergia, dysmetria, and dysdiadochokinesia
Ipsilateral action tremor
Dysarthria (scanning speech)
Ipsilateral horizontal or rotatory nystagmus
Cerebellar infarction with mass effects
   Same findings as above
   Decreased consciousness
   Ipsilateral facial weakness and sensory loss
   Ipsilateral hearing loss and tinnitus
   Ipsilateral conjugate paresis
   Quadriparesis
Isolated Inferior Cerebellar Infarction
   Vertigo, vomiting, and sense of imbalance
   Truncal and gait ataxia (may be mild)
   Ipsilateral limb ataxia (may be absent)
   Ipsilateral horizontal or rotatory nystagmus

with chronic hypertension or diabetes mellitus. These strokes, which are usually smaller than 1 cm in diameter, are secondary to thrombotic occlusion of the vessels that arise from the proximal segments of the anterior cerebral artery, middle cerebral artery, or posterior cerebral artery, the distal internal carotid artery, or the basilar artery.[87,88] Several distinct clinical (lacunar) syndromes are ascribed to lacunar infarctions.[89–93] While the clinical findings of the lacunar syndromes are usually due to small-artery occlusions (lacunar infarctions), these findings have been described in patients with embolic occlusions of larger arteries (for example, striatocapsular infarction) or strokes in more peripheral locations.[94] The lacunar syndromes are described in Table 6-17 and are also included in the LACI category of

▶ **TABLE 6-17.** FINDINGS OF THE COMMON LACUNAR SYNDROMES

Pure motor hemiparesis
   Locations of infarction
      Internal capsule (anterior limb and posterior limb)
      Pons
      Medullary pyramid
      Corona radiata (centrum semiovale)
   Clinical findings
      Contralateral hemiparesis (involving face, upper limb, and lower limb)
      Dysarthria
      No sensory loss or cognitive impairments
Pure sensory stroke
   Location of infarction
      Lateral thalamus
   Clinical findings
      Contralateral hemisensory loss (involving face, upper limb, and lower limb—involving all sensory modalities)
Sensorimotor stroke
   Location of infarction
      Posterior limb of internal capsule and adjacent thalamus
   Clinical findings
      Contralateral hemiparesis (involving face, upper limb, and lower limb)
      Contralateral hemisensory loss (involving face, upper limb, and lower limb—involving all sensory modalities)
Dysarthria—clumsy hand
   Locations of infarction
      Genu of internal capsule
      Pons
   Clinical findings
      Severe dysarthria
      Contralateral facial weakness
      Contralateral hand clumsiness
Homolateral ataxia and hemiparesis
   Location of infarction
      Pons
   Clinical findings
      Contralateral arm and leg ataxia
      Contralateral paresis (involving the distal lower limb)

the Oxfordshire classification of stroke.[15] Pure motor hemiparesis is the most common of these syndromes. While the motor impairments usually affect the face, upper limb, and lower limb equally, differences in the degree of involvement may be found. Dysarthria may be prominent particularly with a lacunar infarction in the brain stem.

► MICROVASCULAR DISEASE OF THE BRAIN

With the advent of modern brain imaging, a population of patients with extensive changes in the white matter were discovered. Most of these patients are elderly, have hypertension, and have progressive cognitive decline. The presumption is that the imaging abnormalities (*leukoaraiosis*) are secondary to microvascular disease. The white matter lesions are usually extensive and situated in periventricular locations, primarily in the frontal and parietal lobes. These lesions are not in the same pattern as those with small-artery (lacunar) disease and they have been correlated with a slowly progressive dementia. The course is not one of stepwise deterioration or prominent focal noncognitive neurological impairments.

REFERENCES

1. Norris JW, Hachinski VC. Misdiagnosis of stroke. *Lancet* 1982;1:328–331.
2. The Members of the Lille Stroke Program. Misdiagnoses in 1250 consecutive patients admitted to an acute stroke unit. *Cerebrovasc Dis* 1997;7:284–288.
3. Harrison MJ. Clinical distinction of cerebral haemorrhage and cerebral infarction. *Postgrad Med J* 1980;56:629–632.
4. Weir CJ, Murray GD, Adams FG, Muir KW, Grosset DG, Lees KR. Poor accuracy of stroke scoring systems for differential clinical diagnosis of intracranial haemorrhage and infarction. *Lancet* 1994;344:999–1002.
5. Besson G, Robert C, Hommel M, Perret J. Is it clinically possible to distinguish nonhemorrhagic infarct from hemorrhagic stroke? *Stroke* 1995;26:1205–1209.
6. Wallis WE, Donaldson I, Scott RS, Wilson J. Hypoglycemia masquerading as cerebrovascular disease (hypoglycemic hemiplegia). *Ann Neurol* 1985;18:510–512.
7. Parvizi J, Damasio AR. Neuroanatomical correlates of brainstem coma. *Brain* 2003;126:1524–1536.
8. Davalos A, de Cendra E, Molins A, Ferrandiz M, Lopez-Pousa S, Genis D. Epileptic seizures at the onset of stroke. *Cerebrovasc Dis* 1992;2:327–331.
9. Kilpatrick CJ, Davis SM, Tress BM, Rossiter SC, Hopper JL, Vandendriesen ML. Epileptic seizures in acute stroke. *Arch Neurol* 1990;47:157–160.
10. Arboix A, Massons J, Oliveres M, Arribas MP, Titus F. Headache in acute cerebrovascular disease. A prospective clinical study in 240 patients. *Cephalalgia* 1994;14:37–40.
11. Ferro JM, Melo TP, Oliveira V, et al. A multivariate study of headache associated with ischemic stroke. *Headache* 1995;35:315–319.
12. Jorgensen HS, Jespersen HF, Nakayama H, Raaschou HO, Olsen TS. Headache in stroke: the Copenhagen Stroke Study. *Neurology* 1994;44:1793–1797.
13. Fisher CM. The headache and pain of spontaneous carotid dissection. *Headache* 1982;22:60–65.
14. Silbert PL, Mokri B, Schievink WI. Headache and neck pain in spontaneous internal carotid and vertebral artery dissections. *Neurology* 1995;45:1517–1522.
15. Bamford J, Sandercock P, Dennis M, Burn J, Warlow C. Classification and natural history of clinically identifiable subtypes of cerebral infarction. *Lancet* 1991;337:1521–1526.
16. Caplan L, Babikian V, Helgason C, et al. Occlusive disease of the middle cerebral artery. *Neurology* 1985;35:975–982.
17. Lyrer PA, Engelter S, Radu EW, Steck AJ. Cerebral infarcts related to isolated middle cerebral artery stenosis. *Stroke* 1997;28:1022–1027.
18. Heinsius T, Bogousslavsky J, Van Melle G. Large infarcts in the middle cerebral artery territory. Etiology and outcome patterns. *Neurology* 1998;50:341–350.
19. Ghika JA, Bogousslavsky J, Regli F. Deep perforators from the carotid system. Template of the vascular territories. *Arch Neurol* 1990;47:1097–1100.
20. Donnan GA, Norrving B, Bamford J, Bogousslavsky J. Subcortical infarction: classification and terminology. *Cerebrovasc Dis* 1993;3:248–251.
21. Kumral E, Evyapan D, Balkir K. Acute caudate vascular lesions. *Stroke* 1999;30:100–108.
22. Bogousslavsky J, Van Melle G, Regli F. Middle cerebral artery pial territory infarcts: a study of the Lausanne Stroke Registry. *Ann Neurol* 1989;25:555–560.
23. Sindermann F, Dichgans J, Bergleiter R. Occlusion of the middle cerebral artery and its branches: angiographic and clinical correlates. *Brain* 1969;92:607–620.
24. Waddington MM, Ring BA. Syndromes of occlusions of middle cerebral artery branches. *Brain* 1968;91:685–696.
25. Caplan LR, Kelly M, Kase CS, et al. Infarcts of the inferior division of the right middle cerebral artery. Mirror image of Wernicke's aphasia. *Neurology* 1986;36:1015–1020.
26. Bogousslavsky J. Double infarction in one cerebral hemisphere. *Ann Neurol* 1991;30:12–18.
27. Leblanc R, Yamamoto YL, Tyler JL, Diksic M, Hakim A. Borderzone ischemia. *Ann Neurol* 1987;22:707–713.
28. Baird AE, Donnan GA, Saling M. Mechanisms and clinical features of internal watershed infarction. *Clin Exp Neurol* 1991;28:50–55.
29. Momjian-Mayor I, Baron JC. The pathophysiology of watershed infarction in internal carotid artery disease. Review of cerebral perfusion studies. *Stroke* 2005;36:567–577.
30. Sage JI, Van Uitert RL. Man-in-the-barrel syndrome. *Neurology* 1986;36:1102–1103.
31. Leys D, Mounier-Vehier F, Rondepierre P, et al. Small infarcts in the centrum ovale: study of predisposing factors. *Cerebrovasc Dis* 1994;4:83–87.
32. Kumral E, Bayulkem G. Spectrum of single and multiple corona radiata infarcts: clinical/MRI correlations. *J Stroke Cerebrovasc Dis* 2003;12:66–73.

33. Lammie GA, Wardlaw JM. Small centrum ovale infarcts—a pathological study. *Cerebrovasc Dis* 1999;9:82–90.

34. Paroni SG, Agatiello LM, Stocchi A, Solivetti FM. CT of ischemic infarctions in the territory of the anterior choroidal artery: a review of 28 cases. *AJNR Am J Neuroradiol* 1987; 8:229–232.

35. Bruno A, Graff-Radfor NR, Biller J, Adams HP, Jr. Anterior choroidal artery territory infarction: a small vessel disease. *Stroke* 1999;20:616–619.

36. Leys D, Mounier-Vehier F, Lavenu I, Rondepierre P, Pruvo JP. Anterior choroidal artery territory infarcts. Study of presumed mechanisms. *Stroke* 1994;25:837–842.

37. Bogousslavsky J, Regli F. Anterior cerebral artery territory infarction in the Lausanne Stroke Registry. *Arch Neurol* 1990;47:144–150.

38. Webster JE, Gurjian ES, Lindner DW, Hardy WG. Proximal occlusion of the anterior cerebral artery. *Arch Neurol* 1960;2:19–26.

39. Klatka LA, Depper MH, Marini AM. Infarction in the territory of the anterior cerebral artery. *Neurology* 1998;51:620–622.

40. Minagar A, David NJ. Bilateral infarction in the territory of the anterior cerebral arteries. *Neurology* 1999;52:886–888.

41. Giroud M, Dumas R. Clinical and topographical range of callosal infarction: a clinical and radiological correlation study. *J Neurol Neurosurg Psychiatry* 1995;59:238–242.

42. Hommel M, Besson G, Pollak P, Kahane P, Le Bas JF, Perret J. Hemiplegia in posterior cerebral artery occlusion. *Neurology* 1990;40:1496–1499.

43. Georgiadis AL, Yamamoto Y, Kwan ES, Pessin MS, Caplan LR. Anatomy of sensory findings in patients with posterior cerebral artery territory infarction. *Arch Neurol* 1999;56: 835–838.

44. Chambers BR, Brooder RJ, Donnan GA. Proximal posterior cerebral artery occlusion simulating middle cerebral artery occlusion. *Neurology* 1991;41:385–390.

45. Aldrich MS, Alessi AG, Beck RW, Gilman S. Cortical blindness. Etiology, diagnosis, and prognosis. *Ann Neurol* 1987; 21:149–158.

46. Caplan LR. "Top of the basilar" syndrome. *Neurology* 1980;30:72–79.

47. Carrera E, Bogousslavsky J. The thalamus and behavior. Effects of anatomically distinct strokes. *Neurology* 2006;66: 1817–1823.

48. Schmahmann JD. Vascular syndromes of the thalamus. *Stroke* 2003;34:2264–2278.

49. Neau JP, Bogousslavsky J. The syndrome of posterior choroidal artery territory infarction. *Ann Neurol* 1996;39: 779–788.

50. Bassetti C, Mathis J, Gugger M, Lovblad KO, Hess CW. Hypersomnia following paramedian thalamic stroke: a report of 12 patients. *Ann Neurol* 1996;39:471–480.

51. Eslinger PJ, Warner GC, Grattan LM, Easton JD. "Frontal lobe" utilization behavior associated with paramedian thalamic infarction. *Neurology* 1991;41:450–452.

52. Gorelick PB, Hier DB, Benevento L, Levitt S, Tan W. Aphasia after left thalamic infarction. *Arch Neurol* 1984;41: 1296–1298.

53. Annoni JM, Khateb A, Gramigna S, et al. Chronic cognitive impairment following laterothalamic infarcts: a study of 9 cases. *Arch Neurol* 2003;60:1439–1443.

54. Biller J, Sand JJ, Corbett JJ, Adams HP, Jr., Dunn V. Syndrome of the paramedian thalamic arteries. Clinical and neuroimaging correlation. *J Clin Neuroophthalmol* 1985;5:217–223.

55. Gentilini M, De Renzi E, Crisi G. Bilateral paramedian thalamic artery infarcts: report of eight cases. *J Neurol Neurosurg Psychiatry* 1987;50:900–909.

56. Melo TP, Bogousslavsky J, Moulin T, Nader J, Regli F. Thalamic ataxia. *J Neurol* 1992;239:331–337.

57. Masdeu JC, Gorelick PB. Thalamic astasia: inability to stand after unilateral thalamic lesions. *Ann Neurol* 1988; 23:596–603.

58. Kim JS. Pure lateral medullary infarction: clinical-radiological correlation of 130 acute, consecutive patients. *Brain* 2003;126:1864–1872.

59. Sacco RL, Freddo L, Bello JA, Odel JG, Onesti ST, Mohr JP. Wallenberg's lateral medullary syndrome. Clinical-magnetic resonance imaging correlations. *Arch Neurol* 1993;50: 609–614.

60. Fisher CM, Tapia J. Lateral medullary infarction extending to the lower pons. *J Neurol Neurosurg Psychiatry* 1987; 50:620–624.

61. Brazis PW. Ocular motor abnormalities in Wallenberg's lateral medullary syndrome. *Mayo Clin Proc* 1992;67: 365–368.

62. Kameda W, Kawanami T, Kurita K, et al. Lateral and medial medullary infarction. A comparative analysis of 214 patients. *Stroke* 2004;35:694–699.

63. Duncan GW, Parker SW, Fisher CM. Acute cerebellar infarction in the PICA territory. *Arch Neurol* 1975;32:364–368.

64. Kumral E, Afsar N, Kirbas D, Balkir K, Ozdemirkiran T. Spectrum of medial medullary infarction: clinical and magnetic resonance imaging findings. *J Neurol* 2002;249:85–93.

65. Toyoda K, Imamura T, Saku Y, et al. Medial medullary infarction: analyses of eleven patients. *Neurology* 1996;47: 1141–1147.

66. Kim JS, Kim HG, Chung CS. Medial medullary syndrome. Report of 18 new patients and a review of the literature. *Stroke* 1995;26:1548–1552.

67. Chokroverty S, Rubino FA, Haller C. Pure motor hemiplegia due to pyramidal infarction. *Arch Neurol* 1975;32:647–648.

68. Manconi M, Mondini S, Fabiani A, Rossi P, Ambrosetto P, Cirignotta F. Anterior spinal artery syndrome complicated by the Ondine curse. *Arch Neurol* 2003;60:1787–1790.

69. Voetsch B, DeWitt LD, Pessin MS, Caplan LR. Basilar artery occlusive disease in the New England Medical Center Posterior Circulation Registry. *Arch Neurol* 2004;61: 496–504.

70. Fisher CM. Bilateral occlusion of basilar artery branches. *J Neurol Neurosurg Psychiatry* 1977;40:1182–1189.

71. Fisher CM, Caplan LR. Basilar artery branch occlusion: a cause of pontine infarction. *Neurology* 1971;21:900–905.

72. Huang MH, Huang CC, Ryu SJ, Chu NS. Sudden bilateral hearing impairment in vertebrobasilar occlusive disease. *Stroke* 1993;24:132–137.

73. Kumral E, Bayulkem G, Evyapan D. Clinical spectrum of pontine infarction. Clinical-MRI correlations. *J Neurol* 2003;249:1659–1670.

74. Schwarz S, Egelhof T, Schwab S, Hacke W. Basilar artery embolism. Clinical syndrome and neuroradiologic patterns

in patients without permanent occlusion of the basilar artery. *Neurology* 1997;49:1346–1352.

75. Patterson JR, Grabois M. Locked-in syndrome: a review of 139 cases. *Stroke* 1986;17:758–764.

76. Ferbert A, Bruckmann H, Drummen R. Clinical features of proven basilar artery occlusion. *Stroke* 1990;21:1135–1142.

77. Kumral E, Bayulkem G, Akyol A, Yunten N, Sirin H, Sagduyu A. Mesencephalic and associated posterior circulation infarcts. *Stroke* 2002;33:2224–2231.

78. Martin PJ, Chang HM, Wityk R, Caplan LR. Midbrain infarction: associations and aetiologies in the New England Medical Center Posterior Circulation Registry. *J Neurol Neurosurg Psychiatry* 1998;64:392–395.

79. Hommel M, Bogousslavsky J. The spectrum of vertical gaze palsy following unilateral brainstem stroke. *Neurology* 1991; 41:1229–1234.

80. Bogousslavsky J, Maeder P, Regli F, Meuli R. Pure midbrain infarction: clinical syndromes, MRI, and etiologic patterns. *Neurology* 1994;44:2032–2040.

81. Amarenco P, Hauw JJ. Cerebellar infarction in the territory of the anterior and inferior cerebellar artery. *Brain* 1990; 113:139–155.

82. Amarenco P, Hauw JJ, Gautier JC. Arterial pathology in cerebellar infarction. *Stroke* 1990;21:1299–1305.

83. Amarenco P, Levy C, Cohen A, Toubouc PJ, Roullet E, Bousser MG. Causes and mechanisms of territorial and non-territorial cerebellar infarcts in 115 consecutive patients. *Stroke* 1994;25:105–112.

84. Amarenco P, Rosengart A, DeWitt LD, Pessin MS, Caplan LR. Anterior inferior cerebellar artery territory infarcts. Mechanisms and clinical features. *Arch Neurol* 1993;50: 154–161.

85. Amarenco P, Roullet E, Govjoa C, Cheron F, Hauw JJ, Bousser MG. Infarction in the anterior rostral cerebellum (the territory of the lateral branch of the superior cerebellar artery). *Neurology* 1991;41:253–258.

86. Chaves CJ, Caplan LR, Chung CS, et al. Cerebellar infarcts in the New England Medical Center Posterior Circulation Stroke Registry. *Neurology* 1994;44:1385–1390.

87. Fisher CM. Lacunar infarcts—a review. *Cerebrovasc Dis* 1991;1:311–20.

88. Fisher CM. Lacunar strokes and infarcts: a review. *Neurology* 1982;32:871–876.

89. Fisher CM. A lacunar stroke. The dysarthria-clumsy hand syndrome. *Neurology* 1967;17:614–647.

90. Fisher CM. Ataxic hemiparesis. A pathologic study. *Arch Neurol* 1978;35:126–128.

91. Fisher CM. Pure sensory stroke involving face, arm and leg. *Neurology* 1965;15:76–80.

92. Fisher CM, Cole M. Homolateral ataxia and rural paresis. A vascular syndrome. *J Neurol Neurosurg Psychiatry* 1965; 28:48–55.

93. Fisher CM, Curry HB. Pure motor hemiplegia. *Trans Am Neurol Assoc* 1964;89:94–97.

94. Arboix A, Marti-Vilalta JL. Lacunar syndromes not due to lacunar infarcts. *Cerebrovasc Dis* 1992;2:287–292.

CHAPTER 7

Clinical Manifestations of Hemorrhagic Stroke

The clinical features of hemorrhagic stroke are influenced by the location, extent, rate, and cause of bleeding. Classic symptoms include rapid or sudden onset of severe headache accompanied by nausea, vomiting, depressed consciousness with or without seizures, and focal neurological impairments that rapidly worsen. Most hemorrhages occur while the patient is awake.[1] Intracranial hemorrhage is a devastating illness that may lead to sudden death and accounts for approximately 10 percent of causes of sudden death.[2] Nearly 25 percent of patients with intracranial bleeding are dead within the first 24 h.[3,4] It is second only to acute cardiac disease as a nontraumatic cause of death within 24 h of onset of symptoms.

A gradual course or evolution of neurological signs during the first few hours of hemorrhage is seen in a majority of patients with intracerebral hemorrhage. The worsening of neurological signs or decline in consciousness may be secondary to expansion of the hematoma, mass effect with increased intracranial pressure, or acute complications such as hydrocephalus.[5,6] Patients with subarachnoid hemorrhage or primary intraventricular hemorrhage usually have headache, nausea, vomiting, seizures, and decreased consciousness but with absence of subtle focal neurological deficits. Small hemorrhages restricted to one location in the brain may mimic a lacunar or subcortical infarction and may not be associated with headache, nausea, vomiting, or altered consciousness. Differentiating a minor hemorrhagic stroke from an ischemic stroke may be difficult clinically and brain imaging (in particular CT) remains a key diagnostic aid (Fig. 7-1).[7]

▶ INTRACEREBRAL (INTRAPARENCHYMAL) HEMORRHAGE

General Symptoms

Approximately 50 percent of patients with intracerebral hemorrhage will have headache, most commonly at the time of onset of symptoms. While headache is more common with intracerebral hemorrhage than with ischemic stroke, it usually is not as severe as that reported with subarachnoid hemorrhage. The headache may lateralize to the side of bleeding in a patient with a hemispheric hemorrhage or may be located in the occiput or base of the head when bleeding occurs in the posterior fossa. If bleeding extends into the subarachnoid space or the ventricles, the patient might complain of neck or back pain (Fig. 7-2). Although some patients with ischemic stroke also have headache, particularly with lesions in the posterior fossa, headache as a prominent complaint increases the likelihood of hemorrhage as the cause of focal neurological impairments. The presence of nausea, vomiting, photophobia, and phonophobia also increases the likelihood that the patient's stroke is hemorrhagic.[7] These symptoms are prominent in nearly 50 percent of the patients with

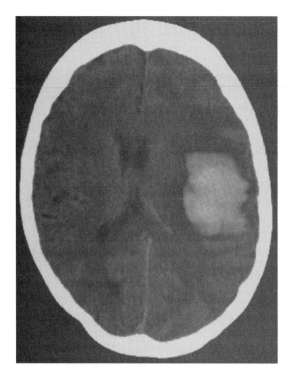

Figure 7-1. Unenhanced CT of the brain shows a large lobar hemorrhage in the left hemisphere.

intracerebral hemorrhage. In particular, the presence of these complaints in a patient whose other findings point to a stroke in the cerebral hemisphere should increase suspicion of a hemorrhagic stroke.

An alteration in consciousness at the time of onset of stroke is a strong clue that the vascular event involves hemorrhage. The initial level of consciousness is a strong prognostic factor; mortality increases rapidly when the patient has a prolonged period of decreased

consciousness.[8–10] Brief or sustained disturbances in consciousness occur in almost one-half of the cases, either at the time of ictus or within the first few hours. Large hematomas (generally >2.5 cm in diameter) or hemorrhages located deep in the hemisphere, brain stem, or cerebellum are most likely to be associated with impaired consciousness (Fig. 7-3). Seizures or seizure-mimicking events may occur at the time of the hemorrhage. Epileptic phenomena are more common with hemorrhagic strokes, particularly those involving the cerebral cortex, than with ischemic lesions, and seizures are more likely to occur with lobar hematomas than with bleeding in the deep hemispheric structures, brain stem, or cerebellum. Some patients with hemorrhagic stroke will act confused or appear to be in a delirium while others complain of agitation and restlessness.

In general, patients with hemorrhagic stroke appear sicker than do patients with ischemic stroke. They often are in distress due to headache, pain, nausea, and vomiting. The presence of depressed consciousness or agitation also adds to the grave nature of the illness. Most patients have abnormalities detected during assessment of the vital signs. Patients may have ventilatory or cardiac arrhythmias secondary to increased intracranial pressure. In addition, hemorrhages in the posterior fossa are associated with high rates of cardiorespiratory dysfunction. Cardiac arrhythmias may be life threatening and the electrocardiogram often demonstrates acute changes consistent with cardiac ischemia. Almost 90 percent of patients with hemorrhagic stroke will have an

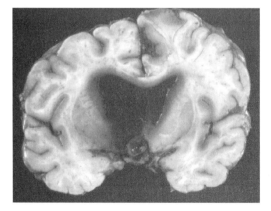

Figure 7-2. Coronal autopsy specimen demonstrates a ruptured anterior communicating artery aneurysm with secondary cerebral and intraventricular hemorrhage. In particular, the bleeding has affected the basal forebrain. (*Courtesy of S.S. Schochet, M.D., Department of Pathology, University of West Virginia, Morgantown WV*)

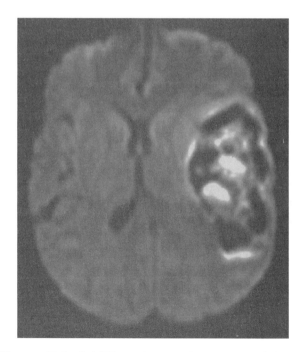

Figure 7-3. A MRI study reveals a large left hemisphere hemorrhage.

elevated blood pressure and in many instances the readings are remarkably high or volatile. In general, the presence of a markedly elevated blood pressure is a poor prognostic sign.[11,12] While it may be a manifestation of either acute or chronic arterial hypertension, which could be the cause of the bleeding, it also may result from the stress of the hemorrhage or increased intracranial pressure. Fever, which generally results from secondary intraventricular or subarachnoid bleeding, generally is considered a poor prognostic sign.[13] Fever may be secondary to neurological dysfunction, an inflammatory reaction to blood in the subarachnoid space, an infectious disease as the cause of the hemorrhagic stroke, or an infectious complication of the bleeding. Nuchal rigidity may be found if the blood reaches the subarachnoid space.

Patients with intraparenchymal hemorrhage will have focal neurological impairments reflecting the location of the bleeding. The likelihood that bleeding is the cause of stroke is increased if focal signs do not reflect those findings associated with occlusion of one artery. The chances of bleeding as the cause of a hemorrhage in the cerebral hemisphere increase if the signs do not point toward a cortical lesion.

Putaminal Hemorrhage

The putamen is the most common site for hemorrhage, particularly among persons with hypertension (Fig. 7-4). Hypertension is the most common etiology of primary putaminal hemorrhage and is the location of approximately one-third of all primary intracerebral hemorrhages. Bleeding usually involves rupture of a lenticulostriate

artery arising from the first portion of the middle cerebral artery. Rupture of the anterior choroidal artery may cause hemorrhage in the posterior limb of the internal capsule and adjacent putamen. In addition, bleeding can extend into the adjacent internal capsule, centrum semiovale, insular region, or temporal lobe. Large putaminal hemorrhages may have secondary intraventricular or subarachnoid extension; the latter may involve the Sylvian fissure. The size of the hematoma affects neurological impairments. Contralateral hemiparesis is the most prominent focal sign and sensory impairments are less obvious.[14] Patients with large hematomas have a flaccid hemiplegia with hemisensory loss (Table 7-1).

▶ **TABLE 7-1.** CLINICAL FINDINGS OF HEMORRHAGES IN THE PUTAMEN AND ADJACENT INTERNAL CAPSULE

Large putaminal hemorrhage
  Decreased consciousness (often coma)
  Contralateral hemiparesis (hemiplegia)
  Contralateral hemisensory loss (not as severe as motor signs)
  Behavioral and cognitive impairments
    Atypical aphasia (dominant hemisphere)
    Neglect or apraxia (nondominant hemisphere)
  Contralateral homonymous visual field defect
  Ipsilateral conjugate gaze deviation (looking toward the lesion)
Internal capsule (posteromedial striatocapsular) hemorrhage
  Contralateral mild-to-moderate hemiparesis
    Pure motor hemiparesis (without sensory loss)
  Dysarthria
  Contralateral hemisensory loss (uncommon)
  Contralateral conjugate gaze deviation
Middle putamen (middle striatocapsular) hemorrhage
  Contralateral mild-to-moderate hemiparesis
    Pure motor hemiparesis (without sensory loss)
  Contralateral hemisensory loss (uncommon)
  Contralateral conjugate gaze deviation
  Behavioral and cognitive impairments
    Aphasia (larger dominant hemisphere)
Posterior putamen (posterior striatocapsular) hemorrhage
  Contralateral moderate-to-severe hemiparesis
  Contralateral hemisensory loss
  Contralateral or ipsilateral conjugate gaze deviation
  Behavioral and cognitive impairments
    Aphasia (dominant hemisphere)
    Neglect (nondominant hemisphere)
Lateral putamen and external capsule (lateral striatocapsular) hemorrhage
  Contralateral mild-to-moderate hemiparesis
  Behavioral and cognitive impairments
    Aphasia (dominant hemisphere)
    Neglect (nondominant hemisphere)
  Contralateral hemisensory loss is uncommon
  Contralateral conjugate gaze deviation is uncommon

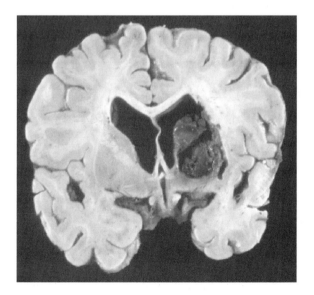

Figure 7-4. Coronal autopsy specimen shows a large left basal ganglion hemorrhage. (*Courtesy of S.S. Schochet, M.D., Department of Pathology, University of West Virginia, Morgantown, WV*)

Most patients with large putaminal hemorrhages have conjugate gaze palsy with the eyes directed toward the lesion but contralateral deviation also can be found.[15] The gaze palsy can be overcome with the doll's eye maneuver. Typically, no pupillary changes are present unless a secondary herniation is occurring. Hemorrhages in the dominant hemisphere can be associated with an atypical nonfluent aphasia, while bleeding in the nondominant putamen may be associated with neglect or apraxia.[16] A contralateral homonymous visual field defect may be detected if bleeding extends posteriorly into the optic radiations.

Striatocapsular Hemorrhage

Chung et al.[14] described patterns of smaller striatocapsular hemorrhages (see Table 7-1). Small hematomas may be detected in the genu or the posterior limb of the internal capsule, while the putamen is spared. Patients have pure motor hemiparesis or contralateral hemiparesis and sensory loss. Consciousness is not impaired and eyes can be deviated toward the side of the hematoma.[14] The prognosis of patients with smaller hemorrhages restricted to the putamen or internal capsule generally is good.

Caudate Hemorrhage

Primary hemorrhages of the caudate nucleus are relatively uncommon. When bleeding occurs, the typical location is the head of the caudate in the distribution of the recurrent artery of Huebner or the more medial lenticulostriate arteries. The leading causes are hypertension or vascular malformations. Intraventricular extension is relatively common and the bleeding may expand to involve the anterior limb of the internal capsule, putamen, or thalamus. In general, the symptoms of caudate hemorrhage mimic those of subarachnoid hemorrhage.[17] Severe headache, nausea, vomiting, and nuchal rigidity are common. These findings are more common with caudate than with putaminal hemorrhage. Consciousness usually is not affected and motor impairments, which are contralateral, usually are mild. Hemisensory loss may also occur. Behavioral and cognitive signs, including neglect, abulia, aphasia, or memory loss, may be detected with larger hematomas.[18]

Thalamic Hemorrhage

Bleeding into the thalamus, most commonly secondary to hypertension, accounts for approximately 20 percent of primary brain hemorrhages (Fig. 7-5). Hemorrhage results from rupture of small penetrating vessels that arise from the basilar, posterior cerebral, or posterior communicating arteries. Bleeding may be restricted to a part of the thalamus or may extend into the midbrain,

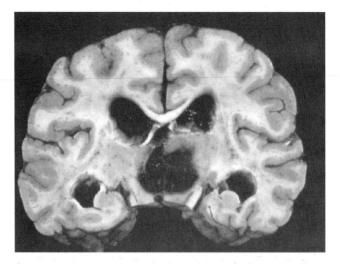

Figure 7-5. Large hemorrhage arising in the left thalamus is found in this coronal autopsy specimen. The bleeding has extended into the third ventricle. Secondary enlargement of both lateral ventricles (acute hydrocephalus) is present. (*Courtesy of S.S. Schochet, M.D., Department of Pathology, University of West Virginia, Morgantown, WV.*)

internal capsule, subthalamic nucleus, or white matter of the parietal lobe.[19] Bleeding may involve the third ventricle and the subarachnoid space. The manifestations of hemorrhage in the thalamus are diverse and reflect the size and primary site of the hematoma. The usual symptoms of large thalamic hematomas (diameter > 3.3 cm) include severe headache, nausea, vomiting, and decreased consciousness.

Focal neurological signs with large hematomas include contralateral hemisensory loss and contralateral hemiparesis. The sensory abnormalities usually are more prominent than the motor impairments (Table 7-2). The sensory loss may be so severe that the patient develops a secondary ataxia.[20] Some patients report sensory loss, including dysesthesias, prior to the development of motor findings. The pattern of weakness appears similar to that found with large putaminal hemorrhages. Less commonly, patients have chorea, ataxia, or abnormal posturing of the upper limb.[20] Behavioral abnormalities including aphasia may be found. Secondary involvement of the rostral and dorsal midbrain may lead to disturbed ocular motility and abnormal pupillary responses. The abnormalities in ocular motility are diverse and may mimic *Parinaud syndrome*. Tonic downward deviation of the eyes (the setting sun sign) may be seen with large thalamic hemorrhages. Impaired upgaze and miotic pupils that do not react to light are suggestive of a large thalamic hemorrhage with secondary compression of the mesencephalic tectum and tegmentum (level of superior colliculus and posterior commissure). Most cases of thalamic hemorrhage induce a tonic deviation of the eyes

▶ **TABLE 7-2.** CLINICAL FINDINGS OF THALAMIC HEMORRHAGE

Large thalamic hemorrhage
  Contralateral hemisensory loss
  Contralateral hemiparesis
  Dysarthria
  Behavioral and cognitive impairments
    Hypersomnolence
    Inattention, unconcern
    Mutism
    Aphasia (dominant hemisphere)
    Anosognosia (nondominant hemisphere)
    Neglect (nondominant hemisphere)
    Visuospatial abnormalities (nondominant hemisphere)
  Disturbances in ocular motility
    Impaired upgaze and tonic downward deviation
    Contralateral or ipsilateral horizontal gaze deviation
    Disconjugate gaze with impaired abduction of one or
      both eyes
    Convergence-retraction nystagmus
    Skew deviation
    Transient opsoclonus
    Ipsilateral ptosis
  Pupillary disturbances
    Light-near dissociation
    Fixed anisocoria
    Anisocoria with ipsilateral miosis
Posterolateral thalamic hemorrhage
  Severe contralateral hemisensory loss
    Pure sensory stroke
    Secondary sensory ataxia
  Contralateral hemiparesis (less than sensory loss)
  Behavioral and cognitive impairments
    Contralateral sensory neglect
    Transcortical aphasia (dominant hemisphere)
    Neglect and anosognosia (nondominant hemisphere)

Neuro-ophthalmological impairments
  Ipsilateral miosis and mild ptosis
  Contralateral horizontal gaze paresis
  Impaired upgaze
  Convergence spasm
  Skew deviation
Anterolateral thalamic hemorrhage
  Moderate-to-severe contralateral hemiparesis
  Moderate-to-severe contralateral hemisensory loss
  Behavioral and cognitive impairments
    Inattention
    Decreased memory
    Aphasia (dominant hemisphere)
  Oculorotatory abnormalities
Medial thalamic hemorrhage
  Contralateral hemiparesis
  Contralateral hemisensory loss
  Behavioral and cognitive impairments
    Inattention
    Decreased spontaneity
    Amnesia
    Confusion
    Aphasia (dominant hemisphere)
    Neglect (nondominant hemisphere)
Dorsal thalamic hemorrhage
  Mild contralateral hemiparesis
  Mild contralateral hemisensory loss
  Behavioral and cognitive impairments
    Amnesia
    Aphasia and apraxia (dominant hemisphere)

toward the lesion (away from the paralysis)—a finding that is important in distinguishing hemorrhages in this location from those arising in the putamen. Unfortunately, some patients with thalamic hemorrhage will have a contralateral horizontal deviation—a finding that can cause confusion in localization.

Smaller thalamic hemorrhages produce discrete neurological impairments reflecting the primary area of the injury.[19,21,22] These hemorrhages may produce symptoms similar to those that occur with small infarctions in the thalamus (see Table 7-2).

Lobar Hemorrhages

Approximately 25 percent of intracerebral hemorrhages involve the subcortical white matter or the gray–white matter junction (Fig. 7-6). Bleeding may occur anywhere in the cerebral hemisphere but typically occurs in the temporoparietal regions. Lobar hemorrhages are less common due to hypertension than deep hemispheric or brain stem hemorrhages. Most lobar hematomas are due to structural diseases including vascular malformations.[23] Amyloid angiopathy preferentially leads to bleeding at the gray–white matter junction in the frontal and occipital poles. The clinical findings correspond to the site and location of the hematoma (Table 7-3). Headache often is unilateral in the ipsilateral fronto-occipital or temporal locations. Seizures are more common with lobar hemorrhages than with bleeding in other locations.[24] Large lobar hematomas also are associated with impaired consciousness including coma[25] (Figs. 7-7 and 7-8). Smaller hemorrhages may cause focal neurological impairments with or without drowsiness. These hemorrhages may mimic infarctions of the cortex or centrum semiovale. The pattern of motor or sensory loss typically includes more involvement of the upper extremity than either the face or lower extremity. With hemorrhages in the anterior aspects of the hemisphere, motor and behavioral signs may be more overt than sensory loss.

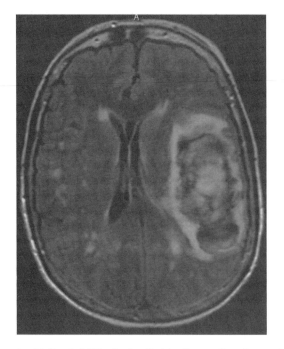

Figure 7-6. A MRI study (fluid attenuation–inversion recovery/FLAIR) sequence demonstrates a left hemisphere hematoma with adjacent adema.

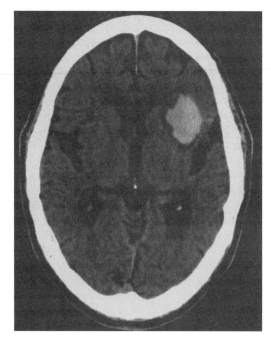

Figure 7-8. Small left frontal hemorrhage is detected on an unenhanced CT of the brain.

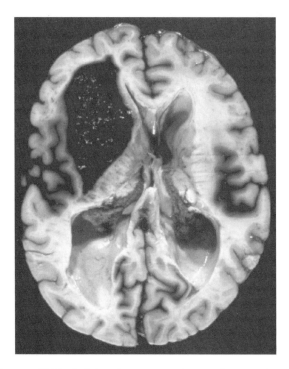

Figure 7-7. Axial autopsy specimen shows a massive lobar hemorrhage in the left basal ganglia and hydrocephalus. In addition blood in the Sylvian fissures (Subarachnoid hemorrhage) also is found. (*Courtesy of S.S. Schochet, M.D., Department of Pathology, University of West Virginia, Morgantown, WV.*)

Hemorrhages in the Brain Stem

While the pons is the primary brain stem site for hemorrhage, bleeding also may occur in the midbrain or medulla. The clinical findings depend upon the site of hemorrhage, its size, and whether intraventricular extension or hydrocephalus complicates the brain stem injury. Larger hemorrhages typically are located in the midline (Fig. 7-9). Smaller dorsolateral pontine hemorrhages also

▶ **TABLE 7-3.** CLINICAL FINDINGS OF LOBAR HEMORRHAGES OF CEREBRAL HEMISPHERES

Frontal lobe
  Contralateral hemiparesis
  Contralateral conjugate gaze palsy
  Aphasia (dominant hemisphere)
  Abulia
Temporal lobe
  Contralateral homonymous hemianopia or superior
    quadrantanopia
Parietal lobe
  Contralateral hemiparesis
  Contralateral hemisensory loss
  Contralateral homonymous hemianopia or inferior
    quadrantanopia
  Aphasia and apraxia (dominant hemisphere)
  Neglect (nondominant hemisphere)
Occipital lobe
  Contralateral homonymous hemianopia

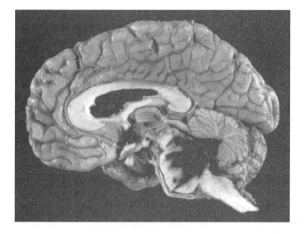

Figure 7-9. Mid-sagittal autopsy specimen shows a large hemorrhage in the base of the pons with extension of blood into the fourth ventricle. (*Courtesy of S.S. Schochet, M.D., Department of Pathology, University of West Virginia, Morgantown, WV.*)

occur. Hypertension is the leading cause of primary brain stem hemorrhage and probably involves the rupture of small penetrating arteries.

Pontine Hemorrhages

The features of major hemorrhages include the rapid development of coma, unstable vital signs, and bilateral severe neurological impairments (Table 7-4). Severe hypertension, cardiac arrhythmias, hyperthermia, and respiratory failure or arrest may occur early in the course.[26] In addition, major pontine hemorrhages may produce quadriplegia or decerebrate posturing. Neuro-ophthalmological abnormalities include paralysis of horizontal eye movements, pinpoint pupils that minimally react to light, and ocular bobbing. While ocular bobbing may be found with acute and large cerebellar lesions, it is a fairly specific localizing sign for an acute pontine hemorrhage. A small hemorrhage involving one side of the basis pontis may present with unilateral signs (see Table 7-4). A contralateral hemiparesis and dysarthria, which mimic the findings of a pure motor lacunar syndrome, are the most prominent symptoms. Ipsilateral facial and abducens nerve palsies may occur if the hemorrhage extends into the pontine tegmentum. Small hemorrhages also arise in the dorsolateral aspects of the pons and produce symptoms that emulate infarctions in the same location[26–29] (see Table 7-4). Patients with these hemorrhages usually are alert and complain of headache, vertigo, and visual symptoms, although sensory, motor, or pain of the contralateral limbs may develop. On examination, patients are found to have contralateral motor and sensory abnormalities, ipsilateral facial weakness or sensory loss, and marked disturbances of ocular motility.

▶ **TABLE 7-4.** CLINICAL FINDINGS OF HEMORRHAGES IN THE PONS

Major pontine hemorrhage
  Coma
  Quadriparesis, contralateral hemiparesis, or decerebrate posturing
  Anarthria
  Dysphagia
  Abnormal vital signs
    Slow and irregular respirations
    Irregular pulse
    Hypertension
    Fever
  Neuro-ophthalmological findings
    Pinpoint pupils (can be minimally reactive)
    Absent horizontal eye movements
    Ocular bobbing
Small pontine hemorrhage involving basis pontis
  Contralateral hemiparesis
  Contralateral hemiparesis and limb ataxia
  Dysarthria
  Ipsilateral facial palsy
  Ipsilateral abducens palsy
Small dorsolateral pontine hemorrhage involving tegmentum
  Contralateral hemisensory loss involving limbs
  Ipsilateral facial sensory loss
  Ipsilateral or bilateral ataxia of the limbs
  Ipsilateral facial palsy
  Contralateral hemiparesis (uncommon)
  Neuro-ophthalmological findings
    Ipsilateral conjugate gaze palsy
    Internuclear ophthalmoplegia
    One-and-one-half syndrome
    Ipsilateral miosis

Mesencephalic Hemorrhages

Midbrain hemorrhages, arising in the cerebral peduncle, tegmentum, or tectum, are much less common than pontine hemorrhages.[30,31] They usually result from rupture of a vascular malformation or hypertension. Large mesencephalic hemorrhages, which produce signs that mimic large pontine hemorrhages, may cause acute hydrocephalus secondary to compression of the cerebral aqueduct. Smaller mesencephalic hemorrhages produce focal neurological signs including an ipsilateral oculomotor nerve palsy and contralateral hemiparesis (*Weber syndrome*) with bleeding primarily in the cerebral peduncle (Table 7-5). Tegmental hemorrhages produce the combination of oculomotor nerve dysfunction and ipsilateral or contralateral tremor, athetosis, or ataxia. Contralateral sensory impairments also may be found. Tectal hemorrhages produce disturbances of ocular motility including Parinaud syndrome, hearing loss, or trochlear nerve palsies.

▶ **TABLE 7-5.** CLINICAL FINDINGS OF HEMORRHAGES OF THE MESENCEPHALON OR MEDULLA

Small mesencephalic hemorrhages
    Cerebral peduncle
        Contralateral hemiparesis
        Ipsilateral oculomotor nerve palsy
    Tegmentum
        Ipsilateral oculomotor nerve palsy
        Contralateral hemisensory loss
        Ipsilateral contralateral tremor, ataxia, athetosis
    Tectum
        Unilateral or bilateral trochlear nerve paresis
        Unilateral or bilateral hearing impairments
        Parinaud syndrome
Small medullary hemorrhages
    Ipsilateral palatal paralysis
    Nystagmus
    Ipsilateral limb ataxia (upper limb)
    Ipsilateral paralysis of one-half of tongue
    Contralateral hemiparesis (upper limb and lower limb)

Medullary Hemorrhages

Primary hemorrhages uncommonly arise in the medulla. Symptoms include headache, vertigo, dysphagia, dysarthria, and loss of balance. Paralysis of the lower cranial nerves may be found in conjunction with paralysis or sensory loss[32] (see Table 7-5). Dorsolateral medullary syndrome of Wallenberg may also occur.

Cerebellar Hemorrhage

Approximately 10 percent of hemorrhages occur in the cerebellum. Hypertension leading to rupture of a penetrating branch of one of the cerebellar arteries is the most common etiology. Bleeding most commonly arises in the deep nuclear structures of the cerebellar hemispheres or the vermis and may extend into the fourth ventricle or brain stem (Figs. 7-10 and 7-11). Large (>3 cm diameter) hematomas produce secondary compression of the brain stem. Hydrocephalus as a result of intraventricular hemorrhage or compression of the fourth ventricle and aqueduct of Sylvius may develop. Large hematomas usually show a rapidly progressive course, while smaller lesions typically cause focal neurological symptoms.

The evolution of symptoms among patients with cerebellar hemorrhage differs from that of patients with brain stem hemorrhages. Most patients initially have severe headache, vertigo, nausea, vomiting, and imbalance.[33] The chief complaint often is the sudden inability to stand or walk. Because hematomas usually arise within a hemisphere, ipsilateral signs of cerebellar dysfunction (limb ataxia) predominate. Subsequently, consciousness may become impaired and cranial nerve palsies appear since the mass effects of a large hematoma cause brain

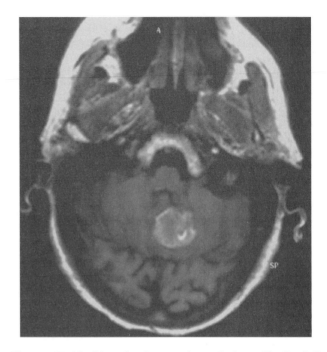

Figure 7-10. Vermian hemorrhage is found in the left cerebellum on a contract-enhanced T1-weighted MRI study.

stem dysfunction.[34] These symptoms evolve over a few minutes to a few hours. Most patients with large hematomas will have worsened by the time they reach medical attention and they will have findings of both cerebellar and brain stem dysfunction (Table 7-6). Disorders of

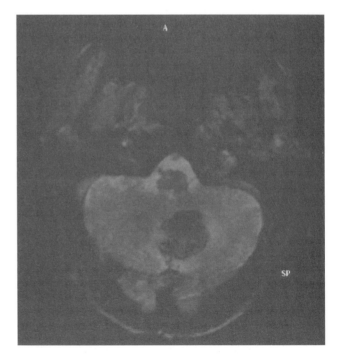

Figure 7-11. A T-2 weighted MRI study shows a hemorrhage in the medial aspect of the left cerebella hemisphere.

▶ **TABLE 7-6.** CLINICAL FINDINGS OF CEREBELLAR HEMORRHAGES

Consciousness can range from alert to coma
Cerebellar signs
   Ipsilateral limb ataxia, dysmetria, dyssynergia, tremor
   Truncal and gait ataxia
   Dysarthria
Neuro-ophthalmological signs
   Nystagmus
   Skew deviation
   Ipsilateral miosis
   Conjugate gaze palsy
   Ipsilateral abducens palsy
   Ocular bobbing
Other brain stem and cranial nerve signs
   Ipsilateral trigeminal dysfunction
   Ipsilateral facial palsy
   Contralateral hemiparesis

extraocular motility and pupillary function often are key findings. With very large hematomas, cardiovascular and respiratory abnormalities appear. Meningeal irritation or tonsillar compression may lead to nuchal rigidity.

▶ PRIMARY INTRAVENTRICULAR HEMORRHAGE

Intraventricular hemorrhage was considered a fatal disease in the era before modern brain imaging because it could be diagnosed only during postmortem examination (Figs. 7-12 and 7-13). Currently, extension of bleeding into the ventricles is recognized as a relatively common

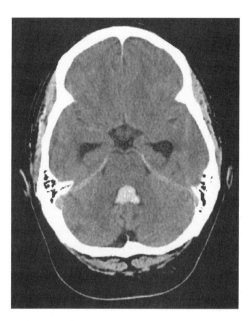

Figure 7-13. Axial CT scan shows a hemorrhage restricted to the fourth ventricle. Hydrocephalic involving both lateral ventricles (dilation of temporal horns) is present.

(approximately 15 percent) complication of both traumatic and spontaneous intracranial hemorrhages. While the presence of intraventricular extension is recognized as not being uniformly fatal, its presence does portend an unfavorable prognosis largely because it is seen primarily among patients with large intracerebral or subarachnoid hemorrhages. Cases of primary intraventricular hemorrhage are rare among adults.[35] The usual cause is rupture of a small vascular malformation located within a subependymal region near the lateral ventricle. In contrast to patients with intraventricular extension with a intracerebral hemorrhage, the prognosis of patients with primary intraventricular hemorrhage is relatively good.

    The findings of primary intraventricular hemorrhage mimic those of subarachnoid hemorrhage[36,37] (Table 7-7). The chief symptoms are sudden onset of severe headache, nausea, vomiting, and confusion. Extensive bleeding may lead to decreased consciousness or seizures. Focal cognitive, motor, or sensory

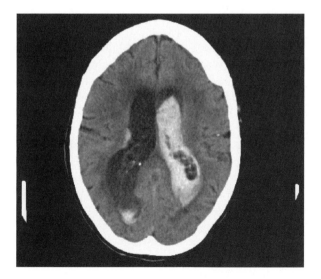

Figure 7-12. Axial CT scan demonstrates a massive intraventricular hemorrhage in the left lateral ventricle. A small amount of blood is found in the right lateral ventricle.

▶ **TABLE 7-7.** CLINICAL FINDINGS OF PRIMARY INTRAVENTRICULAR HEMORRHAGE

Severe headache
Nausea and vomiting
Confusion
Decreased consciousness—coma
Seizures
Focal cognitive, motor, or sensory impairments are subtle

impairments often are subtle. Bilateral Babinski signs and hyperreflexia may be found on examination.

▶ PRIMARY SUBARACHNOID HEMORRHAGE

Trauma is the leading cause of subarachnoid hemorrhage. Therefore, bleeding may complicate rather mild head injuries. Rupture of an intracranial saccular aneurysm is the leading cause of spontaneous subarachnoid hemorrhage. Although the clinical features of subarachnoid hemorrhage are relatively stereotyped, delays in diagnosis are an important problem and despite professional educational efforts the frequency of misdiagnosis has not declined in recent years.[38–42] Because of the nature of the symptoms, in particular the severe headache, patients usually seek medical attention relatively quickly. However, nearly 25 percent of persons with subarachnoid hemorrhage are initially thought to have another illness (Table 7-8). Failure to recognize the nature of the patient's symptoms has the potential for dire consequences because the risk of early recurrent hemorrhage is high (4 percent within 24 h or 20 percent within 1 week) and the aneurysm might be managed successfully if the patient is treated quickly.[42] Delays in diagnosis are most likely to occur among those patients with the mildest symptoms, i.e., those who are actually most likely to respond to early therapy. On the other hand, diagnosis usually is obvious when a patient presents with a devastating subarachnoid hemorrhage leading to coma or severe secondary complications such as intracerebral hemorrhage. Patients with perimesencephalic or pretruncal subarachnoid hemorrhage usually are not as seriously ill as those with ruptured aneurysms.[43–45]

General Symptoms

The history is key to the diagnosis of subarachnoid hemorrhage (Table 7-9). Rupture of an aneurysm can occur at any time but many events happen during exercise or activity. The main complaint is the sudden onset of an unusually severe (thunderclap) headache.[1,46–49] In most

▶ **TABLE 7-8.** MISDIAGNOSES OF SUBARACHNOID HEMORRHAGE

Migraine	Tension headache
Sinusitis	Viral illness (flu)
Viral meningitis	Craniocerebral trauma
Herniated cervical disk	Ischemic stroke
Drug/alcohol abuse	Hypertensive encephalopathy
Myocardial infarction	Brain tumor
Epilepsy	Metabolic encephalopathy
Diabetic III nerve palsy	

▶ **TABLE 7-9.** CLINICAL FINDINGS OF SUBARACHNOID HEMORRHAGE

Sudden onset of an unusually severe headache
Neck, back, eye, ear, chest, or face pain
Nausea, vomiting, photophobia, and phonophobia
Alteration in consciousness
   Syncope or transient loss of consciousness
   Seizures
   Prolonged stupor or coma
   Encephalopathy
Abnormal vital signs
   Severe hypertension
   Cardiac arrhythmias
Nuchal rigidity (Brudzinski sign/Kernig sign)
Intraocular hemorrhages
Focal neurological impairments
   Aneurysm of origin of posterior communicating artery
      Ipsilateral oculomotor nerve palsy
   Aneurysm of the middle cerebral artery
      Contralateral hemiparesis (face, upper limb)
      Contralateral hemisensory loss
      Aphasia (dominant hemisphere)
   Neglect (nondominant hemisphere)
   Aneurysm of the anterior communicating artery
      Paraparesis or contralateral hemiparesis (lower limb)
      Neurogenic bladder
      Abulia or akinetic mutism
      Disinhibition or emotional lability

cases, it is the first symptom and often described as the most severe pain the patient has ever experienced. The complaint of the "worst headache of my life" is an important clue. While the headache may be described as precipitous in onset, it may evolve or worsen over a few minutes.[47] The headache usually occurs instantaneously and reaches a maximal intensity within a few minutes. A severe headache associated with a brief loss of consciousness at the onset of symptoms is highly suggestive of subarachnoid hemorrhage. Less commonly, the headache may increase in severity over a few hours. The diagnosis may be more difficult when the patient has an evolution of the headache and other symptoms. The headache may be generalized or localized. Occipital and nuchal pain can occur with subarachnoid hemorrhage primarily in the posterior fossa. The headache can be described as throbbing, aching, or a severe pressure. The pain may radiate to the eyes, face, and the back of the neck. In addition, patients complain of photophobia, phonophobia, nausea, and vomiting. These symptoms in combination with the headache often prompt the misdiagnosis of migraine.

Sentinel Hemorrhage

A sentinel hemorrhage represents a mild episode of intracranial bleeding.[50–52] These events represent the least severe form of subarachnoid hemorrhage. The headache might not be as cataclysmic as that occurring with a more severe bleeding event but the other qualities often are similar to those that occur with a major subarachnoid hemorrhage. Affected patients usually do not have other symptoms and they do not appear seriously ill. Because of the "mild" nature of the findings, intracranial bleeding often is not considered and the ominous nature of the symptoms is not recognized until the patient has a second, life threatening, hemorrhage.

Perimesencephalic or pretruncal subarachnoid hemorrhage usually is secondary to rupture of a small vascular malformation[43,53] (Fig. 7-14). Affected patients have a headache similar to that occurring with other causes of subarachnoid bleeding. However, these patients usually do not have alteration in consciousness or focal neurological symptoms.

Severe neck pain, often more intense than the headache, may occur, especially when the ruptured aneurysm is located in the posterior fossa. Less commonly, patients may complain of back pain. The presence of blood in the subarachnoid space leads to signs of meningismus. However, meningeal irritative signs can be subtle with minor hemorrhages. In addition, nuchal rigidity might not appear for several hours after the aneurysmal rupture and deeply comatose patients may not have any appreciable nuchal rigidity. The presence or absence of nuchal rigidity is not critical for the diagnosis of subarachnoid hemorrhage and therefore elicitation of this sign should not be performed in a comatose patient until the possibility of a cervical spine injury has been excluded.

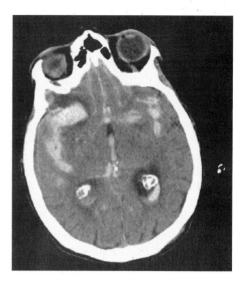

Figure 7-15. Unenhanced CT study reveals subarachnoid and intraventricular hemorrhage. The focal thick collection of blood in the right Sylvian fissuer ruptured suggests a right middle cerebral artery aneurysm.

Many patients with subarachnoid hemorrhage have a disturbance in consciousness[1,49] (Fig. 7-15). Since alterations in consciousness are common following subarachnoid hemorrhage and the history of headache might not be obtainable, a reasonable approach is to consider intracranial bleeding as the potential cause of coma in a patient even if focal motor or sensory impairments are not present. Approximately one-half of patients have a transient episode of loss of consciousness at the time of aneurysmal rupture. Presumably, the loss of consciousness is secondary to a sudden and dramatic increase in intracranial pressure that transiently reduces cerebral perfusion pressure. The event may be a syncopal-like attack marked by unresponsiveness or may be associated with opisthotonus and posturing of the limbs and respiratory arrest. Nearly 25 percent of patients have prolonged stupor or coma.[54] Following the hemorrhage, more severely affected patients may be disoriented, confused, irritable, or delirious.[55] The irritability and agitation may be secondary to the acute brain illness or secondary to meningeal irritation and severe headache. Other behavioral disturbances include abulia or akinetic mutism—findings typically associated with rupture of an anterior communicating artery aneurysm. Approximately 10–25 percent of patients have generalized seizures, which usually occur at the time of aneurysmal rupture.[56,57] Occasionally, patients with subarachnoid hemorrhage will have loss of consciousness followed by trauma. Differentiating traumatic from spontaneous subarachnoid hemorrhage may be problematic.[58–60]

Approximately 15 percent of patients will have subhyloid hemorrhages identified by ophthalmoscopy.[61–63]

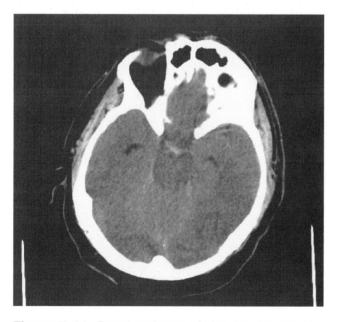

Figure 7-14. Restricted area of blood is detected by CT in the interpeduncular cistern in a patient with a perimesencephalic subarachnoid hemorrhage.

These retinal findings are most commonly among patients with severe hemorrhages (Fig. 7-15).

Focal Neurological Symptoms

Most patients with ruptured aneurysms do not have focal neurological signs. However, the presence of these signs may point to the location of the aneurysm (see Table 7-9). The most common focal sign is an oculomotor nerve palsy that accompanies rupture of an aneurysm at the origin of the posterior communicating artery or at the bifurcation of the basilar artery. Less commonly, an aneurysm of the intracavernous portion of the internal carotid artery produces dysfunction of the oculomotor nerve. A key differentiating point is early involvement of the parasympathetic pupillary constrictive fibers leading to an unreactive mydriasis and preserved ocular motility.[64,65] Persons with a ruptured aneurysm of the middle cerebral artery or distal internal carotid artery may present with a contralateral hemiparesis, contralateral hemisensory loss, and cognitive signs, such as aphasia. Rupture of the anterior communicating artery may cause a transient paraparesis or hemiparesis or a neurogenic bladder. In addition, these aneurysms may be associated with prominent behavioral abnormalities including amnesia, confabulation, or affective changes.

▶ SUBDURAL OR EPIDURAL HEMORRHAGE

Most cases of subdural or epidural bleeding are secondary to acute or recent craniocerebral trauma (Table 7-10). Epidural hematomas usually are due to arterial bleeding and the course is relatively rapid. The usual scenario is laceration of the middle meningeal artery secondary to a fracture of the squamous portion of the temporal bone. In this situation, the patient has a rapidly evolving decline in consciousness and progressively increasing contralateral hemiparesis and ipsilateral oculomotor nerve palsy. While most patients with subdural hematomas have a slowly evolving course of headache, cognitive impairments and waxing–waning motor or sensory loss, some cases have more rapidly evolving symptoms. Most patients have a history of trauma, although the injury may be relatively trivial. Alcoholics are a particularly high-risk group. In addition, patients taking oral anticoagulants have a high risk of a subdural hematoma. Spontaneous subdural hematomas may be associated with the use of anticoagulants and the osmotic shifts that occur during hemodialysis. In addition, subdural hemorrhage may be detected in approximately 5 percent of patients with aneurysmal subarachnoid hemorrhage. Presumably the bleeding extends through the arachnoid membrane into the subdural space. Subdural blood in the

▶ **TABLE 7-10.** FINDINGS OF SUBDRUAL OR EPIDURAL HEMORRHAGES

Subdural hemorrhage
  History of recent (weeks) craniocerebral trauma
  History of trauma—trivial or absent
  Risk factors often present (i.e., alcoholism, oral anticoagulants, hemodialysis)
  Evolving course of gradual or stepwise worsening
  Symptoms can wax and wane (can mimic a TIA)
  Headache
  Confusion or cognitive decline
  Motor or sensory impairments are subtle
  Decreased consciousness occurs late
Epidural hemorrhage
  History of moderate-to-severe craniocerebral trauma
  Transient loss of consciousness at time of trauma
  Rapidly evolving course over hours
  Prominent headache
  Decline in consciousness
  Rapidly evolving contralateral hemiparesis
  Ipsilateral oculomotor nerve palsy

interhemispheric fissure may be confused with subarachnoid hemorrhage.

REFERENCES

1. Fisher CM. Clinical syndromes in cerebral thrombosis, hypertensive hemorrhage and ruptured saccular aneurysm. *Clin Neurosurg* 1975;22:117.
2. Phillips LH, II, Whisnant JP, O'Fallon WM. The unchanging pattern of subarachnoid hemorrhage in a community. *Neurology* 1980;30:1034–1040.
3. Broderick J, Brott T, Tomsick T. Management of intracerebral hemorrhage in a large metropolitan population. *Neurosurgery* 1994;34:882–887.
4. Schievink WI, Wijdicks EFM, Parisi JE. Sudden death from aneurysmal subarachnoid hemorrhage. *Neurology* 1995; 45:871–874.
5. Broderick JP, Brott TG, Tomsick T, Barsan W, Spilker J. Ultra-early evaluation of intracerebral hemorrhage. *J Neurosurg* 1990;72:195–199.
6. Fujii Y, Takeuchi S, Sasaki O, Minakawa T, Tanaka R. Multivariate analysis of predictors of hematoma enlargement in spontaneous intracerebral hemorrhage. *Stroke* 1998;29:1160–1166.
7. Broderick JP, Adams HP, Jr., Barsan W, et al. Guidelines for the management of spontaneous intracerebral hemorrhage: A statement for healthcare professionals from a special writing group of the Stroke Council, American Heart Association. *Stroke* 1999;30:905–915.
8. Franke CL, van Swieten JC, Algra A. Prognostic factors in patients with intracerebral haematoma. *J Neurol Neurosurg Psychiatry* 1992;55:653–657.
9. Rosenow F, Hojer C, Meyer-Lohmann C, et al. Spontaneous intracerebral hemorrhage. Prognostic factors in 896 cases. *Acta Neurol Scand* 1997;96:174–182.

10. Juvela S. Risk factors for impaired outcome after spontaneous intracerebral hemorrhage. *Arch Neurol* 1995;52:1193–1200.

11. Terayama Y, Tanahashi N, Fukuuchi Y, Gotoh F. Prognostic value of admission blood pressure in patients with intracerebral hemorrhage. Keio Cooperative Stroke Study. *Stroke* 1997;28:1185–1188.

12. Fogelholm R, Avikainen S, Murros K. Prognostic value and determinants of first-day mean arterial pressure in spontaneous supratentorial intracerebral hemorrhage. *Stroke* 1997;28:1396–1400.

13. Schwarz S, Hafner K, Aschoff A, Schwab S. Incidence and prognostic significance of fever following intracerebral hemorrhage. *Neurology* 2000;54:354–361.

14. Chung CS, Caplan LR, Yamamoto Y, et al. Straitocapsular haemorrhage. *Brain* 2000;123:1850–1862.

15. Keane JP. Contralateral gaze deviation with supratentorial hemorrhage. *Arch Neurol* 1975;32:119–122.

16. D'Esposito M, Alexander MP. Subcortical aphasia: Distinct profiles following left putaminal hemorrhage. *Neurology* 1995;45:38–41.

17. Kumral E, Evyapan D, Balkir K. Acute caudate vascular lesions. *Stroke* 1999;30:100–108.

18. Waga S, Fujimoto K, Okada M. Caudate hemorrhage. *Neurosurgery* 1986;18:445–450.

19. Kumral E, Kocaer T, Ertubey NO. Thalamic hemorrhage: A prospective study of 100 patients. *Stroke* 1995;26:964–970.

20. Dobato JL, Villanueva JA, Gimenez-Roldan S. Sensory ataxic hemiparesis in thalamic hemorrhage. *Stroke* 1990;21:1749–1753.

21. Shintani S, Tsuruoka S, Shiigai T. Pure sensory stroke caused by a cerebral hemorrhage: Clinical-radiologic correlations in seven patients. *Am J Neuroradiol* 2000;21:515–520.

22. Hirose G, Kosoegawa H, Saeki M. The syndrome of posterior thalamic hemorrhage. *Neurology* 1985;35:998–1002.

23. Toffol GJ, Biller J, Adams HP, Jr. Nontraumatic intracerebral hemorrhage in young adults. *Arch Neurol* 1987;44:483–485.

24. Tanaka Y, Furuse M, Iwasa H. Lobar intracerebral hemorrhage: Etiology and long-term follow-up study of 32 patients. *Stroke* 1986;17:51–57.

25. Weisberg LA. Subcortical lobar intracerebral haemorrhage: Clinical-computed tomographic correlations. *J Neurol Neurosurg Psychiatry* 1985;48:1078–1084.

26. Kushner MJ, Brott TG. The clinical manifestations of pontine hemorrhage. *Neurology* 1985;35:637–643.

27. Kim JS, Lee JH, Lees K. Small primary intracerebral hemorrhage: Clinical presentation in 28 cases. *Stroke* 1994;25:1500–1506.

28. Wijdicks EF, St Louis E. Clinical profiles predictive of outcome in pontine hemorrhage. *Neurology* 1997;49:1342–1346.

29. Pullicino PM, Wong EH. Tonic downward and inward ocular deviation ipsilateral to pontine tegmental hemorrhage. *Cerebrovasc Dis* 2000;10:327–329.

30. Sand JJ, Biller J, Crawley F. Partial dorsal mesencephalic hemorrhages: Report of three cases. *Neurology* 1986;36:529–533.

31. Weisberg LA. Mesencephalic hemorrhages: Clinical and computed tomographic correlations. *Neurology* 1986;36:713–716.

32. Neumann PE, Mehler MF, Horoupian DS. Primary medullary hypertensive hemorrhage. *Neurology* 1985;85:925–928.

33. Fisher CM, Picard EH, Polak A. Acute hypertensive cerebellar hemorrhage: Diagnosis and surgical treatment. *J Nerv Ment Dis* 1966;140:38–57.

34. Ott KH, Kase CS, Ojemann RG. Cerebellar hemorrhage: Diagnosis and treatment. A review of 56 cases. *Arch Neurol* 1974;31:160–167.

35. Darby DG, Donnan G, Saling MA. Primary intraventricular hemorrhage: Clinical and neuropsychological findings in a prospective stroke series. *Neurology* 1988;38:68–75.

36. marti-Fabregas J, Piles S, Guardia E, Marti-Vilalta JL. Spontaneous primary intraventricular hemorrhage: Clinical data, etiology and outcome. *J Neurol* 1999;246:287–291.

37. Gates PC, Barnett HJM, Vinters HV. Primary intraventricular hemorrhage in adults. *Stroke* 1986;17:872–877.

38. Adams HP, Jr., Jergenson DD, Kassell NF. Pitfalls in the recognition of subarachnoid hemorrhage. *JAMA* 1980;244:794–796.

39. Edlow JA, Caplan LR. Avoiding pitfalls in the diagnosis of subarachnoid hemorrhage. *N Engl J Med* 2000;342:29–36.

40. Ferro JM, Melo TP, Oliveira V, Crespo M, Canhao P, Pinto AN. An analysis of the admission delay of acute strokes. *Cerebrovasc Dis* 1994;4:72–75.

41. Neil-Dwyer G, Lang D. 'Brain attack'–aneurysmal subarachnoid haemorrhage: Death due to delayed diagnosis. *J R Coll Physicians Lond* 1997;31:49–52.

42. Kowalski RG, Claassen J, Kreiter KT, et al. Initial misdiagnosis and outcome after subarachnoid hemorrhage. *JAMA* 2004;291:866–869.

43. Schwartz TH, Solomon RA. Perimesencephalic nonaneurysmal subarachnoid hemorrhage: Review of the literature. *Neurosurgery* 1996;39:433–440.

44. Schwartz TH, Mayer SA. Quadrigeminal variant of perimesencephalic nonaneurysmal subarachnoid hemorrhage. *Neurosurgery* 2000;46:584–588.

45. Wijdicks EF, Schievink WI, Miller GM. Pretruncal nonaneurysmal subarachnoid hemorrhage. *Mayo Clin Proc* 1998;73:745–752.

46. Schwedt TJ, Matharu MS, Dodick DW. Thunderclap headache. *Lancet Neurol,* 2006;5:621–631.

47. Linn FH, Rinkel GJ, Algra A, van Gijn J. Headache characteristics in subarachnoid haemorrhage and benign thunderclap headache. *J Neurol Neurosurg Psychiatry* 1998;65:791–793.

48. Morgenstern LB, Luna-Gonzales H, Huber JCJ, et al. Worst headache and subarachnoid hemorrhage: Prospective, modern computed tomography and spinal fluid analysis. *Ann Emerg Med* 1998;32:297–304.

49. Hop JW, Rinkel GJ, Algra A, van Gijn J. Initial loss of consciousness and risk of delayed cerebral ischemia after aneurysmal subarachnoid hemorrhage. *Stroke* 1999;30:2268–2271.

50. Ostergaard JR. Headache as a warning symptom of impeding aneurysmal subarachnoid haemorrhage. *Cephalagia* 1991;11:53–55.

51. Jakobsson KE, saveland H, Hillman J. Warning leak and management outcome in aneurysmal subarachnoid hemorrhage. *J Neurosurg* 1996;85:995–999.

52. Linn FH, Rinkel GJ, Algra A, van Gijn J. The notion of "warning leaks" in subarachnoid haemorrhage: Are such patients in fact admitted with a rebleed? *J Neurol Neurosurg Psychiatry* 2000;68:332–336.

53. Rinkel GJE, Wijdicks EF, Vermeulen M, Hasan D, Brouwers PJAM, van Gijn J. The clinical course of perimesencephalic non-aneurysmal subarachnoid haemorrhage. *Ann Neurol* 1991;29:463–468.

54. Adams HP, Jr., Kassell NF, Torner JC. CT and clinical correlations in recent aneurysmal subarachnoid hemorrhage: A preliminary report of the Cooperative Aneurysm Study. *Neurology* 1983;33:981–988.

55. Reijneveld JC, Wermer M, Boonman Z, van Gijn J, Rinkel GJ. Acute confusional state as presenting feature in aneurysmal subarachnoid hemorrhage: Frequency and characteristics. *J Neurol* 2000;247:112–116.

56. Rhoney DH, Tipps LB, Murry KR, Basham MC, Michael DB, Coplin WM. Anticonvulsant prophylaxis and timing of seizures after aneurysmal subarachnoid hemorrhage. *Neurology* 2000;55:258–265.

57. Pinto AN, Canhao P, Ferro JM. Seizures at the onset of subarachnoid haemorrhage. *J Neurol* 1996;243:161–164.

58. Cummings TJ, Johnson RR, Diaz FG, Michael DB. The relationship of blunt head trauma, subarachnoid hemorrhage, and rupture of pre-existing intracranial saccular aneurysms. *Neurol Res* 2000;22:165–170.

59. Sakas DE, Dias LS, Beale D. Subarachnoid haemorrhage presenting as head injury. *BMJ* 1995;310:1186–1187.

60. Vos PE, Zwienenberg M, O'Hannian KL, Muizelaar JP. Subarachnoid haemorrhage following rupture of an ophthalmic artery aneurysm presenting as traumatic brain injury. *Clin Neurol Neurosurg* 2000;102:29–32.

61. Pfausler B, Belcl R, Metzler R, Mohsenipour I, Schmutzhard E. Terson's syndrome in spontaneous subarachnoid hemorrhage: A prospective study in 60 consecutive patients. *J Neurosurg* 1996;85:392–394.

62. Frizzell RT, Kuhn F, Morris R, Quinn C, Fisher WS. Screening for ocular hemorrhages in patients with ruptured cerebral aneurysms: A prospective study of 99 patients. *Neurosurgery* 1997;41:529–533.

63. Keane JR. Retinal hemorrhages. Its significance in 100 patients with acute encephalopathy of unknown cause. *Arch Neurol* 1979;36:691–694.

64. O'Connor PSTTJ, Green RP. Pupillary-sparing third nerve palsy due to aneurysm: A survey of 249 neurological surgeons. *J Neurosurg* 1983;58:792–793.

65. Jacobson DM. Relative pupil-sharing third nerve palsy: Etiology and clinical variables predictive of a mass. *Neurology* 2001;56:797–798.

CHAPTER 8

Diagnostic Studies in the Evaluation of Patients with Cerebrovascular Diseases

Diagnostic studies are ordered to help assess patients with cerebrovascular diseases. The indications for the tests include (1) confirmation that the patient's neurological findings are secondary to stroke, (2) differentiation of hemorrhagic and ischemic stroke, (3) detection of medical and neurological complications, and (4) determination of the most likely cause of the cerebrovascular event. Because the differential diagnosis of stroke is limited, the number of required tests to confirm the diagnosis of an acute cerebrovascular event is relatively small.[1,2] Some tests are ordered acutely and are aimed at addressing the first three indications listed above, while some studies are performed after the patient's condition is stabilized. The components of the diagnostic evaluation can be further differentiated into tests aimed at assessing the brain and spinal cord and studies that assess the vasculature, the heart, and the blood.

Clinicians need to recognize the advantages and limitations of each of the tests. The usual criteria for useful ancillary tests include the specificity and sensitivity of the study and the resultant positive and negative predictive values. Most tests have not been evaluated using these criteria and, as a result, recommendations usually are made by consensus. Some tests, particularly those that are invasive or semiinvasive, might have specific indications and contraindications. In addition, the results of some tests might be affected by stroke. For example, some of the tests for a prothrombotic disorder might give spurious values if the studies are performed shortly after the vascular event. Several tests are expensive or involve some risk and clinicians need to weigh whether the results will influence the treatment of the patient. For example, the risk of complications of arteriography should be considered in comparison to the potential information about the vasculature, which could affect a decision for surgery. In addition, not all tests need to be done to evaluate a patient for the cause of stroke. A physician does not need to order a panel of tests looking for a prothrombotic disorder when the cause of ischemic stroke already has been diagnosed because the tests' results have a low likelihood of changing antithrombotic treatment. The results of a transesophageal echocardiogram might not affect management if the physician already has strong evidence that a patient has had a cardioembolic stroke and the decision to use anticoagulants already has been made.

▶ EMERGENTLY ORDERED DIAGNOSTIC TESTS

Table 8-1 lists the diagnostic studies that are usually ordered during the initial evaluation of a patient with suspected stroke or transient ischemic attack.[3–6] The tests include brain imaging, most commonly computed tomography (CT), and examination of the cerebrospinal fluid (CSF) if subarachnoid hemorrhage is suspected. Additional studies include electrocardiography to screen for acute cardiac complications of the stroke or the presence of concomitant heart disease and hematological, coagulation, and biochemical studies. These tests can be ordered on an emergency basis at most community hospitals and should be available regardless of the time of the patient's arrival to the emergency department. With the exception of the lumbar puncture, the tests are noninvasive. The examination of the CSF is reserved for those patients with suspected subarachnoid hemorrhage whose CT study does not show hemorrhage.

The role of magnetic resonance imaging (MRI) is expanding; it is replacing CT as the first brain imaging modality at some medical centers. For example, diffusion-weighted imaging (DWI) is becoming a particularly useful tool in the urgent assessment of patients with suspected ischemic stroke. Noninvasive imaging, including transcranial Doppler ultrasonography, CT angiography (CTA), and magnetic resonance angiography (MRA) might become important components of the emergent evaluation. These tests would become important if future research shows that therapies can be selected on the basis of the vascular imaging findings.

▶ **TABLE 8-1.** EMERGENT DIAGNOSTIC STUDIES FOR EVALUATION OF PATIENTS WITH SUSPECTED STROKE

Neurological diagnostic studies
    Computed tomography (CT)
    Magnetic resonance imaging (MRI)
    Cerebrospinal fluid (CSF) examination
    Electroencephalography (EEG) if seizures a consideration
Potential emergency vascular studies
    Computed tomographic angiography (CTA)
    Magnetic resonance angiography (MRA)
    Transcranial Doppler (TCD) ultrasonography
Cardiac diagnostic studies
    Electrocardiography (ECG)
Other diagnostic studies
    Complete blood count
    Platelet count
    Activated partial thromboplastin time (aPTT)
    Prothrombin time/international normalized ratio (INR)
    Blood glucose
    Serum electrolytes
    Pulse oximetry
    Chest x-ray if pulmonary disease is a consideration

▶ SUBSEQUENT DIAGNOSTIC TESTS

Some of the emergently performed diagnostic tests can be repeated during the days following a stroke. These tests are used for screening for acute or subacute neurological or medical complications or evolution of the stroke. Table 8-2 lists tests that are ordered after the patient's medical condition has been stabilized. These tests are used to screen for the cause of stroke or the presence of concomitant diseases, including risk factors for atherosclerosis. These tests include noninvasive or invasive studies of the vasculature, heart, and blood. With advances in genetic research, the role of this testing will likely grow in the evaluation of patients with stroke. Studies such as electroencephalography (EEG) and cardiac monitoring (Holter or King-of-Hearts monitoring) often are done during the evaluation of a patient with recurrent transient ischemic attacks. Although these tests have limited indications as described subsequently.

▶ IMAGING OF THE BRAIN

CT and MRI are core components of the evaluation of patients with suspected cerebrovascular disease.[7] These tests influence the management of patients with stroke primarily because they help differentiate hemorrhagic stroke from ischemic stroke.[8] Physicians should remain cognizant of the strengths and limitations of both tests. The introduction of CT in 1973 was recognized immediately as a revolutionary diagnostic tool and much of the preceding clinical work in stroke became outdated almost immediately. The quality of CT studies has improved markedly during subsequent years. The introduction of MRI a few years later is another major advance in evaluation of patients with neurological disease. Continued development of new MRI equipment and techniques is widening the scope of the test.[9–11] While the availability of MRI continues to increase, CT remains the usual diagnostic test for the rapid evaluation of a patient with ischemic stroke. One of these brain imaging tests is indicated during the assessment of all patients with acute cerebrovascular disease. Imaging of the brain is crucial for helping differentiate hemorrhagic stroke from ischemic stroke.[8,12] The studies are also used to exclude other diseases such as brain tumor, which may cause neurological symptoms, to screen for acute neurological complications, or to monitor the evolution of the vascular lesion.

▶ COMPUTED TOMOGRAPHY

Although studies did not test the specificity and sensitivity of CT in the evaluation of patients with suspected stroke,

▶ **TABLE 8-2.** DIAGNOSTIC STUDIES FOR EVALUATION OF PATIENTS WITH STROKE

Neurological diagnostic studies
    Computed tomography (CT)
    Magnetic resonance imaging (MRI)
    Positron emission tomography (PET)
    Single photon emission computed tomography (SPECT)
    Neuro-ophthalmological evaluation
    Neuropsychological testing
    Electroencephalography (EEG)
    Cerebrospinal fluid (CSF) examination
    Brain and/or meningeal biopsy
Vascular studies
    Carotid ultrasonography (carotid duplex)
    Transcranial Doppler (TCD) ultrasonography
    Computed tomographic (CT) angiography
    Magnetic resonance angiography (MRA)
    Digital subtraction angiography
Cardiac studies
    Electrocardiography (ECG)
    Transthoracic echocardiography (TTE)
    Transesophageal echocardiography (TEE)
    Magnetic resonance imaging (MRI)
    Computed tomography (CT)
    Holter monitoring
    King-of-hearts monitoring
Blood tests
    Hematological
        Complete blood count
        Platelet count
        Hemoglobin electrophoresis
    Coagulation
        Activated partial thromboplastin time (Aptt)
            Russel viper venom time
        Prothrombin time/international normalized ratio (INR)
        Fibrinogen
        Fibrin degradation products, D-dimer
        Thrombin time
        Proteins C and S levels
        Antithrombin levels
        Alpha-2-antiplasmin
        Factor II, V, VII, VIII, IX, X, XI, XII concentrations
        Factor V—Leiden
        Prothrombin gene mutation
    Autoimmune, inflammatory, infectious
        Blood cultures
        Cerebrospinal fluid (CSF) cultures
        Erythrocyte sedimentation rate
        C-reactive protein/high-sensitivity C-reactive protein
        Complement
        Serological tests for syphilis
        Rheumatoid factor
        Antinuclear antibody (ANA)
        Antineuronal cytoplasmic antibody (ANCA)
    Genetic tests
    Risk factors for atherosclerosis
        Blood glucose
        Serum lipids
            Total cholesterol
            HDL cholesterol
            LDL cholesterol
            Triglyceride

the medical community has accepted the utility of the diagnostic test based on its dramatic findings. The utility of CT was self-evident. The findings on CT are correlated with pathological evidence of stroke.[13] Technologic advances greatly increase the diagnostic yield of CT. The test provides detailed anatomic imaging to screen for pathological changes in the brain. When judging the diagnostic sensitivity and specificity of CT, one needs to differentiate the yield of the test itself and the physicians' ability to recognize some of the changes. The latter is particularly important. Some of the imaging changes can be relatively subtle and might be overlooked by physicians.[14,15] CT has several advantages: It is noninvasive, relatively inexpensive, and available at most hospitals. It can be performed rapidly and sequential tests can be done to monitor the course of the illness or to detect the appearance of complications.[16] The results of CT can be used to provide information about the most likely cause of ischemic stroke.[17] Most patients have nonenhanced studies during the initial evaluation but the use of contrast can improve the detection of some diseases that are associated with increased vascularity or inflammation. In addition, contrast-enhanced CT can assess the vasculature. A major limitation of contrast-enhanced CT is allergic reactions to the contrast agent but the use of medications prior to the procedure can lessen the risk. CT does involve an exposure to ionizing radiation and thus should used with caution in women who might be pregnant, although pregnancy is a not a contraindication for the test. It should be done when evaluating a young woman with a suspected stroke. Measures such as covering the abdomen with a lead apron can reduce fetal exposure to the radiation. CT is very useful in the evaluation of patients with suspected stroke, especially because of its ability to distinguish hemorrhagic and ischemic events. The results of CT also can affect decisions about management, including the administration of thrombolytic agents.

CT does have some limitations: It misses small ischemic lesions, especially those in the posterior fossa because of bone artifact. Some of the early changes of ischemic stroke or subarachnoid hemorrhage can be relatively subtle and the findings might be missed.

Intracerebral Hemorrhage

CT is a key component of the evaluation of patients with intracranial bleeding. It provides information about the site and volume of any focal bleeding. Within the first few days, CT can detect blood in almost all cases of intracerebral hemorrhage.[18] It also provides important prognostic information that affects decisions about acute management and the likely cause (Tables 8-3 and 8-4; Fig. 8-1). While CT can detect a hematoma that is only a few millimeters in size, it might miss a small intraparenchymal hemorrhage located adjacent to a bony landmark or bleeding in a patient with severe anemia.

▶ **TABLE 8-3.** COMPUTED TOMOGRAPHY
EVALUATION OF PATIENTS WITH
HEMORRHAGIC STROKE

Detection of hemorrhage
  Intracerebral hemorrhage
    Location of hematoma
    Size of hematoma
    Growth in the size of the hematoma
  Subarachnoid hemorrhage
    Focal, thin collection
    Focal, thick collection
    Diffuse, thin collection
    Diffuse, thick collection
    Recurrent hemorrhage
  Perimesencephalic subarachnoid hemorrhage
  Intraventricular hemorrhage
  Subdural or epidural hemorrhage
Detection of complications of hemorrhagic stroke
  Hydrocephalus
  Brain edema and shift of structures
  Cerebral infarction
Pattern of bleeding points toward the underlying cause

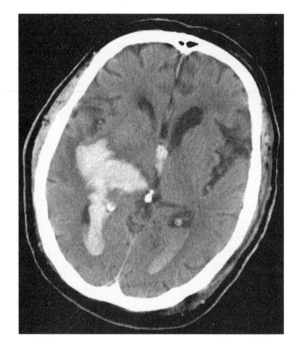

Figure 8-1. An unenhanced CT scan of the brain reveals a large thalamic hemorrhage with intraventricular extension.

Besides finding blood within the brain parenchyma, CT also demonstrates blood in the ventricles or subarachnoid space[4,19–22] (Fig. 8-2). Sequentially performed studies can be used to monitor the progression in the size of a hematoma or the development of other neurological complications such as hydrocephalus, brain edema,

herniation, or infarction (see Table 8-2; Fig. 8-3). CT studies obtained during the first hours after the ictus can show growth of the hematoma presumably due to continued bleeding[23] (Fig. 8-4). This imaging observation changed the common opinion that the actual

▶ **TABLE 8-4.** CLINICAL, COMPUTED
TOMOGRAPHIC, AND ANATOMIC CORRELATIONS
FOR PATIENTS WITH HEMORRHAGE

Multiple cortical hemorrhages in frontal or occipital poles or
  temporal tips
    Craniocerebral trauma
Multiple hemorrhages in different locations in the brain
    Bleeding diathesis, amyloid angiopathy, metastatic tumor
Bilateral parasagittal hemorrhages
    Superosagittal sinus thrombosis
Lobar hemorrhage in a young adult
    Vascular malformation
Lobar hemorrhage (particularly frontal or parietal/occipital)
  in an elderly patient
    Amyloid angiopathy
Hemorrhage in putamen, thalamus, pons, or cerebellum
    Hypertension
Primarily subarachnoid hemorrhage
    Aneurysm
Subarachnoid blood in anterior interhemispheric fissure,
  suprasellar cistern
    Anterior communicating artery aneurysm
Subarachnoid blood in suprasellar cistern and ambient
  cistern
    Posterior communicating artery aneurysm
Subarachnoid blood in Sylvian cistern and Sylvian fissure
    Middle cerebral artery aneurysm

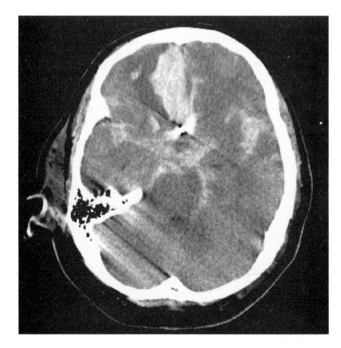

Figure 8-2. An unenhanced CT scan demonstrates a large subarachnoid hemorrhage from an anterior communicating aneurysm. The pattern of subarachnoid bleeding would be rated as diffuse and thick. This pattern of bleeding would predict a high risk for vasospasm.

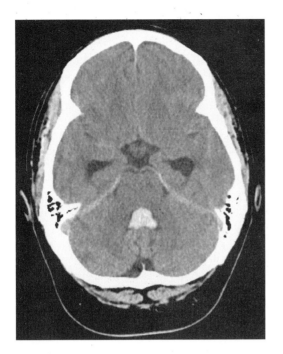

Figure 8-3. An unenhanced CT scan shows a hemorrhage primarily found in the fourth ventricle. Acute hydrocephalus with dilation of the temporal horns of both lateral ventricles also is found.

hemorrhage evolved over a very short time. During the subsequent weeks, CT shows resolution of the hemorrhage with a residual hypodense area in the brain that looks similar to a remote infarction.

The CT location of the hematoma provides hints toward the underlying etiology. A small deep hematoma is most likely to be of hypertensive origin.[24] Hypertensive hemorrhages are located primarily in the putamen, thalamus, brain stem, or cerebellum. Hemorrhages secondary to trauma are usually located at the frontal and occipital poles and the tips of temporal lobes (see Table 8-4). The causes of hemorrhage in lobar white matter are more diverse and include vasculitis, vascular malformations, and bleeding diatheses in addition to hypertension. If the intraparenchymal hemorrhage is adjacent to the circle of Willis or if prominent subarachnoid blood is detected, the possibility of a ruptured saccular aneurysm increases (see Fig. 8-5). Hemorrhages at the gray matter–white matter junction of the cerebral hemispheres are suggestive of amyloid angiopathy particularly if multiple locations or lesions at the frontal and occipital poles are noted. Multiple hemorrhages, especially those located in the frontal and parieto-occipital lobes in an elderly person with preexisting dementia, are hallmarks of amyloid angiopathy.[25] Parasagittal hemorrhages in both hemispheres that are associated with considerable brain edema point toward venous sinus thrombosis[26] (Fig. 8-6). Petechial hemorrhages at the cortical surfaces of the frontal, anterior temporal lobe, or occipital pole are suggestive of trauma. A hemorrhage in any location, particularly in lobar areas, with considerable early adjacent edema suggests an underlying tumor (see Table 8-4). Multiple hemorrhages can be secondary to bleeding diathesis,

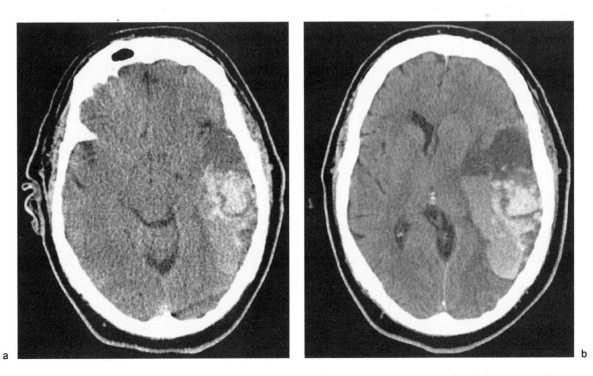

Figure 8-4. Two axial CT scans show progressive enlargement of a left temporal hematoma. The two scans were obtained approximately 9 h apart.

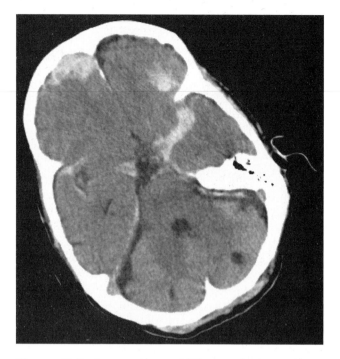

Figure 8-5. An unenhanced CT scan displays a hemorrhage primarily located in the left Sylvian cistern in a patient with ruptured aneurysm of the middle cerebral artery. A small right frontal hemorrhage also is seen.

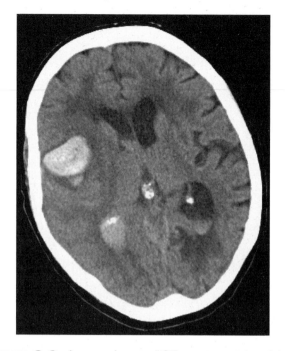

Figure 8-6. An unenhanced CT scan reveals a lobar hemorrhage in an 80-year-old man. The location of the hemorrhage is consistent with the diagnosis of bleeding secondary to amyloid angiopathy. (*Courtesy of Enrique C. Leira, M.D., Department of Neurology, University of Iowa.*)

vasculitis, or metastatic disease. Contrast enhancement may permit detection of an underlying vascular malformation or tumor. In the former, large feeding or draining vessels sometimes can be seen. Contrast-enhanced CT can visualize an aneurysm, particularly if it is >5 mm in size.

The size of a hematoma has a direct effect on management. A hemorrhage >2.5 cm in diameter in the cerebellar hemisphere or >3 cm in diameter in deep cerebral hemispheric structures often portends a poor outcome (Table 8-5). Large (>4 cm diameter or 60 mL) lobar hemorrhages are usually among critically ill patients.[27,28] Patients with these hemorrhages, especially those with posterior fossa bleeding, often need surgical treatment because of the secondary mass-producing effects of the hematoma, with compression of the brain stem and increased intracranial pressure.[29,30] The presence of extensive intraventricular hemorrhage is a predictor of a poor prognosis.[22] In addition, poor outcomes also are more likely among patients with CT evidence of mass effect or hydrocephalus.[28]

Subarachnoid Hemorrhage

In approximately 90–95 percent of patients with SAH, CT detects subarachnoid blood when the test is performed within 24 h of the ictus[4,19,21,31] (see Table 8-4). However, the yield of the test drops dramatically if the procedure is delayed. By 5 days after SAH, CT will demonstrate blood in only 60 percent of patients. The test usually shows blood in the basal cisterns and larger cerebral sulci (see Figs. 8-2 and 8-5). The blood is mostly seen readily on those CT slices that visualize the base of the hemispheres and the area of the circle of Willis. In general, the extent of blood on CT corresponds to the severity of the hemorrhage and the patient's neurological status. CT might miss a small focal collection of blood in an alert patient with minor SAH or a warning leak. CT can detect blood in approximately 75 percent of such patients. In addition, patients with a ruptured aneurysm of the posterior inferior cerebellar artery can have minimal intracranial bleeding and the CT will not detect the blood at base of the skull. The presence of blood on CT obviates the

▶ **TABLE 8-5.** COMPUTED TOMOGRAPHIC PREDICTORS OF POOR OUTCOMES: INTRACRANIAL HEMORRHAGE

Large hematoma
2.5 cm in cerebellum
3.0 cm in cerebral hemisphere
Intraventricular hemorrhage
Hydrocephalus
Mass effect
Focal or diffuse deposits of blood in subarachnoid space

need for a lumbar puncture to make the diagnosis of subarachnoid hemorrhage. Avrahami et al.[32] reported that venous congestion with prominent brain edema might create a hyperintensity along the surface of the brain, which can be confused with subarachnoid hemorrhage.

The patterns of subarachnoid blood vary. Blood can be detected diffusely (either in a thin or thick collection) in the cisterns and sulci or be restricted to one anatomic location (local thin or thick collection). A localized collection of blood points to the most likely site of the ruptured aneurysm[33,34] (see Fig. 8-5). Karttunen et al.[35] found that the pattern of blood on CT within 1 day of subarachnoid hemorrhage is a reliable way to locate a ruptured aneurysm of the middle cerebral or anterior communicating artery. If an adjacent intracerebral hematoma is present, the value of localization is increased. This information is critical for focusing vascular imaging studies. In addition, it provides a clue about which aneurysm might have ruptured if several aneurysms are present. A patient with a ruptured aneurysm of the anterior communicating artery usually has bleeding localized to the anterior interhemispheric fissure, the suprasellar cisterns, and the cistern of the lamina terminalis. A ruptured aneurysm of the middle cerebral artery or internal carotid artery can produce bleeding that is predominantly in the Sylvian fissure and Sylvian cistern. Blood localized to the suprasellar and ambient cisterns can point to a ruptured aneurysm of the posterior communicating artery (see Table 8-4). Aneurysms of the posterior circulation can produce intraventricular hemorrhage or prepontine or ponto-cerebellar cistern bleeding. Perimesencephalic or pre-pontine hemorrhage also can be found with nona-neurysmal subarachnoid hemorrhage. The pattern has been categorized as perimesencephalic subarachnoid hemorrhage (Fig. 8-7).

CT also detects important complications of SAH including extension of blood into the brain or ventricles, subdural hemorrhage, or hydrocephalus. Sequential studies can be used to screen for recurrent hemorrhage and the tests can be used to detect brain edema, mass effect, or infarction. CT also provides prognostic information; patients with complicating intracerebral or intraventricular bleeding and hydrocephalus have poor outcomes. While patients with a focal thin collection of blood or hemorrhage in a perimesencephalic pattern generally have a good prognosis, those persons with more extensive subarachnoid blood have a high rate of serious complications. In particular, a thick collection of blood (either focal or diffuse) is a strong predictor of vasospasm and ischemic stroke.[20,36] Hydrocephalus on the baseline CT or cortical enhancement on a contrast CT also predicts an increased chance of vasospasm.[37]

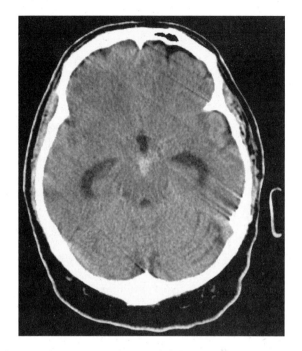

Figure 8-7. An unehanced CT scan shows a small interpedencular hemorrhage in a patient with a benign perimesencephalic subarachnoid hemorrhage. Acute hygrophilous can be seen.

Other Hemorrhages

CT also detects hemorrhages in the subdural and epidural spaces. The shape of the extra-axial hematoma differs between the two locations. In general, subdural hematomas are convex in appearance with epidural collections of blood taking a concave shape. Initially, the hematomas are hyperdense. However, because the interval between the trauma and subdural bleeding and the subsequent clinical presentation can span several weeks, the CT appearance of a subdural hematoma can be isodense or hypodense. At times, findings such as a mass effect or loss of sulci on the hemisphere ipsilateral to the subdural hematoma might be the only CT evidence. A CT performed in a patient with a pituitary hemorrhage can show subarachnoid blood or a hematoma localized to the sella turcica or adjacent area.

Transient Ischemic Attack

While CT often is performed for the assessment of patients with TIA, the primary purposes are to exclude other neurological causes of the symptoms or to confirm the presence of an ischemic stroke. However, CT often shows a hypodensity in the brain following a clinically prolonged TIA, which in fact is a minor stroke.[38] These strokes, which are sometimes called cerebral infarctions with transient symptoms, usually are relatively small and located primarily in deep structures of the hemispheres.

Ischemic Stroke

The CT changes of ischemic stroke are time-linked. Scans performed within the first few hours after stroke usually appear normal.[39,40] In these circumstances, the absence of hemorrhage or other intracranial abnormalities on CT combined with the appropriate clinical features leads to the presumptive diagnosis of acute ischemic stroke. With improvements in CT technology, the ability to find early changes of infarction has expanded (Table 8-6). The usual CT finding of an ischemic stroke is an area of hypodensity. CT information has become increasingly important as decisions about treatment with thrombolytic agents are made[41–45] (Table 8-7; Fig. 8-8). Although the NINDS investigators could not correlate the findings on baseline CT with responses to treatment to rt-PA given within 3 h of stroke, current guidelines still recommend caution if a patient has extensive brain injury noted on imaging.[3, 46] These abnormalities include the appearance of a focal area of decreased density and its size. The age of the ischemic stroke can be estimated by the intensity of the hypodense lesion—the findings gradually evolve during the first 24 h. During the first hours after stroke, the lesion becomes more hypodense than adjacent brain tissue and the degree of hypodensity provides a rough estimate as to the age of the stroke (Fig. 8-9). The lesion generally becomes darker than adjacent brain tissue. CT also can detect clinically silent strokes.[47]

The findings of the CT do influence decisions about administration of thrombolytic agents (Table 8-8). If the area of hypodensity appears to be consistent with a

▶ **TABLE 8-6.** COMPUTED TOMOGRAPHY EVALUATION OF PATIENTS WITH ISCHEMIC STROKE

Screening for intracranial hemorrhage or hemorrhagic transformation
Detect early changes of infarction
Hypodensity
Prominent hypodensity in the lenticulostriate arterial territory
Loss of insular ribbon
Loss of gray–white matter differentiation
Obliteration of sulci
Estimate the age of the infarction (hypodensity)
Estimate the size of the infarction
Multilobar infarction involving more than one-third of hemisphere
Signs of edema or mass effect (shift of midline structures)
Detection of arterial occlusion
Dense artery sign (usually middle cerebral artery)
Dot sign (usually distal middle cerebral artery)

▶ **TABLE 8-7.** POTENTIAL CHANGES IN SEQUTENTIAL COMPUTED TOMOGRAPHIC SCANS OF PATIENTS WITH ISCHEMIC OR HEMORRHAGIC STROKE

Hemorrhagic stroke
Expansion of hematoma
Recurrent hemorrhage
Intraventricular or subarachnoid extension of bleeding
Hydrocephalus
Ischemic stroke secondary to vasospasm
Ischemic stroke
Delineation of infarction (increased hypodensity)
Recurrent infarction
Hemorrhagic transformation of the infarction
Small areas of petechia
Confluent areas of petechia
Small hematoma
Large hematoma
Hemorrhagic or ischemic stroke
Mass effect (including brain edema or hematoma)—hemisphere
Ipsilateral sulci (Sylvian fissure) obliterated
Ipsilateral lateral ventricle compressed
Third ventricle compressed
Contralateral lateral ventricle dilated
Basal cisterns obliterated
Shift of midline structures (herniation)
Cingulate gyrus
Third ventricle
Medial temporal lobe (uncus)
Pineal
Rostral midbrain and diencephalons
Mass effect (including edema or hematoma)—cerebellum
Swelling or mass effect of cerebellar hemisphere
Brain stem compressed and distorted
Prepontine and interpeduncular cisterns obliterated
Fourth ventricle compressed
Third and lateral ventricles dilated

stroke that is older than 3 h, if a large, multilobar lesion is seen, or if mass effect is found, the decision might be made to forego administration of thrombolytic agents. Early hypodensity in the striatocapsular region can predict a major infarction.[40] Some of the findings can be subtle and physicians might not recognize these abnormalities.[14,15,48,49] The pattern of the CT changes (location and size) provides evidence to the location of the arterial occlusion. Several groups have described specific patterns of CT changes that correspond to the vascular territories of the cerebral hemispheres, brain stem, and cerebellum[50–53] (Figs. 8-10 and 8-11). These patterns are helpful for both clinical–anatomic correlations and also provide evidence that affects prognosis and suggests the potential cause of the stroke. For example, small deep infarctions are usually secondary to small artery occlusions, while branch cortical infarctions usually are the

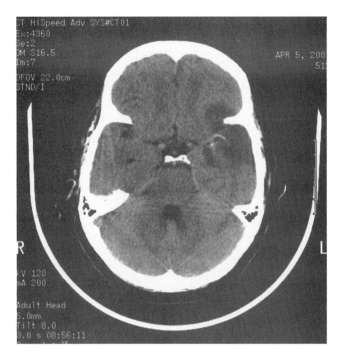

Figure 8-8. An unenhanced CT scan demonstrates an infarction in the left hemisphere in the left hemisphere. A thrombus is found in the middle cerebral artery (dense artery sign).

result of thromboembolic events (Fig. 8-12). A multilobar hemispheric infarction usually is due to either a thrombotic or embolic occlusion of the internal carotid artery or the proximal segment of the middle cerebral artery.[54,55] Cortical or subcortical watershed infarctions

are usually due to recurrent microembolism associated with hypoperfusion.[56]

Pexman et al.[57] reported on a scale that involves the evaluation of several segments of the cerebral hemispheres. It involves assessment of the presence of early signs of infarction in 10 anatomic regions within the cerebral hemispheres. Both superficial and deep structures are examined. They found that this system was very sensitive in predicting outcomes after stroke and the risk of bleeding with medical interventions.[58,59]

Besides assessing the extent of the ischemic brain injury, CT occasionally can detect an embolus or thrombus in the relevant intracranial artery (*dense artery sign* or *dot sign*)[40,60,61] (see Table 8-6 and Fig. 8-8). An area of calcification in an intracranial artery might be confused with the dense artery sign. Follow-up CT examinations also influence management. For example, following administration of thrombolytic agents, another brain imaging study is usually done to exclude major hemorrhagic changes before starting either antiplatelet or anticoagulant medications.

Follow-up CT studies also can be done to assess for the development of complications including hydrocephalus, brain edema, or signs of mass effect and increased intracranial pressure (see Table 8-8[62] and Fig. 8-13). Among the later signs are obliteration of sulci, swelling of the gyri, compression of the ipsilateral lateral ventricle and the Sylvian fissure, and shift of midline structures.[63] Follow-up studies are especially important when treating a patient with a large cerebellar infarction. Obliteration of the prepontine cistern and the fourth ventricle and dilation of the lateral ventricles

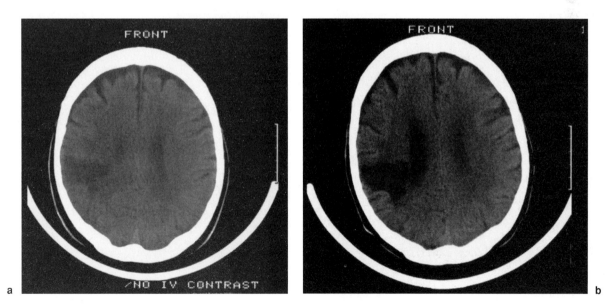

a   b

Figure 8-9. Two unenhanced CT scans show a cortical infarction consistent with a branch (pial) artery occlusion. The two scans demonstrate the change in the appearance of the infarction. The first scan (a) is performed approximately 6 months before the second study (b).

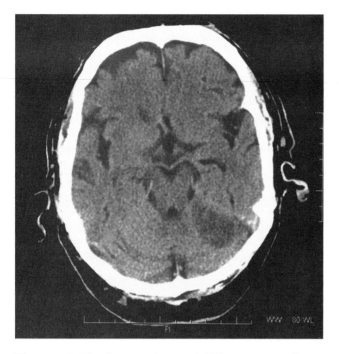

Figure 8-10. An unenhanced CT scan reveals an infarction in the distribution of the left superior cerebellar artery.

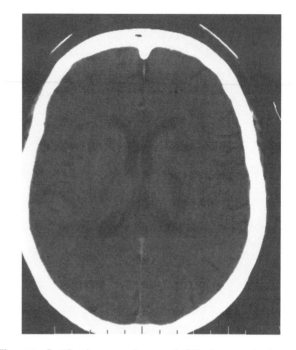

Figure 8-12. An unenhanced CT demonstrates an infarction in the posterior limb of the internal capsule. The imaging finding is compatible with a lacunar infarction in the distribution of the anterior choroidal artery.

often leads to surgical evacuation of the cerebellar mass. Sequential CT studies can detect hemorrhagic transformation of the infarction in 10–40 percent of patients. In most cases, these hemorrhagic changes are not associated with neurological worsening. The findings can be a

localized or confluent area of petechial bleeding or homogenous areas of hemorrhage (hematomas) of variable size.[63] The latter is most commonly associated with neurological deterioration (symptomatic hemorrhagic transformation.)

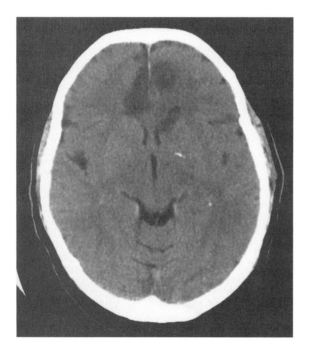

Figure 8-11. An unenhanced CT scan visualizes infarctions in the distribution of both anterior cerebral arteries.

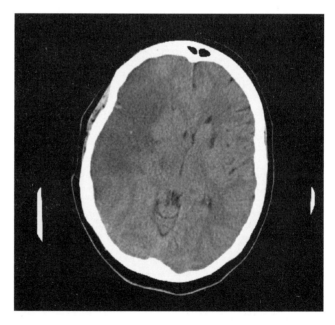

Figure 8-13. An unenhanced CT scan shows a large right hemisphere infarction in the distribution of the middle cerebral artery with secondary obliteration of the ipsilateral sulci and ventricles. Some shift of midline structures also is noted.

▶ **TABLE 8-8.** COMPUTED TOMOGRAPHIC FINDINGS THAT PREDICT UNFAVORABLE OUTCOMES AFTER CEREBRAL INFARCTION OR AN INCREASED RISK OF BLEEDING COMPLICATIONS

Presence of a large area of hypodensity
    Multilobar infarction in hemisphere
    >2. 5 cm in diameter—cerebellum
Signs of brain edema or mass effect
    Cerebral hemisphere
        Swelling of gyri
        Obliteration of sulci
        Obliteration of ipsilateral lateral ventricle
        Dilation of contralateral lateral ventricle
        Shift of midline structures
    Cerebellum or Brainstem
        Obliteration of basal cisterns
        Obliteration of fourth ventricle
        Dilation of lateral ventricles
Dense artery sign
Hemorrhagic transformation—hematoma

Functional Computed Tomography

Advances in technology likely will expand the role of CT in the evaluation of patients with stroke. Among the potential advances are measuring blood flow, determining the sites of hypoperfusion, assessing vascular findings, and possibly evaluating metabolic function.[64] The findings of functional CT correlate with cerebral blood volume in patients with ischemic stroke. Contrast-enhanced, high-resolution CT can be used to assess cerebrovascular physiology.[65] The results of perfusion CT appears to be equivalent to diffusion-weighted and perfusion-weighted MRI in detection of the ischemic penumbra in patients with acute stroke.[66,67] Nonradiolabeled xenon combined with high-resolution CT has been used to assess cerebral blood flow.[20,68] Advantages of these tests include the rapid collection of data because they can be done within a few minutes of the conventional CT study. With the use of additional software programs, expanded CT studies can be performed in more institutions than can MRI studies be. The disadvantage is the requirement to give a bolus of contast agent. At present these studies have not become part of the emergency evaluation of patients with suspected stroke.

▶ MAGNETIC RESONANCE IMAGING

The role of MRI in the assessment of patients with cerebrovascular disease is expanding (Table 8-9). MRI has its limitations: It is less-widely available, more expensive, and takes longer to perform than CT. Although a focused sequence of MRI tests can be done within a few minutes,

▶ **TABLE 8-9.** POTENTIAL ADVANTAGES OF MAGNETIC RESONANCE IMAGING EVALUATION OF PATIENTS WITH CEREBROVASCULAR DISEASES

Multiplanar imaging to assess anatomic location
    Detection of small ischemic or hemorrhagic strokes
    Particularly advantages for lesions in the posterior fossa
Several sequences of studies
    Diffusion-weighted studies—early detection of ischemia
    Perfusion-weighted/diffusion-weighted studies—mismatch
Detection of vascular pathology
    Absence of flow void—arterial occlusion or slow flow
    Dilated feeding arteries or draining veins (vascular malformation)
    Aneurysm
    Arterial pathology—arterial dissection

in other cases, the battery of tests may take up to 45 min to do.[69] While MRI does not involve the use of ionizing radiation, it cannot be done if a patient has a pacemaker, other electronic devices or implanted ferric materials.[69] Confused or agitated patients might need sedation to complete the test. In addition, some patients might develop a sense of claustrophobia that limits the test.

MRI has several advantages (see Table 8-9): It can be used to evaluate patients with either ischemic or hemorrhagic stroke. The axial, sagittal, and coronal images allow a detailed anatomic examination (Fig. 8-14). Three-dimensional mapping of the vascular lesions of the brain can be done.[70] The absence of bone-induced artifacts permits excellent assessment of the cerebellum and brain stem and as a result, MRI can visualize small, deep lesions that might be missed by CT[71–73] (see Table 8-9; Fig. 8-15). Options include T1- weighted, T2-weighted, balanced, fluid attenuation-inversion recovery (FLAIR), gradient-echo T2, diffusion, perfusion, and spectroscopic techniques. While T1- and T2- weighted images often are the primary tests, their utility is limited for assessing stroke. These sequences demonstrate findings of stroke in <50 percent of acute cases.[74] T1 and T2 studies generally are positive within 24 h of stroke.[75] FLAIR imaging demonstrates cortical and periventricular strokes that often are not visualized by T1- and T2-weighted techniques (Fig. 8-16). Still, the findings on FLAIR imaging might be subtle during the first few hours of stroke. DWI can detect brain changes within minutes of onset of infarction[76,77] (Fig. 8-17). It is particularly valuable in the early evaluation of patients who might be treated with rt-PA or other acute interventions. The findings of diffusion MRI also help to differentiate new ischemic lesions from older strokes. In addition, the results provide prognostic information.[78–80] Diffusion-weighted MRI has a high degree of sensitivity (almost 100 percent) and specificity (86–94 percent) with subsequent brain imaging findings.[81–83] Sequential

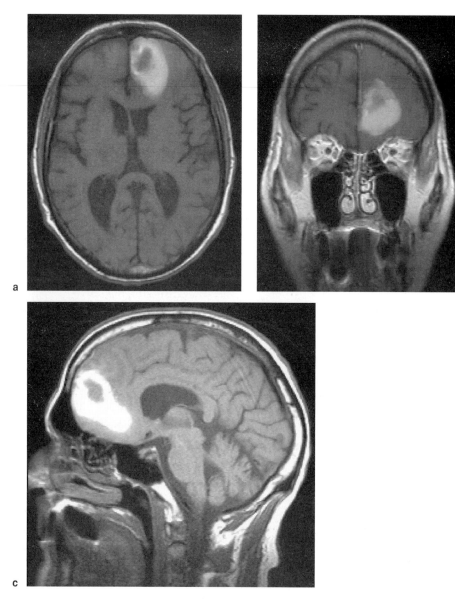

Figure 8-14. (a) Axial, (b) coronal, and (c) sagittal MRI scans demonstrate a left frontal hematoma.

perfusion studies can be used to assess the evolution of an ischemic lesion.[84]

Perfusion imaging allows detection of an area of hypoperfusion including changes in mean transient time, cerebral blood flow, and intravascular volume. A difference in the size of the perfusion and diffusion images (mismatch) is believed to represent the area of the ischemic penumbra[85–87] (Figs. 8-18 and 8-19).

Contrast-enhanced MRI can be used to screen for inflammatory changes in the meninges or the ventricular surface. Contrast-enhanced MRI can detect a reduction in regional cerebral blood volume in advance of the ischemic changes.[88,89] Contrast enhancement can detect an increased mean transit time and increased cerebral blood volume in the brain.[90]

Hemorrhagic Stroke

MRI is useful in the evaluation of patients with hemorrhagic stroke[91] (Fig. 8-20). Intraparenchymal hemorrhage can be detected rapidly using gradient echo techniques.[92–94] In addition, both diffusion-weighted and T2-weighted MRI can be used to differentiate hemorrhage from infarction.[95] MRI can provide information about the age of the hematoma due to the heme components of the hematoma[92] (Table 8-10). Multiplanar capabilities can allow for detailed anatomic definition of the hematoma, which can help the neurosurgeon in surgical management. MRI readily detects complications of hemorrhagic stroke including hydrocephalus or edema. In particular, MRI appears superior to CT in examination of hematomas in the posterior fossa.

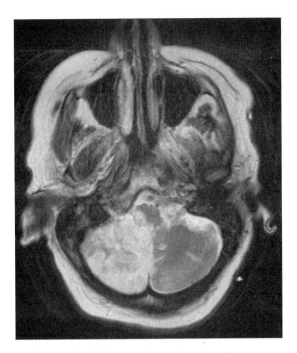

Figure 8-15. A T2-weighted MRI study shows a large infarction in the right dorsolateral medulla and ipsilateral cerebellar hemisphere.

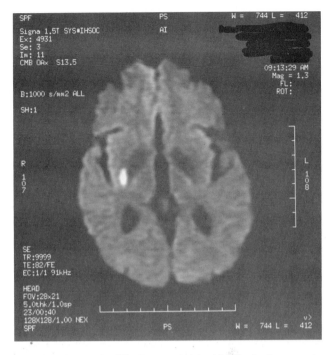

Figure 8-17. A diffusion-weighted MRI study reveals a small lacunar infarction in the posterior aspect of the putamen on the right.

There have been concerns that MRI might not detect small collections of subarachnoid blood as successfully as CT. However, this problem seems to have been overcome largely by the use of higher-strength (1.5 Tesla) machines and the implementation of FLAIR techniques.[96,97] Still, the superiority of MRI in detecting subarachnoid hemorrhage in comparison to CT is not clear. MRI may detect blood density in a patient who is first seen several days after subarachnoid hemorrhage.[98]

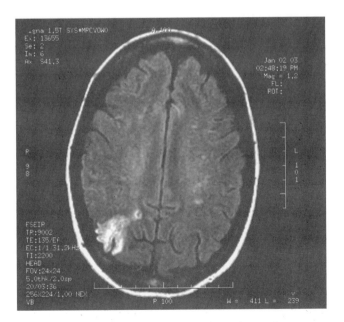

Figure 8-16. A FLAIR MRI study demonstrates a cortical infarction in the right hemisphere. The findings are compatible with a ial (cortical) artery embolic occlusion. Small areas of periventricular white matter changes are seen in both cerebral hemispheres.

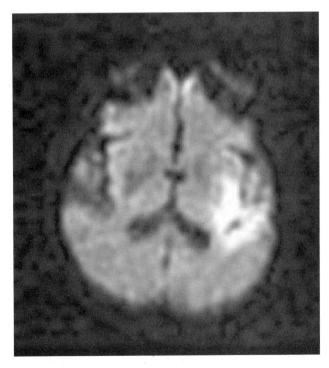

Figure 8-18. A diffusion-weighted MRI performed in a patient with an acute left hemisphere infarction. It shows small areas of infarction in the insula and temporal lobe.

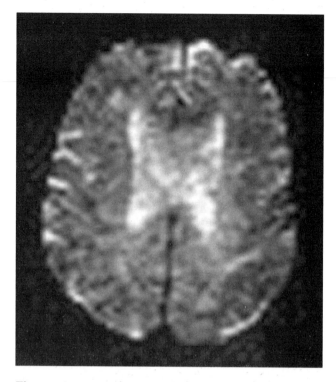

Figure 8-19. A Perfusion MRI performed at the same time as the diffusion-weighted image demonstrated in figure 8-18. The perfusion study demonstrates a large defect consistent with hypoperfusion to a large area of the left hemisphere. The findings in figures 8-18 and 8-19 are compatible with the diagnosis of diffusion-perfusion mismatch.

FLAIR and gradient echo T2 imaging permits detection of small areas of bleeding in the subarachnoid space and the brain.[96,99,100] For example, small punctate clinically silent hemorrhages can be detected in patients with cerebral amyloid angiopathy. MRI can also detect the underlying vascular pathology including an aneurysm or large feeding arteries and draining veins in an arteriovenous malformation. As with CT, MRI too can detect an angiographically occult, slow-flowing vascular malformation such as a cavernous

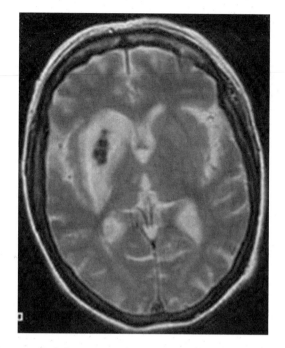

Figure 8-20. A T2-weighted MRI study shows a hemorrhage within an area of infarction in the right basal ganglia. (*Courtesy of Enrique C. Leira, M.D., Department of Neurology, University of Iowa, Iowa City, IA.*)

angioma (Fig. 8-21). Gradient-echo MRI can demonstrate small areas of signal loss, which represent microhemorrhages among patients with cerebral amyloid angiopathy[101,102] (Fig. 8-22). Areas of white matter hyperintensity in patients with an acute cerebral hemorrhage are seen with malignant hypertension.[103] MRI can help diagnose venous disease as a cause of intracranial hemorrhage.[26]

Ischemic Stroke

During the first 24 h, MRI is superior to CT in detecting ischemic stroke. Most ischemic strokes are well defined by T2-weighted MRI (see Table 8-9). In particular, small

▶ **TABLE 8-10.** SEQUENTIAL CHANGES OF INTRACEREBRAL HEMORRHAGE OBSERVED THROUGH MAGNETIC RESONANCE IMAGING

Interval From Time of Hemorrhage	Blood Degradation Product	Comparison to Normal Brain	
		T1 Signal	**T2 Signal**
< 2 h	Center of hematoma	Isointense/hyperintense	
	Periphery of hematoma	—	Hypointense
	Rim	Hypointense	Hyperintense
<24 h	Oxyhemoglobin	Hypointense	Hyperintense
1–3 days	Deoxyhemoglobin	Isointense	Hyperintense or Hypointense
4–7 days	Intracellular methemoglobin	Hyperintense	Hypointense
1–4 weeks	Extracellular methemoglobin	Hyperintense	Hyperintense
>4 weeks	Hemosiderin	Hypointense	Hypointense

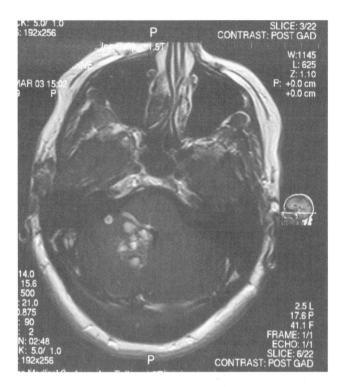

Figure 8-21. A contrast enhanced MRI study shows an arteriovenous malformation in the cerebellum and a dilated vertebral artery.

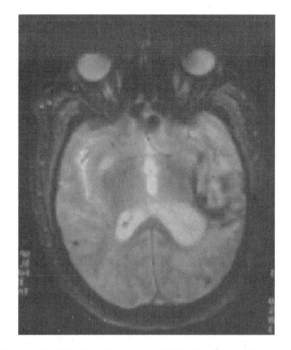

Figure 8-22. Gradient echo MRI shows small area of hemorrhage. Findings are consistent with amyloid angiopathy with small hemorrhage.

and deep hemispheric and brain stem lesions, which might be missed by CT, can be visualized. With the development of diffusion-weighted MRI techniques, the utility of early imaging is increased because changes in the brain can be detected within an hour of onset of stroke. When compared with the ultimate size of a stroke as detected by T2-weighted imaging, diffusion-weighted MRI has a sensitivity and specificity that approaches 100 percent .[104–106] Staaf et al.[107] found that diffusion-weighted MRI can detect small ischemic lesions in the brain stem or basal ganglia (see Fig. 8-17). Diffusion-weighted MRI is especially helpful within the first hours of stroke; its sensitivity and specificity are superior to conventional MRI or CT.[108–110] Recurrent seizures or a brain abscess can give a false positive result on diffusion-weighted MRI. The changes of diffusion-weighted MRI are time-linked. The abnormalities gradually resolve during the first 7–10 days after stroke. Studies done a few weeks after a stroke may not demonstrate any abnormalities on diffusion-weighted MRI.[111] This feature is particularly useful when assessing a patient with a history of previous strokes. The volume of diffusion-weighted MRI acutely often corresponds to the extent of the brain injury found subsequently on T2-weighted images.[81,82] While T2-weighted MRI detects multiple areas of brain injury, the diffusion-weighted image will permit determination as to which stroke is the recent event. Perfusion MRI provides important

information about the area of the brain that is most vulnerable to extension of an acute infarction.[112] A mismatch between the volume of diffusion and perfusion MRI scans might permit improved selection of patients to treat with thrombolytic agents or acute therapies.[113] The usefulness of the finding of "mismatch" in selecting treatment of patients has not been established. Kidwell et al.[114] found that sequential changes on MRI correlated with clinical improvement and recanalization following thrombolytic therapy.

MRI also detects white matter abnormalities in the cerebral hemispheres (Fig. 8-23). These findings are correlated with microvascular causes of dementia such as Binswanger disease.[115,116] Besides imaging the brain, conventional MRI techniques can be used to assess the vasculature. Rapidly flowing blood does not permit acquisition of a signal (flow void phenomenon) and thus the absence of a flow void implies arterial occlusion or sluggish flow[117,118] (Fig. 8-24). Occlusion of the internal carotid artery or proximal portion of the middle cerebral artery can be visualized by the absence of a flow void (see Table 8-9). The absence of flow voids in both internal carotid arteries and both middle cerebral arteries points toward the diagnosis of moyamoya. A loss of the flow void in the prepontine cistern can be found with basilar artery occlusion.[119] The midsagittal view of a sagittal MRI study can demonstrate a thrombus in the basilar artery in the prepontine cistern. Similar loss of a flow void adjacent to the medulla can be found with an occlusion of the vertebral artery. In addition,

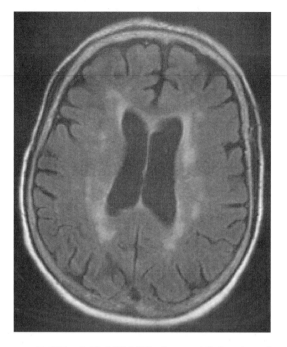

Figure 8-23. A FLAIR MRI shows bilateral periventricular lesions consistent with leukoariosis.

MRI of the neck or base of the skull permits detection of pathology such as an arterial dissection.[120–123] The usual finding is an eccentric area of hyperintensity adjacent to a displaced flow void of a smaller diameter (Fig. 8-25). The area of hyperintensity can be described as curvilinear, band-like, a bamboo-cut, or crescent-shaped. A

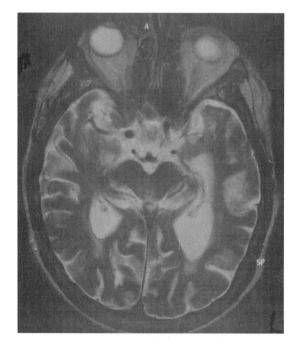

Figure 8-24. A T2-weighted MRI study shows normal flow voids in the carotid arteries and the basilar artery. The proximal segments of the right middle cerebral and posterior cerebral arteries are visualized.

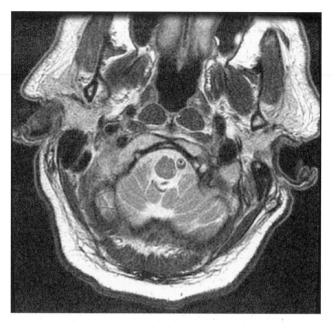

Figure 8-25. A T2-weighted MRI study shows a dissection of the left vertebral artery. An eccentric flow void and an intraluminal thrombus are seen.

large flow void in the prepontine cistern and mass effect with compression of the brain stem are found with a dolichoectatic basilar artery.[124] Contrast-enhanced studies can show a slow flow in cortical arteries consistent with proximal occlusion of a major intracranial artery.

MRI is also useful in the assessment of patients with suspected venous occlusive disease or pituitary apoplexy. Prominent changes in the white and gray matter of both cerebral hemispheres can lead to the diagnosis of *posterior reversible encephalopathy syndrome* (PRES) in a patient with hypertensive encephalopathy or eclampsia[125,126] (Fig. 8-26). The changes of PRES also can be found among patients with hyperperfusion syndrome following carotid endarterectomy.[127]

Magnetic Resonance Spectroscopy

MR spectroscopy can be used to detect metabolic disturbances or biological markers within the first hours after stroke.[128,129] The results of the test can distinguish stroke from brain tumors or other brain diseases; with stroke, rises in lactate and declines in choline and creatine can be found. These studies are particularly useful in evaluating patients with atypical strokes or those with scans that are inconclusive.

▶ POSITRON EMISSION TOMOGRAPHY

Positron emission tomography (PET) is an important research tool for the study of the metabolic consequences

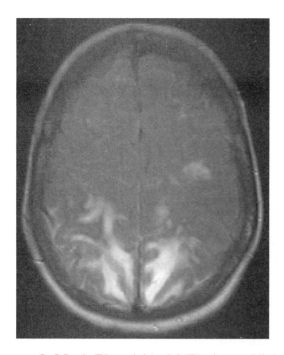

Figure 8-26. A T2-weighted MRI shows bilateral parietal-occipital edema in a patient with hypertensive encephalopathy-posterior reversible encephalopathy syndrome (PRES).

of cerebrovascular disease.[130–133] It gives information about cerebral blood flow, cerebral blood volume, cerebral oxygen consumption, and cerebral metabolism. For example, PET can be used to detect vulnerable areas of metabolism in the ipsilateral hemisphere among patients with carotid occlusion.[134] The information can predict areas of borderline perfusion with a high risk for stroke.[135,136] Following an ischemic lesion, a dissociation occurs between the blood flow and brain metabolism. PET studies demonstrate luxury perfusion in which cerebral blood flow is normal or increased in comparison to brain metabolism. With misery perfusion, the blood flow is decreased in comparison to brain metabolic activity. PET has been used to evaluate the ischemic penumbra and the effects of treatment.[132,137] Heiss et al.[130] concluded that PET was the best method to image the ischemic penumbra. On the other hand, PET is not widely available because of cost. PET also involves an exposure to radiation. Some studies require the creation of a short-lived isotope that must be manufactured on-site. It also lacks the anatomic resolution that is found with CT and MRI. Still, PET is being used in clinical practice. For example, a change in oxygen extraction ratio among symptomatic patients with occlusion of the internal carotid artery predicts a group that is at especially high risk for recurrent ischemic stroke.[135] The results of PET might allow improved selection of patients who could benefit from revascularization procedures.[138] PET can detect secondary metabolic changes of ischemia among persons with hemorrhagic stroke. In addition, because PET can detect hypermetabolic activity such as that found with seizure. The test could be used to differentiate focal seizures from a focal ischemic lesion.

▶ SINGLE PHOTON EMISSION COMPUTED TOMOGRAPHY

Single photon emission computed tomography (SPECT) is used to assess blood flow and metabolic activity in patients with cerebrovascular disease[133,139,140] (Fig. 8-27). This technique, which also involves the injection of a commercially prepared radioisotope, is more widely available than PET. The lack of precise anatomic definition is a limitation of the test. SPECT can be used to distinguish seizures with a secondary Todd paresis from an ischemic locus.[141] The early changes on SPECT are correlated strongly with the severity of neurological impairments, as rated by the NIH Stroke Scale score.[142,143] In addition, SPECT can be used to screen for borderline perfusion in a patient with extensive arterial disease. The administration of adenosine or acetazolamide can be used to augment the ability of SPECT to detect an area of focal hypoperfusion. This information might affect selection of patients who can be treated with a revascularization procedure.[144] The test can be used to detect areas of hypoperfusion in patients with suspected acute ischemic stroke. SPECT has a sensitivity of approximately 80 percent and a specificity of approximately 95 percent in detecting a cortical lesion within 48 h of stroke.[145,146] In the future, the changes on SPECT might be used to select patients who can be treated with thrombolytic agents. For example, Alexandrov et al.[147,148] reported that the results of SPECT could predict the likelihood of bleeding complications from thrombolytic therapy. However, diffusion- and perfusion-weighted MRI appear to provide information that is equal to that obtained from SPECT and the anatomic resolution is superior with MRI.[149] Thus, the use of SPECT might decline with advances in the MRI and CT technology.

▶ EXAMINATION OF THE CEREBROSPINAL FLUID

Lumbar puncture is a time-honored component of the evaluation of patients with suspected stroke. Prior to the introduction of CT, it was the only method to reliably diagnose intracranial bleeding but its role has declined.[150] It is a minimally invasive procedure that does entail some risk. Patients with bleeding diatheses, including those taking oral anticoagulants, cannot have the procedure primarily because of the potential risk for epidural

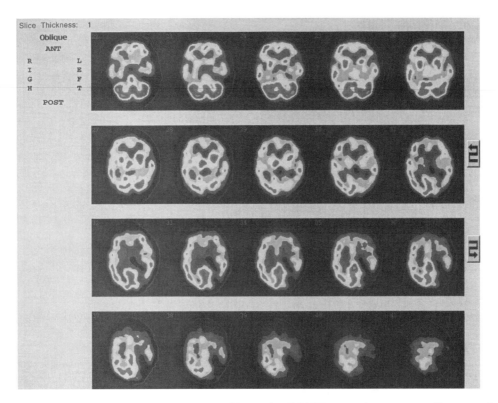

Figure 8-27. A single photon emission CT study (SPECT) reveals an area of hypoperfusion in a patient with a left parietal infarction.

bleeding that could cause cord compression. The procedure is usually avoided among patients with a major hemispheric infarction or hemorrhage. Such strokes are associated with decreased consciousness and increased intracranial pressure. The procedure might cause pressure gradients that lead to herniation. However, lumbar puncture can be done safely in alert patients with severe headache.

Indications—Hemorrhage

In the emergency setting, the primary indication for examination of the CSF is to screen for subarachnoid bleeding.[150] The ability of modern brain imaging studies to detect intracranial hemorrhage has greatly reduced the indications for lumbar puncture. If the diagnosis of hemorrhage already has been made, CSF examination is not needed unless there is some possible information about the etiology of bleeding that can be gleaned. However, examination of the CSF remains critical if a patient has symptoms suggestive of subarachnoid hemorrhage and the CT does not show blood.[4,5] A negative CT scan following subarachnoid hemorrhage is most likely among alert patients. Approximately 2 percent of patients with subarachnoid hemorrhage will have a negative CT study.[151] The risk of complications following lumbar puncture among alert patients appears to be

relatively low, especially in the absence of focal neurological signs. Lumbar puncture can be difficult in obese persons or those with extensive spine disease. In some cases, the procedure will need to be done with fluoroscopic guidance.

The pressure of the CSF is elevated with hemorrhagic strokes and venous thrombosis. The findings of the CSF will be affected by the interval from the stroke. Within the first hours of stroke, bloody CSF will be found in virtually all patients with subarachnoid hemorrhage and in approximately 75 percent of patients with intracerebral hemorrhages. In this situation, the absence of blood means that the hemorrhage did not extend into the ventricles or the subarachnoid space.

Because insertion of the needle might pierce a small spinal epidural vein, the presence of bloody CSF might be secondary to the procedure itself. The risk of iatrogenic bleeding is not necessarily associated with the difficulty in doing the procedure. Thus, it is important to differentiate iatrogenic bloody CSF from that due to subarachnoid hemorrhage. In general, bloody CSF secondary to the procedure will clear during sequential aliquots (tubes). The most reliable way to confirm bleeding from subarachnoid hemorrhage is immediate centrifugation. The presence of xanthochromia points to a subarachnoid hemorrhage.[152] The yellow color is secondary to the release of pigments from the breakdown of the red blood cells and appears within a few hours of subarachnoid hemorrhage.[150] If the fluid is clear after centrifugation, the bloody CSF probably was secondary to the procedure.

The interval from subarachnoid hemorrhage affects the findings on examination of the CSF. Initially the fluid is bloody and the ratio of red blood cells to white blood cells in the CSF is similar to their proportion in the blood. The CSF concentration of protein is elevated while the glucose concentration is normal or slightly reduced. An inflammatory reaction with an increase in white blood cells can predominate when the CSF is analyzed several days after the ictus. At this time xanthochromia, elevated CSF protein levels, and hypoglycorrhachia are present. The findings can mimic viral meningitis. The xanthochromia gradually resolves 2–3 weeks following the hemorrhage.[150] Cytological examination of a CSF sample obtained several days or weeks after subarachnoid hemorrhage might show iron-stained inclusions in the white blood cells. In addition, elevated concentrations of oxyhemoglobin, hemoglobin, or bilirubin are found. Spectroscopic examination of CSF has been used, but the value of this test is not established and it is not widely available.[153,154]

Indications—Ischemic Stroke

Most patients with suspected ischemic stroke do not need examination of the CSF. Lumbar puncture is not needed when the findings are not compatible with subarachnoid hemorrhage. The major reasons for doing the test among persons with ischemic stroke are to screen for an infectious or inflammatory cause of the vascular event. Infections such as meningovascular syphilis can cause CSF leucocytosis, elevated CSF protein, elevated globulins, and hypoglycorrhachia. While a similar inflammatory reaction can occur with multisystem or isolated vasculitis, some patients with vasculitis have normal CSF findings. Microbiological studies can be ordered in cases of suspected stroke secondary to an infectious illness. Although there is some evidence that additional CSF biochemical studies, such as measurement of creatine kinase or lactic acid dehydrogenase, can be performed during the evaluation of patients with ischemic stroke, these tests have not become used widely.[155,156]

► ELECTROENCEPHALOGRAPHY

EEG is of limited utility for assessing patients with suspected stroke. In general, emergency EEG is obtained to look for seizures, to seek an explanation of coma, or to screen for brain death.[157] Periodic lateralized epileptiform discharges or focal or generalized slow activity can be found on an EEG performed following a stroke.[158] These finding are nonspecific for a cerebrovascular event and other acute brain illnesses can produce similar findings. The EEG might help differentiate seizures with a postictal paralysis from a stroke or help distinguish recurrent seizures from repeated TIA. Interictal seizure activity found by EEG would imply a seizure disorder. EEG can be used to screen for seizures complicating either hemorrhagic or ischemic events. EEG, and at times evoked potentials, has been used to monitor patients undergoing cerebrovascular operations such as carotid endarterectomy.[159,160] Changes in the EEG appear to be an early marker of ischemia during the operation and the surgeon should respond accordingly. EEG and evoked potentials have been used as supplements to clinical assessments for monitoring critically ill patients with stroke.[161]

► EXAMINATION OF SUSPECTED VASCULAR EVENTS OF THE SPINAL CORD

Both CT and MRI are used to assess patients with suspected vascular events of the spinal cord. In particular, MRI is effective for screening for a mass or a vascular malformation that could be causing cord dysfunction. Examination of the CSF usually shows blood if the patient has had a primary spinal subarachnoid hemorrhage from a vascular malformation. In general, radiographs of the spine are not particularly helpful in confirming a vascular event of the spinal cord; their primary utility is in excluding a fracture or other spine pathology that is secondarily affecting the spinal cord. Evoked potentials can be used to localize a lesion within the cord.

► EVALUATION OF THE VASCULATURE

Several options are available to assess the patient for the presence of underlying vascular pathology that leads to ischemic or hemorrhagic stroke. The traditional methods for examination are arteriography and ultrasonography. More recently, CTA, MRA, duplex ultrasonographic imaging, and transcranial Doppler ultrasonography have become options. In addition, MR venography (MRV) has become the usual way to assess patients with suspected venous sinus thrombosis. The availability of a large number of noninvasive tests is influencing management of patients with both hemorrhages and infarctions. The vasculature can be rapidly and accurately assessed at the time of the initial evaluation. In the future, the results of these tests might influence decisions about acute management, including the use of thrombolytic therapy for treatment of patients with cerebral infarction.

▶ ARTERIOGRAPHY

Arteriography, including digital subtraction arteriography, is the traditional method for assessing the vasculature. Rothwell et al.[162] found that interrater agreement in interpreting the studies is high. Arteriography has a number of attributes (Table 8-11). It remains the best method to assess both the intracranial and extracranial vasculature. However, the test is invasive and it can be associated with adverse experiences including allergic reactions, myocardial infarction, thromboembolic strokes, or death. Hankey et al.[163] reported complications in 3.4 percent of 382 patients having the study. The rate of complications of arteriography exceeded that associated with carotid endarterectomy among patients enrolled in the Asymptomatic Carotid Atherosclerosis Study.[164] Besides direct thromboembolic events secondary to the

▶ **TABLE 8-11.** ADVANTAGES AND LIMITATIONS OF ARTERIOGRAPHY EVAULATION OF PATIENTS WITH CEREBROVASCULAR DISEASE

Advantages
  Accurately defines atherosclerotic arterial lesions
    Arterial stenosis
    Arterial occlusion
    Differentiates high-grade stenosis from occlusion
    Detects ulceration of atherosclerotic plaque
    Detects intraluminal thrombus on atherosclerotic
      plaque
    Detects both intracranial and extracranial disease
    Provides evidence of collateral circulation
    Used to select patients for surgical or endovascular
      treatment
  Detects intraluminal thromboembolism (arterial or cardiac
    origin)
    Used to select patients for thrombolytic treatment
  Detects nonatherosclerotic arterial diseases that cause
    ischemic stroke
    Arterial dissection
    Fibromuscular dysplasia
    Moyamoya syndrome
    Vasculitis
  Detects arterial diseases that cause hemorrhagic stroke
    Saccular aneurysms
    Nonsaccular aneurysms
    Arteriovenous malformations
    Dissecting aneurysms
    Vasculitis
    Can define vascular anatomy to guide surgical treatment
  Detects vasospasm following subarachnoid hemorrhage
  Could be combined with endovascular treatment
Limitations
  Not available at many community hospitals; requires
    expertise
  Invasive procedure that can be associated with adverse
    experiences

catheter, the contrast agent can cause seizures, transient neurological dysfunction, renal dysfunction, or allergic reactions.[165] Potential interactions with oral hypoglycemic agents, such as metformin, present problems. Local arterial injury at the puncture site, most commonly affecting the femoral artery, can lead to the development of a false aneurysm. A hematoma also can compress the femoral nerve. In the past, there were concerns that arteriography was contraindicated among persons with migraine because it might induce a stroke but these reservations seem to have been misplaced.[166]

Indications—Ischemic Vascular Disease

Arteriography remains the best method to define the residual arterial lumen and surface in a patient with atherosclerotic disease. It also is a very effective way to screen for major arterial abnormalities that lead to ischemic or hemorrhagic stroke including fibromuscular dysplasia, arterial dissections, aneurysms, or vascular malformations (Figs. 8-28 and 8-29). Because flow in cavernous or venous malformations is relatively slow, these lesions can be arteriographically occult. Arteriography does not provide information about changes within the arterial wall. Arteriography (venous phase) has limited utility in examining for cerebral venous sinus disease (Fig. 8-30).

Arteriography is the traditional method to examine the severity of arterial narrowing and its results are used

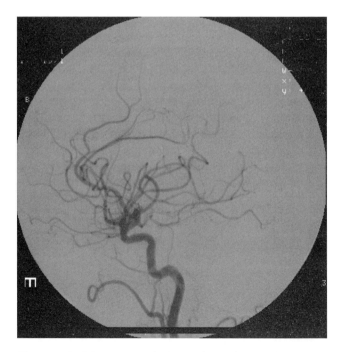

Figure 8-28. A lateral view of a left carotid arteriogram shows an aneurysm arising from the cavernous segment of the internal carotid artery.

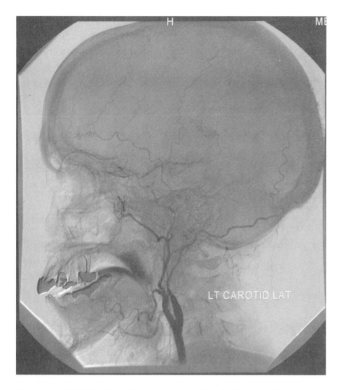

Figure 8-29. A lateral view of a left carotid arteriogram demonstrates a dissection of the cervical segment of the internal carotid artery.

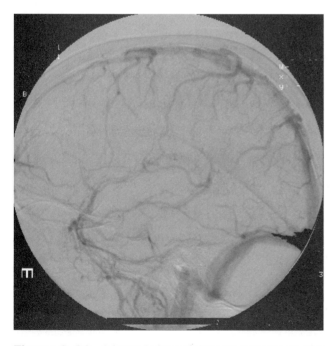

Figure 8-30. A lateral view of the venous phase of a right carotid arteriogram using subtraction techniques reveals normal major cortical veins, the superior sagittal sinus, transverse sinus, and sigmoid sinus.

to determine the need for carotid endarterectomy. The findings of arteriography are correlated strongly with surgical specimens.[167] Investigators in the North American Symptomatic Carotid Endarterectomy Trial (NASCET) developed a method to measure the degree of stenosis demonstrated by arteriography[168]:

Diameter of artery

$$\% \text{ Stenosis} = \frac{\text{Most severe narrowing}}{\text{2 cm distal to narrowing}} \times 100$$

Diameter of artery at approximately 2 cm distal to stenosis.

While the above mathematical calculation is straightforward, physicians often have difficulty determining the diameters especially if digital studies are examined.[169,170] The severity of the stenosis can be both over- and underestimated. At times, a prolonged section of severe narrowing (string sign) can be found distal to a very high-grade stenosis. This area of narrowing probably reflects collapse of the artery secondary to very slow flow. Arteriography can demonstrate ulceration of the atherosclerotic plaque or an intraluminal thrombus.[171–173] Because arteriography does entail some risk, the test should be recommended to only those patients with atherosclerotic disease who could be treated with either surgery or endovascular procedures. The timing of the procedure also is important; arteriography should be done shortly before the planned intervention.

Arteriography remains particularly important for detection of arterial lesions, such as vasculitis or atherosclerosis, which develop in small-to-medium caliber intracranial vessels that cannot be adequately assessed by other techniques.[174] The usual findings of vasculitis are segmental areas of narrowing and dilation (sausage-like appearance) in multiple vessels. Diffuse intracranial atherosclerosis can appear similar. While arteriography is the most definitive imaging method to sustain the diagnosis of cerebral vasculitis, it will be nondiagnostic in approximately 50 percent of patients. Arteriography is the best method to diagnose moyamoya. The arteriographic changes usually are bilateral with the primary changes in the distal (intracranial) segments of the internal carotid arteries and the proximal portions of the middle and anterior cerebral arteries.[175] A meshwork of small caliber vessels appears at the base of the brain in conjunction with the arterial occlusions.

Indications—Hemorrhagic Vascular Disease

Arteriography is included in the evaluation of many patients with hemorrhagic stroke. The procedure probably can be avoided in the case of a deep hemispheric hemorrhage in a patient older than 45 with a strong history of hypertension. However, younger persons, those with lobar hemorrhages, and those without a history of hypertension should have arteriography.[176,177] Arteriography remains a part of the evaluation of patients with hemorrhagic stroke attributed to drug (cocaine) abuse because many of these hemorrhages are secondary to an occult vascular malformation or aneurysm. The risks of arteriography appear to be lower among persons with hemorrhagic stroke than among patients with ischemic stroke. Recurrent rupture of aneurysm has been described during arteriography, especially if the study is done within the first few hours following subarachnoid hemorrhage.[178] Patients with a known coagulopathy leading to intracranial hemorrhage cannot have the test because of the potential risk for bleeding complications.

Unless there is a specific contraindication, arteriography should be a part of the evaluation of patients with subarachnoid hemorrhage (Fig. 8-31). Even those less acutely ill patients with a perimesencephalic pattern of bleeding on CT should be examined. Because of the urgency in treating a ruptured aneurysm, arteriography is done as soon as possible. Based on the pattern of bleeding seen on CT, the relevant artery should be examined first. Still, both carotid territories and the vertebrobasilar circulation are visualized because approximately 25 percent of patients have more than one aneurysm. Most saccular aneurysms are located near the circle of Willis or on the major branches of the vertebral or basilar arteries. Overall, the yield of arteriography is approximately 70 percent among patients with subarachnoid hemorrhage.[179] Occasionally, an arteriogram will produce false-negative results because of the presence of adjacent vasospasm, thrombosis of the aneurysm, a narrow neck that hampers visualization of the aneurysmal sac, or an incomplete examination.[179] Thus, most patients with a negative arteriogram should have a second study done approximately 7–10 days after the first study.[180] The yield of the second study is approximately 5 percent. While this number is relatively low, the ominous nature of aneurysmal subarachnoid hemorrhage means that the second study should be done. A second arteriogram can discover a vascular malformation that is not found by a procedure done shortly after an intracranial hemorrhage.[180,181] Even after two negative studies, a third arteriogram is sometimes done if the clinical suspicion for an aneurysm remains very high.

The type of aneurysm often is predicted by the location of the lesion; arteriographic visualization of an aneurysm on a distal branch cortical artery can be secondary to an infection, tumor, or trauma. Besides helping in determination of the cause of the hemorrhage, arteriography provides information that will affect decisions about surgery, including the anatomy of adjacent vessels. Arteriography also is the most definitive way to detect vasospasm following subarachnoid hemorrhage. However, the development of noninvasive vascular imaging is reducing the role of arteriography in the management of patients with intracranial hemorrhage. Vascular studies, including MRA and CTA, likely will reduce the indications for arteriography in the evaluation of patients with suspected aneurysms or vascular malformations.

► COMPUTED TOMOGRAPHIC ANGIOGRAPHY

Contrast-enhanced spiral CTA is used to evaluate both the intracranial and extracranial vasculature among patients with either hemorrhagic or ischemic cerebrovascular disease (Table 8-12). It can be performed rapidly in conjunction with imaging of the brain. It can provide information about the status of major intracranial vessels. For example, it can detect occlusion of middle cerebral artery.[65,182–184] CTA also is becoming a valuable tool for evaluation of patients with saccular aneurysms or arteriovenous malformations (see Table 8-12). It can be used to evaluate patients with intracranial hemorrhage.[185,186] It generally demonstrates aneurysms larger than 3–5 mm in diameter.[187,188] The sensitivity of CTA is approximately 85–98 percent.[186,189–191] In evaluation of 100 patients with subarachnoid hemorrhage, Dehdashti et al.[192] reported that CTA detected all the ruptured aneurysms and the study was sufficiently diagnostic to

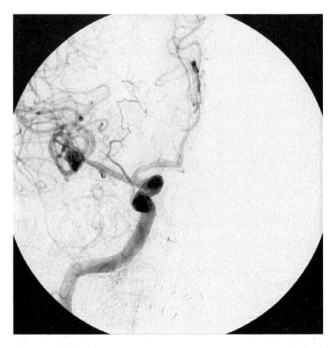

Figure 8-31. An anteroposterior view of an arteriogram illustrates a large aneurysm of the proximal segment of the right middle cerebral artery.

▶ **TABLE 8-12.** ADVANTAGES AND DISADVANTAGES OF NONINVASIVE VASCULAR IMAGING TESTS

Carotid duplex
  Advantages
    Widely available and relatively inexpensive
    Easy to perform
    Information about lumen and arterial wall
      Degree of narrowing
      Ulceration
      Presence of thrombus
      Calcification
      Hemorrhage
      Intimal-medial thickness
    Some information about distal flow
  Disadvantages
    Vulnerable to errors in technique
    Vulnerable to errors in interpretation
    Limited area of vasculature examined
Transcranial Doppler ultrasonography
  Advantages
    Measures flow velocity
      Narrowing of major arteries
      Occlusion of major arteries
    Some imaging of vessels
    Can be done sequentially
      Monitor patient
      Monitor response to therapy
    Can detect microemboli in high-risk patients
  Disadvantages
    Not widely available
    Time consuming
    Vulnerable to errors in technique
    Vulnerable to errors in interpretation
    Can be difficult to find vessels
    Does not evaluate small or distal vessels

Magnetic resonance angiography
  Advantages
    Assesses vasculature bed from chest to brain
    Detects arterial occlusion or stenosis
    Detects aneurysms and vascular malformations
    Can be combined with imaging of the brain
    Gives three dimensional pictures
    Generally low risk for errors in interpretation
  Disadvantages
    Expensive
    No hemodynamic information
    Time consuming
    Limited information on smaller arteries
    Contraindications—pacemaker, metal
    Claustrophobia
    May require sedation
Computed tomographic angiography
  Advantages
    Excellent anatomic resolution
    Can examine multiple segments of vasculature
    Three-dimensional imaging
    Detect arterial occlusion or stenosis
    Detect aneurysm or vascular malformation
    Information about adjacent vasculature
    Image small arteries at base of brain
    Generally low risk for errors in interpretation
  Disadvantages
    Expensive
    Not widely available
    Requires contrast injection
    Exposure to ionizing radiation

permit decisions about endovascular or surgical treatment in 89 cases. There are cases of CTA detecting aneurysms missed by conventional arteriography.[193–195] CTA might detect vasospasm complicating subarachnoid hemorrhage.[196,197] The three-dimensional visualization of the aneurysm and adjacent vascular structures can influence surgical management.[195,198] Detailed examination of the anatomy of the aneurysm and adjacent vascular structures can be obtained. The study can be done to screen for aneurysms in patients with a family history of subarachnoid hemorrhage. Both feeding arteries and draining veins are reliably found during CTA assessment of patients with vascular malformations.[199] The utility of CTA in the management of patients with acute ischemic stroke has not been established. At present, the selection of vascular imaging tests, including CTA, is made on a case-by-case basis.

CTA can visualize the severity of stenosis of extracranial arteries, including the presence of calcification, but can miss an ulcerated plaque.[200] It can be combined with duplex imaging to be an alternative to conventional arteriography to select patients who could be treated with carotid endarterectomy.[184,189,201–204] Its yield is relatively high in detecting occlusions of the basilar or middle cerebral artery. CTA does not appear to be as sensitive or specific as MRA in detecting atherosclerotic disease of the internal carotid artery. At present, the technology to do CTA is not widely available and the requirement for contrast enhancement is a limitation. Comparisons of the relative utility of CTA and MRA are needed.

▶ MAGNETIC RESONANCE ANGIOGRAPHY

The indications for MRA in the assessment of patients with cerebrovascular disease are growing[205–207] (see Table 8-12). This noninvasive test can be performed in conjunction with MRI in patients with both hemorrhagic and ischemic stroke. MRA can assess the intracranial and extracranial vasculature and gadolinium-enhancement improves the ability of the test to accurately

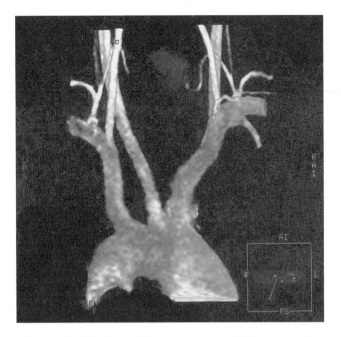

Figure 8-32. An oblique view of a MRA shows the normal anatomy of the arch of the aortic and its major branches. The brachiocephalic artery is on the left side of the image. The origins of the brachiocephalic, left common carotid, left subclavian, right common carotid, and both vertebral arteries are visualized.

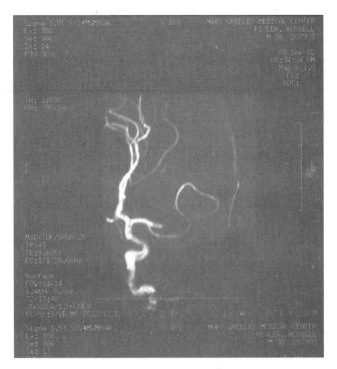

Figure 8-34. An anteroposterior view of an MRA shows an occlusion of the superoanterior division of the left middle cerebral artery. The finding is compatible with an embolic occlusion at the bifurcation of the middle cerebral artery.

examine the vascular anatomy (Fig. 8-32). MRA can be used to assess patients with acute stroke; the test can be used in combination with perfusion and DWI MRI to select patients for acute treatment[113] (Figs. 8-33–8-36). Early detection of arterial occlusion by MRA is associated with the severe strokes.[208,209] MRA has many attributes, but it remains relatively expensive and in some cases it can be time-consuming. MRA may overestimate the

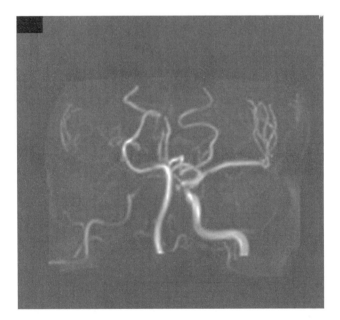

Figure 8-33. An anteroposterior view of MRA reveals narrowing of the right internal carotid artery. In addition, the right middle cerebral artery is not visualized. The findings are consistent with a stenosis or dissection of the internal carotid artery with secondary occlusion of the middle cerebral artery.

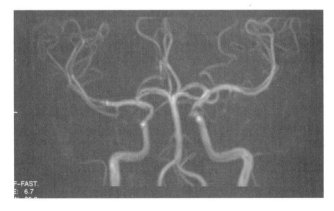

Figure 8-35. An anteroposterior view of MRA reveals the normal vascular anatomy of the distal segments of the vertebral and internal carotid arteries, the basilar artery, and the proximal segment of the posterior cerebral, middle cerebral, and anterior cerebral arteries.

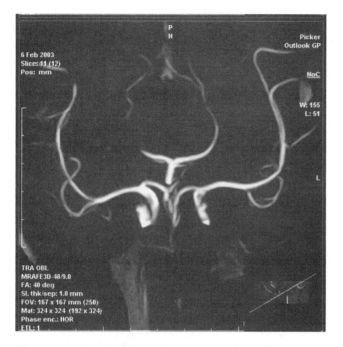

Figure 8-36. An MRA shows narrowing of both posterior cerebral arteries. The stenosis is proximal on the right and more distal on the left.

severity of the arterial narrowing.[210] The test is vulnerable to artifacts such as those induced by swallowing or movement especially when examining the extracranial vasculature. MRA cannot adequately examine medium-to-small caliber intracranial arteries therefore is not helpful for evaluating patients with suspected vasculitis. It is not very successful in imaging the status of the vascular wall.[211] The test could be used to assess the patency of an extracranial-to-intracranial arterial anastomosis.

MRA can readily detect occlusions or high-grade stenoses of major vessels including the internal carotid, middle cerebral, and basilar arteries. In particular, the technique assesses the extracranial vasculature with a high degree of accuracy.[204,212–215] Based on a systemic review, Nederkoorn et al.[210] estimated that the MRA could distinguish a stenosis >70 percent with a sensitivity of approximately 95 percent and a specificity of 90 percent. The use of cross-sectional MRA can be used to predict the severity of stenosis of the proximal segment of the internal carotid artery.[216] Johnston et al.[217] report that contrast-enhanced MRA is highly sensitive for detection of stenoses of the internal carotid artery that can be treated surgically.

The sensitivity and specificity of MRA in detecting intracranial occlusions in the anterior circulation approach 95 percent and its performance in examination of the basilar artery is even higher.[215,218–220] Besides detecting a basilar artery occlusion, MRA may visualize a stenosis or a fusiform aneurysm. MRA may provide evidence for occlusion of major branch arteries in the vertebrobasilar circulations.

MRA provides important information about intracranial aneurysms or vascular malformations, including their size, the presence of an intraluminal thrombus, and their relationships to adjacent vascular or brain structures.[221–224] Sequential MRA studies could be used to monitor the growth of an unruptured aneurysm.[225] While MRA has become an important tool for screening patients for the presence of an intracranial aneurysm, it can miss small lesions. White et al.[190] concluded that MRA has a sensitivity of 70–97 percent and a specificity of 75–100 percent for detecting intracranial aneurysms. MRA has become an effective method for screening persons considered as having a high risk for an intracranial aneurysm, such as persons with autosomal dominant polycystic kidney disease.[226–229] It is a useful method to examine arterial and venous changes in a patient with a vascular malformation.

The presence of occlusions of major intracranial arteries and prominent collateral channels on MRA can point toward the diagnosis of moyamoya as the cause of either hemorrhagic or ischemic stroke.[230] MRA also can be used to screen for dissections of the vertebral or internal carotid arteries. Sequential MRA studies can be used to monitor the evolution of the dissection including the potential development of a false aneurysm.[231] These studies can be used to screen for nonpenetrating, extracranial arterial injuries among persons with craniocerebral trauma.

▶ CAROTID ARTERY DUPLEX ULTRASONOGRAPHY

Duplex ultrasonography is a widely performed noninvasive diagnostic tool for evaluation of the extracranial portion of the internal carotid artery.[232] The test is available in most communities and it can be performed easily. It is relatively inexpensive. Carotid duplex gives information about the anatomy and pathology of the distal common carotid artery, the bifurcation of the common carotid artery, the proximal portion of the internal carotid artery, and the origin of the external carotid artery (Figs. 8-37– 8-39). The technology detects arterial stenosis or occlusion, pathology within the arterial wall and plaque, and the presence of ulceration, or an intraluminal thrombus.[232,233] Among the changes within the plaque are hemorrhage, calcification, or fibrosis.[234,235] Ultrasonography also detects morphologic features that are associated with plaque instability, which in turn probably predicts ischemic stroke or myocardial infarction. These morphologic changes are more commonly found persons with transient ischemic attacks than among persons with asymptomatic atherosclerotic disease of the internal carotid artery.[236,237]

The degree of stenosis is estimated by the direct imaging of the vessel and by the measurement of the

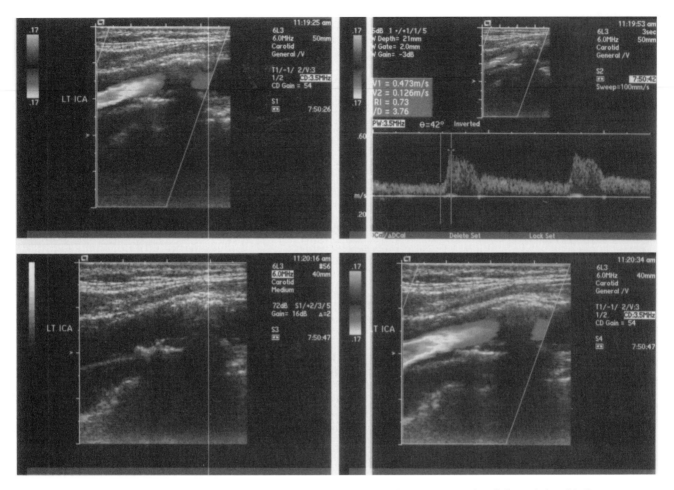

Figure 8-37. Carotid duplex study shows mild to moderate stenosis of the origin of left internal carotid artery.

velocity. Several studies tested the sensitivity and specificity of carotid duplex ultrasonography in predicting the severity of arterial narrowing in comparison to the commonly used measures for rating narrowing by arteriography. Overall, the test has a positive predictive value of approximately 90 percent and a negative predictive value of approximately 95 percent.[204,215,238–240] Duplex ultrasonography has a sensitivity of approximately 98 percent and specificity of nearly 100 percent for detecting occlusion of the internal carotid artery.[215] At times, the test might not be able to differentiate a high-grade stenosis from an occlusion. A severe stenosis or occlusion of the distal internal carotid artery or middle cerebral artery can cause changes in distal flow that can be detected by duplex ultrasonography at the bifurcation. On the other hand, an increase in velocity in one internal carotid artery could be secondary to severe narrowing or occlusion of the contralateral internal carotid artery. The results of the test can be used to screen patients who might be candidates for surgical treatment.[241] Sequential studies can

monitor progression in an atherosclerotic lesion; such progression has been associated with several of the risk factors for accelerated arterial disease.[242,243]

Intimal-Medial Thickness

One of the advances in duplex imaging is the calculation of the intimal-medial thickness (IMT) of the arterial wall.[244–247] Measurement of the depth of the arterial wall in six locations is used to calculate IMT. The findings in the arterial wall also appear before the other changes detected by carotid duplex. An increase in IMT appears to be an early sign of accelerated atherosclerosis and the finding is associated with an increased risk of myocardial infarction and stroke.[248–250] An increase in IMT is associated with the presence of risk factors of atherosclerosis, including hypercholesterolemia.[249]

Carotid duplex ultrasonography could be a component of the emergent evaluation of a patient with a major hemispheric infarction. The test can be used to screen

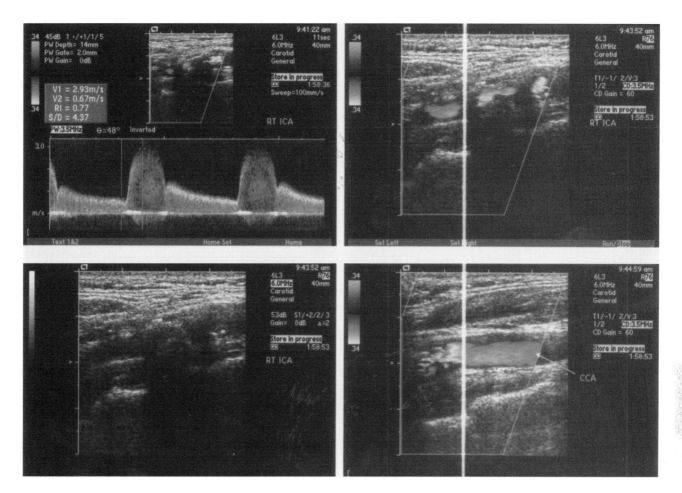

Figure 8-38. Carotid duplex study demonstrates moderate stenosis of the internal carotid artery.

for an acute occlusion of the internal carotid artery—a finding that might influence decisions about acute management.[251] The results of carotid duplex can be complemented by the findings of MRA.[238,252] Many physicians now recommend carotid endarterectomy based on the findings of carotid duplex and MRA.[253] The test also can be used to monitor for growth (increased thickness) of an atherosclerotic plaque in an asymptomatic patient, which might prompt surgical or endovascular treatment. It is also used to screen for postoperative changes in the carotid artery including recurrent stenosis secondary to fibrosis. Besides looking for atherosclerotic disease, duplex ultrasonography can be used to screen for a dissection of the internal carotid artery or fibromuscular dysplasia.

Carotid duplex ultrasonography does have limitations. The test does not visualize the entire vascular circulation from the chest to the brain. It does not provide information about a potential second (tandem) stenosis that may be located in the intracranial portion of the internal carotid artery. Some patients with very severe

arterial narrowing will be misjudged as having an occlusion based on the duplex findings and as a result, a patient who might benefit from a reconstructive procedure might not be referred for surgery. The test's vulnerability to errors in technique is its most important limitation. Major errors that lead to either over- or under-estimation of the degree of arterial stenosis may result and, therefore, clinicians should know about the accuracy of the tests performed in their local laboratory.[254,255] The laboratory should have a strong quality-control program that includes frequent comparisons of their results to the findings on arteriography. Certification programs are available to assure the quality of the local laboratory.

▶ DIRECTIONAL DOPPLER ULTRASONOGRAPHY

Directional Doppler ultrasonography originally was used to assess the carotid circulation, but duplex studies

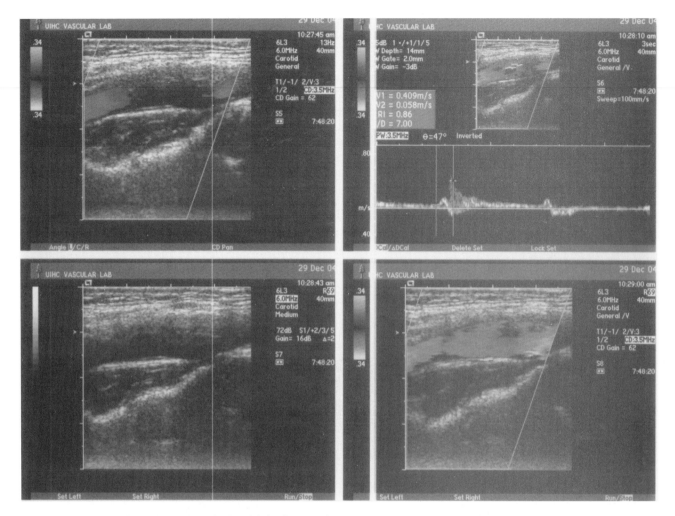

Figure 8-39. Normal carotid duplex study.

have supplanted this test. Directional Doppler studies can be done to assess the direction of flow in the vertebral arteries.[256,257] The results can be used to diagnose a severe stenosis or occlusion of the extracranial portion of the vertebral artery. In the subclavian steal syndrome, the normal cephalad flow is reversed in the ipsilateral vertebral artery. Changes in vertebral flow might be detected with neck rotation and secondary vertebral artery compression. Because the caliber often differs between the two vertebral arteries, caution should be exercised in interpreting results. Rather than being occluded, a vertebral artery might be atretic.

▶ TRANSCRANIAL DOPPLER ULTRASONOGRAPHY

Transcranial Doppler ultrasonography (TCD) uses the same technology as carotid duplex and directional Doppler studies. It is a widely used noninvasive study that can assess the major intracranial arteries in patients with either hemorrhagic or ischemic cerebrovascular disease[258] (Table 8-13). The test detects changes in flow secondary to arterial occlusion or stenosis and assesses for transient signals consistent with embolization.[259] TCD can be used to screen for an acute arterial occlusion, which might guide thrombolytic treatment of a patient with a cerebral infarction[260,261] (Figs. 8-40–8-42). Alexandrov et al.[262] used TCD to monitor for recanalization with intravenous administration of rt-PA. In addition, sequential studies could be screen for reocclusion of the artery after thrombolytic treatment.[263–265] TCD detection of reocclusion is associated with poor neurological outcome. It is used to monitor flow during carotid or cardiac operations and to check the patency of an extracranial-to-intracranial arterial anastomosis.

Detection of Microemboli

The frequency of cerebral microemboli as detected by TCD is associated with the risk of stroke among persons with either cardiac or arterial diseases. A high rate of

▶ **TABLE 8-13.** POTENTIAL INDICATIONS
THROUGH TRANSCRANIAL DOPPLER
ULTRASONOGRAPHY

Detect atherosclerotic stenosis of a major intracranial artery
Detect acute occlusion of a major intracranial artery
Monitor for recanalization following thrombolytic treatment
Monitor for reocclusion following thrombolytic treatment
Monitor for progression of intracranial vascular disease
   Moyamoya syndrome—moyamoya disease
   Sickle cell disease
Monitor for changes in velocity secondary to vasospasm
   Subarachnoid hemorrhage
Detect a medium-to-large arteriovenous malformation
Monitor for changes in velocity during surgery
   Carotid surgery
   Cardiac surgery
Examine for changes of microembolization
   Stenotic disease of extracranial artery
   Cardiac source of emboli

recurrent microembolization correlates with a heightened risk of major stroke.[266–269] Besides monitoring acutely ill patients, TCD is used to evaluate patients with conditions as diverse as sickle cell disease or a patent foramen ovale (PFO).[270–272] While early TCD detection of microemboli is correlated with the presence of a right-to-left shunt, it has not replaced echocardiography as the diagnostic study to screen for the presence of PFO.[273]

Subarachnoid Hemorrhage and Vasospasm

Sequential TCD studies can be performed in patients with recent aneurysmal subarachnoid hemorrhage[274] (see Table 8-13). Changes in flow velocity are associated with the development of vasospasm and increases in velocity precede the appearance of ischemic symptoms.[275–279] Detection of the changes might permit institution of therapies before the patient develops neurological signs.

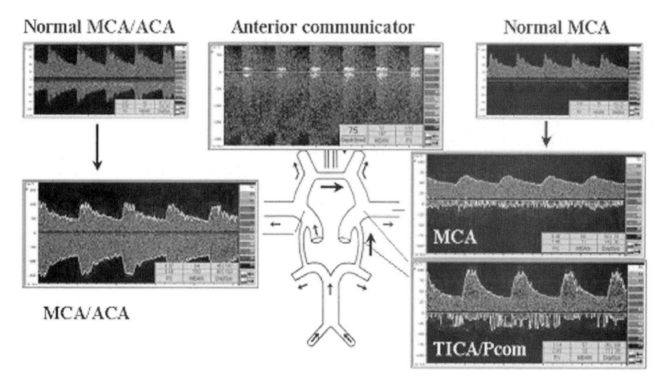

Figure 8-40. A transcranial Doppler ultrasonographic study performed in a patient with an acute right hemisphere infarction. Normal middle cerebral artery (MCA) and anterior cerebral artery (ACA) way forms are shown at the top (right and left). The examination shows a blunted signal in the right MCA (right). This finding is representative of a post-stenotic flow signal with delayed systolic flow acceleration. A signal with more vertical systolic upstroke is seen in the terminal segment of the ipsilateral internal carotid artery (TICA). The signal of TICA also could be originating from the posterior communicating artery (Pcom). Examination of the left MCA and ACA shows normal systolic flow acceleration. Velocities are higher in the ACA than in the MCA suggest flow diversion into this vessel. A stenotic signal below the baseline is labeled anterior communicator in the center waveform. This flow signal indicates the presence of at least partial anterior cross filling via the anterior communicating artery. The findings of delayed systolic flow acceleration of the MCA and two collateral channels at the level of the circle of Willis are indirect signs of hemodynamically significant obstruction or occlusion of the ICA. (*Courtesy of Andrei V. Alexandrov, M.D. University of Texas Health Sciences Center, Houston, TX.*)

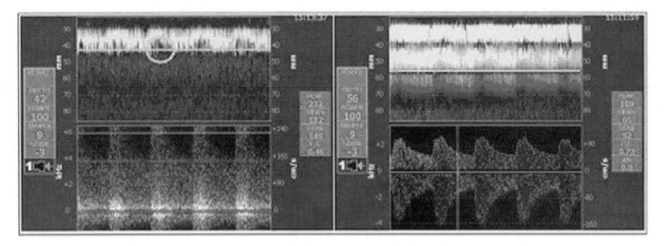

Figure 8-41. A power-motion transcranial Doppler ultrasonographic examination of a patient with an infarction of the right hemisphere shows the presence of a bruit (circle) at the depth of 42 mm. The spectral transcranial Doppler showed mean flow velocities of 182 cm/s (left). Spectral analysis of the signals of the bifurcation of the internal carotid artery shows that the anterior cerebral artery has velocities exceeding those in the middle cerebral artery (right). Velocities were 66 cm/s in the proximal MCA and 182 cm/s for the distal M-1 segment of the MCA. These findings are suggestive of severe intracranial stenosis. (*Courtesy of Andrei V. Alexandrov, M.D., University of Texas Health Sciences Center, Houston, TX.*)

Changes on TCD also can be used to monitor responses to treatment of vasospasm.[280] Mast et al.[281] found that TCD was highly sensitive in detecting medium-to-large arteriovenous malformations. They concluded that TCD could help differentiate vascular malformations from other causes of cerebral hemorrhage. Changes in the pulsatility index detected by TCD also are used to predict outcomes in patients with intracerebral hemorrhage because the findings point to changes in intracranial pressure.[282] Early detection of such changes might prompt early use of medical or surgical interventions to lower intracranial pressure. Unfortunately, the specificity of these changes is not established. The findings on TCD can be influenced by the patient's age and arterial blood pressure.[283–285]

As with other ultrasonographic studies, technical problems limit the utility of TCD.[286] Issues such as the angle of insonation or placement of the probe are important for technical failures and both false-negative and false-positive results can happen. TCD can be nondiagnostic among persons with relatively thick temporal bones. The rates of nondiagnostic TCD studies appear higher in women, African Americans, and older persons. The skill of the operator is important. The injection of contrast can improve the sensitivity of TCD but the usefulness of this approach is yet established.

► EVALUATION OF THE HEART

Because of the strong interaction between cardiovascular and cerebrovascular diseases, diagnostic studies evaluating the heart are a key component of the examination of patients with hemorrhagic or ischemic stroke.[287] The tests look for the cardiac complications of the stroke, serious comorbid heart diseases, or potential sources of the embolization to the brain. While electrocardiography is part of the evaluation of almost all patients with stroke, the other components of the cardiac evaluation should be selected on a case-by-case basis.

► ELECTROCARDIOGRAM

An electrocardiogram (ECG) should be obtained on an emergent basis.[3] The test is noninvasive, inexpensive, and rapidly performed. Besides being obtained in the acute care setting, the ECG also should be part of the assessment of patients with TIA or recent stroke. It is available in all emergency departments. It provides important information about the heart that can affect both acute care and long-term measures to prevent stroke. The 12-lead ECG detects changes consistent with an acute myocardial infarction, other structural heart diseases, cardiac conduction abnormalities, or cardiac arrhythmias[288–291] (Table 8-14).

Myocardial Infarction

The most important findings are those associated with acute myocardial infarction. Acute myocardial injury is a potential cause of early mortality and may be the source of emboli to the brain. An embolic stroke might be the

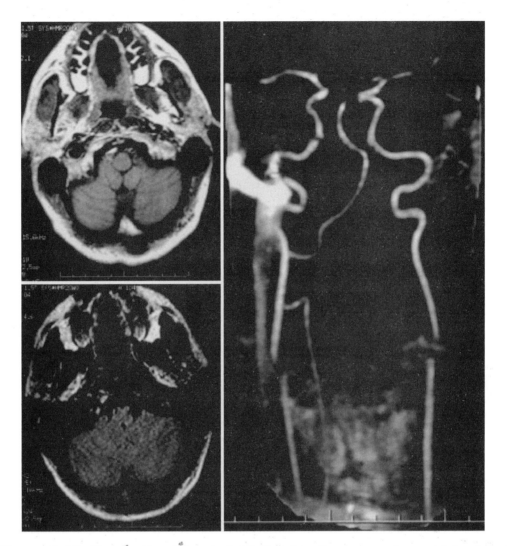

Figure 8-42. The results of transcranial Doppler ultrasonography and lateral and anteroposterior views of vertebral arteriography performed to evaluate a 27-year-old man with a suspected vertebral artery dissection. The transcranial Doppler study shows a high resistance signal at the level of the vertebral confluence with a reversed direction of the systolic component and the absence of diastolic flow in the terminal portion of the left vertebral artery. The findings are consistent with an acute obstruction of the left vertebral artery and not consistent with congenital hypoplasia. (*Courtesy of Andrei V. Alexandrov, M.D., University of Texas Health Sciences Center, Houston, TX.*)

▶ **TABLE 8-14.** ELECTROCARDIOGRAPHIC CHANGES IN THAT MAY OCCUR WITH ISCHEMIC OR HEMORRHAGIC STROKE

Pathological Q waves	Depression of ST segment
Negative T waves	Prolonged QT interval
U waves	Sinus bradycardia
Premature ventricular contractions	Bigeminy or trigeminy
Periods of asystole	Atrial fibrillation
Sinoatrial block	Atrioventricular block
Ventricular tachycardia	Torsades de pointes
Ventricular fibrillation	

initial presentation of a myocardial infarction. ECG evidence of cardiac ischemia portends a high long-term risk of myocardial events and affects plans for long-term care. Myocardial ischemia can be a complication of stroke, in particular subarachnoid hemorrhage. Marked increases in catecholamines secondary to intracranial bleeding can result in coronary artery vasospasm or direct toxicity to the myocardium. Thus, ECG changes of acute myocardial ischemia are detected frequently among patients with acute intracranial hemorrhage. ECG also detects other structural changes of the heart, such as left ventricular hypertrophy.

Cardiac Arrhythmias

Cardiac arrhythmias, such as atrial fibrillation, can be markers of heart disease that lead to embolization and they also can complicate the stroke.[292] The frequency of arrhythmias seems to be increased among elderly persons. In addition, ischemic strokes affecting the insular cortex, particularly on the right, seem to be correlated with an increased risk of serious cardiac arrhythmias. While sinus bradycardia and premature ventricular contractions are the most common disturbances, potentially life-threatening events including torsades de pointes or ventricular tachycardia can develop, especially among patients with intracranial hemorrhages.

▶ CARDIAC MONITORING

Monitoring of the cardiac rate and rhythm is an important component of early management of patients with recent stroke. Some of the early mortality from stroke may be secondary to cardiac arrhythmias, especially among persons with intracranial hemorrhage. Early detection of rhythm disturbances will foster rapid treatment with antiarrhythmic medications. Most of the serious cardiac arrhythmias occur within the first 48 h of stroke. The role of prolonged cardiac monitoring (Holter monitoring or King-of-Hearts monitoring) is restricted primarily to the assessment of patients with suspected syncope or presyncope as the cause of transient neurological symptoms.[293,294] The tests are performed to exclude an intermittent cardiac arrhythmia such an intermittent complete (third degree) heart block or sick sinus (bradycardia-tachycardia) syndrome. Because these cardiac arrhythmias are a potential cause of global ischemia in elderly persons, monitoring remains an important component of evaluation of patients with atypical symptoms of TIA.[294,295]

▶ CHEST X-RAY

A chest x-ray generally is not a recommended component of the emergent evaluation of most patients with suspected stroke.[296] However, it can be used to screen for pulmonary complications of stroke including atelectasis, pneumonia, or pulmonary embolism. Chest x-ray also gives information about changes in the cardiac silhouette or the contour of the aorta. Valuable information about a possible dissection of the aorta can be obtained. It also can be used to detect pulmonary congestion if a patient has congestive heart failure secondary to structural heart disease. Patients with either hemorrhagic or ischemic stroke are at risk for these cardiac or pulmonary complications and repeated chest x-rays are performed.

▶ SCREENING FOR CONCOMITANT CORONARY ARTERY DISEASE

Because of the strong relationship between ischemic stroke and coronary artery disease evaluation for the presence of advanced atherosclerotic disease of the coronary arteries often is recommended.[297,298] The tests, which are not done when a patient is acutely ill neurologically, are especially important for persons with atherosclerosis. Already, evidence exists for a strong relationship between coronary artery disease and IMT or more advanced atherosclerotic lesions of the carotid artery.[299–301] Some patients hospitalized with a TIA or minor stroke could undergo graded exercise testing, radioisotope thallium cardiac scanning, or coronary arteriography as part of their evaluation.[302–305] New tests include screening for coronary artery calcification. In general, the tests for occult coronary artery disease are underutilized and more patients with cerebrovascular disease should be screened for severe atherosclerotic disease of the heart. The results of these tests might influence plans for long-term management including aggressive medical management of the heart disease or local coronary artery interventions.

▶ TRANSTHORACIC AND TRANSESOPHAGEAL ECHOCARDIOGRAPHY

Transthoracic echocardiography (TTE) and transesophageal echocardiography (TEE) are the most commonly performed cardiac imaging studies to look for sources of emboli[287,306] (Figs. 8-43–8-45; Tables 8-15 and Table 8-16).

These tests can be done with contrast enhancement (microbubbles) to screen for an intracardiac right-to-left shunt. While TTE is noninvasive, it has limitations. It does not effectively image the heart among obese persons or those with large chests. It also does not visualize

▶ **TABLE 8-15.** ECHOCARDIOGRAPHIC FINDINGS ASSOCIATED WITH CARDIOEMBOLIC STROKE

Left ventricular thrombus	Left atrial thrombus
Left atrial appendage thrombus	Left atrial enlargement
Akinetic segment	Ventricular aneurysm
Left atrial turbulence	Valvular vegetation/ thrombus
Valvular strands	Lambl's excrescence
Left atrial myxoma	Patent foramen ovale
Atrial septal aneurysm	Mitral valve prolapse
Mitral annulus calcification	Calcific aortic stenosis
Plaque of the aortic arch	Dissection of the aorta

▶ **TABLE 8-16.** CLINICAL VARIABLES FOR SELECTION OF TRANSTHORACIC OR TRANSESOPHAGEAL ECHOCARDIOGRAPHY

Transthoracic	Transesophageal
Suspect left atrial lesion	Suspect left ventricular
Atrial fibrillation	lesion
Prosthetic heart valve	Myocardial infarction
Possible right-to-left shunt	Anterior wall
Patent foramen ovale	Ventricular aneurysm
Atrial septal aneurysm	Dilated cardiomyopathy
Suspected endocarditis	Suspected atrial myxoma
Suspected atrial myxoma	
Suspected aortic	
atherosclerosis	
Stroke of undetermined cause	

the left atrium or left atrial appendage. TEE is a somewhat invasive procedure that requires conscious sedation. Cardiac, bleeding, or pulmonary adverse experiences can complicate the procedure. Patients with bleeding diatheses or esophageal disease should not have the test. In particular, esophageal strictures or varices contraindicate performance of a TEE. Still, the risk of TEE is low.[307] The decision to order these tests is made on a case-by-case basis. TTE and TEE should be done only if the results of the cardiac imaging would affect management. For example, the findings of echocardiography might prompt institution of anticoagulants for treatment of an asymptomatic patient with atrial fibrillation.

Transthoracic Echocardiography

TTE is effective in visualizing the left ventricular wall, the left ventricular cavity, and the mitral valve.[308,309] However, TTE does not clearly image the left atrium or the left atrial appendage. Thus, TTE can be used best to look for an intraventricular thrombus, a dilated cardiomyopathy, a ventricular aneurysm, or an akinetic segment.[310] TTE can be used to screen for the risk of stroke among asymptomatic patients with atrial fibrillation not associated with mitral stenosis[311] (see Table 8-16). Many left ventricular causes of embolic stroke are associated with a history of myocardial infarction and thus, the use of TTE often is restricted to those patients with a history of ischemic heart disease. The yield of TTE in detecting a cardiac source of embolization among older adults with out other cardiac findings is low.[312,313] In most cases, TEE is reserved for evaluation of young adults with cryptogenic stroke.[313,314]

Transesophageal Echocardiography

The yield of TEE is higher than TTE and it now is the most widely used test to examine the heart among patients with stroke.[315–318] The yield of TEE is relatively high; one or more potential cardiac sources for emboli can be found in 35–45 percent of patients.[319–321] The clinical applications for the test include evaluation of native valve disease, dysfunction of prosthetic valves, intracardiac masses, congenital heart disease, presence of intracardiac thrombi, aortic atherosclerosis, aortic dissection, or complications of endocarditis.[306,322] TEE can be used to diagnose coexisting coronary artery disease.[323] The test also can be an adjunct to cardiac endovascular or surgical procedures.[306] For example, TEE can help guide placement of a device to close a patent foramen ovale (PFO). The test assesses the left atrium, the interatrial septum, and the aorta. The test is superior to TTE in detecting cardiac abnormalities that are most prone to embolization including left atrial enlargement, intraatrial thrombi, or vegetations of the mitral and aortic valves. In particular, TEE examines the left atrial appendage, which is a leading site of origin for thromboembolism among persons with atrial fibrillation.[324] Echocardiographic detection of turbulence in the left atrium is associated with a high risk for embolism among patients with atrial fibrillation.[325,326] TEE also can be done to examine the integrity of a bioprosthetic or mechanical cardiac valves. Contrast-enhanced TEE is used to screen for an intracardiac right-to-left shunt, including a PFO.[327,328] The number of bubbles found within a limited number of cardiac contractions provides an estimate of the size of the PFO.[329,330] The diameter of the hole detected by TEE might be useful in ascertaining the risk of paradoxical embolization.[331] Contrast-enhanced TEE also can be used to detect a pulmonary arteriovenous malformation that can cause paradoxical embolism.[332]

TEE is also an effective test for detection of atherosclerotic disease of the ascending aorta or the arch of the aorta.[333–335] Plaques of the aorta are a potential source for embolization among older persons with stroke. The test can detect a spectrum of changes varying from a minor plaque to large mobile lesions with superimposed thrombi. Not surprisingly, the latter plaques are accompanied by the greatest risk for embolization. The presence of plaques in the aorta will affect cardiac surgery; the TEE results can guide the cardiac surgeon's operative techniques including the placement of aortic clamps.[336,337]

▶ OTHER CARDIAC IMAGING TESTS

Ultrafast CT imaging and MRI are alternatives to echocardiography. These tests visualize the left ventricle, left atrium, and aorta. These tests reliably detect intracardiac thrombi or severe atherosclerotic lesions or thrombi of the aorta.[335,338,339] Ohyama et al.[340] showed that MRI of the heart successfully detects thrombi in the left atrial appendage among patients with atrial fibrillation. These studies can demonstrate atherosclerotic ulcers, intramural hematomas, pseudoaneurysm formation, and aortic rupture. While neither study is used widely, they can be ordered if a patient cannot tolerate TEE.

▶ OTHER DIAGNOSTIC TESTS

Most patients with stroke need additional diagnostic tests to screen for medical complications, risk factors for atherosclerosis, or causes of stroke. These tests are ordered on a case-by-case basis for patients with either ischemic or hemorrhagic cerebrovascular disease.

▶ GENERAL SCREENING TESTS AND SCREENING FOR RISK FACTORS FOR ATHEROSCLEROSIS

General screening tests include a complete blood count, serum electrolytes, serum glucose concentration, prothrombin time, and activated partial thromboplastin time (aPTT). The results of these tests provide information about acute complications or potential causes of stroke. For example, hyponatremia is a relatively frequent complication of subarachnoid hemorrhage. The blood glucose level is an important predictor of outcomes following stroke, including subarachnoid hemorrhage. Patients with elevated glucose concentrations generally have poor outcomes. The tests' results also affect acute management of stroke; for example, administration of rt-PA might be aborted because of abnormal baseline coagulation studies. Additional tests, such as examination of the urine, often are needed during management.

Screening for risk factors for stroke also should be done. Besides being important in acute management, the serum glucose concentration is a screen for underlying diabetes mellitus. The hemoglobin A1C level also provides data about the level of control of hyperglycemia. Measurement of a lipid profile (total cholesterol, high density lipoprotein (HDL) cholesterol, low density lipoprotein (LDL) cholesterol and triglycerides) is performed. The timing of the tests is important. If the tests cannot be done within 24–48 h of the onset of stroke, the studies usually are delayed for several weeks because the stroke may cause spuriously low concentrations. Screening of serum levels of homocysteine also is done when evaluating young adults and children with stroke because elevated levels might be markers of accelerated atherosclerosis or a prothrombotic state.

Both hemorrhagic and ischemic stroke can be secondary to infectious or inflammatory disorders. Blood cultures are obtained if infectious endocarditis is a potential diagnosis. While epidemiological studies suggest a potential relationship between recent infection and thrombosis, checking titers for specific infectious usually is not done. General screening inflammatory tests include measurements of the erythrocyte sedimentation rate (ESR) and C-reactive protein (CRP). While an elevation of CRP or an ESR is nonspecific, elevated titers can denote an underlying inflammatory or infectious disease. The stroke, itself, might cause elevation of these tests. High-sensitivity CRP levels can be used to identify persons at high risk of ischemic events. Presumably the elevated levels are markers of instability in the atherosclerotic plaques. Screening for CRP level may become an important component of the future assessment of patients with stroke.

▶ OTHER TESTS LOOKING FOR THE CAUSE OF STROKE

Several tests can be ordered to screen for a cause of either ischemic or hemorrhagic stroke. In general, these tests are categorized as special tests of coagulation, genetic tests, tests for inflammation or infection, and specific tests aimed at uncommon causes of stroke such as drug abuse. Most of these tests involve blood samples. Other tests include screening of the urine for drugs, which might be indicated in young patients with hemorrhagic or ischemic stroke. In some challenging cases, brain or meningeal biopsy might be needed to determine the cause of stroke. The most common indication for biopsy is to establish a diagnosis of vasculitis.

Tests of Coagulation

A large number of tests of coagulation are available and the list of diagnostic studies continues to grow. Before ordering these tests, the physician needs to remember that the frequency of primary disorders of coagulation leading to stroke is relatively low. As a result, the yield from an expensive battery of coagulation tests is limited. Most patients do not need all these tests. Thus, these tests are ordered on a case-by-case basis. In general, the tests are ordered if a patient has an atypical stroke or if the patient has other evidence of thrombosis or bleeding. Among patients with ischemic stroke, a personal or a family history of pulmonary embolism, deep vein thrombosis, or spontaneous abortion in female relatives could point toward an inherited prothrombotic disease. In this situation, an assessment for a coagulopathy would be warranted. The results could help both the patient and his/her relatives. If a child is of either African or Middle Eastern descent, a screening for sickle cell disease, most commonly a hemoglobin electrophoresis is indicated. Medications are the most common disorders of bleeding that lead to intracranial hemorrhage and abnormalities of the initial tests of coagulation (prothrombin time, aPTT, platelet count) usually will detect these conditions. Other inherited or acquired disorders of coagulation are uncommon causes of hemorrhagic stroke. In general, affected patients usually have a strong personal or family history of bleeding. In addition, most patients with coagulopathies will have other evidence of bleeding found on physical examination.

The timing of some of the special coagulation tests is important. The results of some tests (for example, protein C or S levels) are affected by the stroke and the levels of the tests might be spuriously low. These tests can be delayed for a few weeks following the stroke. However, tests for a hemoglobinopathy or a genetic disorder of coagulation usually can be obtained immediately. Prolongation of the aPTT can be found with a lupus anticoagulant and subsequent tests (mixing tests, Russel viper venom time) can be used to confirm the presence of the disorder. Disseminated intravascular coagulation can lead to either hemorrhagic or ischemic stroke and this disorder can be screened by measurements of the concentrations of fibrinogen, fibrin-split products, or D-dimer.

Antiphospholipid (anticardiolipin) antibodies are important screening tools when evaluating a patient with an atypical cerebral infarction, including those with the antiphospholipid antibody syndrome or Sneddon syndrome because an autoimmune endocarditis (Libman-Sacks endocarditis) can be the source of emboli. These antibodies should be measured if a patient has vegetations, which appear not to be of infectious origin, detected on a mitral or aortic valve. The test also should be done when the patient has other evidence of arterial or venous thrombosis. Other tests for an inflammatory disease include rheumatoid factor, antinuclear antibody (ANA), antineuronal cytoplasmic antibody (ANCA), complement, and serum protein electrophoresis. The tests usually are done when the patient's findings are compatible with a multisystem vasculitis or an encephalopathy. Serological studies for syphilis also can be done. This test can be used to screen for the infectious disease and at times, the test will be positive secondary to an autoimmune disease.

Genetic Tests

With the advances in genetic diagnosis, the number of inherited cerebrovascular disorders likely will grow. Besides the inherited disorders of coagulation, genetic causes of stroke, such as cerebral autosomal dominant arteriopathy and subcortical ischemic leukoencephalopathy (CADASIL), are being recognized increasingly. Inherited causes of hemorrhagic vascular disease include familial aneurysms and vascular malformations for example, genetic tests can be done to screen for an inherited protein disorder in a family with intracranial aneurysms. In addition, inherited disorders of lipid metabolism might be the cause of accelerated atherosclerosis. Screening a family with premature atherosclerosis that is symptomatic (myocardial infarction, peripheral vascular disease, or stroke before the age of 60) for a hereditary disorder of lipids is reasonable. Most patients with stroke probably will not need genetic testing. The tests should be ordered if a patient's clinical presentation or family history suggests an inherited disorder. Then, the tests should be restricted to screening for those inherited disorders with phenotypes that correspond to the patient's clinical findings.

REFERENCES

1. Adams HP, Jr. Investigation of the patient with ischemic stroke. *Cerebrovasc Dis* 1991;1:50–54.
2. Donnan GA. Investigation of patients with stroke and transient ischaemic attacks. *Lancet* 1992;339:473–477.
3. Adams HP, Adams RJ, Brott T, et al. Guidelines for the early management of patients with ischemic stroke. A scientific statement from the stroke council of the American Stroke Association. *Stroke* 2003;34:1056–1083.
4. Broderick JP, Adams HP, Jr., Barsan W, et al. Guidelines for the management of spontaneous intracerebral hemorrhage: a statement for healthcare professionals from a special writing group of the Stroke Council, American Heart Association. *Stroke* 1999;30:905–915.
5. Mayberg MR, Batjer HH, Dacey R, et al. Guidelines for the management of aneurysmal subarachnoid hemorrhage. A statement for healthcare professionals from a special writing group of the Stroke Council, American Heart Association. *Stroke* 1994;25:2315–2328.
6. Brainin M, Olsen TS, Chamorro A, et al. Organization of stroke care: education, referral, emergency management and imaging, stroke units and rehabilitation. *Cerebrovasc Dis* 2004;17(suppl 2):1–14.
7. Kidwell C, Villablanca P, Saver JL. Advances in neuroimaging of acute stroke. *Curr Opin Cardiol* 2000;2:126–135.
8. Besson G, Robert C, Hommel M, Perret J. Is it clinically possible to distinguish nonhemorrhagic infarct from hemorrhagic stroke? *Stroke* 1995;26:1205–1209.
9. Hacke W, Warach S. Diffusion-weighted MRI as an evolving standard of care in acute stroke. *Neurology* 2000;54:1548–1549.
10. Zivin JA, Holloway RG. Weighing the evidence on DWI. Caveat emptor. *Neurology* 2000;54:1552.
11. Powers WJ. Testing a test: a report card for DWI in acute stroke. *Neurology* 2000;54:1549–1551.
12. Marik PE, Rakusin A, Sandhu SS. The impact of the accessibility of cranial CT scans on patient evaluation and management decisions. *J Intern Med* 1997;241:237–243.
13. Jacobs L, Kinkel WR, Heffner RR, Jr. Autopsy correlations of computerized tomography: experience with 6,000 CT scans. *Neurology* 1976;26:1111–1118.
14. Schriger DL, Kalafut M, Starkman S, Krueger M, Saver JL. Cranial computed tomography interpretation in acute

stroke: physician accuracy in determining eligibility for thrombolytic therapy. *JAMA* 1998;279:1293–1297.

15. Kalafut MA, Schriger DL, Saver JL, Starkman S. Detection of early CT signs of >1/3 middle cerebral artery infarctions: interrater reliability and sensitivity of CT interpretation by physicians involved in acute stroke care. *Stroke* 2000;31:1667–1671.

16. Pantano P, Caramia F, Bozzao L, Dieler C, von Kummer R. Delayed increase in infarct volume after cerebral ischemia. *Stroke* 1999;30:502–507.

17. Tomura N, Inugami A, Kanno I, et al. Differentiation between cerebral embolism and thrombosis on sequential CT scans. *J Comput Assist Tomogr* 1990;14:26–31.

18. Ruff RL, Dougherty JH, Jr. Evaluation of acute cerebral ischemia for anticoagulant therapy: computed tomography or lumbar puncture. *Neurology* 1981;31:736–740.

19. Adams HP, Jr., Kassell NF, Torner JC. CT and clinical correlations in recent aneurysmal subarachnoid hemorrhage: a preliminary report of the Cooperative Aneurysm Study. *Neurology* 1983;33:981–988.

20. van der Schaaf I, Wermer MJ, van der Graaf Y, et al. CT after subarachnoid hemorrhage: relation of cerebral perfusion to delayed cerebral ischemia. *Neurology,* 2006;66:1533–1538.

21. Morgenstern LB, Luna-Gonzales H, Huber JCJ, et al. Worst headache and subarachnoid hemorrhage: prospective, modern computed tomography and spinal fluid analysis. *Ann Emerg Med* 1998;32:297–304.

22. Tuhrim S, Horowitz D, Sacher M, Godbold J. Volume of ventricular blood is an important determinant of outcome in supratentorial intracerebral hemorrhage. *Crit Care Med* 1999;27:617–621.

23. Broderick JP, Brott TG, Tomsick T, Barsan W, Spilker J. Ultra-early evaluation of intracerebral hemorrhage. *J Neurosurg* 1990;72:195–199.

24. Kim JS, Lee JH, Lees K. Small primary intracerebral hemorrhage: clinical presentation in 28 cases. *Stroke* 1994;25:1500–1506.

25. Miller JH, Wardlaw JM, Lammie GA. Intracerebral haemorrhage and cerebral amyloid angiopathy: CT features with pathological correlation. *Clin Radiol* 1999;54:422–429.

26. Yuh WTC, Simonsen TM, Wang AM. Venous sinus occlusive disease: MR findings. *AJNR Am J Neuroradio* 1994;15:309–316.

27. Weisberg LA. Subcortical lobar intracerebral haemorrhage: clinical-computed tomographic correlations. *J Neurol Neurosurg Psychiatry* 1985;48:1078–1084.

28. Flemming K, Wijdicks E, StLouis E, Li H. Predicting deterioration in patients with lobar haemorrhages. *J Neurol Neurosurg Psychiatry* 1999;66:600–605.

29. Wijdicks EF, St Louis E. Clinical profiles predictive of outcome in pontine hemorrhage. *Neurology* 1997;49:1342–1346.

30. Wijdicks EF, St Louis EK, Atkinson JD, Li H. Clinician's biases toward surgery in cerebellar hematomas: an analysis of decision-making in 94 patients. *Cerebrovasc Dis* 2000;10:93–96.

31. van Gijn J, Van Dongen KJ. The time course of aneurysmal subarachnoid haemorrhage on computed tomography. *Neuroradiology* 1982;23:153–156.

32. Avrahami E, Katz R, Rabin A, Friendman V. CT diagnosis of non-traumatic subarachnoid haemorrhage in patients with brain edema. *Eur J Radiol* 1998;28:222–225.

33. van der Jagt M, Hasan D, Bijvoet HW, et al. Validity of prediction of the site of ruptured intracranial aneurysms with CT. *Neurology* 1999;52:34–39.

34. Hino A, Fujimoto M, Iwamoto Y, Yamaki T, Katsumori T. False localization of rupture site in patients with multiple cerebral aneurysms and subarachnoid hemorrhage. *Neurosurgery* 2000;46:825–830.

35. Karttunen AI, Jartti PH, Ukkola VA, Sajanti J, Haapea M. Value of the quality and distribution of subarachnoid haemorrhage on CT in the localization of a ruptured cerebral aneurysm. *Acta Neurochir (Wien)* 2003;145:655–661.

36. Adams HP, Jr., Kassell NF, Torner JC. Usefulness of computed tomography in predicting outcome after aneurysmal subarachnoid hemorrhage. *Neurology* 1985;35:1263–1267.

37. Black PM. Hydrocephalus and vasospasm after subarachnoid hemorrhage from ruptured intracranial aneurysms. *Neurosurgery* 1986;18:12–16.

38. Dennis M, Bamford J, Sandercock P, Molyneux A, Warlow C. Computed tomography in patients with transient ischaemic attacks: when is a transient ischaemic attack not a transient ischaemic attack but a stroke? *J Neurol* 1990;237:257–261.

39. Horowitz SH, Zito JL, Donnarumma R, Patel M, Alvir J. Computed tomographic-angiographic findings within the first five hours of cerebral infarction. *Stroke* 1991;22:1245–1253.

40. Grond M, von Kummer R, Sobesky J, Schmulling S, Heiss WD. Early computed-tomography abnormalities in acute stroke. *Lancet* 1997;350:1595–1596.

41. Moulin T, Cattin F, Crepin-Leblond T, et al. Early CT signs in acute middle cerebral artery infarction: predictive value for subsequent infarct locations and outcome. *Neurology* 1996;47:366–375.

42. von Kummer R, Allen KL, Holle R, et al. Acute stroke: usefulness of early CT findings before thrombolytic therapy. *Radiology* 1997;205:327–333.

43. von Kummer R, Meyding-Lamade U, Forsting M, et al. Sensitivity and prognostic value of early CT in occlusion of the middle cerebral artery trunk. *AJNR Am J Neuroradiol* 1994;15:9–15.

44. von Kummer R, Bozzao L, Zeumer H, Manelfe C. *Early CT Diagnosis of Hemispheric Brain Infarction.* Heidelberg: Springer Verlag, 1995.

45. von Kummer R, Nolte PN, Schnittger H, Thron A, Ringelstein EB. Detectability of cerebral hemisphere ischaemic infarcts by CT within 6 h of stroke. *Neuroradiology* 1996;38:31–33.

46. Patel SC, Levine SR, Tilley BC, et al. Lack of clinical significance of early ischemic changes on computed tomography in acute stroke. *JAMA* 2001;286:2830–2838.

47. Davis PH, Clarke WR, Bendixen BH, Adams HP, Jr., Woolson RF, Culebras A. Silent cerebral infarction in patients enrolled in the TOAST Study. *Neurology* 1996;46:942–948.

48. Grotta JC, Chiu D, Lu M, et al. Agreement and variability in the interpretation of early CT changes in stroke

patients qualifying for intravenous rtPA therapy. *Stroke* 1999;30:1528–1533.

49. Wardlaw JM, Dorman PJ, Lewis SC, Sandercock PA. Can stroke physicians and neuroradiologists identify signs of early cerebral infarction on CT? *J Neurol Neurosurg Psychiatry* 1999;67:651–653.

50. Damasio H. A computed tomographic guide to the identification of cerebral vascular territories. *Arch Neurol* 1983;40:138–142.

51. Greenberg JO, Smolen A, Cosio L. Computerized tomography in infarctions of the vertebral-basilar system. *Comput Radiol* 1982;6:149–153.

52. Tatu L, Moulin T, Bogousslavsky J, Duvernoy H. Arterial territories of the human brain: cerebral hemispheres. *Neurology* 1998;50:1699–1708.

53. Tatu L, Moulin T, Bogousslavsky J, Duvernoy H. Arterial territories of human brain: brainstem and cerebellum. *Neurology* 1996;47:1125–1135.

54. Kittner SJ, Sharkness CM, Sloan MA, et al. Features on initial computed tomography scan of infarcts with a cardiac source of embolism in the NINDS Stroke Data Bank. *Stroke* 1992;23:1748–1751.

55. Saito I, Segawa H, Shiokawa Y, Taniguchi M, Tsutsumi K. Middle cerebral artery occlusion: correlation of computed tomography and angiography with clinical outcome. *Stroke* 1987;18:863–868.

56. Hennerici M, Daffertshofer M, Jakobs L. Failure to identify cerebral infarct mechanisms from topography of vascular territory lesions. *AJNR Am J Neuroradiol* 1998; 1067–1074.

57. Pexman JH, Barber PA, Hill MD, et al. Use of the Alberta Stroke Program Early CT Score (ASPECTS) for assessing CT scans in patients with acute stroke. *AJNR Am J Neuroradiol* 2001;22:1534–1542.

58. Barber PA, Demchuk AM, Zhang J, et al. Computed tomographic parameters predicting fatal outcome in large middle cerebral artery infarction. *Cerebrovasc Dis* 2003; 16:230–235.

59. Demchuk AM, Tanne D, Hill MD, et al. Predictors of good outcome after intravenous tPA for acute ischemic stroke. *Neurology* 2001;57:474–480.

60. Tomsick T, Brott T, Barsan W, et al. Prognostic value of the hyperdense middle cerebral artery sign and stroke scale score before ultraearly thrombolytic therapy. *AJNR Am J Neuroradiol* 1996;17:79–85.

61. Manelfe C, Larrue V, von Kummer R, et al. Association of hyperdense middle cerebral artery sign with clinical outcome in patients treated with tissue plasminogen activator. *Stroke* 1999;30:769–772.

62. Wardlaw JM, Dennis MS, Lindley RI, Warlow CP, Sandercock PAG, Sellar R. Does early reperfusion of a cerebral infarct influence cerebral infarct swelling in the acute stage or the final clinical outcome? *Cerebrovasc Dis* 1993;3:86–93.

63. Wardlaw JM, Sellar R. A simple practical classification of cerebral infarcts on CT and its interobserver reliability. *AJNR Am J Neuroradiol* 1994;15:1933–1939.

64. Klotz E, Konig M. Perfusion measurements of the brain: using dynamic CT for the quantitative assessment of cerebral ischemia in acute stroke. *Eur J Radiol* 1999;30:170–184.

65. Schramm P, Schellinger P, Feibach JB, et al. Comparison of CT and CT angiography source images with diffusion-weighted imaging in patients with acute stroke within 6 hours after onset. *Stroke* 2002;33:2426–2432.

66. Wintermark M, Reichhart M, Cuisenaire O, et al. Comparison of admission perfusion computed tomography and qualitative diffusion- and perfusion-weighted magnetic resonance imaging in acute stroke patients. *Stroke* 2002;33:2025–2031.

67. Wintermark M, Flanders AE, Velthuis B, et al. Perfusion CT assessment of infarct core and penumbra: receiver operating characteristic curve analysis in 130 patients suspected of acute hemispheric stroke. *Stroke,* 2006;37:979–985.

68. Kaufmann AM, Firlik AD, Fukui MB, Wechsler LR, Jungries CA, Yonas H. Ischemic care and penumbra in human stroke. *Stroke* 1999;30:93–99.

69. von Kummer R, Patel S. Neuroimaging in acute stroke. *J Stroke Cerebrovasc Dis* 1999;8:127–138.

70. Damasio H, Frank R. Three-dimensional in vivo mapping of brain lesions in humans. *Arch Neurol* 1992;49:137–143.

71. Shuaib A, Lee D, Pelz D, Fox A, Hachinski VC. The impact of magnetic resonance imaging on the management of acute ischemic stroke. *Neurology* 1992;42:816–818.

72. Davis SM, Tress BM, Dowling R, Donnan GA, Kiers L, Rossiter SC. Magnetic resonance imaging in posterior circulation infarction: impact on diagnosis and management. *Aust N Z J Med* 1989;19:219–225.

73. Simmons Z, Biller J, Adams HP, Jr., Dunn V, Jacoby CG. Cerebellar infarction: comparison of computed tomography and magnetic resonance imaging. *Ann Neurol* 1986; 19:291–293.

74. Mohr JP, Biller J, Hilal SK, et al. Magnetic resonance versus computed tomographic imaging in acute stroke. *Stroke* 1995;26:807–812.

75. Bryan RN, Levy LM, Whitlow WD, Killian JM, Preziosi TJ, Rosario JA. Diagnosis of acute cerebral infarction: comparison of CT and MR imaging. *AJNR Am J Neuroradiol* 1991;12:611–620.

76. Warach S, Chien D, Li W, Ronthal M, Edelman RR. Fast magnetic resonance diffusion-weighted imaging of acute human stroke. *Neurology* 1992;42:1717–1723.

77. Warach S. Stroke neuroimaging. *Stroke* 2003;34:345–347.

78. Tong DC, Yenari MA, Albers GW, O'Brien M, Marks MP, Moseley ME. Correlation of perfusion- and diffusion-weighted MRI with NIHSS score in acute (<6.5 hour) ischemic stroke. *Neurology* 1998;50:864–870.

79. Tong DC, Adami A, Marks MP, Moseley ME. Relationship between diffusion and perfusion weighted MRI findings and hemorrhagic transformation following acute ischemic stroke: preliminary observations. *Stroke* 2000;31:276.

80. Saver JL, Johnson KC, Homer D, et al. Infarct volume as a surrogate or auxillary outcome measure in ischemic stroke clinical trials. *Stroke* 1999;30:298.

81. Lovblad KO, Laubach HJ, Baird AE, et al. Clinical experience with diffusion-weighted MR in patients with acute stroke. *AJNR Am J Neuroradiol* 1998;19:1061–1066.

82. Lovblad KO. Diffusion-weighted MRI: back to the future. *Stroke* 2002;33:2197–2205.

83. Gonzalez RG, Schaefer PW, Buonanno FS, et al. Diffusion-weighted MR imaging: diagnostic accuracy in patients

imaged within 6 hours of stroke symptom onset. *Radiology* 1999;210:155–162.

84. Baird AE, Benfield A, Schlaug G, et al. Enlargement of human cerebral ischemic lesion volumes measured by diffusion-weighted magnetic resonance imaging. *Ann Neurol* 1997;41:581–589.

85. Kidwell CS, Alger JR, Gobin YP, Sayre J, Duckwiler GR, Vinuela F. MR signatures of infarction vs. salvageable penumbra in acute human stroke: a preliminary model. *Stroke* 2000;31:285.

86. Liebeskind DS, Kidwell CS, UCLA Thrombolysis Investigators. Advanced MR imaging of acute stroke: the University of California at Los Angeles endovascular therapy experience. *Neuroimaging Clin N Amer,* 2005;15:455–466.

87. Kidwell CS, Alger JR, Saver JL. Beyond mismatch. Evolving paradigms in imaging the ischemic penumbra with multimodal magnetic resonance imaging. *Stroke* 2003;34: 2729–2735.

88. Mueller DP, Yuh WT, Fisher DJ, Chandran KB, Crain MR, Kim YH. Arterial enhancement in acute cerebral ischemia: clinical and angiographic correlation. *AJNR Am J Neuroradiol* 1993;14:661–668.

89. Cloft HJ, Murphy KJ, Prince MR, Brunberg JA. 3D gadolinium-enhanced MR angiography of the carotid arteries. *Magn Reson Imaging* 1996;14:593–600.

90. Rother J, Guckel F, Neff W, Schwartz A, Hennerici M. Assessment of regional cerebral blood volume in acute human stroke by use of single-slice dynamic susceptibility contrast-enhanced magnetic resonance imaging. *Stroke* 1996;27:1088–1093.

91. El-Koussy M, Guzman R, Bassetti C, et al. CT and MRI in acute hemorrhagic stroke. *Cerebrovasc Dis* 2000;10: 480–482.

92. Linfante I, Llinas R, Caplan L, Warach S. MRI features of intracerebral hemorrhage within 2 hours from symptom onset. *Stroke* 1999;30:2263–2267.

93. Schellinger P, Jansen O, Fiebach J, Hacke W, Sartor KA. A standardized MRI stroke protocol: comparison with CT in hyperacute intracerebral hemorrhage. *Stroke* 1999;30: 1974–1975.

94. Schellinger PD, Fiebach JB, Hoffmann K, et al. Stroke MRI in intracerebral hemorrhage. Is there a perihemorrhagic penumbra? *Stroke* 2003;34:1674–1680.

95. Ebisu T, Tanaka C, Umeda M, et al. Hemorrhagic and nonhemorrhagic stroke: diagnosis with diffusion-weighted and T2-weighted echo-planar MR imaging. *Radiology* 1997;203:823–828.

96. Noguchi K, Ogawa T, Inugami A, et al. Acute subarachnoid hemorrhage: MR imaging with fluid-attenuated inversion recovery pulse sequences. *Radiology* 1995;196: 773–777.

97. Noguchi K, Seto H, Kamisaki Y, Tomizawa G, Toyoshima S, Watanabe N. Comparison of fluid-attenuated inversion-recovery MR imaging with CT in a simulated model of acute subarachnoid hemorrhage. *AJNR Am J Neuroradiol* 2000;21:923–927.

98. Renowden SA, Molyneux AJ, Anslow P. The value of MRI in angiogram-negative intracranial haemorrhage. *Neuroradiology* 1994;36:422–425.

99. Mitchell P, Wilkinson ID, Hoggard N, et al. Detection of subarachnoid haemorrhage with magnetic resonance imaging. *J Neurol Neurosurg Psychiatry* 2001;70:205–211.

100. Wiesmann M, Mayer TE, Yousry I, Medele R, Hamann GF, Brückmann H. Detection of hyperacute subarachnoid hemorrhage of the brain by using magnetic resonance imaging. *J Neurosurg* 2002;96:684–689.

101. Roob G, Fazekas F. Magnetic resonance imaging of cerebral microbleeds. *Curr Opin Neurol* 2000;13:69–73.

102. Roob G, Schmidt R, Kapeller P, Lechner A, Hartung HP, Fazekas F. MRI evidence of past cerebral microbleeds in a healthy elderly population. *Neurology* 1999;52:991–994.

103. Offenbacher H, Fazekas F, Schmidt R. MR of cerebral abnormalities concomitant with primary intracerebral hematomas. *AJNR Am J Neuroradio* 1996;17:573–578.

104. Lutsep HL, Albers GW, DeCrespigny A, Kamat GN, Marks MP, Moseley ME. Clinical utility of diffusion-weighted magnetic resonance imaging in the assessment of ischemic stroke. *Ann Neurol* 1997;41:574–580.

105. Barber PA, Darby DG, Desmond PM, et al. Identification of major ischemic change. Diffusion-weighted imaging versus computed tomography. *Stroke* 1999;30:2059–2065.

106. Lee YZ, Lee J-M, Vo K, Hsu CY, in W. Rapid perfusion abnormality estimation in acute stroke with temporal correlation analysis. *Stroke* 2003;34:1686–1692.

107. Staaf G, Geijer B, Lindgren A, Norrving B. Diffusion-weighted MRI findings in patients with capsular warning syndrome. *Cerebrovasc Dis* 2004;17:1–8.

108. Mullins ME, Schaefer PW, Sorensen AG, et al. CT and conventional diffusion-weighted MR imaging in acute stroke: study in 691 patients at presentation to the emergency department. *Radiology* 2002;224:353–360.

109. Fiebach J, Schellinger P, Jansen O, et al. CT and diffusion-weighted MR imaging in randomized order: diffusion-weighted imaging results in higher accuracy and lower interrater variability in the diagnosis of hyperacute ischemic stroke. *Stroke* 2002;33:2206–2210.

110. Fiebach JB, Schellinger PD. Comparison of CT with diffusion-weighted MRI in patients with hyperacute stroke. *Neuroradiology* 2002;44:448.

111. Albers GW, Lansberg MG, Norbash AM, et al. Yield of diffusion-weighted MRI for detection of potentially relevant findings in stroke patients. *Neurology* 2000;54:1562–1567.

112. Parsons MW, Yang Q, Barber PA, et al. Perfusion magnetic resonance imaging maps in hyperacute stroke: relative cerebral blood flow most accurately identifies tissue destined to infarct. *Stroke* 2001;32:1581–1587.

113. Staroselskaya IA, Chaves C, Silver B, et al. Relationship between magnetic resonance arterial patency and perfusion-diffusion mismatch in acute ischemic stroke and its potential clinical use. *Arch Neurol* 2001;58:1069–1074.

114. Kidwell CS, Saver JL, Mattiello J, et al. Thrombolytic reversal of acute human cerebral ischemic injury shown by diffusion/perfusion magnetic resonance imaging. *Ann Neurol* 2000;47:621–469.

115. Longstreth WT, Jr., Bernick C, Manolio TA, Bryan N, Jungreis CA, Price TR. Lacunar infarcts defined by magnetic resonance imaging of 3660 eldery people: the cardiovascular health study. *Arch Neurol* 1998;55: 1217–1225.

116. Price TR, Manolio TA, Kronmal RA, et al. Silent brain infarction on magnetic resonance imaging and neurological abnormalities in community-dwelling older adults. The Cardiovascular Health Study. CHS Collaborative Research Group. *Stroke* 1997;28:1158–1164.

117. Yuh WT, Crain MR, Loes DJ, Greene GM, Ryals TJ, Sato Y. MR imaging of cerebral ischemia: findings in the first 24 hours. *AJNR Am J Neuroradiol* 1991;12:621–629.

118. Mead GE, Wardlaw JM. Detection of intraluminal thrombus in acute stroke by proton density MR imaging. *Cerebrovasc Dis* 1998;8:133–134.

119. Knepper L, Biller J, Adams HP, Jr., Yuh W, Ryals T, Godersky J. MR imaging of basilar artery occlusion. *J Comput Assist Tomogr* 1990;14:32–35.

120. Kitanaka C, Tanaka J, Kuwahara M, Teraoka A. Magnetic resonance imaging study of intracranial vertebrobasilar artery dissections. *Stroke* 1994;25:571–575.

121. Mullges W, Ringelstein EB, Leibold M. Non-invasive diagnosis of internal carotid artery dissections. *J Neurol Neurosurg Psychiatry* 1992;55:98–104.

122. Sue DE, Brant-Zawadzki MN, Chance J. Dissection of cranial arteries in the neck: correlation of MRI and arteriography. *Neuroradiology* 1992;34:273–278.

123. Levy C, Laissy JP, Raveau V, et al. Carotid and vertebral artery dissections: three-dimensional time-of-flight MR angiography and MR imaging versus conventional angiography. *Radiology* 1994;190:97–103.

124. Salbeck R, Busse O, Reinbold WD. MRI findings in megadolicho-basilar artery. *Cerebrovasc Dis* 1993;3:309–312.

125. Thambisetty M, Biousse V, Newman NJ. Hypertensive brainstem encephalopathy: clinical and radiographic features. *J Neurol Sci* 2003;208:93–99.

126. Kinoshita T, Moritani T, Shrier DA, et al. Diffusion-weighted MR imaging of posterior reversible leukoencephalopathy syndrome: a pictorial essay. *Clin Imaging* 2003;27:307–315.

127. Naylor AR, Evans J, Thompson MM, et al. Seizures after carotid endarterectomy: hyperperfusion, dysautoregulation or hypertensive encephalopathy? *Eur J Vasc Endovasc Surg* 2003;26:39–44.

128. Parsons MW, Barber PA, Yang Q, et al. Combined 1H MR spectroscopy and diffusion-weighted MRI improves the prediction of stroke outcome. *Neurology* 2000;55:498–505.

129. Rudkin TM, Arnold DL. Proton magnetic resonance spectroscopy for the diagnosis and management of cerebral disorders. *Arch Neurol* 1999;56:919–926.

130. Heiss W-D. Best measure of ischemic penumbra: positron emission tomography. *Stroke* 2003;34:2534–2535.

131. Heiss WD, Podreka I. Role of PET and SPECT in the assessment of ischemic cerebrovascular disease. *Cerebrovasc Brain Metab Rev* 1993;5:235–263.

132. Baron JC. Mapping the ischaemic penumbra with PET: implications for acute stroke treatment. *Cerebrovasc Dis* 1999;9:193–201.

133. Latchaw RE, Yonas H, Hunter GJ, et al. Guidelines and recommendations for perfusion imaging in cerebral ischemia. A scientific statement for healthcare professionals by the Writing Group on Perfusion Imaging, from the Council on Cardiovascular Radiology of the American Heart Association. *Stroke* 2003;1084:1104.

134. Derdeyn CP, Powers WJ, Grubb RL, Jr. Hemodynamic effects of middle cerebral artery stenosis and occlusion. *AJNR Am J Neuroradiol* 1998;19:1463–1469.

135. Derdeyn CP, Grubb RL, Jr., Powers WJ. Cerebral hemodynamic impairment: methods of measurement and association with stroke risk. *Neurology* 1999;53:251–259.

136. Derdeyn CP, Videen TO, Grubb RL, Jr., Powers WJ. Comparison of PET oxygen extraction fraction methods for the prediction of stroke risk. *J Nucl Med* 2001;42:1195–1197.

137. Heiss W-D. Imaging the ischemic penumbra and treatment effects by PET. *Keio J Med* 2001;50:249–256.

138. Grubb RL, Jr. Extracranial-intracranial arterial bypass for treatment of occlusion of the internal carotid artery. *Curr Neurol Neurosci Rep* 2004;4:23–30.

139. Ueda T, Hatakeyama T, Kumon Y, Sakaki S, Uraoka T. Evaluation of risk of hemorrhagic transformation in local intra-arterial thrombolysis in acute ischemic stroke by initial SPECT. *Stroke* 1994;25:298–303.

140. Berrouschot J, Barthel H, von Kummer R, Knapp WH, Hesse S, Schneider. 99m technetium-ethyl-cysteinate-dimer single-photon emission CT can predict fatal ischemic brain edema. *Stroke* 1998;29:2556–2562.

141. Masdeu JC, Brass LM. SPECT imaging of stroke. *J Neuroimaging* 1995;5(suppl 1):S14–S22.

142. Laloux P, Richelle F, Jamart J, De Coster P, Laterre C. Comparative correlations of HMPAO SPECT indices, neurological score, and stroke subtypes with clinical outcome in acute carotid infarcts. *Stroke* 1995;26:816–821.

143. Hanson SK, Grotta JC, Rhoades H, et al. Value of single-photon emission-computed tomography in acute stroke therapeutic trials. *Stroke* 1993;24:1322–1329.

144. Kohno K, Oka Y, Kohno S, Ohta S, Kumon Y, Sakaki S. Cerebral blood flow measurement as an indicator for indirect revascularization procedure for adult patients with moyamoya diesase. *Neurosurgery* 1998;42:752–758.

145. Baird AE, Austin MC, McKay WJ, Donnan GA. Sensitivity and specificity of 99mTc-HMPAO SPECT cerebral perfusion measurements during the first 48 hours for the localization of cerebral infarction. *Stroke* 1997;28:976–980.

146. Brass LM, Walovitch RC, Joseph JL, et al. The role of single photon emission computed tomography brain imaging with 99mTc-bicisate in the localization and definition of mechanism of ischemic stroke. *J Cereb Blood Flow Metab* 1994;14(suppl 1):S91–S98.

147. Alexandrov AV, Masdeu JC, Devous MDS, Black SE, Grotta JC. Brain single-photon emission CT with HMPAO and safety of thrombolytic therapy in acute ischemic stroke. Proceedings of the meeting of the SPECT Safe Thrombolysis Study Collaborators and the members of the Brain Imaging Council of the Society of Nuclear Medicine. *Stroke* 1997;28:1830–1834.

148. Alexandrov AV, Ehrlich LE, Bladin CF, Black SE. Clinical significance of increased uptake of HMPAO on brain SPECT scans in acute stroke. *J Neuroimaging* 1996;6:150–155.

149. Karonen JO, Ostergaard L, Vainio P, et al. Diffusion and perfusion MR imaging in acute ischemic stroke: a

comparison to SPECT. *Comput Methods Programs Biomed* 2001;66:125–128.

150. Vermeulen M, van Gijn J. The diagnosis of subarachnoid hemorrhage. *J Neurol Neurosurg Psychiatry* 1990;53: 365–372.

151. van der Wee N, Rinkel GJE, Hasan D, van Gijn J. Detection of subarachnoid haemorrhage on early CT: is lumbar puncture still needed after negative scan? *J Neurol Neurosurg Psychiatry* 1995;58:357–359.

152. Vermeulen M, Hasan D, Blijenberg B, Hijdra A, van Gijn J. Xanthochromia after subarachnoid haemorrhage needs no revisitation. *J Neurol Neurosurg Psychiatry* 1989;52: 826–828.

153. Cruickshank AM. CSF spectrophotmetry in the diagnosis of subarachnoid haemorrhage. *J Clin Pathol* 2001;54: 827–830.

154. Beetham R, Fahie-Wilson MN, Park D. What is the role of CSF spectrophotometry in the diagnosis of subarachnoid haemorrhage? *Ann Clin Biochem* 1998;35:1–4.

155. Lampl Y, Paniri Y, Eshel Y, Sarova-Pinhas I. Cerebrospinal fluid lactate dehydrogenase levels in early stroke and transient ischemic attacks. *Stroke* 1990;21:854–857.

156. Bell RD, Khan M. Cerebrospinal fluid creatine kinase-BB activity. *Arch Neurol* 1999;56:1327–1328.

157. Quigg M, Shneker B, Domer P. Current practice in administration and clinical criteria of emergent EEG. *J Clin Neurophysiol* 2001;18:162–165.

158. Macdonell RA, Donnan GA, Bladin PF. A comparison of somatosensory evoked and motor evoked potentials in stroke. *Ann Neurol* 1989;25:68–73.

159. Aron KV, Cohen DE, Strobl FT. Effect of intraoperative intervention on neurological outcome based on electroencephalographic monitoring during cardiopulmonary bypass. *Ann Thorac Surg* 1989;48:476–483.

160. Illig KA, Burchfiel JL, Ouriel K, DeWeese JA, Shortell CK, Green RM. Value of preoperative EEG for carotid endarterectomy. *Cardiovasc Surg* 1998;6:490–495.

161. Minahan RE, Bhardwaj A, Williams MA. Critical care monitoring for cerebrovascular disease. *New Horiz* 1997;5: 406–421.

162. Rothwell PM, Gibson RJ, Villagra R, Sellar R, Warlow CP. The effect of angiographic technique and image quality on the reproducibility of measurement of carotid stenosis and assessment of plaque surface morphology. *Clin Radiol* 1998;53:439–443.

163. Hankey GJ, Warlow CP, Molyneux AJ. Complications of cerebral angiography for patients with mild carotid territory ischaemia being considered for carotid endarterectomy. *J Neurol Neurosurg Psychiatry* 1990;53:542–548.

164. Executive Committee for the Asymptomatic Carotid Atherosclerosis Study. Endarterectomy for asymptomatic carotid artery stenosis. *JAMA* 1995;273:1421–1428.

165. Haley EC, Jr. Encephalopathy following arteriography: a possible toxic effect of contrast agents. *Ann Neurol* 1984; 15:100–102.

166. Shuaib A, Hachinski VC. Migraine and the risks from angiography. *Arch Neurol* 1988;45:911–912.

167. Liberopoulos K, Kaponis A, Kokkinis K, et al. Comparative study of magnetic resonance angiography, digital subtraction angiography, duplex ultrasound examination with

surgical and histological findings of atherosclerotic carotid bifurcation disease. *Int Angiol* 1996;15:131–137.

168. Fox AJ. How to measure carotid stenosis. *Radiology* 1993;186:316–318.

169. Pelz DM, Fox AJ, Eliasziw M, Barnett HJM. Stenosis of the carotid bifurcation: subjective assessment compared with strict measurement guidelines. *Can Assoc Radiol J* 1993; 44:247–252.

170. Chang YJ, Golby AJ, Albers GW. Detection of carotid stenosis. From NASCET results to clinical practice. *Stroke* 1995;26:1325–1328.

171. Pelz DM, Buchan A, Fox AJ, Barnett HJM, Vinuela F. Intraluminal thrombus of the internal carotid arteries: angiographic demonstration of resolution with anticoagulant therapy alone. *Radiology* 1986;160:369–373.

172. Streifler JY, Eliasziw M, Fox AJ, et al. Angiographic detection of carotid plaque ulceration. Comparison with surgical observations in a multicenter study. North American Symptomatic Carotid Endarterectomy Trial. *Stroke* 1994; 25:1130–1132.

173. Buchan A, Gates P, Pelz D, Barnett HJM. Intraluminal thrombus in the cerebral circulation. Implications for surgical management. *Stroke* 1988;19:681–687.

174. Alhalabi M, Moore PM. Serial angiography in isolated angiitis of the central nervous system. *Neurology* 1994; 44:1221–1226.

175. Laborde G, Harders A, Klimek L, Hardenack M. Correlation between clinical, angiographic and transcranial Doppler sonographic findings in patients with moyamoya disease. *Neurol Res* 1993;15:87–92.

176. Toffol GJ, Biller J, Adams HP, Jr. The predicted value of arteriography in nontraumatic intracerebral hemorrhage. *Stroke* 1986;17:881–883.

177. Zhu XL, Chan MS, Poon WS. Spontaneous intracranial hemorrhage: which patients need diagnostic cerebral angiography? A prospective study of 206 cases and review of the literature. *Stroke* 1997;28:1406–1409.

178. Saitoh H, Hayakawa K, Nishimura K, et al. Rerupture of cerebral aneurysms during angiography. *AJNR Am J Neuroradiol* 1995;16:539–542.

179. Duong H, Melancon D, Tampieri D. The negative angiogram in subarachnoid hemorrhage. *Neuroradiology* 1996;38:15–19.

180. Griffiths PD, Beveridge CJ, Gholkar A. Angiography in non-traumatic brain haematoma. An analysis of 100 cases. *Acta Radiol* 1997;38:797–802.

181. Hino A, Fujimoto M, Yamaki T, Iwamoto Y, Katsumori T. Value of repeat angiography in patients with spontaneous subcortical hemorrhage. *Stroke* 1998;29: 2517–2521.

182. Verro P, Tanenbaum LN, Borden NM, Sen S, Eshkar N. CT angiography in acute ischemic stroke: preliminary results. *Stroke* 2002;33:276–278.

183. Wildermuth S, Knauth M, Brandt T, Winter R, Sartor K, Hacke W. Role of CT angiography in patient selection for thrombolytic therapy in acute hemispheric stroke. *Stroke* 1998;29:935–938.

184. Brandt T, Knauth M, Wildermuth S, et al. CT angiography and Doppler sonography for emergency assessment in acute basilar artery ischemia. *Stroke* 999;30:606–612.

185. Velthuis BK, van Leeuwen MS, Witkamp TD, Boomstra S, Ramos LM, Rinkel GJE. CT angiography: source images and postprocessing techniques in the detection of cerebral aneurysms. *Am J Roentgenol* 1997;169: 1411–1417.

186. Velthuis BK, Rinkel GJ, Ramos LM, et al. Subarachnoid hemorrhage: aneurysm detection and preoperative evaluation with CT angiography. *Radiology* 1998;208:423–430.

187. Ogawa T, Okudera T, Noguchi K. Cerebral aneurysms: evaluation with three-dimensional CT angiography. *AJNR Am J Neuroradio* 1996;17:447–454.

188. Hope KA, Wilson JL, Thomson FJ. Three-dimensional CT angiography in the detection and characterization of intracranial berry aneurysms. *AJNR Am J Neuroradio* 1996;17:439–445.

189. Velthuis BK, van Leeuwen MS, Witkamp TD, Ramos LMP, van der Sprenkel JWB, Rinkel GJE. Computerized tomography angiography in patients with subarachnoid hemorrhage: from aneurysm detection to treatment without conventional angiography. *J Neurosurg* 1999;91:761–767.

190. White PM, Wardlaw JM, Easton V. Can noninvasive imaging accurately depict intracranial aneurysms? A systematic review. *Radiology* 2000;217:361–370.

191. Zouaoui A, Sahel M, Marro B, et al. Three-dimensional computed tomographic angiography in detection of cerebral aneurysms in acute subarachnoid hemorrhage. *Neurosurgery* 1997;41:125–130.

192. Dehdashti AR, Rufenacht DA, Delavelle J, Reverdin A, De Tribolet N. Therapeutic decision and management of aneurysmal subarachnoid haemorrhage based on computed tomographic angiography. *Br J Neurosurg* 2003; 17:46–53.

193. Hashimoto H, Jun-Ichi I, Hironaka Y, Okada M, Sakaki T. Use of spiral computerized tomography angiography in patients with subarachnoid hemorrhage in whom subtraction angiography did not reveal cerebral aneurysms. *J Neurosurg* 2000;92:278–283.

194. Hirai T, Korogi Y, Ono K, et al. Preoperative evaluation of intracranial aneurysms: usefulness of intraarterial 3D CT angiography and conventional angiography with a combined unit - initial experience. *Radiology* 2001;220: 499–505.

195. Hirai T, Korogi Y, Suginohara K, et al. Clinical usefulness of unsubtracted 3D digital angiography compared with rotational digital angiography in the pretreatment evaluation of intracranial aneurysms. *AJNR Am J Neuroradiol* 2003;24:1067–1074.

196. Anderson GB, Ashforth R, Steinke DE, Findlay JM. CT angiography for the detection of cerebral vasospasm in patients with acute subarachnoid hemorrhage. *AJNR Am J Neuroradiol* 2000;21:1011–1015.

197. Otawara Y, Ogasawara K, Ogawa A, Sasaki M, Takahashi K. Evaluation of vasospams after subarchnoid hemorrhage by use of multislice computed tomographic angiogrphy. *Neurosurgery* 2002;51:939–942.

198. Boet R, Poon WS, Lam JM, Yu SC. The surgical treatment of intracranial aneurysms based on computer tomographic angiography alone—streamlining the acute management of symptomatic aneurysms. *Acta Neurochir (Wien)* 2003;145:101–105.

199. Rieger J, Hosten N, Neumann K. Initial clinical experience with spiral CT and 3D reconstruction in intracranial aneurysms and arteriovenous malformations. *Neuroradiology* 1996;38:245–251.

200. Link J, Brossmann J, Grabener M, et al. Spiral CT angiography and selective digital subtraction angiography of internal carotid artery stenosis. *AJNR Am J Neuroradiol* 1996;17:89–94.

201. Lubezky N, Fajer S, Barmeir E, Karmeli R. Duplex scanning and CT angiography in the diagnosis of carotid artery occlusion: a prospective study. *Eur J Vasc Endovasc Surg* 1998;16:133–136.

202. Anderson GB, Steinke DE, Petruk KC, Ashforth R, Findlay JM. Computed tomographic angiography versus digital subtraction angiography for the diagnosis and early treatment of ruptured intracranial aneurysms. *Neurosurgery* 1999;45:1315–1320.

203. Matsumoto M, Sato M, Nakano M, et al. Three-dimensional computerized tomography angiography-guided surgery of acutely ruptured cerebral anuerysms. *J Neurosurg* 2001;94:718–727.

204. Nonent M, Serfaty J-M, Nighoghossian N, et al. Concordance rate differences of 3 noninvasive imaging techniques to measure carotid stenosis in clinical routine practice. Results of the CARMEDAS Multicenter Study. *Stroke* 2004;35:682–686.

205. Fellner C, Strotzer M, Fraunhofer S, et al. MR angiography of the supra-aortic arteries using a dedicated head and neck coil: image quality and assessment of stenoses. *Neuroradiology* 1997;39:763–771.

206. Yucel EK, Anderson CM, Edelman RR, et al. Magnetic resonance angiography. Update on applications for extracranial arteries. *Circulation* 1999;100:2284–2301.

207. Graves MJ. Magnetic resonance angiography. *Br J Radiol* 1997;70:6–28.

208. Derex L, Hermier M, Adeleine P, Froment JC, Trouillas P, Nighoghossian N. Early detection of cerebral arterial occlusion on magnetic resonance angiography: predictive value of the baseline NIHSS score and impact on neurological outcome. *Cerebrovasc Dis* 2002;13: 225–229.

209. Siewert B, Wielopolski PA, Schlaug G, Edelman RR, Warach S. STAR MR angiography for rapid detection of vascular abnormalities in patients with acute cerebrovascular disease. *Stroke* 1997;28:1211–1215.

210. Nederkoorn PJ, Elgersma OE, Mali WP, Eikelboom BC, Kappelle LJ, Van Der Graaf Y. Overestimation of carotid artery stenosis with magnetic resonance angiography compared with digital subtraction angiography. *J Vasc Surg* 2002;36:806–813.

211. Quick HH, Debatin JF, Ladd ME. MR imaging of the vessel wall. European *Radiology* 2002;12:889–900.

212. Clifton AG. MR angiography. *Br Med Bull* 2000;56:367–377.

213. Fujita N, Hirabuki N, Fujii K, et al. MR imaging of middle cerebral artery stenosis and occlusion: value of MR angiography. *AJNR Am J Neuroradiol* 1994;15:335–341.

214. Korogi Y, Takahashi M, Mabuchi N, et al. Intracranial vascular stenosis and occlusion: diagnostic accuracy of three-dimensional, Fourier transform, time-of-flight MR angiography. *Radiology* 1994;193:187–193.

215. Nederkoorn PJ, Mali WP, Eikelboom BC, et al. Preoperative diagnosis of carotid artery stenosis. Accuracy of noninvasive testing. *Stroke* 2002;33:2003–2008.

216. Morasch MD, Gurjala AN, Washington E, et al. Cross-sectional magnetic resonance angiography is accurate in predicting degree of carotid stenosis. *Ann Vasc Surg* 2002;16:266–272.

217. Johnston D, Eastwood JD, Nguyen T, Goldstein LB. Contrast-enhanced magnetic resonance angioplasty of carotid arteries: utility in routine clinical practice. *Stroke* 2002;33:2834–2838.

218. Kenton AR, Martin PJ, Abbott RJ, Moody AR. Comparison of transcranial color-coded sonography and magnetic resonance angiography in acute stroke. *Stroke* 1997;28:1601–1606.

219. Wentz KU, Rother J, Schwartz A, Mattle HP, Suchalla R, Edelman RR. Intracranial vertebrobasilar system: MR angiography. *Radiology* 1994;190:105–110.

220. Rother J, Wentz KU, Rautenberg W, Schwartz A, Hennerici M. Magnetic resonance angiography in vertebrobasilar ischemia. *Stroke* 1993;24:1310–1315.

221. Mallouhi A, Felber S, Chemelli A, et al. Detection and characterization of intracranial aneurysms with MR angiography: comparison of volume-rendering and maximum-intensity-projection algorithms. *AJR Am J Roentgenol* 2003;180:55–64.

222. Coley SC, Romanowski CA, Hodgson TJ, Griffiths PD. Dural arteriovenous fistulae: noninvasive diagnosis with dynamic MR digital subtraction angiography. *AJNR Am J Neuroradiol* 2002;23:404–407.

223. Anzalone N, Triulzi F, Scotti G. Acute subarachnoid haemorrhage: 3D time-of-flight MR angiography versus intra-arterial digital angiography. *Neuroradiology* 1995;37:257–261.

224. Kurihara N, Takahashi S, Higano. Evaluation of large intracranial aneurysm with three-dimensional MRI. *J Comput Assist Tomogr* 1995;19:707–712.

225. Phan TG, Huston J, III, Brown RB, Jr., Wiebers DO, Piepgras DG. Intracranial accular aneurysm enlargement determined using serial magnetic resonance angiography. *J Neurosurg* 2002;97:1023–1028.

226. Ronkainen A, Hernesniemi J, Tromp G. Special features of familial intracranial aneurysms: report of 215 familial aneurysms. *Neurosurgery* 1995;37:43–47.

227. Kojima M, Nagasawa S, Lee YE, Takeichi Y, Tsuda E, Mabuchi N. Asymptomatic familial cerebral aneurysms. *Neurosurgery* 1998;43:776–781.

228. Raaymakers TW, Rinkel GJ, Ramos LM. Initial and follow-up screening for aneurysms in families with familial subarachnoid hemorrhage. *Neurology* 1998;51:1125–1130.

229. Raaymakers TWM. Aneurysms in relatives of patients with subarachnoid hemorrhage: frequency and risk factors. MARS Study Group. Magnetic Resonance Angiography in relatives of patients with subarachnoid hemorrhage. *Neurology* 1999;53:982–988.

230. Yamada I, Matsushima Y, Suzuki S. Moyamoya disease: diagnosis with three-dimensional time-of-flight MR angiography. *Radiology* 1992;184:773–778.

231. Kasner SE, Hankins LL, Bratina P, Morgenstern LB. Magnetic resonance angiography demonstrates vascular healing of carotid and vertebral artery dissections. *Stroke* 1997;28:1993–1997.

232. Bladin CF, Alexandrov AV, Murphy J, Maggisano R, Norris JW. Carotid Stenosis Index. A new method of measuring internal carotid artery stenosis. *Stroke* 1995;26:230–234.

233. de Bray JM, Glatt B. Quantification of atheromatous stenosis in the extracranial internal carotid artery. *Cerebrovasc Dis* 1995;5:414–426.

234. Falke P, Matzsch T, Sternby NH, Bergqvist D, Stavenow L. Intraplaque haemorrhage at carotid artery surgery—a predictor of cardiovascular mortality. *J Intern Med* 1995;238:131–135.

235. Hatsukami TS, Ferguson MS, Beach KW, et al. Carotid plaque morphology and clinical events. *Stroke* 1997;28:95–100.

236. Kagawa R, Moritake K, Shima T, Okada Y. Validity of B-mode ultrasonographic findings in patients undergoing carotid endarterectomy in comparison with angiographic and clinicopathologic features. *Stroke* 1996;27:700–705.

237. Park AE, McCarthy WJ, Pearce WH, Matsumura JS, Yao JS. Carotid plaque morphology correlates with presenting symptomatology. *J Vasc Surg* 1998;27:872–878.

238. Jackson MR, Chang AS, Robles HA, et al. Determination of 60% or greater carotid stenosis: a prospective comparison of magnetic resonance angiography and duplex ultrasound with conventional angiography. *Ann Vasc Surg* 1998;12:236–243.

239. Moneta GL, Edwards JM, Chitwood RW, et al. Correlation of North American Symptomatic Carotid Endarterectomy Trial (NASCET) angiographic definition of 70% to 99% internal carotid artery stenosis with duplex scanning. *J Vasc Surg* 1993;17:152–157.

240. Lewis RF, Abrahamowicz M, Cote R, Battista RN. Predictive power of duplex ultrasonography in asymptomatic carotid disease. *Ann Intern Med* 1997;127:13–20.

241. Alexandrov AV. Imaging cerebrovascular diseases with ultrasound. *Cerebrovasc Dis* 2003;16:1–3.

242. Olin JW, Fonseca C, Childs MB, Piedmonte MR, Hertzer NR, Young JR. The natural history of asymptomatic moderate internal carotid artery stenosis by duplex ultrasound. *Vasc Med* 1998;3:101–108.

243. Crouse JR, III, Tang R, Espeland MA, Terry JG, Morgan T, Mercuri M. Associations of extracranial carotid atherosclerosis progression with coronary status and risk factors in patients with and without cornary artery disease. *Circulation* 2002;106:2061–2066.

244. Sander D, Klingelhofer J. Early carotid atherosclerosis of the internal and external carotid artery related to twenty-four blood pressure variability. *Cerebrovasc Dis* 1997;7:338–344.

245. Tonstad S, Joakimsen O, Stensland-Bugge E, Ose L, Bonaa KH, Leren TP. Carotid intima-media thickness and plaque in patients with familial hypercholesterolaemia mutations and control subjects. *Eur J Clin Invest* 1998;28:971–979.

246. O'Leary DH, Polak JF, Kronmal RA, et al. Carotid artery intima and media thickness as a risk factor for myocardial infarction and stroke in older adults. *N Engl J Med* 1999;340:14–22.

247. Bots ML, Evans GW, Riley WA, Grobbee DE. Carotid intima-media thickness measurements in intervention studies. Design options, progression rates, and sample size considerations: a point of view. *Stroke* 2003;34:2985–2994.

248. Bots ML, Hoes AW, Koudstaal PJ, Hofman A, Grobbee DE. Common carotid intima-media thickness and risk of stroke and myocardial infarction: the Rotterdam Study. *Circulation* 1997;96:1432–1437.

249. Davis PH, Dawson JD, Mahoney LT, Lauer RM. Increased carotid intimal-medial thickness and coronary calcification are related in young and middle-aged adults. *Circulation* 1999;100:838–842.

250. Espeland MA, Tang R, Terry JG, Davis DH, Mercuri M, Crouse JR, III. Associaion of risk factors with segement-specific intimal-medial thickness of the extracranial carotid artery. *Stroke* 1999;30:1047–1055.

251. Adams HP, Jr., Bendixen BH, Leira EC, et al. Antithrombotic treatment of ischemic stroke among patients with occlusion or severe stenosis of the internal carotid artery. *Neurology* 1999;53:122–125.

252. Guzman RP. Appropriate imaging before carotid endarterectomy. *Can J Surg* 1998;41:218–223.

253. Collier PE. Changing trends in the use of preoperative carotid arteriography: the community experience. *Cardiovasc Surg* 1998;6:485–489.

254. Howard G, Baker WH, Chambless LE, Howard VJ, Jones AM, Toole JF. An approach for the use of Doppler ultrasound as a screening tool for hemodynamically significant stenosis (despite heterogeneity of Doppler performance). A multicenter experience. Asymptomatic Carotid Atherosclerosis Study Investigators. *Stroke* 1996;27:1951–1957.

255. Markus HS, Ackerstaff R, Babikian V, et al. Intercenter agreement in reading Doppler embolic signals. A multicenter international study. *Stroke* 1997;28:1307–1310.

256. Kimura K, Yasaka M, Moriyasu H, Tsuchiya T, Yamaguchi T. Ultrasonographic evaluation of vertebral artery to detect vertebrobasilar axis occlusion. *Stroke* 1994;25:1006–1009.

257. Hoffmann M, Sacco RL, Chan S, Mohr JP. Noninvasive detection of vertebral artery dissection. *Stroke* 1993;24:815–819.

258. Hennerici M, Rautenberg W, Schwartz A. Transcranial Doppler ultrasound for the assessment of intracranial arterial flow velocity–Part 2. Evaluation of intracranial arterial disease. *Surg Neurol* 1987;27:523–532.

259. Baumgartner RW, Mattle HP, Schroth G. Assessment of ≥50% and ≤50% intracranial stenoses by transcranial color-coded duplex sonography. *Stroke* 1999;30:87–92.

260. Goertler M, Kross R, Baeumer M, et al. Diagnostic impact and prognostic relevance of early contrast-enhanced transcranial color-coded duplex sonography in acute stroke. *Stroke* 1998;29:955–962.

261. Alexandrov AV, Demchuk AM, Wein TH, Grotta JC. Yield of transcranial Doppler in acute cerebral ischemia. *Stroke* 1999;30:1604–1609.

262. Alexandrov AV, Grotta JC. Arterial reocclusion in stroke patients treated with intravenous tissue plasminogen activator. *Neurology* 2002;59:862–867.

263. Akopov S, Whitman GT. Hemodynamic studies in early ischemic stroke: serial transcranial Doppler and magnetic resonance angiography evaluation. *Stroke* 2002;33:1274–1279.

264. Christou I, Alexandrov AV, Burgin WS, et al. Timing of recanalization after tissue plasminogen activator therapy determined by transcranial Doppler correlates with clinical recovery from ischemic stroke. *Stroke* 2000;31:1812–1816.

265. Demchuk AM, Burgin WS, Christou I, et al. Thrombolysis in brain ischemia (TIBI) transcranial Doppler flow grades predict clinical severity, early recovery, and mortality in patients treated with intravenous tissue plasminogen activator. *Stroke* 2001;32:89–93.

266. Georgiadis D, Grosset DG, Kelman A, Faichney A, Lees KR. Prevalence and characteristics of intracranial microemboli signals in patients with different types of prosthetic cardiac valves. *Stroke* 1994;25:587–592.

267. Georgiadis D, Uhlmann F, Schorch A, Baumgartner RW, vans DH. Postembolic spectral patterns of Doppler microembolic signals. *Cerebrovasc Dis* 2003;16:253–256.

268. Cullinane M, Wainwright R, Brown A, Monaghan M, Markus HS. Asymptomatic embolization in subjects with atrial fibrillation not taking anticoagulants: a prospective study. *Stroke* 1998;29:1810–1815.

269. Daffertshofer M, Ries S, Schminke U, Hennerici M. High-intensity transient signals in patients with cerebral ischemia. *Stroke* 1996;27:1844–1849.

270. Angeli S, Del Sette M, Beelke M, Anzola GP, Zanette E. Transcranial Doppler in the diagnosis of cardiac patent foramen ovale. *Neurol Sci* 2001;22:253–256.

271. Devuyst G, Darbellay GA, Vesin J-M, et al. Automatic classification of HITS into artifacts or solid or gaseous emboli by a wavelet representation combined with dual-gate TCD. *Stroke* 2001;32:2803–2809.

272. Devuyst G, Despland PA, Bogousslavsky J, Jeanrenaud X. Complementarity of contrast transcranial Doppler and contrast transesophageal echocardiography for the detection of patent foramen ovale in stroke patients. *Eur Neurol* 1997;38:21–25.

273. Baguet J-P, Besson G, Tremel F, Mangin L, Richardot C, Mallion J-M. Should one use echocardiography or contrast transcranial Doppler ultrasound for the detection of a patent foramen ovale after an ischemic cerebrovascualr accident? *Cerebrovasc Dis* 2001;12:318–324.

274. Proust F, Debono B, Gerardin E, et al. Angiographic cerebral vasospasm and delayed ischemic deficit on anterior part of the circle of Willis. Usefulness of transcranial Doppler. *Neurochirurgie* 2002;48:489–499.

275. Grosset DG, Straiton J, McDonald I. Angiographic and Doppler idagnosis or cerebral artery vasospasm following subarachnoid hemorrhage. *Br J Neurosurg* 1993;7:291–298.

276. Laumer R, Steinmeier R, Gonner F. Cerebral hemodynamics in subarachnoid hemorrhage evaluated by transcranial Doppler sonography. *Neurosurgery* 1993;33:11–18.

277. Steinmeier R, Laumer R, Bondar I. Cerebral hemodynamics in subarachnoid hemorrhage evaluated by transcranial Doppler sonography. Part 2. Pulsatility indices normal reference values and characteristics in subarachnoid hemorrhage. *Neurosurgery* 1993;33:10.

278. Boecher-Schwarz HG, Ungersboeck K, Ulrich P, Fries G, Wild A, Perneczky A. Transcranial Doppler diagnosis of

cerebral vasospasm following subarachnoid haemorrhage. Correlation and analysis of results in relation to the age of patients. *Acta Neurochir (Wien)* 1994;127:32–36.

279. Lindegaard KF. The role of transcranial Doppler in the management of patients with subarachnoid haemorrhage–a review. *Acta Neurochir Suppl (Wien)* 1999;72:59–71.

280. Haley EC, Jr, Kassell NF, Torner JC. A randomized trial of nicardipine in subarachnoid hemorrhage: angiographic and transcranial Doppler ultrasound results. A report of the Cooperative Aneurysm Study. *J Neurosurg* 1993;78:548–553.

281. Mast H, Mohr JP, Thompson JL, et al. Transcranial Doppler ultrasonography in cerebral arteriovenous malformations. Diagnostic sensitivity and association of flow velocity with spontaneous hemorrhage and focal neurological deficit. *Stroke* 1995;26:1024–1027.

282. marti-Fabregas J, Belvis R, Guardia E, et al. Prognostic value of Pulsatility Index in acute intracerebral hemorrhage. *Neurology* 2003;61:1051–1056.

283. Ekelund A, Saveland H, Romner B. Transcranial Doppler ultrasound in hypertensive versus normotensive patients after aneurysmal subarachnoid hemorrhage. *Stroke* 1995;26:2071–2074.

284. Giller CA, Batjer HH, Purdy P, et al. Inter-disciplinary evaluation of cerebral hemodynamics in the treatment of arteriovenous fistulae associated with giant varices. *Neurosurgery* 1994;35:778–784.

285. Giller CA, Purdy P, Giller A. Elevated transcranial Doppler ultrasound velocities following therapeutic arterial dilation. *Stroke* 1995;26:123–127.

286. Seidel G, Kaps M, Gerriets T. Potential and limitations of transcranial color-coded sonography in stroke patients. *Stroke* 1995;26:2061–2066.

287. Vandenberg B, Biller J. Cardiac evaulation of the patient with stroke. *Cerebrovasc Dis* 1991;1(suppl 1):73–82.

288. Oppenheimer SM. Neurogenic cardiac effects of cerebrovascular disease. *Curr Opin Neurol* 1994;7:20–24.

289. Oppenheimer SM, Hachinski VC. The cardiac consequences of stroke. *Neurol Clin* 1992;10:167–176.

290. Dimant J, Grob D. Electrocardiographic changes and myocardial damage in patients with acute cerebrovascular accidents. *Stroke* 1977;8:448–455.

291. Norris JW, Froggatt GM, Hachinski VC. Cardiac arrhythmias in acute stroke. *Stroke* 1978;9:392–396.

292. Abboud H, Berroir S, Labreuche J, et al. Insular involvement in brain infarction increases risk for cardiac arrhythmia and death. *Ann Neurol,* 2006;59:691–699.

293. Bell C, Kapral M. Use of ambulatory electrocardiography for the detection of paroxysmal atrial fibrillation in patients with stroke. *Can J Neurol Sci* 2000;27:25–31.

294. Koudstaal PJ, van Gijn J, Klootwijk AP, van der Meche FG, Kappelle LJ. Holter monitoring in patients with transient and focal ischemic attacks of the brain. *Stroke* 1986;17:192–195.

295. Rem JA, Hachinski VC, Boughner DR, Barnett HJM. Value of cardiac monitoring and echocardiography in TIA and stroke patients. *Stroke* 1985;16:950–956.

296. Sagar G, Riley P, Vohrah A. Is admission chest radiography of any clinical value in acute stroke patients? *Clin Radiol* 1996;51:499–502.

297. Chimowitz MI, Poole RM, Starling MR, Schwaiger M, Gross MD. Frequency and severity of asymptomatic coronary disease in patients with different causes of stroke. *Stroke* 1997;28:941–945.

298. Adams RJ, Chimowitz MI, Alpert JS, et al. Coronary risk evaluation in patients with transient ischemic attack and ischemic stroke: a scientific statement of healthcare professionals from the Stroke Council and the Council on Clinical Cardiology of the American Heart Association/American Stroke Association. *Circulation* 2003;108:1278–1290.

299. Hertzer NR, Young JR, Beven EG, et al. Coronary angiography in 506 patients with extracranial cerebrovascular disease. *Arch Intern Med* 1985;145:849–852.

300. Hertzer NR, Loop FD, Beven EG, O'Hara PJ, Krajewski LP. Surgical staging for simultaneous coronary and carotid disease: a study including prospective randomization. *J Vasc Surg* 1989;9:455–463.

301. Rihal CS, Gersh BJ, Whisnant JP, et al. Influence of coronary heart disease on morbidity and mortality after carotid endarterectomy: a population-based study in Olmsted County, Minnesota (1970–1988). *J Am Coll Cardiol* 1992;19:1254–1260.

302. Garber AM, Solomon NA. Cost-effectiveness of alternative test strategies for the diagnosis of coronary artery disease. *Ann Intern Med* 1999;130:719–728.

303. Macko RF, DeSouza CA, Tretter LD, et al. Treadmill aerobic exercise training reduces the energy expenditure and cardiovascular demands of hemiparetic gait in chronic stroke patients. A preliminary report. *Stroke* 1997;28:326–330.

304. Urbinati S, Di Pasquale G, Andreoli A, et al. Heart-brain interactions in cerebral ischaemia: a non-invasive cardiologic study protocol. *Neurol Res* 1992;14:112–117.

305. Urbinati S, Di Pasquale G, Andreoli A, et al. Preoperative noninvasive coronary risk stratification in candidates for carotid endarterectomy. *Stroke* 1994;25:2022–2027.

306. Peterson GE, Brickner ME, Reimold SC. Transesophageal echocardiography: clinical indications and applications. *Circulation* 2003;107:2398–2402.

307. Daniel WG, Erbel R, Kasper W, et al. Safety of transesophageal echocardiography. A multicenter survey of 10,419 examinations. *Circulation* 1991;83:817–821.

308. Urbinati S, Di Pasquale G, Andreoli A, et al. Role and indication of two-dimensional echocardiography in young adults with cerebral ishcemia: a prospective study in 125 patients. *Cerebrovasc Dis* 1992;2:14–21.

309. Hart RG. Cardiogenic embolism to the brain. *Lancet* 1992;339:589–594.

310. Bikkina M, Levy D, Evans JC, et al. Left ventricular mass and risk of stroke in an elderly cohort. *JAMA* 1994;272:33–36.

311. Atrial Fibrillation Investigators. Echocardiographic predictors of stroke in patients with atrial fibrillation: a prospective study of 1066 patients from 3 clinical trials. *Arch Intern Med* 1998;158:1316–1320.

312. Sansoy V, Abbott RD, Jayaweera AR, Kaul S. Low yield of transthoracic echocardiography for cardiac source of embolism. *Am J Cardio* 1995;75:166–169.

313. Beattie JR, Cohen DJ, Manning WJ, Douglas PS. Role of routine transthoracic echocardiography in evaluation and management of stroke. *J Intern Med* 1998;243:281–291.

314. Biller J, Johnson MR, Adams HP, Jr., Kerber RE, Toffol GJ, Butler MJ. Echocardiographic evaluation of young adults with nonhemorrhagic cerebral infarction. *Stroke* 1986;17: 608–612.

315. Cohen A, Chauvel C. Transesophageal echocardiography in the management of transient ischemic attack and ischemic stroke. *Cerebrovasc Dis* 1996;6(suppl 1):15–25.

316. Censori B, Colombo F, Valsecchi MG, et al. Early transoesophageal echocardiography in cryptogenic and lacunar stroke and transient ischaemic attack. *J Neurol Neurosurg Psychiatry* 1998;64:624–627.

317. Husain AM, Alter M. Transesophageal echocardiography in diagnosing cardioembolic stroke. *Clin Cardio* 1995; 18:705–708.

318. Stollberger C, Finsterer J. Transesophageal echocardiography: which stroke patients benefit most from this investigation? *J Neurol Neurosurg Psychiatry* 2003;74:283–284.

319. Warner MF, Momah KI. Routine transesophageal echocardiography for cerebral ischemia. Is it really necessary? *Arch Intern Med* 1996;156:1719–1723.

320. Rauh R, Fischereder M, Spengel FA. Transesophageal echocardiography in patients with focal cerebral ischemia of unknown cause. *Stroke* 1996;27:691–694.

321. Meissner I, Whisnant J, Khandheria BK, et al. Prevalence of potential risk factors for stroke assessed by transesophageal echocardiography and carotid ultrasonography: the SPARC Study. *Mayo Clin Proc* 1999;74:862–869.

322. Palazzuoli A, Ricci D, Lenzi C, Lenzi J, Palazzuoli V. Transesphogeal echocardiography for identifying potential cardiac sources of embolism in patients with stroke. *Neurol Sci* 2000;21:195–202.

323. Voros S, Nanda NC, Samal AK, et al. Transesophageal echocardiography in patients with ischemic stroke accurately detects significant coronary artery stenosis and often changes management. *Am Heart J* 2001;142: 916–922.

324. Stollberger C, Chnupa P, Kronik G, et al. Transesophageal echocardiography to assess embolic risk in patients with atrial fibrillation. ELAT Study Group. Embolism in Left Atrial Thrombi. *Ann Intern Med* 1998;128:630–638.

325. Briley DP, Giraud GD, Beamer NB, et al. Spontaneous echo contrast and hemorheologic abnormalities in cerebrovascular disease. *Stroke* 1994;25:1564–1569.

326. Jones EF, Calafiore P, McNeil JJ, Tonkin AM, Donnan GA. Atrial fibrillation with left atrial spontaneous contrast detected by transesophageal echocardiography is a potent risk factor for stroke. *Am J Cardio* 1996;78:425–429.

327. Tanus-Santos JE, Moreno JH. Pulmonary embolism and impending paradoxical embolism: a role for transesophageal echocardiography? Clinical Cardiology 1999;22:158–159.

328. Klotzsch C, Janssen G, Berlit P. Transesophageal echocardiography and contrast-TCD in the detection of a patent foramen ovale: experiences with 111 patients. *Neurology* 1994;44:1603–1606.

329. Serena J, Segura T, Perez-Ayuso MJ, Bassaganyas J, Molins A, Davalos. The need to quantify right-to-left shunt in acute ischemic stroke: a case-control study. *Stroke* 1998;29:1322–1328.

330. Stone DA, Godard J, Corretti MC, et al. Patent foramen ovale: association between the degree of shunt by contrast transesophageal echocardiography and the risk of future ischemic neurologic events. *Am Heart J* 1996; 131:158–161.

331. Schuchlenz HW, Weihs W, Beitzke A, Stein J-I, Gamillscheg A, Rehak P. Transesophageal echocardiography for quantifying size of patent foramen ovale in patients with cryptogenic cererovascular events. *Stroke* 2002;33:293–296.

332. Ahmed S, Nanda NC, Nekkanti R, Yousif AM. Contrast transesophageal echocardiographic detection of a pulmonary arteriovenous malformation draining into left lower pulmonary vein. *Echocardiography* 2003;20:391–394.

333. Schwammenthal E, Schwammenthal Y, Tanne D, et al. Transcutaneous detection of aortic arch atheromas by suprasternal harmonic imaging. *J Am Coll Cardiol* 2002;39:1127–1132.

334. Marschall K, Kanchuger M, Kessler K, et al. Superiority of transesophageal echocardiography in detecting aortic arch atheromatous disease: identification of patients at increased risk of stroke during cardiac surgery. *J Cardiothorac Vasc Anesth* 1994;8:5–13.

335. Tenenbaum A, Garniek A, Shemesh J, et al. Dual-helical CT for detecting aortic atheromas as a source of stroke: comparison with transesophageal echocardiography. *Radiology* 1998;208:153–158.

336. Ribakove GH, Katz ES, Galloway AC, et al. Surgical implications of transesophageal echocardiography to grade the atheromatous aortic arch. *Ann Thorac Surg* 1992;53:758–761.

337. Choudhary SK, Bhan A, Sharma R, et al. Aortic atherosclerosis and perioperative stroke in patients undergoing coronary artery bypass: role of intra-operative transesophageal echocardiography. *Int J Cardiol* 1997;61:31–38.

338. Krinsky GA. Diagnostic imaging of aortic atherosclerosis and its complications. *Neuroimaging Clin N Am* 2002;12:437–443.

339. Love BB, Struck LK, Stanford W, Biller J, Kerber R, Marcus M. Comparison of two-dimensional echocardiography and ultrafast cardiac computed tomography for evaluating intracardiac thrombi in cerebral ischemia. *Stroke* 1990;21:1033–1038.

340. Ohyama H, Hosomi N, Takahashi T, et al. Comparison of magnetic resonance imaging and transesophageal echocardiography in detection of thrombus in the left atrial appendage. *Stroke* 2003;34:2436–2439.

CHAPTER 9

Atherosclerotic Disease

► GENERAL COMMENTS

Atherosclerosis is the most common arterial disease in the United States and most other parts of the world. This slowly progressive arteriopathy, which seems to be a disease of affluence, evolves over a lifetime.[1] The presence of risk factors in childhood predicts the development of carotid artery atherosclerosis in latter life.[2,3] Virtually, all middle-aged and elderly Americans have some pathological evidence of atherosclerosis. While atherosclerosis is diagnosed most commonly among persons older than 60, accelerated disease can become symptomatic among younger men and women. In general, the disease progresses more rapidly among men. Several factors including a family history of premature atherosclerosis, hypertension, diabetes mellitus, hypercholesterolemia, hyperhomocysteinemia, or smoking are associated with accelerated course for the arterial disease. A number of genetic mutations and polymorphisms are related to premature development of atherosclerosis.[4] The importance of genetic disorders promoting the development of atherosclerosis likely will grow in the future. Based on a series of sequential studies of changes found in the internal carotid arteries, Van der Meer[5] correlated progression of atherosclerosis in men and women with advancing age, smoking, total serum cholesterol, hypertension, and an elevated systolic blood pressure. Depending upon the arteries that are involved preferentially, an affected person initially present with a myocardial infarction, symptomatic peripheral vascular disease, an aortic aneurysm, or a transient ischemic attack (TIA) or ischemic stroke. Atherosclerotic disease involves the aorta, major intracranial or extracranial arteries, smaller cortical vessels, or short penetrating arteries that perfuse the brain. In addition, atherosclerotic disease of the coronary arteries is a leading cause of structural heart disease, which might be complicated by myocardial dysfunction or atrial fibrillation that serves as a nidus for thromboembolism to the brain. Finally, patients with extensive atherosclerotic disease are often treated with surgical or endovascular procedures that can be associated with thromboembolic complications.

► CORONARY ARTERY DISEASE AND PERIPHERAL ARTERY DISEASE

Coronary artery disease generally becomes symptomatic approximately one decade before atherosclerotic cerebrovascular disease produces neurological symptoms. As a result, persons with stroke are usually older than patients with heart or peripheral vascular disease. Many patients with stroke have a history of ischemic heart disease, congestive heart failure, or major cardiovascular operations. On the other hand, the presence of symptomatic intracranial or extracranial atherosclerotic disease (TIA or stroke) also denotes a patient who is at high risk of myocardial infarction or sudden cardiac death. Within 5 years following the neurological event, the chances of dying from heart disease are approximately double of those of having a fatal cerebrovascular event. Patients with stroke also have a high risk of peripheral vascular disease or disease of the abdominal aorta. Conversely, persons with peripheral vascular disease causing intermittent claudication of the lower extremities have an increased risk of stroke.[6]

► EVOLUTION OF ATHEROSCLEROSIS

The first changes of atherosclerosis can be found in the coronary arteries or aorta in young men in the second or third decades. In general, similar changes appear a decade later in young women. The initial insult appears to be some "trauma" to the arterial wall, which leads to an infiltration of inflammatory cells, proliferation of smooth cells, and thickening of the arterial wall.[7] These insults can include physical effects of diseases such as arterial hypertension or toxic phenomena from factors such as smoking or hyperhomocysteinemia. Because flow is turbulent at vascular bifurcations or other arterial stress points, the local arterial changes of atherosclerosis preferentially develop at these points.[8] The "traumatic" event can be self-limited and the artery can recover completely. However, the artery might not heal and lipids accumulate within the wall. The resultant pathological finding, the fatty streak, is the first hallmark of atherosclerosis.[9] With aging, the fatty streak evolves into a fibrous plaque. The plaque has a core that primarily consists of extracellular lipids and cholesterol crystals.[9] In addition, the plaque can contain areas of calcification and hemorrhage. It is covered by a cap, less than 100 μ in thickness, which consists primarily of connective tissue and endothelial cells. The cap can be relatively thin and is vulnerable to fracturing or fissuring. Minor disruptions in the cap promote growth of the atheromatous lesion within the arterial wall. The role of lipids also appears to be critical for growth of the plaque. Passage of low-density lipoprotein (LDL) cholesterol through the surface of the plaque speeds up the enlargement of the lipid core. On the other hand, high-density lipoprotein (HDL) cholesterol reduces oxidation of the LDL cholesterol and the deposition of lipids within the arterial wall. Decreasing serum concentrations of LDL cholesterol reduces the intra-arterial content of lipids, which in turn could stabilize the arterial lesion. Preventing fracture of the atherosclerotic plaque appears to be a key factor in forestalling acute thromboembolic occlusions.[10]

Role of Inflammation

Inflammation also plays a key role in the evolution of atherosclerosis.[7,11] Changes in interleukins, interferons, tumor necrosis factor, and other inflammatory markers and the activity of lymphocytes, mast cells, and macrophages are correlated with progression or destabilization of atherosclerotic plaques.[7] The stability of atherosclerotic plaques can be affected by tumor necrosis factor-α, interleukin-1β, matrix metalloproteinase, tenascin, transforming growth factor-β, tissue factors, and insulinlike growth factor-δ.[10] Infection with *Chlamydia pneumoniae*, *Porphymonas gingivalis*, *Helicobacter pylori*, herpes simplex viruses, influenza, cytomegalovirus, or other organisms might directly or indirectly lead to instability of the atherosclerotic plaque. Ridker et al.[12,13] have shown a strong correlation between levels of high-sensitivity C-reactive protein and the risk of ischemic events among persons with atherosclerotic disease. In a study of more than 14,000 healthy women, Ridker et al.[14] found that elevated C-reactive protein levels added predictive value to the findings of the metabolic syndrome in forecasting ischemic vascular events. Arenillas et al.[15] correlated elevated C-reactive protein levels and the risk of TIA or stroke among patients with extracranial or intracranial atherosclerosis. The elevated C-reactive protein may be a nonspecific marker. A cause-and-effect relationship between the elevated C-reactive protein and the vascular events is not established. Elevations of other inflammatory proteins also denote persons at high risk for ischemic events including stroke. The impact of inflammation on the course of atherosclerosis needs additional research but its effects might be as great as those that accompany hypercholesterolemia. Part of the efficacy of aspirin in preventing arterial thromboembolic events might be secondary to its anti-inflammatory effects.

Endothelial Function

Endothelial cells produce substances, such as nitric oxide, which help maintain vascular tone, promote hemostasis, limit inflammatory responses, or slow down the course of atherosclerosis. Arteries with a denuded endothelial surface do not have normal physiological responses to vasoactive stimuli. The role of endothelial cell in promoting hemostasis and normal vascular function likely is considerable. Additional research probably will lead to important discoveries about endothelial function.

Plaque Morphology

Structural changes in the plaque (active plaque/unstable plaque) appear critical for the development of secondary arterial occlusions.[16] An active plaque is denuded of its endothelial covering and its irregular borders are marked by evidence of active inflammation. Macrophages, the cellular hallmark of the inflammation, release metalloproteinases that cause further changes in the arterial wall.[7] In addition, an active plaque can have other pathological changes including a superficial calcified nodule or an intraplaque hemorrhage (Fig. 9-1). Using high-resolution magnetic resonance imaging (MRI), Yuan et al.[17] found that rupture of the fibrous cap of carotid atherosclerotic lesions was strongly associated with a history of TIA or recent stroke. Surgical specimens obtained at carotid endarterectomy for symptomatic or asymptomatic carotid stenoses correlate the presence of intraplaque hemorrhage and other acute changes with the occurrence of neurological symptoms.

Plaque Instability

The stability of the plaque appears to be more important than the degree of arterial narrowing in predicting acute

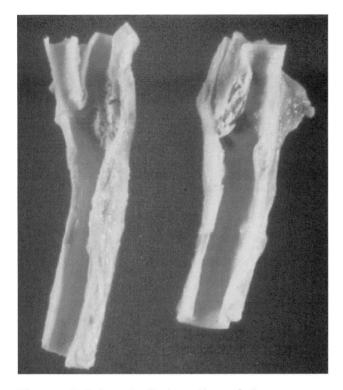

Figure 9-1. Longitudinal section of the common carotid artery, the carotid bifurcation, and the origins of the internal carotid and external carotid arteries shows an atherosclerotic plaque with ulceration and hemorrhage within the plaque at the origin of the internal carotid artery. (*Courtesy of S.S. Schochet, M.D., Department of Pathology, University of West Virginia, Morgantown, WV*)

coronary artery thrombosis as a complication of atherosclerosis. The vulnerable plaque is now recognized as a leading cause of acute occlusions of the coronary arteries.[18] A similar phenomenon might be present among persons with atherosclerotic cerebrovascular disease. On examination of plaques removed during carotid endarterectomy, Carr et al.[19] found a high rate of plaque rupture among patients with recent symptoms. A mildly stenotic plaque could become active, which induces a thrombus that leads to secondary embolism to the brain. Such scenario might be an explanation for some to the thromboembolic ischemic strokes of undetermined etiology—especially among persons older than 50. In addition, activation of plaques in multiple vascular territories could occur simultaneously and patients have both stroke and myocardial infarction within a few days or weeks of each other. Rather than being due to cardioembolism, some strokes following myocardial infarction might be secondary to atherosclerotic artery-to-artery embolization.

Minor fissures frequently develop within the atherosclerotic cap and are usually not associated with ischemic symptoms. The relatively minor fissures, which do not extend through the cap, subsequently heal and the patient is not aware of the event. However, more serious fissuring (a fracture) of the atherosclerotic cap appears to be the key factor in the development of acute arterial thromboembolism. The fracture exposes the underlying lipid core, which is highly thrombogenic, to the circulation. Platelet aggregation is stimulated and markedly elevated levels of thrombin occur. Ischemic symptoms develop when the thrombus becomes sufficiently large to produce arterial occlusion or if distal embolization occurs. This sequence of events suggests that a TIA or other ischemic symptoms should be considered as a potential sign that an atherosclerotic plaque has become active.

Plaque Ulceration

Ulceration of the plaque at the origin of the internal carotid artery is a relatively common finding among patients with TIA or amaurosis fugax. Major fractures can lead to ulceration of the plaque's surface. The soft underlying core is exposed to the circulation. Pieces of plaque are dislodged and the atherosclerotic debris (cholesterol embolism) travel downstream (Fig. 9-2). Atherosclerotic debris (cholesterol embolus/Hollenhorst plaque) can be seen within retinal arteries by direct ophthalmoscopy.[20] Fracture of an atherosclerotic plaque of the aorta during a major cardiac operation can also be the source of debris. This is a direct complication of the surgical procedure and is a leading cause of perioperative stroke following coronary artery bypass grafting. Manipulation of an intra-arterial catheter can also be the source of atherosclerotic debris that embolize to the

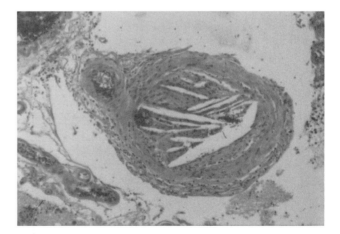

Figure 9-2. Microscopic examination of a cerebral artery shows evidences of embolization of atherosclerotic (cholesterol) debris within the arterial lumen. The most likely source would be either an extracranial artery or the aorta. (*Courtesy of S.S. Schochet, M.D., Department of Pathology, University of West Virginia, Morgantown, WV*)

limbs (trash toes), following arteriography, endovascular procedures, or cardiac catheterization. Extensive aortic atherosclerosis can be the source of cholesterol embolization to the lower extremities (purple toe syndrome).

General Management of Atherosclerosis

A future strategy in management of patients with atherosclerotic disease would include methods to examine the morphology of plaques in an effort to identify lesions that are most prone to rupture. Local interventions could be aimed at these lesions. In addition, management could include interventions to reduce inflammation in the arterial plaque, promote regression or the atherosclerotic lesion, stimulate function of endothelial cells, and stabilization of the plaque.[7] These measures include changes in lifestyle and the use of medications. The interventions to treat risk factors for accelerated atherosclerosis and stroke are discussed in Chapter 4.

Flow-Related Causes of Stroke

Besides being a source of emboli, severe atherosclerotic disease that leads to high-grade stenoses or occlusions can produce ischemia secondary to hypoperfusion. Patients with borderline hypoperfusion secondary to occlusion of the internal carotid artery can be identified by technologies such as positron-emission tomography. In some cases, the borderline hypoperfusion can augment the effects of embolization. Patients with relatively normal perfusion might not have symptoms secondary to embolization, while low flow might not permit rapid restoration of perfusion. Patients with severe intracranial or extracranial atherosclerotic disease can have brain ischemia in a watershed (border zone) pattern secondary to hypotension during cardiac operations. The most common locations for watershed infarctions are at the junctions of the terminal branches of the anterior, middle, and posterior cerebral arteries.

▶ SPECTRUM OF ATHEROSCLEROTIC CEREBROVASCULAR DISEASE

Patients with atherosclerotic cerebrovascular disease can have an ischemic stroke, TIA, amaurosis fugax, ischemic oculopathy, or an audible cranial bruit. In addition, a physician can auscultate a cervical or cranial bruit in an asymptomatic patient. Asymptomatic atherosclerotic disease also can be detected by a diagnostic study, such as vascular imaging.

Atherosclerotic disease usually involves multiple intracranial or extracranial vessels, although the severity of the arterial changes can vary considerably (Table 9-1).

▶ **TABLE 9-1.** MOST COMMON LOCATIONS OF ADVANCED CEREBROVASCULAR ATHEROSCLEROSIS

Aorta
  Ascending
  Arch
  Descending
Brachiocephalic or subclavian arteries
Common carotid arteries
Internal carotid arteries
  Origin
  Intracavernous portion (siphon)
  Distal
Vertebral arteries
  Origin
  Distal portion
Midportion of the basilar artery
Middle cerebral arteries
  Proximal portion
Posterior cerebral arteries
  Proximal portion
Disseminated intracranial
Penetrating arteries

For example, finding a severe stenosis of the origin of one internal carotid artery and minimal disease in the contralateral internal carotid artery is a relatively common situation. The reasons for one artery being more severely affected than other arteries are not obvious. In addition, atherosclerotic disease of the aorta can produce ischemic symptoms in the brain or spinal cord. Atherosclerosis can also affect small arteries penetrating the brain leading to lacunar infarction. While pathological correlations are lacking, microvascular disease of the brain also might be associated with atherosclerosis.

The anatomic locations of the arterial lesions affect the clinical presentations.

▶ AORTA

Atherosclerotic disease of the aorta (ascending, arch, and descending segments) is increasingly recognized as an important cause of ischemic disease of the brain and spinal cord, especially among older persons.[21] Severe atherosclerosis of the aorta is relatively common among elderly patients with stroke, and the proximal (ascending) portion of the aorta can be an occult source for cerebral embolization. Smoking and hyperhomocysteinemia are identified as leading factors that promote atherosclerosis of the aorta. In addition, elevation of fibrinogen, C-reactive protein, and other hemostatic parameters is associated with advanced atherosclerosis of the aortic arch.[22] The use of transesophageal echocardiogram (TEE) or helical computed tomograpgy (CT) has increased physicians' ability to detect atherosclerotic plaques in the aorta. These tests also differentiate the extent of the arteriopathy.[23] Such nuances are important clinically. The presence of a simple atherosclerotic lesion in the aorta increases the risk of stroke by a factor of 2.3.[24] A French study reported that aortic plaque thickness greater than 4 mm is associated with a stroke risk of 11.9 per 1000 patient-years.[25,26] The presence of aortic calcification also is a strong predictor of stroke.[27] Extensive atherosclerotic disease of the aorta can thicken the aortic wall or cause the formation of mobile plaques (*shagbark aorta*). The atherosclerotic lesions can be the nidus for either thromboembolism or embolization of cholesterol debris. Pedunculated and mobile plaques appear to be associated with the greatest risk for embolization. A complex atherosclerotic plaque of the aorta is associated with an increase in the risk of ischemic stroke by a factor of approximately 7.[28] Extensive plaque formation of the aorta is identified as a risk factor for ischemic cerebrovascular complications during cardiovascular operations.[29] Placement of a clamp across an aortic plaque can cause fracturing and release of atherosclerotic debris (*cholesterol embolism*). Surgical repair of the aorta prior to or during cardiac surgery has been proposed as a method to lower the risk of stroke. However, Stern et al.[29] found that aortic arch endarterectomy is a high-risk procedure.

▶ DISSECTION OF THE AORTA AND AORTIC ANEURYSM

In the past, dissection of the ascending portion and the arch of the aorta usually was attributed to *syphilitic aortitis*. This cause of aortic disease has declined since the introduction of modern antibiotics. While connective tissue diseases such as *Marfan syndrome* can cause aortic dissection, atherosclerosis now is the most common cause (Fig. 9-3). Dissections in the proximal segment of the aorta can lead to occlusion of the brachiocephalic, left common carotid, or left subclavian artery. Dissection of the ascending portion or the arch of the aorta usually presents with intense chest and back pain. Stroke can occur and it can be the most prominent or the initial symptom in some patients.[30–32] Because the left subclavian artery is the most distal major branch, it is the vessel most likely to be affected by dissection. Thus, ischemic symptoms often reflect dysfunction in the vertebrobasilar territory. In addition, patients may have hypotension, unstable vital signs, and absent pulses in the upper extremities. Chest X-ray or CT usually demonstrates widening of the aortic silhouette or a double lumen in the aorta.[32] TEE can detect the double lumen of the aorta.[33] In general, management focuses on treatment of the aortic lesion and includes aggressive lowering of

blood pressure and surgical repair. Thrombolytic therapy could prove to be catastrophic if the stroke is secondary to an aortic dissection. Thus, dissection should be a consideration if a patient has clinical findings of the aortic disease in addition to the stroke. Although an aneurysm of the sinus of Valsalva (a portion of the aorta adjacent to the aortic valve) is a potential source for thromboemboli, it appears to be an uncommon cause of stroke.

Atherosclerotic disease of the descending thoracic and abdominal aorta is relatively common among persons with cerebrovascular disease. For example, an abdominal aortic aneurysm is a potential cause of morbidity or mortality among patients with stroke. While atherosclerotic disease in these aortic locations is not associated directly with brain ischemia, it is an important etiology of spinal cord ischemia. Dissection of the aorta secondary to atherosclerosis is a leading cause of spinal cord infarction. The dissection obliterates the ostia of intercostal arteries, which are the parent vessels for radicular branches that send blood to the anterior spinal artery. The midthoracic cord is usually the most

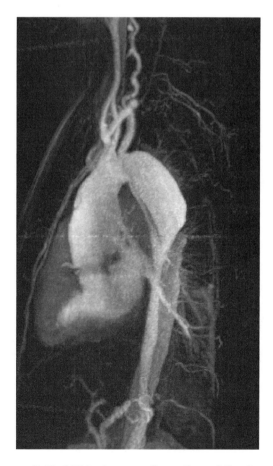

Figure 9-3. MRA shows a dissection of the thoracic aorta in a patient with Marfan syndrome. Similar dissection can occur with atherosclerosis.

vulnerable location. Affected patients usually have severe back, interscapular and abdominal pain, and the sudden development of spinal cord dysfunction. The neurological signs usually reflect a midthoracic cord lesion. The clinical findings of spinal cord infarction are described in Chapter 18.

▶ GREAT BRANCHES OF THE ARCH OF THE AORTA

Atherosclerosis can affect the proximal portions of the brachiocephalic, left common carotid, and left subclavian arteries. The left subclavian artery appears to be involved more frequently than do the other two major cervical vessels (Fig. 9-4). Besides the traditional risk factors, accelerated atherosclerosis of the subclavian artery also can be associated with prolonged hemodialysis for treatment of renal failure.[34] Presumably, the changes are secondary to the increased blood flow through the arteries of the upper extremity, which supply the dialysis fistula. The presence of severe disease of the great branches is often detected on examination. Prominent supraclavicular and cervical bruits can often be auscultated. In addition, differences in pulses or blood pressure levels can often be found between the two upper extremities. In general, subclavian artery atherosclerosis is suspected if a discrepancy of 25 mm Hg

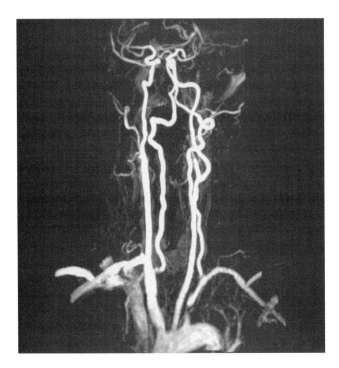

Figure 9-4. Arteriogram demonstrates a high-grade stenosis of the left subclavian artery. In addition, the left vertebral artery is occluded. The ascending vessel is the thyrocervical trunk.

or 25 percent is detected between the two limbs. Lesions of the great vessels also produce ischemic symptoms in the cerebral hemispheres or the posterior circulation.

Subclavian Steal Syndrome

While *subclavian steal syndrome* is the clinical syndrome most often attributed to atherosclerotic disease of the great vessels, it is an uncommon cause of vertebrobasilar TIA or stroke.[35] In subclavian steal, the proximal portion of one subclavian artery is either highly stenotic or occluded, and as a result blood ascends the contralateral vertebral artery and descends through the ipsilateral vertebral artery with resultant decreased perfusion to the posterior circulation. With use of the arm, blood is diverted from the brain stem to meet the metabolic demands of the limb and the patient has neurological symptoms.[36] Most atherosclerotic lesions should involve the left subclavian artery. Patients with severe atherosclerotic disease of the major branches of the aorta can be treated with endovascular procedures, endarterectomies, or surgical revascularization operations.[37-39]

Common Carotid Artery

While atherosclerosis can involve the common carotid arteries, this artery is usually less severely affected than is the origin of the internal carotid arteries. The leading location is the proximal segment of the common carotid artery. Clinical findings of severe atherosclerotic disease of the common carotid artery mimic that seen with lesions of the internal carotid artery.

▶ INTERNAL CAROTID ARTERY

The importance of internal carotid atherosclerosis as a cause of TIA or ischemic stroke has been known for more than 50 years. Because of the strong correlation between atherosclerosis of the origin of the internal carotid artery and stroke, considerable research has focused on methods to evaluate and treat this disease (Fig. 9-5). Among persons of European ancestry, the most common extracranial location for severe atherosclerotic disease is the origin of the internal carotid artery (carotid bifurcation). The plaque may extend from the distal common carotid artery and involve the ostium of the external carotid artery. Advanced atherosclerosis is most common among persons with diabetes mellitus, hypertension, hypercholesterolemia, or tobacco use.[40-41] Radiation may accelerate the course of atherosclerosis because the carotid artery is located relatively superficially and because the vessel is within the field of radiation. Radiation-induced carotid atherosclerosis can be extensive and severe. Because of its location, imaging

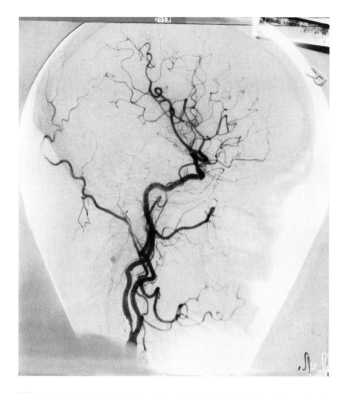

Figure 9-5. Lateral view of a right carotid arteriogram using subtraction techniques demonstrates a moderately severe stenosis at the origin of the internal carotid artery.

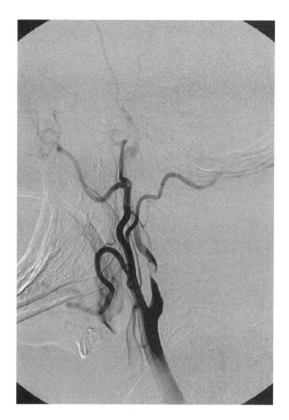

Figure 9-6. Lateral view of a left carotid arteriogram using subtraction techniques shows a severe stenosis at the origin of the internal carotid artery with secondary thrombus.

of the morphology of carotid artery atherosclerosis can be achieved by noninvasive tests. Detection of the early changes of carotid atherosclerosis (*intimal-medial thickness*) by duplex imaging is associated with an increased risk of myocardial infarction and stroke.[27]

Clinical Findings

The clinical manifestations of severe atherosclerotic disease of the internal carotid artery range from an asymptomatic narrowing that is incidentally found to be a major stroke secondary to occlusion. Severe stenosis of internal carotid artery can produce a cervical bruit that can be auscultated in an asymptomatic patient (see Chapter 5). In addition, patients with carotid artery atherosclerosis can have ischemia of the retina or cerebral hemisphere secondary to embolization or hypoperfusion (see Chapters 5 and 6). Severe atherosclerotic disease of the internal carotid artery also has been associated with cognitive decline.[42]

Diagnostic Studies and Treatment

The carotid artery bifurcation can be assessed by carotid duplex, magnetic resonance angiography (MRA), computerized tomographic angiography (CTA), or arteriography

(see Chapter 8; Figs. 9.6 and 9.7). The choice of diagnostic tests is selected on a case-by-case basis. Usually, noninvasive tests are performed prior to a procedure such as arteriography. With improvement in the sensitivity and specificity of the noninvasive vascular imaging studies, the role of arteriography is declining. Many surgeons now are making decisions about carotid endarterectomy based on the results of the noninvasive tests. In the future, arteriographic evaluation of the internal carotid artery might be limited to the setting of angioplasty and stenting. Medical measures to prevent stroke, complemented by surgical or endovascular therapies, are used to treat symptomatic or asymptomatic carotid stenoses. Widely performed procedures include carotid endarterectomy and, more recently, angioplasty and stenting (see Chapter 20).

Other Sites for Atherosclerosis of Internal Carotid Artery

The distal extracranial portion of the internal carotid artery is less commonly affected by atherosclerosis. While atherosclerotic stenosis does develop at this location, fibromuscular dysplasia and arterial dissections are more common pathologies. Severe atherosclerotic

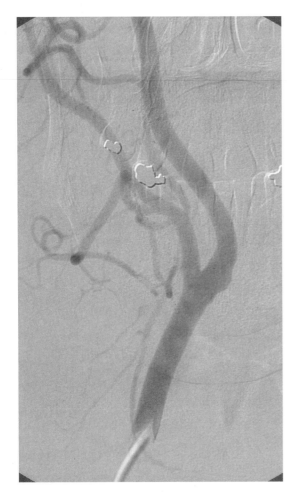

Figure 9-7. Lateral view of a left carotid arteriogram using subtraction techniques reveals a shallow ulcerated plaque at the origin of the internal carotid artery.

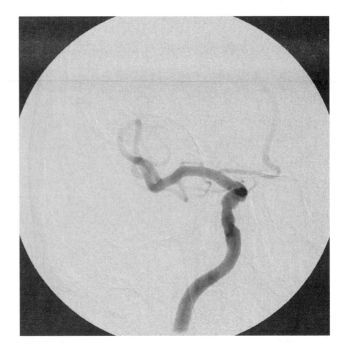

Figure 9-8. Anteroposterior view of a right carotid arteriogram using subtraction techniques shows a moderate stenosis of the cavernous segment (siphon stenosis) of the internal carotid artery.

and MRA are the usual methods for detecting the distal narrowing. Duplex ultrasonography of the neck might show slow flow, which is circumstantial evidence that a high-grade narrowing is present distally. The presence

disease of the distal extracranial portion of the internal carotid artery cannot be treated with carotid endarterectomy. In this situation, angioplasty with stenting is a potential local intervention.

Atherosclerosis of the Intracavernous Segment

The second most frequent site for atherosclerosis of the internal carotid artery is in its intracavernous portion (Figs. 9.8 and 9.9). The relatively high potential for severe narrowing of this portion of the internal carotid artery is one of the reasons for evaluation of the entire carotid vasculature. For example, Rouleau et al.[43] found severe distal stenosis ipsilateral to a high-grade narrowing of the origin of the internal carotid artery in approximately 10 percent of cases. A second lesion, which is located with the cranium (a *tandem stenosis*), sometimes can be more severe than that discovered extracranially. The lesion might be suspected by auscultation of an ipsilateral temporal or orbital bruit. Arteriography

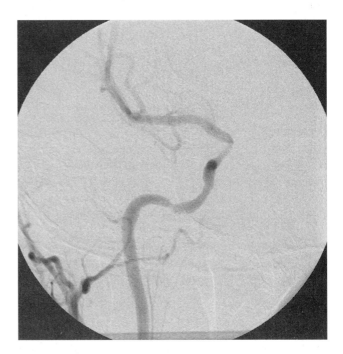

Figure 9-9. Oblique view of a right carotid arteriogram using subtraction techniques reveals an ulcerated plaque in the intracavernous portion (siphon) of the internal carotid artery.

of a plexus of veins forming the cavernous sinus limits direct surgical treatment of lesions of this portion of the internal carotid artery. However, atherosclerotic narrowing of the intracavernous portion of the internal carotid artery can be treated successfully with angioplasty and stenting.

Occlusion of the Internal Carotid Artery

The consequences of an occlusion of the internal carotid artery can vary from no symptoms to a major hemispheric infarction. The wide spectrum of responses reflects the adequacy of collateral channels via branches of the ipsilateral external carotid artery, the circle of Willis, and contralateral carotid circulation (Figs. 9-10 to 9-12).[44,45] Ischemia among persons with occlusions of the internal carotid artery can be secondary to hypoperfusion. Patients with a poor vascular reserve appear to be at high risk for ischemic stroke.[46] The reports about the risk of stroke subsequent to an asymptomatic carotid occlusion vary. Powers et al.[45] reported that their prognosis was good. On the other hand, Hankey and Warlow[47] found that the risk of recurrent stroke ipsilateral to a carotid occlusion is approximately 7 percent per year. Patients with impaired collateral flow secondary to a symptomatic carotid occlusion have even

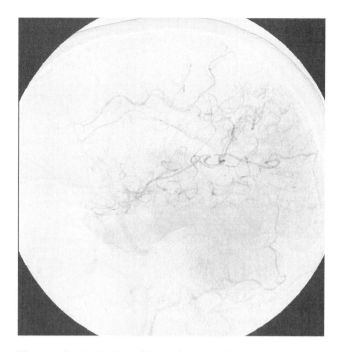

Figure 9-11. Delayed lateral view of a vertebral arteriogram shows branches of the anterior and middle cerebral arteries. Flow into these vessels is delayed. A capillary phase/branch is noted in the cerebellum and occipital pole. The findings suggest retrograde flow via pial (cortical) collaterals in a patient with an occlusion of the internal carotid artery.

higher rates of recurrent brain ischemia.[46] Patients with poor perfusion might benefit from surgical procedures, such as a superficial temporal artery-to-middle cerebral artery anastomosis, which could improve

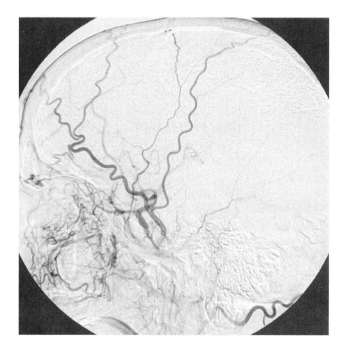

Figure 9-10. Lateral view of a left common carotid arteriogram in a patient with an occlusion of the extracranial internal carotid artery demonstrates filling of the distal internal carotid artery via collateral vessels of the external carotid artery. Retrograde flow of the ophthalmic artery is present.

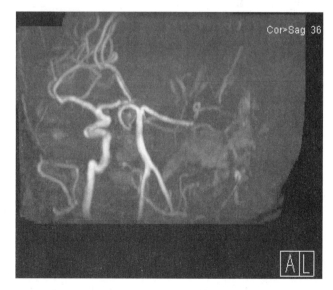

Figure 9-12. Anteroposterior cranial view of an MRA shows an occlusion of the left internal carotid artery. Secondary occlusion of the left middle cerebral artery (artery-to-artery embolism) also is found.

collateral blood flow. Research on this intervention is under way[48] (see Chapter 20).

Stump Syndrome

In addition, an acute thrombotic occlusion of the internal carotid artery can be associated with distal embolization. On the other hand, embolization appears not to be a common mechanism of stroke among persons with chronic occlusions. Emboli could arise from a stump of the internal carotid artery that is proximal to the occlusion. In this situation, thrombosis of stagnant blood can lead to emboli that reach the brain via collateral channels arising from the external carotid artery (*stump syndrome*)[49] (Fig. 9-13). While the number of operations is small, some patients have had successful plication of the stump.

Tortuosity, Kinking, and Coiling

Elderly, hypertensive persons with extensive atherosclerosis of the extracranial portion of the internal carotid artery can lead to tortuosity, kinking, and coiling[50]

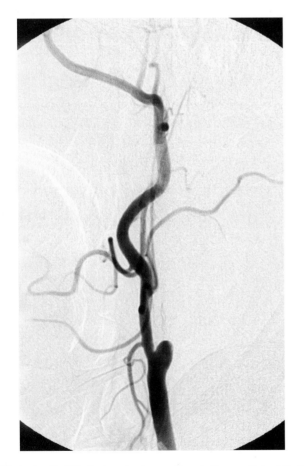

Figure 9-13. Lateral view of a left carotid arteriogram using subtraction techniques visualizes occlusion of the internal carotid artery. A residual proximal segment of the artery (stump) is seen.

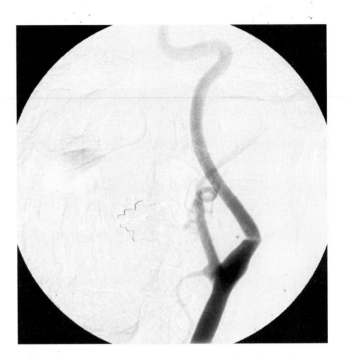

Figure 9-14. Oblique view of a left carotid arteriogram displays a kink in the proximal segment of the internal carotid artery.

(Fig. 9-14). The importance of these arterial changes, in the absence of a stenosis or occlusion, is not known.

▶ VERTEBRAL ARTERY

The most common location for atherosclerosis of the vertebral artery is in its first segment (from its origin from the subclavian artery until it enters the transverse process of the sixth cervical vertebra), typically at the ostium.[51] Scattered atherosclerotic lesions can be found in the second segment as the vertebral artery ascends via the lateral foramina of the sixth to the second cervical vertebrae. The distal segment of the vertebral artery (from the second cervical vertebra to its union with the other vertebral artery to form the basilar artery) can be the site of atherosclerotic lesions, although dissection remains an important alternative diagnosis for stenosis or occlusion at this location.

Clinical Findings

Patients with vertebral atherosclerosis can have TIA or ischemic stroke secondary to hemodynamic factors or embolism.[52,53] Symptoms manifest brain stem, cerebellar, or posterior hemispheric dysfunction. Occasionally, ischemic symptoms are provoked by changes in head posture or rotation, during which one vertebral artery is compressed and flow in the other vessel is inadequate to maintain perfusion.[54] Thrombotic occlusion of the vertebral artery can extend to the posteroinferior cerebellar artery or basilar artery.

Diagnostic Studies

The usual methods for visualizing the vertebral artery include CTA, MRA, and arteriography. Ultrasonography can detect cephalad flow in one or both vertebral arteries. Because the caliber of the two vertebral arteries often varies considerably, an atherosclerotic occlusion or stenosis of an artery needs to be differentiated from congenital findings. Rarely, a physician can hear a bruit over the affected vertebral artery. Surgical resection of an atherosclerotic stenosis of the origin of the vertebral artery can be performed, but operative repairs of the artery have been replaced by endovascular procedures.

▶ MIDDLE CEREBRAL ARTERY

Intracranial atherosclerosis can affect the first portion (M (1 segment) of the middle cerebral artery.[55] This section of the artery extends from the origin of the artery at the terminal bifurcation of the internal carotid artery to the first major division of the middle cerebral artery. The M (1 segment is the origin of the penetrating arteries to the basal ganglia and internal capsule (Fig. 9-15). Severe symptomatic stenosis of the middle cerebral artery appears to be more common among persons of African and Asian ancestry than among persons of European heritage. Advanced atherosclerosis of the middle cerebral artery also is more common among persons with diabetes mellitus or hypertension.

Clinical Findings

Ischemic symptoms result from hypoperfusion, occlusion, or distal embolization, and include TIA, a subcortical infarction, a striatocapsular infarction, a branch cortical infarction, or a major multilobar infarction[56,57] (Fig. 9-16). The symptoms mimic those that occur secondary to atherosclerosis of the internal carotid artery.

Diagnostic Studies

CT of the brain might demonstrate a dense artery sign corresponding to an acute thrombosis. However, this finding is not specific for local disease. CT can also detect calcification in the arterial walls, which can be confused with the dense artery sign. The absence of a flow void in the middle cerebral artery on MRI also corresponds with severe disease; this finding can be secondary to local thrombosis or embolism. Severe middle cerebral artery stenosis usually can be detected by arteriography, MRA, or CTA. Increases in flow velocities detected by transcranial Doppler ultrasonography also occur with severe stenoses. Differentiating a de novo

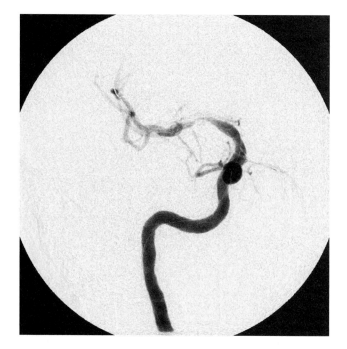

Figure 9-15. Anteroposterior view of a right carotid arteriogram using subtraction techniques demonstrates moderately severe narrowing of the first portion (M – 1 segment) of the left middle cerebral artery. This study was obtained prior to angioplasty.

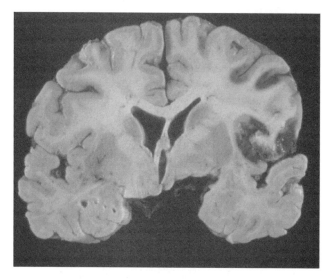

Figure 9-16. Infarction with hemorrhagic changes is seen within the left hemisphere on this coronal autopsy specimen. The findings would be consistent with artery-to-artery embolization to a branch cortical artery. In addition, multiple small cystic lesions consistent with old lacunar infarctions are found in the right temporal lobe. (*Courtesy of S.S. Schochet, M.D., Department of Pathology, University of West Virginia, Morgantown, WV*)

stenosis of the middle cerebral artery from partial recanalization of the artery following thromboembolism is an important issue. At present, no sound rules exist for making the distinction.

Treatment

Some evidence exists that anticoagulants are superior to antiplatelet aggregating agents for preventing stroke secondary to intracranial atherosclerosis. Most data are from nonrandomized studies and additional research is needed.[58,59] Creation of an extracranial-to-intracranial arterial anastomosis to improve flow distal to a middle cerebral artery stenosis was not successful.[60] There is some potential for hemorrhage because the hemodynamic changes might promote occlusion of the proximal segment of the artery. Endovascular procedures are a promising option for treatment of middle cerebral artery stenosis (see Chapter 20).

▶ BASILAR ARTERY

The middle segment of the basilar artery is a relatively common location for intracranial atherosclerosis (Fig. 9-17). It is the section of the vessel that lies imme-diately anterior to the pons and midbrain. The disease can be relatively isolated or produce a long section of narrowing.

Clinical Findings

Severe stenosis can cause recurrent TIA secondary to hypoperfusion or distal embolization.[61,62] In addition, ischemia secondary to occlusion of penetrating branches arising from the basilar artery can lead to ischemia in the pons or midbrain that produces lacunar or isolated brain stem infarctions (Fig. 9-18). Acute occlusion of the basilar artery usually leads to a massive infarction of the brain stem that can cause coma or the locked-in syndrome (Fig. 9-19).

Diagnostic Studies

CT of the brain may demonstrate calcification or a thrombus in the artery. A midsagittal MRI image can visualize a thrombus in the basilar artery, and the corresponding flow void may be absent (Fig. 9-20). MRA is relatively sensitive in detecting severe stenosis or occlusion of the basilar artery. Transcranial Doppler ultrasonography (TCD) also can be done.

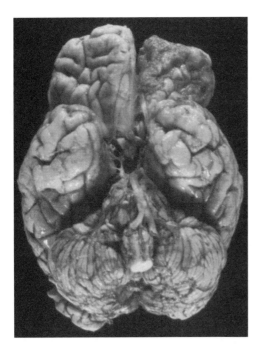

Figure 9-17. The base of the brain examined at autopsy demonstrates an old right frontal lobe infarction. In addition, areas of atherosclerotic plaque are seen in the basilar artery. The plaquing is seen as scattered in patches in the arterial wall from the external examination. (*Courtesy of S.S. Schochet, M.D., Department of Pathology, University of West Virginia, Morgantown, WV*)

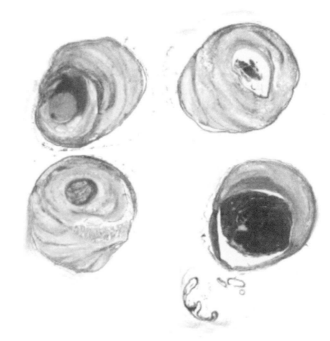

Figure 9-18. Cross section of the basilar artery using trichrome staining shows an acute occlusion of the basilar artery. Extensive atherosclerotic disease also is present. (*Courtesy of S.S. Schochet, M.D., Department of Pathology, University of West Virginia, Morgantown, WV*)

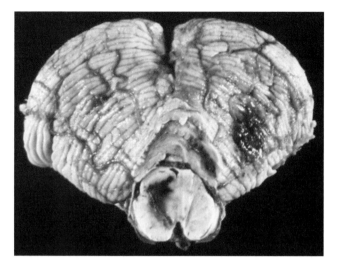

Figure 9-19. Axial autopsy specimen demonstrates hemorrhagic infarctions in the cerebellum and midbrain. Occlusion of the basilar artery also is present. The findings are consistent with occlusion of the distal segment of the basilar artery. (*Courtesy of S.S. Schochet, M.D., Department of Pathology, University of West Virginia, Morgantown, WV*)

Treatment

Treatment of severe atherosclerotic disease of the basilar artery is a challenge (Fig. 9-21). Surgery is usually not an option but endovascular procedures are being performed.[63] The risk of morbidity and mortality from these procedures is considerable.

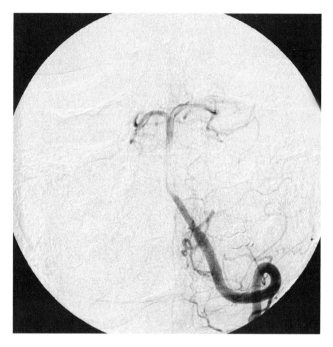

Figure 9-20. Anteroposterior view of an MRA demonstrates a high-grade stenosis of the midportion of the basilar artery.

▶ DOLICHOECTASIA

The term dolichoectasia is used to designate an elongated, enlarged, and tortuous artery. Dolichoectasia can also produce a focal fusiform change. The basilar artery

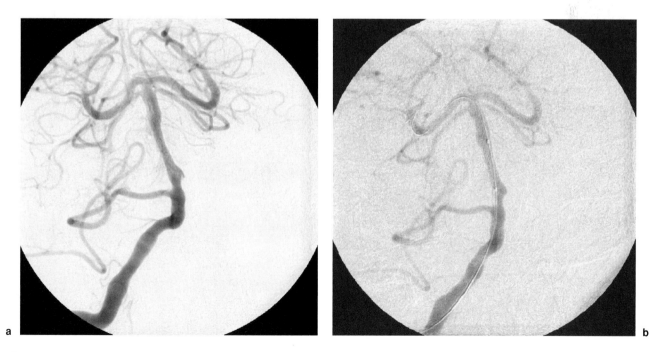

a

b

Figure 9-21. Anteroposterior views of right vertebral arteriogram show a severe stenosis of the basilar artery (a) during and (b) after angioplasty.

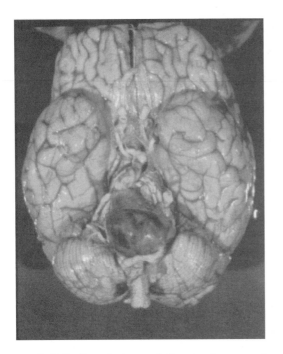

Figure 9-22. Basal view of the brain on autopsy reveals a dolichoectatic aneurysm of the basilar artery. The artery is enlarged and elongated. It is compressing adjacent structures including cranial nerves and the brain stem. (*Courtesy of S.S. Schochet, M.D., Department of Pathology, University of West Virginia, Morgantown, WV*)

is most commonly affected intracranial vessel[64,65] (Fig. 9-22). The cause of dolichoectasia is not established. While dolichoectasia can occur with *Marfan disease*, *Fabry–Anderson disease*, other inherited disorders, and *arterial dissection*, atherosclerosis also is a potential cause.[66–68] Most instances of dolichoectasia are in persons with other evidence of atherosclerosis. Much of the appearance of dolichoectasia resembles those of fusiform atherosclerotic disease elsewhere in the body. Two pathological types of dolichoectasia have been described. With classic dissecting dolichoectasia, the internal elastic lamina is damaged. In the segmental ectasia variety of dolichoectasia, abnormalities affect both the intima and the internal elastic lamina.

Clinical Findings

Because the affected artery is enlarged and elongated, it can present as a mass lying in the prepontine cistern. The long artery means that the bifurcation of the basilar artery might extend above the brain stem and it can be located in the posterior aspect of the third ventricle. The serpentine course of the artery may lead to compression of the brain stem or cranial nerves.[69] The trigeminal and facial nerves, which are most commonly affected, can cause trigeminal neuralgia, facial weakness, or hemifacial

spasm. The mass of the aneurysm might lead to recurrent headaches. Ischemia is secondary to stretching or occlusion of penetrating branches of the basilar artery, dissection of the arterial wall, or intramural or intraluminal thrombosis with embolization.[70,71] The basilar artery can also become occluded.[72] Besides recurrent TIA or ischemic stroke, intracranial hemorrhage secondary to rupture of the vessel also can occur. Occasionally, patients with dolichoectatic basilar arteries also have enlargement of the distal internal carotid arteries or the proximal segments of the middle cerebral arteries.

Diagnostic Studies

A dolichoectatic artery can be recognized as a calcified large, round lesion that is located in the prepontine cistern. The serpentine course of an enlarged artery is a characteristic finding on both MRI and CT[73,74] (Fig. 9-23). The lesion usually moves from one side of the brain stem to the other. A large or displaced flow void with an adjacent area of increased intensity (thrombus) can be detected on MRI. MRA and CTA also can readily visualize the lesion. Arteriography confirms the findings of other imaging tests and it might visualize intraluminal flaps or a double lumen. However, the need for an invasive study is not clear. Some reports suggest that the chance for morbidity secondary to the procedure is high.

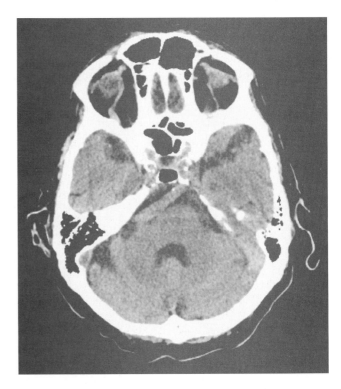

Figure 9-23. Unenhanced CT shows a linear mass in the preparation cistern. The findings are compatible with a dolichoetatic basilar artery.

Treatment

Treatment of patients with dolichoectatic basilar arteries is problematic. Surgical and endovascular procedures have been attempted.[64]

► OTHER SITES FOR ATHEROSCLEROSIS OF INTRACRANIAL ARTERIES

Approximately one-third of persons with symptomatic extracranial atherosclerosis also have intracranial disease.[75] Lesions of segmental narrowing can often be detected in the proximal portions of the posterior cerebral arteries, the proximal portions of the anterior cerebral arteries, and superficial (cortical-pial) branches. Such arterial changes are most common among diabetic persons. These changes can be detected by high-resolution MRA or CTA, but arteriography is the usual method for visualizing disseminated intracranial atherosclerosis. Because of the widespread nature of the atherosclerotic changes, the primary alternative diagnosis is intracranial vasculitis. Management of these lesions usually centers on antithrombotic medications.

► PENETRATING VESSEL OCCLUSIVE DISEASE

Occlusions of small penetrating arteries account for approximately 10–20 percent of ischemic strokes (lacunar infarctions). The clinical findings of the lacunar infarctions are described in Chapter 6. In addition, TIA can be secondary to a transient occlusion of a penetrating artery. These infarctions are generally 15–20 mm in diameter and located primarily in the basal ganglia, internal capsule, thalamus, and brain stem. Some lesions can be in the deep white matter of the hemispheres. The size of the infarction reflects the location and the size of the arterial occlusion.

On brain imaging, small subcortical infarctions (lacunes) can be readily detected. In many patients, these events are not associated with clinical symptoms (clinically silent strokes) (Fig. 9-24). The pathological hallmarks are lipohyalinosis, fibrinoid necrosis, or a small atherosclerotic plaque at the origin of the small penetrating artery (Fig. 9-25). Occlusions can be secondary to a local thrombosis or hemodynamic impairment in the microcirculation.[76]

While many clinicians think of lacunar infarctions as being secondary to a completely independent vascular disease, the clinical profile of affected patients is similar to those found among persons with large-artery atherosclerosis. In particular, the prevalence of diabetes mellitus and hypertension is particularly high. Persons

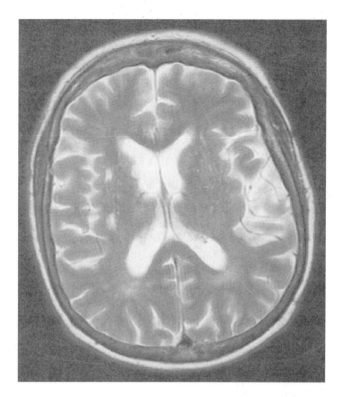

Figure 9-24. T-2-weighted MRI study shows multiple lacunar infarctions in the basal ganglia on the right.

with lacunar infarction are at high risk for thromboembolism from large-artery atherosclerosis.[77] A clinical relationship exists between occlusive penetrating artery disease (lacunar infarction) and hypertensive brain hemorrhage. Multiple lacunar infarctions are associated with vascular dementia (multi-infarct dementia).

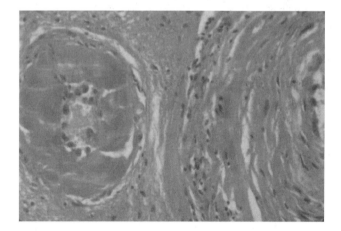

Figure 9-25. Pathological findings of disease of the small penetrating arteries of the brain are found in a patient with chronic severe hypertension. The vessel on the right shows findings of atherosclerosis, while the vessel on the left demonstrates lipohyalinosis. (*Courtesy of S.S. Schochet, M.D., Department of Pathology, University of West Virginia, Morgantown, WV*)

▶ MICROVASCULAR DISEASE OF THE BRAIN

Disseminated disease of the periventricular white matter of the cerebral hemispheres (leukoareosis) is often detected on brain imaging (CT or MRI). The lesions can be found with or without other evidence of stroke. These findings might be indirectly related to atherosclerosis because there is a relatively strong association with hypertension. While these imaging findings might not be associated with ischemic symptoms, these abnormalities can be associated with a subcortical encephalopathy (*Binswanger disease*).[78,79] Patients with this form of vascular dementia have a subacute course of neurological symptoms causing cognitive impairments, bilateral motor signs, and a pseudobulbar palsy.

▶ ATHEROSCLEROTIC DISEASE IN OTHER VASCULAR TERRITORIES

The interaction between cerebrovascular disease and atherosclerotic disease in other vascular territories is strong. Symptomatic or asymptomatic atherosclerotic cerebrovascular disease immediately identifies a patient as having a high risk for myocardial infarction and vice versa.[80] Because coronary artery disease generally becomes symptomatic at a younger age than does intracranial or extracranial atherosclerosis, most patients with severe disease of the coronary arteries already will have had symptoms of angina pectoris or myocardial infarction. In addition, many patients with stroke have a history of endovascular treatment of the coronary arteries or coronary artery bypass surgery.[81] Cardioembolic stroke is a leading complication of ischemic heart disease and its treatment (see Chapter 13). Similarly, many patients have symptomatic vascular disease in other vascular circulations including intermittent claudication, peripheral vascular reconstructive operations, or an abdominal aortic aneurysm. Patients with symptomatic peripheral vascular disease have an especially high risk for severe intracranial or extracranial atherosclerotic disease.[6,82,83] Conversely, patients with symptomatic atherosclerotic disease of the brain have an increased risk for disease of the aorta or peripheral arteries.[84]

Assessment and treatment of codeveloping coronary artery disease and peripheral vascular disease is especially important among patients with atherosclerotic disease of the central nervous system. Treatment of the risk factors predisposing to vascular disease is the first step (see Chapter 4). Management of a patient's heart disease should be included in a plan for prevention of recurrent ischemic events. In patients without cardiac symptoms, this management plan should include an evaluation to detect otherwise occult heart disease.[80]

REFERENCES

1. Falk E. Pathogenesis of atherosclerosis. *J Am Coll Cardiol* 2006;47(8 Suppl):C7–C12.
2. Li S, Chen W, Srinivasan SR, et al. Childhood cardiovascular risk factors and carotid vascular changes in adulthood. The Bogalusa Heart Study. *JAMA* 2003;290:2271–2276.
3. Raitakari OT, Juonala M, Kähönen M, et al. Cardiovascular risk factors in childhood and carotid artery intima-media thickness in adulthood. The Cardiovascular Risk in Young Finns Study. *JAMA* 2003;290:2277–2283.
4. Voetsch B, Loscalzo J. Genetic determinants of arterial thrombosis. *Arterioscler Thromb Vasc Biol* 2003;24:216–229.
5. van der Meer IM, del Sol AI, Hak AE, Bots ML, Hofman A, Witteman JCM. Risk factors for progression of atherosclerosis measured at multiple sites in the arterial tree. The Rotterdam Study. *Stroke* 2003;34:2374–2379.
6. Alexandrova NA, Gibson WC, Norris JW, Maggisano R. Carotid artery stenosis in peripheral vascular disease. *J Vasc Surg* 1996;23:645–649.
7. Stoll G, Bendszus M. Inflammation and atherosclerosis: novel insights into plaque formation and destabilization. *Stroke* 2006;37:1923–1932.
8. Cheng C, Tempel D, van Haperen R, et al. Atherosclerosis lesion size and vulnerability are determined by patterns of fluid sheer stress. *Circulation* 2006;113:2744–2753.
9. Navab M, Fogelman AM, Berliner JA, et al. Pathogenesis of atherosclerosis. *Am J Cardiol* 1995;76:18C–23C.
10. Forrester JS. Prevention of plaque rupture: a new paradigm of therapy. *Ann Intern Med* 2002;137:823–833.
11. Chamorro A. Role of inflammation in stroke and atherothrombosis. *Cerebrovasc Dis* 2004;17(suppl 3):1–5.
12. Ridker PM, Hennekens C, Buring JE, Rifai N. C-reactive protein and other markers of inflammation in the prediction of cardiovascular disease in women. *N Engl J Med* 2002;342:836–843.
13. Ridker PM. Inflammatory biomarkers, statins, and the risk of stroke: cracking a clinical conundrum. *Circulation* 2002;105:2583–2585.
14. Ridker PM, Buring JE, Cook NR, Rifai N. C-reactive protein, the metabolic syndrome, and risk of incident cardiovascular events. An 8-year follow-up of 14,719 initially healthy American women. *Circulation* 2003;107:391–397.
15. Arenillas JF, Alvarez-Sabín J, Molina CA, et al. C-reactive protein predicts further ischemic events in first-ever transient ischemic attack or stroke patients with intracranial large-artery occlusive disease. *Stroke* 2003;34:2463–2468.
16. Hennerici MG. The unstable plaque. *Cerebrovasc Dis* 2004;17(suppl 3):17–22.
17. Yuan C, Zhang SX, Polissar NL, et al. Identification of fibrous cap rupture with magnetic resonance imaging is highly associated with recent transient ischemic attack or stroke. *Circulation* 2002;105:181–185.
18. Virmani R, Burke AP, Farb A, Kolodgie FD. Pathology of the vulnerable plaque. *J Am Coll Cardiol* 2006;47(8 Suppl): C13–C18.
19. Carr S, Farb A, Pearce WH, Virmani R, Yao JS. Atherosclerotic plaque rupture in symptomatic carotid artery stenosis. *J Vasc Surg* 1996;23:755–765.

20. Bruno A, Russell PW, Jones WL, Austin JK, Weinstein ES, Steel SR. Concomitants of asymptomatic retinal cholesterol emboli. *Stroke* 1992;23:900–902.

21. Geraci A, Weinberger J. Natural history of aortic arch atherosclerotic plaque. *Neurology* 2000;54:749–751.

22. Ehlermann P, Mirau W, Jahn J, Remppis A, Sheikhzadeh A. Predictive value of inflammatory and hemostatic parameters, atherosclerotic risk factors, and chest x-ray for aortic arch atheromatosis. *Stroke* 2004;35:34–39.

23. Schwammenthal E, Schwammenthal Y, Tanne D, et al. Transcutaneous detection of aortic arch atheromas by suprasternal harmonic imaging. *J Am Coll Cardiol* 2002;39:1127–1132.

24. Jones EF, Donnan GA. The proximal aorta: a source of stroke. *Baillieres Clin Neurol* 1995;4:207–220.

25. Cohen A, Tzourio C, Bertrand B, Chauvel C, Bousser MG, Amarenco P. Aortic plaque morphology and vascular events: a follow-up study in patients with ischemic stroke. FAPS Investigators. French Study of Aortic Plaques in Stroke. *Circulation* 1997;96:3838–3841.

26. The French Study of Aortic Plaques in Stroke Group. Atherosclerotic disease of the aortic arch as a risk factor for recurrent ischemic stroke. *N Engl J Med* 1999;334:1216–1221.

27. Hollander M, Hak AE, Koudstaal PJ, et al. Comparison between measures of atherosclerosis and risk of stroke. The Rotterdam Study. *Stroke* 2003;34:2367–2372.

28. Jones EF, Kalman JM, Calafiore P, Tonkin AM, Donnan GA. Proximal aortic atheroma. An independent risk factor for cerebral ischemia. *Stroke* 1995;26:218–224.

29. Stern A, Tunick PA, Culliford AT, et al. Protruding aortic arch atheromas: risk of stroke during heart surgery with and without aortic arch endarterectomy. *Am Heart J* 1999;138:746–752.

30. Crawford ES. The diagnosis and management of aortic dissection. *JAMA* 1990;264:2537–2541.

31. Spittell PC, Spittell JAJ, Joyce JW, et al. Clinical features and differential diagnosis of aortic dissection: experience with 236 cases (1980 through 1990). *Mayo Clin Proc* 1993;68:642–651.

32. Flemming KD, Brown RD, Jr. Acute cerebral infarction caused by aortic dissection. Caution in the thrombolytic era. *Stroke* 1999;30:477–478.

33. Kimura BJ, Phan JN, Housman LB. Utility of contrast echocardiography in the diagnosis of aortic dissection. *J Am Soc Echocardiogr* 1999;12:155–159.

34. Jungers P, Massy ZA, Khoa TN, et al. Incidence and risk factors of atherosclerotic cardiovascular accidents in predialysis chronic renal failure patients: a prospective study. *Nephrol Dial Transplant* 1997;12:2597–2602.

35. Fields WS, Lemak NA. Joint Study of Extracranial Arterial Occlusion. VII. Subclavian steal—a review of 168 cases. *JAMA* 1972;222:1139–1143.

36. de Bray JM, Zenglein JP, Laroche JP, et al. Effect of subclavian syndrome on the basilar artery. *Acta Neurol Scand* 1994;90:174–178.

37. Zelenock GB, Cronenwett JL, Graham LM, et al. Brachiocephalic arterial occlusions and stenoses. Manifestations and management of complex lesions. *Arch Surg* 1985;120:370–376.

38. Law MM, Colburn MD, Moore WS, Quinones-Baldrich WJ, Machleder HI, Gelabert HA. Carotid-subclavian bypass for brachiocephalic occlusive disease. Choice of conduit and long-term follow-up. *Stroke* 1995;26:1565–1571.

39. Ogino M, Nagumo M, Nakagawa T, Nakatsukasa M, Murase I. Axilloaxillary bypass for the treatment of subclavian artery stenosis complicated by bilateral common artery occlusion: technical case report. *Neurosurgery* 2003;53:444–447.

40. Prati P, Vanuzzo D, Casaroli M, et al. Prevalence and determinants of carotid atherosclerosis in a general population. *Stroke* 1992;23:1705–1711.

41. Fine-Edelstein JS, Wolf PA, O'Leary DH, et al. Precursors of extracranial carotid atherosclerosis in the Framingham Study. *Neurology* 1994;44:1046–1050.

42. Johnston SC, O'Meara ES, Manolio TA, et al. Cognitive impairment and decline are associated with carotid artery disease in patients without clinical evident cerebrovascular disease. *Ann Intern Med* 2004;140:237–247.

43. Rouleau PA, Huston J, Gilbertson J, et al. Carotid artery tandem lesions: frequency of angiographic detection and consequences for endarterectomy. *AJNR Am J Neuroradiol* 1999;20:621–625.

44. van Everdingen KJ, Visser GH, Klijn CJ, Kappelle LJ, van der Grond J. Role of collateral flow on cerebral hemodynamics in patients with unilateral internal carotid artery occlusion. *Ann Neurol* 1998;44:167–176.

45. Powers WJ, Derdeyn CP, Fritsch SM, et al. Benign prognosis of never-symptomatic carotid occlusion. *Neurology* 2000;54:878–882.

46. Grubb RL, Jr., Derdeyn CP, Fritsch SM, et al. Importance of hemodynamic factors in the prognosis of symptomatic carotid occlusion. *JAMA* 1998;280:1055–1060.

47. Hankey GJ, Warlow CP. Prognosis of symptomatic carotid artery occlusion. *Cerebrovasc Dis* 1991;1:245–256.

48. Adams HP, Jr., Powers WJ, Grubb RLJ, Clarke WR, Woolson RF. Preview of a new trial of extracranial-to-intracranial arterial anastomosis: the carotid occlusion surgery study. *Neurosurg Clin N Am* 2000;12:613–624.

49. Ryan PG, Day AL. Stump embolization from an occluded internal carotid artery. Case report. *J Neurosurg* 1987;67:609–611.

50. Del Corso L, Moruzzo D, Conte B, et al. Tortuosity, kinking, and coiling of the carotid artery: expression of atherosclerosis or aging? *Angiology* 1998;49:361–371.

51. Wityk RJ, Chang HM, Rosengart A, et al. Proximal extracranial vertebral artery disease in the New England Medical Center Posterior Circulation Registry. *Arch Neurol* 1998;55:470–478.

52. Koroshetz WJ, Ropper AH. Artery-to-artery embolism causing stroke in the posterior circulation. *Neurology* 1987;37:292–295.

53. Caplan LR, Amarenco P, Rosengart A, et al. Embolism from vertebral artery origin occlusive disease. *Neurology* 1992;42:1505–1512.

54. Kuether TA, Nesbit GM, Clark WM, Barnwell SL. Rotational vertebral artery occlusion: a mechanism of vertebrobasilar insufficiency. *Neurosurgery* 1997;41:427–432.

55. Ueda S, Fujitsu K, Inomori S, Kuwabara T. Thrombotic occlusion of the middle cerebral artery. *Stroke* 1992;23:1761–1766.

56. Caplan L, Babikian V, Helgason C, et al. Occlusive disease of the middle cerebral artery. *Neurology* 1985;35:975–982.

57. Lyrer PA, Engelter S, Radu EW, Steck AJ. Cerebral infarcts related to isolated middle cerebral artery stenosis. *Stroke* 1997;28:1022–1027.

58. Benesch CG, Chimowitz MI, for the WASID Investigators. Best treatment of intracranial arterial stenosis? 50 years of uncertainty. *Neurology* 2000;55:465–466.

59. Thijs VN, Albers GW. Symptomatic intracranial atherosclerosis. Outcome of patients who fail antithrombotic therapy. *Neurology* 2000;55:490–497.

60. The EC/IC Bypass Study Group. Failure of extracranial-intracranial arterial bypass to reduce the risk of ischemic stroke. Results of an international randomized trial. *N Engl J Med* 1985;313:1191–1200.

61. Muller-Kuppers M, Graf KJ, Pessin MS, DeWitt LD, Caplan LR. Intracranial vertebral artery disease in the New England Medical Center Posterior Circulation Registry. *Eur Neurol* 1997;37:146–156.

62. Pessin MS, Gorelick PB, Kwan ES, Caplan LR. Basilar artery stenosis: middle and distal segments. *Neurology* 1987;37:1742–1746.

63. Nakatsuka H, Ueda T, Ohta S, Sakaki S. Successful percutaneous transluminal angioplasty for basilar artery stenosis: technical case report. *Neurosurgery* 1996;39:161–164.

64. Anson JA, Lawton MT, Spetzler RF. Characteristics and surgical treatment of dolichoectatic and fusiform aneurysms. *J Neurosurg* 1996;84:185–193.

65. Nakatomi H, Segawa H, Kurata A, et al. Clinicopathological study of intracranial fusiform and dolichoectatic aneurysms. Insight on the mechanism of growth. *Stroke* 2000;31:896–900.

66. Maisey DN, Cosh JA. Basilar artery aneurysm and Anderson–Fabry disease. *J Neurol Neurosurg Psychiatry* 1980;43:85–87.

67. Mizutani T. A fatal, chronically growing basilar artery: a new type of dissecting aneurysm. *J Neurosurg* 1996;84:962–971.

68. Mizutani T, Miki Y, Kojima H, Suzuki H. Proposed classification of nonatherosclerotic cerebral fusiform and dissecting aneurysms. *Neurosurgery* 1999;45:253–260.

69. Echiverri HC, Rubino FA, Gupta SR, Gujrati M. Fusiform aneurysm of the vertebrobasilar arterial system. *Stroke* 1989;20:1741–1747.

70. Kumral E, Kisabay A, Atac C, et al. The mechanism of ischemic stroke in patients with dolichoectactic basilar artery. *Eur J Neurol* 2005;12:437–444.

71. Besson G, Bogousslavsky J, Moulin T, Hommel M. Vertebrobasilar infarcts in patients with dolichoectatic basilar artery. *Acta Neurol Scand* 1995;91:37–42.

72. Watanabe T, Sato K, Yoshimoto T. Basilar artery occlusion caused by thrombosis of atherosclerotic fusiform aneurysm of the basilar artery. *Stroke* 1994;25:1068–1070.

73. Aichner FT, Felber SR, Birbamer GG, Posch A. Magnetic resonance imaging and magnetic resonance angiography of vertebrobasilar dolichoectasia. *Cerebrovasc Dis* 1993;3:280–284.

74. Vishteh AG, Spetzler RF. Evolution of a dolichoectatic aneurysm into a giant serpentine aneurysm during long-term follow up. *J Neurosurg* 1999;91:346.

75. Kappelle LJ, Eliaziw M, Fox AJ, Sharpe BL, Barnett HJM, for the North American Symptomatic Carotid Endarterectomy Trial (NASCET) Group. Importance of intracranial atherosclerotic disease in patients with symptomatic stenosis of the internal carotid artery. *Stroke* 1999;30:282–286.

76. Terai S, Hori T, Miake S, Tamaki KSA. Mechanism in progressive lacunar infarction: a case report with magnetic resonance imaging. *Arch Neurol* 2000;57:225–232.

77. Kappelle LJ, Koudstaal PJ, van Gijn J, Ramos LM, Keunen JE. Carotid angiography in patients with lacunar infarction. A prospective study. *Stroke* 1988;19:1093–1096.

78. Caplan L, Schoene WC. Clinical features of subcortical arteriosclerotic encephalopathy (Binswanger disease). *Neurology* 1978;28:1206–1215.

79. Kinkel WR, Jacobs L, Polachini I, Bates V, Heffner RR, Jr. Subcortical arteriosclerotic encephalopathy (Binswanger's disease). Computed tomographic, nuclear magnetic resonance, and clinical correlations. *Arch Neurol* 1985;42:951–959.

80. Adams RJ, Chimowitz MI, Alpert JS, et al. Coronary risk evaluation in patients with transient ischemic attack and ischemic stroke: a scientific statement of healthcare professionals from the Stroke Council and the Council on Clinical Cardiology of the American Heart Association/American Stroke Association. *Circulation* 2003;108:1278–1290.

81. Whisnant JP, Brown RD, Petty GW, O'Fallon WM, Sicks JD, Wiebers DO. Comparison of population-based models of risk factors for TIA and ischemic stroke. *Neurology* 1999;53:532–536.

82. Ogren M, Hedblad B, Isacsson SO, Janzon L, Jungquist G, Lindell SE. Non-invasively detected carotid stenosis and ischaemic heart disease in men with leg arteriosclerosis. *Lancet* 1993;342:1138–1141.

83. Smith FB, Rumley A, Lee AJ, Leng GC, Fowkes FG, Lowe GD. Haemostatic factors and prediction of ischaemic heart disease and stroke in claudicants. *Br J Haematol* 1998;100:758–763.

84. Karanjia PN, Madden KP, Lobner S. Coexistence of abdominal aortic aneurysm in patients with carotid stenosis. *Stroke* 1994;25:627–630.

CHAPTER 10

Nonatherosclerotic, Noninflammatory Arteriopathies Causing Ischemic Stroke

While atherosclerosis is the most common arterial pathology among persons with cerebrovascular disease, several nonatherosclerotic arteriopathies can cause ischemic stroke. Less commonly, some of these arteriopathies are associated with hemorrhagic events. Although these arteriopathies account for a small percentage of strokes, their importance as a cause of stroke in children and young adults is considerable. In addition, some of these arterial diseases should be considered when a patient has an atypical presentation for stroke. The nonatherosclerotic vasculopathies can be acquired or be secondary to an inherited disease. The genetic arterial diseases leading to brain ischemia are described in Chapter 12. The acquired arteriopathies are divided into inflammatory (vasculitis) or noninflammatory diseases. The inflammatory arteriopathies can be subdivided into diseases that are secondary to infectious or noninfectious (autoimmune) causes. These diseases are described in Chapter 11. A smaller number of acquired, noninflammatory arteriopathies that cause stroke are discussed in this chapter (Table 10-1).

▶ ARTERIAL DISSECTION

Dissection of an intracranial or extracranial artery is recognized increasingly as a leading cause of cerebral ischemia in either the anterior or posterior circulation. Arterial dissection probably is second only to atherosclerosis as a cause of large-artery stroke. The incidence of symptomatic extracranial or intracranial arterial dissection is estimated as approximately 2.6 (0.9 – 4.2) per 100,000.[1] Arterial dissection is most commonly diagnosed in children, adolescents, and young adults.[2] Some of the high rate of arterial dissection in younger persons probably is secondary to the high rate of trauma secondary to sports or other strenuous activities. In particular, the disease is an important consideration if the neurological symptoms have occurred in close proximity to trauma or if a young person does not have any of the traditional risk factors for premature atherosclerosis. In addition, the diagnosis of arterial dissection is considered as a possible cause of stroke or transient ischemic attack (TIA) in a young adult more readily than in older persons. A classical scenario is a stroke occurring in a young person who has intense neck or head pain that corresponds to the symptomatic artery. Besides ischemic stroke, other clinical presentations include TIA, ocular ischemia, cranial nerve palsies, headache, face or neck pain, or subarachnoid hemorrhage.

Pathophysiology

Arterial dissection can follow cranial or cervical trauma in which there is hyperrotation or hyperextension of

► **TABLE 10-1.** NONATHEROSCLEROTIC, NONINFLAMMATORY ARTERIOPATHIES THAT CAUSE ISCHEMIC STROKE

Arterial dissection
   Traumatic
   Spontaneous (nontraumatic)
Arterial injuries
   Blunt
   Penetrating
   Posttraumatic vasospasm
Compressive arterial occlusion
Radiation-induced vasculopathy
Fibromuscular dysplasia
Buerger disease
Saccular aneurysm
Moyamoya syndrome

► **TABLE 10-2.** LOCATIONS OF ARTERIAL DISSECTIONS

Internal carotid artery
   1.5–2 cm above the carotid bifurcation
   At base of skull or penetration of dura
Vertebral artery
   Penetrates the dura at the C – 1 vertebra—foramen magnum
   Proximal segment (C – 6)
Middle cerebral artery
   Proximal segment adjacent to base of skull
Basilar artery
   Middle segment

the neck (Table 10-2). The injury usually involves the stretching of the artery against a bony prominence, during which the artery is tethered by structures such as a foramen at the base of the skull, the dura, soft tissue of the neck, or the vertebra. The intimal surface of the artery is torn and blood enters the wall (Fig. 10-1(a) and 10-1(b)). The blood tears (dissects) through the tissue of the medial layer of the arterial wall. The accumulation of the blood within the arterial wall usually leads to compression of the lumen that produces a long area of stenosis or an occlusion. The cephalad dissection of the blood can cause a distal tear in the intimal surface, and a new (false) lumen can develop. A large collection of blood leads to formation of a false aneurysm. In addition, the dissection can cause occlusion of the orifices of small branches. Thus, an ischemic event can be secondary to artery-to-artery embolism, hypoperfusion, or local thrombosis. While a dissection may traverse all three layers of the arterial wall leading to an extravascular hematoma, this scenario is most likely to occur with an intracranial dissection that causes a subarachnoid hemorrhage. The mechanisms of arterial pathology and stroke among persons with spontaneous dissection probably are similar to those that occur with traumatic dissections. Spontaneous dissections usually are secondary to an underlying arterial pathology that weakens the arterial intima. Presumably, very subtle or occult trauma or some other incident might promote the spontaneous tear in the intimal surface. The anatomic relationships of the cervical arteries and the other neck structures, and the wide range of mobility of the neck are the major explanations for the finding that most arterial dissections involve the extracranial arteries. However, not all segments of the extracranial arteries are equally vulnerable.[3] The most common locations of arterial dissections are given in Table 10-2.

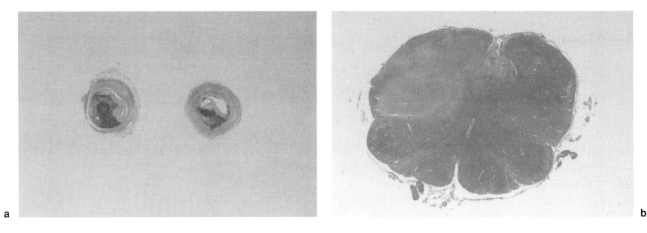

a   b

Figure 10-1. (a) Cross section of the right vertebral artery shows an arterial dissection. The residual lumen is displaced lateral and is compressed by an intramural thrombus located within the dissection. (b) Cross section of the medulla reveals an infarction in the dorsolateral aspect of the medulla. The infarction was secondary to the dissection. (*Courtesy of S. S. Schochet, M.D., Department of Pathology, University of West Virginia, Morgantown, WV*)

Traumatic Dissections

Traumatic dissections can complicate major craniocervical trauma, including falls or motor vehicle crashes.[4] Either the extracranial carotid or vertebral artery is the most commonly affected location. Besides causing infarction in the brain, a vertebral artery dissection that complicates cervical trauma might lead to infarction of the spinal cord. An arterial dissection should be suspected if a patient has major focal neurological impairments following craniocerebral trauma but brain imaging does not demonstrate hemorrhage. In addition, the infarction might not occur in conjunction with the arterial injury—a lag of a few hours or days might occur. Presumably, this lag is secondary to subsequent formation of a thrombus that is then dislodged to go to the brain. Growth of the intramural thrombus also may lead to compression of the lumen and secondary ischemia.

Dissection of cervical arteries (carotid or vertebral) also may complicate sporting activities that involve sudden or brief rotational, torsional, or hyperextension movements of the neck[5–7] (Table 10-3). For example, dissection is a potential complication of a whiplash injury.[8] Sports associated with frequent falls, such as skiing, are most often complicated by arterial dissections. Dissection of the vertebral artery has complicated self-manipulation of the neck or yoga exercises. Chiropractic manipulation of the neck also is described as a cause of vertebral artery dissection.[9,10] A study from California supports a cause-and-effect relationship between cervical manipulation and the arterial lesion.[11] Dissection has followed hyperextension of the neck during endotracheal intubation, surgical procedures, or labor or delivery.[12] Dissection of the internal carotid artery has followed attempted strangulation during domestic violence. Malek et al.[13] described three young women who developed arterial dissections

▶ **TABLE 10-3.** ACTIVITIES ASSOCIATED WITH TRAUMATIC DISSECTIONS

Sports	
Treadmill	Motor cross
Skiing	Cycling
Wrestling	Golf
Basketball	Football
Volleyball	Archery
Martial arts	Baseball
Equestrian	Softball
Other activities	
Sneezing	Coughing
Playing instruments	Yoga
Self-manipulation	Attempted strangulation
Medical procedures	
Needle aspiration	
Chiropractic manipulation	Endotracheal intubation
Surgical procedures	Labor and delivery

▶ **TABLE 10-4.** CONDITIONS PREDISPOSING TO SPONTANEOUS ARTERIAL DISSECTION

Fibromuscular dysplasia	Cystic medial necrosis
Osteogenesis imperfecta	α-1-antitrypsin deficiency
Marfan syndrome	Ehlers–Danlos III collagen deficiency
Dilation of the aortic root	Mitral dystrophy
Mitral valve prolapse	Aortic valve dystrophy

3 months to 1 year following attempted strangulation by their spouses. Dissections also have complicated playing of a wind instrument or violent coughing or sneezing.[14]

Spontaneous Dissections and Associated Conditions

Some of the traumatic dissections probably reflect an underlying arterial lesion that predisposes to the response. In addition, some patients with dissection do not have any history of trauma and these events are called spontaneous dissection. In these cases, an underlying acquired or inherited predisposition is assumed (Table 10-4). While some of the associations (for example, migraine) probably do not represent a cause-and-effect relationship, other arteriopathies such as fibromuscular dysplasia (FMD) and cystic medial necrosis probably are predisposing factors.[15,16] Dissection can complicate infections in the neck or throat.[17–19] Familial clustering of some cases has raised consideration of disorders such as Marfan syndrome or Ehlers–Danlos type III.[16,20–22] Research on the connections between inherited or acquired arterial diseases and dissections is ongoing. For example, Vila et al.[23] recently reported on the potential relationship between α-1-antitrypsin and spontaneous cervical dissection. In the latter, a gap defect in the internal elastic lamina is speculated to be the underlying pathological finding that leads to the vulnerability to dissection. An underlying arteriopathy should be sought if a patient has more than one arterial dissection. This information may affect the patient's prognosis or decisions about medical treatment.

Clinical Findings of Carotid Artery Dissection

The interval from the time of arterial dissection until the appearance of symptoms can range from a few minutes to 1 month but most patients have symptoms within 1 week of the arterial injury.[24] Most cases of infarction secondary to arterial dissection probably are on the basis of thromboembolism.[25] Dissections of the *extracranial portion of the internal carotid artery* can produce ocular or cerebral ischemia in addition to cranial nerve palsies, Horner syndrome, and intense pain[26–29] (Table 10-5). The presence of an ipsilateral Horner syndrome in combination with a contralateral hemiparesis, sensory

▶ **TABLE 10-5.** CLINICAL FEATURES OF DISSECTION OF THE EXTRACRANIAL PORTION OF THE INTERNAL CAROTID ARTERY

Hemispheric ischemia
    Transient ischemic attack
    Cerebral infarction
        Entire middle cerebral artery territory
        Lenticulostriate territory
        Branch cortical artery territory
        Watershed territory
Ocular ischemia
    Amaurosis fugax
    Anterior or posterior ischemic optic neuropathy
    Branch retinal artery infarction
Intense ipsilateral eye, ear, or face pain
Ipsilateral headache
Intense neck pain or carotidynia
Horner syndrome
Pulsatile tinnitus and cranial or cervical bruit
Isolated or multiple cranial nerve palsies
    Ophthalmoparesis (III, IV, or VI)
    Other (VII, IX, X, XI, or XII)

loss, and cognitive impairments is highly suggestive of a dissection of an internal carotid artery—especially if these findings are accompanied by ipsilateral neck pain and if they are found in a young adult.[30] Besides ischemia and Horner syndrome, other ocular findings include proptosis, chemosis, optic disk edema, and ophthalmoparesis.[26,29,31,32] The cranial nerve palsies are due to compression by the arterial lesion or from ischemia because of secondary involvement of penetrating arteries.[33] Approximately 5–40 percent of patients with carotid dissections can have a secondary false aneurysm, which can present as a pulsatile mass in the neck or with compression of the extracranial segments of the lower cranial nerves. Headache or neck pain is a prominent symptom, and in some cases pain may be the chief complaint.[27,34,35] The pain usually is along the sternocleidomastoid muscle (carotidynia).

Clinical Findings of Vertebral Artery Dissection

Vertebral artery dissection (Table 10-6) most commonly leads to an infarction of the dorsolateral medulla (*Wallenberg syndrome*)[36–38] (see Fig. 1-1(a) and 1-1(b)). Dissection probably is the leading cause of Wallenberg syndrome in young adults and is a leading alternative diagnosis for atherosclerosis in older persons. Isolated cerebellar infarction, in the territory of the posteroinferior cerebellar artery, is less common. Progression of the arterial lesion or the intraluminal thrombus can lead to occlusion of the basilar artery, with a major brain stem infarction or distal embolization. Besides the ischemic symptoms, patients usually have intense ipsilateral

▶ **TABLE 10-6.** CLINICAL FEATURES OF DISSECTION OF THE VERTEBRAL ARTERY

Brain stem and cerebellar ischemia
    Transient ischemic attack
    Infarction
        Dorsolateral medullary
        Pontine
        Inferior cerebellar
        Top of the basilar
Spinal cord ischemia
Occipital or nuchal pain
Subarachnoid hemorrhage
Cranial nerve palsies

nuchal or occipital pain.[35] The pain usually precedes the ischemic symptoms. Subarachnoid hemorrhage and mass effects causing compression of cranial nerves are less common symptoms. The features of secondary subarachnoid hemorrhage are similar to those associated with bleeding from other sources.

Clinical Findings of Other Arteries

Dissections of the intracranial arteries are much less common; the most common sites are the basilar artery and the middle cerebral artery.[39–41] Intracranial dissections can cause subarachnoid hemorrhage or infarction in the respective vascular bed.[42] Basilar artery dissection can lead to brain stem infarction, and the lesion can mimic a fusiform or dolichoectatic aneurysm.

Diagnostic Studies

Brain imaging, especially magnetic resonance imaging (MRI), of the base of the skull or neck can image the arterial lesion (Table 10-7). MRI has a sensitivity and

▶ **TABLE 10-7.** RESULTS OF DIAGNOSTIC IMAGING OF ARTERIAL DISSECTIONS

MRI/CT
    Eccentric flow void or lumen
    Intramural deposit of blood density
    Patterns
        Curvilinear
        Bandlike
        Crescentic
        Bamboo-cut
Carotid duplex
    Absent flow
    High-resistance pattern
Arteriography
    Tapered narrowing—occlusion
    Sting sign
    Intimal flap
    False aneurysm—either globular or fusiform in shape
    Double lumen

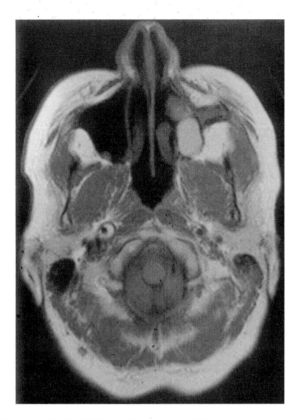

Figure 10-2. MRI of the base of the brain demonstrates a dissection of the right internal carotid artery. The normal lesion is displaced by the intramural hematoma.

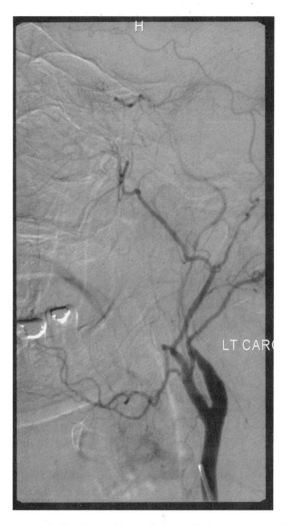

Figure 10-3. Dissection of the left internal carotid artery is shown on a lateral view of an arteriogram. The vessel tapers and then becomes occluded approximately 1.5 cm above the bifurcation.

specificity of approximately 85–99 percent respectively for detecting dissections of the internal carotid artery[43] (Fig. 10-2). However, the yield is slightly lower for finding vertebral artery lesions.[44] While the yield of computed tomography (CT) is lower than that of MRI, the test can demonstrate the arterial abnormality. The classic finding is an eccentric flow void of decreased caliber in the artery with an adjacent semilunar hyperdensity.[38,44] The latter finding is secondary to the blood sequestered within the arterial wall. The area of the hyperdensity has been described as curvilinear, band-like, crescentic, or bamboo-cut in appearance. The flow void might be absent if the artery is occluded. Because the brain imaging findings are very specific for arterial dissection, additional vascular imaging studies might not be needed.

Evaluation of the vasculature, including digital arteriography, can be done to confirm the arterial lesion (see Table 10-7). The usual finding is a tapered narrowing of the artery that can progress to an occlusion. The long area of narrowing is often described as the string sign (Figs. 10-3 and 10-4). Other patterns can include a flap, a false aneurysm, or a double lumen. The latter occurs when the flow of blood exits the arterial wall distally. The false aneurysms usually are fusiform and

globular in appearance. When the aneurysms are intracranial, they can be differentiated from saccular aneurysms primarily by their location, which is usually not at an arterial bifurcation.[39] Although carotid duplex usually cannot directly image a dissection of the internal carotid artery distal to the bifurcation, it can detect distal decreases in flow.[45,46] The types of diminished flow including an absent signal, a biphasic pattern, or a high-resistance pattern have a sensitivity and specificity of approximately 80 percent in diagnosing a dissection. Transcranial Doppler ultrasonography can be used to detect dissections of the vertebral or basilar artery. Sequential imaging studies can be used to monitor the course of the arterial lesion.[47–49]

Prognosis

In general, the patient's prognosis reflects the severity of the neurological injury.[40] The prognosis of patients with

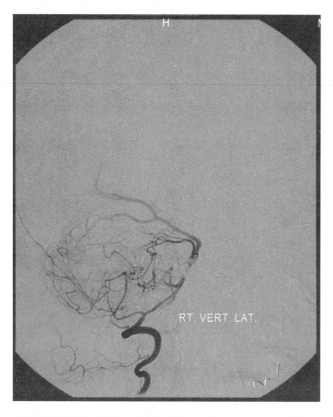

Figure 10-4. Dissection of the distal right vertebral artery is found on a lateral view of an arteriogram. The dissection involves the segment of the artery as it penetrates the dura at the level of the foramen magnum.

subarachnoid hemorrhage is poorer than that of patients with ischemic events; approximately 75 percent of patients with intracranial bleeding die. As with infarctions of other arterial causes, patients with severe neurological impairments have a relatively high risk for death or serious neurological residuals. Patients with minor stroke, TIA, ocular ischemia, or local signs have a favorable prognosis.[28]

The long-term prognosis of patients with arterial dissection is usually good. Some of the favorable prognosis probably reflects the overall good health of the affected young adults. Recanalization of the artery usually occurs within the first few months.[48] Recurrent ischemic events are relatively uncommon. Recurrent arterial dissection also is relatively uncommon.[49,50] Recurrent dissection seems to be more likely among patients with familial arteriopathies.

Treatment

Clinical trials have not tested any specific therapy for treatment of patients with stroke secondary to arterial dissection. Some patients with arterial dissection have been treated with thrombolytic agents, although some risk of promoting the arterial injury might occur. Urgent

anticoagulation is often recommended with the goal of limiting the intraluminal thrombus or distal embolism, but no data are available to support this intervention. As with thrombolytic therapy, anticoagulation might promote the arterial dissection. Both anticoagulation and thrombolytic therapy might be dangerous when treating a patient with a vertebral dissection because of the potential for subarachnoid hemorrhage. Long-term oral anticoagulant therapy also has been recommended but data are not available to buttress this treatment. The necessity for anticoagulants seems weak because the overall long-term prognosis of patients with arterial dissections is relatively good. Antiplatelet agents might be as effective. In addition, issues related to compliance and trauma-associated bleeding in a group of physically active young adults probably are less with antiplatelet agents. A systemic review noted that no trials have tested the utility of either anticoagulants or antiplatelet agents in prevention of recurrent stroke and that a trial testing medical therapies is needed.[51]

Revascularization procedures include ligation, resection, or reconstruction of the artery.[52–54] The surgical procedures have been usually directed at the extracranial portions of the vertebral or internal carotid arteries. Muller et al.[55] reported on surgical treatment of 48 patients with dissections of the extracranial portion of the internal carotid artery. Resection and vein graft replacement with restoration of flow was achieved in 40 cases. One patient died from a hemorrhagic stroke and five others had minor ischemic strokes. Cranial nerve injuries developed in 29 cases. Bypass operations and surgical treatment of an aneurysm also can be considered. Although dissection is a potential complication of angioplasty and stenting, endovascular treatment of an arterial dissection also can be done.[56] The utility of these surgical procedures has not been tested.

▶ ARTERIAL INJURIES

Besides arterial dissections, blunt or penetrating arterial injuries of the extracranial arteries can lead to cerebral or spinal cord infarction.[57] Such injuries could complicate motor vehicle crashes, falls, sports-related injuries, or neck trauma[4,58–60] (Table 10-8). In addition, trauma can cause intracranial arterial injuries. Subarachnoid hemorrhage following craniocerebral trauma also can induce vasospasm to produce brain ischemia.

Carotid artery injury can result from a brief violent movement or sustained pressure on the artery by a postural change.[4,61] A blow to the neck could cause the fracture of an atherosclerotic plaque of the internal carotid artery in an older person, which promotes a local thrombosis. Blunt trauma to the carotid artery in the tonsillar fossa also can lead to occlusion.[62] A potential

► **TABLE 10-8.** STROKE RELATED TO TRAUMA

Craniocerebral trauma
  Contusion
  Subarachnoid hemorrhage
  Subdural hematoma
  Epidural hematoma
  Vasospasm
Penetrating arterial injury
Blunt arterial injury
Dissection
Fractured plaque
Pseudoaneurysm
Carotid-cavernous fistula

scenario would be puncture or compression of the artery if a child falls while having a stick in his/her mouth—lollypop palsy. Severe bleeding during tonsillectomy can prompt placement of a suture that could cause carotid occlusion. Trauma to the base of the skull also can cause the development of a pseudoaneurysm or a carotid-cavernous fistula.[61] The clinical features of a carotid-cavernous fistula are as follows: Penetrating carotid injuries can occur secondary to stabbing or gunshot wounds. Less commonly, the vertebral artery can be affected.[63,64] Occasionally, an intracranial artery can be injured during trauma.[65]

Patients with penetrating arterial injuries are seriously ill. In a series of 151 patients with extracranial penetrating arterial injuries, du Toit et al.[66] reported a mortality of 21.2 percent and strokes in 15.1 percent of survivors. Most deaths were related to strokes. Because severe bleeding often results from the arterial puncture, urgent surgical treatment, including potentially ligation, is needed. The presence of hypovolemic shock secondary to the blood loss, injury to the internal carotid artery, complete transection of the artery, or the need for arterial ligation to control the hemorrhage is associated with an unfavorable outcome.[66]

The vertebral artery also can be damaged during craniocerebral trauma, and frequency of injuries probably is greater than that previously assumed. Besides dissection due to stretching, the vertebral artery can also be injured secondarily by vertebral fracture and dislocation.[67,68] The trauma may damage short collateral arteries, which are arising from the cervical portion of the vertebral artery and which supply the anterior spinal artery. Thus, besides causing an infarction in the posterior circulation, the vertebral artery injury can also promote spinal cord infarction. Infarction might be one of the leading explanations for spinal cord dysfunction following a closed neck injury. In some cases, the infarction may not occur for several days following the injury. Evaluation of the vertebral artery should be performed if a patient develops signs of posterior circulation or spinal

cord infarction following a neck injury. Management of the underlying cervical and arterial injuries usually involves neurosurgical procedures.

Patients with severe subarachnoid hemorrhage following craniocerebral trauma are at risk for symptomatic vasospasm at approximately 5–10 days following the head injury. The symptoms are similar to those that occur with vasospasm complicating a ruptured aneurysm (see Chapter 15). Cerebral infarction is the potential outcome. The diagnosis, evaluation, and treatment of patients with posttraumatic vasospasm is similar to that used in management of patients with ruptured aneurysms.

► **COMPRESSIVE VASCULOPATHY**

Compressive vasculopathies are a relatively uncommon cause of brain ischemia and usually reflect involvement of the vertebral arteries. Compression by an osteophytic spur of a vertebra can occur with rotation of the head. Severe osteoarthritis or rheumatoid arthritis appears to be a predisposing factor. Patients with laxity of the ligaments of the odontoid secondary to rheumatoid arthritis also can have compression of the vertebral artery. Affected patients can develop symptoms of posterior circulation ischemia in addition to brain stem compression. Compression of the vertebral artery should be suspected if a patient's symptoms of vertebrobasilar ischemia stereotypically occur with head rotation. Most of these patients will also have symptoms of neck and radicular pain.

► **RADIATION-INDUCED VASCULOPATHY**

Therapeutic radiation for treatment of patients with malignancies of the brain, head, or neck can lead to secondary arterial changes.[69–72] The frequency of carotid, subclavian, and coronary artery lesions among persons who received radiation therapy for treatment of Hodgkin disease is markedly increased 15–20 years after the radiation exposure.[73] The arteriopathy appears to be secondary to toxic effects of the radiation on endothelial cells and occlusion of the vasa vasorum of the larger intracranial or extracranial arteries. The arteriopathy can progress to high-grade stenosis or occlusion. In addition, radiation-induced necrosis of the arterial wall can lead to rupture. The diagnosis of radiation-induced arteriopathy usually is considered when a patient with a history of prior radiation exposure develops ischemic symptoms. Narrowing of the affected artery is usually found during evaluation.[74] Management typically is with antiplatelet agents and anticoagulants. Surgical treatment can be problematic because the radiation changes in soft tissue can hamper healing. Following carotid endarterectomy, blood pressure can be volatile because of radiation-induced changes in the carotid bodies. However, Kashyap et al.[75] reported that carotid endarterectomy could be done safely among patients with prior radiation therapy to the neck. Endovascular interventions appear to be superior to surgery in management of severe stenoses of major intracranial or extracranial arteries.

▶ BUERGER DISEASE

The usual features of Buerger disease include digital ischemia, Raynaud phenomenon, limb claudication, and superficial thrombophlebitis.[76,77] Although cerebral ischemia is rare, a few cases of TIA or cerebral infarction have been reported.[78] Most affected patients are young or middle-aged men. Buerger disease is strongly correlated with heavy and long-term use of tobacco products. Treatment focuses on cessation of smoking.

▶ SUSAC SYNDROME

Susac syndrome is a relatively rare arteriopathy that occurs primarily in young women (Table 10-9). The key findings of this condition are retinopathy, encephalopathy, deafness, and microangiopathy.[79–81] Affected women often have a progressive dementing syndrome secondary to presumed small arterial occlusions.[82] While focal motor or sensory deficits are uncommon, the cognitive symptoms can wax and wane. Deafness can be unilateral or bilateral. The hearing loss can recover in some cases. Visual impairments secondary to retinal ischemia also are found. The visual loss can be partial or complete in one or both eyes. Visualization of the ocular fundus demonstrates a segmental arteriopathy. Recently, Susac et al.[83] found that the images on MRI are relatively

distinct, including multifocal supratentorial white matter lesions involving the corpus callosum. The lesions are often found in the basal ganglia and the thalamus. Occasionally, leptomeningeal enhancement can be detected. The cause of Susac syndrome has not been established, although an inflammatory vasculitis is speculated. Patients have been treated with antiplatelet aggregating agents, anticoagulants, calcium channel blockers, and immunosuppressive medications.[84–86]

▶ FIBROMUSCULAR DYSPLASIA

FMD is a relatively uncommon arteriopathy that is discovered most frequently among young-to-middle-aged women (Table 10-10). The cause of this arteriopathy is unknown. FMD most commonly affects the renal artery and causes hypertension. The extracranial portion of the internal carotid artery is the second most common location.[87–89] While the intracranial portion of the internal carotid artery does not seem to be involved, FMD has been detected in the vertebral or basilar artery.[90]

Clinical Findings

Ischemic stroke, TIA, and retinal ischemia are the most common complaints.[89] Other presentations include pulsatile tinnitus or an asymptomatic carotid bruit. FMD is one of the underlying arteriopathies predisposing to spontaneous arterial dissection, which is the presumed underlying mechanism for many of the ischemic symptoms. Although a potential relationship between FMD and intracranial saccular aneurysms is speculated, this correlation is not established. FMD can be incidentally found during a vascular evaluation for another neurological illness, such as subarachnoid hemorrhage.

▶ **TABLE 10-9.** FEATURES OF SUSAC SYNDROME

Young women
  Encephalopathy
    Multifocal cognitive impairments
    Absence of motor or sensory loss
    Dementia
  Retinopathy
    Visual field impairments
    Blindness
    Segmental arteriopathy visualized
  Hearing loss
  Imaging
    Multifocal white matter changes
    Involvement of the corpus callosum
    Meningeal enhancement

▶ **TABLE 10-10.** FEATURES OF FMD

Most commonly found in young-to-middle-age women
  Segmental arterial involvement
    Renal artery
    Extracranial segment internal carotid artery
  Neurological symptoms
    Transient ischemic attack
    Ischemic stroke
    Amaurosis fugax
    Pulsatile tinnitus
    Auscultated cervical bruit
  Associations
    Dissection of the internal carotid artery
    Intracranial saccular aneurysm
  Vascular imaging findings
    String-of-beads appearance
    String sign
    False aneurysm

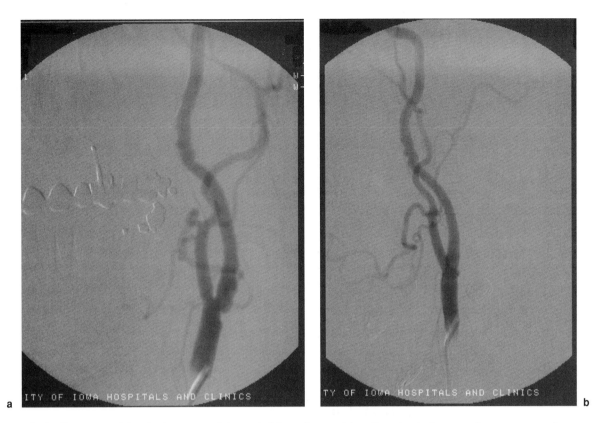

Figure 10-5. Two carotid arteriograms (a) and (b), using subtraction techniques, show areas of segmental changes consistent with FMD. Both studies show a coin (beaded) appearance of the internal carotid artery in the extracranical segment of the internal carotid artery above the bifurcation.

Diagnostic Studies

Arteriography is the usual method for diagnosing FMD (Fig. 10-5(a) and 10-5(b)). The most common and specific arteriographic finding is a string-of-beads pattern of segmental narrowing and dilation of the internal carotid artery approximately 1.5–2 cm above the origin of the internal carotid artery.[88] Other changes include a long tapered segment or a false aneurysm. Differentiating FMD from an arterial dissection is difficult because the arteriographic findings can appear similar in both conditions.

Treatment

In general, patients with FMD have a favorable prognosis; the frequency of recurrent ischemic symptoms seems to be much lower than that among persons with extracranial atherosclerotic disease. Most patients with FMD, including those with complicating arterial dissection, are treated with antiplatelet agents. Endovascular treatment and surgical resection can be performed. The relatively distal location of the FMD makes surgery difficult. The operation might require dislocation or fracture of the jaw in order for the surgeon to reach the involved arterial segment. Graduated dilation of the artery has also been performed.[91]

▶ INTRACRANIAL SACCULAR ANEURYSMS

Cerebral infarction and TIA are uncommon presentations of large intracranial saccular aneurysms.[92–94] Most instances are associated with aneurysms large than 1–2.5 cm in diameter. The large aneurysmal sac serves as a source of emboli that arise from an intracavitary thrombus. A laminar intra-aneurysmal thrombus usually develops secondary to slow flow and turbulence. The diagnosis and management of patients with saccular aneurysms are discussed in Chapter 15.

▶ MOYAMOYA SYNDROME

Moyamoya disease was first diagnosed in Japan. This inherited vasculopathy, which occurs most commonly among persons of East Asian ancestry, is described in Chapter 12. Moyamoya syndrome encompasses an acquired intracranial vasculopathy that produces occlusions of the distal portions of both internal carotid arteries (Fig. 10-6) and the proximal portions of the anterior and middle cerebral arteries[95] (Fig. 10-7). As the major intracranial arteries disappear, a mesh of small caliber

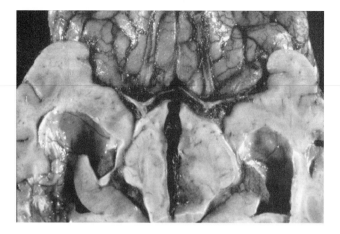

Figure 10-6. Basal view of the brain from a patient dying of moyamoya disease shows the reduction in the caliber of the anterior cerebral and middle cerebral arteries. In addition, small vessels can be seen bilaterally in the Sylvian cisterns. (*Courtesy of S.S. Schochet, M.D., Department of Pathology, University of West Virginia, Morgantown, WV*)

vessels grows at the base of both hemispheres. The appearance of these small vessels, which resembles a puff of a smoke, is the hallmark of moyamoya syndrome and gives the name to the arteriopathy (Table 10-11). Electron microscopic findings of biopsied vessels show endothelial cell degeneration with vacuoles and membrane blebs.[96] Collateral vessels arising from the posterior cerebral arteries or the ethmoidal arteries at the base of the skull help maintain perfusion to the involved areas. The course of the vasculopathy is progressive, and the collateral channels often fail.[97,98] The course of the illness varies widely among persons. While the find-

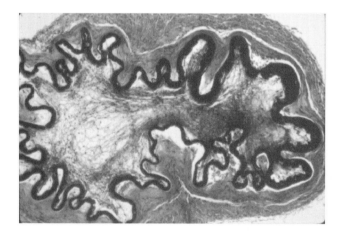

Figure 10-7 Cross section of the middle cerebral artery from a patient with moyamoya disease is stained with elastin stain. Thickening of the elastin-stained components of the arterial wall is seen. (*Courtesy of S.S. Schochet, M.D., Department of Pathology, University of West Virginia, Morgantown, WV*)

▶ **TABLE 10-11.** RADIOLOGICAL FEATURES OF MOYAMOYA SYNDROME

Vascular imaging
  Usually bilateral involvement of intracranial arteries
  Stenosis or occlusion of distal internal carotid arteries
  Stenosis or occlusion of proximal middle cerebral arteries
  Stenosis or occlusion of proximal anterior cerebral arteries
  Delayed involvement of the posterior cerebral arteries
  Basilar artery relatively unaffected
  Prominent meshwork of fine vessels deep in cerebral hemispheres
  Prominent leptomeningeal vessels
  Prominent collateral ethmoidal vessels
  Saccular aneurysms
Brain imaging
  Multiple small (lacunar infarctions) in hemispheres
  Watershed infarctions
  Frontal hemispheric or white matter infarctions
  Absence of flow voids of major arteries on MRI

ings may be unilateral or asymmetrical early in the course, both hemispheres become involved.

Clinical Findings

Moyamoya syndrome is most commonly diagnosed in children and young adults. Most North American studies of stroke in young adults report that women constitute the majority of affected patients.[99,100] A large number of potential risk factors for or associated with moyamoya syndrome have been reported[101,102] (Table 10-12). The relationships between these conditions and moyamoya

▶ **TABLE 10-12.** POTENTIAL RELATIONSHIPS (CAUSES) OF MOYAMOYA SYNDROME

Inherited diseases
  Neurofibromatosis, Turner syndrome, Down syndrome
  Tuberous sclerosis, retinitis pigmentosa, sickle-cell disease
  Pseudoxanthoma elasticum, polycystic kidney disease
  Glycogen storage disease type I, osteogenesis imperfecta
  Cardio-facio-cutaneous syndrome, Alagille syndrome
Infectious diseases
  Anaerobic meningitis, tuberculous meningitis, tonsillitis
  Ebstein–Barr infection, pharyngitis, proprionibacterium acne
Autoimmune diseases
  Systemic lupus erythematosus, Sjögren syndrome
  Polyarteritis nodosa, Kawasaki disease
Other factors
  Oral contraceptive use, tobacco use, alcohol use
  Parasellar neoplasm, craniocerebral trauma
  Atherosclerosis, renal artery stenosis, arterial dissection
  Saccular aneurysm, arteriovenous malformation
  Fibromuscular dysplasia, radiation therapy

syndrome are not established. The potential interaction with use of oral contraceptives and tobacco abuse appears to be relatively strong.[103] Patients with moyamoya syndrome usually have recurrent TIA or cerebral infarction. Most of the infarctions are small and subcortical in location. In addition, bilateral watershed or frontal infarctions can be found. With recurrent stroke, adults develop signs consistent with vascular dementia and affected children might have mental retardation. Other symptoms of moyamoya include movement disorders, such as hemichorea, or seizures. A case of vascular Parkinsonism secondary to moyamoya has been described.[96] These findings are more common among children.

In addition, the presence of small aneurysmal dilations on the basal vessels or saccular aneurysms, particularly located in the posterior circulation, predispose to intracranial hemorrhage.[104] Hemorrhage is a particularly common presentation for adults with moyamoya.[105] Patients with hemorrhagic moyamoya disease have a high risk for rebleeding.[106] Morioka et al.[107] reported that 61 percent of their patients had recurrent hemorrhages. In particular, the risk of hemorrhages increased when patients were older than 45.

Diagnostic Studies

Brain imaging usually demonstrates multiple small subcortical or bilateral watershed infarctions. Extensive white matter or anterior hemispheric ischemic changes also can be found on CT or MRI.[108] The brain imaging studies may also show the absence of flow voids in the major intracranial arteries (internal carotid, middle cerebral, and anterior cerebral arteries). Moyamoya syndrome is usually diagnosed by the detection of the characteristic arteriographic findings (Figs. 10-8 to 10-11; see Table 10-11). The distal portions of both internal carotid arteries and the proximal segments of both middle cerebral and anterior cerebral arteries are occluded. Prominent collaterals arise from the deep basal skull branches of the external carotid artery. The collateral arteries are often small and tortuous. Small aneurysmal enlargements are seen. The mesh of small vessels is found in the region of the basal ganglia. While the disease is present bilaterally, asymmetries in the vascular changes are often found. Magnetic resonance angiography and computerized tomographic angiography also can be used to detect the occlusions of the major

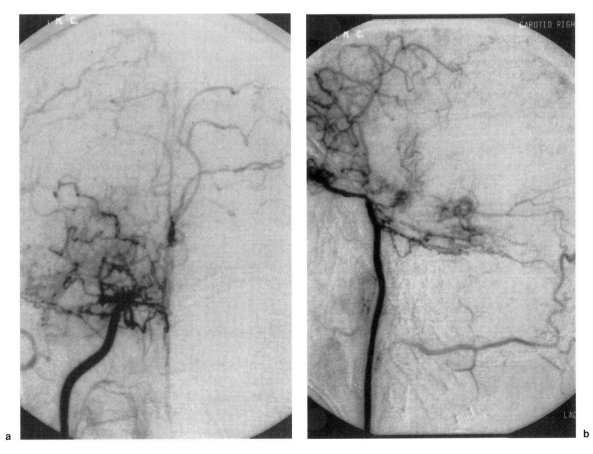

Figure 10-8. (a) Anteroposterior and (b) lateral views of a right carotid arteriogram using subtraction techniques show changes consistent with moyamoya disease (or syndrome). The middle cerebral artery is absent and prominent pial and basal collateral vessels are visualized.

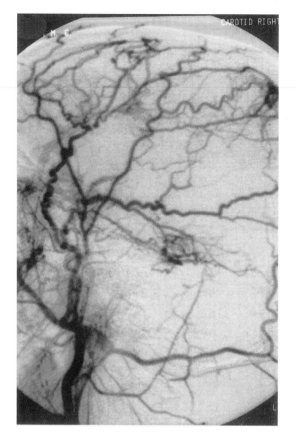

Figure 10-9. Prominent collateral vessels from the external carotid circulation are visualized in this lateral view of a left external carotid arteriogram. The collateral vessels are anastomosed to pial vessels on the surface of the brain. In addition, prominent ethmoidal collateral vessels are present.

intracranial arteries.[109,110] Cerebral blood flow studies will show hypoperfusion most marked in a watershed pattern. Transcranial Doppler ultrasonography can detect changes in velocity in the major arteries of the anterior circulation.[111] The velocities increase as the arterial narrowing evolves and are lost as the arteries become obliterated. The results of such studies can be used to help decide about revascularization operations.[112]

Treatment

Patients with moyamoya syndrome usually have a high risk for recurrent ischemic events. Abstaining from tobacco use by both young men and women, and halting use of oral contraceptives by women are recommended (Table 10-13). Patients are often prescribed antiplatelet agents. Because of the potentially increased risk for intracranial hemorrhage, oral anticoagulants are often avoided. Surgical procedures are employed to restore or improve perfusion. Among the options are creations of a superficial temporal artery-to-middle cerebral artery anastomosis or indirect revascularization

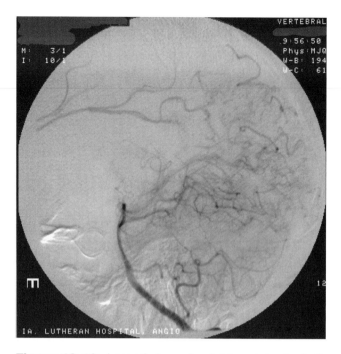

Figure 10-10. Lateral view of a right vertebral arteriogram using subtraction techniques shows prominent collateral vessels in a patient with moyamoya syndrome. The anterior cerebral artery is receiving flow via collateral vessels from the posterior cerebral artery. This pattern of blood supply may be seen in patients with advanced moyamoya disease (or syndrome).

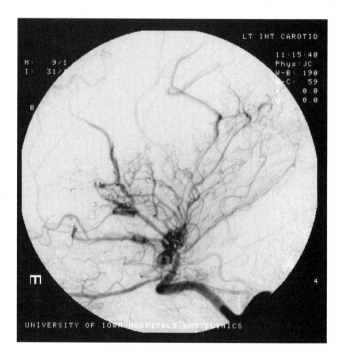

Figure 10-11. Prominent basal collateral vessels (puff of smoke) at the base of the brain is shown on the lateral view of a left carotid arteriogram using subtraction techniques.

▶ **TABLE 10-13.** MANAGEMENT OF PATIENTS WITH MOYAMOYA SYNDROME

Control risk factors
    Avoid use of oral contraceptives
    Smoking cessation
Antiplatelet agents
Surgical revascularization
    Extracranial-to-intracranial bypass
    Encephaloduroarteriosynangiosis
    Encephaloduromyosynagiosis
    Omental transposition

(encephaloduroarteriosynangiosis) procedures including placement of muscle, tissue, or blood vessels on the cortical surface.[113–115] In particular, these operations are recommended for children with moyamoya syndrome.[116,117] The associated aneurysms, which are located on major intracranial vessels, particularly in the posterior circulation, can be treated with either surgical or endovascular interventions.[118] Overall, the prognosis of patients with moyamoya syndrome is not good. Patients are at risk for both recurrent ischemic and hemorrhagic stroke.

REFERENCES

1. Schievink WI, Mokri B, Whisnant JP. Internal carotid artery dissection in a community. Rochester, Minnesota, 1987–1992. *Stroke* 1993;24:1678–1680.
2. Schievink WI, Mokri B, Piepgras DG. Spontaneous dissections of cervicocephalic arteries in childhood and adolescence. *Neurology* 1994;44:1607–1612.
3. Bartels E, Flugel KA. Evaluation of extracranial vertebral artery dissection with duplex color-flow imaging. *Stroke* 1996;27:290–295.
4. Thie A, Hellner D, Lachenmayer L, Janzen RWC, Kunze K. Bilateral blunt traumatic dissections of the extracranial internal carotid artery; report of eleven cases and review literature. *Cerebrovasc Dis* 1993;3:295–303.
5. Noelle B, Clavier I, Besson G, Hommel M. Cervicocephalic arterial dissections related to skiing. *Stroke* 1994;25:526–527.
6. Zimmerman AW, Kumar AJ, Gadoth N, Hodges FJ. Traumatic vertebrobasilar occlusive disease in childhood. *Neurology* 1978;28:185–188.
7. Schievink WI, Atkinson JL, Bartleson JD, Whisnant JP. Traumatic internal carotid artery dissections caused by blunt softball injuries. *Am J Emerg Med* 1998;16:179–182.
8. Chung YS, Han DH. Vertebrobasilar dissection: a possible role of whiplash injury in pathogenesis. *Neurol Res* 2002;24:129–138.
9. Peters M, Bohl J, Thomke F, et al. Dissection of the internal carotid artery after chiropractic manipulation of the neck. *Neurology* 1995;45:2284–2286.
10. Reuter U, Hamling M, Kavuk I, et al. Vertebral artery dissections after chiropractic neck manipulation in Germany over three years. *J Neurol* 2006;253:724–730.
11. Lee KP, Carlini WG, McCormick GF, Albers GW. Neurologic complications following chiropractic manipulation: a survey of California neurologists. *Neurology* 1995;45:1213–1215.
12. Van de Kelft E, Kunnen J, Truyen L, Heytens L. Postpartum dissecting aneurysm of the basilar artery. *Stroke* 1992;23:114–116.
13. Malek AM, Higashida RT, Halbach VV, et al. Patient presentation, angiographic features, and treatment of strangulation-induced bilateral dissection of the cervical internal carotid artery. Report of three cases. *J Neurosurg* 2000;92:481–487.
14. Evers S, Altenmuller E, Ringelstein EB. Cerebrovascular ischemic events in wind instrument players. *Neurology* 2000;55:865–867.
15. Wiest T, Hyrenbach S, Bambul P, et al. Genetic analysis of familial connective tissue alterations associated with cervical artery dissections suggests locus heterogeneity. *Stroke* 2006;37:1667–1702.
16. Schievink WI, Michels VV, Piepgras DG. Neurovascular manifestations of heritable connective tissue disorders. A review. *Stroke* 1994;25:889–903.
17. Grau AJ, Brandt T, Buggle F, et al. Association of cervical artery dissection with recent infection. *Arch Neurol* 1999;56:851–856.
18. Grau AJ, Brandt T, Forsting M, Winter R, Hacke W. Infection-associated cervical artery dissection. Three cases. *Stroke* 1997;28:453–455.
19. Guillon B, Berthet K, Benslamia L, Bertrand M, Bousser MG, Tzourio C. Infection and the risk of spontaneous cervical artery dissection: a case-control study. *Stroke* 2003;34:e79–e81.
20. Neau JP, Masson C, Vandermarcq P, et al. Familial occurrence of dissection of the cervical arteries. *Cerebrovasc Dis* 1995;5:310–312.
21. Schievink WI, Mokri B, Piepgras DG, Kuiper JD. Recurrent spontaneous arterial dissections: risk in familial versus nonfamilial disease. *Stroke* 1996;27:622–624.
22. van den Berg JS, Limburg M, Kappelle LJ, Pals G, Arwert F, Westerveld. The role of type III collagen in spontaneous cervical arterial dissections. *Ann Neurol* 1998;43:494–498.
23. Vila N, Millan M, Ferrer X, Riutort N, Escudero D. Level of α-1-antitrypsin in plasma and risk of spontaneous cervical artery dissections: a case-control study. *Stroke* 2003;34:e168–e169.
24. Biousse V, d'Anglejan-Chatillon J, Touboul PJ, Amarenco P, Bousser MG. Time course of symptoms in extracranial carotid artery dissections. A series of 80 patients. *Stroke* 1995;26:235–239.
25. Benninger DH, Georgiadis D, Kremer C, Studer A, Nedeltchev K, Baumgartner RW. Mechanism of ischemic infarct in spontaneous carotid dissection. *Stroke* 2004;35:482–485.
26. Biousse V, Touboul PJ, d'Anglejan-Chatillon J, Levy C, Schaison M, Bousser MG. Ophthalmologic manifestations of internal carotid artery dissection. *Am J Ophthalmol* 1998;126:565–577.
27. Fisher CM, Ojemann RG, Roberson GH. Spontaneous dissection of cervico-cerebral arteries. *Can J Neurol Sci* 1978;5:9–19.

28. Guillon B, Levy C, Bousser MG. Internal carotid artery dissection: an update. *J Neurol Sci* 1998;153:146–158.

29. Galetta SL, Leahey A, Nichols CW, Raps EC. Orbital ischemia, ophthalmoparesis, and carotid dissection. *J Clin Neuroophthalmol* 1991;11:284–287.

30. Leira EC, Bendixen BH, Kardon RH, Adams HP, Jr. Brief, transient Horner's syndrome can be the hallmark of a carotid artery dissection. *Neurology* 1998;50:289–290.

31. Schievink WI, Mokri B, Garrity JA, Nichols DA, Piepgras DG. Ocular motor nerve palsies in spontaneous dissections of the cervical internal carotid artery. *Neurology* 1993;43:1938–1941.

32. Koennecke H, Seyfert S. Mydriatic pupil as the presenting sign of common carotid artery dissection. *Stroke* 1998;29:2653–2655.

33. Mokri B, Schievink WI, Olsen KD, Piepgras DG. Spontaneous dissection of the cervical internal carotid artery. Presentation with lower cranial nerve palsies. *Arch Otolaryngol Head Neck Surg* 1992;118:431–435.

34. Mokri B. Headaches in cervical artery dissections. *Curr Pain Headache Rep* 2002;6:209–216.

35. Silbert PL, Mokri B, Schievink WI. Headache and neck pain in spontaneous internal carotid and vertebral artery dissections. *Neurology* 1995;45:1517–1522.

36. Caplan LR, Baquis GD, Pessin MS, et al. Dissection of the intracranial vertebral artery. *Neurology* 1988;38:868–877.

37. Greselle JF, Zenteno M, Kien P, Castel JP, Caille JM. Spontaneous dissection of the vertebro-basilar system. A study of 18 cases (15 patients). *J Neuroradiol* 1987;14:115–123.

38. Hosoya T, Adachi M, Yamaguchi K, Haku T, Kayama T, Kato T. Clinical and neuroradiological features of intracranial vertebrobasilar artery dissection. *Stroke* 1999;30:1083–1090.

39. Pozzati E, Andreoli A, Padovani R, Nuzzo G. Dissecting aneurysms of the basilar artery. *Neurosurgery* 1995;36:254–258.

40. Bassetti C, Bogousslavsky J, Eskenasy-Cottier AC, Janzen RWC, Regli F. Spontaneous intracranial dissection in the anterior circulation. *Cerebrovasc Dis* 1994;4:170–174.

41. Sharif AA, Remley KB, Clark HB. Middle cerebral artery dissection: a clinicopathologic study. *Neurology* 1995;45:1929–1931.

42. Redekop G, TerBrugge K, Willinsky R. Subarachnoid hemorrhage from vertebrobasilar dissecting aneurysm treated with staged bilateral vertebral artery occlusion: the importance of early follow-up angiography: technical case report. *Neurosurgery* 1999;45:1258–1263.

43. Levy C, Laissy JP, Raveau V, et al. Carotid and vertebral artery dissections: three-dimensional time-of-flight MR angiography and MR imaging versus conventional angiography. *Radiology* 1994;190:97–103.

44. Auer A, Felber S, Schmidauer C, Waldenberger P, Aichner F. Magnetic resonance angiographic and clinical features of extracranial vertebral artery dissection. *J Neurol Neurosurg Psychiatry* 1998;64:474–481.

45. Sidhu PS, Jonker ND, Khaw KT, et al. Spontaneous dissections of the internal carotid artery: appearances on colour Doppler ultrasound. *Br J Radiol* 1997;70:50–57.

46. Sturzenegger M, Mattle HP, Rivoir A, Baumgartner RW. Ultrasound findings in carotid artery dissection: analysis of 43 patients. *Neurology* 1995;45:691–698.

47. Steinke W, Rautenberg W, Schwartz A, Hennerici M. Noninvasive monitoring of internal carotid artery dissection. *Stroke* 1994;25:998–1005.

48. Leys D, Moulin T, Stojkovic T, Begey S, Chavot D. Follow-up of patients with history of cervical artery dissection. *Cerebrovasc Dis* 1995;5:43–49.

49. Kasner SE, Hankins LL, Bratina P, Morgenstern LB. Magnetic resonance angiography demonstrates vascular healing of carotid and vertebral artery dissections. *Stroke* 1997;28:1993–1997.

50. Bassetti C, Carruzzo A, Sturzenegger M, Tuncdogan E. Recurrence of cervical artery dissection. A prospective study of 81 patients. *Stroke* 1996;27:1804–1807.

51. Georgiadis D, Caso V, Baumgartner RW, Acute therapy and prevention of stroke in spontaneous carotid dissection. *Clin Exp Hypertens* 2006;28:365–370.

52. Schievink WI. The treatment of spontaneous carotid and vertebral artery dissections. *Curr Opin Cardiol* 2000;15:316–321.

53. Schievink WI, Piepgras DG, McCaffrey TV, Mokri B. Surgical treatment of extracranial internal carotid artery dissecting aneurysms. *Neurosurgery* 1994;35:809–815.

54. Vishteh AG, Marciano FF, David CA, Schievink WI, Zabramski JM, Spetzler RF. Long-term graft patency rates and clinical outcomes after revascularization for symptomatic traumatic internal carotid artery dissection. *Neurosurgery* 1998;43:761–768.

55. Muller BT, Luther B, Hort W, Neumann-Haefelin T, Aulich A, Sandmann W. Surgical treatment of 50 carotid dissections: indications and results. *J Vasc Surg* 2000;31:980–988.

56. Rabinov JD, Hellinger FR, Morris PP, Ogilvy CS, Putman CM. Endovascular management of vertebrobasilar dissecting aneurysms. *AJNR Am J Neuroradiol* 2003;24:1421–1428.

57. Miller PR, Fabian TC, Bee TK, et al. Blunt cerebrovascular injuries: diagnosis and treatment. *J Trauma* 2001;51:279–285.

58. Prall JA, Brega KE, Coldwell DM, Breeze RE. Incidence of unsuspected blunt carotid artery injury. *Neurosurgery* 1998;42:495–498.

59. Krauss JK, Jankovic J. Hemidystonia secondary to carotid artery gunshot injury. *Childs Nerv Syst* 1997;13:285–288.

60. Rommel O, Niedeggen A, Tegenthoff M, Kiwitt P, Botel U, Malin J. Carotid and vertebral artery injury following severe head or cervical spine trauma. *Cerebrovasc Dis* 1999;9:202–209.

61. Welling RE, Saul TG, Tew JMJ, Tomsick TA, Kremchek TE, Bellamy MJ. Management of blunt injury to the internal carotid artery. *J Trauma* 1987;27:1221–1226.

62. Moriarity JL, Wetzel M, Clatterbuck RE, et al. The natural history of cavernous malformations: a prospective study of 68 patients. *Neurosurgery* 1999;44:1166–1173.

63. Garg BP, Ottinger CJ, Smith RR, Fishman MA. Strokes in children due to vertebral artery trauma. *Neurology* 1993;43:2555–2558.

64. Pryse-Phillips W. Infarction of the medulla and cervical cord after fitness exercises. *Stroke* 1989;20:292–294.

65. De Caro R, Munari PF, Parenti A. Middle cerebral artery thrombosis following blunt head trauma. *Clin Neuropathol* 1998;17:1–5.

66. du Toit DF, van Schalkwyk GD, Wadee SA, Warren BL. Neurologic outcome after penetrating extracranial arterial trauma. *J Vasc Surg* 2003;38:257–262.

67. Willis BK, Greiner F, Orrison WW, Benzel EC. The incidence of vertebral artery injury after midcervical spine fracture or subluxation. *Neurosurgery* 1994;34:435–441.

68. Tulyapronchote R, Selhorst JB, Malkoff MD, Gomez CR. Delayed sequelae of vertebral artery dissection and occult cervical fractures. *Neurology* 1994;44: 1397–1399.

69. Murros KE, Toole JF. The effect of radiation on carotid arteries. *Arch Neurol* 1989;46:449–455.

70. Zuber M, Khoubesserian P, Meder JF, Mas JL. A 34-year delayed and focal postirradiation intracranial vasculopathy. *Cerebrovasc Dis* 1993;3:181–182.

71. Bowen J, Paulsen CA. Stroke after pituitary irradiation. *Stroke* 1992;23:908–911.

72. Bitzer M, Topka H. Progressive cerebral occlusive disease after radiation therapy. *Stroke* 1995;26:131–136.

73. Hull MC, Morris CG, Pepine CJ, Mendenhall NP. Valvular dysfunction and carotid, subclavian, and coronary artery disease in survivors of Hodgkin lymphoma treated with radiation therapy. *JAMA* 2003;290:2831–2837.

74. Chung TS, Yousem DM, Lexa FJ, Markiewicz DA. MRI of carotid angiopathy after therapeutic radiation. *J Comput Assist Tomogr* 1994;18:533–538.

75. Kashyap VS, Moore WS, Quinones-Baldrich WJ. Carotid artery repair for radiation-associated atherosclerosis is a safe and durable procedure. *J Vasc Surg* 1999;29: 90–96.

76. Joyce JW. Buerger's disease (thromboangiitis obliterans). *Rheum Dis Clin North Am* 1990;16:463–470.

77. Olin JW, Young JR, Graor RA, Ruschhaupt WF, Bartholomew JR. The changing clinical spectrum of thromboangiitis obliterans (Buerger's disease). *Circulation* 1990;82:IV3–IV8.

78. Inzelberg R, Bornstein NM, Korczyn AD. Cerebrovascular symptoms in thromboangiitis obliterans. *Acta Neurol Scand* 1989;80:347–350.

79. Susac JO, Hardman JM, Selhorst JB. Microangiopathy of the brain and retina. *Neurology* 1979;29:313–316.

80. Bousser MG, Blousse V. Small vessel vasculopathies affecting the central nervous system. *J Neuroophthalmol* 2004;24:56–61.

81. Papo T, Biousse V, Lehoang P, et al. Susac syndrome. *Medicine* 1998;77:3–11.

82. Bogousslavsky J, Gaio JM, Caplan LR, et al. Encephalopathy, deafness and blindness in young women: a distinct retinocochleocerebral arteriolopathy? *J Neurol Neurosurg Psychiatry* 1989;52:43–46.

83. Susac JO, Murtagh FR, Egan RA, et al. MRI findings in Susac's syndrome. *Neurology* 2003;61:1783–1787.

84. Gordon DL, Hayreh SS, Adams HP, Jr. Microangiopathy of the brain, retina, and ear: improvement without immunosuppressive therapy. *Stroke* 1991;22:933–937.

85. Vila N, Graus F, Blesa R, Santamaria J, Ribalta T, Tolosa E. Microangiopathy of the brain and retina (Susac's

86. Wildemann B, Schulin C, Storch-Hagenlocher B, et al. Susac's syndrome: improvement with combined antiplatelet and calcium antagonist therapy. *Stroke* 1996;27: 149–151.

87. Balaji MR, DeWeese JA. Fibromuscular dysplasia of the internal carotid artery: its occurrence with acute stroke and its surgical reversal. *Arch Surg* 1980;115:984–986.

88. Corrin LS, Sandok BA, Houser OW. Cerebral ischemic events in patients with carotid artery fibromuscular dysplasia. *Arch Neurol* 1981;38:616–618.

89. So EL, Toole JF, Dalal P, Moody DM. Cephalic fibromuscular dysplasia in 32 patients: clinical findings and radiologic features. *Arch Neurol* 1981;38:619–622.

90. Hegedus K, Nemeth G. Fibromuscular dysplasia of the basilar artery. Case report with autopsy verification. *Arch Neurol* 1984;41:440–442.

91. Van Damme H, Sakalihasan N, Limet R. Fibromuscular dysplasia of the internal carotid artery. Personal experience with 13 cases and literature review. *Acta Chir Belg* 1999;99:163–168.

92. Nanda A, Vannemreddy PS. Cerebral ischemia as a presenting feature of intracranial aneurysms. A negative prognostic indicator in the management of aneurysms. *Neurosurgery* 2006;58:831–837.

93. Sakaki T, Kinugawa K, Tanigake T, Miyamoto S, Kyoi K, Utsumi S. Embolism from intracranial aneurysms. *J Neurosurg* 1980;53:300–304.

94. Steinberger A, Ganti SR, McMurtry JG, Hilal SK. Transient neurological deficits secondary to saccular vertebrobasilar aneurysms. Report of two cases. *J Neurosurg* 1984;60: 410–413.

95. Masuda J, Ogata J, Yutani C. Smooth muscle cell proliferation and localization of macrophages and T cells in the occlusive intracranial major arteries in moyamoya disease. *Stroke* 1993;24:1960–1967.

96. Tan E-K, Chan L-L, Yu GX, Rumpel H, Wilder-Smith E, Wong M-C. Vascular Parkinsonism in moyamoya: microvascular biopsy and imaging correlates. *Ann Neurol* 2003;54:836–840.

97. Miyamoto S, Kikuchi H, Karasawa J, Nagata I, Ikota T, Takeuchi S. Study of the posterior circulation in moyamoya disease. Clinical and neuroradiological evaluation. *J Neurosurg* 1984;61:1032–1037.

98. Hojo M, Hoshimaru M, Miyamoto S, et al. Role of transforming growth factor-beta1 in the pathogenesis of moyamoya disease. *J Neurosurg* 1998;89:623–629.

99. Bruno A, Adams HP, Jr., Biller J, Rezai K, Cornell S, Aschenbrener CA. Cerebral infarction due to moyamoya disease in young adults. *Stroke* 1988;19:826–833.

100. Chiu D, Shedden P, Bratina P, Grotta JC. Clinical features of moyamoya disease in the United States. *Stroke* 1998;29:1347–1351.

101. Cramer SC, Robertson RL, Dooling EC, Scott RM. Moyamoya and Down syndrome. Clinical and radiological features. *Stroke* 1996;27:2131–2135.

102. Berg JM, Armstrong D. On the association of moyamoya disease with Down's syndrome. *J Ment Defic Res* 1991;35: 398–403.

103. Levine SR, Fagan SC, Pessin MS, et al. Accelerated intracranial occlusive disease, oral contraceptives, and cigarette use. *Neurology* 1991;41:1893–1901.

104. Kawaguchi S, Sakaki T, Morimoto T, Kakizaki T, Kamada K. Characteristics of intracranial aneurysms associated with moyamoya disease. *Acta Neurochir (Wien)* 1996; 138:1287–1294.

105. Sun JCL, Yakimov M, Al-Badawi I, Honey CR. Hemorrhagic moyamoya disease during pregnancy. *Can J Neurol Sci* 2000;27:73–76.

106. Kobayashi E, Saeki N, Oishi H, Hirai S, Yamaura A. Long-term natural history of hemorrhagic moyamoya disease in 42 patients. *J Neurosurg* 2000;93:976–980.

107. Morioka M, Hamada J, Todaka T, Yano S, Kai Y, Ushio Y. High-risk age for rebleeding in patients with hemorrhagic moyamoya disease: long-term follow-up study. *Neurosurgery* 2003;52:1049–1054.

108. Bruno A, Yuh WT, Biller J, Adams HP, Jr., Cornell SH. Magnetic resonance imaging in young adults with cerebral infarction due to moyamoya. *Arch Neurol* 1988;45:303–306.

109. Houkin K, Aoki T, Takahashi A, Abe H. Diagnosis of moyamoya disease with magnetic resonance angiography. *Stroke* 1994;25:2159–2164.

110. Barboriak DP, Provenzale JM. MR arteriography of intracranial circulation. *AJR Am J Roentgenol* 1998;171: 1469–1478.

111. Laborde G, Harders A, Klimek L, Hardenack M. Correlation between clinical, angiographic and transcranial Doppler sonographic findings in patients with moyamoya disease. *Neurol Res* 1993;15:87–92.

112. Kohno K, Oka Y, Kohno S, Ohta S, Kumon Y, Sakaki S. Cerebral blood flow measurement as an indicator for indirect revascularization procedure for adult patients with moyamoya disease. *Neurosurgery* 1998;42:752–758.

113. Kim SK, Wang KC, Kim IO, Lee DS, Cho BK. Combined encephaloduroarteriosynangiosis and bifrontal encephalogaleo (periosteal) synangiosis in pediatric moyamoya disease. *Neurosurgery* 2002;50:88–96.

114. Isono M, Ishii K, Kobayashi H, Kaga A, Kamida T, Fujiki M. Effects of indirect bypass surgery for occlusive cerebrovascular diseases in adults. *J Clin Neurosci* 2002;9: 644–647.

115. Iwama T, Hashimoto N, Miyake H, Yonekawa Y. Direct revascularization to the anterior cerebral artery territory in patients with moyamoya disease: report of five cases. *Neurosurgery* 1998;42:1157–1161.

116. Golby AJ, Marks MP, Thompson RC, Steinberg GK. Direct and combined revascularization in pediatric moyamoya disease. *Neurosurgery* 1999;45:50–60.

117. Caldarelli M, Di Rocco C, Gaglini P. Surgical treatment of moyamoya disease in pediatric age. *J Neurosurg Sci* 2001;45:83–91.

118. Arita K, Kurisu K, Ohba S, et al. Endovascular treatment of basilar tip aneurysms associated with moyamoya disease. *Neuroradiology* 2003;45:441–444.

CHAPTER 11

Infectious and Inflammatory Vasculitides Causing Ischemic or Hemorrhagic Stroke

The vasculitides (inflammatory diseases of arteries) of the central nervous system can be secondary to either an infectious or a primary autoimmune process. A number of terms, which can be used interchangeably, are used to describe the vasculitides including vasculitis, arteritis, or angiitis. Lie[1] defined vasculitis as an inflammatory disease of blood vessels that results in histologically apparent structural injury to the vessel wall. Vasculitis occurs with thrombosis and secondary organ ischemia. The vasculitides can potentially involve arteries of any caliber including the aorta and major extracranial vessels, moderately sized intracranial or extracranial arteries, or small arterioles. The vasculitis can be acute, such as those occurring with hypersensitivity reactions, or subacute-to-chronic, in which healing lesions might be intermixed with acute vascular changes.[2]

A vasculitis can be primary when it is not associated with a specific underlying cause or secondary when it is a feature of another illness, such as an infection, malignancy, or adverse experience to a medication.[1,3] While vasculitis can complicate several types of malignancy, hairy cell leukemia is most commonly implicated. It can be associated with small vessel vasculitis and periarteritis nodosa.[3] Several drugs of abuse are associated with the development of a vasculitis that can lead to either hemorrhagic or ischemic stroke. Heroin and the stimulants

are most commonly implicated. Stroke complicating the abuse of drugs is discussed in Chapter 17. Most cases of medication-induced vasculitis occur within the first 3 weeks of initiating treatment. Medication-associated autoimmune reactions might explain up to 10 percent of cases of cutaneous vasculitis.[3] Most affected patients are adults who have palpable purpura or skin eruptions.[4] Besides cutaneous reactions, elevated levels of autoimmune markers can be found. For example, the development of antineutrophil cytoplasmic antibodies (ANCA) has been linked to the use of propylthiouracil or hydralazine.[3] Involvement of the central nervous system is uncommon with medication-associated immune reactions.

While the initial presentations of the inflammatory vasculitides might be either hemorrhagic or ischemic stroke, patients can have other neurological symptoms. In particular, many of the primary vasculitides have signs of peripheral nerve or muscle dysfunction. The course of the neurological illness of patients with vasculitides often is subacute with a stepwise course of deterioration and often with signs of involvement of multiple locations within the central nervous system. In addition, nonneurological findings frequently are prominent. In many cases, the clinical findings of specific vasculitides are relatively stereotyped.

▶ INFECTIOUS VASCULITIDES

Several acute or subacute bacterial, viral, fungal, or parasitic infectious diseases affect intracranial arteries or veins and lead to either hemorrhagic or ischemic stroke (Table 11-1). Suppurative or granulomatous infections of the meninges at the base of the brain can induce inflammation of penetrating arteries. In addition, the organisms invade the vessel itself, causing formation of an aneurysm or stagnation of the blood supply to the brain or spinal cord. The presence of fever and other systemic manifestations of an infectious illness, signs of meningeal irritation, existence of multifocal neurological impairments, and signs of increased intracranial pressure often are present. The clinical picture, brain imaging findings, and the results of other diagnostic studies vary by the underlying infectious illness. The CSF usually shows leucocytosis with a predominance of either lymphocytes or polymorphonuclear leucocytes, elevated levels of protein, and hypoglycorrhachia. Cultures of blood or cerebrospinal fluid often provide the diagnosis. In other instances, serological studies are needed to confirm the infectious disease. Management focuses on treatment of the underlying infection. Infective endocarditis, which is an important underlying cause of both ischemic and hemorrhagic stroke, is discussed in Chapter 13.

▶ SYPHILIS

Cerebral infarction is a well-recognized neurological complication of syphilis (*Treponema pallidum*). Since the advent of modern antibiotic treatment, the frequency of tabes dorsalis and general paresis has declined and as result, the relative importance of *meningovascular syphilis* (Huebner arteritis) has increased. Meningovascular syphilis involves inflammation of large to medium-sized intracranial arteries, most commonly the middle cerebral artery[5,6] (Table 11-2). The basilar or anterior spinal artery also can be affected preferentially. The inflammation leads to narrowing of the lumen and secondary thrombosis.

Clinical Features

Stroke usually occurs several years after the primary syphilitic infection. Most patients have a low-grade fever, headache, and signs of meningeal irritation that precede the development of seizures or focal impairments. If the anterior spinal artery is occluded, the patient shows signs of a transverse myelopathy. *Syphilitic aortitis* can involve the origins of the great vessels that perfuse the brain or cause a spinal cord infarction. Luetic involvement of the basilar meninges and vessels can cause cranial nerve abnormalities including bilateral hearing loss (*Cogan syndrome*).[7,8]

▶ **TABLE 11-1.** INFECTIOUS VASCULITIC CAUSES OF STROKE

Bacterial infections
  Syphilis
    Meningovascular syphilis
    Syphilitic aortitis
  Cogan syndrome
  Tonsillar and paratonsillar abscess
  Suppurative infections of head and face
    Cavernous sinus thrombosis
    Transverse sinus thrombosis
  Acute bacterial meningitis
  Tuberculous meningitis
  Brucellosis
  Rocky Mountain spotted fever
  Lyme disease
  Cat scratch disease
  Whipple disease
  Typhoid fever
Viral infections
  Acquired immune deficiency syndrome
  Herpes zoster-varicella
  Behcet disease
Fungal infection
  Cryptococcal meningitis
  Coccidioidal meningitis
  Candida
  Aspergillosis
  Mucormycosis
Parasitic infections
  Cysticercosis
  Gnathostomiasis
  Schistosomiasis
  Sparganosis
  Malaria

▶ **TABLE 11-2.** SYPHILIS AND STROKE

Meningovascular syphilis
  Medium-to-large caliber arteritis
  Basilar, middle cerebral, anterior spinal arteries
Syphilitic aortitis dissection and spinal cord infarction
Vascular symptoms usually occur in secondary or early tertiary stages of syphilis
Clinical presentations
  Fever and headache
  Signs of meningeal irritation
  Seizures
  Focal impairments
  Bilateral hearing loss (Cogan syndrome)
Diagnostic tests
  Cerebrospinal fluid
    Lymphocytosis
    Elevated protein concentration
    Reduced glucose concentration
    Serological tests positive in blood and CSF

▶ **TABLE 11-3.** TREATMENT OF INFECTIOUS DISEASES LEADING TO STROKE

Disease	Treatment
Meningovascular syphilis	Penicillin Erythromycin Antiplatelet agents
Tuberculous meningitis	Isoniazid Rifampin Ethambutol Streptomycin
Rocky Mountain spotted fever	Doxycycline
Herpes zoster arteritis	Corticosteroids Acyclovir Antiplatelet agents
Fungal meningitis	Amphotericin B Flucytosine Ambisome Fluconazole
Cysticercosis	Albendazole Praziquantel Corticosteroids
Malaria	Chloroquine Quinine Doxycycline Mefloquine

Diagnostic Studies

Examination of the CSF usually shows leucocytosis (lymphocytes), elevated protein content, and decreased glucose concentration. Serological tests for syphilis in the blood and CSF are positive.

Treatment

Besides antiplatelet agents, most patients with meningovascular syphilis are treated with penicillin (Table 11-3). Many patients with syphilis also have HIV infection; these patients require a prolonged course of antibiotic therapy. The course of neurosyphilis among persons with HIV appears to be accelerated.

▶ RETROPHARYNGEAL SUPPURATIVE INFECTIONS

Tonsillitis or a paratonsillar abscess can cause an arteritis of the adjacent internal carotid artery that leads to occlusion of the artery. Because of the swelling of the sheath, ipsilateral Horner syndrome can be detected.[9] A retropharyngeal infection can spread to involve the jugular vein and lead to thrombosis of the vessel at the level of the jugular foramen. This location for the thrombosis is suspected when palsies of the ipsilateral glossopharyngeal, vagal, and accessory nerves are found. Occasionally, an ipsilateral hypoglossal nerve palsy or Horner syndrome is found.

▶ SUPPURATIVE VENOUS THROMBOSIS

Suppurative infections of the face and head are important causes of venous thrombophlebitis. Bacterial infections of the nose, orbit, sinuses, and maxilla are associated with *cavernous sinus thrombosis* (see Chapter 18). Patients with cavernous sinus thrombosis usually have severe headache and fever followed by the development of ipsilateral orbital edema. Exophthalmos, chemosis, ocular congestion, ophthalmoplegia, and visual loss that initially appear ipsilaterally and then become bilateral are prominent. Patients can have evidence of pituitary failure. Examination of the CSF usually demonstrates lymphocytosis, elevated protein, and mildly depressed glucose. The cavernous sinus can be visualized by venography. Infections of the middle or inner ear or the mastoid or petrous portions of the temporal bone can lead to secondary *thrombosis of the transverse sinus*. The time course often is more prolonged than with cavernous sinus thrombosis, and in the past, the illness was described as otitic hydrocephalus. Patients usually have a course of increasing headache followed by signs of increased intracranial pressure, including papilledema. Focal neurological impairments, such as a cranial nerve palsy or hemiparesis, are uncommon. Brain imaging studies, including magnetic resonance venography, can be done to establish the diagnosis. Treatment of infectious venous sinus thrombophlebitis centers on antibiotics. Both heparin and oral anticoagulants can be prescribed.

▶ ACUTE BACTERIAL MENINGITIS

Arterial occlusion leading to infarction is a relatively uncommon complication of bacterial meningitis.[10,11] Presumably an inflammatory arteritis occurs secondary to the purulent material in the subarachnoid space. Cortical vein thrombophlebitis probably is more common than arteritis. The appearance of focal neurological impairments in a person with bacterial meningitis should prompt consideration of a secondary cortical vein thrombosis leading to infarction or secondary cortical hemorrhage.

▶ TUBERCULOUS MENINGITIS

Tuberculosis (*Mycobacterium tuberculosis*) affecting the nervous system causes proliferative and exudative meningitis that is located predominantly at the base of the brain. A secondary tuberculous endarteritis can cause either infarction or hemorrhage. Infarctions usually are in the pattern of the small penetrating arteries that arise from the basilar artery or the circle of Willis. Besides stroke, the pachymeningitis leads to multiple cranial nerve palsies and hydrocephalus. Tuberculous meningitis should be suspected as a cause of stroke among persons living in endemic areas, particularly if multiple cranial nerve palsies that appear to be of extra-axial origin are found. Persons from lower socioeconomic groups or who have an immunocompromised state (in particular HIV) are at risk. Chest X-ray should be done to look for a pulmonary cavitary lesion. Examination of the CSF usually detects a lymphocytic pleocytosis, depressed glucose level, low chloride level, and elevated protein concentration. The CSF protein level can be extraordinarily high. Cultures and staining for acid-fast bacilli are required. Treatment involves isoniazid, rifampin, ethambutol, and streptomycin (see Table 11-3).

▶ OTHER BACTERIAL INFECTIONS

Stroke has also been described as a complication of *brucellosis* of the central nervous system. In the United States, neurobrucellosis is rare and occurs among persons who deal with infected animals (veterinarians, farmers, or packing house employees). A cerebral arteritis usually occurs in the setting of a subacute or chronic granulomatous meningoencephalitis.

Rocky Mountain Spotted Fever

Patients with *Rocky Mountain spotted fever* (*Rickettsia rickettsii*) or *ehrlichiosis* can have prominent neurological impairments that are due to secondary vascular involvement. The vasculitis of small arterioles and venules can lead to multiple small infarctions in the brain. These tick-born illnesses usually present with fever, prostration, headache, nausea, vomiting, and myalgias within a few days of the bite. Rocky Mountain spotted fever usually has a maculopapular skin eruption that begins on the ankles and wrists and becomes generalized. The appearance of the skin eruption becomes petechial or purpuric. The dermatological features are less prominent with ehrlichiosis. Patients with ehrlichiosis usually have the triad of leucopenia, thrombocytopenia, and abnormal liver enzymes. The neurological signs include seizures, confusion, delirium, or coma. The CSF usually is consistent with an infectious process. Serological studies can detect increasing titers to Rickettsia rickettsii in Rocky Mountain spotted fever, while Giemsa stained blood smears can detect Ehrlichia inclusion bodies (morulae) within leucocytes. Doxycycline is the key antibiotic agent. Stroke is a rare complication of *Lyme disease* (*Borrelia burgdorferi*).[12]

Cat Scratch Disease

Cat scratch disease is secondary to infection with *Bartonella henselae*. Affected patients usually have fever, constitutional symptoms, and lymphadenopathy. Stroke secondary to an arteritis has been described.

Although *Whipple disease* (*Tropheryma whippelii*) does not produce an arteritis, it is among the alternative diagnoses in patients with suspected vasculitis of the central nervous system.[13] Patients usually have a history of chronic diarrhea complicated by multifocal neurological signs including dementia and oculomasticatory movements. *Typhoid fever* (salmonella typhi) can cause an endocarditis but strokes are uncommon.

▶ VIRAL ILLNESSES

Acquired Immune Deficiency Syndrome

Stroke is a potential complication of acquired immune deficiency syndrome (AIDS).[14,15] The viral illness is associated with an increased likelihood of both ischemic and hemorrhagic stroke.[15] Qureshi et al.[16] estimate that HIV infection increases the risk of cerebral infarction by a factor of 3.4. Inflammatory vascular disease is relatively common among children or adults with AIDS.[3] Evers et al.[17] found that strokes are secondary to an HIV-associated vasculitis or vasculopathy. Manifestations include silent stroke, clinically overt large or small artery occlusions or vascular dementia. Strokes can be the direct result of the HIV infection or be secondary to complicating viral or other opportunistic infections, endocarditis, or a prothrombotic state such as nonbacterial thrombotic endocarditis or thrombotic thrombocytopenia purpura. Hyperlipidemia also results from use of the protease inhibitor medications. In addition, some patients with AIDS will have meningovascular syphilis.

Hepatitis

A strong association exists between *hepatitis B* and periarteritis nodosa. In addition, *hepatitis C* can be linked to mixed cryoglobulinemia and vasculitis.[3]

Herpes Zoster

An intense arteritis of the intracranial (intracavernous) portion of the internal carotid artery can complicate herpes zoster infection involving the ophthalmic division of the trigeminal nerve.[18,19] The intense perivascular inflammation can lead to thrombosis and secondary retinal or cerebral ischemia. The ischemic symptoms usually develop several weeks after the overt cutaneous signs. The clinical scenario is a cerebral infarction that is compatible with an occlusion of the ipsilateral internal carotid artery than follows the herpetic infection. The affected patient might have residuals from the cutaneous vesicles. Vascular imaging shows severe stenosis or occlusion of the internal carotid artery. Treatment usually involves corticosteroids and antiplatelet aggregating agents. An antiviral agent, such as acyclovir, can be prescribed. A vasculitis or post-varicella angiopathy can complicate chickenpox in children. Disseminated varicella-zoster virus infections can lead to a vasculitis complicating HIV or other immuno-compromised states. In addition, there might be a relationship between varicella-zoster virus and the development of primary central nervous system vasculitis.

Herpes simplex encephalitis can cause hemorrhagic lesions within the temporal lobe. Rarely, the infection can produce a large symptomatic hemorrhage.[20]

Behçet Disease

The cause of Behçet disease has not been established; it could be either an infectious or inflammatory process. The usual symptoms are migratory arthralgias, oral and genital mucosal ulcerations, and meningitis. In addition, patients can have ischemic stroke, cerebral vasculitis, or cerebral venous thrombosis.[21]

► FUNGAL DISEASES

While sporadic cases of fungal infections leading to neurological dysfunction can be described, most infections are found among immunocompromised persons. The most common settings are patients with HIV infection or persons who have had transplantation. Both venous and arterial occlusions leading to hemorrhagic or ischemic strokes occur secondary to *candidiasis, mucormycosis, aspergillosis, coccidioidomycosis, cryptococcosis, histoplasmosis, nocardiosis,* and *actinomycosis.* Overall, the prognosis of patients with fungal causes of stroke is unfavorable, in part due to the patients' poor underlying health.

An arteritis can complicate fungal meningitis, including *cryptococcal meningitis.* Occlusion of larger intracranial arteries, including the vertebral artery, can occur. Vasculitis has been described as a complication of *coccidioidal meningitis.*

Candida fungemia can lead to meningoencephalitis, microabscesses, cerebral vasculitis, and infective aneurysms of the brain.[22] Cerebral infarction, intracerebral hemorrhage, and subarachnoid hemorrhage can be the result.

Aspergillosis

Aspergillosis can invade the intracranial vessels and produce a septic arteritis, progressive arterial occlusion, or infective aneurysm that leads to cerebral infarction or subarachnoid hemorrhage.[23,24] In addition, aspergillosis can produce a progressively enlarging intracranial mass with signs of increased intracranial pressure.

Mucormycosis

Mucormycosis usually involves the paranasal sinuses.[25,26] The infection can spread to the cavernous sinus leading to thrombosis and secondary occlusion of the internal carotid artery. Signs of cavernous sinus thrombosis usually are superimposed on the findings the sinus infection. Mucormycosis is most commonly detected among patients with diabetes mellitus.

Treatment focuses on intravenous or occasionally intrathecal administration of amphotericin B. Flucytosine, AmBisome, and fluconazole are also used to treat fungal infections (see Table 11-3). Surgical interventions or corticosteroids also might be needed.

► PARASITIC INFECTIONS

Stroke is a potential complication of helminthic infections.

Cysticercosis

Cysticercosis (taenia solium) usually presents with seizures, headache, decreased consciousness, or signs of increased intracranial pressure (Table 11-4). In addition, an inflammatory reaction secondary to brain or meningeal cysticerci involvement can lead to a proliferative endarteritis and a secondary infarction.[27] Associated severe basilar meningitis can induce occlusion of major arteries of the anterior or posterior circulation.[28] Strokes have been reported in 2–12 percent of patients with neurocysticercosis.[29] Brain imaging usually shows multiple intracranial calcifications. The presence of a cystic lesion with a scolex is a diagnostic CT finding. CSF examination usually shows leucocytosis and antibodies to the parasite.

► **TABLE 11-4.** CYSTICERCOSIS AND STROKE

Inflammatory reaction—brain/meningeal cysticerci
   Basilar meningitis
Clinical features
   Headache
   Seizures
   Decreased consciousness
   Signs of increased intracranial pressure
Diagnostic studies
   Multiple intracranial calcifications
   Cystic lesions with scolex
   Antibodies to parasite in CSF

Treatment includes albendazole and praziquantel and corticosteroids.

Malaria

Cerebral *malaria* usually is secondary to infection with *plasmodium falciparum.* Newton et al.[30] concluded that cerebral malaria might be the most common non-traumatic encephalopathy in the world. The neurological symptoms are secondary to stagnation of erythrocytes containing plasmodium trophozoites and meronts within the capillaries and venules in the brain.[31] Secondary ischemia and hemorrhage occur. Clavier et al.[32] could not find hypoperfusion among patients with cerebral malaria. Affected patients usually are natives of visitors to areas of the world where plasmodium falciparum is found. Patients have recurrent and episodic severe fevers associated with headache, sweats, malaise, and arthralgias. The neurological symptoms include seizures, papilledema, retinal hemorrhages, and decreased consciousness. The multifocal neurological impairments include ataxia, hemiparesis, and cortical blindness. Hypoglycemia can be a complication of severe malaria and a low blood glucose concentration should be excluded as an explanation for the neurological impairments. Thick blood smears obtained during a period of high fever and stained with Giemsa stain usually will detect the parasite. On occasion, several blood smears may need to be performed. Chloroquine and intravenously administered quinine are the primary therapies for treatment of cerebral malaria[30] (see Table 11-3). Quinine combined with doxycycline or mefloquine is prescribed to a patient who is infested with chloroquine-resistant plasmodium falciparum. Because increased intracranial pressure is a major cause of neurological morbidity, management also involves measures to control cerebral edema. Many patients will have relatively severe neurological sequelae.[30]

Other Parasitic Diseases

Neurological symptoms secondary to migration of the nematode *Gnathostoma spinigerum* (*gnathostomiasis*) can include intracranial hemorrhage. Damage of leptomeningeal or parenchymal blood vessels can result in hemorrhagic or ischemic stroke among persons infested with schistosomiasis. Parasitic involvement with *Schistosoma japonicum* (*schistosomiasis*) can cause intracranial hemorrhage while infarction of the spinal cord secondary to occlusion of the anterior spinal artery usually is due to infestation with either *Schistosoma mansoni* or *Schistosoma haematobium.*

A vasculitis has been described as a complication of *sparganosis,* which is secondary to the migration of the larva of the Spirometra cestodes. Large artery occlusions can be secondary to meningoencephalitis secondary to free living amebae such as acanthamoeba.

▶ NONINFECTIOUS INFLAMMATORY VASCULOPATHIES

Noninfectious vasculopathies that lead to ischemic or hemorrhagic stroke can be isolated to the central nervous system or can involve multiple organs in the body. The latter, called multisystem vasculitides, are more common and these vasculopathies usually are categorized by their pathological findings or presumed cause (Table 11-5). Vasculitis can be associated with collagen vascular disease, other systemic diseases, or hypersensitivity diseases, including reactions to medications.

Clinical Findings

Inflammatory vasculitis of the central nervous system can cause either hemorrhagic or ischemic vascular events. In general, patients with vasculitis of the central nervous system have clinical findings that are subacute or indolent in onset or symptoms that reflect involvement of multiple areas of the brain.[33,34] Rarely, vasculitis can affect the spinal cord.[35] In addition, many patients will have headaches, seizures, meningitis, cranial nerve palsies, peripheral neuropathy, or muscle dysfunction. Either mononeuropathy multiplex or polyneuropathy can be detected.[36–38] Patients with multisystem vasculitides also have findings reflecting involvement of other organs, the most common being the skin, kidney, lungs, and joints. In addition, many patients with multisystem vasculitides have abnormal serological findings.

▶ **TABLE 11-5.** NONINFECTIOUS INFLAMMATORY VASCULOPATHIES

Giant cell vasculitides
  Giant cell (temporal) arteritis
  Takayasu arteritis
Necrotizing vasculitides
  Polyarteritis (periarteritis) nodosa
  Wegener disease
  Churg–Strauss angiitis
  Microscopic polyangiitis
  Lymphomatoid granulomatosis
Collagen vascular diseases
  Systemic lupus erythematosus
  Rheumatoid arthritis
  Scleroderma
  Sjögren syndrome
Isolated vasculitis of the central nervous system
Other vasculitides
  Henoch–Schönlein purpura
  Cogan syndrome
  Eale disease
  Kawasaki disease
  Inflammatory bowel disease
  Sarcoidosis
Drug-induced vasculitis

► **TABLE 11-6.** NEUROLOGICAL MANIFESTATIONS OF MULTISYSTEM VASCULITIDES

Stroke
   Hemorrhagic stroke
   Ischemic stroke
   Encephalopathy
Headaches
Seizures
Psychiatric diseases
Dementia
Meningitis
Neuropathy
   Cranial nerve palsy
   Mononeuropathy
   Mononeuropathy multiplex
   Polyneuropathy
Myositis

Most patients with inflammatory vasculitides of the central nervous system have symptoms and signs that reflect involvement of multiple areas of the brain, which evolve or progress over a time course of several weeks (Table 11-6). Patients usually do not have symptoms or signs of a vascular event that affects only one area of the brain. Besides recurrent ischemic or hemorrhagic stroke, patients often have headaches, personality changes, psychiatric symptoms, cognitive decline, seizures, or decreased consciousness. Besides neurological impairments that reflect the multifocal nature of the illness, signs of meningeal irritation or cranial nerve palsies often are present.

Diagnostic Studies

While some patients' brain imaging tests are normal, most studies show multiple small lesions in both the gray and white matter (Fig. 11-1). Larger cerebral infarctions or parenchymal hemorrhages also can be found (Table 11-7). Less common findings include cortical atrophy or

► **TABLE 11-7.** RESULTS OF DIAGNOSTIC TESTS THAT SUGGEST A VASCULITIS

Brain imaging
   Multiple small areas of infarction
   Hemorrhages
Electroencephalography
   Diffuse slow activity
Cerebrospinal fluid examination
   Elevated lymphocytes
   Normal or slightly reduced glucose
   Elevated protein concentration
   Elevated immune globulins
Vascular imaging (arteriography)
   Segmental areas of narrowing
   Usually medium or small caliber vessels

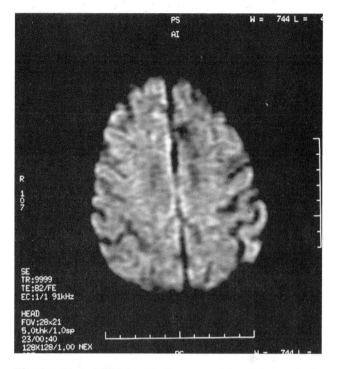

Figure 11-1. Multiple small areas of hyperintensity in both cerebral hemispheres are noted on a diffusion-weighted magnetic resonance imaging in a patient with suspected vasculitis.

hydrocephalus. An electroencephalogram commonly demonstrates diffuse slow activity consistent with global or multifocal brain dysfunction. Findings on CSF examination include lymphocytosis and a moderately elevated concentration of protein. A protein electrophoresis can show an inflammatory pattern of proteins. Because most vasculitides affect medium-caliber or smaller arteries, noninvasive vascular imaging studies, including MRA, usually are nondiagnostic. Arteriography remains the most effective method to screen for a vasculitis.[36,37] (Fig. 11-2). Several segmental areas of sausage-like narrowing that affect multiple intracranial arteries are the usual findings. While arteriography usually detects arteritis of a moderate-caliber vessel, the test might miss changes in smaller arteries. As a result, the study is nondiagnostic in approximately 50 percent of cases. The results of serological testing help define a multisystem vasculitis but these tests usually are normal when a patient has an isolated central nervous system angiitis. Brain and meningeal biopsy often is required to establish a diagnosis in a particularly challenging case. However, even this aggressive step can be nondiagnostic because an affected vessel might not be included in the biopsy specimen. Overall, the rate of false-negative biopsies can be as high as 50 percent. Trying to focus the biopsy on areas that show extensive involvement by brain or vascular imaging might improve the diagnostic yield.

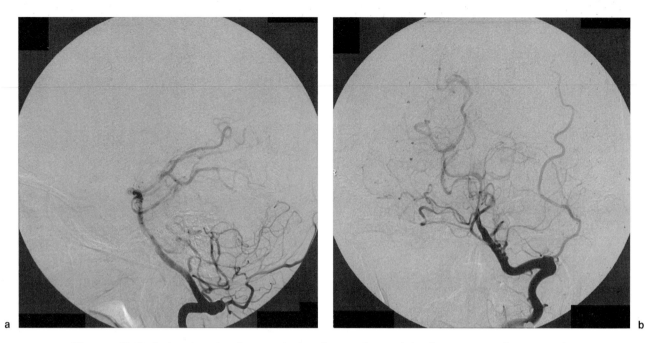

a   b

Figure 11-2. Lateral and anteroposterior views of a vertebral artery arteriogram using subtraction techniques demonstrate multiple areas of segmental narrowing in the cerebellar arteries. The findings are consistent with the diagnosis of vasculitis.

Treatment

While patients with ischemia secondary to an inflammatory vasculitis often are prescribed antiplatelet agents, the propensity for bleeding complications limits the use of anticoagulants. Medical treatment emphasizes the use of immunosuppressive agents including corticosteroids, cyclophosphamide, methotrexate, or azathioprine. Rarely, patients might be treated with reconstructive surgical procedures or endovascular interventions. The prognosis of persons with vasculitis has improved dramatically with the advent of modern immunosuppressive therapy.[4]

▶ GIANT CELL VASCULITIDES

The pathological finding of giant cells within the arterial wall is the hallmark of Takayasu disease and giant cell (temporal) arteritis.[39,40] The underlying pathology is an increase in the production of interleukin 1 and interleukin 6. These cytokines combined with gamma interferon activate the macrophages within the arterial wall.[39] The acute arterial injury promotes thrombosis and secondary ischemia, including stroke. In addition, these vasculitides can present as an isolated polymyalgia rheumatica with myalgias and signs of systemic inflammation.[39]

▶ TAKAYASU ARTERITIS

Takayasu disease leads to continuous or patchy granulomatous changes with lymphocytes, histiocytes, and multinucleated giant cells in all layers of the arterial wall and produces giant cells in the medial and adventitial layers.[2,33,41] The wall of the affected artery becomes thickened and the vascular lumen is impinged. Aneurysmal dilatations can also develop. It preferentially affects the aorta and its major branches.[42] It also affects the proximal portions of the mesenteric and renal arteries. Secondary thrombosis of the inflamed vessels occurs.

In North America, the incidence of Takayasu disease is estimated as 2.6 per million people.[43] It is most commonly detected among women younger than 40.[43,44] The prevalence of Takayasu disease is highest in eastern Asia and Mexico.

Clinical Findings

Early involvement of the subclavian arteries leads to absence of pulses in the upper extremities (Table 11-8). Some patients will be asymptomatic with only decreased pulses being found. However, secondary hypoperfusion can lead to limb claudication or rarely the symptoms of subclavian steal syndrome.[4] Asymmetrical involvement of the major arteries can produce an asymmetry of pulses or blood pressure readings between the two arms. These

▶ **TABLE 11-8.** TAKAYASU ARTERITIS

Granulomatous changes in aorta and major arteries
    Involve subclavian and common carotid arteries
Clinical features
    Age < 40
    Women more frequent than men
    Persons of Asian or Mexican ancestry
    Fever, chills, malaise, weight loss
    Carotidynia
    Limb claudication
    Decreased pulses in upper extremities
    Asymmetrical blood pressure values in upper extremities
    Pain with chewing
Cerebrovascular features
    Cerebral infarction
    TIA
    Seizures
    Vascular dementia
    Amaurosis fugax
    Ischemic oculopathy
Diagnostic studies
    Anemia
    Elevated erythrocyte sedimentation rate
    Elevated C-reactive protein
    Progressive stenosis or occlusion of major arteries

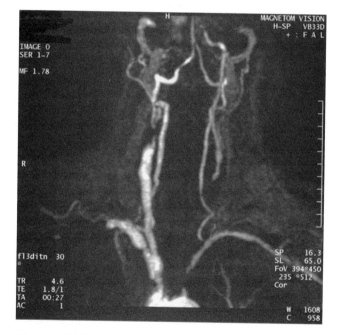

Figure 11-3. An aortiogram demonstrates occlusions of the left common carotid and left sublavian arteries in young women with Takayasu disease. A stenosis of the brachiophalic artery is visualized.

findings mimic those seen with severe extracranial atherosclerosis. Arterial hypertension with higher levels in the lower extremities than in the arms or multiple cervical bruits can be detected.

Most patients with Takayasu arteritis have headache, fever, malaise, weight loss, carotidynia, myalgias, or arthralgias.[2,44] Some patients can have ischemic muscle pain with chewing or atrophy of the muscles of the face. Dilation of the aorta can cause aortic regurgitation. Involvement of the abdominal aorta can affect the origins of the renal arteries, which in turn leads to hypertension. Patients with pulmonary involvement can have cough, dyspnea, chest pain, or pulmonary hypertension.[43] Stroke is the most serious complication of Takayasu disease. Ischemic symptoms also include amaurosis fugax, TIA, cerebral infarction, seizures, or vascular dementia. Hypertensive retinopathy, ischemic oculopathy, ischemic optic neuropathy, or retinal hemorrhages can be found.

Diagnostic Studies

Laboratory abnormalities include anemia, leucocytosis, and increases in erythrocyte sedimentation rate (ESR) and C-reactive protein (CRP). Other serological studies usually are normal. Narrowing, occlusion, or aneurysms of the major arteries can be detected by arteriography, CTA, or MRA (Figs. 11-3 and 11-4). Wall thickening, calcification, and mural thrombosis also can be imaged. A *double ring pattern* in the arterial wall can be detected by CT.[3]Ultrasonography of the common carotid artery

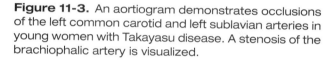

Figure 11-4. A magnetic resonance angiogram obtained in a young woman with Takayasu disease shows absence of the left common carotid artery. Stenosis of the brachiocephalia and right subclavian artery are present. The left subclavian aretery, which is occluded proximally, is perfused via retrograde flow in the vertebral artery (subclavian steal).

detects a homogenous increase in the thickness of the arterial wall. A long continuous circumferential and homogenous thickening of the wall (*macaroni sign*) of the common carotid artery can be detected by high-resolution ultrasonography.[3]

Treatment

The prognosis generally is influenced by the presence of congestive heart failure, hypertension, aortic regurgitation, and a dilated cardiomyopathy.[43] Medical management usually involves a course of steroids combined with antiplatelet agents (Table 11-9). Cyclophosphamide or methotrexate has been administered in combination with steroids.[2] Reconstructive operations and endovascular interventions have been used to improve flow, although Hunder[2] reported that angioplasty was not particularly useful.

▶ **TABLE 11-9.** MANAGEMENT OF PATIENTS WITH INFLAMMATORY VASCULITIDES

Disease	Treatment
Takayasu arteritis	Corticosteroids
	Cyclophosphamide
	Revascularization operations
	Antiplatelet agents
Giant cell (temporal) arteritis	Corticosteroids
Periarteritis (polyarteritis) nodosa	Cyclophosphamide
	Corticosteroids
Wegener disease	Cyclophosphamide
	Corticosteroids
	Azathioprine
	Methotrexate
Churg–Strauss angiitis	Corticosteroids
	Cyclophosphamide
	Azathioprine
	Intravenous immune globulin
	Interferon-alpha
	Cyclosporine
Systemic lupus erythematosus	Corticosteroids
	Cyclophosphamide
	Azathioprine
Antiphospholipid antibodies/ Sneddon syndrome	Anticoagulants
	Antiplatelet agents
Rheumatoid arthritis	Corticosteroids
	Cyclophosphamide
Sjögren syndrome	Corticosteroids
	Cyclophosphamide
	Methotrexate
	Cyclosporine
Isolated vasculitis of the central nervous system	Corticosteroids
	Cyclophosphamide

▶ GIANT CELL ARTERITIS

Giant cell arteritis (temporal arteritis, cranial arteritis) is one of the more common forms of vasculitis in the United States.[2] It causes a segmental granulomatous inflammation of medium-caliber arteries of the head.[42] The disease most commonly affects the superficial temporal, ophthalmic, posterior ciliary, and vertebral arteries. The inflammatory disease can also affect the aorta and several branches.[43] The classic pathological finding on arterial biopsy is the presence of intramural giant cells within the artery (Fig. 11-5). The inflammatory changes are seen along the internal elastic lamina of the arterial wall.[2] The changes are segmental and a temporal biopsy can be falsely negative.

Clinical Findings

Giant cell arteritis rarely affects persons younger than 60 (Table 11-10). Women are much more commonly affected than men. The disease is more commonly diagnosed among persons of Northern European ancestry than among persons of Asian or African heritage. Most patients have malaise, low-grade fever, weight loss, and muscle aches.[34,45] *Polymyalgia rheumatica*, which is marked by pain and stiffness in the neck and proximal muscles of the upper and lower extremities, is strongly associated with giant cell arteritis.[39] Polymyalgia rheumatica is more common than giant cell arteritis and not all patients with the muscle symptoms will develop other evidence of the arterial disease.[2] The diagnosis of polymyalgia requires muscle pain and stiffness, particularly prominent in the morning, in the shoulders, hips, neck, or trunk and an elevated erythrocyte sedimentation rate. Jaw pain (jaw claudication) occurs with chewing and this symptom presumably is

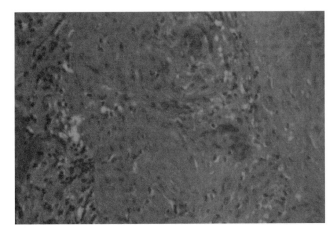

Figure 11-5. A biopsy from the superficial temporal artery in a patient with giant cell arteritis shows marked inflammatory changes, obliteration of the vascular lumen, and giant cells. (*Courtesy of S.S. Schoche, M.D., Department of Pathology, University of West Virginia.*)

► **TABLE 11-10.** GIANT CELL (TEMPORAL) ARTERITIS

Granulomatous inflammation of medium-caliber arteries of head
  Superficial temporal
  Ophthalmic and posterior ciliary
  Vertebral
Clinical features
  Age > 60
  Women more frequent than men
  Persons of Northern European ancestry
  Polymyalgia rheumatica
  Jaw claudication
  Severe unilateral (temporal) headache
  Palpably enlarged, tortuous, and tender artery
  Myocardial infarction
Cerebrovascular features
  Monocular or binocular blindness
  Posterior ciliary artery occlusion
  Central retinal artery occlusion
  Cerebral infarction
  TIA
Diagnostic studies
  Elevated erythrocyte sedimentation rate
  Elevated C-reactive protein
  Anemia and leucocytosis
  Temporal artery biopsy

due to ischemia of the muscles secondary to arteritis involving branches of the external carotid artery.[4] A severe headache, which usually is unilateral and often described as throbbing, is the most important symptom. Because of the importance of headache as a presentation of giant cell arteritis, the illness should be suspected whenever an elderly patient complains of the recent onset of persisting unilateral headaches. On examination, the superficial temporal artery often is palpably enlarged, tortuous, and tender.[4] Occasionally, a cervical bruit or decreased pulse is detected when the arteritis involves extracranial vessels.

Giant cell arteritis is a leading cause of visual loss in the elderly. Ocular ischemia, secondary to occlusion of an affected posterior ciliary, can lead to monocular or rarely binocular blindness. Less frequently, blindness can be secondary to occlusion of a central retinal artery. Cerebral infarction, most commonly in the distribution in the posterior circulation, is another complication.[46,47] Myocardial infarction and aortic disease also are potential complications of giant cell arteritis. The aortitis can lead to formation of an aneurysm, aortic dissection, or aortic rupture.[43]

Diagnostic Studies

Almost all patients have markedly increased levels of the ESR and CRP. Occasionally, a patient will have a normal ESR level but increased levels of CRP. As a result, the CRP may be a more sensitive screening test. An elevated plasma level of interleukin-6 or other cytokines is associated with the degree of disease activity.[3] Most patients will have a normocytic, normochromic anemia, and leucocytosis. Temporal artery biopsy usually is recommended. Because it is a segmental arteritis, the biopsy should include a long segment of the artery on the symptomatic side. On occasion, bilateral resections are necessary. A second biopsy is done when the first specimen is negative and the index of suspicion for giant cell arteritis is strong. Still, some patients with giant cell arteritis have negative temporal artery biopsies.

Treatment

Treatment with large doses of corticosteroids is the mainstay of management (see Table 11-9). Because of the high risk of visual loss, patients with suspected giant cell arteritis should be treated with corticosteroids even while awaiting the results for the temporal artery biopsy. The usual treatment is 40–60 mg of oral prednisone given daily and then tapered as the patient's symptoms improve. Alternative day administration of medication usually is not effective. Patients generally have a dramatic response to corticosteroids—not only does the headache improve but the other symptoms also resolve. Most patients require a prolonged course of treatment with a gradual tapering dosage regimen. An increase in constitutional symptoms or a recurrent elevation of CRP or ESR usually mandates an increase in the corticosteroids. The usual course of the illness is 2–3 years.

► NECROTIZING VASCULITIDES

The multisystem necrotizing vasculitides can cause neurological symptoms secondary to involvement of medium-caliber or smaller arteries. The most common are Wegener disease, Churg–Strauss angiitis, and polyarteritis (periarteritis) nodosa. Other illnesses include microscopic polyangiitis, necrotizing systemic vasculitis-overlap syndrome, and lymphomatoid granulomatosis.

► POLYARTERITIS (PERIARTERITIS) NODOSA

Polyarteritis nodosa (PAN), which affects medium-to-small arterioles, capillaries, and venules, occurs in people of all ages although the peak ages are 40–60.[33,34,42] Men are more commonly affected than women and the disease occurs in all ethnic groups.[2] Approximately 10 percent of cases seem to be associated with hepatitis B virus infections.[2] Central nervous system disease is second to renal failure as a cause of death among persons with

▶ **TABLE 11-11.** POLYARTERITIS (PERIARTERITIS) NODOSA

Necrotizing Vasculitis of Small Caliber Arteries

Clinical features
  All ages, but peak at 40–60
  Men more frequent than women
  Fever, malaise, arthralgias, and weight loss
  Asthma
  Hypertension
  Hematuria
  Myocardial infarction
  Congestive heart failure
  Abdominal pain
  Nausea, vomiting, and anorexia
  Diarrhea including melena
  Hepatomegaly
  Cutaneous hemorrhages and ulcers
  Livedo reticularis
Cerebrovascular features
  Lobar hemorrhage
  Cerebral infarction including lacunar infarctions
  Encephalopathy
  Seizures
  Headaches
  Spinal cord infarction or hemorrhage
Diagnostic studies
  Abnormal urinalysis (red blood cells and casts)
  Leucocytosis and eosinophilia
  Elevated erythrocyte sedimentation rate
  Abnormal hepatitis B antigen
  Antiphospholipid antibodies
  Stenosis or aneurysmal dilation of arteries
  Renal, muscle, or peripheral nerve biopsy

PAN. In particular, children and young adults appear vulnerable to central nervous system involvement.[1]

Clinical Findings

Most patients with PAN are acutely ill (Table 11-11). Fevers, malaise, arthralgias, and weight loss often are prominent. Most patients have evidence of gastrointestinal, pulmonary, renal, or dermatological dysfunction. Male patients can complain of testicular pain or tenderness.[4] Skin changes include ulcers and livedo reticularis. Renal involvement, secondary to local vasculitis leading to multiple infarctions, can progress to renal failure or malignant hypertension.[42] Renal failure and gastrointestinal ischemia are the leading causes of death.[2] Skin or mucosal ulcerations are found. Cardiac signs are less frequent. Mononeuropathy multiplex, secondary to vasculitic induced ischemia, is the most common neurological complication.[4]

Ocular ischemia or hemorrhage results from retinal vasculitis. Central nervous system symptoms include headache, seizures, encephalopathy, spinal cord ischemia,

and hemorrhagic or ischemic strokes of the brain. Multiple lacunar infarctions secondary to a microangiopathy have been reported.[48] However, hemorrhagic stroke is more frequent than ischemic stroke largely because of the necrotizing nature of the vasculitis.[48] Most hemorrhages are lobar in location. Rarely, intracranial bleeding can be the presenting feature of PAN.

Diagnostic Studies

Laboratory abnormalities include increased protein and the presence of red blood cells in the urinalysis reflecting renal involvement. Renal arteriography can demonstrate microaneurysms in the kidneys. Mesenteric arteriography can demonstrate focal stenosis or aneurysmal dilation in a patient with abdominal symptoms.[2] Chest X-ray usually is normal. Other findings include eosinophilia, an elevated ESR, antiphospholipid antibodies, and abnormal serological studies including hepatitis B antigen.[49] Some patients will have antiphospholipid antibodies. Renal, cutaneous, muscle, or peripheral nerve biopsy usually is required to demonstrate the changes of arteritis.

Treatment

Cyclophosphamide is the primary therapy (see Table 11-9). The agent can be given in a daily oral dose program or an intravenous pulse regimen. Maintenance of adequate hydration helps lessen the complication of hemorrhagic cystitis. Administration of mesna can less the bladder toxicity from cyclophosphamide. Other potential complications of cyclophosphamide are gonadal dysfunction, alopecia, or malignancies. Corticosteroids usually are given in conjunction with cyclophosphamide. Interferon alpha-2 has been used to treat patients with hepatitis-B associated arteritis.[2]

▶ WEGENER DISEASE

Clinical Findings

Wegener disease is a fulminating necrotizing disease that usually causes granulomas of the sinuses and airway leading to prominent pulmonary and sinus symptoms. The peak incidence of Wegener disease is the fourth and fifth decades and it has a slightly higher frequency in men than in women[2] (Table 11-12). The disease is associated with a necrotizing glomerulonephritis. Fulminant Wegener disease can be rapidly fatal. Nasal and oral inflammation is not unique to Wegener disease, the same symptoms can occur among patients who have microscopic polyangiitis.[4]

Ocular findings include uveitis, retinal hemorrhages, retinal infarction, ocular myositis, or orbital pseudotumor.[50–52] Neurological symptoms usually involve an isolated cranial or peripheral mononeuropathy or

► **TABLE 11-12.** WEGENER DISEASE

Necrotizing Vasculitis of Small-to-Medium Caliber Arteries

Clinical features
  Nasal discharge and sinusitis
  Nasal mucosal ulceration
  Cough
  Weight loss
  Hematuria
  Arthritis
Ocular features
  Uveitis
  Corneal ulcers
  Ocular myositis
  Orbital pseudotumor
Cerebrovascular features
  Retinal hemorrhage or infarction
  Intracranial hemorrhage
  Venous thrombosis
  Arterial thrombosis
Diagnostic studies
  Eosinophilia
  Elevated erythrocyte sedimentation rate
Presence of cytoplasmic antineutrophil cytoplasmic
  antibodies (c-ANCA)

mononeuropathy multiplex.[52] The neuropathies are secondary to ischemic vasculitis or granuloma formation. Other neurological complications include a myopathy, cerebritis, or myelopathy. Involvement of the central nervous system is much less common than the peripheral neuropathies. Central nervous system vasculitis usually involves small-to-moderate vessels (Fig. 11-6). Stroke is the result of intracranial hemorrhage, venous thrombosis,

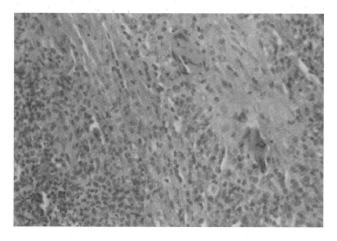

Figure 11-6. An orbital tissue specimen reveals marked inflammatory changes found with a necrotizing vasculitis. The pathological findins are supportive of the diagnosis of Wegener disease. (*Courtesy of S.S. Schochett, M.D., Department of Pathology, University of West Virginia.*)

or arterial thrombosis.[53] Arteritis of the basilar artery leading to brain stem infarction has been reported.[54]

Diagnostic Studies

Patients usually have eosinophilia, an elevated ESR, and the presence of cytoplasmic-ANCA (c-ANCA).[3] The presence of c-ANCA is strongly associated with active Wegener disease. Because of the strong relationship to high c-ANCA levels, the diagnosis of Wegener disease should be questioned if c-ANCA titers are not elevated. Imaging (CT) of the chest can demonstrate nodular or cavitary lesions or areas of segmental narrowing of airways.[2] CT of the skull also can detect involvement of the bony sinuses or areas behind the orbits.

Treatment

Administration of corticosteroids in combination with cyclophosphamide is the foundation of medical treatment[2] (see Table 11-9). Remission can be achieved in more than 90 percent of patients. In order to reduce toxic side effects, a pulse intravenous administration of cyclophosphamide is often recommended. However, a daily oral regimen of cyclophosphamide might be more effective.[2] Azathioprine and methotrexate are alternatives to treatment with cyclophosphamide. The combination of trimethoprim and sulfamethoxazole also has been recommended.

► CHURG–STRAUSS ANGIITIS

Clinical Findings

Churg–Strauss angiitis (syndrome) is a relatively rare multisystem allergic vasculitis that causes asthma, eosinophilia, sinusitis, prominent pulmonary infiltrates on chest X-ray, and neurological symptoms.[55] The frequency of Churg–Strauss syndrome is estimated as approximately 2.4–6.8/100,000 although the incidence is significantly higher among a population of persons with asthma.[55] Pathologically, the disease is marked by eosinophilic-rich granulomatous inflammation and a necrotizing vasculitis affecting small-to-medium sized vessels.[4,42] The most common neurological symptoms are mononeuropathy, mononeuropathy multiplex, or polyneuropathy presumably secondary vasculitis-induced ischemia (Table 11-13). Cranial neuropathy, anterior ischemic optic neuropathy, or retinal vasculitis occurs rarely.[56] Central nervous system involvement is limited but intraventricular hemorrhage can be secondary to a necrotizing vasculitis of the choroid plexus.

Churg–Strauss angiitis is most commonly diagnosed in middle-aged women. The course of the illness can be fulminant with a neurological course than can mimic an acute inflammatory polyradiculoneuropathy. Cardiac

▶ **TABLE 11-13.** CHURG–STRAUSS ANGIITIS

Multisystem Allergic Vasculitis

Clinical features
  Most commonly among ages 40–60 years
  Women more frequent then men
  Asthma
  Sinusitis
  Abdominal pain
  Congestive heart failure
  Myocarditis or pericarditis
  Palpable purpura of skin
  Cerebrovascular features
  Anterior ischemic optic neuropathy
  Retinal vasculitis
  Intraventricular hemorrhage
Diagnostic studies
  Eosinophilia
  Pulmonary infiltrates
  Sinus abnormalities
  Presence of antineutrophil cytoplasmic antibodies

involvement can lead to death. The presence of a strong history of asthma and the laboratory finding of eosinophilia are required for diagnosis.

Diagnostic Studies

While all patients have eosinophilia, in some cases, the eosinophil count can be extremely high. The chest X-ray usually demonstrates multiple areas of parenchymal consolidation in the lung parenchyma. Approximately two-thirds of the patients have perinuclear-ANCA (p-ANCA).[55] While the p-ANCA pattern can respond to several antigens, the antibodies develop especially against myeloperoxidase in polymorphonuclear leukocytes and monocytes.

The overall prognosis of patients with Churg–Strauss syndrome is relatively good. Most deaths are secondary to cardiac involvement.

Treatment

The combination of corticosteroids and cyclophosphamide is the usual management (see Table 11-9). Azathioprine also has been given to some patients. Alternative therapies include intravenous immune globulin, interferon-alpha, mycophenolate mofetil, and cyclosporine.[55]

▶ OTHER NECROTIZING VASCULITIDES

Microscopic Polyangiitis

Microscopic polyangiitis is a rare multisystem necrotizing vasculitis, which is distinct from PAN because it affects primarily small vessels such as arterioles, capillaries, and

venules.[42] The primary clinical manifestation is renal failure secondary to a severe necrotizing glomerulonephritis. Pulmonary involvement can occur. While neurological symptoms are relatively uncommon, small artery occlusions leading to stroke could be a potential complication. Findings on diagnostic evaluation include hematuria, proteinuria, and the presence of p-ANCA. Corticosteroids and cyclophosphamide are the primary therapies.

Lymphomatoid Granulomatosis

Lymphomatoid granulomatosis affects the central nervous system, respiratory tract, and skin.

▶ COLLAGEN VASCULAR DISEASES

Systemic lupus erythematosus, rheumatoid arthritis, scleroderma, and Sjögren syndrome are the collagen vascular diseases most commonly associated with neurological complications, including stroke. The ischemic and hemorrhagic events presumably are secondary to vasculitis.

▶ SYSTEMIC LUPUS ERYTHEMATOSUS

Systemic lupus erythematosus (SLE) is the most common collagen vascular disease. It is diagnosed in young women with evidence of multisystem involvement.

Clinical Findings

Fever, malaise, arthralgias, renal dysfunction, pulmonary symptoms, and prominent dermatological changes occur (Table 11-14). Peripheral neuropathy is relatively uncommon. Signs of central nervous system dysfunction are relatively common. Psychiatric disturbances, cognitive impairments, or mental status changes are the most common abnormalities presumably on the basis of a multifocal process.[34,57] Headaches, seizures, or a myelopathy also can occur. Hemorrhagic or ischemic stroke are potential complications. Recent reports suggest that the inflammatory process of SLE can promote the development of atherosclerosis at a young age.[58,59]

While vasculitis can affect the skin and other organs, vasculitic involvement of intracranial arteries is relatively uncommon. Rather than generalized ischemia secondary to small artery vasculitis, some of the encephalopathic symptoms may be secondary to the primary immunological disease. Strokes in the setting in the SLE are relatively uncommon and probably are secondary to nonvasculitic causes.[57,60,61] Most patients with SLE and stroke will not have evidence of a vasculitis on arteriography.

▶ **TABLE 11-14.** SYSTEMIC LUPUS ERYTHEMATOSUS

Multisystem Inflammatory Disease

Clinical features
  Age < 40
  Women more frequent than men
  Malar erythema (butterfly rash)
  Erythematous raised discoid patches
  Photosensitivity
  Mucosal or nasal ulcers
  Renal dysfunction
  Pleuritis or pericarditis
Cerebrovascular features
  Psychiatric symptoms
  Cognitive impairments
  Encephalopathy
  Headaches
  Seizures
  Cerebral infarction
  Hypertensive brain hemorrhage
Diagnostic studies
  Abnormal urinalysis (hematuria and casts)
  Leucocytosis
  Thrombocytopenia
  Anemia
  Presence of antinuclear antibodies
  Elevated erythrocyte sedimentation rate
  Elevated C-reactive protein
  Presence of cryoglobulins

Lupus Anticoagulants

Ischemic strokes among persons with SLE often are secondary to the presence of circulating anticoagulants (*lupus anticoagulants*) or antiphospholipid antibodies[61,62,63] (Table 11-15). These serological changes lead to the intravascular deposition of platelets and clotting proteins leading to venous or arterial occlusion. As a result, affected patients can have deep vein thrombosis, pulmonary embolism, myocardial ischemia, or recurrent ischemic stroke.

▶ **TABLE 11-15.** SYSTEMIC LUPUS ERYTHEMATOSUS AND ANTIPHOSPHOLIPID ANTIBODIES

Sneddon syndrome
  Digital ischemia
  Livedo reticularis
  Recurrent ischemic stroke
  Seizures
Libman–Sacks endocarditis
Presence of a lupus anticoagulant
  Prolonged activated partial thromboplastin time
  Presence of antiphospholipid antibodies

Sneddon Syndrome

Some patients will have the presence of livedo reticularis, digital ischemia, and stroke (*Sneddon syndrome*).[64] The presence of antiphospholipid antibodies in a patient with SLE is associated with the development of *Libman–Sacks endocarditis*. The vegetations, which are most commonly detected on the mitral valve, are secondary to the immune prothrombotic state can be the source of recurrent cerebral embolization. In addition, some patients with SLE will have evidence of *thrombotic thrombocytopenic purpura* or the *hemolytic uremic syndrome*, which can be complicated by an encephalopathy or recurrent ischemic stroke.[65] Because of the renal involvement with secondary hypertension, persons with SLE have an increased risk of large or small artery atherosclerotic disease leading to cerebral infarction or hypertensive hemorrhage.

Diagnostic Studies

Serological studies usually are abnormal, including an elevated ESR, CRP, and cryoglobulins. Both C-3 and C-4 complement levels can be low. Antinuclear antibodies are present. The urinalysis usually is abnormal. Some patients will have leucocytosis or thrombocytopenia. Anemia also can be found. The presence of a lupus anticoagulant can be detected by the finding of a prolonged activated partial thromboplastin time that can be corrected. Elevated IgM and IgG antiphospholipid antibodies often are found among patients with stroke and SLE.

Treatment

Most patients with SLE, including those with evidence of vasculitis, are treated with corticosteroids (see Table 11-9). Some patients require more aggressive immunosuppressive therapy including cyclophosphamide or azathioprine. Patients with circulating antiphospholipid antibodies or lupus anticoagulants usually are treated with anticoagulants. However, the superiority of anticoagulants over antiplatelet aggregating agents is not established.

▶ RHEUMATOID ARTHRITIS

Rheumatoid arthritis is most commonly diagnosed in young adult men and women; as denoted by the name, inflammation of the joints is the most common clinical finding. The most common neurological problems are a compressive mononeuropathy or mononeuropathy multiplex, the later due to a panarteritis involving small- to medium-caliber vessels (Table 11-16). Spine involvement (*ankylosing spondylitis*) is diagnosed most commonly in young men. Rheumatologic involvement of the spine can cause a compressive myelopathy. In addition, severe

▶ **TABLE 11-16.** NEUROLOGICAL MANIFESTATIONS OF RHEMATOID ARTHERITIS AND SJÖGREN SYNDROME

Rheumatoid arthritis
   Compressive mononeuropathy
   Mononeuropathy multiplex
   Myelopathy
   Atlanto-occipital subluxation
   Vertebral artery compression
   Vasculitis
      Infarction
      Hemorrhage
Sjögren syndrome
   Trigeminal neuropathy
   Dry eyes and dry mouth
   Vasculitis

---

arthritis of the cervical spine can cause secondary compression of a vertebral artery. Laxity of the longitudinal ligament of the cervical spine can cause *subluxation of the atlantooccipital junction* leading to secondary brainstem or vertebral artery compression.[66,67] Patients with vertebral artery compression have transient symptoms reflecting posterior circulation ischemia provoked by head movements. A vasculitis of the central nervous system is relatively rare.[34,68] However, some patients can have multiple small infarctions, cerebritis, subarachnoid hemorrhage, or intracerebral hemorrhage. An elevated rheumatoid factor usually is found on serological examination. Corticosteroids usually are the primary therapy but when the medication is ineffective, cyclophosphamide usually is given (see Table 11-9).

▶ SCLERODERMA

Scleroderma is diagnosed most commonly among middle-aged women. Rarely scleroderma or *CREST (calcinosis, Raynaud phenomenon, esophageal dysfunction, sclerodactyly, and telangiectasia)* can be complicated by neurological symptoms, including a vasculitis[69] (see Table 11-16).

▶ SJÖGREN SYNDROME

Stroke can be the initial finding of Sjögren (sicca) syndrome. The cerebrovascular events usually are ascribed to vasculitis of small- to medium-caliber arteries.[70,71] However, cranial neuropathies, especially trigeminal neuropathy, are the most common neurological complications of the illness (see Table 11-16). Sjögren syndrome occurs in isolation or in combination with other autoimmune disorders including rheumatoid arthritis or SLE. The illness should be suspected when a patient has dryness of the eyes and mouth in conjunction to other evidence of a multisystem vasculitis. Corticosteroids are the mainstay of treatment. Other therapies include cyclophosphamide, methotrexate, and cyclosporine.

▶ ISOLATED VASCULITIS OF THE CENTRAL NERVOUS SYSTEM

Isolated (primary) central nervous system vasculitis (*granulomatous angiitis*) occurs in men and women of any age. This relatively rare necrotizing arteriopathy, which affects medium-sized and small arteries, does not involve other organs or produce systemic serological abnormalities (Table 11-17).[1,33,34,72]

Clinical Findings

While some patients can have fever, malaise, or uveitis, most have findings reflecting only dysfunction of the central nervous system. Most patients with isolated vasculitis of the central nervous system do not have evidence of major arterial involvement; as a result, a major hemorrhagic or ischemic stroke is uncommon. Rather, the multifocal inflammatory arteriopathy usually is restricted to medium- or small-caliber arteries. Patients have headache, seizures, a delirium, or cognitive changes that evolve over several days to weeks. While focal motor, sensory, or visual impairments occur, most patients have an encephalopathy that evolves into a decline in consciousness. Occasionally, the symptoms can mimic those of an intracranial mass.

▶ **TABLE 11-17.** ISOLATED VASCULITIS OF THE CENTRAL NERVOUS SYSTEM

Necrotizing Vasculitis of Medium-Caliber Arteries

Clinical features
   All age groups
   Women and men
   Nonneurological symptoms are uncommon
Cerebrovascular features
   Headache
   Seizures
   Encephalopathy
   Delirium
   Cognitive changes
   Ischemic stroke
Diagnostic studies
   Elevated erythrocyte sedimentation rate
   Multiple areas of infarction on brain imaging
   Contrast enhancement of meninges
   Cerebrospinal fluid—lymphocytosis, increased protein, elevated immune globulins, decreased glucose
   Segmental narrowing on arteriography
   Brain and meningeal biopsy

Diagnostic Studies

Most serological studies are normal although sometimes an elevated ESR is seen. Brain imaging studies usually show multiple areas of ischemia. Contrast-enhanced imaging studies show enhancement of the meninges or small penetrating arteries of the brain. The electroencephalographic findings include generalized slow activity. The CSF usually is abnormal; findings include lymphocytosis, elevated protein level, elevated immune globulins, and normal glucose concentration. Arteriography remains the most important diagnostic test but the study can be normal in up to 50 percent of cases.[73] The usual findings are segmental areas of narrowing in multiple intracranial arteries, arterial occlusions, peripheral aneurysms, and sluggish flow (see Fig. 11-2). Brain and leptomeningeal biopsy often is needed but because of the focal nature of the vasculitis, the biopsy can give a false negative diagnosis (Fig. 11-7). The classical histopathological findings are a segmental granulomatous vasculitis with Langhans or multinucleated giant cells.[1]

Treatment

Long-term administration of corticosteroids is the mainstay of treatment. Some patients also are treated with cyclophosphamide (see Table 11-9).

▶ OTHER VASCULITIDES

Ischemic or hemorrhagic stroke can be a complication of other autoimmune diseases such as hypersensitivity vasculitis, reactions to medications, inflammatory bowel disease, sarcoidosis, Cogan syndrome, Eale disease, Kawasaki disease, cryoglobulinemia, or dermatomyositis.

Henoch–Schönlein Purpura

Henoch–Schönlein purpura is a hypersensitivity vasculitis that is most commonly diagnosed in children. Pathologically, IgA dominant immune deposits affecting small vessels are found primarily in the skin, bowel, and kidneys.[4] Clinical features include purpura, arthritis, gastrointestinal disease, renal disease, and neurological problems. Both intracranial hemorrhage and cerebral infarction are potential complications.

Cogan Syndrome

Cogan syndrome is secondary to a vasculitis that has features consistent with periarteritis nodosa (Table 11-18). It is usually diagnosed in young adults and is more common in men.[7,8] Bilateral hearing loss secondary to ischemia usually occurs suddenly. Uveitis, conjunctivitis, ocular ischemia, and episcleritis also are found. Patients also have fever, headache, weight loss, malaise, psychiatric disease, arthralgias, and aortic insufficiency. Thrombocytopenia and abnormal CSF, including leucocytosis and an elevated protein, are found during assessment. Treatment focuses on corticosteroids.

Eale Disease

Eale disease usually is diagnosed in young men who have recurrent ocular symptoms including retinal perivasculitis and vitreous hemorrhage. Ischemic stroke can complicate this illness.[74]

Kawasaki Disease

Kawasaki disease can be complicated by stroke in children. Approximately 80 percent of the affected patients are under the age of 5.[75] It is more common among boys and among children of Asian ancestry. The highest incidence of Kawasaki disease in the United States is in Hawaii.[75] This vasculitis, which can lead to formation of aneurysms, can affect the coronary arteries and other vessels. Patients have fever, mucosal inflammation, and lymphadenopathy.[4]

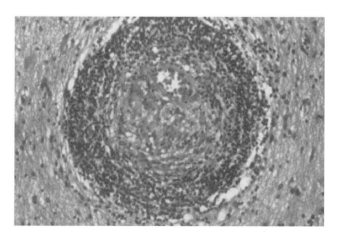

Figure 11-7. Results of brain biopsy demonstrates marked perivascular inflammatory changes consistent with vasculitis. Note that the lumen of the vessel is almost completely obliterated. (*Courtesy of S.S. Schochett, M.D., Department of Pathology, University of West Virginia.*)

▶ **TABLE 11-18.** NEUROLOGICAL MANIFESTATIONS OF COGAN SYNDROME

Bilateral hearing loss
Ocular manifestations
    Uveitis
    Conjunctivitis
    Ocular ischemia
    Episcleritis
Constitutional symptoms

Inflammatory Bowel Disease

Cerebral infarction is a rare complication of inflammatory bowel disease (either *regional enteritis* or *ulcerative colitis*). Other complications include ischemic oculopathy. A vasculitis of the central nervous system has been described among patients with ulcerative colitis.[76] However, the ischemic events probably are more likely due to changes in coagulation.[77,78] These enteropathies can lead to a loss of proteins including a reduction in clotting factors, such as protein S. In addition, malabsorption of vitamin B-12 in the terminal ileum among patients with regional enteritis can lead to an increase in the concentration of homocysteine, which in turn, accelerates the course of atherosclerosis.

Sarcoidosis

Sarcoidosis is a relatively uncommon inflammatory disease of undetermined cause. A secondary vasculitis, which is a rare complication, can lead to TIA or ischemic stroke.[79] Meningeal sarcoidosis could lead to secondary changes in penetrating arteries. Both spinal cord and brain dysfunction can occur. The CSF usually demonstrates lymphocytosis, elevated protein and immune globulin concentrations, and a depressed glucose level. Other findings on evaluation include hilar lymphadenopathy, hypocalcemia, and anergy. The angiotensin converting enzyme level also is abnormal. Corticosteroids are the usual method of medical management.

▶ MEDICATION-INDUCED VASCULITIS

The use of a large number of medications can be complicated by a multisystem vasculitis (Table 11-19). In general, dermatological manifestations are the most prominent. However, patients also can have neurological complications including cerebrovascular events. Patients with presumed vasculitis as the cause of neurological abnormalities should be asked about the use of the medications that are most commonly implicated.

▶ **TABLE 11-19.** MEDICATIONS THAT CAN INDUCE A SECONDARY VASCULITIS

Hydralazine	Propylthiouracil
Methimazole	Minocycline
Penicillamine	Allopurinol
Thiazide diuretics	Captopril
Azathioprine	Cimetidine
Methotrexate	Penicillin
Sulfonamides	Streptokinase

REFERENCES

1. Lie JT. Classification and histopathologic spectrum of central nervous system vasculitis. *Neurol Clin* 1997;15:805–819.
2. Hunder G. Vasculitis: diagnosis and therapy. *Am J Med* 1996;100:37S–45S.
3. Mohan N, Kerr GS. Diagnosis of vasculitis. *Best Pract Res Clin Rheumatol* 2001;15:203–223.
4. Luqmani RA, Robinson H. Introduction to, and classification of, the systemic vasculitides. *Best Pract Res Clin Rheumatol* 2001;15:187–202.
5. Holmes MD, Brant-Zawadzki MM, Simon RP. Clinical features of meningovascular syphilis. *Neurology* 1984;34:553–556.
6. Landi G, Villani F, Anzalone N. Variable angiographic findings in patients with stroke and neurosyphilis. *Stroke* 1990;21:333–338.
7. Bicknell JM, Holland JV. Neurologic manifestations of Cogan syndrome. *Neurology* 1978;28:278–281.
8. Vollertsen RS, McDonald TJ, Younge BR, et al. Cogan's syndrome: 18 cases and a review of the literature. *Mayo Clin Proc* 1986;61:344–361.
9. Bollen AE, Krikke AP, de Jager AEJ. Painful Horner syndrome due to arteritis of the internal carotid artery. *Neurology* 1998;51:1471–1472.
10. Ries S, Schminke U, Fassbender K, Daffertshofer M, Steinke W, Hennerici M. Cerebrovascular involvement in the acute phase of bacterial meningitis. *J Neurol* 1997;244:51–55.
11. Muller M, Merkelbach S, Huss GP, Schimrigk K. Clinical relevance and frequency of transient stenoses of the middle and anterior cerebral arteries in bacterial meningitis. *Stroke* 1995;26:1399–1403.
12. Schmiedel J, Gahn G, von Kummer R, Reichmann H. Cerebral vasculitis with multiple infarcts caused by lyme disease. *Cerebrovasc Dis* 2004;17:79–80.
13. Knox DL, Green WR, Troncoso JC, Yardley JH, Hsu J, Zee DS. Cerebral ocular Whipple's disease: a 62-year odyssey from death to diagnosis. *Neurology* 1995;45:617–625.
14. Pinto AN. AIDS and cerebrovascular disease. *Stroke* 1996;27:538–543.
15. Cole JW, Pinto AN, Hebel JR, et al. Acquired immunodeficiency syndrome and the risk of stroke. *Stroke* 2004;35:51–56.
16. Qureshi AI, Janssen RS, Karon JM, et al. Human immunodeficiency virus infection and stroke in young patients. *Arch Neurol* 1997;54:1150–1153.
17. Evers S, Nabavi A, Rahmann A, Heese C, Reichelt D, Husstedt IW. Ischaemic cerebrovascular events in HIV infection: a cohort study. *Cerebrovasc Dis* 2003;15:199–205.
18. Eidelberg D, Sotrel A, Horoupian DS, Neumann PE, Pumarola-Sune T, Price RW. Thrombotic cerebral vasculopathy associated with herpes zoster. *Ann Neurol* 1986;19:7–14.
19. Hilt DC, Buchholz D, Krumholz A, Weiss H, Wolinsky JS. Herpes zoster ophthalmicus and delayed contralateral hemiparesis caused by cerebral angiitis: diagnosis and management approaches. *Ann Neurol* 1983;14:543–553.
20. Erdem G, Vanderford PA, Bart RD. Intracranial hemorrhage in herpes simplex encephalitis: an unusual presentation. Pediatric *Neurology* 2002;27:221–223.

21. Shakir RA, Sulaiman K, Kahn RA, Rudwan M. Neurological presentation of neuro-Behcet's syndrome: clinical categories. *Eur Neurol* 1990;30:249–253.

22. Grimes DA, Lach B, Bourque PR. Vasculitic basilar artery thrombosis in chronic Candida albicans meningitis. *Can J Neurol Sci* 1998;25:76–78.

23. Walsh TJ, Hier DB, Caplan LR. Aspergillosis of the central nervous system: clinicopathological analysis of 17 patients. *Ann Neurol* 1985;18:574–582.

24. Sila CA. Spectrum of neurologic events following cardiac transplantation. *Stroke* 1989;20:1586–1589.

25. Galetta SL, Wulc AE, Goldberg HI, Nichols CW, Glaser JS. Rhinocerebral mucormycosis: management and survival after carotid occlusion. *Ann Neurol* 1990;28:103–107.

26. Wilson WB, Grotta JC, Schold C, Fisher LE. Cerebral mucormycosis: an unusual case. *Arch Neurol* 1979;36:725–726.

27. Monteiro L, Almeida-Pinto J, Leite I, Xavier J, Correia M. Cerebral cysticercus arteritis: five angiographic cases. *Cerebrovasc Dis* 1994;4:125–133.

28. McCormick GF, Giannotta S, Zee C, Fisher M. Carotid occlusion in cysticercosis. *Neurology* 1983;33:1078–1080.

29. Cantu C, Barinagarrementeria F. Cerebrovascular complications of neurocysticercosis. Clinical and neuroimaging spectrum. *Arch Neurol* 1996;53:233–239.

30. Newton CRJC, Tinh Hien T, White N. Cerebral malaria. *J Neurol Neurosurg Psychiatry* 2000;69:433–441.

31. Toro G, Roman G. Cerebral malaria. A disseminated vasculomyelinopathy. *Arch Neurol* 1978;35:271–275.

32. Clavier N, Rahimy C, Falanga P, Ayivi B, Payen D. No evidence for cerebral hypoperfusion during cerebral malaria. *Crit Care Med* 1999;27:628–632.

33. Ferro JM. Vasculitis of the central nervous system. *J Neurol* 1998;245:766–776.

34. Sigal LH. The neurologic presentation of vasculitic and rheumatologic syndromes. A review. *Medicine* 1987;66:157–180.

35. Ropper AH, Ayata C, Adelman L. Vasculitis of the spinal cord. *Arch Neurol* 2003;60:1791–1794.

36. Moore PM, Cupps TR. Neurological complications of vasculitis. *Ann Neurol* 1983;14:155–167.

37. Moore PM, Richardson B. Neurology of the vasculitides and connective tissue diseases. *J Neurol Neurosurg Psychiatry* 1998;65:10–22.

38. Berlit P, Moore PM, Bluestein HG. Vasculitis, rheumatic disease and the neurologist: the pathophysiology and diagnosis of neurologic problems in systemic disease. *Cerebrovasc Dis* 1993;3:139–145.

39. Weyand CM, Goronzy JJ. Giant-cell arteritis and polymyalgia rheumatica. *Ann Intern Med* 2003;138:505–515.

40. Nolfe G, D'Aniello AM, Muschera R, Giaquinto S. The aftermath of rehabilitation for patients with severe stroke. *Acta Neurol Scand* 2003;107:281–284.

41. Kerr GS, Hallahan CW, Giordano J, et al. Takayasu arteritis. *Ann Intern Med* 1994;120:919–929.

42. Guillevin L, Lhote F. Classification and management of necrotising vasculitides. *Drugs* 1997;53:805–816.

43. Weyand CM, Goronzy JJ. Medium- and large-vessel vasculitis. *N Engl J Med* 2003;349:160–169.

44. Hall S, Barr W, Lie JT, Stanson AW, Kazmier FJ, Hunder GG. Takayasu arteritis. A study of 32 North American patients. *Medicine* 1985;64:89–99.

45. Turnbull J. Temporal arteritis and polymyalgia rheumatica: nosographic and nosologic considerations. *Neurology* 1996;46:901–906.

46. Caselli RJ, Hunder GG, Whisnant JP. Neurologic disease in biopsy-proven giant cell (temporal) arteritis. *Neurology* 1988;38:352–359.

47. Reich KA, Giansiracusa DF, Strongwater SL. Neurologic manifestations of giant cell arteritis. *Am J Med* 1990;89:67–72.

48. Hevener AL, Reichart D, Janez A, Olefsky J. Thiazolidinedione treatment prevents free fatty acid-induced insulin resistance in male wistar rats. *Diabetes* 2001;50:2316–2322.

49. Morelli S, Perrone C, Paroli M. Recurrent cerebral infarctions in polyarteritis nodosa with circulating antiphospholipid antibodies and mitral valve disease. *Lupus* 1998;7:51–52.

50. Nishino H, Rubino FA, DeRemee RA, Swanson JW, Parisi JE. Neurological involvement in Wegener's granulomatosis: an analysis of 324 consecutive patients at the Mayo Clinic. *Ann Neurol* 1993;33:4–9.

51. Fauci AS, Haynes BF, Katz P, Wolff SM. Wegener's granulomatosis: prospective clinical and therapeutic experience with 85 patients for 21 years. *Ann Intern Med* 1983;98:76–85.

52. Seror R, Mahr A, Ramanoelina J, et al. Central nervous system involvement in Wegener granulomatosis. *Medicine* 2006;85:54–65.

53. Nardone R, Lochner P, Tezzon F. Wegener's granulomatosis presenting with intracerebral hemorrhages. *Cerebrovasc Dis* 2004;17:81–82.

54. Savitz JM, Young MA, Ratan RR. Basilar artery occlusion in a young patient with Wegener's granulomatosis. *Stroke* 1994;25:214–216.

55. Noth I, Strek ME, Leff AR. Churg-Strauss syndrome. *Lancet* 2003;361:587–594.

56. Kattah JC, Chrousos GA, Katz PA, McCasland B, Kolsky MP. Anterior ischemic optic neuropathy in Churg-Strauss syndrome. *Neurology* 1994;44:2200–2202.

57. Wong KL, Woo EK, Yu YL, Wong RW. Neurological manifestations of systemic lupus erythematosus: a prospective study. *Q J Med* 1991;81:857–870.

58. Roman MJ, Shanker B-A, Davis A, et al. Prevalence and correlates of accelerated atherosclerosis in systemic lupus enrythematosus. *N Engl J Med* 2003;349:2399–2406.

59. Asanuma Y, Oeser A, Shintani AK, et al. Premature coronary-artery atherosclerosis in systemic lupus erythematosus. *N Engl J Med* 2003;349:2407–2415.

60. D'Cruz D. Vasculitis in systemic lupus erythematosus. *Lupus* 1998;7:270–274.

61. Kitagawa Y, Gotoh F, Koto A, Okayasu H. Stroke in systemic lupus erythematosus. *Stroke* 1990;21:1533–1539.

62. Trimble M, Bell DA, Brien W, et al. The antiphospholipid syndrome: prevalence among patients with stroke and transient ischemic attacks. *Am J Med* 1990;88:593–597.

63. Verro P, Levine SR, Tietjen GE. Cerebrovascular ischemic events with high positive anticardiolipin antibodies. *Stroke* 1998;29:2245–2253.
64. Tourbah A, Piette JC, Iba-Zizen MT, Lyon-Caen O, Godeau P, Frances C. The natural course of cerebral lesions in Sneddon syndrome. *Arch Neurol* 1997;54:53–60.
65. Asherson RA, Khamashta MA, Gil A, et al. Cerebrovascular disease and antiphospholipid antibodies in systemic lupus erythematosus, lupus-like disease, and the primary antiphospholipid syndrome. *Am J Med* 1989;86:391–399.
66. Shim SC, Yoo DH, Lee JK, et al. Multiple cerebellar infarction due to vertebral artery obstruction and bulbar symptoms associated with vertical subluxation and atlanto-occipital subluxation in ankylosing spondylitis. *J Rheumatol* 1998;25:2464–2468.
67. Robinson BP, Seeger JF, Zak SM. Rheumatoid arthritis and positional vertebrobasilar insufficiency. Case report. *J Neurosurg* 1986;65:111–114.
68. Ramos M, Mandybur TI. Cerebral vasculitis in rheumatoid arthritis. *Arch Neurol* 1975;32:271–275.
69. Estey E, Lieberman A, Pinto R, Meltzer M, Ransohoff J. Cerebral arteritis in scleroderma. *Stroke* 1979;10:595–597.
70. Bragoni M, Di P, V, Priori R, Valesini G, Lenzi GL. Sjogren's syndrome presenting as ischemic stroke. *Stroke* 1994;25:2276–2279.
71. Alexander E. Central nervous system disease in Sjogren's syndrome. New insights into immunopathogenesis. *Rheum Dis Clin N Am* 1992;18:637–672.
72. Moore PM. Diagnosis and management of isolated angiitis of the central nervous system. *Neurology* 1989;39:167–173.
73. Woolfenden AR, Tong DC, Marks MP, Ali AO, Albers GW. Angiographically defined primary angiitis of the CNS: is it really benign? *Neurology* 1998;51:183–188.
74. Gordon MF, Coyle PK, Golub B. Eales' disease presenting as stroke in the young adult. *Ann Neurol* 1988;24:264–266.
75. American Heart Association. Heart disease and stroke statistics - 2004 update. 2004. (GENERIC) Ref Type: Pamphlet
76. Nelson J, Barron MM, Riggs JE, Gutmann L, Schochet SS, Jr. Cerebral vasculitis and ulcerative colitis. *Neurology* 1986;36:719–721.
77. Vaezi MF, Rustagi PK, Elson CO. Transient protein S deficiency associated with cerebral venous thrombosis in active ulcerative colitis. *Am J Gastroenterol* 1995;90:313–315.
78. Weber P, Husemann S, Vielhaber H, Zimmer KP, Nowak-Gottl U. Coagulation and fibrinolysis in children, adolescents, and young adults with inflammatory bowel disease. *J Pediatr Gastroenterol Nutr* 1999;28:418–422.
79. Brown MM, Thompson AJ, Wedzicha JA, Swash M. Sarcoidosis presenting with stroke. *Stroke* 1989;20:400–405.

CHAPTER 12
Genetic Causes of Stroke

Because of the high prevalence of both hemorrhagic and ischemic cerebrovascular disease in the American population, many affected patients report a history of stroke in one or more relatives.[1] Familial aggregations of stroke might also be ascribed to behavioral or environmental factors, including lifestyle, diet, and socioeconomic status. While most familial cases of stroke are probably not inherited, some cases of stroke are secondary to genetic diseases. A genetic predisposition to diseases, such as diabetes mellitus, also can lead to a familial aggregation of stroke. Caution should be exercised in diagnosing a genetic cause of stroke if only one or two family members are affected, particularly if they had their vascular events ascribed to common types of vascular diseases such as atherosclerosis.

▶ CLINICAL FINDINGS POINTING TO A GENETIC CAUSE OF STROKE

A genetic disease should be considered when the affected persons are young or have clinical features that raise suspicion for one of the described inherited syndromes (Table 12-1). In particular, genetic diseases are an important cause of stroke in children and young adults.[2] Careful screening of the family history for cerebrovascular disease is important. For example, history of family members having myocardial infarction or stroke before the age of 60 might point to an inherited predisposition to premature atherosclerosis. In addition, the history of deep vein thrombosis, pulmonary embolism, miscarriages, or ischemic cerebrovascular events should raise consideration of an inherited disorder of coagulation. A family history of other diseases, such as polycystic kidney disease, should increase consideration of a genetic cause predisposing to cerebrovascular disease. However, because of considerable heterogeneity of the inherited disorders, much more epidemiological and bench research will be needed to determine the effects of genetic diseases on the incidence of ischemic stroke.[3]

▶ INHERITED PROTHROMBOTIC DISEASES

Inherited prothrombotic diseases are potential causes of cerebral infarction.[4–6] Genetic disorders leading to a bleeding diathesis are among the causes of hemorrhagic stroke.[7] These disorders of coagulation are discussed in detail in Chapter 14.

▶ GENETIC FACTORS PREDISPOSING TO ATHEROSCLEROSIS

Advances in our understanding of the human genome mean that the genetic underpinnings for a number of diseases, including vascular disease and stroke, will grow considerably in the future.[6,8–12] New genetic factors that predispose to all types of vascular diseases, including atherosclerosis, likely will lead to major changes in the diagnosis and treatment of patients with stroke.[4,13–15] The number of genetic polymorphisms that promote development of atherosclerosis is already increasing (Table 12-2). Inherited disorders of lipid metabolism that lead to premature atherosclerosis include familial

▶ **TABLE 12-1.** GENETIC CAUSES OF STROKE

Mitochondrial disorders
    Mitochondrial encephalopathy, lactic acidosis, and
      strokelike episodes
    Kearns–Sayre syndrome
    Myoclonus epilepsy with ragged red fibers
Mendelian disorders
    X-linked
      Fabry–Anderson disease
    Autosomal dominant
      Cerebral autosomal-dominant arteriopathy with
        subcortical ischemic leukoencephalopathy
      Hereditary cerebroretinal vasculopathy
      Hereditary endotheliopathy with retinopathy,
        nephropathy, and stroke
      Moyamoya disease
      Hereditary hemorrhage telangiectasia (types I and II)
      Polycystic kidney disease
      Familial cavernous malformation
      Hereditary cerebral hemorrhage with amyloidosis
        (Dutch or Icelandic)
    Autosomal recessive
      Homocystinuria
      Methylenetetrahydrofolate reductase deficiency
      Saguenay Lac St. Jean syndrome
    Other genetic diseases that can be complicated by
    stroke
      Marfan syndrome
      Ehlers–Danlos syndrome (types III and IV)
      Osteogenesis imperfecta
      Pseudoxanthoma elasticum
      Systemic elastorrhexis
      Von Hippel–Lindau disease
      Neurofibromatosis
      Tuberous sclerosis
      Cobb syndrome
      Klippel–Trénaunay syndrome
      Parkes–Weber syndrome
      Propionic acidemia
      Methylmalonic acidemia
      Isovaleric acidemia
      Glutaric acidemia
      Ornithine transcarbamoylase deficiency
      Carbamoyl phosphate synthetase deficiency
      Williams syndrome
      Carbohydrate-deficient glycoprotein syndrome

▶ **TABLE 12-2.** GENETIC PREDISPOSTION TO ATHEROSCLEROSIS

Familial disorders of lipid metabolism
    Familial hypercholesterolemia type II
    Familial hypercholesterolemia type IV
    Hypoalphalipoproteinemia
    Familial disturbances of apolipoprotein A
Other inherited disorders
    Angiotensin-converting enzyme
    Methylenetetrafolate reductase
    Platelet glycoprotein IIIa
    Apolipoprotein E
    Hyperhomocysteinemia

calcification within the arterial wall. {Doherty, Fitzpatrick, et al. 2004 ID: 10485} Disorders of apolipoprotein E alleles have been correlated with the development of amyloid angiopathy, which is associated with both hemorrhagic and ischemic stroke. In addition, the apolipoprotein E4 allele also linked to poor outcomes following subarachnoid hemorrhage. Hyperhomocysteinemia also can be inherited. Polymorphisms of the angiotensin-converting enzyme gene also might be correlated with leukoaraiosis. Abnormalities in the nitric oxide synthase system altering endothelial cell function also predispose to atherosclerosis and stroke. Additional genetic abnormalities can be anticipated. This chapter focuses on Mendelian and mitochondrial genetic disorders that cause cardiac or nonatherosclerotic arterial diseases that cause brain or spinal cord ischemia or hemorrhage. The Mendelian disorders can show an autosomal-dominant, autosomal-recessive, or X-linked pattern.[7]

▶ **MITOCHONDRIAL DISORDERS**

Because mitochondrial DNA is inherited only from the mother, a pattern of maternal transmission is a key component of the family history. Several inherited mitochondrial disorders produce neurological symptoms, including stroke.[6,16] Affected patients may have both normal and abnormal mitochondrial DNA (heteroplasmy). During division, the amount of normal or abnormal mitochondrial DNA into cells can vary greatly. Some organs may have a considerable amount of abnormal mitochondrial DNA and others have very little. Because not all cells might be equally affected by the genetic abnormality, phenotypic expression of the mitochondrial disorders varies greatly. Still, some clinical features are common among most affected individuals. For example, most patients with mitochondrial disorders are of short stature and have prominent hearing loss.

hypoalphalipoproteinemia (Tangier disease), familial hypercholesterolemia types II and IV, and familial disturbances of apolipoprotein A. Genetic abnormalities in angiotensin-converting enzyme, methylenetetrafolate reductase, platelet glycoprotein IIIa, and apolipoprotein E are being correlated with subtypes of ischemic stroke.[4] Several of these potential genetic determinants have also been described to be associated with the development of

► MITOCHONDRIAL ENCEPHALOPATHY, LACTIC ACIDOSIS, AND STROKELIKE EPISODES

Mitochondrial encephalopathy, lactic acidosis, and stroke-like episodes (MELAS) is a relatively uncommon cause of neurological problems in children and young adults[17–19] (Table 12-3). It is caused by a translational point mutation of A3243G, which affects the transfer RNA for leucine. Approximately 10 percent of persons with MELAS have a point T3271C mutation. Secondary changes in smooth muscle and epithelial cells can affect capillaries and vessels. Because of heteroplasmy, pathological findings can vary considerably between tissues in affected patients.

Clinical Findings

While the strokelike episodes might be secondary to arterial occlusion and ischemia, the neurological symptoms are probably secondary to mitochondrial dysfunction in neurons and glia. The mechanism for the episodes of transient and partially reversible cerebral dysfunction is not established.

Affected persons usually are short and have progressive hearing loss. Nonneurological findings include episodic ileus and congestive heart failure. Manouvrier et al.[20] also described hypertrophic cardiomyopathy and renal failure in a family with this mutation. Other symptoms include headache, seizures, fatigue, and cognitive decline. In addition, episodic motor, sensory, visual, or language disturbances that mimic stroke also occur. The events, which are often accompanied by severe headache, can last from a few hours to several days.

► **TABLE 12-3.** MITOCHONDRIAL ENCEPHALOPATHY, LACTIC ACIDOSIS, AND STROKELIKE EPISODES

Translational mutation A3243G or point mutation T3271C
  Clinical features
    Short stature
    Progressive hearing loss
    Episodic ileus
    Congestive heart failure
  Cerebrovascular features
    Episodic motor, sensory, language, or visual
      disturbances
    Headaches
    Seizures
    Cognitive decline
  Diagnostic studies
    Cortical lesions that mimic ischemic stroke
    Lesions often do not fit a specific vascular territory
    Lesions can resolve
    Elevated lactate levels

Diagnostic Studies

Magnetic resonance imaging (MRI) studies can visualize abnormalities, most commonly in cortical regions of the parietal, temporal, and occipital lobes, which mimic those of ischemic stroke. However, these lesions may not respect specific vascular territories, and sequential studies will show resolution of the changes. On sequential studies, new lesions can appear as other lesions are resolving. Elevated lactate concentrations in the lesions can be found by MRI spectroscopy. Elevated blood and cerebrospinal fluid (CSF) levels of lactic acid are found, especially when the patient is having acute neurological symptoms. CSF protein levels are usually moderately elevated. Muscle biopsy can demonstrate ragged red fibers. Coenzyme Q or L-carnitine has been prescribed to limit the mitochondrial abnormality.

Treatment

At present, no treatment has been established as effective. Anticonvulsants are prescribed to patients with seizures, although valproate is avoided because it can induce convulsions.

► OTHER MITOCHONDRIAL DISEASES

Kearns–Sayre Syndrome

Kearns–Sayre syndrome, which is secondary to a mitochondrial deletion syndrome, causes a progressive myopathy, leading to external ophthalmoplegia, retinitis pigmentosa, and cardiac disease.[21,22] Other abnormalities include ataxia and an elevated CSF protein level. Less commonly, patients are of short stature and have deafness, dementia, limb weakness, and endocrine disorders. The pathological hallmark on muscle biopsy is the presence of ragged red fibers on Gomori trichrome stain. Cardioembolic stroke is a potential complication of the heart disease.[23] Cardiac conduction defects, which can lead to sudden death, can be treated with a pacemaker.

Myoclonus Epilepsy with Ragged Red Fibers

Myoclonus epilepsy with ragged red fibers (*MERRF*) is associated with structural heart disease, leading to conduction disturbances.[24] Cardioembolic stroke can be a complication. Other features include a short stature, generalized epilepsy, ataxia, and ragged red fibers detected by muscle biopsy. It is secondary to a mutation in mitochondrial DNA.

The *Saguenay Lac St. Jean syndrome* is inherited in an autosomal-recessive pattern, but it is associated with a deficiency of cytochrome oxidase and lactic acidosis.

The illness can evolve into a syndrome that mimics Leigh disease, but it can also be a cause of strokelike episodes in children.

▶ FABRY–ANDERSON DISEASE

Fabry–Anderson disease (alpha-galactosidase A deficiency) is caused by a point mutation in the long arm of the X chromosome (Xq22.1) that leads to a deficiency in the lysosomal enzyme, alpha-galactosidase A. Less commonly, the disorder can be secondary to a deletion or insertion at the same site. The incidence of Fabry–Anderson disease is approximately 1 in 40,000–60,000 men.[25] The deficiency leads to an accumulation of sphingolipids in vascular endothelium, smooth muscle cells, renal epithelium, myocardium, dorsal root ganglia, autonomic nerves, and brain.

Clinical Findings

Female carriers may become symptomatic with pain, proteinuria, stroke or heart disease. Affected men usually develop clinical findings in their late teens or early twenties (Table 12-4). A milder variant can present with cardiovascular disease after the age of 40 years. Most young men have a painful polyneuropathy with burning dysesthesias (acroparesthesias) in the limbs and hypohidrosis.[25] In addition, they have findings of renal dysfunction, corneal opacities, and heart disease causing both valvular changes and arrhythmias. The corneal opacity, which can be found only on slit-lamp microscopy, is found in almost all affected men and in 70 percent of female carriers and is fairly specific of the

▶ TABLE 12-4. FABRY–ANDERSON DISEASE

X-linked point mutations—deficiency of
alpha-galactosidase A
  Clinical features
    Painful polyneuropathy
    Renal dysfunction
    Corneal opacities
    Heart disease including myocardial infarction
    Purple-red skin lesions (angiokeratoma diffusum)
  Cerebrovascular features
    Cerebral infarction
      Large-artery occlusion
      Small-artery occlusion
      Cardioembolism
    Dolichoectasia of the basilar artery
  Diagnostic studies
    Abnormal blood levels of the alpha-galactosidase A
    Genetic testing
    Maltese cross crystals in urinary sediment
    Slow nerve conduction velocities

disease.[25] The secondary kidney disease can lead to renal failure that requires dialysis or transplantation. Relatively specific cutaneous abnormalities described as purple-red punctate lesions on the groin, anterior abdominal wall, and scrotum (angiokeratoma diffusum universalis) can be found. The young men have a high risk for myocardial infarction or cerebral infarction.[26] In some cases, the infarctions might be secondary to cardioembolism. However, most strokes are secondary to occlusion of both large and small intracranial arteries. A predominance of events in the posterior circulation and dolichoectasia of the basilar artery have been described.[27] Female carriers also have had transient ischemic attack or stroke.[25]

Diagnostic Studies

Imaging of the brain demonstrates multiple deep white matter lesions, particularly in periventricular regions. Other strokes can be found in the brain stem, cerebellum, and cortical gray matter. Abnormalities in blood levels of alpha-galactosidase A or the genetic abnormality can be detected on examination. Examination of the urine shows multiple crystals that have a Maltese cross pattern. Nerve conduction velocities demonstrate slowing.

Treatment

Treatment involves antiplatelet aggregating agents. Intravenous infusions of alpha-galactosidase are a promising therapy that reduces blood levels of glycophospholipid, lessens neuropathic pain, and possibly limits the vascular injury. The medication is relatively safe but it is very expensive.[28]

▶ PHOSPHODIESTERASE 4D

Genetic studies describe a strong link between stroke and hypertension and the gene-encoding phosphodiesterase 4D.[29] They found that approximately 16 percent of the Icelandic population had at least one copy of the at-risk haplotype and that 0.8 percent of persons were homozygous. The mechanism of increased stroke risk is speculated, with this genetic abnormality. However, it might be related to disturbances in signal transduction and regulation.

▶ HOMOCYSTINURIA

Homocystinuria is inherited in an autosomal-recessive pattern. The most common form of the disease results from a homozygous defect in the gene that encodes cystathionine beta-synthetase, which results in increased concentrations of methionine and homocysteine in blood.

The accumulation of homocysteine appears to cause endothelial cell dysfunction, changes in the extracellular matrix, smooth muscle proliferation, and changes in lipoprotein oxidation.[30,31] The elevated levels of homocysteine promote the development of premature and advanced atherosclerosis. Pathological changes include disruption of the internal elastic lamina, fibrosis, and fibrous intimal plaques. Carotid duplex studies can show increased intimal-medial thickness at a young age. The patients also have abnormalities in coagulation that promote arterial or venous thrombosis.[32]

Clinical Findings

Affected patients are usually mentally retarded (Table 12-5). They also have dislocated lens and skeletal abnormalities including scoliosis and dolichostenomelia. Many of the patients are tall and thin or have a Marfanoid appearance. Recurrent ischemic vascular events, including myocardial infarction, peripheral artery occlusion, or cerebral infarction, usually occur before the age of 30.[33]

Diagnostic Studies

Increased levels of homocysteine can be measured in the blood. Urinary screening for amino acids also is abnormal.

Treatment

Treatment focuses on vitamin supplementation to the diet to lower the protein concentrations. The usual treatment is with pyridoxine (25–500 mg/day), folic acid (1–5 mg/day), or vitamin B-12 (250 μg–2 mg/day). Some patients are particularly responsive to the administration of pyridoxine. A methionine-deficient diet has also been prescribed.

Homocystinuria also has been a complication of a deficiency of methylenetetrahydrofolate reductase. This rare inherited disorder has an autosomal-recessive pattern. Affected children have mental retardation, seizures,

and multiple vascular events. Vitamin supplementation appears not to be effective in treating this genetic disorder.

► CEREBRAL AUTOSOMAL-DOMINANT ARTERIOPATHY AND SUBCORTICAL ISCHEMIC LEUKOENCEPHALOPATHY

Approximately 90 percent of cases of cerebral autosomal-dominant arteriopathy and subcortical ischemic leukoencephalopathy (CADASIL) are secondary to a notch 3 gene mutation located on chromosome 19.[34,35] While rare de novo mutations occur, most cases are inherited on an autosomal-dominant manner. The genetic defect leads to an arteriopathy that affects small caliber vessels in the brain, meninges, muscles, skin, and peripheral nerves. The arteriopathy leads to multiple thrombotic occlusions of penetrating vessels of the brain. The disease is relentlessly progressive, and extensive vascular changes in deep structures of the cerebral hemispheres are found.

Clinical Findings

Most affected patients become symptomatic between the ages of 20 and 40[36,37] (Table 12-6). Patients usually become bedridden or demented before the age of 50, and they require long-term institutionalized care. Patients have multiple infarctions with pseudobulbar palsy and a progressive dementia. Psychiatric and behavioral disturbances are prominent.[38] Gait disturbances and pseudobulbar palsy are found.[39] The dementing syndrome might not be associated with motor or sensory impairments. Seizures occur in 10 percent of patients. The genetic mutation for CADASIL is close to that seen among persons with

---

► **TABLE 12-5.** HOMOCYSTINURIA

Autosomal recessive-encoding cystathionine beta-synthase
  Clinical features
    Tall stature with Marfanoid appearance
    Mental retardation
    Dislocation of lens
    Skeletal anomalies
    Myocardial infarction
    Peripheral vascular disease
  Cerebrovascular features
    Cerebral infarction
  Diagnostic studies
    Blood levels of homocysteine
    Urinary screening for amino acids

► **TABLE 12-6.** CEREBRAL AUTOSOMAL-DOMINANT ARTERIOPATHY WITH SUBCORTICAL ISCHEMIC LEUKOENCEPHALOPATHY

Autosomal-dominant notch 3 gene mutation on chromosome 19
  Cerebrovascular features
    Multiple thrombotic occlusions of penetrating arteries
    Recurrent ischemic stroke
    Hemiplegic migraine
    Dementia
    Seizures
  Diagnostic studies
    Genetic testing
    Biopsy—osmiophilic deposits in the vascular smooth muscle
    Multiple ischemic lesions in deep hemispheric structures
    Multiple periventricular white lesions

familial hemiplegic migraine. As a result, many patients with CADASIL have a strong history of migraine, with or without aura. In general, both the stroke and the migraine will be clinically obvious before the age of 35.

Diagnostic Studies

Brain imaging shows multiple ischemic lesions in the thalamus and basal ganglia. In addition, diffuse changes in the periventricular white matter are also seen on MRI. The pattern of lesions on MRI appear similar to those found with plaques that occur among persons with multiple sclerosis.[40–43] The imaging findings in conjunction with multifocal neurological dysfunction in a young adult often lead to the misdiagnosis of demyelinating disease. The severity of brain imaging changes correlates with the extent of the neurological impairments. Symptomatic patients usually have more extensive brain imaging abnormalities than do asymptomatic relatives. Lesnik Oberstein et al.[34] reported that the characteristic white matter changes could be detected on imaging in otherwise asymptomatic adults as early as the age of 21. Skin biopsy can lead to the diagnosis.[44,45] On microscopic examination, osmiophilic deposits can be seen adjacent to vascular smooth muscle. Genetic testing can detect the abnormality on chromosome 19. While testing symptomatic patients is appropriate, caution should be exercised when evaluating asymptomatic relatives. Consultation by a genetics service is recommended. Family members can have the appropriate consultation about the implications for the testing.

Prognosis and Treatment

At present, the prognosis of patients affected by CADASIL is very poor. Patients have a relentless course with progressive neurological worsening leading to dementia and debility. No specific therapeutic interventions are available. Most patients are treated with antiplatelet aggregating agents.

▶ HEREDITARY CEREBRORETINAL VASCULOPATHY AND HEREDITARY ENDOTHELIOPATHY WITH RETINOPATHY, NEPHROPATHY, AND STROKE

Hereditary cerebroretinal vasculopathy (HCRV) and hereditary endotheliopathy with retinopathy, nephropathy, and stroke (HERNS) are rare autosomal-dominant diseases that usually produce neurological symptoms in adulthood. HERNS appears to be localized to a defect on chromosome 3p21. Both conditions have capillary telangiectases and microinfarctions of the retina. In addition, the vasculopathy, which involves small and medium caliber arteries, leads to small infarctions in the brain. Renal involvement occurs in HERNS. The neurological symptoms of these disorders can mimic those of a brain tumor. Vahedi et al.[46] reported another distinct syndrome called *hereditary retinal arteriolar tortuosity*, which presents with infantile hemiparesis, migraine with aura, and retinal hemorrhages. Affected patients also have leukoencephalopathy found on brain imaging. The genetic defect appears to be distinct from HERNS.

▶ MOYAMOYA DISEASE

Although persons in other ethnic groups can be affected, moyamoya disease is recognized as an inherited intracranial vasculopathy that is most commonly diagnosed in Japanese, Korean, and Taiwanese populations. At least three genetic defects have been reported. The disease has been correlated with genetic changes in chromosomes 3, 6, or 17. Moyamoya disease usually causes recurrent cerebral infarction and mental retardation among children younger than 10 (Table 12-7). The disease can also cause recurrent stroke or intracranial hemorrhage in young adults. The pathological findings of moyamoya disease include thickening of the intima, smooth muscle cell proliferation, and abnormalities in the internal elastic lamina.[47] The radiological findings of moyamoya disease are similar to those reported with moyamoya syndrome (see Chapter 10).

Moyamoya syndrome has been reported as a potential complication of inherited diseases including sickle-cell disease, neurofibromatosis, Down syndrome, and Fanconi anemia.

▶ TABLE 12-7. MOYAMOYA DISEASE

Genetic mutations on chromosomes 3, 6, or 17
  Clinical features
    Most common in Japanese, Korean, and Taiwanese populations
    Symptoms in children or young adults
  Cerebrovascular features
    Children
      Recurrent ischemic stroke
      Seizures
      Mental retardation
      Dementia
    Young adults
      Recurrent ischemic stroke
      Subarachnoid hemorrhage
  Diagnostic studies
    Arteriopathy demonstrated by arteriography
      Bilateral, progressive
      Major arterial occlusions
      Minor collaterals
      Aneurysms

► HEREDITARY HEMORRHAGIC TELANGIECTASIA

Hereditary hemorrhagic telangiectasia (HHT/Rendu–Osler–Weber disease) is an autosomal-dominant inherited arteriopathy that predisposes to development of multiple vascular abnormalities throughout the body (Table 12-8). Although the clinical features are similar, two genetic variations HHT1 and HHT2 have been described. HHT1 is secondary to mutation at chromosome 9 that alters the protein endoglin.[48–50] In HHT2, a disturbance in protein activin is secondary to a mutation of chromosome 12. Affected patients have telangiectasia in the mucosa as well as larger vascular malformations most commonly located in the brain and lungs. Multiple vascular malformations can be found.[51] Arteriovenous malformations of the spinal cord can also be detected.[52]

Clinical Findings

On examination, patients have multiple small telangiectases in the nose, lips, and under the tongue. Approximately one-third of affected persons have pulmonary vascular malformations. Patients with a pulmonary arteriovenous malformation can have a thoracic bruit and some evidence of cyanosis. The pulmonary lesions can serve as a conduit for paradoxical embolization that causes cerebral infarction or a brain abscess.[53] Mucosal telangiectases often produce recurrent epistaxis and gastrointestinal bleeding. Cerebrovascular malformations are found in approximately 10 percent of cases. The intracerebral lesions can rupture, causing intracranial hemorrhage. The risk of hemorrhage from vascular malformations among patients with hereditary hemorrhagic telangiectasia is estimated as approximately 1.4–2.0 percent per year.[54] Surgical or endovascular

► **TABLE 12-8.** HEREDITARY HEMORRHAGIC TELANGIECTASIA

Multiple telangiectases
  Lips
  Tongue
  Nose
  Gastrointestinal mucosa
Arteriovenous malformations
  Brain
  Lung
Symptoms
  Recurrent epistaxis
  Recurrent gastrointestinal bleeding
  Intracranial hemorrhage
  Pulmonary bruit
  Paradoxical embolization
  Brain abscess

treatment of the pulmonary or cerebrovascular malformations is often recommended.

► POLYCYSTIC KIDNEY DISEASE

Autosomal-dominant polycystic kidney disease (ADPKD) is associated with the development of intracranial saccular aneurysms[55,56] (see Chapter 15). Two genetic loci have been described—ADPKD1 is located on chromosome 16 and ADPKD2 on chromosome 4. Approximately 2–5 percent of patients with PKD have aneurysms detected on screening. The frequency approaches 10 percent if another member of the family has had a subarachnoid hemorrhage. Subarachnoid hemorrhage is the most feared complication. Because of the relatively high prevalence of intracranial lesions among persons of families with PKD, screening with magnetic resonance angiography or computerized tomographic angiography is often recommended. In general, patients older than 30 or who have at least one close relative with an aneurysm are evaluated.

► FAMILIAL CAVERNOUS MALFORMATIONS

The first type of familial cavernous malformations is attributed to an autosomal-dominant trait with incomplete penetrance, which is localized to a mutation on chromosome 7. This condition, which is characterized by multiple intracerebral lesions that can cause intracerebral hemorrhage, has been detected primarily among Hispanic Americans. However, affected non-Hispanic families have been described. A linkage to a genetic change in chromosome 3 also has been described in non-Hispanic families. An important nuance between incidental and familial cases of cavernous malformations is the presence of multiple intracranial malformations, which is usually found in the inherited disease.

► STROKE AS A COMPLICATION OF OTHER INHERITED DISEASES

Familial Cerebral Amyloid Angiopathy

Some cases of cerebral amyloid angiopathy are inherited. The pathological findings of amyloidosis appear similar to acquired cases. The familial predisposition to Alzheimer disease and amyloid angiopathy has been correlated with E2/E3 genotype and E4 alleles. Interest in the potential relationships between different alleles of apolipoprotein and the development of amyloid angiopathy is considerable. Affected patients have a high risk for both ischemic stroke and intraparenchymal hemorrhages. The relationship between cerebral amyloid angiopathy and brain hemorrhage is discussed in more detail in Chapter 16. Patients with the *Dutch type of hereditary cerebral hemorrhage with amyloidosis* (HCHWA-D) have a very high rate of intracerebral hemorrhage. Affected patients also develop vascular dementia. The *Icelandic type of hereditary cerebral hemorrhage with amyloidosis* (HCHWA-I) is the result of a different genetic mutation. Patients have a high risk of brain hemorrhage or other stroke before the age of 30. In Iceland, HCHWA-I is a leading cause of stroke in young adults. A British variant of amyloid angiopathy, which is inherited in an autosomal-dominant pattern, can cause recurrent ischemic strokes and progressive dementia.

Marfan Syndrome

Several inherited diseases have been implicated as the underlying etiologies of aortic, extracranial, or intracranial arterial dissections, which in turn cause stroke. *Marfan syndrome*, which is secondary to a mutation in chromosome 15q21.1 that leads to an accumulation of fibrillin in the arterial wall, is usually inherited in an autosomal-dominant pattern. Approximately one-fourth of cases are the result of a new mutation. Affected persons are usually tall and thin with long digits (Table 12-9). A cardiac murmur and dislocation of the lens can be detected. Stroke is usually secondary to dissection of the aorta or extracranial arteries. Some patients will require replacement of the aortic valve, and surgical repair of the aortic lesion can be performed. A potential relationship between Marfan syndrome and intracranial aneurysms has been proposed but data are conflicting.

Several families with thoracic aortic aneurysms, with or without dissection, have also been reported. Inheritance of *familial thoracic aortic aneurysms* appears to be primarily autosomal dominant. At least three

▶ **TABLE 12-9.** MARFAN SYNDROME

Tall and thin
Long digits
Reduced upper-to-lower segment ratio
  (arm span to height ratio)
Reduced extension of the elbow
Pectus carinatum or pectus excavatum
Dislocation of the lens (ectopic lens)
Spontaneous pneumothorax
Cardiac murmur
Mitral valve prolapse
Dilation of the ascending aorta
Dissection of aorta
  Cerebral infarction
  Spinal cord infarction
Intracranial aneurysms

genetic loci have been identified. An association with intracranial disease, such as dolichoectatic basilar artery disease, might exist.

Ehlers–Danlos Syndrome

Dissection of the cerebral vessels, carotid-cavernous fistula, and intracranial aneurysms are described as manifestations of *Ehlers–Danlos syndrome, type III*. Other manifestations of this disorder, which is secondary to an autosomal-dominant mutation on chromosome 2q31 leading to changes in type III collagen, include thin translucent skin, laxity of the skin, and skeletal changes. Affected patients have thin lips, small chin and nose, and large eyes. They are at risk for intestinal or uterine rupture. Vascular rupture with bleeding also occurs. *Ehlers–Danlos syndrome, type IV*, also has been complicated by the development of intracranial aneurysms in childhood and carotid-cavernous fistulas. Multiple genetic mutations can produce this syndrome. Most patients are symptomatic before the age of 40, and the median age of death among patients with Ehlers–Danlos syndrome is 48.

Osteogenesis Imperfecta

Arterial dissection and carotid-cavernous fistula are a potential complication of *osteogenesis imperfecta*. The term probably designates several inherited disorders. The hallmarks include bony fragility leading to fractures following trivial trauma, dental anomalies, hearing loss, and bluish discoloration of the sclerae. Mitral valve prolapse and aortic valve abnormalities, which could be potential sources for cardioembolism, have also been described. A deficiency of alpha-1-antitrypsin has been detected in a small number of patients with extracranial arterial dissections; presumably, this metabolic abnormality is on an inherited basis.

Pseudoxanthoma Elasticum

Pseudoxanthoma elasticum is secondary to a variety of genetic mutations that cause an accumulation of proteoglycans and changes in elastic fibers. Ocular, vascular, and skin changes result. Irregular wrinkling of the skin in flexion areas is found. Premature vascular changes that mimic atherosclerosis have been described.

Systemic elastorrhexis (*Gronblad–Strandberg–Touraine syndrome*) has been associated with ischemic heart disease, hypertension, and premature peripheral vascular disease. Some cases of fibromuscular dysplasia also might be on an inherited basis.

Vascular disease, which can cause intracranial bleeding, has been reported as a potential complication of *von Hippel–Lindau syndrome*. This inherited disorder is complicated by renal cell carcinoma or pheochromocytoma.

Both can lead to hypertension. In addition, the hemangioblastoma, most commonly located in the cerebellar hemisphere, can bleed. Stroke, independent of moyamoya syndrome, also is described as a rare event among persons with *neurofibromatosis* or *tuberous sclerosis*. Posterior reversible encephalopathy syndrome, which causes headache, seizures, blindness, and mental status changes in children, can complicate familial hypertensive syndromes. Vascular malformations of the central nervous system are found among patients who have *Cobb syndrome, Klippel–Trénaunay syndrome,* or *Parkes–Weber syndrome.*[52] These syndromes are presumably secondary to an inherited abnormality.

Because of the strong familial clustering of intracranial saccular aneurysm, a genetic predisposition or mutation is presumed. Studies looking at abnormalities in collagen, matrix metalloproteinases, and tissue inhibitors of the metalloproteinases are under way. Multiple differing genetic mutations likely are responsible.

Cerebrovascular events have been described as manifestations of a number of relatively uncommon inherited disorders of metabolism. Intracranial hemorrhage is a complication of acidosis among patients affected with *propionic, methylmalonic,* or *isovaleric acidemia. Glutaric acidemia* might be associated with strokelike episodes. In addition, deficiencies of *ornithine transcarbamoylase* and *carbamoyl phosphate synthetase* can be complicated with cerebral infarction. *Williams syndrome,* which is secondary to a microdeletion of chromosome 7, causes cardiac lesions, mental retardation, and dysmorphism. Stroke could be secondary to the supraventricular aortic stenosis, although an intracranial vasculopathy has also been described. Cerebrovascular disease has been described in the *carbohydrate-deficient glycoprotein syndrome.* Other features include ataxia, mental retardation, hypotonia, peripheral neuropathy, and retinitis pigmentosa. Stroke has been described as a complication in patients with deficiencies of carnitine.

REFERENCES

1. Tentschert S, Greisenegger S, Wimmer R, Lang W, Lalouschek W. Association of parental history of stroke with clinical parameters in patients with ischemic stroke or transient ischemic stroke. *Stroke* 2003;34:2114–2119.
2. Pavlakis SG, Kingsley PB, Bialer MG. Stroke in children: genetic and metabolic issues. *J Child Neurol* 2003;15:308–315.
3. Flossmann E, Schulz UGR, Rothwell PM. Systematic review of methods and results of studies of the genetic epidemiology of ischemic stroke. *Stroke* 2004;35:212–227.
4. Voetsch B, Loscalzo J. Genetic determinants of arterial thrombosis. *Arterioscler Thromb Vasc Biol* 2003;24:216–229.
5. Petrovic D, Milanez T, Kobal J, Bregar D, Potisk KP, Peterlin B. Prothrombotic gene polymorphisms and atherothrombotic cerebral infarction. *Acta Neurol Scand* 2003;108:109–113.
6. Meschia JF. Ischemic stroke as a complex genetic disorder. *Semin Neurol* 2006;26:49–56.
7. Natowicz M, Kelley RI. Mendelian etiologies of stroke. *Ann Neurol* 1987;22:175–192.
8. Read SJ, Parsons AA, Harrison DC, et al. Stroke genomics: approaches to identify, validate, and understand ischemic stroke gene expression. *J Cereb Blood Flow Metab* 2001;21:755–778.
9. Rosand J, Altshuler D. Human genome sequence variation and the search for genes influencing stroke. *Stroke* 2003;34:2512–2516.
10. Alberts MJ. Stroke genetics update. *Stroke* 2003;34:342–344.
11. Majersik JJ, Skalabrin EJ. Single-gene stroke disorders. *Semin Neurol* 2006;26:33–48.
12. Alberts MJ. Genetics of cerebrovascular disease. *Stroke* 2004;35:342–344.
13. Hassan A, Markus HS. Genetics and ischaemic stroke. *Brain* 2000;123:1784–1812.
14. Hassan A, Sham PC, Markus HS. Planning genetic studies in human stroke: sample size estimates based on family history data. *Neurology* 2002;58:1483–1488.
15. Jerrard-Dunne P, Cloud G, Hassan A, Markus HS. Evaluating the genetic component of ischemic stroke subtypes. A family history study. *Stroke* 2003;34:1364–1369.
16. Chinnery PF. Mitochondrial disorders come full circle. *Neurology* 2003;61:878–880.
17. Liou CW, Huang CC, Chee EC, et al. MELAS syndrome: correlation between clinical features and molecular genetic analysis. *Acta Neurol Scand* 1994;90:354–359.
18. Ohno K, Isotani E, Hirakawa K. MELAS presenting as migraine complicated by stroke: case report. *Neuroradiology* 1997;39:781–784.
19. Gilchrist JM, Sikirica M, Stopa E, Shanske S. Adult-onset MELAS. Evidence for involvement of neurons as well as cerebral vasculature in strokelike episodes. *Stroke* 1996;27:1420–1423.
20. Manouvrier S, Rotig A, Hannebique G, et al. Point mutation of the mitochondrial tRNA (Leu) gene (A 3243 G) in maternally inherited hypertrophic cardiomyopathy, diabetes mellitus, renal failure, and sensorineural deafness. *J Med Genet* 1995;32:654–656.
21. Provenzale JM, VanLandingham K. Cerebral infarction associated with Kearns–Sayre syndrome-related cardiomyopathy. *Neurology* 1996;46:826–828.
22. Sakuta R, Nonaka I. Vascular involvement in mitochondrial myopathy. *Ann Neurol* 1989;25:594–601.
23. Kosinski C, Mull M, Lethen H, Topper R. Evidence for cardioembolic stroke in a case of Kearns–Sayre syndrome. *Stroke* 1995;26:1950–1952.
24. Chinnery PF, Howell N, Lightowlers RN, Turnbull DM. MELAS and MERRF. The relationship between maternal mutation load and the frequency of clinically affected offspring. *Brain* 1998;121:1889–1894.
25. Desnick RJ, Brady R, Barranger J, et al. Fabry disease, an under-recognized multisystemic disorder: expert recommendations for diagnosis, management, and enzyme replacement therapy. *Ann Intern Med* 2003;138:338–346.

26. Mitsias P, Levine SR. Cerebrovascular complications of Fabry's disease. *Ann Neurol* 1996;40:8–17.

27. Maisey DN, Cosh JA. Basilar artery aneurysm and Anderson–Fabry disease. *J Neurol Neurosurg Psychiatry* 1980;43: 85–87.

28. Eng CM, Guffon N, Wilcox WR, et al. Safety and efficacy of recombinant human α-galactosidase: a replacement therapy in Fabry's disease. *N Engl J Med* 2001;345:9–16.

29. Brophy VH, Ro SK, Rhees BK, et al. Association of phosphodiesterase 4D polymorphisms with ischemic stroke in a US population stratified by hypertension status. *Stroke* 2006;37:1385–1390.

30. Bellamy MF, McDowell IF. Putative mechanisms for vascular damage by homocysteine. *J Inherit Metab Dis* 1997; 20:307–315.

31. Megnien JL, Gariepy J, Saudubray JM, et al. Evidence of carotid artery wall hypertrophy in homozygous homocystinuria. *Circulation* 1998;98:2276–2281.

32. Lobo CA, Millward SF. Homocystinuria: a cause of hypercoagulability that may be unrecognized. *J Vasc Interv Radiol* 1998;9:971–975.

33. Wilcken DE, Wilcken B. The natural history of vascular disease in homocystinuria and the effects of treatment. *J Inherit Metab Dis* 1997;20:295–300.

34. Lesnik Oberstein SAJ, van den Boom R, Middelkoop HAM, et al. Incipient CADASIL. *Arch Neurol* 2003;60:707–712.

35. Joutel A, Corpechot C, Ducros A, et al. Notch3 mutations in CADASIL, a hereditary adult-onset condition causing stroke and dementia. *Nature* 1996;383:707–710.

36. Sabbadini G, Francia A, Calandriello L, et al. Cerebral autosomal dominant arteriopathy with subcortical infarcts and leucoencephalopathy (CADASIL). Clinical, neuroimaging, pathological and genetic study of a large Italian family. *Brain* 1995;118:207–215.

37. Dichgans M, Mayer M, Uttner I, et al. The phenotypic spectrum of CADSIL: clinical findings in 102 cases. *Ann Neurol* 1998;44:731–739.

38. Charlton RA, Morris RG, Nitkunan A, Markus HS. The cognitive profiles of CADASIL and sporadic small vessel disease. *Neurology* 2006;66:1523–1526.

39. Abe K, Murakami T, Matsubara E, Manabe Y, Nagano I, Shoji M. Clinical features of CADASIL. *Ann N Y Acad Sci* 2002;977:266–272.

40. Chabriat H, Levy C, Taillia H, et al. Patterns of MRI lesions in CADASIL. *Neurology* 1998;51:452–457.

41. Chabriat H, Mrissa R, Levy C, et al. Brain stem MRI signal abnormalities in CADASIL. *Stroke* 1999;30:457–459.

42. Dichgans M, Filippi M, Bruning R, et al. Quantitative MRI in CADASIL. *Neurology* 1999;52:1361–1367.

43. Dichgans M, Holtmannspotter M, Herzog J, Peters N, Bergmann M, Yousry TA. Cerebral microbleeds in CADASIL: a gradient-echo magnetic resonance imaging and autopsy study. *Stroke* 2002;33:67–71.

44. Ebke M, Dichgans M, Bergmann M, et al. CADASIL: skin biopsy allows diagnosis in early stages. *Acta Neurol Scand* 1997;95:351–357.

45. Ruchoux MM, Maurage CA. Endothelial changes in muscle and skin biopsies in patients with CADASIL. *Neuropathol Appl Neurobiol* 1998;24:60–65.

46. Vahedi K, Massin P, Guichard J-P, et al. Hereditary infantile hemiparesis, retinal arteriolar tortuosity, and leukoencephalopathy. *Neurology* 2003;60:57–63.

47. Fukui M, Kono S, Sueishi K, Ikezaki K. Moyamoya disease. *Neuropathology* 2000;20:S61–S64.

48. Harrison RE, Flanagan JA, Sankelo M, et al. Molecular and functional analysis identifies ALK-1 as the predominant cause of pulmonary hypertension related to hereditary haemorrhagic telangiectasia. *J Med Genet* 2003;40:865–871.

49. Berg J, Porteous M, Reinhardt D, et al. Hereditary haemorrhagic telangiectasia: a questionnaire based study to delineate the different phenotypes caused by endoglin and ALK1 mutations. *J Med Genet* 2003;40:585–590.

50. Lenato GM, Guanti G. Hereditary hemorrhagic telangiectasia (HHT): genetic and molecular aspects. *Curr Pharm Des* 2006;12:1173–1193.

51. Jessurun G, Kamphuis DJ, van der Zande FH, Nossent JC. Cerebral arteriovenous malformations in the Netherlands Antilles. High prevalence of hereditary hemorrhagic telangiectasia-related single and multiple cerebral arteriovenous malformations. *Clin Neurol Neurosurg* 1993; 95:193–198.

52. Rodesch G, Hurth M, Alvarez H, Tadie M, Lasjaunias P. Classification of spinal cord arteriovenous shunts: proposal for a reappraisal—the Bicetre experience with 155 consecutive patients treated between 1981 and 1999. *Neurosurgery* 2002;51:374–379.

53. Retnakaran RR, Faughnan ME, Chan RP, Pugash RA, O'Connor PW, Chow CM. Pulmonary arteriovenous malformation: a rare, treatable cause of stroke in young adults. *Int J Clin Pract* 2003;57:731–733.

54. Easey AJ, Wallace GM, Hughes JM, Jackson JE, Taylor WJ, Shovlin CL. Should asymptomatic patients with hereditary haemorrhagic telangiectasia (HHT) be screened for cerebral vascular malformations? Data from 22,061 years of HHT patient life. *J Neurol Neurosurg Psychiatry* 2003;74:743–748.

55. Watnick T, Phakdeekitcharoen B, Johnson A, et al. Mutation detection of PKD1 identifies a novel mutation common to three families with aneurysms and/or very-early-onset disease. *Am J Hum Genet* 1999;65:1561–1571.

56. Pirson Y, Chauveau D, Torres V. Management of cerebral aneurysms in autosomal dominant polycystic kidney disease. *J Am Soc Nephrol* 2002;13:269–276.

CHAPTER 13
Cardiogenic Embolism

▶ RELATIONSHIP BETWEEN HEART DISEASE AND STROKE

Approximately 20–25 percent of ischemic strokes are secondary to emboli that arise within the heart.[1] Cardioembolic strokes affect children and men and women of all ethnic groups. While cardioembolic strokes occur in persons of all ages, the rapid increase in the frequency of stroke secondary to atherosclerosis among persons older than 55 years decreases the relative importance of cardioembolic events. However, a high frequency of cardioembolism reemerges among the very elderly. Among persons older than 80 years, especially women, the presence of atrial fibrillation is recognized as a premier factor that identifies a high risk for stroke. The cardiac sources of embolism vary between the elderly and younger persons. Among persons younger than 45 years, most cardioembolic strokes are secondary to congenital heart diseases or acquired valvular abnormalities. Among older persons, the leading causes of embolic stroke are coronary artery disease (including recent myocardial infarction) and atrial fibrillation.

Emboli arising in the heart can lodge in any cerebral vessel. Thus, cardioembolism is among the potential causes of an ischemic stroke or TIA that occurs in both the internal carotid and vertebrobasilar arterial territories. It also is a possible cause of spinal cord infarction. Recurrent ischemic events in different cerebrovascular territories happening in close proximity to each other suggest cardioembolism as do the development of stroke and embolization to other organs (Figs. 13-1 to 13-3). Cardioembolic strokes appear to have a high propensity for hemorrhagic transformation (Fig. 13-4). Thus, an occasional "hemorrhage" might be a cardioembolic stroke. Although stroke can be the initial presentation of heart disease, most patients with cardioembolic stroke have a history of symptomatic heart disease including chest pain, palpitations, fatigue, dyspnea, or ankle edema. Affected patients often have a cardiac murmur, cyanosis, cardiomegaly, or signs of heart failure. Constitutional symptoms, such as fever or malaise, also might be seen in patients with cardioembolic stroke. The presence of a high fever can point to infective endocarditis as a cause of stroke. In some instances, the neurological symptoms immediately follow a major cardiovascular procedure.

▶ HIGH- AND LOWER-RISK CARDIAC SOURCES FOR EMBOLI

Several cardiac diseases are associated with a risk of thromboembolism. These conditions usually are categorized as higher or lower risk based on currently available epidemiological data. (Tables 13-1 and 13-2). These conditions include disturbances of cardiac rhythm, most commonly atrial fibrillation, and structural heart diseases. Many patients have more than one cardiac abnormality. The most common scenario is the presence of a cardiac arrhythmia, especially atrial fibrillation, associated with a structural lesion.

The list of potential cardiac sources for embolization has grown during the last two decades, partially because of improvements in imaging of the heart. Still, information about the risks of stroke associated with some of the newly described changes is limited. Long-term natural history data often are not available and with the absence of such information, decisions about treatment become murky. Some of these conditions, which presumably are associated with a low risk of embolization, are common in the population. Because of their high prevalence in normal persons, these cardiac lesions often are detected frequently among

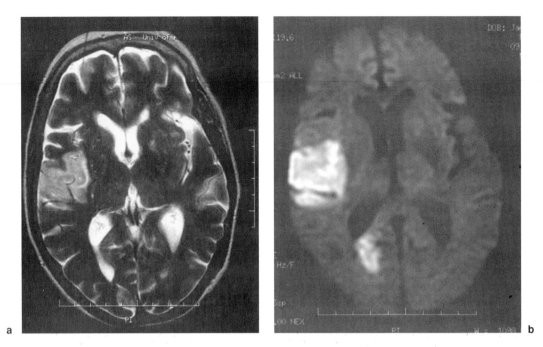

a   b

Figure 13-1. Axial T-2 and diffusion weighted MRI studies show infarction in two different vascular territories in a patient with atrial fibrillation.

patients with stroke or TIA and a cause-and-effect relationship between the cardiac finding and the neurological symptoms can be difficult to establish. Future research might clarify some of the controversies about the interactions between some of these cardiac changes and embolization to the nervous system.

In addition, embolization to the brain can complicate several invasive cardiovascular procedures (Table 13-3). With the advances in interventional cardiology and cardiovascular surgery, the number of procedures that might be associated with thromboembolic events to the brain will likely grow. Cardiovascular procedures also can be complicated with hypoperfusion or vascular compromise to the spinal cord. Cardiovascular therapies, especially the administration of agents that affect coagulation, also can be complicated by hemorrhagic

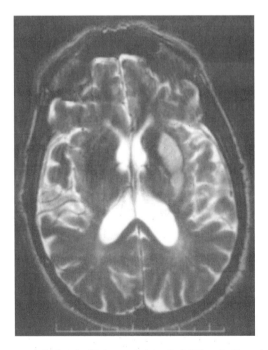

Figure 13-2. A T-2 weighted MRI of the brain demonstrates a striatocapsular infarction. This finding suggests an embolic occlusion of the first segment of the middle cerebral artery.

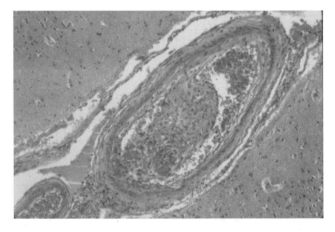

Figure 13-3. An embolus is demonstrated in a cortical (pial) artery on this autopsy specimen. (*Courtesy of S.S. Schochet, M.D., Department of Pathology, University of West Virginia.*) Morgantown, WV

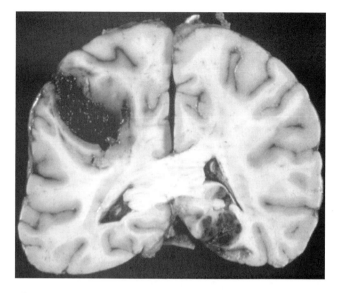

Figure 13-4. Two areas of hemorrhagic infarction are shown on this coronal autopsy specimen. The disseminated pattern of the infarctions involving both hemispheres is consistent with the diagnosis of cardioembolism. (*Courtesy of S.S. Schochet, M.D., Department of Pathology, University of West Virginia.*)

strokes. For example, intracranial hemorrhage is a leading noncardiac cause of major morbidity or mortality following thrombolytic treatment of patients with acute myocardial ischemia.

▶ ATRIAL FIBRILLATION

Approximately 10–16 percent of patients with ischemic stroke have atrial fibrillation; it is the most commonly implicated finding for the diagnosis of cardioembolic stroke.[2,3] In comparison to sinus rhythm, atrial fibrillation is associated with a five to seven times increase risk

▶ **TABLE 13-1.** HEART DISEASES CATEGORIZED AS HAVING A HIGH RISK FOR EMBOLIZATION

Structural heart disease complicated by atrial fibrillation
Acute myocardial infarction
Dilated cardiomyopathy
Rheumatic stenosis of mitral valve
Infective endocarditis
Nonbacterial thrombotic (marantic) endocarditis
Libman—Sacks endocarditis
Mechanical prosthetic valve (particularly in mitral position)
Left atrial myxoma
Intracavitary thrombus
    Left ventricle
    Left atrium
    Left atrial appendage

▶ **TABLE 13-2.** HEART DISEASES CATEGORIZED AS HAVING LOW OR UNCERTAIN RISK FOR EMBOLIZATION

Atrial fibrillation (lone) without structural heart disease
Sick sinus syndrome
Akinetic or hypokinetic segment of left ventricle
Aneurysm of left ventricle
Rheumatic stenosis of aortic valve
Bicuspid aortic valve
Calcification of annulus of mitral valve
Calcific stenosis of aortic valve
Mitral valve prolapse
Atrial septal aneurysm
Patent foramen ovale
Atrial septal defect
Bioprosthetic mitral valve
Mechanical prosthetic aortic valve
Idiopathic hypertrophic subaortic stenosis
Aneurysm of the sinus of Valsalva
Mitral valve strands
Lambl excrescences
Turbulence in left atrium

in embolic stroke.[4,5] The arrhythmia usually complicates most structural diseases of the heart (Table 13-4). In some circumstances, the arrhythmia is the first overt finding of the heart disease. For example, new onset atrial fibrillation may be the first manifestation of a clinically silent myocardial infarction. In addition, atrial fibrillation occurs among patients without other serious heart disease (lone atrial fibrillation). Still, the effects of the arrhythmia are additive. The combination of the arrhythmia and an underlying pathological change in the left atrium, left ventricle, or mitral valve is associated with a higher risk of embolization that the presence of either the arrhythmia or the structural heart disease alone.

Pathogenesis of Emboli

The thromboembolic risk of atrial fibrillation appears to be secondary to reduced contractility of the left

▶ **TABLE 13-3.** CARDIOVASCULAR PROCEDURES COMPLICATED BY EMBOLIZATION

Coronary artery bypass graft surgery
Valvular replacement
Valvuloplasty
Cardiac transplantation
Cardiac assist devices
Cardiac catheterization
Electrophysiological studies of the heart
Placement of pacemaker
Obliteration of atrioventricular node
Placement of intracardiac devices

▶ **TABLE 13-4.** STRUCTURAL HEART DISEASES MOST COMMONLY ASSOCIATED WITH ATRIAL FIBRILLATION

Recent myocardial infarction
Ischemic cardiomyopathy
Dilated cardiomyopathy
Hypertensive heart disease
Rheumatic mitral stenosis
Prosthetic cardiac valve

atrium and increased turbulence with the atrial cavity. Secondary dilation of the left atrium and left atrial appendage develops (Fig. 13-5). In particular, stagnation of low in the left atrial appendage is associated with thrombosis.[6] A majority of emboli among patients with atrial fibrillation appear to arise from the left atrial appendage rather from the remainder of the left atrial cavity.[3] Dysfunction of the left atrial appendage is associated with an increased risk of recurrent stroke.[7] Embolization to the brain can be clinically occult and it might be detected only by transcranial Doppler ultrasonography or brain imaging studies.[8,9] Such clinically

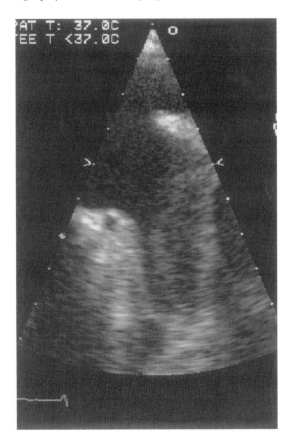

Figure 13-5. A transesophageal echocardiogram obtained in a patient with chronic atrial fibrillation visualizes a thrombus within the left atrial appendage. (*Courtesy of R.E. Kerber, M.D., Department of Internal Medicine, University of Iowa, City, IA University of Iowa.*)

covert stroke is not benign; recurrent ischemic lesions predispose to cognitive decline or dementia. The risk of embolization generally is similar whether the arrhythmia is sustained or intermittent.[10] However, a particular high-risk period for embolization can follow the return to a sinus rhythm following a period of atrial fibrillation.

In some patients, the arrhythmia is detected at the time of a cerebrovascular event. Establishing a cause-and-effect relationship can be difficult because the arrhythmia can be a complication rather than a predisposing cause of an infarction. The arrhythmia might be secondary to acute cardiac ischemia or to the release of neurotransmitters at the time of stroke. This scenario is most common with subarachnoid hemorrhage. Thus, new onset atrial fibrillation in a patient with an intracranial hemorrhage is considered as a complication of the intracranial event.[11,12] In most cases of infarction, the atrial fibrillation should be deemed as a flag for a cardioembolic etiology of the stroke.

Epidemiology

Approximately two million Americans have atrial fibrillation.[5] Atrial fibrillation is a risk factor for stroke in all age groups.[13] The prevalence of the cardiac arrhythmia is approximately 0.4 percent in the general population. The arrhythmia is relatively uncommon among children and young adults. The risk of embolization among persons younger than 65 who have atrial fibrillation but no structural heart disease (lone atrial fibrillation) is relatively low. The prevalence of atrial fibrillation increases rapidly after the age of 65 and it is found in 6–8 percent in persons older than 70.[3,14,15] Approximately 10 percent of persons 80 years of age or older have atrial fibrillation.[5] While heart disease and atrial fibrillation are more common in men, the strong age-relationship of the arrhythmia makes atrial fibrillation a particular potent risk factor for women. Atrial fibrillation is the single most important forecaster of cerebral infarction among elderly women. Besides an important predictor of cerebrovascular disease, the presence of atrial fibrillation has a major impact on prognosis; both early and long-term mortality following stroke is high among persons with the arrhythmia.[16,17] Most deaths are due to the underlying severe heart disease.

Associated Heart Diseases

Atrial fibrillation most commonly occurs among persons who have a history of hypertension, diabetes mellitus, smoking, or congestive heart failure[14] (see Table 13-4). In particular, the presence of arterial hypertension is strongly associated with atrial fibrillation and an associated risk of embolism.[18] Several cardiac diseases are complicated by the arrhythmia including coronary artery disease, recent myocardial infarction, cardiovascular procedures, congestive heart failure, valvular heart disease, congenital heart disease, hypertrophic or dilated cardiomyopathies, or thyrotoxicosis[14] (see Table 13-4). The increased risk of atrial fibrillation among patients with hypertension might be secondary to left ventricular hypertrophy, impaired ventricular filling, left atrial enlargement, and slowing of atrial conduction velocity.[18] Atrial fibrillation complicating thyrotoxicosis is accompanied by an especially high risk of embolization[19] (Table 13-5). Both clinical and imaging findings can help predict the frequency of embolization.[10,20,21] For example, Benjamin et al.[22] reported that each 10 mm increase in size of the left atrium increased risk of stroke by a factor of 2.4 in men and 1.4 in women. Recently, Wang et al.[23] developed a risk score based on the following factors: advancing age, female sex, increasing systolic blood pressure, diabetes, or previous neurological symptoms. Patients with these factors have a considerably higher risk of embolic stroke than persons with atrial fibrillation that did not have these findings. The highest risk group of patients is those who have had previous neurological symptoms—TIA or stroke.[24,25]

▶ **TABLE 13-5.** RISK OF EMBOLIZATION SUBGROUPS OF PATIENTS WITH ATRIAL FIBRILLATION

Clinical Findings
  Highest risk
    Prior neurological symptoms or embolization
    Rheumatic mitral stenosis
    Prosthetic mitral valve
    New onset atrial fibrillation
      Acute myocardial infarction
      Cardiovascular procedures
      Cardioversion
  Higher risk
    History of diabetes mellitus
    History of hypertension
    Systolic blood pressure >160 mm Hg
    Coronary artery disease
    Congestive heart failure
    Women
    Age >75 years
  Intermediate risk
    Men or women >65 but no other changes
  Lower risk
    Persons <65 with no other changes
Cardiac imaging findings
  Highest risk
    Intra-atrial thrombus
    Intraventricular thrombus
    Spontaneous left atrial contrast
  Higher risk
    Left ventricular enlargement
    Left atrial enlargement
  Lower risk
    Normal

Treatment of Atrial Fibrillation

Guidelines for the management of newly detected atrial fibrillation are available.[26] One of the goals of treatment of either the cardiac rate or rhythm among patients with atrial fibrillation is to lower the risk of embolization. There is considerable uncertainty about the best strategy to treat the arrhythmia.[27] Electrical or chemical cardioversion can be used to achieve sinus rhythm. However, cardioversion can be accompanied by embolization because the sudden increase in left atrial contractility might prompt release of thrombi.[28] For acute conversion of atrial fibrillation, ibutilide, flecainide, dofetilide, propafenone, amiodarone, and quinidine are effective.[29] The risk of embolization following cardioversion is approximately 1 percent.[30] Based on an analysis of four clinical trials, Gronefeld and Hohnloser[31] concluded that rate control was as effective as measures to control cardiac rhythm. Saxonhouse and Curtis[32] concluded that rate control is an acceptable primary strategy for treatment of patients with recurrent atrial fibrillation. A review of management options found that verapamil, diltiazem, atenolol, and metoprolol are superior to digoxin in controlling ventricular rate.[29] Maintenance of sinus rhythm is best achieved with amiodarone, propafenone, disopyramide, and sotalol.[29]

Despite measures to control the cardiac rate and rhythm, antithrombotic therapy remains a cornerstone in preventing stroke among persons with the arrhythmia.[3,33–36] The effects of these medications in lowering the risk of stroke are dramatic. Despite robust data showing efficacy, a large number of eligible patients with atrial fibrillation unfortunately are not treated with warfarin.[37,38] Aspirin can be prescribed to patients who cannot be treated with anticoagulants (see Chapter 19). Percutaneous placement of an occlusive device within the left atrial appendage might prevent recurrent embolization among persons with atrial fibrillation.[39] This procedure could be used as a therapeutic alternative to long-term oral anticoagulation. However, experience is limited. Additional information is needed to determine the safety and efficacy of such devices.

▶ OTHER CARDIAC ARRHYTHMIAS

While atrial fibrillation is the primary cardiac arrhythmia identified as associated with an increased risk of thromboembolism, other cardiac conduction disturbances can produce recurrent syncope or transient neurological symptoms. Common episodic cardiac arrhythmias are *sick sinus syndrome (tachycardia–bradycardia syndrome)* or *intermittent complete heart block*. While some cases of stroke are associated with these arrhythmias, most patients have global symptoms (Stokes-Adams syncope). These arrhythmias are found most commonly among older persons with ischemic heart disease. Occasionally, ventricular or other atrial arrhythmias can be complicated by hypoperfusion or syncope. Cardiac conduction defects leading to embolization have been reported among persons with neuromuscular diseases including *Kearns-Sayre syndrome, mitochondrial encephalopathy with lactic acidosis and stroke-like episodes (MELAS), myoclonus epilepsy with ragged red fibers (MERRF), limb girdle dystrophies, myotonic dystrophy,* and *scapuloperoneal dystrophy.*

► CONGENITAL HEART DISEASES

Approximately 1,000,000 Americans have a history of a congenital heart defect.[5] *Cyanotic congenital heart disease* remains an important underlying mechanism for ischemic stroke in children (Table 13-6). Among the cardiac lesions are an *interatrial septal defect*, an *interventricular septal defect, transposition of the great vessels, patent ductus arteriosus, pulmonary artery atresia* or the *Tetralogy of Fallot*.[40] Affected children often have hypoxia, cyanosis, and polycythemia. In addition, the presence of a right-to-left intracardiac shunt allows for paradoxical embolism. Because some emboli are infected, children with cyanotic heart disease also have a high risk for development of brain abscess secondary to an anaerobic infection. Strokes are a potential complication of cardiovascular operations to treat these lesions. The frequency of neurological sequelae following a major cardiac operation in childhood is estimated as high as 30 percent. Stroke has been associated with a *bicuspid aortic valve*, although the risk apparently is very low.

Occasionally, adults with an *atrial septal defect* will be identified. Because the defect involves a persistent channel between the right and left atria, the risk of paradoxical embolism probably is greater than that which occurs with a patent foramen ovale (PFO).

► ATRIAL SEPTAL ANEURYSM

An atrial septal aneurysm is defined as displacement and bowing of the interatrial septum during cardiac

► **TABLE 13-6.** CONGENITAL HEART DISEASES ASSOCIATED WITH CEREBRAL INFARCTION

Interatrial septal defect
Patent foramen ovale
Patent ductus arteriosus
Interventricular septal defect
Transposition of the great vessels
Pulmonary artery atresia
Tetralogy of Fallot

contraction.[41,42] The average amount of bowing is approximately 3.8 mm.[43] This change is relatively common in asymptomatic people. Mattioli et al.[43] found an atrial septal aneurysm in 28 percent of 215 patients with stroke and normal carotid arteries. The vast majority of persons with stroke identified with an atrial septal aneurysm are young adults and in some cases it is the only potential cause for stroke.[44,45] Some of the association of atrial septal aneurysm and stroke might be secondary to a more extensive cardiac evaluation performed in young adults with otherwise cryptogenic stroke. It can be an isolated finding or can be detected in conjunction with a PFO. The risk of embolization appears to be low when this cardiac change occurs in isolation. In a French study, none of the patients with atrial septal aneurysm and previous stroke had recurrent neurological symptoms during treatment with aspirin.[46] The combination of an atrial septal aneurysm and PFO may be more dangerous. Mattioli et al.[47] reported a relationship between atrial septal aneurysm and mitral valve prolapse (MVP). Carerj et al.[48] found an increased frequency of atrial septal aneurysm among persons with migraine with aura. They concluded that the aura of migraine might be related to the presence of the septal change. Further research is needed to determine if a relationship exists between atrial septal aneurysm alone or in combination with other cardiac conditions with either stroke or migraine.

► PATENT FORAMEN OVALE

During pregnancy, a fetus has a hole in the interatrial septum, which permits the movement of blood from the venous to systemic circulation and bypasses the lungs. At birth, a fibrous membrane closes the hole but in up to 20 percent of normal adults, the membrane does not completely fuse and small potential channel persists (PFO).[49–51] Based on this figure, one could estimate that 60–70 million Americans have a PFO. Thus, a PFO is a relatively common finding detected during the evaluation of the heart in a patient with a stroke (see Chapter 8).

Pathogenesis of Paradoxical Embolism

The membrane is located on the left side of the interatrial septum. Because intra-atrial pressure is higher in the left atrium than on the right, the membrane is pushed against the septum and no channel is open. On the other hand, if right-sided cardiac pressure exceeds that on the left, a small hole could open. A right-to-left movement of blood and potentially paradoxical embolism could result. Transient increases in right cardiac pressure, such as with Valsalva maneuver, could lead to a temporary right-to-left shunt. For embolization to occur, a thrombus or embolus would need to be in the right atrium at the time when the right-to-left shunt is present. Cases of a clot traversing the atrial septum via a PFO have been described.[52] Presumably, the embolus would be of venous origin and be secondary to thrombosis of veins in the pelvis or lower extremity. Cases of stroke occurring among persons taking long-distance airplane flights have been attributed to deep vein thrombosis in the leg leading to paradoxical embolization via a PFO.[53] Still, the frequency of deep vein thrombosis in the lower extremities among persons with stroke and PFO is relatively low.[54] In a relatively small case-control study, Cramer et al.[55] found that possible thrombi in pelvic veins were detected by magnetic resonance venography in 20 percent of 46 patients with cryptogenic stroke and in 4 percent of 49 patients with stroke of a determined cause. This observation is interesting and needs to be confirmed.

Specific anatomic-pathological or physiological changes within the PFO might forecast a high risk of embolic stroke. A large aperture or volume of blood traversing the PFO might be predictive of an increased risk for embolization.[56] While direct imaging would assess the former finding, the volume of bubbles that are seen in the left atrium during contrast echocardiography also could be a surrogate for the size of the shunt.[57] Unfortunately, current data do not support any specific relationship between either the size of the PFO or the amount of the shunt with the risk of cerebral embolism. In addition, interrater agreement and intrarater reproducibility in interpreting the echocardiographic findings of PFO and ASA are relatively low and means that the diagnosis of the cardiac abnormalities can be uncertain.[58]

A French study concluded that the presence of an atrial septal aneurysm is associated with a heightened risk of embolic events among persons with PFO.[46] Additional research is needed to substantiate this observation. In general, no specific feature of PFO has consistently identified those persons who have the greatest risk for thromboembolic events.[59]

Clinical Findings

Most patients with PFO are asymptomatic and the abnormality is found as an incidental finding. Some patients, especially women, might have a family trait that predisposes to development of PFO.[60] While most patients do not have cyanosis or symptoms of hypoxia, occasional cases are diagnosed with the *platypnea-orthodeoxia syndrome* in which severe symptoms of shortness of breath are associated with postural changes.[61] No cardiac murmurs or other abnormalities are detected on physical examination. A PFO can be suspected if an electrocardiogram demonstrates an "M" shaped notch in

the "R" wave on leads II, III, and AVF. The possibility of paradoxical embolization as the cause of the neurological symptoms might be increased if the event occurs in close proximity to a Valsalva maneuver. The usual scenario is detection of the PFO during cardiac evaluation searching for the cause of TIA or stroke, especially among younger persons.

Relationship of PFO and Stroke

The cause-and-effect relationship between PFO (paradoxical embolism) and ischemic stroke is unclear in part because of the high prevalence of cardiac lesion in the general population.[59] While approximately 20 percent of healthy adults have a PFO, rates are approximately twice as high among persons with stroke, especially among young persons without another obvious explanation for the ischemic symptoms. Based on a meta-analysis of several case-control studies, Overell et al.[62] concluded that either atrial septal aneurysm or PFO alone or in combination was associated with an increased risk of stroke, particularly among persons younger than 55. Part of the presumed relationship between PFO and cryptogenic stroke in young adults might be the result of selection bias. An aggressive cardiac evaluation is more likely to be done when a young adult has an unexplained stroke than when an older person has an otherwise obvious cause already discovered. There is no obvious reason for a PFO to close with advancing age and thus, it should be found among elderly persons with stroke. In fact, Lewis et al.[63] showed that PFO can be found when screening elderly persons with stroke. However, Jones et al.[64] concluded that PFO was not associated with stroke in older adults. This conclusion probably is based on the high prevalence of other possible explanations for stroke. These observations support the contention that the potential interactions between PFO and stroke should be viewed with caution. Detection of a PFO should not preclude evaluation for another cause including an arterial lesion or prothrombotic disorder. In some patients, the PFO likely is an incidental finding that has no relationship to the stroke. Conversely, there is ample evidence that some strokes are secondary to paradoxical embolism via a PFO; for example, case reports demonstrate a clot traversing the cardiac lesion.[52] In addition, neurological symptoms secondary to Caisson disease or decompression sickness following diving can be secondary to paradoxical embolism via a PFO.[61] A potential interaction between PFO and migraine also has been reported.[65] The explanation for this interaction is not obvious. Still, Sztajzel et al.[66] found a PFO in 44 of evaluated 74 patients with cryptogenic stroke. Sixteen of these patients had a history of migraine with aura. They concluded that the septal defect could play a pathogenic role in migraine with aura in young adults. Because the data about PFO and neurological symptoms are unclear, additional epidemiological research is needed to define these relationships. While closure of the PFO has been recommended to prevent recurrent migraine, better data are needed to establish a cause-and-effect relationship before this therapy is recommended.

Risk of Recurrent Stroke

Controversy will continue until strong data are available about the associations between PFO and ischemic cerebrovascular disease. The risk of stroke or recurrent stroke among patients with PFO also is not well established.[67] While some researchers report a high risk of recurrent embolic events, a French study showed that the likelihood of recurrent ischemia was lower among persons with PFO than among a cohort of patients who did not have the cardiac lesion.[46] This same study found an increased risk among patients that had both PFO and an atrial septal aneurysm but the number of followed patients was relatively small and these data need to be substantiated. Another trial did not find any significant difference in the rate of recurrent stroke between patients with PFO and those who did not have the cardiac finding.[68]

Treatment

Because of the uncertainty about the risk of recurrent events, the best management of patients with PFO and stroke is in doubt.[51,59,69] The choices include antiplatelet agents, oral anticoagulants, endovascular placement of a device to occlude the hole, or direct surgical closure.[70] Mas et al.[46] found that aspirin was as effective in preventing recurrent ischemia among patients with PFO as it was among persons who did not have the cardiac lesion. A substudy of the Warfarin–Aspirin Recurrent Stroke Study (WARSS) found that aspirin and warfarin were of equal efficacy in preventing recurrent stroke.[68] Direct surgical closure has been recommended for treatment of some patients with PFO.[71,72] Still, such a strategy involves a major cardiac operation that can be complicated by stroke.[73] Because the risk of neurological complications with major open-heart surgery is considerable, it might exceed the likelihood of ischemic stroke. Thus, such operations would seem to be indicated for only exceptional cases. Enthusiasm for endovascular placement of PFO occlusive devices is considerable. These devices can be placed with a reasonable degree of safety and anecdotal experience and uncontrolled studies suggest that they are effective.[74–78] Still, trials have not directly compared the usefulness of placement of such a device to best medical treatment. Such research is underway. One can assume that some

patients will benefit from placement of a PFO closure device while other patients probably will not need the procedure. At present, none of the treatment options have been established as effective in preventing stroke among persons with PFO.[69,79,80]

▶ VALVULAR HEART DISEASES

▶ RHEUMATIC VALVULAR DISEASE

Since the introduction of antibiotics to treat streptococcal diseases leading to rheumatic fever, the frequency of rheumatic (mitral) valvular disease has declined greatly in the United States and most other industrialized countries. However, despite the advances in care, rheumatic fever remains a public health problem. It is more common in minority groups in the United States than in whites.[5] Persons living in developing countries, where antibiotics might not be readily available, also can have the valvular complications of rheumatic fever. In addition, some older persons, who were children in the preantibiotic era, have rheumatic valvular heart disease. Secondary stenosis of either the mitral and aortic valve results from the infection and autoimmune disease.

Pathogenesis of Emboli

Rheumatic stenosis of the mitral valve is the most serious. Because of secondary enlargement of the left atrium, atrial fibrillation often develops. The combination of rheumatic mitral stenosis and atrial fibrillation is particularly dangerous. Coulshed et al.[81] found that embolic events occurred in 8 percent of their patients with mitral stenosis alone and in 32 percent of the patients who had the mitral valve lesion complicated by atrial fibrillation. In comparison to age-matched healthy persons, the relative risk of embolic stroke among persons with the combination of mitral stenosis and the arrhythmia is increased by a factor of 13.[82] Other factors associated with an increased risk of embolization include advancing age, reduced cardiac output, decreased area of the mitral valve, mitral regurgitation, and aortic regurgitation.[83,84] The abnormal mitral valve also is associated with an increased risk of infective endocarditis, which could follow an operation such as a dental procedure.

Clinical Findings

The diagnosis of rheumatic mitral stenosis usually is made on the basis of the relevant history of rheumatic fever or streptococcal infections and the presence of cardiac murmurs, cardiomegaly, or signs of heart failure.

Treatment

Management of patients with rheumatic mitral stenosis includes perioperative prescription of antibiotics to prevent infective endocarditis during most surgical procedures and anticoagulants to lower the risk of thromboembolism. Other options include mitral valvuloplasty or surgical placement of a bioprosthetic or mechanical valve. These procedures can be complicated by embolization. Most patients with mitral valve replacement will require long-term anticoagulant treatment.[85]

▶ MITRAL VALVE PROLAPSE

Mitral valve prolapse (MVP) is another common valvular lesion that might be a substrate for thromboembolism to the brain. MVP is detected in approximately 2.5 percent of adults of all ages, with the prevalence being higher in women than in men.[86] While MVP is more commonly diagnosed in young adults than in older persons, this relationship might reflect the more widespread use of echocardiography in the evaluation in younger persons. MVP can be found during the evaluation of persons older than 65. Besides being the site of thrombi, a redundant and prolapsing mitral valve also is associated with an increased risk of infective endocarditis following surgical procedures. Most patients with MVP are asymptomatic. Physical findings include a cardiac murmur and click. Affected persons usually are thin and some have pectus excavatum.

In the past, MVP was considered as an important cause of cerebral infarction among young adults.[87,88] However, the preponderance of the subsequence evidence suggests that the risk of thromboembolic stroke among persons with MVP is relatively low.[89,90] The frequency of MVP among young persons with cryptogenic stroke is not elevated and most patients with MVP and stroke have another explanation for their neurological symptoms. Thus, detection of MVP should not forestall additional evaluation for the cause of stroke. The risk of recurrent stroke among persons with MVP does not appear to be excessively high. Treatment emphasizes antiplatelet aggregating agents. Anticoagulants do not seem to be necessary. Prophylactic antibiotics should be given prior to dental or surgical procedures. Surgical replacement of the valve is not needed unless a complication, such as infectious endocarditis, develops.

▶ MITRAL ANNULUS CALCIFICATION AND CALCIFICATION OF THE AORTIC VALVE

Calcification of the annulus of the mitral valve is commonly found among elderly persons, especially women.[91]

It is found in approximately 20 percent of persons older than 65 and its prevalence among persons with stroke is slightly higher.[92,93] A potential relationship of mitral annulus calcification to chronic renal disease or hyperparathyroidism exists. Presumably the mitral annulus calcification can be the source of thromboemboli or pieces of calcified spicules. Still, the risk of stroke directly attributable to mitral annulus calcification is unclear because the lesion is most commonly found among persons who have hypertension, atrial fibrillation, atherosclerotic vascular disease, and congestive heart failure.[94] Because of the uncertainty about the significance of mitral annulus calcification as a cause of stroke, other explanations for the ischemic symptoms should be sought. Because of the apparent low risk of stroke secondary to the valvular abnormality, it should not be considered as a heart disease that warrants long-term anticoagulation for stroke prophylaxis unless other cardiac lesions are found.

While calcification of the aortic valve with or without secondary stenosis can lead to turbulent flow or to the formation of small thrombi, it appears to be an uncommon cause of embolization.[95]

▶ MECHANICAL PROSTHETIC VALVES

Since the introduction of mechanical prosthetic valves to treat patients with severe valvular heart disease, embolism has been a well-established complication. The likelihood of clot formation is extremely high and in the absence of long-term anticoagulant therapy, the frequency of embolic events from a mechanical mitral valve might be as high as 25 percent per year. The valves are associated with both an acute and long-term increase in the risk of stroke. The recurrent events can lead to cognitive impairments. Deklunder et al.[96] found that cognitive impairments are relatively common among persons with prosthetic heart valves. The risk is even higher if a patient has both mechanical mitral and aortic valve prostheses or if the patient also has atrial fibrillation. While the chances of embolization from a mechanical aortic prosthesis are considerable, the risks are lower than that reported with a mitral valve replacement. The risk of embolization varies with the type of prosthesis; Medtronic and Carpentier valves appear to be associated with a lower risk than Bjork-Shiley valves.[97–99] Besides being a nidus for thrombi, the prosthetic valve also is vulnerable to infective endocarditis.[100] Valve malfunction or failure or a secondary prothrombotic state is additional potential causes of thromboembolic events among persons with prosthetic valves.

Because of the associated high risk for embolism, any stroke occurring in a patient with a mechanical prosthetic valve initially should be considered as of cardioembolic origin. Most strokes are related directly to the prosthesis. Although not formally tested in clinical trials, the medical community has accepted the utility of long-term anticoagulation for treatment of patients with mechanical valves.[101,102] Anticoagulants are the traditional intervention to prevent stroke (see Chapter 19). However, even with the use of anticoagulants, the risk of embolism is considerable. Because of the perceived high risk of thromboembolic events, the desired level of anticoagulation is higher for patients with prosthetic valves than it is for persons with other potential cardiac sources of embolism. In addition, many patients are treated with the combination of an antiplatelet agent and the oral anticoagulant. Combination therapy usually is instituted after a patient has ischemic symptoms despite treatment with anticoagulants alone. Because of the higher levels of anticoagulation and the use of a combination of oral anticoagulants and antiplatelet agents, the risk of intracerebral and subdural hemorrhages is considerable. As a result, intracranial bleeding is an important alternative diagnosis to ischemic stroke as an explanation for the acute onset of neurological symptoms in a patient with a prosthetic valve. Oral anticoagulants are contraindicated during pregnancy because of their teratogenic effects, and a pregnant woman with a mechanical prosthetic valve should receive either unfractionated heparin or a low molecular weight heparin.[103]

▶ BIOPROSTHETIC VALVES

The likelihood of thromboembolism among persons with bioprosthetic valves is lower than among patients who have mechanical valve replacements.[104] In particular, the chances of embolism are relatively low with bioprosthetic aortic valves.[105] Most patients with either mitral or aortic bioprosthetic valves often receive a short course (3 months) of oral anticoagulants following surgery before being switched to treatment with antiplatelet agents. Subsequently, most patients do well with treatment with aspirin. However, delayed neurological symptoms usually are secondary to deterioration of the bioprosthetic valves or infective endocarditis.

▶ INFECTIVE ENDOCARDITIS

Even in the modern antibiotic era, infectious endocarditis remains a highly fatal disease (Fig. 13-6). Most cases are secondary to bacterial infection but fungal endocarditis can occur especially among immunocompromised individuals. Approximately 20,000 people are hospitalized with infectious endocarditis annually in the

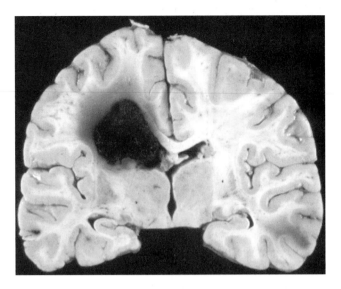

Figure 13-6. A coronal autopsy specimen of the brain of a patient dying of infective endocarditis shows a hemorrhagic infarction of the right hemisphere. The blood has extended into the right lateral ventricle. (*Courtesy of S.S. Schochet, M.D., Department of Pathology, University of West Virginia, Morgantown, WV*)

United States.[5] A recent study from Connecticut found that the 6-month mortality is approximately 25 percent.[106] Anderson et al.[107] reported that the 1-year mortality was more than 50 percent. The infection causes the formation of vegetations on the valves. Involvement of the mitral value is a special concern.

Clinical Findings

Approximately 10–15 percent of patients develop focal neurological symptoms or an altered mental status as complications of left-sided infective endocarditis.[106–108] The symptoms occur with either acute or subacute infective endocarditis affecting either the mitral or aortic valve (Table 13-7). Anderson et al.[107] reported that the risk of embolization was greater with endocarditis of the mitral valve (17 percent) than with aortic valve involvement (9 percent). Infective endocarditis usually develops in a patient who has an underlying valvular abnormality. In particular, patients with mechanical or bioprosthetic valves have a high risk for this complication.[100] A transient bacteremia following an invasive ("dirty") medical procedure, such as dental care, or trauma is often an underlying contributing cause. Because of the high risk of infectious endocarditis among persons with valvular heart disease, prophylactic antibiotics are given in the perioperative period when these surgical procedures are performed. Acute infectious endocarditis is a potential complication of intravenous abuse of illegal drugs.

Most cases of infective endocarditis have a subacute course of malaise, intermittent fever, and constitutional

▶ **TABLE 13-7.** CLINICAL FEATURES OF INFECTIVE ENDOCARDITIS

General features
  Fever
  Malaise
  Nausea and vomiting
  Abdominal pain
  Hematuria
  Changing cardiac murmur
  New onset congestive heart failure
  Splinter hemorrhages
  Janeway lesions
  Osler nodes
  Roth spots
  Conjunctival hemorrhages
Neurological features
  Cerebral infarction
  Cerebral hemorrhage
  Infective aneurysm
  Meningitis
  Encephalitis (cerebritis)
  Brain abscess

symptoms (see Table 13-7). Abdominal pain and/or hematuria can be secondary to splenic, visceral, or renal embolization. On examination, a changing murmur, signs of heart failure, and skin lesions, including splinter hemorrhages, Janeway lesions, and Osler nodes can be found. Ocular abnormalities include Roth spots in the retina and conjunctival telangiectases. Fulminant cardiac failure can be the presentation of patients with acute infectious endocarditis, most commonly due to staphylococcus aureus. Besides cardioembolic stroke, patients can have intracranial hemorrhage, a septic aneurysm, encephalitis, meningitis, or brain abscess.[109] Rupture of a secondary infective intracranial aneurysm can cause subarachnoid hemorrhage.

Diagnostic Studies

Laboratory abnormalities include leucocytosis and an elevated erythrocyte sedimentation rate. Signs of infection can be found in examination of the cerebrospinal fluid. Echocardiography often demonstrates vegetations on the value. Aerobic and anaerobic blood cultures are the most definitive tests. On occasion, several blood cultures will need to be obtained over several days in order to screen for infectious endocarditis. Cerebral arteriography to screen for the presence of secondary infective aneurysms usually is performed when a patient has neurological symptoms.[110] Sequential cerebral arteriograms often are performed when the initial study demonstrates an aneurysm. The studies are looking for growth in the aneurysm, a finding that might portend a high risk for rupture.

Treatment

Antibiotics are the mainstay of management. Most patients require a several week course of intravenously administered antibiotics, which are selected on the basis of the blood cultures. A severely damaged native valve might need to be replaced surgically. Vikram et al.[111] found that surgical replacement of serious affected left-sided valves was associated with a reduction in mortality within 6 months following endocarditis. An infected prosthetic valve also might need to have operative treatment. Because of the perceived high risk of intracranial bleeding, most patients with stroke secondary to infective endocarditis are not treated with anticoagulants. The exception is the patient who has an infection of a prosthetic valve. Surgical or endovascular treatment of an infective aneurysm is a consideration, especially if the aneurysm shows expansion on sequential examinations.

▶ NONBACTERIAL THROMBOTIC ENDOCARDITIS

Nonbacterial thrombotic endocarditis (NBTE/marantic endocarditis) is secondary to changes in coagulation that leads to a disseminated intravascular coagulation (DIC) (Table 13-8).[112,113] As a result of the DIC, thrombocytopenia, decreased fibrinogen concentration, elevated D-dimer and fibrinogen degradation productions, and prolongations of the aPTT and prothrombin time are found. The decline in clotting factors and

▶ **TABLE 13-8.** CLINICAL AND LABORATORY FINDINGS FOR NONBACTERIAL THROMBOTIC ENDOCARDITIS

Associated diseases
  Malignancy (pancreas, ovary, lung, bowel)
  Dehydration
  AIDS
  Pregnancy
  Diabetes mellitus
  Surgery
Clinical findings
  Cerebral infarction
  Abdominal pain
  Hematuria
  Deep vein thrombosis
  Cardiac failure
Laboratory findings
  Thrombocytopenia
  Prolonged prothrombin time
  Prolonged activate partial thromboplastin time
  Decreased fibrinogen level
  Elevated fibrin split products
  Elevated D-dimer levels

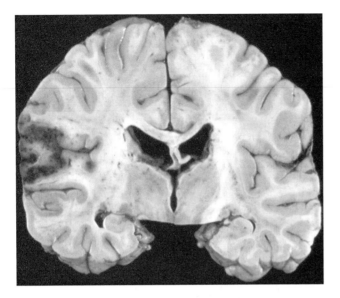

Figure 13-7. A coronal autopsy specimen demonstrates a cortical infarction in the right hemisphere consistent with the diagnosis of cardio embolic occlusion of a cortical branch of the middle cerebral artery. (*Courtesy of S.S. Schochet, M.D., Department of Pathology, University of West Virginia, Morgantown WV*)

platelets are secondary to their consumption by diffuse intravascular microthrombosis. The coagulation disturbance leads to formation of vegetations and thickening of the mitral and aortic valves. These vegetations, which consist of platelets and fibrinogen, detach and form emboli that go to the brain or other organs (Figs. 13-7 and 13-8).

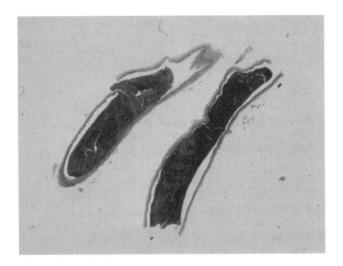

Figure 13-8. An organized embolus found within the lumen of the middle cerebral artery. The findings would be consistent with cardioembolism. (*Courtesy of S.S. Schochet, M.D., Department of Pathology, University of West Virginia, Morgantown WV*)

Associated Diseases

NBTE is a potential explanation of cerebral infarction, especially among persons with debilitating diseases and especially those with mucin-producing adenocarcinomas.[114–117] NBTE is a relatively rare complication of malignancy, dehydration, pregnancy, AIDS, surgery, or diabetes mellitus.[118] Presumably, the malignancy is producing a protein or antibody that induces changes in the coagulation cascade that leads to formation of microthrombi and the consumption of coagulation factors.

Clinical Findings

The risk of secondary cerebral embolism is approximately one in three. Besides cerebral infarction, patients with NBTE also have a high risk for embolism to the kidneys, spleen, and abdominal viscera. Patients also have a high risk for deep vein thrombosis and hemorrhagic events. Clinical features include mental status changes, focal or multifocal neurological impairments, abdominal or flank pain, an acute abdomen, hematuria, or cardiac symptoms. The multifocal and evolving nature of the neurological symptoms often can be confused with those associated with cerebral vasculitis.[117] Stroke often is the initial presentation of NBTE and it can be the first symptom of an underlying malignancy. NBTE should be considered when a patient has ischemic neurological symptoms in conjunction with either abdominal complaints or deep vein thrombosis.

Diagnostic Studies

Changes in the platelet count or coagulation studies provide an important initial clue. Subsequent blood tests screen for DIC. Echocardiography might demonstrate the valvular changes although the yield of the test is relatively low and the diagnosis of NBTE should not be refuted by a normal study.[119–121] Evaluation for an underlying malignancy arising in the pancreas, ovary, lung, or bowel should be performed when NBTE is diagnosed.

Treatment

While anticoagulants are prescribed to slow the DIC, the key to management involves interventions to treat the underlying disease. Because NBTE often occurs in the setting of an advanced malignancy and DIC, the prognosis of most patients is relatively poor.

▶ LIBMAN–SACKS ENDOCARDITIS

Libman–Sacks endocarditis is secondary to antibody–antigen complexes forming small vegetations on the mitral valve.[122] It usually occurs in the setting of systemic lupus erythematosus and Libman–Sacks endocarditis is strongly associated with the presence of lupus anticoagulants or the antiphospholipid antibody syndrome (see Chapter 14). The diagnosis of a cerebral infarction in a patient with systemic lupus erythematosus should prompt cardiac evaluation looking for the valvular vegetations. In addition, patients with *Sneddon syndrome* (cerebral infarction, digital ischemia, and generalized livedo reticularis) often have underlying antiphospholipid antibodies and Libman–Sacks endocarditis.[123] The cardiac lesions also can complicate polyarteritis nodosa.[124] The endocarditis can lead to cerebral embolization and microemboli can produce an encephalopathy or multifocal neurological impairments. Patients usually have evidence of systemic lupus erythematosus including abnormal serological and coagulation studies. An echocardiogram usually demonstrates the valvular vegetations. Treatment focuses on long-term administration of oral anticoagulants.

▶ MYOCARDIAL DISEASES

▶ CORONARY ARTERY DISEASE AND ACUTE MYOCARDIAL INFARCTION

Cerebral infarction is the most important noncardiac complication of acute myocardial infarction. Spencer et al.[125] recently reported that 1.5 percent of patients with acute myocardial infarction have a stroke during their initial hospitalization and that the rate of stroke might be increasing. In some cases of clinically occult myocardial infarction, especially among diabetic patients, stroke may be the initial symptom of the acute cardiac lesion. Most cases of secondary cerebral embolization occur within the first days or weeks after the myocardial infarction.[126–128,129] The risk returns to baseline levels at approximately 3–6 months following the cardiac injury. The embolic events reflect the acute cardiac injury and cardiac instability. Embolism is secondary to ventricular dysfunction, formation of intraventricular thrombi, or changes in the coagulation cascade. In addition, cardiac complications including congestive heart failure, reduced cardiac ejection fraction, or atrial fibrillation may be contributing factors for the thromboembolism. Patients with complicating stroke have a higher mortality during the initial hospitalization than do other patients with myocardial infarction.[125]

While the overall risk of cerebral embolism is estimated to be approximately 1–6 percent, risks are highest among those patients who have a large anterior wall myocardial infarction.[130] The chances of thromboembolic events among persons with inferior wall myocardial infarction are <1 percent. Echocardiographic

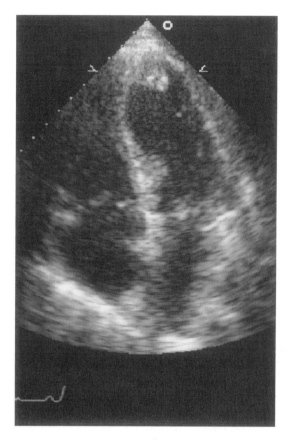

Figure 13-9. A transthoracic echocardiogram demonstrates a thrombus within the left ventricular apex. (*Courtesy of R.E. Kerber, M.D., University of Iowa. Department of Internal Medicine, University of Iowa, Iowa City, IA*)

detection of an intraventricular or a mural thrombus identifies patients at high risk.[131,132] The thrombus usually is located adjacent to a hypokinetic or akinetic segment of the left ventricle (Fig. 13-9). The advent of modern thrombolytic and antithrombotic therapies to treat patients with acute myocardial ischemia might lower the risk of secondary thromboembolic events.[133] Presumably, the treatment lessens the extent of myocardial injury with a resultant lowering in embolization. Still, high-risk patients should receive interventions to lower the likelihood of emboli. The success of anticoagulants seems to be superior to that achieved with antiplatelet aggregating agents.[134,135] Anticoagulants usually are prescribed for 6 months following the acute myocardial injury.

▶ VENTRICULAR ANEURYSM

Ischemic cardiomyopathy and a *ventricular aneurysm* are long-term sequelae of recurrent episodes of myocardial ischemia or a severe myocardial infarction. In general, affected patients have a reduced left ventricular ejection fraction and signs of congestive heart failure. In general, the risk of cerebral embolism seems to be low unless the patient has atrial fibrillation or congestive heart failure.[136] Because of the perceived relatively low risk of embolization among patients with ventricular aneurysms, anticoagulants usually are not prescribed. Patients are generally treated with aspirin or aspirin and clopidogrel.

▶ DILATED CARDIOMYOPATHIES

Approximately 85 percent of the persons hospitalized with cardiomyopathies have dilated cardiomyopathy.[5] The prognosis of patients with dilated cardiomyopathy is poor, more than 75 percent are dead within 10 years of diagnosis. A dilated cardiomyopathy in adults usually is secondary to ischemic heart disease, chronic alcohol abuse, pregnancy, or a viral illness.[137] Cardiomyopathy in children might be a complication of mitochondrial diseases or primary muscular diseases including Kearns-Sayre syndrome, MELAS, MERRF, myotonic dystrophy, scapuloperoneal dystrophy, and limb-girdle syndromes.[138,139] Poor left ventricular contraction leads to symptoms of congestive heart failure. The dilated left ventricular cavity serves as a nidus for thrombus formation. Cardiac imaging studies usually show a poor ejection fraction and often an intraventricular clot is found. Although data from clinical trials are lacking, the risk of embolization appears to be high and oral anticoagulants often are recommended.[140] Hypertrophic cardiomyopathy more commonly leads to sudden cardiac death than to cerebrovascular events.

▶ IDIOPATHIC HYPERTROPHIC SUBAORTIC STENOSIS

While cerebral infarction can be a presenting finding of idiopathic hypertrophic subaortic stenosis (IHSS), neurological complications are relatively uncommon.[141,142] Most thromboembolic events are reported among patients with IHSS in combination with another cardiac factor such as atrial fibrillation.

▶ ATRIAL MYXOMA

Myxomas are rare intracardiac tumors that most commonly arise in the left atrium[143,144] (Fig. 13-10). The tumors are more common in women than in men but occur in all age groups including children.[145] Embolization

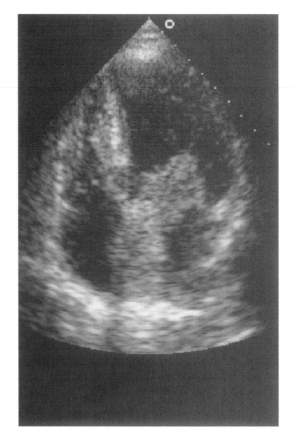

Figure 13-10. An atrial myxoma is demonstrated on this transesophageal echocardiogram. (*Courtesy of R.E. Kerber, M.D., University of Iowa. Department of Internal Medicine, University of Iowa, Iowa City, IA*)

of pieces of tumor tissue or secondary thrombi can lead to ischemic stroke. Approximately one-third of patients have neurological symptoms and ischemic stroke can be the initial clinical symptom. The embolic tumor material lodged in an intracranial artery can lead to the formation of a neoplastic intracranial aneurysm[146–148] (see Chapter 15). Subarachnoid hemorrhage is a potential complication. Patients often have symptoms of a subacute fever, skin eruptions, and arthralgias, which are associated with an elevated erythrocyte sedimentation rate or abnormal C-reactive protein, which presumably are secondary to the shedding of tumor tissue. These findings can lead to the misdiagnosis of a multisystem inflammatory disease such as systemic lupus erythematosus. In addition, the tumor mass can obstruct the mitral orifice resulting in sudden heart failure or death. Many patients have normal cardiac examinations but a cardiac murmur that changes in response to alterations in posture might provide a clue. The tumor usually is diagnosed by echocardiography. Treatment focuses on surgical resection of the tumor. Neither anticoagulants nor antiplatelet agents have a major role in stroke prophylaxis.

▶ PAPILLARY FIBROELASTOMA AND OTHER TUMORS

A papillary fibroelastoma is a rare, histologically benign tumor that most commonly affects the cardiac valves.[149] Gowda et al.[150] reported on a series of 725 patients with cardiac papillary fibroelastoma. Most patients were older than 70 and a majority of patients were men. Pieces of the tumor can embolize to the cerebral vessels or other arteries. These tumors can cause brain ischemia, pulmonary embolism, myocardial infarction, peripheral embolization, or sudden death. A highly mobile tumor is associated with an increased likelihood of embolization. In general, symptomatic patients should be treated with surgical removal of the tumor.

Malignant tumors of the heart are very uncommon but could be the potential source of emboli. These tumors will be detected on cardiac imaging and need to be differentiated from other cardiac masses including thrombi. The treatment focuses on surgical resection of the mass.

▶ OTHER CARDIAC LESIONS

Primary oxalosis, which can lead to intracardiac calcification, has been complicated by thromboembolism.[151]

Echocardiography permits discovery of a number of cardiac abnormalities that might be associated with thromboembolism. The significance of some of these changes is uncertain; some of these, in isolation, might not forecast a high risk for embolism. Considerable research is needed to determine the risk associated with each of these findings. Additional data are needed to guide decisions about prescription of long-term stroke prophylaxis therapies.

Spontaneous echocardiographic contrast (smoke) is secondary to turbulence within the left atrial cavity. It has been correlated with an increased risk of embolization among persons with either atrial fibrillation or mitral stenosis.[152,153] *Valvular strands*, which are thin pieces of material attached to the mitral or aortic valve, also appear to be associated with an increased risk of embolic stroke.[154-156] The nature of these lesions, which are most commonly found during echocardiographic evaluation of younger patients, is not known. Valvular strands are most commonly found in conjunction with mitral valve dystrophy or among persons with mechanical mitral valve prostheses. They do not seem to be associated with MVP, mitral annulus calcification, or other valvular abnormalities. Echocardiography also can detect a *Lambl excrescence*.[157] The significance of this finding, which is best described as an outgrowth on the mitral valve, is not known. *Myxomatous changes* of the mitral valve also can be found.

▶ STROKE COMPLICATING CARDIOVASCULAR PROCEDURES AND THERAPIES

Both hemorrhagic and ischemic stroke are potential complications of cardiovascular procedures. For example, intracranial hemorrhage is a rare (<1 percent) complication of thrombolytic treatment of patients with acute coronary artery occlusions.[158-161] In addition, many patients with myocardial infarction also receive potent antiplatelet aggregating agents and anticoagulants, which can be complicated by intracranial or spinal bleeding. Some patients with the cardiovascular interventions, such as left ventricular assist devices, also have bleeding secondary to the concomitant use of medications prescribed to prevent thromboembolic complications.[162] Still, most cerebrovascular events complicating cardiovascular treatments are ischemic and are secondary to either hypotension or cardioembolism.

▶ ENDOVASCULAR PROCEDURES

Ischemic neurological complications usually occur immediately following the cardiac procedure (see Table 13-3). The frequency of ischemic stroke following *cardiac catheterization* or *coronary arteriography* are estimated to be <0.1–1 percent.[163] Most are due to embolization of clots that develop on the catheter tip. Local arterial trauma, air embolism, or neurotoxicity secondary to the contrast agent also can cause neurological symptoms. Other cardiac interventions that can be complicated by stroke include *coronary artery angioplasty and stenting, endovascular closure of a PFO, placement of a pacemaker, ablation procedures, electrophysiological studies, right ventricular endomyocardial biopsy, retrograde catheterization of the aortic valve,* and *transmyocardial laser revascularization* procedures.[164-169] Fortunately, the risk of cerebral embolism seems to be very low. Embolization also can complicate *percutaneous balloon valvoplasty*.[170] Silaruks et al.[171] reported on 219 cases in which left atrial thrombi were detected following transvenous mitral commissurotomy. Approximately one-fourth of the patients had resolution of their clots with 6 months of treatment with oral anticoagulants. Presumably, this group of patients would have been at high risk for thromboembolic events without anticoagulant treatment following the procedure.

▶ CORONARY ARTERY BYPASS GRAFT SURGERY AND OTHER MAJOR CARDIAC OPERATIONS

Neurological disease is an important cause of disability following coronary artery bypass graft (CABG) operations or other major cardiac operations requiring cardiopulmonary bypass.[172–174] Most neurological complications occur within the first 24–48 hours following the operation.[175] The risk of major stroke following coronary artery bypass operations is estimated to be as high as 6 percent and similar or higher risks are associated with valvular replacement surgery.[176,177] In addition to obvious ischemic strokes, subtler neuropsychological impairments are found in approximately 20–50 percent of patients.[178,179] These impairments include a delirium, visual field defects, decreased visual acuity, cortical blindness, memory loss, or psychiatric disturbances.[174,180,181] Fortunately, many of these impairments resolve in the months following the operation. Retinal ischemia also is a potential complication.

Risk of Neurological Complications

The risk of major neurological complications appears to be considerable in adults, especially those persons older than 70. Factors that identify a high risk of ischemia include the presence of diabetes mellitus, peripheral vascular disease, or congestive heart failure.[182] Patients who are unstable medically, those required prolonged use of the extracorporeal device, those who need combined valvular and coronary artery surgery, and those persons with extensive intracranial or extracranial atherosclerosis also have a high risk. Severe stenosis of the origin of the internal carotid artery probably is associated with a higher risk of stroke. Interest has focused on the utility of carotid endarterectomy in limiting the risk of stroke associated with CABG.[183] Still, Safa et al.[184] found that prophylactic carotid surgery did not lessen the risk of stroke. Brown[185] reviewed the surgical management options for patients with concomitant severe coronary and carotid artery disease. No data are available about the utility of staged or combined surgical procedures. In particular, no data are available about the utility of prophylactic carotid endarterectomy in lowering the likelihood of neurological complications during CABG surgery.

Pathophysiology

The mechanisms of ischemic stroke in adults include hypotension or embolization of atherosclerotic debris, air, fat, or thrombotic material.[186–189] Likosky et al.[175] found that embolization accounted for approximately 60 percent of strokes complicating bypass procedure. Fracturing of an atherosclerotic plaque by intraoperative placement of an aortic clamp can cause massive embolization of atherosclerotic debris.[189,190] This scenario appears to be an important cause of neurological complications among elderly patients. Careful placement of the clamp, guided by TEE to evaluate the aortic disease, may lower the risk of this complication. Small

thrombi can develop within the extracorporeal device. In addition, complications of surgery including atrial fibrillation can lead to embolization. Endocarditis also is a potential etiology of stroke. Several strategies have been developed to reduce the risk of neurological complications of CABG.[191] Among patients having cardiopulmonary bypass, hypothermic cerebral perfusion, careful acid–base management, and slow rewarming might lessen neurological sequelae. Performing CABG without cardiopulmonary bypass appears to reduce the risk of stroke, especially among elderly patients. Sharony et al.[192] showed that off-pump CABG is associated with a reduced risk of stroke among patients with severe atherosclerotic disease of the aorta. An international study found that intra-aortic filtration might prevent emboli from reaching the brain.[193]

Approximately 30 percent of children having major cardiac operations have neurological complications including stroke[194,195] (see Chapter 17).

▶ LEFT VENTRICULAR ASSIST DEVICES

Left or right ventricular assist devices, which often are located in the descending aorta, are used to treat patients with intractable congestive heart failure. Approximately 20 percent of patients have thromboembolic complications including either spinal cord or cerebral infarction.[196–199] Spinal cord infarction also can result from local arterial trauma or occlusion. Vascular complications can occur any time during the use of the device and the risk persists as long as the device is used.

▶ CARDIAC TRANSPLANTATION

Patients with intractable heart failure can undergo cardiac transplantation. This procedure, which is used to treat a group of extraordinarily sick patients, is associated with a high rate of cerebrovascular complications. Embolic or hypoxic events occur with the surgical procedure. Patients have a high risk for metabolic encephalopathy, seizures, opportunistic central nervous system infections, or peripheral nerve palsies.[200–203] These complications usually occur in months following the transplantation.

REFERENCES

1. Murtagh B, Smalling RW. Cardioembolic stroke. Curr Atheroscler Rep. 2006;8:310–316.
2. Sandercock P, Bamford J, Dennis M, et al. Atrial fibrillation and stroke: prevalence in different types of stroke and influence on early and long term prognosis

(Oxfordshire Community Stroke Project). *BMJ* 1992;305: 1460–1465.

3. Mattle HP. Long-term outcome after stroke due to atrial fibrillation. *Cerebrovasc Dis* 2003;16(suppl):3–8.

4. Petersen P. Thromboembolic complications in atrial fibrillation. *Stroke* 1990;21:4–13.

5. American Heart Association. Heart disease and stroke statistics—2004 update. 2004.

6. Shively BK, Gelgand EA, Crawford MH. Regional left atrial stasis during atrial fibrillation and flutter: determinants and relation to stroke. *J Am Coll Cardiol* 1996;27: 1722–1729.

7. Panagiotopoulos K, Toumanidis S, Vemmos K, Saridakis N, Stamatelopoulos S. Secondary prognosis after cardioembolic stroke of atrial origin: the role of left atrial and left atrial appendage dysfunction. *Clin Cardiol* 2003;26:269–274.

8. Cullinane M, Wainwright R, Brown A, Monaghan M, Markus HS. Asymptomatic embolization in subjects with atrial fibrillation not taking anticoagulants: a prospective study. *Stroke* 1998;29:1810–1815.

9. EAFT Study Group. Silent brain infarction in nonrheumatic atrial fibrillation. European Atrial Fibrillation Trial. *Neurology* 1996;46:159–165.

10. van Latum JC, Koudstaal PJ, Venables GS, van Gijn J, Kappelle LJ, Algra A. Predictors of major vascular events in patients with a transient ischemic attack or minor ischemic stroke and with nonrheumatic atrial fibrillation. European Atrial Fibrillation Trial (EAFT) Study Group. *Stroke* 1995;26:801–806.

11. DiPasquale G. Andreoli A, Lusa AM et al. Cardiac complications of subarachnoid hemorrhage. J Neurosurg Sci, 1998;43:33–36

12. Di Pasquale G, Andreoli A, Lusa AM, et al. Cardiologic complications of subarachnoid hemorrhage. *J Neurosurg Sci* 1998;42:33–36.

13. You RX, McNeil JJ, Farish SJ, O'Malley HM, Donnan GA. The influence of age on atrial fibrillation as a risk factor for stroke. *Clin Exp Neurol* 1991;28:37–42.

14. Kannel WB, Wolf PA, Benjamin EJ, Levy D. Prevalence, incidence, prognosis, and predisposing conditions for atrial fibrillation: population-based estimates. *Am J Cardiol* 1998;82:2N-9N.

15. Furberg CD, Psaty BM, Manolio TA, Gardin JM, Smith VE, Rautaharju PM. Prevalence of atrial fibrillation in elderly subjects (the Cardiovascular Health Study). *Am J Cardiol* 1994;74:236–241.

16. Lin HJ, Wolf PA, Benjamin EJ, Belanger AJ, D'Agostino RB. Newly diagnosed atrial fibrillation and acute stroke. The Framingham Study. *Stroke* 1995;26:1527–1530.

17. Kaarisalo MM, Immonen-Raiha P, Marttila RJ, et al. Atrial fibrillation and stroke. Mortality and causes of death after the first acute ischemic stroke. *Stroke* 1997;28:311–315.

18. Healey JS, Connolly SJ. Atrial fibrillation: hypertension as a causative agent, risk factor for complications, and potential therapeutic target. *Am J Cardiol* 2003;91:9G–14G.

19. Presti CF, Hart RG. Thyrotoxicosis, atrial fibrillation, and embolism, revisited. *Am Heart J* 1989;117:976–977.

20. Atrial Fibrillation Investigators. Echocardiographic predictors of stroke in patients with atrial fibrillation: a prospective study of 1066 patients from 3 clinical trials. *Arch Intern Med* 1998;158:1316–1320.

21. The Stroke Prevention in Atrial Fibrillation Investigators Committee on Echocardiography. Transesophageal echocardiographic correlates of thromboembolism in high-risk patients with nonvalvular atrial fibrillation. *Ann Intern Med* 1998;128:639–647.

22. Benjamin EJ, D'Agostino RB, Belanger AJ, Wolf PA, Levy D. Left atrial size and the risk of stroke and death. *Circulation* 1995;92:835–841.

23. Wang TJ, Massaro JM, Levy D, et al. A risk score for predicting stroke or death in individuals with new-onset atrial fibrillation in the community: the Framingham Heart Study. *JAMA* 2003;290:1049–1056.

24. Hart RG, Halperin JL. Atrial fibrillation and thromboembolism: a decade of progress in stroke prevention. *Ann Intern Med* 1999;131:492–501.

25. Hart RG, Palacio S, Pearce LA. Atrial fibrillation, stroke and acute antithrombotic therapy: analysis of randomized clinical trials. *Stroke* 2002;33:2722–2727.

26. Snow V, Weiss KB, LeFevre M, et al. Management of newly detected atrial fibrillation: a clinical practice guideline from the American Academy of Family Physician and the American College of Physicians. *Ann Intern Med* 2003;139:1009–1017.

27. Mehta NN, Greenspon AJ. Atrial fibrillation. Rhythm versus rate control. *Geriatrics* 2003;58:39–44.

28. Weigner MJ, Caulfield TA, Danias PG, Silverman DI, Manning WJ. Risk for clinical thromboembolism associated with conversion to sinus rhythm in patients with atrial fibrillation lasting less than 48 hours. *Ann Intern Med* 1997;126:615–620.

29. McNamara RL, Tamariz LJ, Segal JB, Bass EB. Management of atrial fibrillation: review of the evidence for the role of pharmacologic therapy, electrical cardioversion, and echocardiography. *Ann Intern Med* 2003;139:1018–1033.

30. Zeiler AA, Mick MJ, Mazurer RP, Loop FD, Trohman RG. Role of prophylactic anticoagulation for direct current cardioversion in patients with atrial fibrillation or atrial flutter. *J Am Coll Cardiol* 1992;19:851–855.

31. Gronefeld G, Hohnloser SH. Rhythm or rate control in atrial fibrillation: insights from the randomized controlled trials. *J Cardiovasc Pharmacol Ther* 2003;8:S39–S44.

32. Saxonhouse SJ, Curtis AB. Risks and benefits of rate control versus maintenance of sinus rhythm. *Am J Cardiol* 2003;91:27D–32D.

33. Go AS, Hylek EM, Chang Y, et al. Anticoagulation therapy for stroke prevention in atrial fibrillation. How well do randomized trials translate into clinical practice? *JAMA* 2003;290:2685–2692.

34. Albers GW, Easton JD, Sacco RL, Teal P. Antithrombotic and thrombolytic therapy for ischemic stroke. *Chest* 1998;114:683S–698S.

35. Albers GW. Choice of antithrombotic therapy for stroke prevention in atrial fibrillation. *Arch Intern Med* 1998; 158:1487–1491.

36. Sudlow M, Thomson R, Thwaites B, Rodgers H, Kenny RA. Prevalence of atrial fibrillation and eligibility for anticoagulants in the community. *Lancet* 1998;352: 1167–1171.

37. Brass LM, Krumholz HM, Scinto JD, Mathur D, Radford M. Warfarin use following ischemic stroke among Medicare patients with atrial fibrillation. *Arch Intern Med* 1998;158:2093–2100.

38. Brass LM, Krumholz HM, Scinto JM, Radford M. Warfarin use among patients with atrial fibrillation. *Stroke* 1997; 28:2382–2389.

39. Sievert H, Lesh MD, Trepels T, et al. Percutaneous left atrial appendage transcatheter occlusion to prevent stroke in high-risk patients with atrial fibrillation: early clinical experience. *Circulation* 2002;105:1887–1889.

40. Kowalski M, Hoffman P, Rozanski J, Rydlewska-Sadowska W. Ischemic neurologic event in a child as a result of ventricular septal aneurysm. *J Am Soc Echocardiogr* 1998;11: 1161–1162.

41. Nater B, Bogousslavsky J, Regli J, Stauffer JC. Stroke patterns with atrial septal aneurysm. *Cerebrovasc Dis* 1992;2: 342–346.

42. Mugge A, Daniel WG, Angermann C, et al. Atrial septal aneurysm in adult patients. A multicenter study using transthoracic and transesophageal echocardiography. *Circulation* 1995;91:2785–2792.

43. Mattioli AV, Aquilina M, Oldani A, Longhini C, Mattioli G. Frequency of atrial septal aneurysm in patients with recent stroke: preliminary results from a multicenter study. *Clin Cardiol* 2001;24:297–300.

44. Mattioli AV, Aquilina M, Oldani A, Longhini C, Mattioli G. Atrial septal aneurysm as a cardioembolic source in adult patients with stroke and normal carotid arteries. A multicentre study. *Eur Heart J* 2001;22:261–268.

45. Agmon Y, Khandheria BK, Meissner I, et al. Frequency of atrial septal aneurysms in patients with cerebral ischemic events. *Circulation* 1999;99:1942–1944.

46. Mas JL, Arquizan C, Lamy C, et al. Recurrent cerebrovascular events associated with patent foramen ovale, atrial septal aneurysm, or both. *N Engl J Med* 2001;345:1740–1746.

47. Mattioli AV, Bonetti L, Aquilina M, et al. The association between atrial septal aneurysm and mitral valve prolapse in patients with recent stroke and normal carotid arteries. *Ital Heart J* 2003;4:602–606.

48. Carerj S, Narbone MC, Zito C, et al. Prevalence of atrial septal aneurysm in patients with migraine: an echocardiographic study. *Headache* 2003;43:725–728.

49. Schneider B, Zienkiewicz T, Jansen V, Hofmann T, Noltenius H, Meinertz T. Diagnosis of patent foramen ovale by transesophageal echocardiography and correlation with autopsy findings. *Am J Cardiol* 1996;77:1202–1209.

50. Fisher DC, Fisher EA, Budd JH, Rosen SE, Goldman ME. The incidence of patent foramen ovale in 1,000 consecutive patients. A contrast transesophageal echocardiography study. *Chest* 1995;107:1504–1509.

51. Rodriguez CJ, Homma S. Management of patients with stroke and a patent foramen ovale. *Curr Neurol Neurosci Rep* 2004;4:19–22.

52. Rinaldi CA, Stewart AJ, Blauth CI. Intracardiac thrombus traversing a patent foramen ovale: impending paradoxical embolism demonstrated by transesophageal echocardiography. *Int J Clin Pract* 2002;56:230–231.

53. Isayev Y, Chan RKT, Pullicino PM. "Economy Class" stroke syndrome? *Neurology* 2002;58:960–961.

54. Lethen H, Flachskampf FA, Schneider R, et al. Frequency of deep vein thrombosis in patients with patent foramen ovale and ischemic stroke or transient ischemic attack. *Am J Cardiol* 1997;80:1066–1069.

55. Cramer SC, Rordorf G, Maki JH, et al. Increased pelvic vein thrombi in cryptogenic stroke. Results of the Paradoxical Emboli from Large Veins in Ischemic Stroke (PELVIS) Study. *Stroke* 2004;35:46–50.

56. Kerut EK, Norfleet WT, Plotnick GD, Giles TD. Patent foramen ovale: a review of associated conditions and the impact of physiological size. *J Am Coll Cardiol* 2001;38: 613–623.

57. Serena J, Segura T, Perez-Ayuso MJ, Bassaganyas J, Molins A, Davalos. The need to quantify right-to-left shunt in acute ischemic stroke: a case-control study. *Stroke* 1998;29:1322–1328.

58. Cabanes L, Coste J, Derumeaux G, et al. Interobserver and intraobserver variability in detection of patent foramen ovale and atrial septal aneurysm with transesophageal echocardiography. *J Am Soc Echocardiogr* 2002;15:441–446.

59. Mas JL. Specifics of patent formane ovale. *Adv Neurol* 2003;92:197–202.

60. Arquizan C, Coste J, Touboul PJ, Mas JL. Is patent foramen ovale a family trait? A transcranial Doppler sonographic study. *Stroke* 2001;32:1563–1566.

61. Wahl A, Windecker S, Meier B. Patent foramen ovale: pathophysiology and therapeutic options in symptomatic patients. *Minerva Cardioangiol* 2001;49:403–411.

62. Overell JR, Bone I, Lees KR. Interatrial septal abnormalities and stroke: a meta-analysis of case-control studies. *Neurology* 2000;55:1172–1179.

63. Lewis RR, Hussain A, Rashed KA, Cooke RA, cNabb WR, hambers J. Patent foramen ovale in elderly stroke patients. *Int J Clin Pract* 2001;55:596–598.

64. Jones EF, Calafiore P, Donnan GA, Tonkin AM. Evidence that patent foramen ovale is not a risk factor for cerebral ischemia in the elderly. *Am J Cardiol* 1994;74:596–599.

65. Lamy C, Giannesini C, Zuber M, et al. Clinical and imaging findings in cryptogenic stroke patients with and without patent formamen ovale; the PFO-ASA study. *Stroke* 2002;33:706–711.

66. Sztajzel R, Genoud D, Roth S, Mermillod B, Le Floch-Rohr J. Paten foramen ovale, a possible cause of symptomatic migraine: a study of 74 patients with acute ischemic stroke. *Cerebrovasc Dis* 2002;13:102–106.

67. Bogousslavsky J, Garazi S, Jeanrenaud X, Aebischer N, Van Melle G. Stroke recurrence in patients with patent foramen ovale: the Lausanne Study. Lausanne Stroke with Paradoxal Embolism Study Group. *Neurology* 1996;46:1301–1305.

68. Homma S, Sacco RL, Di Tullio MR, Sciacca RR, Mohr JP. Effect of medical treatment in stroke patients with patent foramen ovale: patent foramen ovale in cryptogenic stroke study. *Circulation* 2002;105:2625–2631.

69. Adams HP, Jr. Patent foramen ovale: paradoxical embolism and paradoxical data. *Mayo Clin Proc* 2004;79:15–20.

70. Nendaz MR, Sarasin FP, Junod AF, Bogousslavsky J. Preventing stroke recurrence in patients with patent foramen ovale: antithrombotic therapy, foramen closure,

or therapeutic abstention? A decision analytic perspective. *Am Heart J* 1998;135:532–541.

71. Ruchat P, Bogousslavsky J, Hurni M, Fischer AP, Jeanrenaud X, von Segesser LK. Systematic surgical closure of patent foramen ovale in selected patients with cerebrovascular events due to paradoxical embolism. Early results of a preliminary study. *Eur J Cardiothorac Surg* 1997;11:824–827.

72. Dearnai JA, Ugurlu BS, Danielson GK, et al. Surgical patent foramen ovale closure for prevention of paradoxical embolism-related cerebrovascular ischemic events. *Circulation* 1999;100:II171–II175.

73. Rodriguez CJ, Di Tullio MR, Sacco RL, Homma S. Intra-atrial thrombus after surgical closure of patent foramen ovale. *J Am Soc Echocardiogr* 2001;14:63–66.

74. Braun MU, Fassbender D, Schoen SP, et al. Transcatheter closure of patent foramen ovale in patients with cerebral ischemia. *J Am Coll Cardiol* 2002;39:2019–2025.

75. Pinto FF, Sousa L, Abreu J, et al. Percutaneous occlusion of patent foramen ovale in patients with paradoxical embolism. *Rev Port Cardiol* 2001;20:747–757.

76. Sievert H, Horvath K, Zadan E, et al. Patent foramen ovale closure in patients with transient ischemia attack/stroke. *J Interv Cardiol* 2001;14:261–266.

77. Horton SC, Bunch TJ. Patent foramen ovale and stroke. *Mayo Clin Proc* 2004;79:79–88.

78. Khositseth A, Cabalka AK, Sweeney JP, et al. Transcatheter amplatzer device closure of atrial septal defect and patent foramen ovale in patients with presumed paradoxical emoblism. *Mayo Clin Proc* 2004;79:35–41.

79. Rosin L. Neurological aspects of patent foramen ovale: in search of the optimal treatment. *J Interv Cardiol* 2001;14: 197–201.

80. Halperin JL, Fuster V. Patent foramen ovale and recurrent stroke: another paradoxical twist. *Circulation* 2002;105: 2580–2582.

81. Coulshed N, Epstein EJ, McKendrick CS, Galloway RW, Walker E. Systemic embolism in mitral valve disease. *Br Heart J* 1970;32:26–34.

82. Aronow WS, Ahn C, Kronzon I, Gutstein H. Risk factors for new thromboembolic stroke in patients > or = 62 years of age with chronic atrial fibrillation. *Am J Cardiol* 1998;82:119–121.

83. Chiang CW, Lo SK, Ko YS, Cheng NJ, Lin PJ, Chang CH. Predictors of systemic embolism in patients with mitral stenosis. A prospective study. *Ann Intern Med* 1998;128: 885–889.

84. Dewar HA, Weightman D. A study of embolism in mitral valve disease and atrial fibrillation. *Br Heart J* 1983;49: 133–140.

85. Adams GF, Merrett JD, Hutchinson WM, Pollock AM. Cerebral embolism and mitral stenosis. Survival with and without anticoagulants. *J Neurol Neurosurg Psychiatry* 1974;37:378–383.

86. Freed LA, Levy D, Levine RA, et al. Prevalence and clinical outcome of mitral-valve prolapse. *N Engl J Med* 1999;341:1–7.

87. Jackson AC, Boughner DR, Barnett HJM. Mitral valve prolapse and cerebral ischemic events in young patients. *Neurology* 1984;34:784–787.

88. Barnett HJM, Boughner DR, Taylor DW, Cooper PE, Kostuk WJ, Nichol PM. Further evidence relating mitral-valve prolapse to cerebral ischemic events. *N Engl J Med* 1980;302:139–144.

89. Petty GW, Orencia AJ, Khandheria BK, Whisnant JP. A population-based study of stroke in the setting of mitral valve prolapse: risk factors and infarct subtype classification. *Mayo Clin Proc* 1994;69:632–634.

90. Gilon D, Buonanno F, Joffe MM, et al. Lack of evidence of an association between mitral-valve prolapse and stroke in young adults. *N Engl J Med* 1999;341:8–13.

91. Savage DD, Garrison RJ, Castelli WP, et al. Prevalence of submitral (annular) calcium and its correlates in a general population-based sample (the Framingham Study). *Am J Cardiol* 1983;51:1375–1378.

92. Fulkerson PK, Beaver BM, Auseon JC, Graber HL. Calcification of the mitral annulus: etiology, clinical associations, complications and therapy. *Am J Med* 1979; 66:967–977.

93. Benjamin EJ, Plehn JF, D'Agostino RB, et al. Mitral annular calcification and the risk of stroke in an elderly cohort. *N Engl J Med* 1992;327:374–379.

94. Adler Y, Koren A, Fink N, et al. Association between mitral annulus calcification and carotid atherosclerotic disease. *Stroke* 1998;29:1833–1837.

95. Boon A, Lodder J, Cheriex E, Kessels F. Risk of stroke in a cohort of 815 patients with calcification of the aortic valve with or without stenosis. *Stroke* 1996;27:847–851.

96. Deklunder G, Roussel M, Lecroart JL, Prat A, Gautier C. Microemboli in cerebral circulation and alteration of cognitive abilities in patients with mechanical prosthetic heart valves. *Stroke* 1998;29:1821–1826.

97. Georgiadis D, Grosset DG, Kelman A, Faichney A, Lees KR. Prevalence and characteristics of intracranial microemboli signals in patients with different types of prosthetic cardiac valves. *Stroke* 1994;25:587–592.

98. Baudet EM, Oca CC, Roques XF, et al. A 5 1/2 year experience with the St. Jude Medical cardiac valve prosthesis. Early and late results of 737 valve replacements in 671 patients. *J Thorac Cardiovasc Surg* 1985;90:137–144.

99. Hutchinson K, Hafeez F, Woods TD, et al. Recurrent ischemic strokes in a patient with Medtronic-Hall prosthetic aortic valve and valve strands. *J Am Soc Echocardiogr* 1998;11:755–757.

100. Keyser DL, Biller J, Coffman TT, Adams HP, Jr. Neurologic complications of late prosthetic valve endocarditis. *Stroke* 1990;21:472–475.

101. Tiede DJ, Nishimura RA, Gastineau DA, et al. Modern management of prosthetic valve anticoagulation. *Mayo Clin Proc* 1998;73:665–680.

102. Cannegieter SC, Rosendal FR, Wintzen AR, van der Meer FJM, Vandenbroucke JP, Briet E. Optimal oral anticoagulant therapy in patients with mechanical heart valves. *N Engl J Med* 1995;333:11–17.

103. Ginsberg JS, Barron WM. Pregnancy and prosthetic heart valves. *Lancet* 1994;344:1170–1172.

104. Cohn LH, Collins JJJ, Rizzo RJ, Adams DH, Couper GS, Aranki SF. Twenty-year follow-up of the Hancock modified orifice porcine aortic valve. *Ann Thorac Surg* 1998; 66:S30–S34.

105. Moinuddeen K, Quin J, Shaw R, et al. Anticoagulation is unnecessary after biological aortic valve replacement. *Circulation* 1998;98:II95–II98.

106. Hasbun R, Vikram HR, Barakat LA, Buenconsejo J, Quagliarello VJ. Complicated left-sided native valve endocarditis in adults. Risk classification for mortality. *JAMA* 2003;289:1933–1940.

107. Anderson DJ, Goldstein LB, Wilkinson WE, et al. Stroke location, characterization, severity, and outcome in mitral vs aortic valve endocarditis. *Neurology* 2003;61:1341–1346.

108. Bitsch A, Nau R, Hilgers RA, Verheggen R, Werner G, Prange HW. Focal neurologic deficits in infective endocarditis and other septic diseases. *Acta Neurol Scand* 1996;94:279–286.

109. Shetty PC, Krasicky GA, Sharma RP, Vemuri BR, Burke MM. Mycotic aneurysms in intravenous drug abusers: the utility of intravenous digital subtraction angiography. *Radiology* 1985;155:319–321.

110. van der Meulen JH, Weststrate W, van Gijn J, Habbema JD. Is cerebral angiography indicated in infective endocarditis? *Stroke* 1992;23:1662–1667.

111. Vikram HR, Buenconsejo J, Hasbun R, Quagliarello VJ. Impact of valve surgery on 6-month mortality in adults with complicated, left-sided native valve endocarditis. A propensity analysis. *JAMA* 2003;290:3207–3214.

112. Schwartzman RJ, Hill JB. Neurologic complications of disseminated intravascular coagulation. *Neurology* 1982;32:791–797.

113. Lopez JA, Ross RS, Fishbein MC, Siegel RJ. Nonbacterial thrombotic endocarditis: a review. *Am Heart J* 1987;113:773–784.

114. Kooiker JC, MacLean JM, Sumi SM. Cerebral embolism, marantic endocarditis, and cancer. *Arch Neurol* 1976;33:260–264.

115. Rogers LR. Cerebrovascular complications in cancer patients. *Neurol Clin* 1991;9:889–899.

116. Rogers LR, Cho ES, Kempin S, Posner JB. Cerebral infarction from non-bacterial thrombotic endocarditis. Clinical and pathological study including the effects of anticoagulation. *Am J Med* 1987;83:746–756.

117. Vassallo R, Remstein ED, Parisi JE, Huston J, Brown RD. Multiple Cerebral Infarctions From Nonbacterial Thrombotic Endocarditis Mimicking Cerebral Vasculitis. *Mayo Clin Proc* 1999;74:798–802.

118. Pinto AN. AIDS and cerebrovascular disease. *Stroke* 1996;27:538–543.

119. Dutt T, Karas MG, Segal AZ, Kizer JR Yield of transesophageal echocardiography for nonbacterial thrombotic endocarditis and other cardiac sources of embolism in cancer patients with cerebral ischemia. Am J Cardiol, 2006;97:894–898

120. Blanchard DG, Ross RS, Dittrich HC. Nonbacterial thrombotic endocarditis. Assessment by transesophageal echocardiography. *Chest* 1992;102:954–956.

121. Edoute Y, Haim N, Rinkevich D, Brenner B, Reisner SA. Cardiac valvular vegetations in cancer patients: a prospective echocardiographic study of 200 patients. *Am J Med* 1997;102:252–258.

122. Galve E, Ordi J, Barquinero J, Evangelista A, Vilardell M, Soler-Soler J. Valvular heart disease in the primary antiphospholipid syndrome. *Ann Intern Med* 1992;116:293–298.

123. Sitzer M, Sohngen D, Siebler M, et al. Cerebral microembolism in patients with Sneddon's syndrome. *Arch Neurol* 1995;52:271–275.

124. Morelli S, Perrone C, Paroli M. Recurrent cerebral infarctions in polyarteritis nodosa with circulating antiphospholipid antibodies and mitral valve disease. *Lupus* 1998;7:51–52.

125. Spencer FA, Gore JM, Yarzebski J, Lessard D, Jackson EA, Goldberg RJ. Trends (1986 to 1999) in the incidence and outcomes of in-hospital stroke complicating acute myocardial infarction (The Worchester Heart Attack Study). *Am J Cardiol* 2003;92:383–388.

126. Tanne D, Goldbourt U, Zion M, Reicher-Reiss H, Kaplinsky E, Behar S. Frequency and prognosis of stroke/TIA among 4808 survivors of acute myocardial infarction. The SPRINT Study Group. *Stroke* 1993;24: 1490–1495.

127. Moore T, Eriksson P, Stegmayr B. Ischemic stroke after acute myocardial infarction. A population-based study. *Stroke* 1997;28:762–767.

128. Moore T, Olofsson B-O, Stegmayr B, Eriksson P. Ischemic Stroke. Impact of a Recent Myocardial Infarction. *Stroke* 1999;30:997–1001.

129. Maggioni AP, Franzosi MG, Santoro E, White H, Van de Werf F, Tognoni. The risk of stroke in patients with acute myocardial infarction after thrombolytic and antithrombotic treatment. Gruppo Italiano per lo Studio della Sopravvivenza nell'Infarto Miocardico II (GISSI-2), and The International Study Group. *N Engl J Med* 1992; 327:1–6.

130. Bodenheimer MM, Sauer D, Shareef B, Brown MW, Fleiss JL, Moss AL. Relation between myocardial infarct location and stroke. *J Am Coll Cardiol* 1994;24:61–66.

131. Vaitkus PT, Barnathan ES. Embolic potential, prevention and management of mural thrombus complicating anterior myocardial infarction: a meta-analysis. *J Am Coll Cardiol* 1993;22:1004–1009.

132. Johannessen KA, Nordrehaug JE, von der L. Left ventricular thrombosis and cerebrovascular accident in acute myocardial infarction. *Br Heart J* 1984;51:553–556.

133. Longstreth WT, Jr., Litwin PE, Weaver WD. Myocardial infarction, thrombolytic therapy, and stroke. A community-based study. The MITI Project Group. *Stroke* 1993;24:587–590.

134. Smith P. Oral anticoagulants are effective long-term after acute myocardial infarction. *J Intern Med* 1999;245:383–387.

135. Anand SS, Yusuf S. Oral anticoagulant therapy in patients with coronary artery disease: a meta-analysis. *JAMA* 1999;282:2058–2067.

136. Lapeyre AC, Steele PM, Kazmier FJ, Chesebro JH, Vlietstra RE, Fuster V. Systemic embolism in chronic left ventricular aneurysm: incidence and the role of anticoagulation. *J Am Coll Cardiol* 1985;6:534–538.

137. Hodgman MT, Pessin MS, Homans DC, et al. Cerebral embolism as the initial manifestation of peripartum cardiomyopathy. *Neurology* 1982;32:668–671.

138. Provenzale JM, VanLandingham K. Cerebral infarction associated with Kearns-Sayre syndrome-related cardiomyopathy. *Neurology* 1996;46:826–828.

139. Karande SC, Kulthe SG, Lahiri KR, Jain MK. Embolic stroke in a child with idiopathic dilated cardiomyopathy. *J Postgrad Med* 1996;42:84–86.

140. Pullicino PM, Halperin JL, Thompson JLP. Stroke in patients with heart failure and reduced left ventricular ejection fraction. *Neurology* 2000;54:288–294.

141. Furlan AJ, Craciun AR, Raju NR, Hart N. Cerebrovascular complications associated with idiopathic hypertrophic subaortic stenosis. *Stroke* 1984;15:282–284.

142. Russell JW, Biller J, Hajduczok ZD, Jones MP, Kerber RE, Adams HP, Jr. Ischemic cerebrovascular complications and risk factors in idiopathic hypertrophic subaortic stenosis. *Stroke* 1991;22:1143–1147.

143. Swartz MF, Lutz CJ, Chandan VS, et al. Atrial myxomas. Pathologic types, tumor location, and presenting symptoms. J Card Surg, 2006;21:435–440.

144. Knepper LE, Biller J, Adams HP, Jr., Bruno A. Neurologic manifestations of atrial myxoma. A 12-year experience and review. *Stroke* 1988;19:1435–1440.

145. Al-Mateen M, Hood M, Trippel D, Insalaco SJ, Otto RK, Vitikainen KJ. Cerebral embolism from atrial myxoma in pediatric patients. *Pediatrics* 2003;112:E162–E167.

146. Damasio H, Seabra-Gomes R, da Silva JP, Damasio AR, Antunes JL. Multiple cerebral aneurysms and cardiac myxoma. *Arch Neurol* 1975;32:269–270.

147. Furuya K, Sasaki T, Yoshimoto Y, Okada Y, Fujimaki T, Kirino T. Histologically verified cerebral aneurysm formation secondary to embolism from cardiac myxoma. Case report. *J Neurosurg* 1995;83:170–173.

148. Suzuki T, Nagai R, Yamazaki T, et al. Rapid growth of intracranial aneurysms secondary to cardiac myxoma. *Neurology* 1994;44:570–571.

149. Brown RD, Jr., Khandheria BK, Edwards WD. Cardiac papillary fibroelastoma: a treatable cause of transient ischemic attack and ischemic stroke detected by transesophageal echocardiography. *Mayo Clin Proc* 1995;70: 863–868.

150. Gowda RM, Khan IA, Nair CK, Mehta NJ, Vasavada BC, Sacchi TJ. Cardiac papillary fibroelastoma: a comprehensive analysis of 72 cases. *Am Heart J* 2003;146:404–410.

151. Di Pasquale G, Ribani M, Andreoli A, Zampa GA, Pinelli G. Cardioembolic stroke in primary oxalosis with cardiac involvement. *Stroke* 1989;20:1403–1406.

152. Chimowitz MI, DeGeorgia MA, Poole RM, Hepner A, Armstrong WM. Left atrial spontaneous echo contrast is highly associated with previous stroke in patients with atrial fibrillation or mitral stenosis. *Stroke* 1993;24: 1015–1019.

153. Karatasakis GT, Gotsis AC, Cokkinos DV. Influence of mitral regurgitation on left atrial thrombus and spontaneous echocardiographic contrast in patients with rheumatic mitral valve disease. *Am J Cardiol* 1995;76: 279–281.

154. Orsinelli DA, Pearson AC. Detection of prosthetic valve strands by transesophageal echocardiography: clinical significance in patients with suspected cardiac source of embolism. *J Am Coll Cardiol* 1995;26:1713–1718.

155. Freedberg RS, Goodkin GM, Perez JL, Tunick PA, Kronzon I. Valve strands are strongly associated with systemic embolization: a transesophageal echocardiographic study. *J Am Coll Cardiol* 1995;26:1709–1712.

156. Roberts JK, Omarali I, Di Tullio MR, Sciacca RR, Sacco RL, Homma S. Valvular strands and cerebral ischemia. Effect of demographics and strand characteristics. *Stroke* 1997;28:2185–2188.

157. Nighoghossian N, Derex L, Loire R, et al. Giant Lambl excrescences. An unusual source of cerebral embolism. *Arch Neurol* 1997;54:41–44.

158. Zahger D, Weiss AT, Anner H, Waksman R. Systemic embolization following thrombolytic therapy for acute myocardial infarction. *Chest* 1990;97:754–756.

159. Gore JM, Granger CB, Simoons ML, et al. Stroke after thrombolysis. Mortality and functional outcomes in the GUSTO-I trial. Global Use of Strategies to Open Occluded Coronary Arteries. *Circulation* 1995;92:2811–2818.

160. Gore JM, Sloan M, Price TR, et al. Intracerebral hemorrhage, cerebral infarction, and subdural hematoma after acute myocardial infarction and thrombolytic therapy in the Thrombolysis in Myocardial Infarction Study. Thrombolysis in Myocardial Infarction, Phase II, pilot and clinical trial. *Circulation* 1991;83:448–459.

161. Uglietta JP, O'Connor CM, Boyko OB, Aldrich H, Massey EW, Heinz ER. CT patterns of intracranial hemorrhage complicating thrombolytic therapy for acute myocardial infarction. *Radiology* 1991;181:555–559.

162. Wolman R, Nussmeier N, Aggarwal A, et al. Cerebral injury after cardiac surgery. *Stroke* 1999;30:514–522.

163. Dawson DM, Fischer EG. Neurologic complications of cardiac catheterization. *Neurology* 1977;27:496–497.

164. Fischer A, Ozbek C, Bay W, Hamann GF. Cerebral microemboli during left heart catheterization. *Am Heart J* 1999;137:162–168.

165. Wijman CA, Kase CS, Jacobs AK, Whitehead RE. Cerebral air embolism as a cause of stroke during cardiac catheterization. *Neurology* 1998;51:318–319.

166. Dimarco JP, Garan H, Ruskin JN. Complications in patients undergoing cardiac electrophysiologic procedures. *Ann Intern Med* 1982;97:490–493.

167. Bladin CF, Bingham L, Grigg L, Yapanis AG, Gerraty R, Davis SM. Transcranial Doppler detection of microemboli during percutaneous transluminal coronary angioplasty. *Stroke* 1998;29:2367–2370.

168. Wong SC, Minutello R, Hong MK. Neurological complications following percutaneous coronary interventions. A report form the 2000-2001 New York State Angioplasty Registry. Am J Cardiol, 2005;96:1248–1250.

169. Omran H, Schmidt H, Hackenbroch M, et al. Silent and apparent cerebral embolism after retrograde catheterisation of the aortic valve in valvular stenosis: a prospective, randomised study. *Lancet* 2003;361:1241–1246.

170. Davidson CJ, Skelton TN, Kisslo KB, et al. The risk for systemic embolization associated with percutaneous balloon valvuloplasty in adults. A prospective comprehensive evaluation. *Ann Intern Med* 1988;108:557–560.

171. Silaruks S, Thinkhamrop B, Kiatchoosakun S, Wongvipaporn C, Tatsanavivat P. Resolution of left atrial thrombus after 6 months of anticoagulation in candidates for percutaneous transvenous mitral commissurotomy. *Ann Intern Med* 2004;140:101–105.

172. Libman RB, Wirkowski E, Neystat M, Barr W, Gelb S, Graver M. Stroke associated with cardiac surgery. Determinants, timing, and stroke subtypes. *Arch Neurol* 1997;54:83–87.

173. Barbut D, Caplan LR. Brain complications of cardiac surgery. *Curr Probl Cardiol* 1997;22:449–480.

174. Barbut D, Grassineau D, Lis E, Heier L, Hartman GS, Isom OW. Posterior distribution of infarcts in strokes related to cardiac operations. *Ann Thorac Surg* 1998;65:1656–1659.

175. Likosky DS, Marrin CAS, Caplan LR, et al. Determination of etiologic mechanisms of strokes secondary to coronary artery bypass graft surgery. *Stroke* 2003;34:2830–2834.

176. Borger MA, Ivanov J, Weisel RD, et al. Decreasing incidence of stroke during valvular surgery. *Circulation* 1998;98:II137–II143.

177. Roach GW, Kanchuger M, Mangano CM, et al. Adverse cerebral outcomes after coronary bypass surgery. Multicenter Study of Perioperative Ischemia Research Group and the Ischemia Research and Education Foundation Investigators. *N Engl J Med* 1996;335:1857–1863.

178. Savageau JA, Stanton BA, Jenkins CD, Frater RW. Neuropsychological dysfunction following elective cardiac operation. II. A six-month reassessment. *J Thorac Cardiovasc Surg* 1982;84:595–600.

179. Savageau JA, Stanton BA, Jenkins CD, Klein MD. Neuropsychological dysfunction following elective cardiac operation. I. Early assessment. *J Thorac Cardiovasc Surg* 1982;84:585–594.

180. Shaw PJ, Bates D, Cartlidge NE, et al. Neuro-ophthalmological complications of coronary artery bypass graft surgery. *Acta Neurol Scand* 1987;76:1–7.

181. Carrascal Y, Guerrero AL, Maroto LC, et al. Neurological complications after cardiopulmonary bypass: an update. *Eur Neurol* 1999;41:128–134.

182. Hogue CWJ, Murphy SF, Schechtman KB, Davila-Roman VG. Risk factors for early or delayed stroke after cardiac surgery. *Circulation* 1999;100:642–647.

183. Borger MA, Fremes SE. Management of patients with concomitant coronary and carotid vascular disease. *Semin Thorac Cardiovasc Surg* 2001;13:192–198.

184. Safa TK, Friedman S, Mehta M, et al. Management of coexisting coronary artery and asymptomatic carotid artery disease: report of a series of patients treated with coronary bypass alone. *Eur J Vasc Endovasc Surg* 1999;17:249–252.

185. Brown KR. Treatment of concomitant carotid and coronary artery disease. Decision-making regarding surgical options. *J Cardiovasc Surg* 2003;44:395–399.

186. Mills NL, Ochsner JL. Massive air embolism during cardiopulmonary bypass. Causes, prevention, and management. *J Thorac Cardiovasc Surg* 1980;80:708–717.

187. Brown WR, Moody DM, Challa VR. Cerebral fat embolism from cardiopulmonary bypass. *J Neuropathol Exp Neurol* 1999;58:109–119.

188. Brooker RF, Brown WR, Moody DM, et al. Cardiotomy suction: a major source of brain lipid emboli during cardiopulmonary bypass. *Ann Thorac Surg* 1998;65:1651–1655.

189. Masuda J, Yutani C, Ogata J, Kuriyama Y, Yamaguchi T. Atheromatous embolism in the brain: a clinicopathologic analysis of 15 autopsy cases. *Neurology* 1994;44:1231–1237.

190. Choudhary SK, Bhan A, Sharma R, et al. Aortic atherosclerosis and perioperative stroke in patients undergoing coronary artery bypass: role of intra-operative transesophageal echocardiography. *Int J Cardiol* 1997;61:31–38.

191. Scarborough JE, White W, Derilus FE, Mathew JP, Newman MF, Landolfo KP. Neurologic outcomes after coronary artery bypass grafting with and without cardiopulmonary bypass. *Semin Thorac Cardiovasc Surg* 2003;15:52–62.

192. Sharony R, Bizekis CS, Kanchuger M, et al. Off-pump coronary artery bypass grafting reduces mortality and stroke in patients with atheromatous aortas: a case control study. *Circulation* 2003;108:II15–II20.

193. Wimmer-Greinecker G, International Council of Emboli Management (ICEM) Study Group. Reduction of neurologic complications by intra-aortic filtration patients undergoing combined intracardiac and CABG procedures. *Eur J Cardiothorac Surg* 2003;23:159–164.

194. Kirkham FJ. Recognition and prevention of neurological complications in pediatric cardiac surgery. *Pediatr Cardiol* 1998;19:331–345.

195. Pua HL, Bissonnette B. Cerebral physiology in paediatric cardiopulmonary bypass. *Can J Anaesth* 1998;45:960–978.

196. Goldstein DJ, Oz MC, Rose EA. Implantable left ventricular assist devices. *N Engl J Med* 1998;339:1522–1533.

197. Schmid C, Weyand M, Nabavi DG, et al. Cerebral and systemic embolization during left ventricular support with the Novacor N100 device. *Ann Thorac Surg* 1998;65:1703–1710.

198. Moazami N, Roberts K, Argenziano M, et al. Asymptomatic microembolism in patients with long-term ventricular assist support. *ASAIO J* 1997;43:177–180.

199. Lazar HL, Bao Y, Rivers S, Treanor PR, Shemin RJ. Decreased incidence of arterial thrombosis using heparin-bonded intraaortic balloons. *Ann Thorac Surg* 1999;67:446–449.

200. Sila CA. Spectrum of neurologic events following cardiac transplantation. *Stroke* 1989;20:1586–1589.

201. Adair JC, Call GK, O'Connell JB, Baringer JR. Cerebrovascular syndromes following cardiac transplantation. *Neurology* 1992;42:819–823.

202. Andrews BT, Hershon JJ, Calanchini P, Avery GJ, II, Hill JD. Neurologic ecomplications of cardiac transplantation. *West J Med* 1991;153:146–148.

203. Patchell RA. Neurological complications of organ transplantation. *Ann Neurol* 1994;36:688–703.

CHAPTER 14

Disorders of Coagulation That Cause Hemorrhagic or Ischemic Stroke

Patients with inherited or acquired diseases that induce thrombosis (prothrombotic or hypercoagulable states) or bleeding (bleeding diatheses) are associated with a high risk of neurological symptoms. Both the brain and the spinal cord can be affected from venous and arterial occlusions or bleeding secondary to the blood disorder. With advances in understanding of the coagulation cascade and its disturbances, the number of coagulation disorders, which might lead to stroke, has increased. Additional inherited or acquired coagulation diseases likely will be identified in the future. In particular, the number of genetic mutations or polymorphisms that are associated with blood diseases leading to cerebral infarction or cerebral hemorrhage likely will grow dramatically.[1,2] Still, the number of strokes secondary to a coagulation disorder is relatively small; most cases are diagnosed in children and young adults.[3,4] Still, in these cohorts, the importance of coagulation disorders is considerable.[5-7] In addition, the likelihood of an underlying coagulation disorder is high among persons with stroke of an otherwise undetermined cause.

The most common hemorrhagic diatheses leading to central nervous system bleeding are antithrombotic or thrombolytic medications, leukemia, thrombocytopenia, disseminated intravascular coagulation (DIC), hemophilia, hypoprothrombinemia, afibrinogenemia, and sickle-cell disease (Table 14-1). A large number of disorders

of the cellular elements or coagulation factors also can induce a hypercoagulable syndrome (prothrombotic state) (Table 14-2). Also, a disorder of coagulation presumably leads to thrombosis or less commonly bleeding among persons with a broad spectrum of serious medical illnesses (Table 14-3).

In general, a disorder of coagulation is suspected in a patient with stroke if there is other evidence of either bleeding or thromboembolism. Coagulation disorders can cause stroke in children, men, and women of all ages and ethnic groups. Because some of these disorders are inherited, a family history of recurrent bleeding or thromboembolism can provide important clues. Other features of the history also provide hints. For example, an intracranial hemorrhage is a consideration whenever a patient develops acute neurological symptoms while taking oral anticoagulants, antiplatelet agents, or thrombolytic agents. Similarly, a bleeding diathesis should be sought if the patient has other evidence of bleeding, including retinal or ocular hemorrhages, petechiae or purpura, or visceral bleeding. A likelihood of a hypercoagulable cause of infarction increases if the patient has recurrent or recent venous, or arterial thromboembolism. In particular, history of recurrent, spontaneous deep vein thrombosis or pulmonary embolism in a young person is an important feature. A female patient also might have a history of recurrent fetal demise and spontaneous abortion. Evidence of simultaneous arterial and venous thrombosis also suggests a prothrombotic disorder. In some patients with coagulation disturbances, evidence of both bleeding and thrombosis will be found. Because of the expense of a large battery of special tests for coagulation disturbances, most patients should not have all of these studies obtained unless there is other evidence of either a bleeding diathesis or a thrombophilia (Table 14-4). On the other hand, almost all patients should have some general screening of the blood and coagulation, including complete blood count, platelet count, prothrombin time, and activated partial thromboplastin time (aPTT) (see Chapter 8). If these tests are normal and if the clinical findings support either a hypercoagulable or bleeding diathesis, additional testing should be ordered.

► HEMORRHAGIC DIATHESES

► DISORDERS OF CELLULAR ELEMENTS

Leukemia

Intracranial bleeding is an important, often terminal, complication of *leukemia* (Table 14-5). The chance of hemorrhage is greatest among persons with either *acute lymphoblastic leukemia* or *acute myeloblastic leukemia* and is most likely during a blastic crisis or when the leukemia is not responding to chemotherapy.[8–12] Bleeding can be the result of secondary thrombocytopenia, hyperviscosity, infections, or DIC. Hemorrhages usually are multifocal and arise in the white matter of the cerebral hemispheres. Bleeding can be restricted to the central nervous system or can be part of multisystem hemorrhages. Intracranial bleeding can be forecasted by the presence of retinal hemorrhages in patients with leukemia.[13]

Primary Eosinophilia Syndrome

Intracranial hemorrhage also is a potential complication of the *primary eosinophilia syndrome.*[14] Other neurological symptoms of hypereosinophilia include an encephalopathy, neuropathy, and recurrent cerebral infarction. Intracranial bleeding is a less common complication of polycythemia than is ischemic stroke; the causes of secondary hemorrhage include vascular distension, impaired platelet activity, or abnormal clot formation.[15,16]

Thrombocytopenia

Thrombocytopenia is the most common cellular disorder associated with a high risk of bleeding. While bleeding usually does not affect inherited disorders of platelets, hemorrhage is an important complication of acquired thrombocytopenia—especially when the platelet count drops below 30,000. Patients with hemorrhages secondary to thrombocytopenia usually have other evidence of multisystem bleeding, including purpura or petechia. A decline in platelet count can be secondary to depression of bone marrow or an increase in the destruction or utilization of the platelets (Table 14-6). Secondary thrombocytopenia can be secondary to leukemia or the administration of chemotherapeutic agents that treat leukemia or other forms of cancer. Intracranial bleeding secondary to thrombocytopenia can complicate aplastic anemia, myelofibrosis, transfusion disorders, acute infections, hypersplenism, DIC, or immune disorders.

Idiopathic Thrombocytopenic Purpura

Idiopathic thrombocytopenic purpura can be associated with intracranial bleeding or fluctuating neurological signs. Most cases of bleeding occur with the first 2 weeks of the onset of illness.[17,18] The other findings are renal insufficiency, a hemolytic anemia, and fever.

Other Platelet Disorders

Intracranial bleeding can complicate *HELLP syndrome* (hemolysis, elevated liver enzymes, and low platelets), which can occur during pregnancy.[19] *Thrombotic thrombocytopenia purpura* (TTP) is more commonly associated with ischemic stroke than with bleeding.

► **TABLE 14-1.** INHERITED OR ACQUIRED HEMORRHAGIC DIATHESES LEADING TO STROKE

Thrombolytic agents
Defibrinogenating agents
Oral anticoagulants
Heparin, low-molecular-weight heparins, heparinoid
Thrombin inhibitors
Platelet glycoprotein IIb/IIIa receptor blockers
Antiplatelet agents
Leukemia
Thrombocytopenia
Afibrinogenemia/hypofibrinogenemia
Hypoprothrombinemia
Hemophilia
Disseminated intravascular coagulation
Hyperviscosity syndromes
Sickle-cell disease

► **TABLE 14-2.** INHERITED OR ACQUIRED HYPERCOAGULABLE DISORDERS LEADING TO STROKE

Polycythemia	Anemia
Sickle-cell disease	Thrombocytosis
Thrombotic thrombocytopenia purpura	Leukemia
Heparin-associated thrombocytopenia	Decreased protein C
Decreased protein S	Antithrombin deficiency
Disseminated intravascular coagulation	Prothrombin G20210A
Deficiency of heparin cofactor II	Deficiency of plasminogen
Antiphospholipid antibody syndrome	Thalassemia
Carbohydrate-deficient glycoprotein	Factor V Leiden
Waldenström macroglobulinemia	

Heparin-associated thrombocytopenia usually is not associated with bleeding complications. Heparin-associated thrombocytopenia usually appears after several days of treatment. However, patients with a previous exposure to heparin can have an early decline in platelets with secondary thrombosis. In the series of Pohl et al.[20,21], 9 percent of patients with heparin-associated thrombocytopenia had neurological complications, including both arterial and venous thrombotic events. Patients with neurological symptoms had a higher risk of death or disability than did those persons who did not have strokes. Patients with intracranial hemorrhage complicating thrombocytopenia are usually treated with transfusions of platelets. Neurosurgical management of the hematoma will require correction of the coagulopathy. Long-term management of patients with autoimmune or idiopathic thrombocytopenia can include plasma exchange, splenectomy, or immunosuppressive agents.

Disseminated Intravascular Coagulation

Subarachnoid or massive intracerebral hemorrhage is a complication of DIC, which can occur in patients with malignancies, AIDS (acquired immmuno deficiency syndrome), severe infections, severe trauma, pregnancy,

► **TABLE 14-3.** DISEASES ASSOCIATED WITH A DISORDER OF COAGULATION THAT MIGHT INDUCE STROKE

Pregnancy and puerperium
Oral contraceptives
Cancer and chemotherapy
Dehydration
Inflammatory bowel disease
Nephrotic syndrome
Hemolytic-uremic syndrome
Sepsis
Inflammation
Trauma
Surgery

shock, renal failure, or hepatic failure[9,22,23] (Table 14-7; Fig. 14-1). While less frequent than ischemic cerebrovascular complications, bleeding is secondary to consumption of clotting factors and platelets. Laboratory findings include thrombocytopenia, hypofibrinogenemia, elevated fibrin-split products and D-dimer, and prolongation of the prothrombin time and aPTT. Treatment involves replacement of the coagulation factors and treatment of the underlying severe illness. Although heparin often is given to a patient with DIC and ischemic symptoms, this therapy is usually withheld if the patient has serious bleeding complications.

Sickle-Cell Disease

While infarction is the most common cerebrovascular event among persons with *sickle-cell disease*, brain hemorrhage is relatively common complication—especially among adolescents and young adults[24–26] (see Chapter 17). A potential relationship may occur between sickle-cell disease and intracranial saccular aneurysms. However, some of the symptoms of a sickle crisis, including severe headache or altered consciousness, can mimic intracranial hemorrhage. Cerebral arteriography can be dangerous because the contrast agent can induce sickling, and magnetic resonance angiography should be performed to screen for an aneurysm. Exchange transfusions to maintain a hemoglobin S level greater than 30 percent should be performed prior to an arteriogram or neurosurgical procedure to treat the hemorrhage.

► **TABLE 14-4.** TESTING FOR HYPERCOAGULABLE STATES

Activated protein C resistance	Clotting assay
Factor V Leiden	Polymerase chain reaction
Prothrombin gene mutation	Polymerase chain reaction
Deficiency of antithrombin	Functional assay
Deficiency of protein C	Functional assay
Deficiency of protein S	Functional assay
Deficiency of plasminogen	Functional assay
Dysfibrinogenemia	Functional assay

▶ **TABLE 14-5.** CEREBROVASCULAR COMPLICATIONS OF LEUKEMIA

Events
  Cerebral infarction
  Cerebral hemorrhage
  Cerebral venous thrombosis
Results from
  Thrombocytopenia
  Hyperviscosity
  Disseminated intravascular coagulation
  Infections
  Side effects from medications
Bleeding can be restricted to nervous system
Most common scenarios
  Blastic crisis
  Disease not responding to therapy

▶ **NONCELLULAR COAGULOPATHIES**

Hyperviscosity Syndromes

Patients with hyperviscosity syndromes secondary to *Waldenström macroglobulinemia* or other dysproteinemias (*multiple myeloma*) can have either subarachnoid hemorrhage or intracerebral hemorrhage. The bleeding might be secondary to vascular congestion, or secondary to abnormalities in platelets or coagulation factors.

Inherited Deficiencies of Coagulation Factors

A subdural hematoma, subarachnoid hemorrhage, or intracerebral hemorrhage is a potentially life-threatening complication of inherited deficiencies of coagulation factors including *classic hemophilia (factor VIII deficiency)*, *Christmas disease (factor IX deficiency)*, or *factor V deficiency*.[27–29] The hemorrhages can be spontaneous or can follow trivial trauma and most events occur during childhood. While most affected patients will have been already diagnosed as having hemophilia, spontaneous intracranial hemorrhage in a child (especially a boy) should prompt consideration of an inherited coagulopathy, particularly if the child has other evidence of bleeding.

▶ **TABLE 14-6.** CAUSES OF THROMBOCYTOPENIA

Leukemia
Aplastic anemia
Myelofibrosis
Hypersplenism
Disseminated intravascular coagulation
Idiopathic thrombocytopenia purpura
Thrombotic thrombocytopenia purpura
Heparin-associated thrombocytopenia
Chemotherapy

▶ **TABLE 14-7.** DISSEMINATED INTRAVASCULAR COAGULATION

Events
  Cerebral infarction
  Cerebral hemorrhage
  Subarachnoid hemorrhage
Associated conditions
  Malignancy
  Severe infection
  AIDS
  Multisystem trauma
  Pregnancy
  Diabetes mellitus
  Renal failure
  Hepatic failure
Laboratory findings
  Thrombocytopenia
  Decreased level of fibrinogen
  Increased level of D-dimer
  Increased levels of fibrin-split products
  Increased prothrombin time
  Increased aPTT

Recurrent episodes of bleeding can occur, and central nervous system hemorrhage is a leading cause of death among children with hemophilia. Treatment involves immediate infusion of the coagulation factor to a goal of 80–100 percent of normal levels. Replacement of the coagulation factors must be done prior to any surgical intervention. Continued replacement of the coagulation factors is needed during postoperative management. A *deficiency of factor XIII* can also cause neonatal hemorrhages (see Chapter 17). *Congenital afibrinogenemia* is a rare cause of severe umbilical, gastrointestinal, cutaneous,

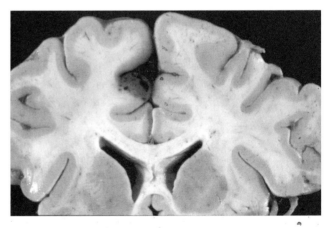

Figure 14-1. Coronal autopsy specimen obtained from a patient dying of promyelocytic leukemia and DIC. A small hemorrhagic infarction is seen in the right parasagittal frontal cortex. (*Courtesy of S.S. Schochet, M.D., Department of Pathology, University of West Virginia, Morgantown, WV*)

nasal, or intracranial bleeding.[30] Brain hemorrhage is a common cause of death.

Congenital factor II deficiency is a potential cause of serious bleeding. *Hypoprothrombinemia* also is a cause of severe neonatal bleeding. Low levels of thrombin can be the result of inadequate transplacental transport of vitamin K or the absence of flora in the infant's gut. Maternal use of anticonvulsants can lead to infantile vitamin K deficiency.[31] Aspirin also can lead to neonatal bleeding. Hypoprothrombinemia in adults can be secondary to malnutrition, malabsorption, or severe liver disease. The latter probably is the most common. A number of medications, other than the oral anticoagulants, also can affect metabolism of vitamin K. Among these medications are the broad-spectrum antibiotics or vitamin E.

Other causes of intracranial bleeding in adults include *deficiencies of factor VII, factor X, factor XII,* or *factor XIII.* Patients with *von Willebrand disease* also can have bleeding, particularly if they have been taking an antiplatelet agent such as aspirin. Hemorrhage also has been described as a complication of uremia or scurvy. While the lupus anticoagulant results in abnormal results on aPTT testing, patients with antiphospholipid antibodies appear not to be associated with a high risk of intracranial bleeding.

▶ MEDICATIONS THAT AFFECT COAGULATION

Hemorrhage into the cranial vault is the most common location for fatal bleeding following administration of a medication that affects coagulation[32] (see Table 14-1; see Chapter 19). The most common sites, in descending order, are the subdural space, the brain, the subarachnoid space, and the epidural space. Intracranial hemorrhage is a feared complication of acutely administered *antithrombotic* or *thrombolytic medications* to treat patients with cerebral infarction, myocardial infarction, or other acute ischemic illnesses. Serious neurological bleeding also is a potentially life-threatening complication of *antiplatelet agents* and *oral anticoagulants* given to patients who are at high risk for ischemic events.[33–37] Acute intraspinal bleeding leading to cord compression or cord dysfunction also is a complication of these medications. Both intracranial and intraspinal bleeding can be spontaneous or be secondary to trauma. The trauma that can induce major bleeding is often relatively trivial and not that which would lead to a major hematoma in a person who is not receiving such medications. Because of the potential for hemorrhagic complications, bleeding should be considered whenever a patient develops new focal neurological impairments while being treated with a medication that affects coagulation. In general, the risk of bleeding is greatest following administration of thrombolytic

agents. Anticoagulants are associated with a higher risk than are antiplatelet agents.

The risk of bleeding with antiplatelet agents is relatively low, and no major difference in the rates of serious hemorrhage has been reported among persons who receive *aspirin, ticlopidine, clopidogrel,* or *dipyridamole.* The use of a combination of aspirin and clopidogrel appears to be associated with an increased risk of bleeding that with either medication prescribed as a monotherapy (see Chapter 19). No relationship between the dose of aspirin and the likelihood of serious intracranial bleeding has been described. The risk of major hemorrhage appears to be increased when an antiplatelet agent is combined with an oral anticoagulant. While hemorrhagic stroke is a complication of aspirin or other antiplatelet agents administered for primary or secondary prevention of ischemic stroke, myocardial infarction, or other ischemic events, the risk is considerably less than the benefit in preventing the ischemic events.

Although some modest increase in serious bleeding is reported, aspirin has been administered with a reasonable degree of safety within the first 48 h following ischemic stroke.[38,39] Administration of aspirin following streptokinase is associated with a marked increase in serious bleeding complications following the use of the thrombolytic agent for treatment of patients with acute ischemic stroke.[40] Although previous treatment with antiplatelet agents is not a contraindication for thrombolytic therapy for treatment of acute ischemic stroke, the medications are not initiated within 24 h of administration of recombinant tissue plasminogen activator (rtPA), primarily because of the risk of serious neurological bleeding.

The *glycoprotein IIb/IIIa receptor blockers,* including abciximab, have been used to manage patients with acute ischemic cardiovascular and cerebrovascular diseases. These medications appear to increase the risk of neurological bleeding complications (see Chapter 19). Several oral glycoprotein IIb/IIIa receptors were tested alone or in combination for long-term management of patients with ischemic vascular disease. Unfortunately, these potent agents were accompanied by a high rate of bleeding complications, including intracranial hemorrhage (see Chapter 19).

Oral anticoagulants are used to prevent cerebral infarction among persons with atrial fibrillation or other high-risk cardiac lesions or hypercoagulable states. In addition, these medications can be used to prevent deep vein thrombosis and pulmonary embolism. While bleeding is the primary complication of oral anticoagulants, the overall risk is low (see Chapter 19). It is not clear whether the anticoagulants are the primary reason for the hemorrhage or whether their presence potentiates bleeding from other causes. The hemorrhage is potentially life threatening and the physician prescribing oral anticoagulants needs to be aware of this complication. The most common sites are in the subdural space or within the brain. Bleeding can occur spontaneously or be secondary to trauma. Intraspinal hemorrhage usually follows trauma and is a potential complication of lumbar puncture (see Chapter 18). The hematoma will often demonstrate enlargement within the first few hours of the initial bleeding.

Hemorrhage can occur at any level of anticoagulation, but avoidance of excessive levels of anticoagulation is the most effective way to prevent serious bleeding complications (see Chapter 19). Prior to the development of the international normalized ratio (INR), many patients received excessive doses of medication because of inconsistencies in laboratory monitoring. In general, the risk of bleeding escalates rapidly when the INR exceeds 3. In addition, concomitant administration of medications or changes in diet can lead to excessive anticoagulation. In order to improve safety, patients need to understand the importance of compliance with the treatment regimen. Because of the high risk of bleeding, patients with poor balance, dementia, or alcohol abuse usually are not treated with oral anticoagulants. The likelihood of hemorrhage is greater among the elderly and those who have had a stroke. One trial testing oral anticoagulants in preventing recurrent stroke, which had a desired INR of 3–4.5, was halted prematurely because of the high risk of fatal intracranial hemorrhagic complications.[41] On the other hand, a second clinical trial, which had a lower desired INR, demonstrated that the medications could be given safely to prevent recurrent ischemic stroke.[42] Intracranial hemorrhage is an indication for immediate reversal of the oral anticoagulants. Discontinuance of the medication alone is not sufficient; patients usually are treated with vitamin K or replacement of clotting factors. The goal is to lower the INR to less than 1.4 before surgical treatment is recommended.

Serious intracranial bleeding can also complicate parenteral administration of *heparin* and other rapidly acting anticoagulants (see Chapter 22). While hemorrhage can complicate either intravenous or subcutaneous treatment, the risks of bleeding appear to be greater with intermittent intravenous injections than with a continuous infusion. Unlike the oral anticoagulants, the risk of bleeding does not appear to be strongly related to the level of anticoagulation.[43] Intracranial bleeding can complicate the use of heparin in treatment of serious medical illnesses such as a recent pulmonary embolism or myocardial infarction. Intracranial hemorrhage is a leading complication of the use of parenteral anticoagulants in treatment of patients with acute ischemic stroke. The chances of bleeding are greatest among persons with multilobar infarctions or major embolic events. The anticoagulant should be discontinued if the patient develops a hemorrhage. A slow infusion of *protamine sulfate* can be given as an antidote to heparin. There are no specific antidotes when hemorrhage occurs secondary to a *low-molecular-weight heparins* or *heparinoid*. Cerebral hemorrhage is a potential complication of treatment with *hirudin* or *argatroban*.

Intracranial hemorrhage is a major complication of thrombolytic agents used to treat patients with acute myocardial infarction, pulmonary embolism, deep vein thrombosis, or peripheral artery disease. Hemorrhage is the leading noncardiac cause of death following thrombolytic therapy for treatment of acute myocardial ischemia. Approximately 0.5–1.1 percent of patients given thrombolytic agents for treatment of nonneurological ischemia will have a complicating brain hemorrhage (see Chapter 22). Most hemorrhages complicating thrombolytic therapy are lobar in location and can be multiple. Symptomatic hemorrhagic transformation is a leading complication of thrombolytic therapy for treating patients with ischemic cerebrovascular disease. Trials of streptokinase were stopped prematurely because of excessively high rates of fatal hemorrhages.[40,44,45] While rtPA is effective in improving outcomes following acute cerebral infarction when administered within 3 h of onset of stroke, symptomatic bleeding complications occur in approximately 6 percent of cases.[46] Hemorrhages are more common among persons with multilobar infarctions and the elderly.[47] Bleeding also occurs when the guidelines for administration of rtPA are not followed. Intracranial hemorrhage also is a complication of intra-arterial administration of thrombolytic agents for treatment of stroke. Bleeding can complicate thrombolytic therapy for treatment of cerebral venous occlusive disease. Newer thrombolytic agents might be associated with a lower risk of intracranial hemorrhage. Hemorrhage complicating thrombolytic agents requires discontinuance of the medication. Replacement of clotting factors may be needed.

▶ HYPERCOAGULABLE STATES

Several studies have reported a broad range in the frequency of hypercoagulable states as a cause of ischemic stroke; rates have ranged from 1 to 25 percent.[5,6] The higher frequency is reported among studies that have focused on the etiologies of stroke in children and young adults. The significance of these percentages is debated because approximately 10–15 percent of the population might have a potential procoagulant abnormality found on evaluation. Most of these persons live their entire life without any symptoms secondary to a thrombophilia. Arterial or venous occlusions have been ascribed to disorders of either cellular elements or coagulation factors that are acquired or inherited. Although specific coagulation disturbances have not been described, stroke complicating pregnancy and several serious diseases is often attributed to a prothrombotic state. With advances in understanding of the biology of thrombosis, the number of hypercoagulable diseases that lead to ischemia likely will grow.

▶ DISORDERS OF CELLULAR ELEMENTS

Polycythemia

An increase in the concentration of red blood cells can increase viscosity and decrease cerebral blood flow.[48] An elevated hematocrit (polycythemia) is recognized as a marker of a high risk for ischemia and a potential cause of stroke.[49,50] In general, a hematocrit exceeding 50 percent is associated with an escalation in the chances of ischemia. Polycythemia can be a component of a *myeloproliferative syndrome, cyanotic congenital heart disease,* or *pulmonary disease.*[51] A tumor that produces *erythropoietin* or administration of *alfa epoetin* also can lead to an elevated hematocrit.[52] Reducing the hematocrit by periodic removal of 500 mL of blood can lower the hematocrit level to approximately 40 percent in order to reduce viscosity and improve blood flow. Radioactive phosphorus is administered to treat myeloproliferative diseases. Hypervolemic hemodilution can be prescribed to lower viscosity and to improve blood flow to treat patients with stroke.

Anemia

A marked reduction of oxygen-carrying capacity secondary to severe anemia (hematocrit < 30 percent) can lead to cerebral ischemia. Anemia can be secondary to blood loss, hemolysis, or suppression of bone marrow function. Rather than stroke, most patients with anemia will have syncope or symptoms of global ischemia. A secondary increase in blood flow can produce a cervical or cranial bruit. *Iron-deficiency anemia* is very prevalent in infants, especially in underdeveloped countries. Severe anemia appears to be a contributing factor for ischemic stroke or venous thrombosis in infants and young children (see Chapter 17).

Sickle-Cell Disease

Sickle-cell disease is most commonly diagnosed among persons of African or Arab descent. It is inherited on an autosomal-recessive basis and is very common in West Africa, where up to 120,000 babies with the disease are born annually. Approximately 8 percent of African Americans have *SA hemoglobinopathy* (*sickle-cell trait*), while *SS hemoglobinopathy* (*sickle-cell disease*) is found in approximately 0.2 percent. Almost 70 percent of the

▶ **TABLE 14-8.** SICKLE-CELL DISEASE—SS HEMOGLOBINOPATHY

Attacks provoked by hypoxia or acidosis
  Increased viscosity
  Arterial occlusion
Symptoms usually appear in childhood
  Pain—joints, limb, chest, back, and abdomen
  Anemia
  Splenic infarction-pneumococcal meningitis
Ischemic stroke in childhood
  Clinical silent strokes
  Cognitive decline
  Seizures
  Moyamoya syndrome
Hemorrhagic stroke in young adults
  Aneurysm

cases of sickle-cell disease in the United States are due to SS hemoglobinopathy (Table 14-8). *SC hemoglobinopathy* and the D-Punjab and D-Arab variants also occur. The abnormal hemoglobin structure causes changes in the red blood cells, which are aggravated by either hypoxia or acidosis. The sickled red cells lead to increased viscosity or arterial occlusion.[53] Children with sickle-cell disease are usually symptomatic at a very young age. Patients with sickle-cell trait often do not have ischemic symptoms until adolescence or young adulthood. Attacks are often provoked by hypoxia.

Clinical manifestations vary considerably among affected individuals. Pain is the most frequent complain and results from venous occlusions leading to ischemia. The pain is located primarily in the limbs in children but older persons also have headache, and chest, back, or abdominal pain. Patients have splenic sequestration leading to anemia. Because of the secondary splenic dysfunction, pneumococcal meningitis can occur. Less common complications include lung disease, cardiomyopathy, avascular necrosis of the femoral head, and delayed growth. The incidence of ischemic stroke among children with sickle-cell disease is estimated as 0.6 per 1000 patient-years (see Chapter 17). A recent report looking at brain and vascular imaging among children with sickle-cell disease found changes of infarction, ischemic damage, or atrophy in 46 percent of cases.[54] Vascular changes involve large and small arteries in a sizable percentage of patients. It is among the leading causes of stroke in childhood.[55] The risk of stroke is high when the concentration of hemoglobin S is greater than 30 percent.[56] Sickle-cell disease is a leading cause of stroke among African-American children. Many patients have clinically silent strokes found on brain imaging.[54,57] Recurrent ischemic strokes lead to neuropsychological impairments.[58] Seizures also occur. Affected persons often have evidence of occlusions of major intracranial arteries, which can be detected by magnetic resonance arteriopathy. Moyamoya syndrome is a potential complication. Using angiography or magnetic resonance angiography, Dobson et al.[59] found the vascular changes of moyamoya in 19 of 44 patients with stroke and sickle-cell disease. Patients with the moyamoya collaterals had a high risk for recurrent ischemic strokes. Positron emission tomography and magnetic resonance imaging can detect areas of hypoperfusion and influence treatment decisions. Transcranial Doppler ultrasonography can detect changes in blood flow that portend a high risk for stroke.[62–65] Changes in blood flow velocities can be used as an indicator for exchange transfusion to lower the concentration of hemoglobin S.[62,63] The utility of recurrent blood transfusions to prevent stroke among persons with sickle-cell disease was examined in another study.[64] While there is evidence that transfusions do lower the risk of ischemic cerebrovascular events, concerns persist about the safety of repeated blood transfusions in this population of children and young adults. Additional research is needed to learn about the long-term usefulness of repeated blood transfusions.

Thrombocytosis

Thrombocytosis is usually diagnosed when the platelet count exceeds 600,000. Occasionally, the platelet count can be greater than 1 million. The incidence of thrombocytosis is very low. Thrombocytosis usually results from myeloproliferative disorders, including *polycythemia, chronic myelogenous leukemia,* or *essential thrombocythemia.*[66] While thrombocytosis can lead to venous or arterial occlusion, the platelets may be dysfunctional in some patients with elevated platelet counts. Abnormal platelet function also can lead to thromboembolic events. *Sticky platelet syndrome* is a potential cause of stroke.[67,68] Ongoing platelet activation, denoted by elevations in platelet factor 4 or beta-thromboglobulin, can also be associated with stroke. The usual management is with antiplatelet agents.[69]

Thrombotic Thrombocytopenia Purpura/Hemolytic-Uremic Syndrome

Purpura, bleeding, hemolysis, fever, renal failure, and neurological symptoms are the hallmarks of the microangiopathy associated with TTP/ hemolytic-uremic syndrome[70,71] (Fig. 14-2). The neurological symptoms include seizures, an encephalopathy, or decreased mental status (Table 14-9). Focal neurological signs usually are not prominent. It can occur in persons of all ages, though a majority of affected persons are women. Brain imaging findings include edema in a pattern that mimics that seen with posterior reversible encephalopathy syndrome.

Endothelial cell dysfunction interacts with the platelets and leads to arterial occlusion.[72] TTP is ascribed

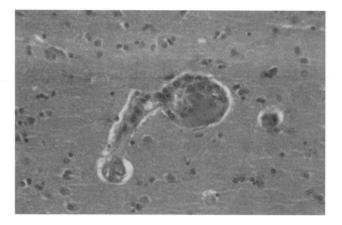

Figure 14-2. Microscopic specimen shows arteriolar occlusions in a patient dying of TTP. (*Courtesy of S.S. Schochet, M.D., Department of Pathology, University of West Virginia, Morgantown, WV*)

to an autoimmune process, and antibodies to von Willebrand metalloproteinase may lead to increased circulating von Willebrand factor proteins, which in turn leads to platelet aggregation.[73,74] TTP is associated with systemic lupus erythematosus (SLE), pregnancy, AIDS, transplantation, and infection. A potential relationship with antiphospholipid antibodies has been speculated.

TTP is also a complication of the antiplatelet agents, ticlopidine or clopidogrel. *Ticlopidine-associated TTP* has been described in approximately 0.02–0.5 percent of patients who are treated with the medication[75,76] (see Chapter 19). The complication, which appears to be an idiosyncratic autoimmune reaction, usually appears

▶ **TABLE 14-9.** THROMBOTIC THROMBOCYTOPENIA PURPURA— HEMOLYTIC-UREMIC SYNDROME

Autoimmune illness—antibody to von Willebrand metalloproteinases
Neurological symptoms
Seizures
Encephalopathy
Decreased consciousness
Associated diseases
Systemic lupus erythematosus
Pregnancy
AIDS
Transplant
Complication of ticlopidine or clopidogrel
Laboratory findings
Thrombocytopenia
Hemolytic anemia
Renal dysfunction
Brain imaging (posterior reversible encephalopathy syndrome)

during the first 3–4 months of treatment. Approximately 80 percent of the events occur within 1 month of treatment. The risk of TTP is sufficiently high and so the patients treated with ticlopidine should have platelet counts checked regularly. Clopidogrel is associated with a lower risk of TTP than is ticlopidine.[77]

TTP is a potentially fatal disease; approximately 50 percent of patients die without treatment. Therapeutic options include aspirin, corticosteroids, vincristine, and plasma exchange. Some patients need several plasma exchanges. Some patients with medication-associated TTP have had recurrent episodes that mandate repeated courses of treatment. TTP also has been treated successfully with cyclophosphamide and rituximab.[78]

Heparin-Associated Thrombocytopenia

Approximately 40 percent of patients treated with heparin will develop a decline in platelet count (<100,000)[79] (Table 14-10; see Chapter 22). In most cases, these declines are asymptomatic. However, heparin also induces elevations of IgG and IgM antibodies that can lead to a severe autoimmune thrombocytopenia.[80–82] The dosage, duration, and route of administration of heparin are not predictive of the development of this hematological complication. In general, the severe autoimmune thrombocytopenias do not appear within the first week of treatment with heparin.[83] However, prior administration of heparin might sensitize a patient, and the autoimmune reaction can occur with hours of starting treatment with heparin. The risk of a similar autoimmune reaction is less with low-molecular-weight heparin or heparinoids than with unfractionated heparin. Because of the potential risk of thrombocytopenia, physicians prescribing heparin should monitor the platelet count every 2–3 days during treatment. A decline in the platelet count to less than

▶ **TABLE 14-10.** HEPARIN-ASSOCIATED THROMBOCYTOPENIA

IgG or IgM antibodies
  Usually >1 week of treatment
  Prior heparin sensitization
  Platelet count <50,000
Risk
  Unfractionated heparin > low-molecular-weight heparin
  Occur with either subcutaneous or intravenous therapy
Neurological findings
  Seizures
  Encephalopathy
  Cerebral infarction
Other findings—white clot syndrome
  Deep vein thrombosis
  Myocardial infarction
  Limb ischemia

100,000 is concerning. A level less than 50,000 should prompt discontinuance of the medication.

The autoimmune thrombocytopenia can lead to arterial occlusion, which results in myocardial or cerebral ischemia. Neurological symptoms often mimic those seen among persons with TTP.[20,21,81] Venous thrombosis, myocardial infarction, and limb ischemia can also be found. Heparin-associated thrombocytopenia can lead to arterial occlusion following a vascular operation or endovascular procedure.[84,85] Treatment involves discontinuance of the heparin. Because of the potential for cross-reactivity between low-molecular-weight heparins and unfractionated heparin, the former medications are not a therapeutic alternative. Low-molecular-weight heparinoid and argatroban can be prescribed.[86–88]

Leukemia

An increase in the number of white blood cells or in their functional activity can lead to thromboembolism. Stroke is a potential complication of acute leukemia, especially in children[89] (see Table 14-4). Stroke is an uncommon complication of leukemia in adults. The marked leukocytosis is associated with increased viscosity, and it impairs blood flow. *Acute lymphoblastic leukemia* has been associated with thrombosis and *acute promyelocytic leukemia* can be associated with DIC. Stroke is a complication of the *hypereosinophilia syndrome*, a neoplastic proliferation of eosinophils, which can induce a microangiopathy and a multifocal ischemic encephalopathy.[14] Venous thrombosis has been attributed to *L-asparaginase*, which is often used to treat children with leukemia.[90]

▶ PROTHROMBOTIC DISORDERS OF CLOTTING PROTEINS

The inherited causes of thrombosis have gained importance with the discovery of factor V Leiden and the prothrombin gene mutation.[91,92] Most of these disorders are primarily associated with venous thrombosis. Patients with congenital deficiencies of protein C, protein S, and antithrombin usually have symptoms prior to the age of 60. Patients with the other disorders usually become symptomatic at older ages.[91]

Decreased Protein C Activity

Protein C is a natural anticoagulant that inhibits the actions of activated factors V and VIII.[93] An inherited deficiency of protein C has been reported.[94,95] The frequency of protein C deficiency is estimated as 0.2 percent of the general population and approximately 2.5–6 percent of persons with venous thrombosis[91] (Table 14-11). Ethnic differences in levels of protein C have been described,

▶ **TABLE 14-11.** PROTEIN C DEFICIENCY

Inherited deficiency
    Heterozygous—low levels
    Homozygous—neonatal purpura fulminans
Acquired deficiency
    Hepatic disease
    Nephrotic syndrome
    Protein-losing enteropathy
    Malignancy
    Disseminated intravascular coagulopathy
    Infectious disease
Transient decline in levels
    Acute cerebral infarction
    Acute myocardial infarction
    Other acute ischemic events
Medication-induced declines
    Oral anticoagulants (warfarin-induced skin necrosis)

with lower levels of the antithrombotic factor found in healthy persons of African ancestry than in other racial groups. A homozygous deficiency of protein C can cause *neonatal purpura fulminans*. It produces diffuse venous thrombosis in infancy, which usually results in death[91] (see Chapter 17). Affected children need to receive protein C as soon as possible. Most cases of deficiency of protein C are secondary liver disease, malignancy, infectious disease, DIC, nephrotic syndrome, or organ failure.[96] The concentration of protein C also drops following acute ischemic event, including stroke. Administration of warfarin also can be associated with a transient decline in protein C levels. Secondary digital ischemia, *warfarin-induced skin necrosis*, usually occurs when the anticoagulant is prescribed to a patient with a preexisting deficiency of protein C. Venous thrombosis, including cerebral venous thrombosis, is the most common vascular occlusive complication of protein C deficiency. A few children and young adults probably have cerebral infarction secondary to protein C deficiency. Protein C deficiency is not a common cause of stroke in middle-aged adults or the elderly.

Protein S Deficiency

A deficiency of protein S is a relatively uncommon cause of ischemic stroke among children or young adults. The frequency of protein S deficiency is not known.[91] Protein S deficiency is not an important cause of stroke in middle-aged adults or the elderly. It can result from an inherited disturbance or be acquired in situations such as a protein-losing enteropathy or nephrotic syndrome.[97] Disturbances of both antigenic and functional protein S can be found. In general, the causes of protein S deficiency are similar to those that induce protein C deficiency. A decline in protein S concentration can be secondary to venous or arterial thrombosis. In addition, the administration of warfarin also can lower protein S levels.

Antithrombin Deficiency

Decreased antithrombin (antithrombin III) activity results from an acquired deficiency or an inherited abnormality in the development of the polypeptide. Both reduced antigenic and functional antithrombin deficiencies have been described. For example, the level of antithrombin can drop following a stroke. The inherited deficiency appears to be more common. The frequency of antithrombin deficiency is low—approximately 0.2 percent of the general population and 0.5–7.5 percent of the persons with venous thromboembolism.[91] Overall, the risk of thrombosis is higher than that seen with other inherited or acquired hypercoagulable disorders. Persons with a heterozygous deficiency have a high risk of venous occlusions, while both arterial and venous thromboses have been described among persons with a homozygous deficiency. Antithrombin deficiency as a potential explanation for ischemic cerebrovascular events in children, and a few young adults have been described. Antithrombin deficiency appears not to be an important cause of stroke in persons older than 45.

Factor V Leiden

A1691 G-A point mutation (Arg 506Glu) in the nucleotides in the factor V gene can lead to resistance to the inactivation of factor V by activated protein C (factor V Leiden).[98,99] A homozygous state, which is rare, leads to a profound coagulopathy that causes multiple arterial thromboses in infancy and childhood. The heterozygous gene mutation can be found in approximately 5 percent of Americans of European ancestry, and as such it appears to be the most common inherited coagulopathy in the United States.[100,101] This genetic defect is rare among populations of Asian or African ancestry. It is an important cause of both venous and arterial occlusions, especially in young adults. Ruggeri et al.[102] reported that factor V Leiden was found in approximately 5 percent of patients with venous thromboembolism and that the risk for recurrent thromboembolic events was higher among patients with the gene mutation. Its presence increases the risk of venous thromboembolism by a factor of 3–6.[100] Factor V Leiden can promote venous thrombosis, which in turn serves as a source for paradoxical embolism in a patient with a patent foramen ovale.[103] Kartunnen et al.[103] concluded that factor V Leiden was an important contributing factor in otherwise cryptogenic stroke. While factor V Leiden is most commonly diagnosed among young adults with stroke, it has been implicated as a contributing cause for myocardial infarction and cerebral infarction in older persons.[98,101] A potential relationship between factor V Leiden and migraine has also been proposed. The use of oral contraceptives might increase resistance to protein C, and the medication might increase the risk of venous thrombosis among women with factor V Leiden.[100,104] A possible relationship with high homocysteine levels or thalassemia has also been speculated. A syndrome that includes recurrent stroke, cutis marmorata, telangiectasia, and factor V Leiden has been described.[105]

Genetic testing for factor V Leiden is available commercially. The study should be performed if a possible hypercoagulable state for stroke is entertained. Because the genetic test is not affected by a recent thromboembolic event, the assessment for factor V Leiden can be done soon after the stroke. Oral anticoagulants usually are given to lower the risk of recurrent arterial or venous thromboembolic events, although no trials have tested the utility of these medications. However, Baglin et al.[106] concluded that anticoagulants should be reserved for treatment of those patients with factor V Leiden who have recurrent thromboembolic events.

Prothrombin G20210A Mutation

A hypercoagulable state, which is associated with increased concentrations of thrombin, prothrombin, thrombin–antithrombin complex, and prothrombin fragment 1 + 2, can occur with the genetic prothrombin G20210A mutation.[107,108] This genetic abnormality is relatively common among persons of European ancestry and relatively rare among persons of Asian or African heritage. While the risk of thrombotic complications is greatest among persons with a homozygous defect, persons with a heterozygous state probably have some risk of ischemic events.[109] The data about the associated risk of arterial thrombosis are less than that seen for venous occlusive events. Secondary venous thrombosis in a patient with a patent foramen ovale could lead to paradoxical embolization.[103] Cases of myocardial infarction and stroke have been reported, although some epidemiological studies have not been able to confirm a relationship. While uncertainty remains about the significance of the prothrombin G20210A mutation, it appears that it is the second most important inherited hypercoagulable disorder.[110] The risk might be less than that seen with factor V Leiden. Anticoagulants usually are recommended for long-term prophylaxis in patients with the prothrombin G20210A mutation, but no clinical trials are available to support this treatment approach.

Hyperfibrinogenemia

Hyperfibrinogenemia is associated with an increased risk of myocardial infarction and ischemic stroke. The relative risk of ischemic events increases by a factor of 1.78 when the concentration of fibrinogen exceeds 3.6 g/L.[111,112] While modest elevations of fibrinogen are detected in a sizable number of patients, cases of true hyperfibrinogenemia seem to be relatively rare. The elevation of fibrinogen leads to an increase in viscosity and a decline in cerebral blood flow. The hyperfibrinogenemia may also stimulate formation of thrombi. Men, the elderly, African Americans, and persons with peripheral vascular disease have higher fibrinogen concentrations than do other groups in the population. Inactivity, a recent infectious illness, smoking, and the use of oral contraceptives also appear to be associated with an elevation of fibrinogen levels.[113] Volume expansion, plasma exchange, and removal of one or more units of blood are potential therapies for lowering the fibrinogen level.

Paraproteinemias

Increases in immune globulins can lead to increases in blood viscosity, decreases in blood flow, and a heightened risk of arterial occlusions.[114,115] The risk seems to be greatest for patients with *Waldenström macroglobulinemia*, which leads to high levels of IgM. Stroke also is a potential complication of *cryoglobulinemia*.

► ANTIPHOSPHOLIPID ANTIBODIES

The potential role of antiphospholipid antibodies in the pathogenesis of venous or arterial occlusion has received considerable attention (Table 14-12). The presence of

► **TABLE 14-12.** FEATURES OF ANTIPHOSPHOLIPID ANTIBODY SYNDROME

Recurrent arterial or venous thrombosis
Myocardial infarction
Deep vein thrombosis—pulmonary embolism
Peripheral artery thrombosis
Fetal demise—spontaneous abortion
Cerebral infarction
Cerebral venous thrombosis
Other neurological findings
Migraine
Cognitive decline
Seizures
Movement disorders
Acute neuropathy
Acute myelopathy
Sensorineural hearing loss
Associated conditions
Systemic lupus erythematosus—lupus anticoagulant
Arthritis
Thrombocytopenia
Neutropenia
Sneddon syndrome
Livedo reticularis
Digital ischemia and pain
Recurrent stroke
Libman–Sacks endocarditis

these antibodies appears to be the most common type of acquired thrombophilia leading to stroke. Abnormal IgG or IgM antiphospholipid antibodies may be a potential cause of stroke in children, young adults, or older persons. Men and women of all ethnic groups can be affected, although a recent large study from Europe found that women are more commonly affected.[116] The thrombogenic mechanism of these antibodies has not been established, but it appears to relate to the presence of cardiolipins in endothelial cells. These antibodies might also affect concentrations or activity of protein C, fibrinogen, factor VII, or factor VIII.[117,118] Antibodies to cardiolipin, prothrombin, or phosphatidylinositol have been found in patients with ischemic stroke.[119] At present, a correlation between the level of antibodies and the risk of thromboembolic events has not been made. The risk of ischemic events seems to be higher among patients with IgG antibodies than it is among those with elevated levels of IgM antibodies.[120] Changes in levels of the antibodies have not been associated with the development of ischemic neurological symptoms.[121] Increased IgG titers of anticardiolipin antibodies are not associated with the occurrence of cerebrovascular events in children.[122]

Although the relationship is not uniform, the presence of the *lupus anticoagulant* is associated with antiphospholipid antibodies.[123–125] Although the lupus anticoagulant is associated with a prolongation of the aPTT, this laboratory finding does not predict bleeding. Rather, patients with the lupus anticoagulant also have an increased risk of ischemic events. The addition of normal plasma to the patient's specimen usually reverses the aPTT. In addition, confirmatory tests include the dilute Russel pit viper time or kaolin clotting time.[126] Some patients will have the lupus anticoagulant with or without the presence of the antiphospholipid antibodies. As the name implies, a sizable percentage of patients with antiphospholipid antibodies and lupus anticoagulant also have other findings consistent with SLE. Approximately one-third of patients with antiphospholipid antibody syndrome will have other evidence of SLE.[125,127] Another 5 percent will have a lupuslike illness, while approximately one-half will have *primary antiphospholipid antibody syndrome*.[116] The mechanism of stroke in most patients with SLE probably involves the presence of antiphospholipid antibodies. In addition, a falsely positive test for syphilis can be detected among persons with antiphospholipid antibodies.[128]

A fairly stereotyped clinical syndrome has been described in patients with antiphospholipid antibodies. Affected persons often have recurrent arterial or venous thrombotic occlusions, leading to deep vein thrombosis, pulmonary embolism, myocardial infarction, or stroke.[129] Both arterial and venous cerebrovascular events can occur.[130] The risk of stroke appears greater among persons who develop antibodies after the age of 50.[116] Men

appear to have an increased risk of myocardial infarction, seizures, and peripheral arterial thrombosis, while affected women have a higher risk for arthritis, livedo reticularis, and migraine. Affected women who become pregnant have a high risk for fetal demise.[131,132] Thus, many women report recurrent spontaneous abortion. Besides stroke, other neurological symptoms include migraine, chorea, seizures, cognitive, multiple sclerosis-like disease, Guillain–Barré syndrome, sensorineural hearing loss, behavioral changes, or transverse myelitis.[133] Children with elevated antiphospholipid can have migraine, pseudotumor cerebri, hemichorea, or hemidystonia.[134] Patients with antiphospholipid antibodies and SLE often have arthritis, livedo reticularis, leukopenia, and thrombocytopenia. Patients with antiphospholipid antibodies can have vegetations on cardiac valves (*Libman–Sacks endocarditis*) that embolized to occlude major intracranial arteries.[135] Antiphospholipid antibodies also are associated with *Sneddon syndrome*, which presents with recurrent ischemic stroke, digital ischemia, and prominent livedo reticularis that also involves the trunk.[136–138] Sneddon syndrome also can occur without the presence of antiphospholipid antibodies.[138] Sneddon syndrome has been described as a cause of cognitive decline in young adults.[139,140]

Because of the perceived high risk for recurrent thromboembolic events, oral anticoagulants are usually prescribed on a long-term basis.[125,141,142] In general, the desired level of INR exceeds 3. A recent trial compared aspirin to a lower level of anticoagulation, and no major differences in recurrences were noted.[143] This trial did not find a disparity in responses among patients who had elevated antiphospholipid antibodies, the presence of lupus anticoagulant, or the both. While this trial did not test the higher level of INR, it did raise doubts about the utility of anticoagulants among persons with antiphospholipid antibodies. Additional research is needed to determine the best long-term therapy. Possible alternatives to anticoagulants include antiplatelet agents or immunosuppressive medications. No information is available about the utility of immunosuppressive therapy in treatment of patients with antiphospholipid antibodies.

▶ DISSEMINATED INTRAVASCULAR COAGULATION

While DIC is associated with the potential risk for serious bleeding including intracranial hemorrhage, most patients have ischemic symptoms from occlusion of multiple small or large arteries and veins.[23] Clinical findings include mental status changes and multifocal neurological impairments. Large-artery occlusions can be secondary to cardioembolism with *nonbacterial thrombotic endocarditis*, which is associated with the coagulation disorders that highlight DIC.[144,145] The laboratory findings were described previously. The prognosis of patients with DIC is very poor, in part because of the severe nature of the underlying disease. In the absence of bleeding, heparin is often prescribed in an effort to slow the consumption of the platelets and clotting factors.

► OTHER PROTHROMBOTIC DISTURBANCES

Rare cases of stroke have been ascribed to other inherited and acquired disturbances of coagulation factors. Because of the uncommon nature of these conditions, screening for these disorders is not indicated during the evaluation of most persons with ischemic cerebrovascular disease, including children. A *deficiency of heparin cofactor II* has been described as a cause of stroke.[91] Abnormalities in or low levels of *plasminogen* have been associated with venous or arterial occlusions, including stroke, in young adults or children.[146] Thromboembolism has been a complication of *beta-thalassemia, thalassemia major,* or *thalassemia intermedia.* Seizures, hypotonia, bleeding, and thrombotic strokelike events have been reported as part of the autosomal-recessive-inherited *carbohydrate-deficient glycoprotein syndrome.*[147] The hemorrhagic and ischemic events are secondary to abnormalities in either prothrombotic or antithrombotic glycoproteins. Abnormally high or low levels in *plasminogen activator inhibitor* have been associated with the promotion of atherosclerosis or thromboembolism.[148] Elevated *tissue plasminogen activator antigen* also is a potential contributing factor for stroke in young adults.[149,150] Stroke is also a potential complication of an inherited *abnormality in factor XII.* Increased levels of coagulation *factors VIII, IX,* or *XI* also can be complicated by thrombosis.[91] Abnormalities in levels of *fibrinopeptide A, von Willebrand factor,* D-*dimer, factor V activity, prekallikreins,* or *prothrombin fragment 1.2* also are described in some patients with ischemic strokes.[151]

► HYPERCOAGULABILITY SECONDARY TO OTHER CONDITIONS OR DISEASES

Arterial or venous thromboembolism of the brain is a potential complication of *pregnancy*[152] (see Table 14-3). The highest risk period for these vascular events, which are often ascribed to a disturbance in clotting factors, is during the *puerperium* (see Chapter 17). Some of the perceived high risk of ischemic stroke among women taking *oral contraceptives* or *postmenopausal* use of *estrogen* medications may be secondary to medication-induced changes in coagulation.[153] *Dehydration,* complicating surgery, infectious diseases, malignancy, multisystem diseases, or decreased fluid intake can cause increased viscosity and increases in levels of blood clotting factors, which in turn promote ischemic stroke. In addition, severe infections can lead to cause stroke secondary to reductions in protein C, protein S, or antithrombin. A hypercoagulable state has been described among persons with *AIDS, paroxysmal nocturnal hemoglobinuria, acute respiratory distress syndrome, prolonged hyperglycemia, heart failure, liver disease, prolonged bed rest, burns, multisystem trauma, surgery,* use of *anabolic steroids,* or *alcohol* consumption.[154–159] Ischemic stroke is a potential complication of *ulcerative colitis* or *regional enteritis.*[160] Both of these inflammatory bowel diseases can cause a reduction in protein C or protein S levels, increased fibrinogen, thrombocytosis, and increased thrombomodulin. A deficiency of factor VII has also been described.[161] Some relationship between inflammatory bowel disease and antiphospholipid antibodies has also been reported. Stroke is a potential complication among persons with *nephritic syndrome.*[162] The proteinuria leads to reduction in concentrations of protein C and protein S, which leads to hypercoagulability.

REFERENCES

1. Petrovic D, Milanez T, Kobal J, Bregar D, Potisk KP, Peterlin B. Prothrombotic gene polymorphisms and atherothrombotic cerebral infarction. *Acta Neurol Scand* 2003;108:109–113.
2. Voetsch B, Loscalzo J. Genetic determinants of arterial thrombosis. *Arterioscler Thromb Vasc Biol* 2003;24:216–229.
3. Habel RL, Biniasch O, Ott M, Peinemann A, Wick M, Kempter B. Infrequency of stroke caused by specific coagulation disorders. *Cerebrovasc Dis* 1995;5:391–396.
4. Pilarska E, Lemka M, Bakowska A. Prothrombotic risk factors in ischemic stroke and migraine in children. *Acta Neurol Scand* 2006;114:13–16.
5. Barinagarrementeria F, Cantu-Brito C, De La Pena A, Izaguirre R. Prothrombotic states in young people with idiopathic stroke. A prospective study. *Stroke* 1994;25:287–290.
6. Gobel U. Inherited or acquired disorders of blood coagulation in children with neurovascular complications. *Neuropediatrics* 1994;25:4–7.
7. Bonduel M, Sciuccati G, Hepner M, Torres AF, Pieroni G, Frontroth JP. Prethrombotic disorders in children with arterial ischemic stroke and sinovenous thrombosis. *Arch Neurol* 1999;56:967–971.
8. Gore RM, Weinberg PE, Anandappa E, Shkolnik A, White H. Intracranial complications of pediatric hematologic disorders: computed tomographic assessment. *Invest Radiol* 1981;16:175–180.
9. Graus F, Rogers LR, Posner JB. Cerebrovascular complications in patients with cancer. *Medicine* 1985;64:16–35.

10. Groch SN, Sayre GP, Heck FJ. Cerebral hemorrhage in leukemia. *Arch Neurol* 1960;2:439–451.

11. Pochedly C. Neurologic manifestations in acute leukemias. I. Symptoms due to increased cerebrospinal fluiod pressure and hemorrhage. *N Y State J Med* 1975;75:575–580.

12. Gralnich HR, Abrell E. Studies on the procoagulant and fibrinolytic activity of promyelocytes in acute promyelocytic leukemia. *Br J Haematol* 1973;24:89–99.

13. Jackson N, Reddy SC, Harun MH, Quah SH, Low HC. Macular haemorrhage in adult acute leukaemia patients at presentation and the risk of subsequent intracranial haemorrhage. *Br J Haematol* 1997;98:204–209.

14. Rothenberg ME. Eosinophilia. *N Engl J Med* 1998;338:1592–1600.

15. Wasserman LR, Gilbert HS. Complications of polycythemia vera. *Semin Hematol* 1986;3:199–208.

16. Silverstein A, Gilbert H, Wasserman LR. Neurologic complications of polycythemia. *Ann Emerg* 1962;57:909–915.

17. Medeiros D, Buchanan GR. Major hemorrhage in children with idiopathic thrombocytopenic purpura: immediate response to therapy and long-term outcome. *J Pediatr* 1998;133:334–339.

18. Cohen YC, Djulbegovic B, Shamai-Lubovitz O, Mozes B. The bleeding risk and natural history of idiopathic thrombocytopenic purpura in patients with persistent low platelet counts. *Arch Intern Med* 2000;160:1630–1638.

19. Isles C, Norrie J, Paterson J, Ritchie L. Risk of major gastrointestinal bleeding with aspirin. *Lancet* 1999;353:148–150.

20. Pohl C, Klockgether T, Greinacher A, Hanfland P, Harbrecht U. Neurological complications in heparin-induced thrombocytopenia. *Lancet* 1999;353:1678–1679.

21. Pohl C, Harbrecht U, Greinacher A, et al. Neurologic complications in immune-mediated heparin-induced thrombocytopenia. *Neurology* 2000;54:1240–1245.

22. Collins RC, Al-Mondhiry H, Chernik NL, Posner JB. Neurologic manifestations of intravascular coagulation in patients with cancer. A clinicopathologic analysis of 12 cases. *Neurology* 1975;25:795–806.

23. Schwartzman RJ, Hill JB. Neurologic complications of disseminated intravascular coagulation. *Neurology* 1982;32:791–797.

24. Batjer HH, Adamson TE, Bowman GW. Sickle cell disease and aneurysmal subarachnoid hemorrhage. *Surg Neurol* 1991;36:145–149.

25. Preul MC, Cendes F, Just N, Mohr G. Intracranial aneurysms and sickle cell anemia: multiplicity and propensity for the vertebrobasilar territory. *Neurosurgery* 1998;42:971–977.

26. Oyesiku NM, Barrow DL, Eckman JR, et al. Intracranial aneurysms in sickle-cell anemia: clinical features and pathogenesis. *J Neurosurg* 1991;75:356–363.

27. Alaani WS, Awidi AS. Spontaneous intracranial bleeding in hemorrhagic diathesis. *Surg Neurol* 1982;17:137–140.

28. Papa ML, Schisano G, Franco A, et al. Congenital deficiency of factor VII in subarachnoid hemorrhage. *Stroke* 1994;25:508–510.

29. Cahill MR, Colvin BT. Haemophilia. *Postgrad Med J* 1997;73:201–206.

30. Henselmans J, Meijer K, Haaxma R, Hew J, van der Meer J. Recurrent spontaneous intracerebral hemorrhage in a congenitally afibrinogenemic patient: diagnostic pitfalls and therapeutic options. *Stroke* 1999;30:2479–2482.

31. Sutherland J, Glucek H, Gleser G. Hemorrhagic disease of the newborn: breast feeding is a necessary factor in the pathogenesis. *Am J Dis Child* 1967;113:524–533.

32. Levine MN, Raskob G, Landefeld S, Kearon C. Hemorrhagic complications of anticoagulant treatment. *Chest* 1998;114:511S–523S.

33. Hart RG, Benavente O, Pearce J. Increased risk of intracranial hemorrhage when aspirin is combined with warfarin: a meta-analysis and hypothesis. *Cerebrovasc Dis* 1999;9:215–217.

34. Thrift AG, McNeil JJ, Forbes A, Donnan GA. Risk of primary intracerebral haemorrhage associated with aspirin and non-steroidal anti-inflammatory drugs: case-control study. *BMJ* 1999;318:759–764.

35. Chen ZM, Sandercock P, Pan HC, et al. Indications for early aspirin use in acute ischemic stroke : a combined analysis of 40 000 randomized patients from the Chinese acute stroke trial and the international stroke trial. On behalf of the CAST and IST collaborative groups. *Stroke* 2000;31:1240–1249.

36. Wong KS, Mok V, Lam WW, et al. Aspirin-associated intracerebral hemorrhage: clinical and radiologic features. *Neurology* 2000;54:2298–2301.

37. Iso H, Hennekens CH, Stampfer MJ, et al. Prospective study of aspirin use and risk of stroke in women. *Stroke* 1999;30:1764–1771.

38. CAST (Chinese Acute Stroke Trial) Collaborative Group. CAST: randomised placebo-controlled trial of early aspirin use in 20,000 patients with acute ischaemic stroke. *Lancet* 1997;349:1641–1649.

39. International Stroke Trial Collaborative Group. The International Stroke Trial (IST): a randomised trial of aspirin, subcutaneous heparin, both, or neither among 19435 patients with acute ischaemic stroke. *Lancet* 1997;349:1569–1581.

40. Multicentre Acute Stroke Trial–Italy (MAST-I) Group. Randomised controlled trial of streptokinase, aspirin, and combination of both in treatment of acute ischaemic stroke. *Lancet* 1995;346:1509–1514.

41. The Stroke Prevention in Reversible Ischemia Trial (SPIRIT) Study Group. A randomized trial of anticoagulants versus aspirin after cerebral ischemia of presumed arterial origin. *Ann Neurol* 1997;42:857–865.

42. Mohr JP, Thompson JLP, Lazar RM, et al. A comparison of warfarin and aspirin for the prevention of recurrent ischemic stroke. *N Engl J Med* 2001;345:1444–1451.

43. The Publications Committee for the Trial of ORG 10172 in Acute Stroke Treatment (TOAST) Investigators. Low molecular weight heparinoid, ORG 10172 (danaparoid), and outcome after acute ischemic stroke: a randomized controlled trial. *JAMA* 1998;279:1265–1272.

44. Donnan GA, Davis SM, Chambers BR, et al. Streptokinase for acute ischemic stroke with relationship to time of administration: Australian Streptokinase (ASK) Trial Study Group. *JAMA* 1996;276:961–966.

45. Multicenter Acute Stroke Trial–Europe Study Group. Thrombolytic therapy with streptokinase in acute ischemic stroke. *N Engl J Med* 1996;335:145–150.

46. The National Institute of Neurological Disorders and Stroke rt-PA Stroke Study Group. Tissue plasminogen activator for acute ischemic stroke. *N Engl J Med* 1995;333:1581–1587.

47. The NINDS t-PA Stroke Study Group. Intracerebral hemorrhage after intravenous t-PA therapy for ischemic stroke. *Stroke* 1997;28:2109–2118.

48. Lowe GD, Lee AJ, Rumley A, Price JF, Fowkes FG. Blood viscosity and risk of cardiovascular events: the Edinburgh Artery Study. *Br J Haematol* 1997;96:168–173.

49. Tatlisumak T, Fisher M. Hematologic disorders associated with ischemic stroke. *J Neurol Sci* 1996;140:1–11.

50. Finazzi G, Brancaccio V, Moia M, et al. Natural history and risk factors for thrombosis in 360 patients with antiphospholipid antibodies: a four-year prospective study from the Italian Registry. *Am J Med* 1996;100:530–536.

51. Ruggeri M, Tosetto A, Frezzato M, Rodeghiero F. The rate of progression to polycythemia vera or essential thrombocythemia in patients with erythrocytosis or thrombocytosis. *Ann Intern Med* 2003;139:470–475.

52. Finelli PF, Carley MD. Cerebral venous thrombosis associated with epoetin alfa therapy. *Arch Neurol* 2000;57: 260–262.

53. French JA, Kenny D, Scott JP, et al. Mechanisms of stroke in sickle cell disease: sickle erythrocytes decrease cerebral blood flow in rats after nitric oxide synthase inhibition. *Blood* 1997;89:4591–4599.

54. Steen RG, Xiong X, Langston JW, Helton KJ. Brain injury in children with sickle cell disease: prevalence and etiology. *Ann Neurol* 2003;54:564–572.

55. Prengler M, Pavlakis SG, Prohovnik I, Adams RJ. Sickle cell disease: the neurological complications. *Ann Neurol* 2002;51:543–552.

56. Pegelow CH, Adams RJ, McKie V, et al. Risk of recurrent stroke in patients with sickle cell disease treated with erythrocyte transfusions. *J Pediatr* 1995;126:896–899.

57. Pegelow CH, Wang W, Granger S, et al. Silent infarcts in children with sickle cell anemia and abnormal cerebral artery velocity. *Arch Neurol* 2001;58:2017-2021.

58. Steen RG, Xiong X, Mulhern RK, Langston JW, Wang WC. Subtle brain abnormalities in children with sickle cell disease. Relationship to blood hematocrit. *Ann Neurol* 1999; 45:279–286.

59. Dobson SR, Holden KR, Nietert PJ, et al. Moyamoya syndrome in childhood sickle cell disease: a predictive factor for recurrent cerebrovascular events. *Blood* 2002;99:3144–3150.

60. Adams RJ, McKie VC, Nichols FT, et al. The use of transcranial ultrasonography to predict stroke in sickle cell disease. *N Engl J Med* 1992;326:605–610.

61. Adams RJ. Stroke prevention in sickle cell disease. *Curr Opin Hematol* 2000;7:101–105.

62. Adams RJ, Pavlakis S, Roach ES. Sickle cell disease and stroke: primary prevention and transcranial Doppler. *Ann Neurol* 2003;54:559–563.

63. Adams RJ, McKie VC, Hsu L, et al. Prevention of a first stroke by transfusions in children with sickle cell anemia and abnormal results on transcranial Doppler ultrasonography. *N Engl J Med* 1998;339:5–11.

64. Riddington C, Wang W. Blood transfusion for preventing stroke in people with sickle cell disease. *Cochrane Database Syst Rev* 2002.

65. Casto L, Caverni L, Camerlingo M, et al. Intra-arterial thrombolysis in acute ischaemic stroke: experience with a superselective catheter embedded in the clot. *J Neurol Neurosurg Psychiatry* 1996;60:667–670.

66. Arboix A, Besses C, Acin P, et al. Ischemic stroke as first manifestation of essential thrombocythemia. Report of six cases. *Stroke* 1995;26:1463–1466.

67. Chaturvedi S, Dzieczkowski JS. Protein S deficiency, activated protein C resistance and sticky platelet syndrome in a young woman with bilateral strokes. *Cerebrovasc Dis* 1999;9:127–130.

68. Chaturvedi S, Dzieczkowski J. Multiple hemostatic abnormalities in young adults with activated protein C resistance and cerebral ischemia. *J Neurol Sci* 1998;159:209–212.

69. Griesshammer M, Bangerter M, van Vliet HH, Michiels JJ. Aspirin in essential thrombocythemia: status quo and quo vadis. *Semin Thromb Hemost* 1997;23:371–377.

70. George JN, Gilcher RO, Smith JW, Chandler L, Duvall D, Ellis C. Thrombotic thrombocytopenic purpura-hemolytic uremic syndrome: diagnosis and management. *J Clin Apheresis* 1998;13:120–125.

71. Sarode R, Gottschall JL, Aster RH, McFarland JG. Thrombotic thrombocytopenic purpura: early and late responders. *Am J Hematol* 1997;54:102–107.

72. Ruggenenti P, Remuzzi G. Pathophysiology and management of thrombotic microangiopathies. *J Nephrol* 1998; 11:300–310.

73. Tsai HM, Rice L, Sarode R, Chow TW, Moake JL. Antibody inhibitors to von Willebrand factor metalloproteinase and increased binding of von Willebrand factor to platelets in ticlopidine-associated thrombotic thrombocytopenic purpura. *Ann Intern Med* 2000;132:794–799.

74. Eldor A. Thrombotic thrombocytopenic purpura: diagnosis, pathogenesis and modern therapy. *Baillieres Clin Haematol* 1998;11:475–495.

75. Bennett CL, Weinberg PD, Rozenberg-Bendror K, Yarnold PR, Kwaan HC, Green D. Thrombotic thrombocytopenia purpura associated with ticlopidine. *Ann Intern Med* 1998;128:541–544.

76. Steinhubl SR, Tan WA, Foody JM, Topol EJ. Incidence and clinical course of thrombotic thrombocytopenic purpura due to ticlopidine following coronary stenting. EPISTENT investigators. Evaluation of platelet IIb/IIIa inhibitor for stenting. *JAMA* 1999;281:806–810.

77. Bennett CL, Connors JM, Carwile MJ, et al. Thrombotic thrombocytopenic purpura associated with clopidogrel. *N Engl J Med* 2000;325:1371–1372.

78. Zheng X, Pallera AM, Goodnough LT, Sadler E, Blinder MA. Remission of chronic thrombotic thrombocytopenic purpura after treatment with cyclophosphamide and rituximab. *Ann Intern Med* 2003;138:105–108.

79. Ramirez-Lassepas M, Cipolle RJ, Rodvold KA, et al. Heparin induced thrombocytopenia in patients with cerebrovascular ischemic disease. *Neurology* 1986;34:736–740.

80. Kappers-Klunne MC, Boon DM, Hop WC, et al. Heparin-induced thrombocytopenia and thrombosis: a prospective analysis of the incidence in patients with heart and cerebrovascular diseases. *Br J Haematol* 1997;96:442–446.

81. Boon DM, Michiels JJ, Tanghe HL, Kappers-Klunne MC. Heparin-induced thrombocytopenia with multiple cerebral infarctions simulating thrombotic thrombocytopenic purpura. A case report. *Angiology* 1996;47:407–411.

82. Horne MK, Alkins BR. Platelet binding of IgG from patients with heparin-induced thrombocytopenia. *J Lab Clin Med* 1996;127:435–442.

83. Gupta AK, Kovacs MJ, Sauder DN. Heparin-induced thrombocytopenia. *Ann Pharmacother* 1998;32:55–59.

84. Atkinson JL, Sundt TMJ, Kazmier FJ, Bowie EJ, Whisnant JP. Heparin-induced thrombocytopenia and thrombosis in ischemic stroke. *Mayo Clin Proc* 1988;63:353–361.

85. Calaitges JG, Liem TK, Spadone D, Nichols WK, Silver D. The role of heparin-associated antiplatelet antibodies in the outcome of arterial reconstruction. *J Vasc Surg* 1999;29:779–785.

86. Magnani HN. Heparin-induced thrombocytopenia (HIT): an overview of 230 patients treated with orgaran (Org 10172). *Thromb Haemost* 1993;70:554–561.

87. Lewis BE, Walenga JM, Wallis DE. Anticoagulation with novastan (argatroban) in patients with heparin-induced thrombocytopenia and heparin-induced thrombocytopenia and thrombosis syndrome. *Semin Thromb Hemost* 1997;23:197–202.

88. Kanagasabay RR, Unsworth-White MJ, Robinson G, et al. Cardiopulmonary bypass with danaparoid sodium and ancrod in heparin-induced thrombocytopenia. *Ann Thorac Surg* 1998;66:567–569.

89. Gore JM, Sloan M, Price TR, et al. Intracerebral hemorrhage, cerebral infarction, and subdural hematoma after acute myocardial infarction and thrombolytic therapy in the Thrombolysis in Myocardial Infarction Study. Thrombolysis in myocardial infarction, phase II, pilot and clinical trial. *Circulation* 1991;83:448–459.

90. Alberts SR, Bretscher M, Wiltsie JC, O'Neill BP, Mokri B, Witzig TE. Thrombosis related to the use of L-asparaginase in adults with acute lymphoblastic leukemia: a need to consider coagulation monitoring and clotting factor replacement. *Leuk Lymphoma* 1999;32:489–496.

91. Crowther MA, Kelton JG. Congenital thrombophilic states associated with venous thrombosis: a qualitative overview and proposed classification system. *Ann Intern Med* 2003;138:128–134.

92. Austin H, Chimowitz MI, Hill H, et al. Cryptogenci stroke in relation to genetic variation in clotting factors and other genetic polymorphism among young men and women. *Stroke* 2002;33:2762–2769.

93. Sagripanti A, Carpi A. Natural anticoagulants, aging, and thromboembolism. *Exp Gerontol* 1998;33:891–896.

94. Aiach M, Gandrille S, Emmerich J. A review of mutations causing deficiencies of antithrombin, protein C, and protein S. *Thromb Haemost* 1995;74:81–89.

95. Camerlingo M, Finazzi G, Casto L, Laffranch C, Barbui T, Mamoli A. Inherited protein C deficiency and nonhemorrhagic arterial stroke in young adults. *Neurology* 1991;41:1371–1373.

96. Bick RL. Hypercoagulability and thrombosis. *Med Clin North Am* 1994;78:635–665.

97. Vaezi MF, Rustagi PK, Elson CO. Transient protein S deficiency associated with cerebral venous thrombosis in active ulcerative colitis. *Am J Gastroenterol* 1995;90:313–315.

98. Press RD, Liu XY, Beamer N, Coull BM. Ischemic stroke in the elderly. Role of the common factor V mutation causing resistance to activated protein C. *Stroke* 1996;27:44–48.

99. Sanchez J, Roman J, de la Torre MJ, Velasco F, Torres A. Low prevalence of the factor V Leiden among patients with ischemic stroke. *Haemostasis* 1997;27:9–15.

100. Price DT, Ridker PM. Factor V Leiden mutation and the risks for thromboembolic disease: a clinical perspective. *Ann Intern Med* 1997;127:895–903.

101. Eskandari MK, Bontempo FA, Hassett AC, Faruki H, Makaroun MS. Arterial thromboembolic events in patients with the factor V Leiden mutation. *Am J Surg* 1998;176:122–125.

102. Ruggeri M, Gisslinger H, Tosetto A, et al. Factor V Leiden mutation carriership and venous thromboembolism in polycythemia vera and essential thrombocythemia. *Am J Hematol* 2002;71:1–6.

103. Karttunen V, Hiltunen L, Rasi V, Vahtera E, Hillbom M. Factor V Leiden and prothrombin gene mutation may predispose to paradoxical embolism in subjects with patent foramen ovale. *Blood Coagul Fibrinolysis* 2003;14:261–268.

104. Martinelli I, Sacchi E, Landi G, Taioli E, Duca F, Mannucci PM. High risk of cerebral-vein thrombosis in carriers of a prothrombin-gene mutation and in users of oral contraceptives. *N Engl J Med* 1998;338:1793–1797.

105. Gruppo RA, DeGrauw TJ, Palasis S, Kalinyak KA, Bofinger MK. Strokes, cutis marmorata telangiectatica congenita, and factor V Leiden. *Pediatr Neurol* 1998;18:342–345.

106. Baglin C, Brown K, Luddington R, Baglin T. Risk of recurrent venous thromboembolism in patients with the factor V Leiden (FVR506Q) mutation: effect of warfarin and prediction by precipitating factors. East Anglian Thrombophilia Study Group. *Br J Haematol* 1998;100:764–768.

107. Franco RF, Trip MD, ten Cate H, et al. The 20210 G—>A mutation in the 3'-untranslated region of the prothrombin gene and the risk for arterial thrombotic disease. *Br J Haematol* 1999;104:50–54.

108. Vicente V, Gonzalez-Conejero R, Rivera J, Corral J. The prothrombin gene variant 20210A in venous and arterial thromboembolism. *Haematologica* 1999;84:356–362.

109. Eikelboom JW, Ivey L, Ivey J, Baker RI. Familial thrombophilia and the prothrombin 20210A mutation: association with increased thrombin generation and unusual thrombosis. *Blood Coagul Fibrinolysis* 1999;10:1–5.

110. Young G, Manco-Johnson M, Gill JC, et al. Clinical manifestations of the prothrombin G20210A mutation in children: a pediatric coagulation consortium study. *J Thromb Haemost* 2003;1:958–962.

111. Ernst E, Resch KL. Fibrinogen as a cardiovascular risk factor: a meta-analysis and review of the literature. *Ann Intern Med* 1993;118:956–963.

112. Qizilbash N, Jones L, Warlow C, Mann J. Fibrinogen and lipid concentrations as risk factors for transient ischaemic attacks and minor ischaemic strokes. *BMJ* 1991;303:605–609.

113. Ernst E. Fibrinogen as a cardiovascular risk factor—inter-relationship with infections and inflammation. *Eur Heart J* 1993;14(suppl K):82–87.

114. Di Perri T, Guerrini M, Pasini FL, et al. Hemorheological factors in the pathophysiology of acute and chronic cerebrovascular disease. *Cephalalgia* 1985;5(suppl 2):71–77.

115. Elwan O, al-Ashmawy S, el-Karaksy S, Hassan AA. Hemorheology, stroke and the elderly. *J Neurol Sci* 1991; 101:157–162.

116. Cervera R, Piette JC, Font J, et al. Antiphospholipid syndrome: clinical and immunologic manifestations and patterns of disease expression in a cohort of 1,000 patients. *Arthritis Rheum* 2002;46:1019–1027.

117. Aznar J, Villa P, Espana F, Estelles A, Grancha S, Falco C. Activated protein C resistance phenotype in patients with antiphospholipid antibodies. *J Lab Clin Med* 1997;130: 202–208.

118. Coull BM, Goodnight SH. Antiphospholipid antibodies, prethrombotic states, and stroke. *Stroke* 1990;21:1370–1374.

119. Toschi V, Motta A, Castelli C, Paracchini ML, Zerbi D, Gibelli A. High prevalence of antiphosphatidylinositol antibodies in young patients with cerebral ischemia of undetermined cause. *Stroke* 1998;29:1759–1764.

120. Tanne D, D'Olhaberriague L, Schultz LR, Salowich-Palm L, Sawaya L, Levine SR. Anticardiolipin antibodies and their associations with cerebrovascular risk factors. *Neurology* 1999;52:1368–1373.

121. Greaves M. Antiphospholipid antibodies and thrombosis. *Lancet* 1999;353:1348–1353.

122. Lanthier S, Kirkham FJ, Mitchell LG, et al. Increased anticardiolipin antibody IgG titers do not predict recurrent stroke or TIA in children. *Neurology* 2004;62:194–200.

123. de Groot PG, Horbach DA, Simmelink MJ, van Oort E, Derksen RH. Anti-prothrombin antibodies and their relation with thrombosis and lupus anticoagulant. *Lupus* 1998;7(suppl 2):S32–S36.

124. Kalashnikova LA, Korczyn AD, Shavit S, Rebrova O, Reshetnyak T, Chapman J. Antibodies to prothrombin in patients with Sneddon's syndrome. *Neurology* 1999;53: 223–225.

125. Verro P, Levine SR, Tietjen GE. Cerebrovascular ischemic events with high positive anticardiolipin antibodies. *Stroke* 1998;29:2245–2253.

126. Exner T, Triplett DA, Taberner D, Machin SJ. Guidelines for testing and revised criteria for lupus anticoagulants. SSC Subcommittee for the Standardization of Lupus Anticoagulants. *Thromb Haemost* 1991;65:320–322.

127. Tanne D, Bates VE, Verro P, et al. Initial clinical experience with IV tissue plasminogen activator for acute ischemic stroke: a multicenter survey. The t-PA Stroke Survey Group. *Neurology* 1999;53:424–427.

128. Asherson RA, Khamashta MA, Gil A, et al. Cerebrovascular disease and antiphospholipid antibodies in systemic lupus erythematosus, lupus-like disease, and the primary antiphospholipid syndrome. *Am J Med* 1989;86: 391–399.

129. Vaarala O, Manttari M, Manninen V, et al. Anti-cardiolipin antibodies and risk of myocardial infarction in a prospective cohort of middle-aged men. *Circulation* 1995;91: 23–27.

130. Christopher R, Nagaraja D, Dixit NS, Narayanan CP. Anticardiolipin antibodies: a study in cerebral venous thrombosis. *Acta Neurol Scand* 1999;99:121–124.

131. Miesbach W, Gilzinger A, Gokpinar B, et al. Prevalence of antibodies in patients with neurological symptoms. *Clin Neurol Neurosurg* 2006;108:135–142.

132. Brey RL. Antiphospholipid antibodies in young adults with stroke. *J Thromb Thrombolysis* 2005;20:105–112.

133. Chapman J, Rand JH, Brey RL, et al. Non-stroke neurological symptoms associated with antiphospholipid antibodies: evaluation of clinical and experimental studies. *Lupus* 2003;12:514–517.

134. Angelini L, Zibordi F, Zorzi G, et al. Neurological disorders, other than stroke, associated with antiphospholipid antibodies in childhood. *Neuropediatrics* 1996;27:149–153.

135. Galve E, Ordi J, Barquinero J, Evangelista A, Vilardell M, Soler-Soler J. Valvular heart disease in the primary antiphospholipid syndrome. *Ann Intern Med* 1992;116: 293–298.

136. Fetoni V, Grisoli M, Salmaggi A, Carriero R, Girotti E. Clinical and neuroradiological aspects of Sneddon's syndrome and primary antiphospholipid antibody syndrome. A follow-up study. *Neurol Sci* 2000;21:157–164.

137. Gantcheva M, Tsankov N. Livedo reticularis and cerebrovascular accidents (Sneddon's syndrome) as a clinical expression of antiphospholipid syndrome. *J Eur Acad Dermatol Venereol* 1999;12:157–160.

138. Frances C, Papo T, Wechsler B, Laporte JL, Biousse V, Piette JC. Sneddon syndrome with or without antiphospholipid antibodies. A comparative study in 46 patients. *Medicine* 1999;78:209–219.

139. Adair JC, Digre KB, Swanda RM, et al. Sneddon's syndrome: a cause of cognitive decline in young adults. *Neuropsychiatry Neuropsychol Behav Neurol* 2001;14: 197–204.

140. Boesch SM, Plorer AL, Auer AJ, et al. The natural course of Sneddon syndrome: clinical and magnetic resonance imaging findings in a prospective six year observation study. *J Neurol Neurosurg Psychiatry* 2003;74:542–544.

141. Khamashta MA, Cuadrado MJ, Mujic F, Taub NA, Hunt BJ, Hughes GR. The management of thrombosis in the antiphospholipid-antibody syndrome. *N Engl J Med* 1995; 332:993–997.

142. Lim W, Crowther MA, Eikelboom JW. Management of antiphospholipid antibody syndrome. A systematic review. *JAMA* 2006;295:1050–1057.

143. The APASS Investigators. Antiphospholipid antibodies and subsequent thrombo-occlusive events in patients with ischemic stroke. *JAMA* 2004;291:576–584.

144. Biller J, Challa VR, Toole JF, Howard VJ. Nonbacterial thrombotic endocarditis. *Arch Neurol* 1982;39:95–98.

145. Kooiker JC, MacLean JM, Sumi SM. Cerebral embolism, marantic endocarditis, and cancer. *Arch Neurol* 1976;33: 260–264.

146. Demarmels BF, Sulzer I, Stucki B, Wuillemin WA, Furlan M, Lammle B. Is plasminogen deficiency a thrombotic risk factor? A study on 23 thrombophilic patients and their family members. *Thromb Haemost* 1998;80: 167–170.

147. Young G, Driscoll MC. Coagulation abnormalities in the carbohydrate-deficient glycoprotein syndrome: case report and review of the literature. *Am J Hematol* 1999;60:66–69.

148. Salomaa V, Stinson V, Kark JD, Folsom AR, Davis CE, Wu KK. Association of fibrinolytic parameters with early atherosclerosis. The ARIC Study. Atherosclerosis Risk in Communities Study. *Circulation* 1995;91:284–290.

149. Macko RF, Kittner SJ, Epstein A, et al. Elevated tissue plasminogen activator antigen and stroke risk: the Stroke Prevention in Young Women Study. *Stroke* 1999;30:7–11.

150. Lindgren A, Lindoff C, Norrving B, Astedt B, Johansson BB. Tissue plasminogen activator and plasminogen activator inhibitor-1 in stroke patients. *Stroke* 1996;27:1066–1071.

151. Qizilbash N, Duffy S, Prentice CR, Boothby M, Warlow C. Von Willebrand factor and risk of ischemic stroke. *Neurology* 1997;49:1552–1556.

152. Ballem P. Acquired thrombophilia in pregnancy. *Semin Thromb Hemost* 1998;24(suppl 1):41–47.

153. Martinelli I, Battaglioli T, Burgo I, et al. Oral contraceptive use, thrombophilia, and their interaction in young women with ischemic stroke. *Haematologica* 2006;91: 844–847.

154. Pinto AN. AIDS and cerebrovascular disease. *Stroke* 1996;27:538–543.

155. Macko RF, Ameriso SF, Gruber A, et al. Impairments of the protein C system and fibrinolysis in infection-associated stroke. *Stroke* 1996;27:2005–2011.

156. Rao AK, Chouhan V, Chen X, Sun L, Boden G. Activation of the tissue factor pathway of blood coagulation during prolonged hyperglycemia in young healthy men. *Diabetes* 1999;48:1156–1161.

157. Lip GY, Gibbs CR. Does heart failure confer a hypercoagulable state? Virchow's triad revisited. *J Am Coll Cardiol* 1999;33:1424–1426.

158. Ansell JE, Tiarks C, Fairchild VK. Coagulation abnormalities associated with the use of anabolic steriods. *Am Heart J* 1993;125:367–371.

159. Hendriks HF, Veenstra J, Velthuis-te WE, Schaafsma G, Kluft C. Effect of moderate dose of alcohol with evening meal on fibrinolytic factors. *BMJ* 1994;308:1003–1006.

160. Weber P, Husemann S, Vielhaber H, Zimmer KP, Nowak-Gottl U. Coagulation and fibrinolysis in children, adolescents, and young adults with inflammatory bowel disease. *J Pediatr Gastroenterol Nutr* 1999;28:418–422.

161. Morello F, Ronzani G, Cappellari F. Migraine, cortical blindness, multiple cerebral infarctions and hypocoagulopathy in celiac disease. *Neurol Sci* 2003;24:85–89.

162. Marsh EE, Biller J, Adams HP, Jr., Kaplan JM. Cerebral infarction in patients with nephrotic syndrome. *Stroke* 1991;22:90–93.

CHAPTER 15

Intracranial Aneurysms and Vascular Malformations

Intracranial aneurysms and vascular malformations are important causes of intracranial hemorrhage in persons of all ages, including childhood (Tables 15-1 and 15-2). Ruptured saccular aneurysms are the most common cause of spontaneous subarachnoid hemorrhage and a leading cause of intracerebral hemorrhage. Ruptured vascular malformations are among the most common etiologies of primary intracerebral hemorrhage, especially when bleeding involves the lobar white matter. Besides leading to bleeding, these vascular lesions also can cause ischemic stroke, recurrent headache, an audible bruit, seizures, or focal neurological symptoms because of compression of adjacent structures. In infants, a large vascular malformation also can cause an enlarging head or congestive heart failure. The former is from the mass effect of the vascular lesion. The latter is due to a high cardiac output to maintain flow through a large fistula.

▶ SACCULAR ANEURYSMS

Rupture of a saccular aneurysm accounts for approximately 85 percent of cases of subarachnoid hemorrhage and approximately 10 percent of cases of intracerebral hemorrhage. As a result approximately 30,000 people in North America have a catastrophic stroke secondary to aneurysmal rupture—approximately 5 percent of all strokes. Approximately one-half of persons are within 1 month of rupture of an aneurysm, a statistic that emphasizes the highly lethal nature of this intracranial vascular lesion. Many of the deaths occur before the patient could be brought to medical attention. Unlike some of the other forms of acute stroke, the incidence of subarachnoid hemorrhage did not decline during the latter third of the twentieth century.

Size and Locations

Saccular aneurysms are found in approximately 2–5 percent of persons; in most cases, these aneurysms are asymptomatic and are found incidentally.[1] Most people live their entire life not knowing that they have this potentially life-threatening vascular lesion. Aneurysms usually are globular in shape, an appearance that leads to the other term to describe these lesions—berry. Some can be lobulated or have a small outpouching. Aneurysms are classified on the basis of their greatest diameter—small <10 mm, large 10–25 mm, and giant >25 mm. Often the neck (orifice) is small. In addition, patients can have an infundibulum, which is a small area of dilation of the artery or an outpouching. Approximately 25 percent of affected persons have more than one aneurysm; in some cases multiple aneurysms can be found. Mirror aneurysms are two aneurysms located at approximately the same location in the right and left internal carotid artery circulations. These vascular abnormalities usually develop at the bifurcations of the major intracranial arteries on or near the circle of Willis (Fig. 15-1). While aneurysms usually are found at the origin of the major arteries, they can be found on proximal portions of any intracranial vessel. Saccular aneurysms usually are not located on

▶ **TABLE 15-1.** CLASSIFICATION OF ANEURYSMS

Saccular
Nonsaccular
   Fusiform
   Dissection
   Infective
   Neoplastic
   Posttraumatic

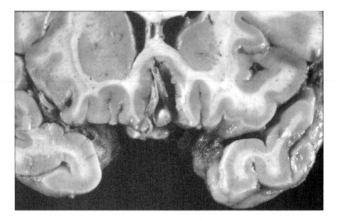

Figure 15-1. An unruptured aneurysm of the anterior communicating artery is visualized on this autopsy specimen. (*Courtesy of S.S. Schochet, M.D., Department of Pathology, University of West Virginia, Morgantown WV*)

terminal pial arteries. Approximately 85 percent of the aneurysms are located in the carotid circulation with the region of the anterior communicating artery, the origin of the posterior communicating artery, and the bifurcation of the middle cerebral artery being the most common sites (Fig. 15-2). Less common locations include the intracavernous portion of the internal carotid artery, the origin of the ophthalmic artery, or distal segments of the anterior cerebral artery. The most common locations for aneurysms arising in the posterior circulation are the basilar bifurcation (apex) or the origin of the posterior inferior cerebellar artery.

Pathogenesis

Aneurysms arise at the bifurcation of arteries largely because of hemodynamic stresses at this location. The absence of the second elastic lamina in the intracranial arteries, which is found in extracranial arteries, appears to be a critical factor for the development of the aneurysm. Fragmentation of the arterial internal elastic lamina is a feature leading to the development of the aneurysm. The neck of the aneurysm usually demonstrates smooth muscle and intima but the elastic layer is absent. These are true aneurysms with elements of the intimal, medial, and adventitial layers within the wall of the aneurysm. The wall of the aneurysmal sac often is very thin and the elastic lamina is absent. The dome of the aneurysm usually points in the direction of the blood flow of the parent artery. Many larger aneurysms will have an outpouching (bleb) along the dome. This area has a very thin wall and is the usual location for aneurysmal rupture. In most other cases, the apex of the dome is the site of rupture.

In general, the risk of bleeding is associated with the size of the aneurysm.[2] The risk of rupture is relatively low

when an aneurysm is <5 mm in diameter. The average size of ruptured aneurysms is approximately 6–8 mm. Unruptured aneurysms >10 mm in diameter have the highest risk for bleeding. Giant intracranial aneurysms can have areas of calcification or atherosclerotic plaquing

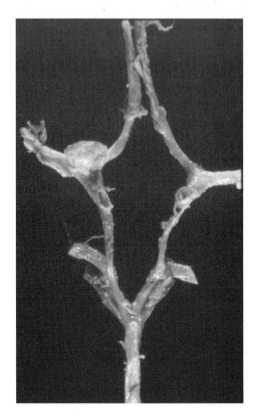

Figure 15-2. A dissection of the circle of Willis shows a large unruptured aneurysm located at the distal portion of the left internal carotid artery. (*Courtesy of S.S. Schochet, M.D., Department of Pathology, University of West Virginia, Morgantown WV*)

▶ **TABLE 15-2.** CLASSIFICATION OF VASCULAR MALFORMATIONS

Arteriovenous
Venous
Cavernous
Telangiectasis
Arteriovenous fistula

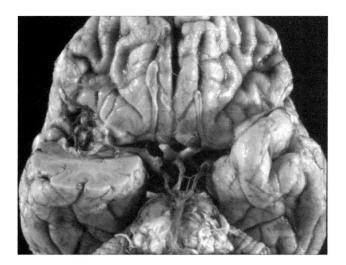

Figure 15-3. A dissection of the brain with visualization of the right middle cerebral artery shows an aneurysm at the bifurcations of the middle cerebral artery. (*Courtesy of S.S. Schochet, M.D., Department of Pathology, University of West Virginia, Morgantown WV*)

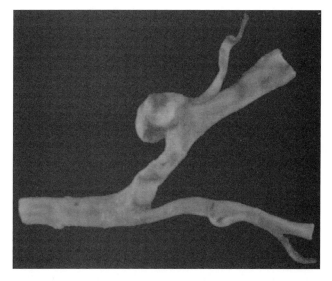

Figure 15-4. A dissection of the vertebral arteries and the proximal portion of the basilar artery shows an aneurysm arising from the origin of the posterior inferior cerebellar artery. (*Courtesy of S.S. Schochet, M.D., Department of Pathology, University of West Virginia, Morgantown WV*)

in the wall. Because of laminar flow leads to stagnation, an intramural thrombus also can be found in giant aneurysms. These clots can be the source of emboli to the brain. Giant aneurysms also can compress adjacent intracranial structures, such as cranial nerves.

Epidemiology

Aneurysms are found in men and women of all ages and of all ethnic groups (Figs. 15-3 and 15-4). Saccular aneurysms are not diagnosed frequently in children or adolescents. This relationship suggests some evolution or growth of the aneurysm during life. Approximately 80 percent of the children who have symptomatic saccular aneurysms are boys. With advancing age the male to female ratio changes and by the fifth decade both sexes are equally affected. The average of age of patients with subarachnoid hemorrhage is approximately 55. While aneurysms might be found slightly more frequently among men, women account for approximately 60 percent of the cases of aneurysmal subarachnoid hemorrhage. In general, women are older than men at the time of the bleeding. The locations of aneurysms differ slightly between men and women. Women more frequently have aneurysms at the origin of the posterior communicating artery, while the anterior communicating artery is a more common location in men.

Associated Diseases and Familial Aneurysms

Approximately 10–20 percent of patients with aneurysmal subarachnoid hemorrhage will report a history of a relative

with a similar illness[3–6] (Table 15-3). Kim et al.[7] found that the incidence of familial intracranial aneurysms was similar among persons of Hispanic, African, or European ancestry. The diagnosis of *familial aneurysms* is entertained when patient has two or more first-degree (parent, child, sibling) affected relatives. Overall, the chances that a first-degree relative will have an aneurysm increase by a factor of approximately 4 when another family member is diagnosed with an aneurysm.[8] The likelihood is approximately 4 percent that a sibling of a patient with a subarachnoid hemorrhage has an aneurysm.[6,9–11]

▶ **TABLE 15-3.** DISEASES ASSOCIATED WITH SACCULAR ANEURYSMS

Autosomal dominant polycystic kidney disease
Moyamoya disease/syndrome
Coarctation of the aorta
Arteriovenous malformation of the brain
Type III collage deficiency
Ehlers–Danlos syndrome
Marfan syndrome
Elastin polymorphisms
Endoglin genetic defect
Klinefelter syndrome
Tuberous sclerosis
Sickle cell disease
Acid maltase deficiency
Pompe disease
Beçhet disease
Diamond–Blackfan syndrome
Klippel–Trenaunay–Weber syndrome

Connolly et al.[12] suggest that in women the presence of hypertension or smoking associated with an increased likelihood that a relative would also have an aneurysm. Aneurysms are more common among relatives who smoke or who have hypertension.[12] This finding suggests some contribution of environmental factors to the promotion of growth of an aneurysm. Kissela et al.[13] concluded that stopping smoking, treating hypertension, and reducing alcohol use could lower the risk of subarachnoid hemorrhage among families with a genetic predisposition to aneurysms.

Although a specific genetic defect has not been discovered, the clustering of familial aneurysms is consistent with autosomal dominant, autosomal recessive, or multifactorial inheritance patterns[14] (see Chapter 12). In general, most families seem to have an autosomal dominant pattern of inheritance. Japanese studies have suggested an elastin polymorphism, possibly located on 7q11, or the endoglin gene might be key but other research has suggested greater genetic heterogeneity.[15–17] Keramatipour et al.[18] reported that I allele at the ACE locus is associated with ruptured intracranial aneurysms. Yoneyama[19] found a genetic abnormality in collage type I as a potential cause for saccular aneurysms.

In general, persons with familial aneurysms become symptomatic at a younger age than do patients with a negative family history. In addition, the chances of multiple aneurysms seem to be increased in familial aneurysms. Because most aneurysms are sporadic, the yield of screening relatives of a patient with a symptomatic saccular aneurysm is relatively low. However, noninvasive screening of the vasculature can be performed if a patient has two or more first-degree relatives who are affected and is concerned about the potential for subarachnoid hemorrhage.[6,9] The utility of screening patients for aneurysm is debated. The absence of an aneurysm will be reassuring. However, an asymptomatic patient must be prepared to deal with the consequences of finding an aneurysm. The patient might need surgery.

A strong relationship exists between *autosomal dominant polycystic kidney disease* (ADPKD) and intracranial saccular aneurysms[20,21] (see Chapter 12). Approximately 10 percent of patients with ADPKD have aneurysms and subarachnoid hemorrhage is a leading cause of death in this group. Gieteling and Rinkel[22] found that the middle cerebral artery and the anterior communicating artery were the most common locations and that the average age at the time of subarachnoid hemorrhage was 41 years. Because of the high risk of intracranial aneurysms among families with ADPKD, especially if other family members have had subarachnoid hemorrhage, screening of asymptomatic persons often is recommended. Intracranial aneurysms also have been reported in persons with *Type III collagen deficiency*.

An association between intracranial aneurysms and *fibromuscular dysplasia* is reported (see Chapter 10). The arteriopathy is most commonly diagnosed in young women. The arteriographic change can be mimicked by arterial vasospasm secondary to the arteriographic procedure. While fibromuscular dysplasia is associated with arterial dissection including the formation of a dissecting aneurysm, the relationship between fibromuscular dysplasia and saccular aneurysms needs clarification. It is possible that fibromuscular dysplasia is an incidental finding discovered during the evaluation of a young woman with subarachnoid hemorrhage.

A link between saccular aneurysms and *coarctation of the aorta* also is speculated. While the population of patients with coarctation is relatively small and thus its impact on the frequency of subarachnoid hemorrhage is minimal. Data suggest that the chances of an intracranial aneurysm are considerably increased among the population of patients with aortic lesion. A possible common underlying predisposition might be present. Recently, Connolly et al.[23] found intracranial aneurysms in 10 of 277 adult patients with coarctation of the aorta; the relatively risk was estimated as five times higher than that found in the general population. The strong relationship between coarctation and high blood pressure might lead to secondary effects on the intracranial vasculature, which promotes growth of aneurysms.

Subarachnoid hemorrhage is a common presentation among young adults with *moyamoya disease* or moyamoya syndrome (see Chapters 10 and 12). The hallmarks of moyamoya disease are bilateral occlusion of the proximal portions of the major intracranial arteries, especially in the anterior circulation, and development of a network of fine collateral vessels in the region of the basal ganglia. Important collateral vessels arise from the external carotid circulation via ethmoidal branches and the posterior circulation. Because of hemodynamic changes, a relatively high frequency of intracranial aneurysms is found on the collateral vessels or the moyamoya network. Saccular aneurysms are predominately found in the vertebrobasilar circulation. Small microaneurysms can arise on the small caliber vessels.

Intracranial saccular aneurysms are reported as an associated finding among persons with *sickle cell disease, Marfan syndrome, Ehlers–Danlos syndrome type IV, neurofibromatosis, tuberous sclerosis, Diamond–Blackfan syndrome, Klippel–Trénaunay–Weber syndrome, Klinefelter syndrome, Behçet's disease, acid maltase deficiency*, or *Pompe disease*.[24–28] Approximately 5 percent of patients with large intracranial *arteriovenous malformations* can have aneurysms.[29,30] The aneurysms, which are more likely to bleed than the vascular malformation, usually are found at close proximity on major feeding vessels.

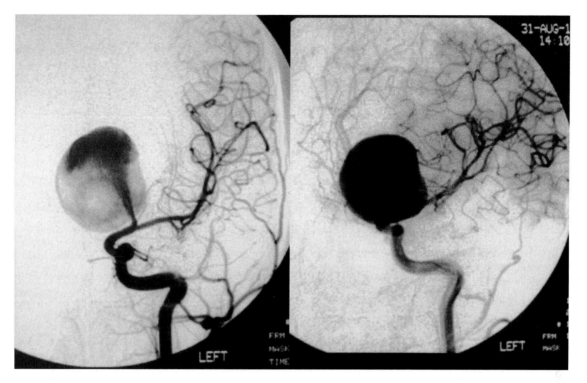

Figure 15-5. Two anterior posterior views of a giant aneurysm arising from the internal carotid artery demonstrates laminar flow within the aneurysm. (*Courtesy of Duke Samson, M.D., Department of Neurological Surgery, University of Texas Southwestern School of Medicine, Dallas, TX*)

Clinical Presentations

Intracranial hemorrhage is the most common presentation of a ruptured aneurysm. Bleeding usually is restricted to the subarachnoid space but secondary intracerebral or intraventricular hemorrhage each occurs in approximately 15 percent of patients. Occasionally, bleeding from a saccular aneurysm can extend into the subdural space. The usual symptoms are an unusually severe headache, transient loss of consciousness, seizures, nausea, and vomiting (see Chapter 7). Focal neurological symptoms also can be detected. A ruptured aneurysm of the anterior communicating artery can produce a paraparesis and a hemiparesis or aphasia can accompany a hemorrhage of an aneurysm of the middle cerebral artery. The most common focal neurological is an oculomotor nerve palsy (with pupillary involvement) secondary to rupture of an aneurysm of the posterior communicating artery or the basilar tip. A sizable percentage of patients with subarachnoid hemorrhage have warning symptoms, usually a headache.[31,32] These symptoms, which usually are not recognized as being an omen for a serious hemorrhage, occur on an average approximately 1–3 weeks before the major aneurysmal rupture.

Large or giant aneurysms can compress adjacent structures—the most common are the oculomotor nerve in the subarachnoid space secondary to an aneurysm of the posterior communicating artery or the basilar bifurcation and multiple cranial nerves when the aneurysm is in the cavernous sinus. A thrombus can arise inside a giant aneurysm and pieces of the clot can embolize to the brain and lead to either a TIA or ischemic stroke (Fig. 15-5). In addition, an incidental aneurysm can be found on brain or vascular imaging during an evaluation for another neurological problem.[33] Most commonly, either CT or MRI will visualize an aneurysm; these lesions usually are >5 mm in size. Recurrent headache or seizures usually are not the symptoms of saccular aneurysms.

Risk of Rupture

The risk of rupture of an intact saccular aneurysm is estimated as approximately 0.2–3 percent per year[34] (Table 15-4). The risk of bleeding seems to be greatest among those patients who already have had a subarachnoid hemorrhage from another aneurysm (Fig. 15-6). In addition, patients whose aneurysms are larger than 10 mm in diameter seem to have an increased risk. Wiebers et al.[35,36] found that the 5-year cumulative risks for rupture of aneurysms in the anterior circulation were 0 percent for aneurysms <7 mm in diameter, 2.6 percent for aneurysms 7–12 mm, 14.5 percent for aneurysms 13–24 mm, and 40 percent for aneurysms >24 mm. Among patients with aneurysms in the vertebrobasilar circulation or

▶ **TABLE 15-4.** FACTORS ASSOCIATED WITH RUPTURE OF INTRACRANIAL ANEURYSM

Women > men
Aneurysm > 6 mm in diameter
Arterial hypertension
Smoking
Heavy alcohol use
Oral contraceptive use
Sympathomimetic drug use/abuse

posterior communicating artery, the 5-year rate for hemorrhages was 2.5 percent for aneurysms <7 mm, 14.5 percent for aneurysms 7–12 mm, 18.4 percent when the aneurysm was 13–24 mm, and 50 percent for aneurysms >24 mm. The management of unruptured aneurysms is uncertain. Conservative measures, such as treatment of arterial hypertension, probably are not sufficient. Juvela et al.[37] recommended that unruptured aneurysms in young-to-middle age adults be treated regardless of the size of the aneurysm. Tuffiash et al.[38] reported that cognitive impairments following clipping of an intact aneurysm were uncommon. Brilstra et al.[39] found that neurosurgical

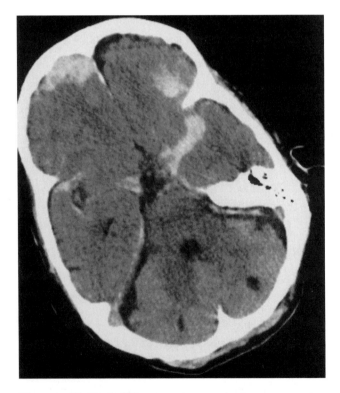

Figure 15-6. A CT scan demonstrates a massive subarachnoid hemorrhage with a focal thick collection of blood in the left Sylvian cistern. The findings are consistent with a ruptured aneurysm. Frontal bleed also is present.

treatment of unruptured aneurysms was associated with a decline in quality of life. A large international trial did not demonstrate a benefit from surgical clipping for most patients.[40] To the consternation of both physicians and patients, the study found that the risk of complications of surgery appeared to be greater than the risk of bleeding. No age relationship was reported to either the risk of aneurysmal rupture or the frequency of operative complications. Another trial compared the utility of endovascular occlusion of the aneurysm to surgical treatment; the endovascular intervention appeared to be superior. Still, the recent study of Wiebers et al.[36] demonstrated that the risks of endovascular or surgical treatment of the aneurysm were worse than the natural history. They noted that the patient's age and the location and size of the aneurysm influenced the outcomes of endovascular or surgical therapies. Endovascular treatment had a lower negative impact on outcomes. Endovascular treatment of unruptured aneurysms appears to be associated with less morbidity that surgical clipping.[39] For patients with intact aneurysms, endovascular treatment by skilled physicians at institutions with a high volume is associated with significant declines in morbidity and mortality.[41,42] Complete obliteration of the aneurysm might not be achieved by endovascular interventions. Selection of the patients who should be treated needs to be refined. Management of intracranial saccular aneurysms that have not ruptured will remain an important issue and additional information about the natural history of these vascular lesions is needed.[43]

A number of factors have been associated with an increased risk of aneurysmal rupture including smoking, poorly treated hypertension, or heavy alcohol use.[44–47] While hypertension usually is not considered as a risk factor for aneurysmal subarachnoid hemorrhage, a sudden rise in blood pressure might precipitate rupture. A marked increase in blood pressure might explain subarachnoid hemorrhage associated with vigorous exercise, lifting, or coitus. A sudden surge in blood pressure might be an explanation for aneurysmal rupture secondary to the use of stimulants such as cocaine or amphetamines.[48,49] Heavy consumption of alcohol is associated with an increased rate of subarachnoid hemorrhage on weekends. This relationship seems to be greatest among young persons. Cigarette smoking also is described as a factor associated with an increased likelihood of aneurysmal rupture, particularly in younger persons.[45] The frequency of subarachnoid hemorrhage is higher among women than men.[2] A potential relationship between the use of oral contraceptives and subarachnoid hemorrhage has been reported.[50,51] While many patients report the onset of subarachnoid hemorrhage in close proximity to vigorous exercise, no definite relationship to physical activity has been established. Aneurysmal rupture has been described as a potential complication of coitus, a Valsalva maneuver, or straining. No relationship to the time of day, season, or weather has been established.

Diagnostic Studies

CT has a high diagnostic yield for intracranial blood[52] (see Fig. 15-6; see Chapter 8). The findings on CT are influenced by the interval from aneurysmal rupture, the severity of the patient's hemorrhage, and the patient's neurological status. Almost all patients with altered consciousness will have blood detected by CT. Brain imaging can miss bleeding if the test is done several days after the ictus or if the patient has a very mild hemorrhage. MRI does not appear to be more sensitive than CT. Because most aneurysms arise near the circle of Willis, the blood is found predominantly in the cisterns at the base of the brain. In a patient with multiple aneurysms, the location of a focal collection of subarachnoid blood points to the aneurysm that ruptured. The pattern and severity of bleeding also forecasts outcomes and the likelihood of complications. In addition, imaging also can demonstrate complicating intracerebral or intraventricular hemorrhage, hydrocephalus, or secondary infarction. Aneurysms (>5 mm) often are detected on contrast-enhanced CT or MRI. The MRI can show a large flow void within the aneurysm. These tests could be performed following subarachnoid hemorrhage or to assess another neurological condition. Angiography, CTA, or MRA can be used to evaluate the presence of an aneurysm, adjacent vascular anatomy, or

arterial complications of subarachnoid hemorrhage, including vasospasm (Figs. 15-7 and 15-8).

Prognosis

Aneurysmal subarachnoid hemorrhage remains a life-threatening disease.[53–56] Fortunately, the mortality from subarachnoid hemorrhage has declined in the last 30 years.[57,58] Still, approximately 80 percent of deaths occur within the first week following the hemorrhage.[59,60] The severity of the subarachnoid hemorrhage, as denoted by the level of consciousness, strongly predicts the outcome.[61] The 30-day mortality among alert patients is approximately 15 percent and among comatose patients, it exceeds 75 percent.[62] Patients with large amounts of blood on CT also have a poor prognosis.[62] Patients with ruptured aneurysms of the posterior circulation have a poor prognosis.[63] Approximately 50 percent of survivors have residual neurological impairments including cognitive abnormalities.[64–68]

The leading causes of death and disability are the effects of the initial hemorrhage, vasospasm causing infarction, and recurrent hemorrhage.[53,69] Other causes of

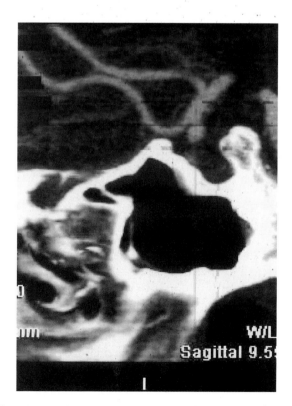

Figure 15-8. A lateral view of a CT angiography reveals an aneurysm of the anterior communicating artery.

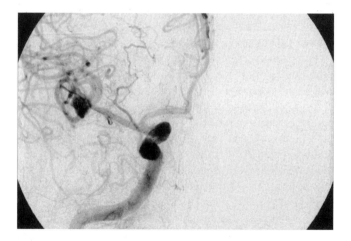

Figure 15-7. An anteroposterior view of a right carotid arteriogram reveals a large aneurysm of the middle cerebral artery.

morbidity include hydrocephalus, hyponatremia, seizures, and complications of medical or surgical interventions.

Treatment

Details about the management of aneurysmal subarachnoid hemorrhage are included in Chapter 23. Prevention of recurrent rupture of a saccular aneurysm is a key component of management of a patient with aneurysmal subarachnoid hemorrhage.[53] The likelihood of recurrent bleeding is approximately 20 percent within 10 days of the initial hemorrhage and the risk within 24 hours is approximately 4 percent.[70] Thereafter the chances of a second hemorrhage decline to approximately 2–3 percent per year, with this rate being noted after 6 months following subarachnoid hemorrhage. The differential diagnosis of rebleeding as a cause of neurological worsening include ischemia secondary to vasospasm, brain edema, seizures, infections, electrolyte disturbances, or hydrocephalus.[71]

Prolonged bed rest, sedation, and treatment of hypertension are used to lower the transmural pressure gradients that might provoke recurrent aneurysmal rupture.[52] This regimen is not particularly successful and it should not be considered as an effective therapy to prevent recurrent aneurysmal rupture. Antifibrinolytic agents (aminocaproic acid or tranexamic acid) are administered to prevent early lysis of the perianeurysmal clot in the subarachnoid space.[72–76] While the short-term administration of these medications does lower the risk of rebleeding, these agents do not improve outcomes. In addition, the concomitant administration of antifibrinolytic and antihypertensive medications appears to increase the risk of ischemic complications of vasospasm.

Surgical clipping of the neck of the aneurysm is the traditional method to prevent recurrent rupture.[27,52,77] In the past, neurosurgical treatment of the aneurysm was delayed for approximately 2 weeks following subarachnoid hemorrhage because of the perceived high risk for complications.[78,79] More recently with advances in surgical techniques, the use of the operating microscope, and improvements in neuroanesthesia, neurosurgeons have moved to clipping of the aneurysm within the first few days of subarachnoid hemorrhage. Although a large international trial was unable to demonstrate definitive data for the superiority of early surgery, operations now are recommended within 48 hours following hemorrhage.[80,81] Premature recurrent rupture is a potential complication of manipulation of the aneurysm. In addition, dissection of the aneurysm and adjacent tissue can lead to occlusion of adjacent arteries. Because the aneurysms are located at the base of the brain, occlusion of these small penetrating arteries can cause infarctions that produce serious neurological sequelae. Other neurological complications include brain hemorrhage, cerebral infarc-

tion, or severe cerebral edema. Most neurosurgeons do intraoperative or postoperative angiograms to assess the adequacy of occlusion; on occasion, the clip will not have completely occluded the aneurysmal neck. Fracture or slippage of the clip is a potential but rare long-term cause of treatment failure. Modern aneurysm clips are not ferromagnetic and thus, follow-up MRI can be performed. Occasionally, the surgeon is unable to clip the aneurysm and wrapping of the aneurysm will be performed. The goal of the wrapping is to buttress the aneurysmal wall. This procedure does not eliminate communication between the aneurysmal sac and the arterial circulation.

Endovascular placement of a balloon, coil, or a thrombogenic agent is used to occlude the aneurysm or parent artery.[82–84] Technical advances are increasing the role of endovascular therapy. Endovascular procedures now are recommended to occlude aneurysms that are not easy to treatment with direct clipping of the aneurysm. In particular, aneurysms of the middle cerebral artery and posterior circulation, especially the basilar bifurcation, are treated with coiling.[85–88] A recent clinical trial demonstrated that endovascular treatment is superior to surgical clipping for management of most patients with ruptured aneurysms.[84] The role of endovascular treatment likely will expand during the next few years and it may become the intervention of choice to prevent recurrent rupture.

▶ OTHER INTRACRANIAL ANEURYSMS

With the exception of dissecting and dolichoectatic aneurysms, nonsaccular aneurysms usually are located on superficial branches of either the major cerebral arteries or the basilar artery (see Table 15-1). Other than dolichoectatic or dissecting aneurysms, most of these abnormalities are smaller is size than saccular aneurysms. Most of these aneurysms are fusiform in shape although a saccular component can be visualized. Multiple aneurysms might be found. Nonsaccular aneurysms are classified as false aneurysms in that all three layers of the arterial wall might not be present within the lesion. For example, the external wall of a dissecting aneurysm does not have a tunica intima. In addition, aneurysms secondary to an infection or tumor are the result of an ongoing destruction of the arterial wall. Because these aneurysms usually have major intramural structural abnormalities, the risk of rupture is high. Still, because of their relative infrequency, rupture of a nonsaccular aneurysm is an uncommon cause of intracranial hemorrhage. However, bleeding due to a nonsaccular aneurysm should be suspected if the patient's clinical presentation is atypical or if the patient has other evidence pointing to an infection, tumor, or recent trauma. In addition, a nonsaccular aneurysm should be suspected if the bleeding is primarily located in peripheral subarachnoid spaces.

Infective Aneurysms

Infections probably are the most common cause of nonsaccular aneurysms. The aneurysms presumably develop at the site of a septic embolus that lodges in a distal intracranial artery.[89] A local suppurative process weakens the arterial wall and leads to development of the aneurysm. Because of the destructive nature of the infection, the risk of bleeding is considerable. Most infective (mycotic) aneurysms are secondary to bacteria and usually are in the setting of infective endocarditis. Streptococcal and staphylococcal infections are the most commonly implicated bacterial organisms. Fungal aneurysms also can occur; aspergillus is the most likely organism. Evaluation of the intracranial vasculature will demonstrates aneurysms in as many as 4–15 percent of persons with infective endocarditis.[90,91] Ischemic stroke is the most common neurological presentation of infective endocarditis but headaches or seizures can be the other presenting symptoms. Hemorrhage usually does not occur early in the course of infective endocarditis. However, as the result of the high risk of bleeding, most patients with infective endocarditis are not treated with anticoagulants. Because of the potential for complicating aneurysms, arteriography is recommended to evaluate a patient who develops neurological symptoms secondary to infective endocarditis. Sequential studies might be needed to assess the evolution of the aneurysm; enlargement of the lesion usually prompts endovascular or neurosurgical treatment. In addition, antibiotics are the key medical therapy to treat infective aneurysms.

Besides infective endocarditis, infective aneurysms can complicate bacterial meningitis, cavernous sinus thrombosis, cortical thrombophlebitis, skull osteomyelitis, pneumonia, or other septic disease. Infective aneurysms of several microbiological causes also can be found among persons intravenously injecting illegal drugs. Fungal aneurysms are found among persons who have immune deficiencies including those who have had renal or other organ transplantation, malignancy, or AIDS.

Tumor Aneurysms

Neoplastic aneurysms are most commonly detected among patients who have either metastatic choriocarcinoma or an atrial myxoma.[92–94] In the latter situation, some cases are diagnosed after discovery of the cardiac tumor. Less commonly, aneurysmal formation can complicate other metastatic tumors. Presumably, neoplastic cells are shed in the arterial circulation and these cells become implanted in the distal intracranial arteries. The tumor grows within the artery to form the aneurysm. Surgical resection of the aneurysm is the usual management. On occasion, the neoplastic aneurysm might regress after management of the primary tumor. The utility of either radiation therapy or chemotherapy for the management of neoplastic intracranial aneurysms is not established.

Traumatic Aneurysms

Most patients with traumatic aneurysms are children or young men who have had closed head injury. In addition, aneurysms can complicate a penetrating head injury or follow nasal or transsphenoidal surgery.[95] Traumatic aneurysms are described as an important complication of gunshot wounds or other missile injuries. The usual location is on a pial branch cortical artery. They also can be located on the meningeal branches of the external carotid artery. Traumatic aneurysms are uncommon in the posterior circulation. The mechanism of the aneurysm formation presumably involves a direct injury to the arterial wall that forms an area of weakness, which serves as the nidus for the aneurysm. Rupture of a traumatic aneurysm can explain an intracranial hemorrhage that occurs several days or weeks after the original head injury. Rupture of a traumatic aneurysm of a meningeal artery might produce an acute epidural hematoma. Besides causing intracranial hemorrhage, enlargement of a traumatic aneurysm might lead to cranial nerve palsies. Recurrent epistaxis has been described as a complication of a traumatic aneurysm at the base of skull. Because of the high risk for aneurysm formation and bleeding, arteriography often is recommended as part of the evaluation of a patient with a penetrating head injury. As with other nonsaccular aneurysms, endovascular or neurosurgical obliteration is the main treatment option.

Fusiform Aneurysms

Most fusiform (dolichoectatic) aneurysms do not produce intracranial bleeding (see Chapter 9). However, the rare cases of hemorrhage usually are catastrophic. While the basilar artery is most commonly affected, the distal portions of the internal carotid arteries and the proximal segments of the middle cerebral arteries often are implicated (Figs. 15-9 and 15-10). While many of these lesions probably are secondary to atherosclerosis, fusiform aneurysms also have been described as complications of diseases of collagen metabolism. Fusiform aneurysms usually can be identified as a large mass in the prepontine cistern, which can be readily visualized by CT or MRI. Arteriography, CTA, and MRA also can be used to examine the abnormality. Treatment has focused on medical management but surgical resection has been applied. Endovascular treatment involves placement of a stent to recreate a normal caliber arterial lumen and possibly combined with coiling to promote extraluminal thrombosis.

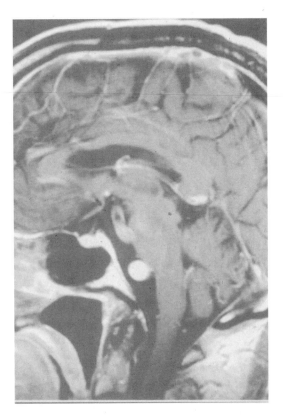

Figure 15-9. A mid sagittal T-1 weighted MRI shows a fusiform aneurysm of the basilar artery.

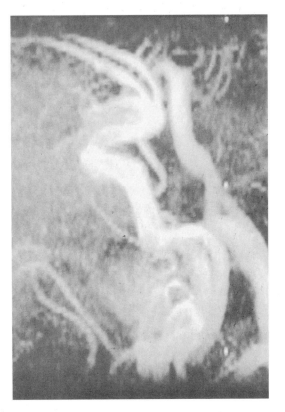

Figure 15-10. An axial CT angiography shows a large basilar artery. The finding is compatible with a fusiform aneurysm.

Dissecting Aneurysms

While dissection of intracranial arteries can cause ischemic stroke, subarachnoid hemorrhage can be secondary to a dissecting aneurysm that arises on the vertebral, basilar, distal internal carotid, or middle cerebral arteries[96–99] (see Chapter 10). These lesions often arise in locations close to those where saccular aneurysms usually are found. Features that help differentiate the dissecting aneurysm include its smaller diameter, fusiform appearance, and location other than at vascular bifurcations. The prognosis of patients with subarachnoid hemorrhage is poor. While intracranial dissection can occur spontaneously, most cases follow mild closed craniocerebral trauma. Dissection of the distal vertebral artery, which leads to the subarachnoid hemorrhage, can occur with chiropractic manipulation or other maneuvers that involve hyperextension or rotation of the neck. Overall, management is similar to that prescribed to persons with hemorrhage secondary to ruptured saccular aneurysms.

Other Causes of Intracranial Aneurysms

Aneurysms have been reported as a rare complication of radiation therapy, Behçet disease, and inflammatory vasculopathies. Exceptional cases of aneurysms developing years following radiation treatment of medulloblastoma or craniopharyngioma have been reported. Rarely, patients with systemic lupus erythematosus, Takayasu disease, giant cell arteritis, Wegener granulomatosis, or primary central nervous system vasculitis can have an intracranial aneurysm and subarachnoid hemorrhage. Both saccular and nonsaccular aneurysms can be found among patients with moyamoya disease.

▶ VASCULAR MALFORMATIONS

Vascular malformations are a leading cause of intracranial hemorrhage. Stapf et al.[100] estimated that the incidence of hemorrhage from a vascular malformation among adults is 0.55 per 100,000 person-years. Bleeding from a ruptured vascular malformation occurs in children and men and women of any age. However, vascular malformations are an especially important cause of hemorrhage in children and young adults.[30] The frequency of hemorrhage secondary to a vascular malformation peaks in the fourth decade of life.

Pathogenesis and Pathological Classification

These lesions are presumed to be congenital in origin. Vascular malformations are classified based on the nature of the vessels including in the lesion[101] (see Table 15-2).

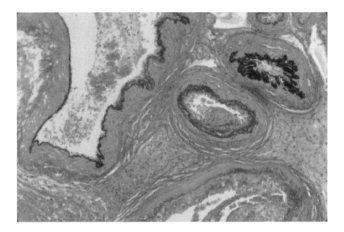

Figure 15-11. Elastic stained surgical specimen demonstrates both arterial and venous structures. The findings are consistent with an arteriovenous malformation. (*Courtesy of S.S. Schochet, M.D., Department of Pathology, University of West Virginia, Morgantown WV*)

Arteriovenous Malformation

The most common is the *arteriovenous malformation*, which includes arterial elements, a node of dysplastic vessels, which is intermixed with gliotic brain tissue, and dilated, arterialized veins (Fig. 15-11). The prevalence of arteriovenous malformations is estimated to be approximately 1.12/100,000.[102] The size of these lesions can vary from <1 cm in diameter to a malformation that affects most of a cerebral hemisphere. In some patients, multiple arterial branches arising from both the carotid and vertebrobasilar circulations can be found (Fig. 15-12). Branches of the external carotid artery also can supply the malformation. Todaka et al.[103] recently demonstrated that a high mean-transient time detected by blood flow tests could demonstrate a dysequilibrium between flow into the nidus from outflow. These lesions usually have a high flow and venous drainage usually is via one dilated vein. Bleeding usually occurs on the venous side of the lesion and it probably reflects increased pressure within the draining vein.[103] Hemorrhage may be more frequent among those arteriovenous malformations that are small or located deep in the cerebral hemispheres.[104] Arteriovenous malformations can grow during life and thrombosis can occur within the lesion.

Venous Malformation

Venous malformations have only venous elements and have a relatively slow flow (Fig. 15-13). These lesions usually are located in the white matter of the cerebral hemispheres. Their prevalence is estimated to be 0.43/100,000.[102,105]

Cavernous Malformation

A *cavernous malformation* consists primarily of dilated venous structures (Figs. 15-14 to 15-17). The prevalence of this vascular anomaly is estimated to be 0.56/100,000.[102,105] Flow is slow in these lesions and as a result they often are described as arteriographically occult. Bleeding from a venous or cavernous malformation is relatively low.

Telangiectasis

Telangiectases are primarily of capillary origin and are very small. Many patients will have multiple venous or cavernous malformations or telangiectases but arteriovenous malformations usually are solitary.

Other Malformations

A vein of Galen aneurysm is a vascular malformation that is associated with dilation of the vessel, which produces symptoms in primarily infancy and childhood. While vascular malformations can be located anywhere in the central nervous system, approximately 90 percent are found in the cerebral hemispheres. These lesions can extend into the ventricles or the subarachnoid space. *Dural fistulas or vascular malformations* can

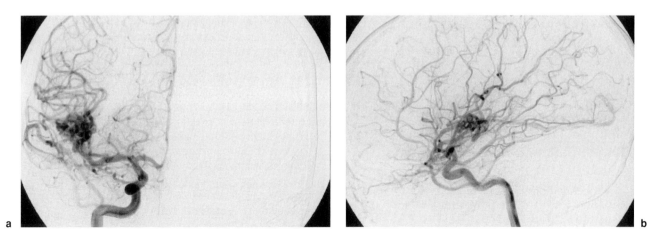

Figure 15-12. Lateral and anterior posterior views of a right carotid arteriogram reveal a large temporal arteriovenous malformation.

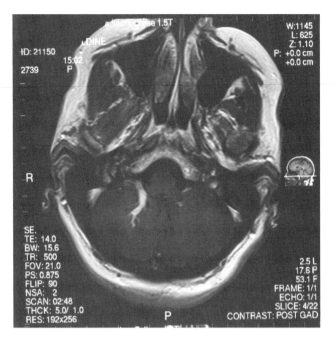

Figure 15-13. Axial view of a contrast-enhanced T-1 weighted MRI study of the posterior fossa reveals a large draining vein in a patient with a venous malformation of the cerebellum.

arise in the meninges (Fig. 15-18). The location of vascular malformation, the number of feeding vessels, and the size of the lesion are using in systems that help neurosurgeons decide about surgical resection.

Associated Diseases

Familial aggregations of vascular malformations have been reported. An especially high rate of vascular mal-

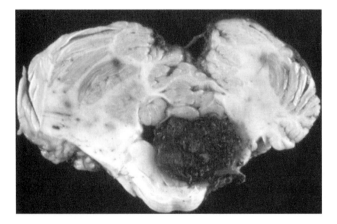

Figure 15-14. Sagittal autopsy specimen of the pons and cerebellum shows a large cavernous vascular malformation arising in the pontine tegmentum of the left. (*Courtesy of S.S. Schochet, M.D., Department of Pathology, University of West Virginia, Morgantown WV*)

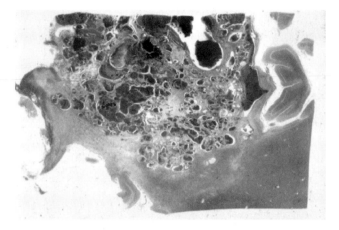

Figure 15-15. Microscopic findings of the cavernous malformation (shown in Fig. 14) demonstrate multiple dilated veins. (*Courtesy of S.S. Schochet, M.D., Department of Pathology, University of West Virginia, Morgantown WV*)

formations has been reported in Hispanic Americans.[106] Families of other ethnic groups also have been reported. In general, familial vascular malformations are associated with symptoms at a younger age and multiple lesions often are found. Multiple, small vascular malformations of the brain can occur in *hereditary hemorrhagic telangiectasia (Rendu–Osler–Weber disease)* or *Klippel—Trenaunay–Weber* disease[107–109] (see Chapter 12).

Clinical Presentations

Intracranial hemorrhage is the presenting symptom of a vascular malformation in almost one-half of cases[30] (Table 15-5). The average age of persons with hemorrhage from a vascular malformation is approximately 30.[110] The annual risk of bleeding from an intact arteriovenous malformation is estimated to be 2–4 percent.[111–113] The annual mortality from ruptured vascular malformations is approximately 1 percent and the combined morbidity and mortality is approximately 2.7 percent. The chances of hemorrhage from an intact venous or cavernous malformation are much lower for an arteriovenous malformation. The risk of bleeding appears to

▶ **TABLE 15-5.** PRESENTATIONS OF VASCULAR MALFORMATIONS

Intracranial hemorrhage
   Intracerebral hemorrhage
   Intraventricular hemorrhage
Recurrent migraine
Seizures
Progressive worsening—focal neurological impairments
Audible bruit—pulsatile tinnitus
Enlarging head (infants)
High-output cardiac failure (infants)

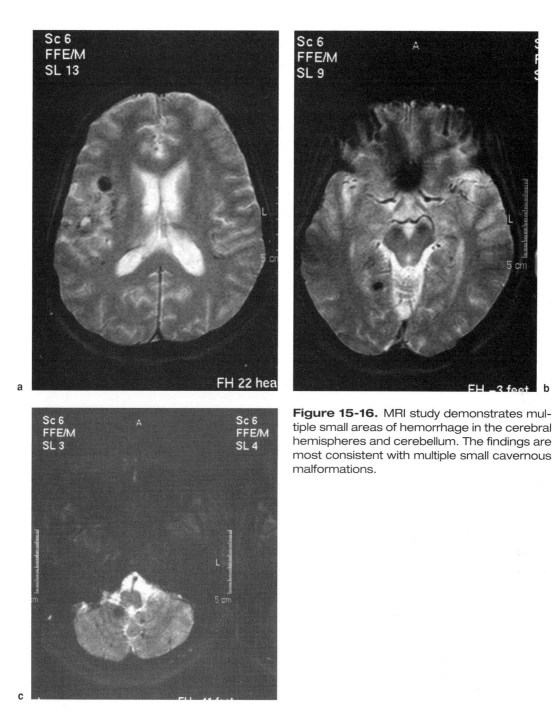

Figure 15-16. MRI study demonstrates multiple small areas of hemorrhage in the cerebral hemispheres and cerebellum. The findings are most consistent with multiple small cavernous malformations.

be greater among persons with posterior fossa vascular malformations, those with large deep draining veins, and those with associated aneurysms. The risk of hemorrhage appears to be increased during pregnancy and childbirth.

Bleeding from a vascular malformation is located primarily within the parenchyma but subarachnoid hemorrhage or primary intraventricular hemorrhage also occurs.[114] A ruptured vascular malformation also should be sought whenever a hemorrhage is located in the deep white matter of the cerebral hemisphere, particularly if

the patient does not have a history of hypertension. The likelihood of a vascular malformation as a cause of hemorrhage is increased if the patient has a past history of headaches or seizures.

The likelihood of a second rupture within the first days following hemorrhage is relatively low. The overall risk of a second hemorrhage is approximately 6–10 percent during the first year and subsequently, the annual risk of rebleeding is approximately 3 percent.[111] Mast et al.[111] noted that the risk of recurrent hemorrhage was higher among men than among women. The risk of

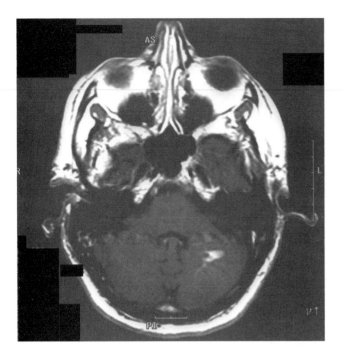

Figure 15-17. Enhanced MRI study reveals a cavernous malformation of the cerebellum.

recurrent bleeding seems to be increased if the malformation involves the basal ganglia or the thalamus.

Recurrent headaches, which have many of the features of migraine, can be the initial symptom of a vascular malformation or fistula.[110] In differentiation to migraine, the unilateral headaches are persistently on one side of the head. Presumably the headaches are due to vascular congestion or increased flow through the malformation. Approximately 30 percent of patients have generalized seizures and 10 percent have focal seizures either as the initial symptom or subsequently in the course of the illness.[110] Seizures are secondary to scarring cerebral tissue adjacent to the malformation. Some patients with a high-flow malformation will report hearing a pulsatile sound (audible tinnitus) in their heads. They will report that the swishing sound is in synchrony with their pulse. The bruit usually can be auscultated and depending upon the location of the malformation, it can be heard over the neck, orbit, temple, occiput, or mastoid region. A large arteriovenous malformation with high flow can steal blood from normal neural tissue, which can cause focal neurological signs that gradually progress. The focal neurological worsening presumably is secondary to ischemia. In addition, infants with large, high-flow, vascular malformations can have increase in head circumference or intractable heart failure.[115]

Diagnostic Studies

While hemorrhages secondary to a ruptured vascular malformation can be located anywhere in the brain, imaging usually demonstrates the bleeding to be close to the cortical rim in the lobar white matter of the cerebral hemispheres (Fig. 15-19; see Chapter 8). Contrast-enhanced CT often visualizes the large feeding and draining vessels, especially if the malformation is larger than 2.5 cm. Smaller vascular malformations, including venous or cavernous malformations, also can be shown

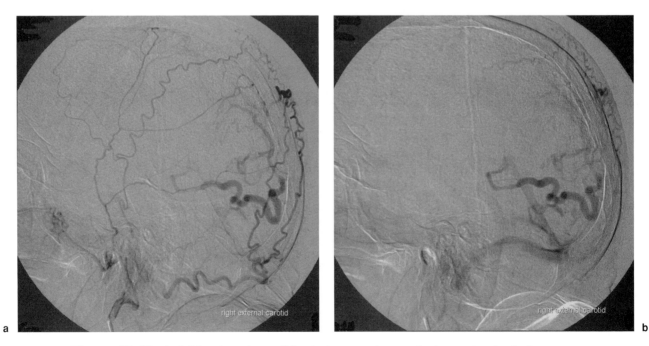

Figure 15-18. A right external carotid arteriogram demonstrates a dural arteriovenous fistula.

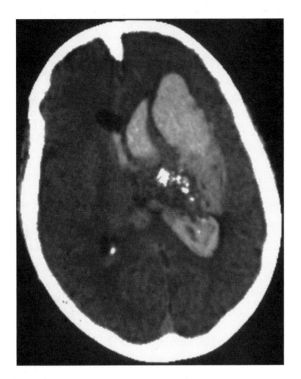

Figure 15-19. A CT scan obtained in a patient with a major left hemisphere hemorrhage. The areas of calcification suggest an underlying vascular malformation.

on CT. The yield of MRI generally is greater (Fig. 15-20). Besides displaying a hematoma, MRI usually visualizes the large flow voids representing the arteries and veins associated with the malformation. MRI also readily detects cavernous and venous malformations. Neither

CT nor MRI is particularly successful in finding small telangiectases.

Single photon emission computed tomography or positron emission tomography might be used to measure the degree of blood flow through the lesion and in adjacent areas of the brain. The vascular malformation often is found as an area of hyperdynamic flow and hyperperfusion with adjacent areas of hypoperfusion, which might represent areas of steal. Arteriography, CTA, or MRA are used to evaluate the vascular anatomy (Fig. 15-21). Because of the high flow of some of the arteriovenous anomalies or fistulas, rapid sequence studies usually are performed to evaluate the size and location of the malformation and the number and types of feeding arteries (see Fig. 15-12). Slow-flow lesions, such as a cavernous malformation, might be occult to arteriography and CT or MRI often better detects them. In some patients, the vascular malformation might be obliterated at the time of the hemorrhage.

Treatment

Depending upon the clinical findings, options for treatment include surgical resection, endovascular interventions, or focused radiation therapy with the goal of achieving complete obliteration of the vascular lesion[116] (see Chapter 23). In addition, medical measures include anticonvulsants and symptomatic medications. No medical therapy is available to reduce the size of a vascular malformation. While no evidence exists that antihypertensive medications lessen the risk of hemorrhage, lowering the blood pressure probably is reasonable, especially if

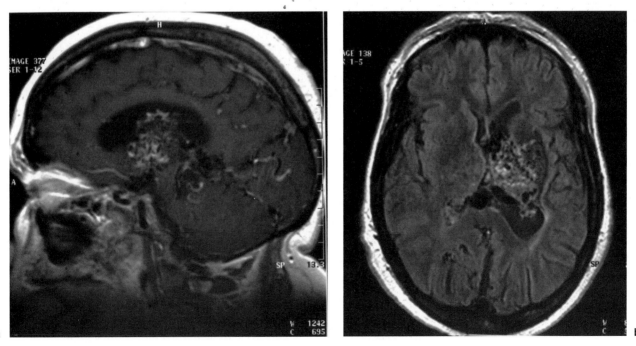

Figure 15-20. (a) Sagittal and (b) axial views of the MRI reveal a large deep left hemisphic vascular malformation primarily located in the thalamus.

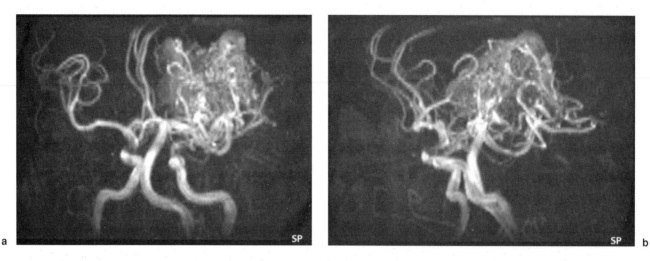

Figure 15-21. (a) Anteroposterior and (b) lateral views of an MRA demonstrate a large left hemisphere arteriovenous malformation.

the patient has hypertension. The presumed pathological type, size, and location of the malformation and the number of feeding and draining vessels influence decisions[117] (Table 15-6). The components of commonly used rating scales used by neurosurgeons to decide about surgery are listed in Table 15-6. In general, surgery becomes more difficult when a patient has 2 or more points calculated on this scale. Because of the relatively low risk for early recurrent bleeding, most interventions aimed at obliterating the malformation are not prescribed immediately after the initial hemorrhage. In addition, a lag permits improvement in the patient's condition and allows for resolution of the hematoma; which makes surgical excision somewhat easier.

The desired surgical treatment has been operative resection of the malformation (see Chapter 23). It has the advantage of immediate cure and eliminating the risk of hemorrhage. A postoperative arteriogram is performed to ascertain whether any remnant of the malformation is present. In general, surgery is recommended for small-to-moderate sized malformations located near the cortical surface, especially if they are located at the poles. Operative treatment of malformations located deep in the hemisphere or the brain stem is difficult. Factors that are important in influencing a decision for operative resection include the (1) the patient's age and overall health, (2) the presence of a concomitant saccular aneurysm, (3) the pattern of flow in the lesion, (4) the availability of a skilled surgeon, and (5) the wishes of the patient.

Alternatives to surgery include endovascular administration of sclerotic or thrombophilic agents (cyanoacrylate or polyvinyl alcohol), placement of coils or particles that serve as nidus for thrombosis, or insertion of balloons that occlude the major feeding arteries[118–125] (see Chapter 23). In general this intervention should be considered as adjunctive. Endovascular treatment can be done in conjunction with surgery or focused irradiation.

Focused, high-intensity radiation can be administered to cause sclerosis of a small vascular malformation[126–129] (see Chapter 23). A lag of approximately 2 years from the radiation until the vascular malformation is obliterated means the patient is at risk for recurrent hemorrhage during this interval. Some instances of recurrent AVM following radiation therapy have been reported.[130]

▶ ARTERIOVENOUS FISTULAS

The prevalence of arteriovenous fistulas is estimated as 0.16/100,000.[102] They can be either congenital or acquired. In the latter circumstances, a puncture wound allows a direct arterial-venous connection. A spontaneous

▶ **TABLE 15-6.** SCORING SYSTEM FOR DECISIONS ABOUT SURGICAL RESECTION OF VASCULAR MALFORMATIONS

Size of vascular malformation	
<3 cm	1 point
3–6 cm	2 points
>6 cm	3 points
Draining veins	
Superficial veins present	0 point
Deep veins present	1 point
Location of vascular malformation	
Noneloquent location	0 point
Eloquent location	1 point

Adapted from Spetzler and Martin.[117]

tear in an artery leading to a direct connection with an adjacent vein also can occur. These vascular abnormalities most commonly arise in the cavernous sinus, anterior fossa, tentorium, or the posterior fossa. Dural arteriovenous fistulas can drain into cortical veins or directly into the major sinuses—the most common being the transverse or sigmoid sinuses. Intracerebral, subarachnoid, or subdural hemorrhage can occur. These lesions can produce recurrent headaches, seizures, an audible bruit, or focal neurological impairment. Cranial and vascular imaging will detect a fistula. Because dural fistulas often receive blood primarily via meningeal collaterals, a selective injection of the external carotid artery often is needed to ascertain the extent of the lesion. Management options include surgical resection of the lesion or endovascular obliteration using techniques similar to those applied to arteriovenous malformations.

Carotid-cavernous Fistula

A *carotid-cavernous fistula* usually presents with a unilateral throbbing headache, proptosis, and conjunctival injection (Table 15-7). Paralysis of the oculomotor, trochlear, abducens, and ophthalmic branch of the trigeminal nerve can be detected along with a pulsatile orbital bruit. Because the progressive orbital edema, patients also can have visual loss. In most cases, the lesion follows a closed head injury. Spontaneous fistulas also can happen. The abnormality is detected readily by CTA, MRA, or arteriography. Because of the prominent symptoms and the potential for visual loss, obliteration of the carotid-cavernous fistula by endovascular procedures is recommended. Balloons may be placed in the internal carotid artery above and below the fistula to isolate the lesion. The resultant occlusion can be complicated by an ipsilateral cerebral infarction.

▶ **TABLE 15-7.** CLINICAL FINDINGS
CAROTID-CAVERNOUS FISTULA

Unilateral throbbing headache
Eye findings
   Proptosis
   Conjunctival injection
   Orbital edema
   Visual loss
Cranial nerve palsies
   Oculomotor (III, IV, and VI)
   Ophthalmic division of V
Orbital or cranial bruit (pulsatile tinnitus)
   Beçhet disease
   Diamond–Blackfan syndrome
   Klippel–Trenaunay–Weber syndrome

REFERENCES

1. McCormick WF, Schochet SS, Jr. *Atlas of Cerebrovascular Disease.* Philadelphia, PA: WB Saunders Co; 1976:
2. Miyazawa N, Akiyama I, Yamagata Z, Risk factors for growth of unruptured intracranial aneurysms. Follow-up study by serial 0.5 T magnetic resonance angiography. *Neurosurgery* 2006;58:1047–1053.
3. Krischek B, Inoue I. The genetics of intracranial aneurysms. *J Hum Genet* 2006;51:587–594.
4. Leblanc R. Familial cerebral aneurysms: a bias for women. *Stroke* 1996;27:1050–1054.
5. Ronkainen A, Hernesniemi J, Puranen M, et al. Familial intracranial aneurysms. *Lancet* 1997;349:380–384.
6. Raaymakers TWM. Aneurysms in relatives of patients with subarachnoid hemorrhage: frequency and risk factors. MARS Study Group. Magnetic Resonance Angiography in relatives of patients with subarachnoid hemorrhage. *Neurology* 1999;53:982–988.
7. Kim DH, Van Ginhoven G, Milewicz DM. Incidence of familial intracranial aneurysms in 200 patients: comparison among Caucasian, African-American, and Hispanic populations. *Neurosurgery* 2003;53:302–308.
8. Gaist D, Vaeth M, Tsiropoulos I, et al. Risk of subarachnoid haemorrhage in first degree relatives of patients with subarachnoid haemorrhage: follow up study based on national registries in Denmark. *BMJ* 2000;320:141–145.
9. Raaymakers TW, Rinkel GJ, Ramos LM. Initial and follow-up screening for aneurysms in families with familial subarachnoid hemorrhage. *Neurology* 1998;51:1125–1130.
10. Raaymakers TW, Buys PC, Verbeeten BJ, et al. MR angiography as a screening tool for intracranial aneurysms: feasibility, test characteristics, and interobserver agreement. *Am J Roentgenol* 1999;173:1469–1475.
11. Ronkainen A, Niskanen M, Piironen R, Hernesniemi J. Familial subarachnoid hemorrhage. Outcome study. *Stroke* 1999;30:1099–1102.
12. Connolly ES, Jr., Choudhri TF, Mack WJ, et al. Influence of smoking, hypertension, and sex on the phenotypic expression of familial intracranial aneurysms in siblings. *Neurosurgery* 2001;48:64–69.
13. Kissela BM, Sauerbeck L, Woo D, et al. Subarachnoid hemorhage: a preventable disease with a heritable component. *Stroke* 2002;33:1321–1326.
14. Wills S, Ronkainen A, van der Voet M, et al. Familial intracranial aneurysms. An analysis of 346 multiplex Finnish families. *Stroke* 2003;34:1370–1374.
15. Hofer A, Hermans M, Kubassek N, et al. Elastin polymorphism haplotype and intracranial aneurysms are not associated in Central Europe. *Stroke* 2003;34:1207–1211.
16. Yamada S, Utsunomiya M, Inoue K, et al. Absence of linkage of familial intracranial aneurysms to 7q11 in highly aggregated Japanese families. *Stroke* 2003;34:892–900.
17. Krex D, Ziegler A, Schackert HK, Schackert G. Lack of association between endoglin intron 7 insertion polymorphism and intracranial aneurysms in a white population: evidence of racial/ethnic differences. *Stroke* 2001;32:2689–2694.
18. Keramatipour M, McConnell RS, Kirkpatrick P, Tebbs S, Furlong RA, Rubinsztein DC. The ACE I allele is associated

with increased risk for ruptured intracranial aneurysms. *J Med Genet* 2000;37:498–500.

19. Yoneyama T, Kasuya H, Onda H, et al. Collagen type α 2 (COL1A2) is the susceptible gene for intracranial aneurysms. *Stroke* 2004;35:443–448.

20. Pirson Y, Chauveau D, Torres V. Management of cerebral aneurysms in autosomal dominant polycystic kidney disease. *J Am Soc Nephrol* 2002;13:269–276.

21. Watnick T, Phakdeekitcharoen B, Johnson A, et al. Mutation detection of PKD1 identifies a novel mutation common to three families with aneurysms and/or very-early-onset disease. *Am J Hum Genet* 1999;65:1561–1571.

22. Gieteling EW, Rinkel GJ. Characteristics of intracranial aneurysms and subarachnoid haemorrhage in patients with polycystic kidney disease. *J Neurol* 2003;250:418–423.

23. Connolly HM, Huston J, III, Brown RD, Jr., Warnes CA, Ammash NM, Tajik AJ. Intracranial aneurysms in patients with coarctation of the aorta: a prospective magnetic resonance angiographic study of 100 patients. *Mayo Clin Proc* 2003;78:1491–1499.

24. Schievink WI, Parisi JE, Piepgras DG, Michels VV. Intracranial aneurysms in Marfan's syndrome: an autopsy study. *Neurosurgery* 1997;41:866–870.

25. Hashimoto T, Meng H, Young WL. Intracranial aneurysms: links among inflammation, hemodynamics and vascular remodeling. *Neurol Res* 2006;28:372–380.

26. Schievink WI, Kaufman JA, Piepgras DG, Schaid DJ. Alpha 1-antitypsin phenotypes among patients with intracranial aneurysms. *J Neurosurg* 1996;84:781–784.

27. Schievink WI. Intracranial aneurysms. *N Engl J Med* 1997; 336:25–40.

28. Preul MC, Cendes F, Just N, Mohr G. Intracranial aneurysms and sickle cell anemia: multiplicity and propensity for the vertebrobasilar territory. *Neurosurgery* 1998; 42:971–977.

29. Brown RD, Jr, Wiebers DO, Forbes GS. Unruptured intracranial aneurysms and arteriovenous malformations: frequency of intracranial hemorrhage and relationship of lesions. *J Neurosurg* 1990;73:859–863.

30. Brown RD, Jr., Wiebers DO, Torner JC, O'Fallon WM. Frequency of intracranial hemorrhage as a presenting symptom and subtype analysis: a population-based study of intracranial vascular malformation in Olmsted County, Minnesota. *J Neurosurg* 1996;85:29–32.

31. Ostergaard JR. Headache as a warning symptom of impeding aneurysmal subarachnoid haemorrhage. *Cephalagia* 1991;11:53–55.

32. Jakobsson KE, Saveland H, Hillman J. Warning leak and management outcome in aneurysmal subarachnoid hemorrhage. *J Neurosurg* 1996;85:995–999.

33. Raps EC, Rogers JD, Galetta SL. The clinical spectrum of unruptured intracranial aneurysms. *Arch Neurol* 1993;50: 265–268.

34. Wiebers DO, Whisnant JP, Sundt TM, Jr. The significance of unruptured intracranial saccular aneurysms. *J Neurosurg* 1987;66:23–29.

35. Wiebers DO, Piepgras DG, Brown RD, Jr., et al. Unruptured aneurysms. *J Neurosurg* 2002;96:50–51.

36. Wiebers DO, Whisnant JP, Huston J, III, et al. Unruptured intracranial aneurysms: natural history, clinical outcome,

and risks of surgical and endovascular treatment. *Lancet* 2003;362:103–110.

37. Juvela S. Unruptured aneurysms. *J Neurosurg* 2002;96: 58–60.

38. Tuffiash E, Tamargo RJ, Hillis AE. Craniotomy for treatment of unruptured aneurysms is not associated with long-term cognitive dysfunction. *Stroke* 2003;34:2195–2199.

39. Brilstra EH, Rinkel GJE, Van Der Graaf Y, et al. Quality of life after treatment of unruptured intracranial aneurysms by neurosurgical clipping or by emolisation with coils. A prospetive, observational study. *Cerebrovasc Dis* 2004;17: 44–52.

40. International Study of Unruptured Intracranial Aneurysms Investigators. Unruptured intracranial aneurysms–risk of rupture and risks of surgical intervention. *N Engl J Med* 1998;339:1725–1733.

41. Hoh BL, Rabinov JD, Pryor JC, Carter BS, Barker FG, II. In-hospital morbidity and mortality after endovascular treatment of unruptured intracranial aneurysms in the United States, 1996–2000: effect of hospital and physician volume. *Am J Neuroradiol* 2003;24:1409–1420.

42. Barker FG 2nd, Amin-Hanjani S, Butler WE, Ogilvy CS, Carter BS. In-hospital morality and morbidity after surgical treatment of unruptured intracranial aneurysms in the united states, 1996–2000: the effect of hospital and surgeon volume. *Neurosurgery* 2003;52:995–1009.

43. Rasmussen PA, Mayberg MR. Defining the natural history of unruptured aneurysms. *Stroke* 2004;35:232–233.

44. Thrift A, Donnan G, McNeil J. Heavy drinking, but not moderate or intermediate drinking, increases the risk of intracerebral hemorrhage. *Epidemiology* 1999;10: 307–312.

45. Weir BK, Kongable GL, Kassell NF, Schultz JR, Truskowski LL, Sigrest A. Cigarette smoking as a cause of aneurysmal subarachnoid hemorrhage and risk for vasospasm: a report of the Cooperative Aneurysm Study. *J Neurosurg* 1998;89:405–411.

46. Juvela R, Hillborn M, Palomaki H. Risk factors for spontaneous intracerebral hemorrhage. *Stroke* 1995;26:1558–1564.

47. Leppala JM, Paunio M, Virtamo J, et al. Alcohol consumption and stroke incidence in male smokers. *Circulation* 1999;100:1209–1214.

48. Oyesiku NM, Colohan ART, Barrow DL, Etal X. Cocaine-induced aneurysmal rupture: an emergent negative factor in the natural history of intracranial aneurysms. *Neurosurgery* 1993;32:518–526.

49. Nanda A, Vannemreddy PS, Polin RS, Willis BK. Intracranial aneurysms and cocaine abuse: analysis of prognostic indicators. *Neurosurgery* 2000;46:1063–1067.

50. Schwartz SM, Petitti DB, Siscovick DS, et al. Stroke and use of low-dose oral contraceptives in young women: a pooled analysis of two US studies. *Stroke* 1998;29:2277–2284.

51. Johnston SC, Colford JMJ, Gress DR. Oral contraceptives and the risk of subarachnoid hemorrhage: a meta-analysis. *Neurology* 1998;51:411–418.

52. Mayberg MR, Batjer HH, Dacey R, et al. Guidelines for the management of aneurysmal subarachnoid hemorrhage. A statement for healthcare professionals from a special writing group of the Stroke Council, American Heart Association. *Stroke* 1994;25:2315–2328.

53. Broderick JP, Adam SA, Mann JI. Initial and recurrent bleeding are the major causes of death following subarachnoid hemorrhage. *Stroke* 1994;25:1342–1347.

54. Ostbye T, Levy AR, Mayo NE. Hospitalization and case-fatality rates for subarachnoid hemorrhage in Canada from 1982 through 1991. The Canadian Collaborative Study Group of Stroke Hospitalizations. *Stroke* 1997;28: 793–798.

55. Truelsen T, Bonita R, Duncan J, Anderson NE, Mee E. Changes in subarachnoid hemorrhage mortality, incidence, and case fatality in New Zealand between 1981–1983 and 1991–1993. *Stroke* 1998;29:2298–2303.

56. Olafsson E, Hauser WA, Gudmundsson G. A population-based study of prognosis of ruptured cerebral aneurysm: mortality and recurrence of subarachnoid hemorrhage. *Neurology* 1997;48:1191–1195.

57. Hop JW, Rinkel GJ, Algra A, van Gijn J. Case-fatality rates and functional outcome after subarachnoid hemorrhage: a systematic review. *Stroke* 1997;28:660–664.

58. Cesarini KG, Hardemark H-G, Persson L. Improved survival after aneurysmal subarachnoid hemorrhage: review of case management during a 12-year period. *J Neurosurg* 1999;90:664–672.

59. Schievink WI, Wijdicks EFM, Parisi JE. Sudden death from aneurysmal subarachnoid hemorrhage. *Neurology* 1995; 45:871–874.

60. Arboix A, Marti-Vilalta JL. Predictive clinical factors of very early in-hospital mortality in subarachnoid hemorrhage. *Clin Neurol Neurosurg* 1999;101:100–105.

61. LeRoux PD, Elliott JP, Newell DW. Predicting outcome in poor-grade patients with subarachnoid hemorrhage: a retrospective review of 159 aggressively managed cases. *J Neurosurg* 1996;85:39–49.

62. Adams HP, Jr., Kassell NF, Torner JC. CT and clinical correlations in recent aneurysmal subarachnoid hemorrhage: a preliminary report of the Cooperative Aneurysm Study. *Neurology* 1983;33:981–988.

63. Schievink WI, Wijdicks EFM, Piepgras DG. The poor prognosis of ruptured intracranial aneurysms of the posterior circulation. *J Neurosurg* 1995;82:791–795.

64. Torner JC, Kassell NF, Wallace RB. Preoperative prognostic factors for rebleeding and survival in aneurysm patients receiving fibrinolytic therapy: report of the Cooperative Aneurysm Study. *Neurosurgery* 1981;9: 506–513.

65. Hellawell DJ, Taylor R, Pentland B. Persisting symptoms and carers' views of outcome after subarachnoid haemorrhage. *Clin Rehabil* 1999;13:333–340.

66. Hutter BO, Kreitschmann-Andermahr I, Gilsbach JM. Cognitive deficits in the acute stage after subarachnoid hemorrhage. *Neurosurgery* 1998;43:1054–1065.

67. Hutter BO, Kreitschmann-Andermahr I, Mayfrank L, Rohde V, Spetzger U, Gilsbach JM. Functional outcome after aneurysmal subarachnoid hemorrhage. *Acta Neurochir Suppl* 1999;72:157–174.

68. Hackett ML, Anderson CS. Health outcomes 1 year after subarachnoid hemorrhage: an international population-based study. The Australian Cooperative Research on Subarachnoid Hemorrhage Study Group. *Neurology* 2000; 55:658–662.

69. Franke CL, van Swieten JC, Algra A. Prognostic factors in patients with intracerebral haematoma. *J Neurol Neurosurg Psychiatry* 1992;55:653–657.

70. Fujii Y, Takeuchi S, Sasaki O. Ultra-early rebleeding in spontaneous subarachnoid hemorrhage. *Neurosurgery* 1996;84:35–42.

71. Vermuelen M, van Gijn J, Hijdra A. Causes of acute deterioration inpatients with a ruptured intracranial aneurysm. *J Neurosurg* 1984;60:935–939.

72. Vermuelen M, Lindsay KW, Murray GD. Antifibrinolytic treatment in subarachnoid hemorrhage. *N Engl J Med* 1984;311:432–437.

73. Kassell NF, Torner JC, Adams HP, Jr. Antifibrinolytic therapy in the acute period following aneurysmal subarachnoid hemorrhage. Preliminary observations form the Cooperative Aneurysm Study. *J Neurosurg* 1984;61: 225–230.

74. Roos Y, Rinkel G, Vermeulen M, Algra A, van Gijn J. Antifibrinolytic therapy for aneurysmal subarachnoid hemorrhage. A major update of a Cochrane review. *Stroke* 2003;34:2308–2309.

75. Roos Y, for the STAR Study Group. Antifibrinolytic treatment in subarachnoid hemorrhage. A randomized placebo-controlled trial. *Neurology* 2000;54:77–82.

76. Leipzig TJ, Redelman K, Horner TG. Reducing the risk of rebleeding before early aneurysm surgery: a possible role for antifibrinolytic therapy. *J Neurosurg* 1997;86: 220–225.

77. Roos YB, Beenen LF, Groen RJ, Albrecht KW, Vermeulen M. Timing of surgery in patients with aneurysmal subarachnoid haemorrhage: rebleeding is still the major cause of poor outcome in neurosurgical units that aim at early surgery. *J Neurol Neurosurg Psychiatry* 1997;63: 490–493.

78. Maurice-Williams RS, Wadley JP. Delayed surgery for ruptured intracranial aneurysms: a reappraisal. *Br J Neurosurg* 1997;11:104–109.

79. Lafuente J, Maurice-Williams RS. Ruptured intracranial aneurysms: the outcome of surgical treatment in experienced hands in the period prior to the advent of endovascular coiling. *J Neurol Neurosurg Psychiatry* 2003;74: 1680–1684.

80. Kassell NF, Torner JC, Jane JA, Haley EC, Jr, Adams HP, Jr. The International Cooperative Study on the Timing of Aneurysm Surgery. Part 2: surgical results. *J Neurosurg* 1990;73:37–47.

81. Kassell NF, Torner JC, Haley EC, Jr., Jane JA, Adams HP, Jr., Kongable GL. The International Cooperative Study on the Timing of Aneurysm Surgery. Part 1: overall management results. *J Neurosurg* 1990;73:18–36.

82. Pouratian N, Oskouian RJ Jr, Jensen ME, Kassell NF, Dumont AS. Endovascular management of unruptured intracranial aneurysms. *J Neurol Neurosurg Psych* 2006; 77:572–578.

83. Grunwald IQ, Papanangiotou P, Politi M, et al. Endovascular treatment of unruptured intracranial aneurysms. Occurrence of thromboembolic events. *Neurosurgery* 2006;58:612–618.

84. International Subarchnoid Aneurysm Trial (ISAT) Collaborative Group. International subarachnoid aneurysm trial (ISAT) of neurosurgical clipping versus endovascular

coiling in 2143 patients with ruptured intracranial aneurysms: a randomised trial. *Lancet* 2002;360:1267–1274.

85. Eskridge J, Song J. Endovascular embolization of 150 basilar tip aneurysms with Guglielmi detachable coils: results of the Food and Drug Administration multicenter clinical trial. *J Neurosurg* 1998;89:81–86.

86. Henkes H, Reinartz J, Preiss H, et al. Endovascular treatment of small intracranial aneurysms. Three alternatives to coil occlusion. *Minim Invasive Neurosurg* 2006:49:65–69.

87. Raymond J, Roy D, Leblanc P, et al. Endovascular treatment of intracranial aneurysms with radioactive coils. Initial clinical experience. *Stroke* 2003;34:2801–2806.

88. Tascher CA, Leclerc X, Rachdi H, Barros AM, Pruvo JP. Matrix detachable coils for the endovascular treatment of intracranial aneurysms. Analysis of early angiographic and clinical outcomes. *Stroke* 2005;36:2176–2180.

89. Bakshi R, Wright PD, Kinkel PR, et al. Cranial magnetic resonance imaging findings in bacterial endocarditis: the neuroimaging spectrum of septic brain embolization demonstrated in twelve patients. *J Neuroimaging* 1999;9:78–84.

90. Bohmfalk GL, Story JL, Wissinger JP, et al. Bacterial intracranial aneurysm. *J Neurosurg* 1978;49:369–382.

91. Morawetz RB, Acker JD, Harsh GR, III. Management of mycotic (bacterial) intracranial aneurysms. *Contemp Neurosurg* 1981;3:1–6.

92. Branch CL, Laster W, Kelly DL. Left atrial myxoma with cerebral emboli. *Neurosurgery* 1985;16:675–680.

93. Weir B, Macdonald N, Mielki B. Intracranial vascular complications of choriocarcinoma. *Neurosurgery* 1978;2:138–142.

94. Helmer FA. Oncotic aneursym: case report. *J Neurosurg* 1976;45:98–100.

95. Asari S, Nakamura S, Yamada O, et al. Traumatic aneurysm of peripheral cerebral arteries. *J Neurosurg* 1977;46:795–803.

96. Hosoda K, Fujita S, Kawaguchi T, et al. Spontaneous dissecting aneurysms of the basilar artery presenting with a subarachnoid hemorrhage: report of two cases. *J Neurosurg* 1991;75:628–633.

97. Guridi J, Gallego J, Monzon F, et al. Intracrebral hemorrhage caused by transmural dissection of the anterior cerebral artery. *Stroke* 1993;24:1400–1402.

98. Kaplan SS, Ogilvy CS, Gonzalez R, et al. Extra-cranial vertebral artery pseudoaneurysm presenting as subarachnoid hemorrhage. *Stroke* 1993;24:1397–1399.

99. Sakata N, Takebayashi S, Kojima M, Masawa N, Suzuki K, Takatama M. Pathology of a dissecting intracranial aneurysm. *Neuropathology* 2000;20:104–108.

100. Stapf C, Labowitz DL, Sciacca RR, Mast H, Mohr JP, Sacco RL. Incidence of adult brain arteriovenous malformation hemorrhage in a prospective population-based stroke survey. *Cerebrovasc Dis* 2002;13:43–46.

101. McCormick WF. The pathology of vascular "arteriovenous" malformation. *J Neurosurg* 1966;24:807–816.

102. Al-Shahi R, Bhattacharya JJ, Currie DG, et al. Prospective, population-based detection of intracranial vascular malformations in adults: the Scottish Intracranial Vascular Malformation Study (SIVMS). *Stroke* 2003;34:1163–1169.

103. Todaka T, Hamada J-I, Kai Y, Morioka M, Ushio Y. Analysis of mean transit time of contrast medium in ruptured and unruptured arteriovenous malformations. A digital subtraction angiographic study. *Stroke* 2003;34:2410–2414.

104. Langer DJ, Lasner TM, Hurst RW, Flamm ES, Zager EL, King JT, Jr. Hypertension, small size, and deep venous drainage are associated with risk of hemorrhagic presentation of cerebral arteriovenous malformations. *Neurosurgery* 1998;42:481–486.

105. Al-Shahi R, Warlow CP. Quality of evidence for management of arteriovenous malformations of the brain. *Lancet* 2002;360:1022–1023.

106. Bicknell JM. Familial cavernous angioma of the brain stem dominantly inherited in Hispanics. *Neurosurgery* 1989;24:102–105.

107. Sadick H, Sadick M, Gotte K, et al. Hereditary hemorrhagic telangiectasia. An update on clinical manifestations and diagnostic measures. *Wien Klin Wochenschr* 2006:118:72–80.

108. Petzold A, Bischoff C, Conrad B. Repetitive cerebral bleeding in an adult with Klippel-Trenaunay syndrome. *J Neurol* 2000;247:389–391.

109. Willemse RB, Mager JJ, Westermann CJ, et al. Bleeding risk of cerebrovascular malformations in hereditary hemorrhagic telangiectasia. *J Neurosurg* 2000;92:779–784.

110. Hofmeister C, Stapf C, Hartmann A, et al. Demographic, morphological, and clinical characteristics of 1289 patients with brain arteriovenous malformation. *Stroke* 2000;31:1307–1310.

111. Mast H, Young WL, Koennecke HC, et al. Risk of spontaneous haemorrhage after diagnosis of cerebral arteriovenous malformation. *Lancet* 1997;350:1065–1068.

112. Stapf C, Mast H, Sciacca RR, et al. Predictors of hemorrhage in patients with untreated brain arteriovenous malformations. *Neurology* 2006;66:1350–1355.

113. McLaughlin MR, Kondziolka D, Flickinger JC, Lunsford S, Lunsford LD. The prospective natural history of cerebral venous malformations. *Neurosurgery* 1998;43:195–200.

114. Choi JH, Mast H, Sciacca RR, et al. Clinical outcome after first and recurrent hemorrhage in patients with untreated brain arteriovenous malformation. *Stroke* 2006;37:1243–1247.

115. Fullerton HJ, Aminoff AR, Ferriero DM, Gupta N, Dowd CF. Neurodevelopmental outcome after endovascular treatment of vein of Galen malformations. *Neurology* 2003;61:1386–1390.

116. Stapf C Mohr JP, Choi JH, Hartmann A, Mast H. Invasive treatment of unruptured brain arteriovenous malformations is experimental therapy. *Curr Opin Neurol* 2006;19:63–68.

117. Spetzler RF, Martin NA. A proposed grading system for arteriovenous malformations. *J Neurosurg* 1986;65:476–483.

118. Haw CS, terBrugge K, Willinsky R, Tomlinson G. Complications of embolization of arteriovenous malformations of the brain. *J Neurosurg* 2006;104:226–232.

119. Sugita M, Takahashi A, Ogawa A, et al. Improvement of cerebral blood flow and clinical symptoms associated

with embolization of a large arteriovenous malformation: case report. *Neurosurgery* 1993;33:748–752.

120. Redekop GJ, Elisevich KV, Gaspar LE, et al. Conventional radiation therapy of intracranial arteriovenous malformations: long-term results. *J Neurosurg* 1993;78:413–422.

121. Pollock BE, Lunsford LD, Kondziolka D, et al. Stereotactic radiosurgery for post-geniculate visual pathway arteriovenous malformations. *J Neurosurg* 1996; 84:437–441.

122. Pollock BE, Flickinger JC. A proposed radiosurgery-based grading system for arteriovenous malformations. *J Neurosurg* 2002;96:79–85.

123. Yamamoto M, Jimbo M, Hara M, et al. Gamma knife radiosurgery for arteriovenous malformations: long-term follow-up results focusing on complications occurring more than 5 years after irradiation. *Neurosurgery* 1996;38: 906–914.

124. Gallina P, Merienne L, Meder J, Schlienger M, Lefkopoulos D, Merland J. Failure in radiosurgery treatment of cerebral arteriovenous malformations. *Neurosurgery* 1998;42: 996–1002.

125. Chang HS, Nihei H. Theoretical comparison of surgery and radiosurgery in cerebral arteriovenous malformations. *J Neurosurg* 1999;90:709–719.

126. Kurita H, Kawamoto S, Sasaki T, et al. Results of radiosurgery for brain stem arteriovenous malformations. *J Neurol Neurosurg Psychiatry* 2000;68:563–570.

127. Nakamura N, Shin M, Tago M, et al. Gamma knife radiosurgery for cavernous hemangiomas in the sinus. Report of three cases. *J Neurosurg* 2002;97:477–480.

128. Maruyama K, Shin M, Kurita H, Tago M, Krinio T. Stereotactic radiosurgery for dural arteriovenous fistula involving the superior sagittal sinus. Case report. *J Neurosurg* 2002;97:481–483.

129. Shin M, Kawamoto S, Kurita H, et al. Retrospective analysis of a 10-year experience of stereotactic radiosurgery for arteriovenous malformations in children and adolescents. *J Neurosurg* 2002;97:779–784.

130. Lindqvist M, Karlsson B, Guo WY, Kihlstrom L, Lippitz B, Yamamoto M. Angiographic long-term follow-up data for arteriovenous malformations previously proven to be obliterated after gamma knife radiosurgery. *Neurosurgery* 2000;46:803–808.

CHAPTER 16
Causes of Intracranial Hemorrhage

Intracranial hemorrhages account for approximately 15 percent of all strokes.[1-3] As with cerebral infarctions, the list of causes of bleeding within or adjacent to the brain is extensive (Table 16-1). A number of epidemiological and clinical features influence the differential diagnosis for the cause of the patient's hemorrhage. This list of causes of intracranial bleeding in the elderly differs from the etiologies of hemorrhage in children and young adults.[4-6] For example, cerebral amyloid angiopathy is a leading cause of intracerebral hemorrhage in persons older than 75, while vascular malformations and inherited coagulopathies are relatively more important diagnostic considerations for bleeding in a child. In general, the causes of hemorrhage are similar in men and women, although hemophilia-associated bleeding occurs only in boys while pregnancy-related hemorrhage happens in young women. Some ethnic differences for the causes of hemorrhage also occur; subarachnoid hemorrhage secondary to moyamoya disease is most commonly diagnosed among young adults of Asian heritage, while sickle-cell disease is a potential etiology of subarachnoid hemorrhage in African Americans.[7]

Lifestyle and behavioral activities, which are associated with an increased risk for brain hemorrhage, include alcohol, tobacco, or drug abuse; these conditions are most common among young adults.[8-11] Cases of intracranial hemorrhage complicating vigorous physical activity are reported.[12-15] Sports, work, heavy lifting, and straining at stool, coitus, or an argument are described as provoking events. However, many cases of hemorrhage occur when a person is quiet or inactive. Craniocerebral trauma, which can be relatively occult, is an important potential explanation for hemorrhage in a person for whom no history is available. Acute or chronic hypertension is recognized as a leading risk factor for hemorrhage. The elevated blood pressure can directly lead to rupture of an intracranial artery or the arterial hypertension can prompt bleeding from another pathological process, such as a vascular malformation or aneurysm. Unlike ischemic stroke, some epidemiological evidence shows that the risk of major intracranial bleeding is lower in diabetic patients than in nondiabetic persons. The risk of hemorrhage also might be higher among persons with hypocholesterolemia than among persons with normal-to-high levels of cholesterol.[16,17] Some causes of hemorrhage might be recognized immediately because of a time-related intervention or event, such as administration of a thrombolytic agent, a surgical procedure, or a medical illness, such as leukemia. Acquired or inherited disorders of coagulation that predispose to intracranial bleeding are discussed in Chapter 14. Aneurysms and vascular malformations, which are among the most common causes of bleeding, are described in Chapter 15. Intracranial bleeding can be an important finding of venous sinus thrombosis (see Chapter 18). The other important causes of brain hemorrhage are reviewed in this chapter. Hemorrhages of the spinal cord are described in Chapter 18.

▶ **TABLE 16-1.** CAUSES OF INTRACRANIAL HEMORRHAGE

Craniocerebral trauma	Arterial hypertension
Aneurysm	Chronic
Saccular	Acute
Infective	Eclampsia
Neoplastic	Cerebral amyloid angiopathy
Traumatic	Moyamoya disease
Dissecting	Vasculitis
Fusiform	Multisystem vasculitis
Vascular malformation	Coagulation disorders
Arteriovenous	Leukemia
Cavernous	Thrombocytopenia
Venous	Sickle-cell disease
Telangiectasis	DIC
Arteriovenous fistula	Hemophilia
Venous thrombosis	Antiplatelet agents
Sympathomimetic agents	Anticoagulants

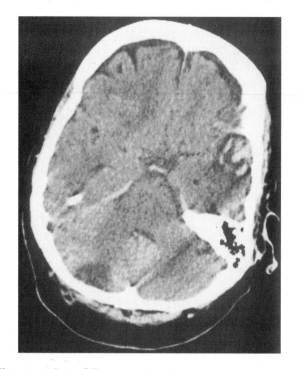

Figure 16-1. CT scan obtained in a young man who had a recent head injury. A traumatic intracerebral hemorrhage is present in the tip of the left temporal lobe. The hematoma represents a contrecoup lesion.

▶ CRANIOCEREBRAL TRAUMA

While craniocerebral trauma is a leading cause of intracranial hemorrhage, bleeding secondary to major head injury usually is not included in the category of hemorrhagic cerebrovascular disease. In most cases, the evidence for trauma is obvious. However, information about an injury might be lacking if the patient has an impaired level of consciousness and if no witnesses are available to give a history. Thus, trauma remains an important consideration in the differential diagnosis of spontaneous intracranial hemorrhage (Fig. 16-1). Some patients have both spontaneous and traumatic intracranial bleeding. For example, a patient may have a stroke leading to a head injury. Separating the scenario of subarachnoid hemorrhage followed by loss of consciousness and a head injury from the sequence of loss of consciousness, head injury, and secondary subarachnoid hemorrhage is difficult. Both traumatic and spontaneous hemorrhages can have bleeding within the brain, ventricles, subarachnoid space, subdural space, or epidural space (Fig. 16-2). In general, the evaluation and treatment of patient with intracranial hemorrhage should be aimed at the potentially most ominous situation, for example, aneurysmal subarachnoid hemorrhage.

Occasionally, a hemorrhage can be a delayed consequence of a head injury. In this situation, which is called spat apoplexy, the interval from trauma to bleeding can range from a few hours to several days or weeks. In general, the delayed hemorrhage occurs within the first week. The hemorrhage probably is secondary to a neurological or vascular injury, which results in localized bleeding. In addition, vasospasm can complicate severe subarachnoid hemorrhage following craniocerebral trauma. Ischemic neurological symptoms

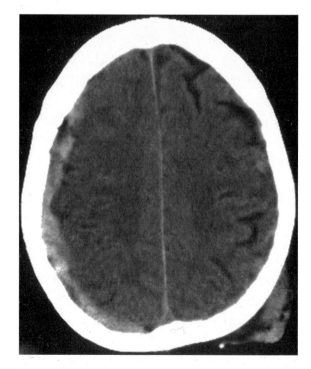

Figure 16-2. CT scan obtained in a patient taking oral anticoagulants who has had a mild head injury. An acute subdural hematoma is demonstrated.

can develop secondary to the vasospasm. Traumatic subarachnoid hemorrhage is second only to aneurysmal rupture as a cause of cerebral vasospasm. Arterial dissections, which could be spontaneous or secondary to trauma, also can cause hemorrhage.[18–20]

The types of neurological impairments and the patterns of hemorrhage found by brain imaging help differentiate bleeding due to craniocerebral trauma from hemorrhagic stroke. If the patient has decreased consciousness, confusion, or headache without focal neurological impairments, diffuse subarachnoid hemorrhage can be secondary to trauma. Trauma is the most likely cause if the bleeding is primarily located in the subdural or epidural space. It is also the likely diagnosis if the pattern of cerebral bleeding is compatible with coup and contrecoup lesions (see Fig. 16-1). In such circumstances, bleeding is primarily located at the cortical portions of the temporal tips or the frontal or occipital poles. Petechial bleeding along the anterior and medial portions of the temporal lobes also is suggestive of trauma. On the other hand, prominent subarachnoid blood to one cistern or an intracerebral hematoma in the deep structures of the cerebral hemispheres, brain stem, or cerebellum usually points to a nontraumatic cause. In particular, primary brain stem hemorrhage is rarely due to trauma. If there is doubt about the etiology of a hemorrhage, further evaluation for a nontraumatic cause should be done.

The presence of a coagulopathy can increase the likelihood of severe intracranial bleeding as a consequence of minor trauma. For example, a minor blow to the head of a patient taking an oral anticoagulant can lead to formation of a subdural hematoma (see Chapter 19). Intracerebral or subarachnoid bleeding following minimal trauma also could occur among patients taking oral anticoagulants.

▶ HYPERTENSION

Hypertension is often described as the primary cause of spontaneous bleeding into the brain (see Fig. 16-2). Arterial hypertension is recognized as a leading contributing factor to or the primary cause of intracerebral hemorrhage.[5,21] Overall, approximately one-half of all nonlobar hemorrhages in the brain are secondary to hypertension.[22] Effective management of elevated blood pressure is the most effective measure to prevent brain hemorrhage.[16,23] Both elevated diastolic blood pressure and an isolated high systolic blood pressure are associated with an increased risk of intracranial bleeding. Both sustained hypertension and acute elevations of blood pressure lead to intracerebral hemorrhage. A chronically elevated blood pressure increases the risk of bleeding especially among persons younger than 55, those who are not compliant with their medications, or

those who smoke. Systolic hypertension also is a risk factor for hemorrhage in the elderly.[5] Chronic hypertension is an especially important cause of hemorrhage in African Americans.[24,25] Some of the association of intracerebral hemorrhage with cold weather probably is secondary to an increased prevalence of hypertension.[26] Indirectly, chronic hypertension can induce rupture of other vascular lesions. For example, the combination of smoking and hypertension appears to increase the risk of aneurysmal subarachnoid hemorrhage[11,27] (Table 16-2).

Chronic Hypertension

Chronic hypertension can lead to hemorrhage involving the deep structures of the cerebral hemispheres or brain stem. Acute hypertensive crises can induce rupture of an abnormal vascular structure, for example, the scenario of a ruptured aneurysm following abuse of a sympathomimetic agent. A hypertensive crisis also can cause rupture of normal blood vessels. Hemorrhage also is a potential complication of the hypertensive effects of *pheochromocytoma*.

While hypertensive hemorrhage is diagnosed commonly, some cases of intracerebral bleeding among patients with an elevated blood pressure are probably due to other causes. In effect, a hemorrhage might be attributed to hypertension incorrectly, primarily because a patient's blood pressure is elevated. The elevated blood pressure might be an epiphenomenon secondary to the stress of the neurological event, severe headache

▶ **TABLE 16-2.** CAUSES OF ACUTE HYPERTENSIVE REACTIONS THAT CAN BE COMPLICATED BY INTRACRANIAL HEMORRHAGE

Pheochromocytoma
Acute glomerulonephritis
Acute renal failure
Eclampsia
Medications—drugs
   Cocaine
   Amphetamines
   Phenylpropanolamine
   Ephedrine
   Ephedra
   Antimigraine medications
Physical or emotional stress
Pain
Labor and delivery
Surgical procedures
Dental procedures
Hyperperfusion syndrome
   Carotid endarterectomy
   Extracranial-to-intracranial bypass
   Endovascular procedures

or nausea, or secondary to increased intracranial pressure. In general, hypertensive hemorrhage should be diagnosed only if a patient has a strong history of hypertension or if the patient has other evidence of hypertension on physical examination. The presence of hypertensive retinopathy, electrocardiographic evidence of left ventricular hypertrophy, or findings of renal dysfunction support the diagnosis of chronic hypertension.

The locations of primary hypertensive hemorrhage are rather stereotyped; the most common site is the putamen secondary to rupture of a lenticulostriate artery[28] (Figs. 16-3 to 16-5). Other common sites are the thalamus, pons, cerebellum, and deep lobar white matter. The areas of brain affected by hypertensive hemorrhage are the same regions that are the locations of lacunar infarctions; another type of stroke is strongly correlated with chronically elevated blood pressure. Bleeding is presumably secondary to rupture of one of small penetrating arteries arising directly from the major vessels of the circle of Willis or the basilar artery. While the bleeding has been attributed to rupture of small dilations of these arterioles (*Charcot–Bouchard aneurysm*), other pathological substrates include fibrinoid necrosis, lipohyalinosis, early atherosclerosis, or medial degeneration.[29–31] Presumably, the chronically elevated blood pressure leads to these arterial pathologies and the secondary weakness of the vessel leads to hemorrhage. Early recurrent bleeding is uncommon but a second

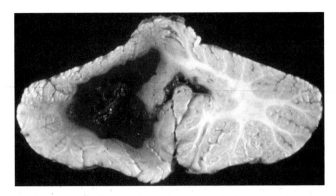

Figure 16-4. Coronal autopsy specimen demonstrates a large hemorrhage of the right cerebellum. The findings would be consistent with a hypertensive hemorrhage arising in the deep nuclei of the cerebellum. (*Courtesy of S.S. Schochet, M.D., Department of Pathology, University of West Virginia, Morgantown, WV*)

hemorrhage can occur if the blood pressure is not adequately controlled.[32–36]

With advances in the management of arterial hypertension, the frequency of secondary hypertensive hemorrhage should decline in the future. Effective treatment of hypertension is the single most important long-term medical therapy that will lower the risk of intracranial hemorrhage. However, many patients with hypertension are not diagnosed or inadequately treated. Thrift et al.[37] noted that stopping antihypertensive medications might be correlated with a subsequent increased likelihood of brain

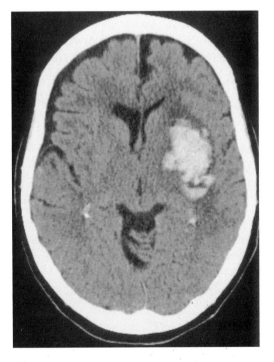

Figure 16-3. CT scan demonstrates a large left putamen hemorrhage on a patient with chronic hypertension.

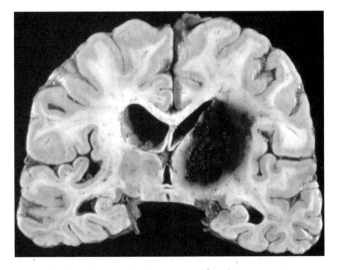

Figure 16-5. Coronal autopsy specimen obtained from a patient dying of a hypertensive hemorrhage. The hemorrhage has arisen in the basal ganglia on the left. (*Courtesy of S.S. Schochet, M.D., Department of Pathology, University of West Virginia, Morgantown, WV*)

hemorrhage. Thus, management of hypertension remains a primary strategy to prevent intracerebral hemorrhage.

Acute Hypertension

Hemorrhage also can complicate acute elevations of blood pressure; common scenarios are acute hypertension secondary to *acute glomerulonephritis, acute renal failure,* or *eclampsia* (see Table 16-2). Eclampsia-associated intracranial bleeding deserves special attention because of the potential for both maternal and fetal morbidity or mortality. The usual findings are hypertension, proteinuria, and peripheral edema, which are followed by seizures and altered alertness (see Chapter 18). The bleeding can be diffuse and petechial in appearance or in a hematoma. Besides hemorrhage, other imaging findings might be compatible with *posterior reversible encephalopathy syndrome* (PRES) (Fig. 16-6). Intracranial bleeding following delivery is a potential complication of postpartum cerebral vasculopathy.[38] In addition, reactions to surgical procedures, psychological stresses, or medications also can lead to hypertensive crises and secondary intracranial hemorrhage (see Table 16-2). The cause-and-effect relationship is obvious in most cases. In some of these events, the findings are compatible with a breakthrough in autoregulation and an acute hypertensive encephalopathy. In other instances, the acute hypertensive response caused bleeding from another arterial pathology or rupture of a normal artery.

The management of acute hypertensive hemorrhage is described in Chapters 21 and 23. Based on observational studies of patients having brain imaging studies performed within a few hours of the ictus and then repeated several hours later, a sizable percentage of patients with hypertensive hemorrhage will have growth in the size of the hematoma during the first few hours.

► CEREBRAL AMYLOID ANGIOPATHY

While cerebral amyloid angiopathy accounts for approximately 2 percent of all intracranial hemorrhages, it is a leading cause of bleeding in older adults.[39] The incidence of hemorrhage secondary to cerebral amyloid angiopathy increases rapidly among elderly persons; this diagnosis is unlikely among persons younger than 65.[40–42] The prevalence of cerebral amyloid angiopathy is estimated as approximately 5 percent among persons aged 60–69, 25–30 percent among persons aged 70–79, and greater than 50 percent among persons older than 80. The pathological hallmark of cerebral amyloid angiopathy is the deposition of amyloid material within the wall or in the perivascular spaces of small-to-medium-sized arterioles and arteries in the cerebral cortex and meninges[41–44] (Fig. 16-7). This protein is stained readily by Congo red stain and this selective staining is the source of the name *congophilic angiopathy,* which is sometimes used to describe this arteriopathy. The deposits have a birefringence that is detected under polarized light and appear similar to those found in systemic amyloidosis, although affected patients do not have other evidence of amyloidosis. This arteriopathy is

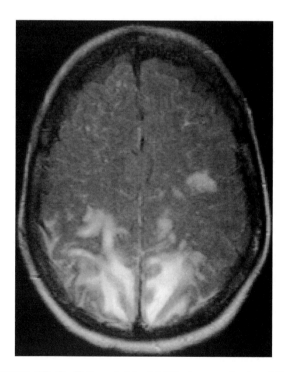

Figure 16-6. T-2-weighted MRI demonstrates bilateral posterior hyperintensities in white matter consistent with PRES.

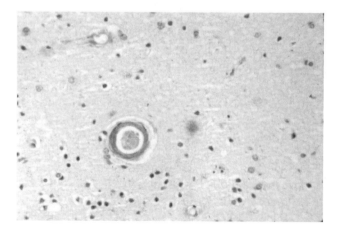

Figure 16-7. Surgical specimen of the brain stained with Congo red shows perivascular amyloid deposits. The findings are those of cerebral amyloid angiopathy. (*Courtesy of S.S. Schochet, M.D., Department of Pathology, University of West Virginia, Morgantown, WV*)

► **TABLE 16-3.** POTENTIAL ASSOCIATED
DISEASES—CEREBRAL AMYLOID ANGIOPATHY

Alzheimer disease	Granulomatous angiitis
Down syndrome	Rheumatoid arthritis
Dementia pugilistica	Giant cell arteritis
Creutzfeldt–Jakob disease	Radiation necrosis
Cerebellar ataxia	Vascular malformations

not part of systemic amyloidosis. Microaneurysmal formation and fibrinoid degeneration also can be found. Bleeding results from any of these secondary arterial changes. The use of anticoagulants or thrombolytic agents also might predispose to bleeding. Some of the high risk of hemorrhage among elderly persons receiving anticoagulants or thrombolytic agents might be secondary to the presence of cerebral amyloid angiopathy.

A history of preexisting dementia, especially that consistent with the diagnosis of Alzheimer disease, is an important clinical finding (Table 16-3). The history of dementia greatly increases the likelihood that a hematoma is secondary to cerebral amyloid angiopathy. While cerebral amyloid angiopathy is often associated with Alzheimer disease, the arteriopathic changes also are found in the brains of nondemented elderly persons. The vascular disease has been associated with the apolipoprotein E4 or E2 alleles.[45–50] These genetic changes appear to be linked with earlier onset and recurrent hemorrhages. Woo et al.[22,48] concluded that approximately one-third of the cases of lobar hemorrhages associated with cerebral amyloid angiopathy are related to the presence of either an apolipoprotein E4 or E2 allele. The chances of recurrent hemorrhage also are increased by the presence of these genetic changes. While the alleles are associated with the amyloid deposit, other potential secondary effects include weakening of the arterial wall, such as through fibrinoid necrosis. Cerebral amyloid angiopathy also has been found in patients with several other neurological conditions (see Table 16-3). Rare inherited forms of cerebral amyloid angiopathy have been reported in the Netherlands and Iceland; both varieties seem to be associated with hemorrhages at younger ages than with the sporadic form of the disease. In the *Icelandic* version (*HCHWA-I*), hemorrhages usually occur in middle-aged adults, while in the *Dutch* form (*HCHWA-D*), most hemorrhages occur among persons aged 50–70. The components of the protein deposited in familial cerebral amyloid angiopathy appear to differ from those seen with the sporadic disease.

Cerebral amyloid angiopathy should be considered whenever an elderly patient has a cerebral hemorrhage (Fig. 16-8). Besides a past history of dementia, a prior history of multiple small strokes or transient ischemic attack also suggests the diagnosis of cerebral amyloid

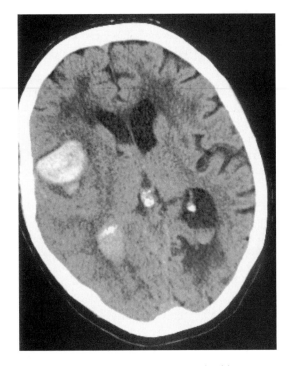

Figure 16-8. CT scan shows a cortical hematoma in the right hemisphere obtained in an elderly patient. The location points toward the diagnosis of the amyloid angiopathy.

angiopathy. The diagnosis should be suspected even if an elderly patient with intracerebral hemorrhage does not have a history of arterial hypertension. Because the likelihood of recurrent bleeding is considerable, many patients have a history of repeated cerebral hemorrhages. Small areas of hemorrhage (microbleeds) can be associated with symptomatic cerebral hemorrhages in the same general region of the brain.[51] When these areas of hemorrhage are located in deep hemispheric structures, they might be associated with hypertensive small-vessel disease. Lobar or cortical hemorrhages are probably a manifestation of amyloid angiopathy.

While the only definitive way to establish the diagnosis is through brain and meningeal biopsy, the clinical and imaging findings can lead to a probable diagnosis. The hemorrhages are usually located in the cortex and adjacent lobar white matter, which are the locations of the arteriopathy[36,52] (see Fig. 16-7). The frontal and occipital lobes seem to be preferentially involved. While rare cases of cerebellar hemorrhage have been reported, hematomas located in the deep structures of the cerebral hemispheres or the brain stem probably are not secondary to cerebral amyloid angiopathy.[53] Subdural hematoma and subarachnoid hemorrhage are potential but rare complications. Some patients may have multiple hematomas located at the gray–white junction—a finding that is suggestive of cerebral amyloid angiopathy.

In addition, many patients have evidence of previous, often asymptomatic, hemorrhages. The use of gradient-echo magnetic resonance imaging (MRI) facilitates the detection of small hemorrhages among persons with cerebral amyloid angiopathy. The lesions, which appear as small black spots, are scattered throughout the gray matter of both cerebral hemispheres. Because of the perceived propensity to recurrent bleeding, there is a reluctance to recommend cerebral biopsy in order to establish a diagnosis. Arteriography is normal because it cannot visualize the small caliber vessels that are affected by cerebral amyloid angiopathy.

Patients with cerebral amyloid angiopathy generally have a poor prognosis in part because of their risk for recurrent hemorrhage. The patients' age and concomitant dementia also portend a poor prognosis. In addition, a risk for recurrent ischemia also exists. No specific intervention is available to treat the arteriopathy other than antihypertensives to lower the risk of arterial rupture. Administration of antiplatelet agents or anticoagulants in an effort to prevent ischemic stroke is accompanied by a possibility of cerebral bleeding complications. While screening a gradient-echo MRI might provide information about previous minor hemorrhages and might influence choices about medications to prevent ischemia, the utility of such a strategy is not known. Surgery can be done for treatment of a major hemorrhage.[54]

▶ MOYAMOYA DISEASE AND MOYAMOYA SYNDROME

Subarachnoid hemorrhage is a potential complication of moyamoya disease, which is an inherited arteriopathy, and moyamoya syndrome, which is an acquired arteriopathy secondary to a large number of causes[55–57] (see Chapters 10 and 12). Most affected patients have recurrent ischemic stroke but hemorrhagic events are an important cause of morbidity, especially among young adults. The high propensity for bleeding affects decisions about management to prevent recurrent infarction. Bleeding is often ascribed to rupture of saccular aneurysms, which are located most frequently in the posterior circulation[55,58] (see Chapter 15). In addition, rupture of the small vessels at the base of the brain or small collaterals of the rete mirabile can lead to hemorrhage.[58,59] Besides subarachnoid hemorrhage, bleeding can occur within the brain. Moyamoya is a potential cause of basal ganglionic hemorrhage in young adults. The presence of multiple small infarctions in the hemispheres and absence of the normal flow voids of the carotid, anterior cerebral, and middle cerebral arteries suggest moyamoya. The arteriographic findings are stereotyped and relatively specific. Medical and surgical

therapies for treatment of patients with moyamoya are primarily aimed at prevention of recurrent cerebral infarction. Because of the relatively high risk of hemorrhage, oral anticoagulants usually are not prescribed. Revascularization procedures (extracranial-to-intracranial artery bypass operations or duromyosynangioses) might be helpful in preventing bleeding because of the modification of flow (see Chapter 20).

▶ VASCULITIS

Although the risk of bleeding is less than ischemia, hemorrhage can occur secondary to either a *multisystem* or *primary central nervous system vasculitis* (*granulomatous angiitis*).[60–63] Subarachnoid hemorrhage, intracerebral hemorrhage, and primary intraventricular hemorrhage are complications of primary central nervous system. Bleeding occurs primarily with necrotizing vasculitis including *periarteritis nodosa*, *Takayasu disease*, *giant cell arteritis*, or *Churg–Strauss angiitis*, but it is uncommon with most other vasculitides[64] (see Chapter 11). Recurrent brain hemorrhage can complicate periarteritis nodosa. Brain imaging usually will not provide any specific clues. In general, examination of the cerebrospinal fluid is not helpful but it might demonstrate signs of inflammation in addition to evidence of bleeding. Magnetic resonance angiography and computerized tomographic angiography help eliminate other arterial causes of stroke but these tests probably will not visualize the arteriographic changes of vasculitis. Arteriography remains the most important diagnostic test; segmental narrowing or occlusions involving medium-to-large arteries can be generalized or relatively localized. Small distal aneurysms also can be found. However, arteriography can miss a medium-to-small inflammatory arteriopathy. In some cases, brain and meningeal biopsies are required but some biopsies will not be diagnostic because of the segmental and scattered nature of the vasculitis. Neurosurgeons should alert the pathologists about the possible diagnosis if a large hematoma is evacuated in a patient who might have vasculitis because examination of the adjacent brain tissue might permit determination of the cause of bleeding. The mainstays of treatment are immunosuppressive therapies including corticosteroids and cyclophosphamide.

▶ ARTERIAL DISSECTIONS

Both spontaneous and traumatic arterial dissections can be associated with subarachnoid hemorrhage[20,65] (see Chapter 10). While hemorrhages have been correlated with dissections of the basilar or vertebral arteries, bleeding also can complicate arterial dissections of the internal carotid artery and its branches.[65–68] The prognosis of patients with bleeding due to an arterial dissection is poor. Rebleeding can occur in 30–70 percent of patients.[18–20] Most recurrent hemorrhages occur within the first few weeks following the initial event, and most rebleeding events are fatal.

▶ INFECTIONS

Intracerebral hemorrhage also can complicate bacterial, fungal, or viral infections of the brain. Besides being a complication of *infectious endocarditis*, infective aneurysms can result from meningitis or thrombophlebitis. Persons with AIDS or other immunocompromised patients can also have a vasculitis secondary to an opportunistic infection. The most common infection leading to intracerebral hemorrhage is *Aspergillus fumigatus*, which can cause a rapidly enlarging mass in the brain that is associated with bleeding or progressive infarction. While antifungal medications are prescribed, the outcomes of patients with hemorrhage secondary to a fulminant fungal infection of the brain are very poor. While cerebral infarction is relatively common complication of *herpes zoster ophthalmicus*, intracerebral hemorrhage also can occur. Bleeding also is reported to complicate *leptospirosis*, *Lyme disease*, or *tuberculous meningitis*. Multiple small areas of petechial bleeding secondary to vascular slugging can complicate *rickettsial infections* but large individually symptomatic hemorrhages are not described. Hemorrhage has been a complication of AIDS, although the bleeding is through opportunistic infections, vasculitis, or tumors including Kaposi sarcoma. Recent infections, especially those affecting the upper respiratory tract, may be associated with an increased risk of aneurysmal subarachnoid hemorrhage.[69]

▶ INTRACRANIAL TUMORS

Intracranial hemorrhage can be the initial presentation of a primary or metastatic tumor of the brain. In the experience of Schrader et al.,[70] brain hemorrhage was often the initial clinical sign of the neoplastic disease. Bleeding can complicate 1–10 percent of all intracranial tumors.[71] Still, tumors are a relatively uncommon cause of hemorrhage, probably accounting for 1–2 percent of cases. Intense vascularity, rapid growth, vascular invasion, or areas of necrosis mark the tumors associated with bleeding (Table 16-4).

Metastatic disease is probably more commonly associated with bleeding than is a malignant primary brain tumor. The frequency of hemorrhage is highest with choriocarcinoma, melanoma, renal cell carcinoma,

▶ **TABLE 16-4.** INTRACRANIAL TUMORS ASSOCIATED WITH HEMORRHAGE

Astrocytoma	Malignant melanoma
Oligodendroglioma	Renal cell carcinoma
Meningioma	Metastatic carcinoma of lung
Hemangioblastoma	Metastatic thyroid malignancies
Spongioblastoma	Choriocarcinoma
Acoustic Schwannoma	Pituitary adenoma
Glioblastoma	Kaposi sarcoma
Medulloblastoma	

bronchogenic carcinoma, and carcinoma of the thyroid.[72–74] In general, hemorrhages secondary to metastatic tumors are located in the subcortical white matter, while glioblastoma can lead to bleeding in the hemisphere, basal ganglia, or corpus callosum. In addition, multiple areas of hemorrhage can occur in metastatic tumors. The presence of edema surrounding the hematoma on a brain imaging study obtained shortly after hemorrhage also points to an underlying tumor. Besides intracerebral bleeding, subarachnoid hemorrhage, subdural hemorrhage, or intraventricular hemorrhage also might occur. An enhanced computed tomography (CT) or MRI study often detects the underlying tumor nodule.

A tumor should be suspected if the patient has a history of progressively worsening neurological problems, such as headache, seizures, personality change, or fluctuating focal signs, before the hemorrhage. Detection of papilledema also suggests preexisting intracranial hypertension, and this evidence could point to an underlying brain tumor. The presence of abundant edema shortly after the ictus or multiple hemorrhagic lesions also increases the likelihood of metastatic disease. *Choriocarcinoma* should be considered if a young woman, who recently was pregnant, has a lobar hemorrhage associated with marked edema.[75,76] The tumor can complicate an abortion, hydatiform mole, ectopic pregnancy, or normal pregnancy.[77] The tumor spreads by an arterial route to the lungs and brain. Measuring levels of beta-human chorionic gonadotropin is an effective way to screen for this tumor. The chest X-ray will usually be abnormal. Multiple lesions are seen in both lungs. Brain hemorrhage can be the initial clinical manifestation of *melanoma*.[78] Multiple tumors and hemorrhages are often found. The bleeding apparently is secondary to tumor invasion of the vasa vasorum. A careful dermatological evaluation might discover the underlying skin lesion, which can be quite small. The prognosis of patients with bleeding secondary to melanoma is very poor. *Renal cell carcinoma* is a highly vascular tumor and, on occasion, a brain metastasis with secondary hemorrhage can be the initial symptom. Because *carcinoma of the lung* with secondary brain involvement is very common, it also is an important cause of bleeding secondary to a tumor. The relative frequency of hemorrhages is lower than that with some of the other metastatic lesions. Intracranial bleeding is an uncommon complication of *intravascular lymphomatosis.* Hemorrhage is relatively uncommon among patients with carcinoma of the breast or other malignancies. Intracranial hemorrhage can also be an exceptional presentation for a cardiac myxoma.[79,80] If tumor is suspected, evaluation should be done for a primary tumor somewhere else in the body. Biopsy of the primary tumor can achieve the diagnosis and brain biopsy can be avoided.

While hemorrhage is a potential complication of several primary tumors of the central nervous system, bleeding is an important presentation among persons with *glioblastoma multiforme.* The associations described with metastatic disease, premonitory neurological symptoms and abundant edema, also are found. Hemorrhages also occur with *hemangioblastoma,* which is most commonly located in the cerebellum. The tumor is usually noted as an eccentric nodule with a cyst. The tumor, which is usually found as part of the autosomal-dominant-inherited *von Hippel–Lindau syndrome,* can be complicated by polycythemia secondary to production of erythropoietin. Examination of the retina can find characteristic vascular changes. Hemorrhage rarely occurs with primary benign tumors of the central nervous system, including *meningiomas.* Other primary tumors associated with hemorrhage are astrocytoma, spongioblastoma, acoustic neuroma, and pituitary adenomas. Pituitary apoplexy is described in Chapter 18. Hemorrhage has been reported in patients with *primary central nervous system lymphoma* and AIDS.[81]

The diagnosis of a neoplastic cause of a brain hemorrhage usually requires biopsy of the hematoma and adjacent brain tissue, particularly if a primary brain tumor is suspected. Neurosurgeons and neuropathologists need to screen the adjacent neurological tissue for the neoplastic tissue when surgical evacuation of a hematoma is performed.

▶ PERIMESENCEPHALIC SUBARACHNOID HEMORRHAGE

With the development of modern brain imaging studies, a subgroup of patients with subarachnoid hemorrhage was identified. These patients had a deposit of blood localized in the cisterns around the midbrain and in front of the pons.[82,83] At times, the bleeding is found primarily in the region of the quadrigeminal cistern and in other patients, the blood is localized in front of the brain stem.[82,83] The clinical features of patients with perimesencephalic subarachnoid hemorrhage are

similar to those with intracranial bleeding due to other causes including ruptured aneurysms. However, this group looks surprisingly well and has an excellent prognosis.[82,84] Patients with perimesencephalic subarachnoid hemorrhage have a much lower risk for vasospasm or recurrent hemorrhage than do persons who have ruptured aneurysms. Other neurological impairments, including cranial nerve palsies, are uncommon. However, affected patients can have hyponatremia, hydrocephalus, or seizures.[85] Because the pattern of bleeding in front of the brain stem can be secondary to a ruptured aneurysm of the posterior circulation, arteriography to screen for an aneurysm should be done.[82,86] The cause of perimesencephalic subarachnoid hemorrhage has not been determined because most affected patients have an excellent outcome and pathological data are not available.[84,87] Data about a relationship to preexisting hypertension are inconclusive.[82,88] Presumably, the bleeding is secondary to rupture of a small vascular malformation or a small vein. Management focuses on symptomatic treatment during the acute illness. The risk of recurrent hemorrhage among this group of patients seems to be virtually nonexistent.

▶ DRUG ABUSE

Intracranial hemorrhage can complicate abuse of drugs, in particular medications with sympathomimetic effects. As a result, drug abuse is a leading cause of brain hemorrhage in adolescents and young adults[89–92] (see Chapter 17). The most commonly implicated medications are *cocaine, amphetamine, methamphetamine, ephedra,* or other stimulants, which are taken via oral, intranasal, or parenteral routes, or through smoking[91,93–95] (see Chapter 17). In particular, hemorrhage has been associated with use of alkaloid form of cocaine (crack).[94,96,97] Bleeding also can complicate the use of *ephedrine, pseudoephedrine,* or *phenylpropanolamine.* The latter medication was withdrawn in the United States because of a perceived high risk of intracranial bleeding when it was taken as a diet suppressant.[98] Ephedra also was removed from food supplements in the United States because of presumed complications including intracranial hemorrhage.

Bleeding is presumably secondary to a hypertensive surge[99] (Table 16-5). The high blood pressure can result in a hemorrhage from rupture of an otherwise occult vascular malformation or aneurysm, or bleeding from normal vessels also could happen.[100,101] In addition, parenteral drug abuse can be complicated by infective endocarditis, which leads to an infective aneurysm that bleeds. Sympathomimetic drugs also can cause a vasculitis or a moyamoyalike vasculopathy.[94,102]

▶ **TABLE 16-5.** CAUSES OF INTRACRANIAL HEMORRHAGE SECONDARY TO DRUGS OF ABUSE

Marked increase in blood pressure
Rupture of aneurysm
Rupture of vascular malformation
Rupture of normal artery
Infective endocarditis with aneurysm
Vasculitis
Moyamoya syndrome

The pathological findings on examination of affected vessels look similar to that found with periarteritis nodosa.[97,102] A moyamoyalike vasculopathy also has been described.[103]

The interval from the use of the drugs until bleeding can range from a few hours to several days. Severe bleeding has complicated either long-term use or a single exposure. The experience of hemorrhage secondary to phenylpropanolamine might be associated with a prolonged use of the medication for weight control.[104] This association is implied because the same medication, when taken as a decongestant, appears not to be complicated by hemorrhage. Most hemorrhages are lobar in location; primary subarachnoid or intraventricular hemorrhage is less common. Screening of the urine or blood for drugs of abuse should be done in these circumstances. The screening tests should be done as soon as possible because of the relatively rapid clearance of these agents or their metabolites. Steroids have been prescribed because of the presumed vasculitic component of the arteriopathy. Calcium-channel-blocking drugs have been used because of the assumed vasospastic nature of the disease. Some success has been described with each therapy. Still, the best therapy is to halt abuse of the agents.

▶ MEDICATIONS

Intracranial bleeding is a potential complication of medications that affect coagulation (see Chapters 19, 21 to 23). Hemorrhages have followed the use of *antimigraine medications*.[105] Presumably, the vasoconstrictive effects lead to an elevation of blood pressure that prompts arterial rupture. Although a potential relationship between hypocholesterolemia and an increased risk of intracranial hemorrhage has been speculated, the administration of cholesterol-lowering medications is not accompanied by any increase in bleeding risk.[106] The risk of subarachnoid hemorrhage appears to be increased among young women taking oral contraceptives, especially those with high estrogen doses.[107,108]

▶ ALCOHOL ABUSE

Alcohol abuse is recognized as a risk factor for both hemorrhagic and ischemic stroke (see Chapter 17). The pattern of subarachnoid hemorrhage in young adults, especially men, corresponds to times of heavy alcohol consumption; more bleeding events occur on weekends.[10,109] The bleeding appears to be secondary to changes in coagulation factors. Alcohol also might affect the integrity of the arterial walls. In addition, heavy alcohol consumption is associated with an increased risk for traumatic intracranial hemorrhages. Modest alcohol consumption does not increase the risk of intracranial bleeding.[110]

▶ HEMORRHAGES ASSOCIATED WITH SURGICAL PROCEDURES

Bleeding can complicate neurosurgical procedures including biopsies, placement of intraventricular catheters, evacuation of a subdural hematoma, or resection of a tumor. Fortunately, major symptomatic hemorrhage is relatively uncommon following neurosurgical procedures. *Pallidotomy* or *placement of deep brain stimulators* has been developed for treatment of movement disorders; hemorrhages seem to be the primary vascular complication. Some of the bleeding is attributed to changes in coagulation or a subtle disseminated intravascular coagulation secondary to consumption of clotting factors. In addition, labile postoperative hypertension or intracranial shifts secondary to treatment of brain edema and increased intracranial pressure also can lead to vascular rupture. Approximately 0.5 percent of *carotid endarterectomies* are complicated by intracranial hemorrhage.[111–113] The average interval from the operation until the hemorrhage is approximately 3.5 days. Affected patients have seizures and decreased consciousness. These hemorrhagic complications seem to be most common when a patient with a severe stenosis and poor collaterals is treated. Elderly patients and those with volatile or elevated blood pressure following surgery also have a high risk of bleeding. The presumed mechanism of hemorrhage is a *hyperperfusion syndrome*, which results from a hyperemia and venous congestion ipsilateral to the operated artery. Perioperative administration of anticoagulants or antiplatelet agents probably also play a role. One of the reasons for delaying operation following a stroke is the risk of bleeding complications. Hemorrhage also is a potential complication of other revascularization operations, including *extracranial-to-intracranial arterial anastomoses*.[114] *Angioplasty* and *stenting* for treatment of an extracranial-or-intracranial stenosis also can be complicated by hemorrhage.[115,116] Endovascular procedures treating intracranial lesions also can be complicated by arterial rupture. Bleeding also can complicate *coiling* or *obliterative endovascular procedures.*[117–120]

Hemorrhage is also a complication of *major cardiovascular operations.*[121] While the frequency of bleeding is much lower than the incidence of infarction, the uses of anticoagulants, volatile blood pressure, venous congestion, or perioperative embolism are probably the mechanisms of stroke. Intracranial bleeding, including acute subdural hematomas, are complications of *hemodialysis.*[122,123] The bleeding probably is secondary to administration of anticoagulants or shifts secondary to osmotic changes. Intracranial hemorrhage is relatively common cause of death among patients having *bone-marrow transplantation.* No specific relationship of the bleeding to underlying disease, preparatory therapies, immunological status, or graft-versus-host disease has been found. Hemorrhages have also complicated *dental procedures, electroconvulsive therapy,* and the use of *extracorporeal membrane oxygenation.*[124–128]

▶ OTHER CAUSES OF HEMORRHAGE

Intracranial hemorrhage is a rare complication of *endometriosis.* Presumably, the ectopic location is secondary to hematogenous spread from the pelvis. Intracranial bleeding is a potential complication of *Zieve Syndrome,* which consists of severe liver disease, hemolytic anemia, and hyperlipidemia. *Pregnancy* and *eclampsia* are factors associated with an increased risk of intracranial bleeding.[129–131] Hemorrhage is a potential complication of *postpartum cerebral angiopathy.*[132,133] This relatively uncommon condition is more commonly correlated with ischemic events and is recognized by segmental arterial narrowing found at arteriography (see Chapter 17). In the presence of intracranial bleeding, the vascular changes could be confused with vasospasm following subarachnoid hemorrhage. Intracranial bleeding has also been associated with *cyclosporine toxicity, fibrous dysplasia of the skull, Menke's kinky hair syndrome, Sturge–Weber syndrome, Klinefelter syndrome, primary aldosteronism, thyrotoxicosis,* or *poststreptococcal acute glomerulonephritis.*[134–138] Hemorrhages also have complicated *heat stroke,* or *lightning strike.* Rare causes of hemorrhage include scorpion or snake bites that lead to a coagulopathy.

Vahedi et al.[139] described *hereditary endotheliopathy* with *retinopathy, nephropathy,* and *stroke.* This autosomal-dominant disorder is associated with retinal arterial tortuosity, retinal hemorrhages, migraine with aura, infantile hemiparesis, leukoencephalopathy, and small brain hemorrhages. The frequency of this genetic disease is not known.

REFERENCES

1. Sacco R, Wolf P, Bharuca N, et al. Subarachnoid and intracerebral hemorrhage: natural history, prognosis, and precursive factors in the Framingham Study. *Neurology* 1984;34:847–856.
2. Broderick JP, Brott TG, Tomsick T. Intra-cerebral hemorrhage more than twice as common as subarachnoid hemorrhage. *J Neurosurg* 1993;78:188–191.
3. Taylor TN, Davis PH, Torner JC. Projected number of strokes by subtype in the year 2050 in the United States. *Stroke* 1998;29:322.
4. Biller J, Toffol GJ, Kassell NF, Adams HP, Jr., Beck DW, Boarini DJ. Spontaneous subarachnoid hemorrhage in young adults. *Neurosurgery* 1987;21:664–667.
5. Broderick J, Brott T, Tomsick T, Leach A. Lobar hemorrhage in the elderly. The undiminishing importance of hypertension. *Stroke* 1993;24:49–51.
6. Broderick JP, Talbot T, Prenger E. Stroke in children within a major metropolitan area: the surprising importance of intracerebral hemorrhage. *J Child Neurol* 1993; 8:250–255.
7. Carey J, Numaguchi Y, Nadell J. Subarachnoid hemorrhage in sickle cell disease. *Childs Nerv Syst* 1990;6:47–50.
8. Thrift AG, McNeil JJ, Forbes A, Donnan GA. Risk of primary intracerebral haemorrhage associated with aspirin and non-steroidal anti-inflammatory drugs: case-control study. *BMJ* 1999;318:759–764.
9. Thrift A, McNeil J, Donnan G. The risk of intracerebral haemorrhage with smoking. The Melbourne Risk Factor Study Group. *Cerebrovasc Dis* 1999;9:34–39.
10. Thrift A, Donnan G, McNeil J. Heavy drinking, but not moderate or intermediate drinking, increases the risk of intracerebral hemorrhage. *Epidemiology* 1999;10:307–312.
11. Weir BK, Kongable GL, Kassell NF, Schultz JR, Truskowski LL, Sigrest A. Cigarette smoking as a cause of aneurysmal subarachnoid hemorrhage and risk for vasospasm: a report of the Cooperative Aneurysm Study. *J Neurosurg* 1998;89:405–411.
12. Lee I, Hennekens C, Berger K, Buring JE, Manson J. Exercise and risk of stroke in male physicians. *Stroke* 1999;30:1–6.
13. Vermeer SE, Rinkel GJ, Algra A. Circadian fluctuations in onset of subarachnoid hemorrhage. New data on aneurysmal and perimesencephalic hemorrhage and a systematic review. *Stroke* 1997;28:805–808.
14. Lammie GA, Lindley R, Keir S, Wiggam MI. Stress-related primary intracerebral hemorrhage: autopsy clues to underlying mechanism. Stroke 2000;31:1426–1428.
15. Nencini P, Basile AM, Sarti C, Inzitari D. Cerebral hemorrhage following a roller coaster ride. *JAMA* 2000;284: 832–833.
16. Leppala JM, Virtamo J, Fogelholm R, Albanes D, Heinonen OP. Different risk factors for different stroke subtypes: association of blood pressure, cholesterol, and antioxidants. *Stroke* 1999;30:2535–2540.
17. Segal AZ, Chiu RI, Eggleston-Sexton PM, Beiser A, Greenberg SM. Low cholesterol as a risk factor for primary intracerebral hemorrhage: a case-control study. *Neuroepidemiology* 1999;18:185–193.

18. Yamaura A, Watanabe Y, Saiki N. Dissecting aneurysms of the intracranial vertebral artery. *J Neurosurg* 1990;72: 183–188.

19. Aoki N, Sakai T. Rebleeding from intracranial dissecting aneurysms in the vertebral artery. *Stroke* 1990;21: 1628–1631.

20. Mizutani T, Aruga T, Kirino T, et al. Recurrent subarachnoid hemorrhage from untreated ruptured vertebrobasilar dissecting aneurysm. *Neurosurgery* 1955;36: 905–913.

21. Brott T, Thalinger K, Hertzberg V. Hypertension as a risk factor for spontaneous intracerebral hemorrhage. *Stroke* 1986;17:1078–1083.

22. Woo D, Sauerbeck LR, Kissela BM, et al. Genetic and environmental risk factors for intracerebral hemorrhage: preliminary results of a population-based study. *Stroke* 2002;33:1190–1195.

23. Perry HMJ, Davis BR, Price TR, et al. Effect of treating isolated systolic hypertension on the risk of developing various types and subtypes of stroke: the systolic hypertension in the elderly program (SHEP). *JAMA* 2000;284:465–471.

24. Broderick JP, Brott T, Tomsick T, Huster G, Miller R. The risk of subarachnoid and intracerebral hemorrhages in blacks as compared with whites. *N Engl J Med* 1992;326: 733–736.

25. Broderick J, Brott T, Kothari R, et al. The Greater Cincinnati/Northern Kentucky Stroke Study: preliminary first-ever and total incidence rates of stroke among blacks. *Stroke* 1998;29:415–421.

26. Passero S, Reale F, Ciacci G, Zei E. Differing temporal patterns of onset in subgroups of patients with intracerebral hemorrhage. *Stroke* 2000;31:1538–1544.

27. Bonita R. Cigarette smoking, hypertension, and the risk of subarachnoid hemorrhage: a population-based case-control study. *Stroke* 1986;17:831–835.

28. Chung CS, Caplan LR, Yamamoto Y, et al. Straitocapsular haemorrhage. *Brain* 2000;123:1850–1862.

29. Takebayashi S. Ultrastructural morphometry of hypertensive medial damage in lenticulostriate and other arteries. *Stroke* 1985;16:449–453.

30. Challa V, Moody DM, Bell MA. The Charcot–Bouchard aneurysm controversy: impact of a new histologic technique. *J Neuropathol Exp Neurol* 1992;51:264–271.

31. Auer RN, Sutherland GR. Primary intracerebral hemorrhage. Pathophysiology. *Can J Neurol Sci* 2005;32 (suppl 2)S3–S12.

32. Passero S, Burgalassi L, D'Andrea P. Recurrence of bleeding in patients with primary intracerebral hemorrhage. *Stroke* 1995;26:1189–1192.

33. Chen ST, Chiang CY, Hsu CY. Recurrent hypertensive intracerebral hemorrhage. *Acta Neurol Scand* 1995;91: 128–132.

34. Arakawa S, Saku Y, Ibayashi S, Nagao T, Fujishima M. Blood pressure control and recurrence of hypertensive brain hemorrhage. *Stroke* 1998;29:1806–1809.

35. Bae H, Jeong D, Doh J, Lee K, Yun I, Byun B. Recurrence of bleeding in patients with hypertensive intracerebral hemorrhage. *Cerebrovasc Dis* 1999;9:102–108.

36. Gonzalez-Duarte A, Cantu C, Ruiz-Sandoval JL, Barinagarrementeria F. Recurrent primary cerebral hemorrhage: frequency, mechanisms, and prognosis. *Stroke* 1998;29:1802–1805.

37. Thrift A, McNeil J, Forbes A, Donnan G. Three important subgroups of hypertensive persons at greater risk of intracerebral hemorrhage. Melbourne Risk Factor Study Group. *Hypertension* 1998;31:1223–1229.

38. Geocadin RG, Razumovsky AY, Wityk RJ, Bhardwaj A, Ulatowski JA. Intracerebral hemorrhage and postpartum cerebral vasculopathy. *J Neurol Sci* 2002;205:29–34.

39. Schutz H, Bodeker RH, Damain M, Krack P, Dorndorf W. Age-related spontaneous intracerebral hematoma in a German community. *Stroke* 1990;21:1412–1418.

40. Kalyan-Raman VP, Kalyan-Raman K. Cerebral amyloid angiopathy causing intracranial hemorrhage. *Ann Neurol* 1986;16:321–329.

41. Yamada M. Cerebral amyloid angiopathy: an overview. *Neuropathology* 2000;20:8–22.

42. Mandybur TI. Cerebral amyloid angiopathy: the vascular pathology and complications. *J Neuropathol Exp Neurol* 1986;45:79–90.

43. Vinters HV. Cerebral amyloid angiopathy: a critical review. *Stroke* 1987;18:311–324.

44. Vonsattel JP, Myers RH, Hedley-Whyte ET, Ropper AH, Bird ED, Richards EP, Jr. Cerebral amyloid angiopathy without and with cerebral hemorrhages: a comparative histological study. *Ann Neurol* 1991;30:637–649.

45. Greenberg SM. Cerebral amyloid angiopathy: prospects for clinical diagnosis and treatment. *Neurology* 1998;51: 690–694.

46. Greenberg SM. Cerebral amyloid angiopathy and dementia: two amyloids are worse than one. *Neurology* 2002;58: 1587–1588.

47. Greenberg SM. Cerebral amyloid angiopathy and vessel dysfunction. *Cerebrovasc Dis* 2002;13(suppl 2):42–47.

48. Woo D, Sekar P, Chakraborty R, et al. Genetic epidemiology of intracerebral hemorrhage. *J Stroke Cerebrovasc Dis* 2006;14:239–243.

49. McCarron MO, Hoffmann KL, DeLong DM, Gray L, Saunders AM, Alberts MJ. Intracerebral hemorrhage outcome: apolipoprotein E genotype, hematoma, and edema volumes. *Neurology* 1999;53:2176–2179.

50. O'Donnell HC, Rosand J, Knudsen KA, et al. Apolipoprotein E genotype and the risk of recurrent lobar intracerebral hemorrhage. *N Engl J Med* 2000;342: 240–245.

51. Lee SH, Bae HJ, Kwon SJ, et al. Cerebral microbleeds are regionally associated with intracerebral hemorrhage. *Neurology* 2004;62:72–76.

52. Finelli PF, Kessimian N, Bernstein PW. Cerebral amyloid angiopathy manifesting as recurrent intracerebral hemorrhage. *Arch Neurol* 1984;41:330–333.

53. Ishihara T, Takahashi M, Yokota T, et al. The significance of cerebrovascular amyloid in the aetiology of superficial (lobar) cerebral haemorrhage and its incidence in the elderly population. *J Pathol* 1991;165: 229–234.

54. Izumihara A, Ishihara T, Iwamoto N, Yamashita K, Ito H. Postoperative outcome of 37 patients with lobar intrac-

erebral hemorrhage related to cerebral amyloid angiopathy. *Stroke* 1999;30:29–33.

55. Hamada JI, Hashimoto N, Tsukahara T. Moya-moya disease with repeated intraventricular hemorrhage due to aneurysm rupture. *J Neurosurg* 1994;80:328–331.

56. Yoshida Y, Yoshimoto T, Shirane R, Sakurai Y. Clinical course, surgical management, and long-term outcome of moyamoya patients with rebleeding after an episode of intracerebral hemorrhage: an extensive follow-up study. *Stroke* 1999;30:2276.

57. Saeki N, Nakazaki S, Kubota M, et al. Hemorrhagic type moyamoya disease. *Clin Neurol Neurosurg* 1997;99(suppl 2):S196–S201.

58. Herreman F, Nathal E, Yasuri N, et al. Intracranial aneurysms in moyamoya disease: report of ten cases and review of the literature. *Cerebrovasc Dis* 1993;4: 329–336.

59. Iwama T, Morimoto M, Hashimoto N, Goto Y, Todaka T, Sawada M. Mechanism of intracranial rebleeding in moyamoya disease. *Clin Neurol Neurosurg* 1997;99(suppl 2):S187–S190.

60. Biller J, Loftus CM, Moore JA, et al. Isolated central nervous system angiitis first presenting as spontaneous intracranial hemorrhage. *Neurosurgery* 1987;20:310–315.

61. Ozawa T, Sasaki O, Sorimachi T, et al. Primary angiitis of the central of the central nervous system: report of two cases and review of the literature. *Neurosurgery* 1995;36: 173–179.

62. Moore PM, Cupps TR. Neurological complications of vasculitis. *Ann Neurol* 1983;14:155–167.

63. Moore PM. Diagnosis and management of isolated angiitis of the central nervous system. *Neurology* 1989;39:167–173.

64. Liou HH, Liu HM, Chiang IP, Yeh TS, Chen RC. Churg–Strauss syndrome presented as multiple intracerebral hemorrhage. *Lupus* 1997;6:279–282.

65. Massoud TF, Anslow P, Molyneux AJ. Subarachnoid hemorrhage following spontaneous intracranial carotid artery dissection. *Neuroradiology* 1992;34:33–35.

66. Ohkuma H, Nakano T, Manabe H, Suzuki S. Subarachnoid hemorrhage caused by a dissecting aneurysm of the internal carotid artery. *J Neurol* 2002;97:576–583.

67. Ohkuma H, Suzuki S, Ogane K. Dissecting aneurysms of intracranial carotid circulation. *Stroke* 2002;33:941–947.

68. Piepgras DG, McGrail KM, Tazelaar HD. Intracranial dissection of the distal middle cerebral artery as an uncommon cause of distal cerebral artery aneurysm. Case report. *J Neurosurg* 1994;80:909–913.

69. Kunze AK, Annecke A, Wigger F, et al. Recent infection as a risk factor for intracerebral and subarachnoid hemorrhages. *Cerebrovasc Dis* 2000;10:352–358.

70. Schrader B, Barth H, Lang EW, et al. Spontaneous intracranial hematomas caused by neoplasms. *Acta Neurochir* 2000;142:979–985.

71. Wakai S, Yamakawa K, Manaka S, et al. Spontaneous intracranial hemorrhage caused by brain tumor: its incidence and clinical significance. *Neurosurgery* 1982;10: 437–444.

72. Mandybur TI. Intracranial hemorrhage caused by metastatic tumors. *Neurology* 1977;27:650–655.

73. Quinn JA, DeAngelis LM. Neurologic emergencies in the cancer patient. *Semin Oncol* 2000;27:311–321.

74. Kalafut M, Vinuela F, Saver JL, Martin N, Vespa P, Verity MA. Multiple cerebral pseudoaneurysms and hemorrhages: the expanding spectrum of metastatic cerebral choriocarcinoma. *J Neuroimaging* 1998;8:44–47.

75. Weir B, Macdonald N, Mielki B. Intracranial vascular complications of choriocarcinoma. *Neurosurgery* 1978;2: 138–142.

76. Helmer FA. Oncotic aneursym: case report. *J Neurosurg* 1976;45:98–100.

77. Pullar M, Blumbergs PC, Phillips GE, et al. Neoplastic cerebral aneurysm from metastatic gestational choriocarcinoma. *J Neurosurg* 1985;63:644–647.

78. Byrne TN, Cascino TL, Posner JB. Brain metastasis from melanoma. *J Neurooncology* 1983;1:313–317.

79. Furuya K, Sasaki T, Yoshimoto Y, Okada Y, Fujimaki T, Kirino T. Histologically verified cerebral aneurysm formation secondary to embolism from cardiac myxoma. Case report. *J Neurosurg* 1995;83:170–173.

80. Branch CL, Laster W, Kelly DL. Left atrial myxoma with cerebral emboli. *Neurosurgery* 1985;16:675–680.

81. Pinto AN. AIDS and cerebrovascular disease. *Stroke* 1996;27:538–543.

82. Rinkel GJE, Wijdicks EF, Vermeulen M, Hasan D, Brouwers PJAM, van Gijn J. The clinical course of perimesencephalic non-aneurysmal subarachnoid haemorrhage. *Ann Neurol* 1991;29:463–468.

83. Schwartz TH, Solomon RA. Perimesencephalic nonaneurysmal subarachnoid hemorrhage: review of the literature. *Neurosurgery* 1996;39:433–440.

84. Brilstra EH, Hop JW, Rinkel GJE. Quality of life after perimesencephalic haemorrhage. *J Neurol Neurosurg Psychiatry* 1997;63:382–384.

85. Rinkel GJE, Wijdicks EFM, Vermeulen M, Tans JTJ, Hasan D, van Gijn J. Acute hydrocephalus in nonaneurysmal perimesencephalic hemorrhage: evidence of CSF block at the tentorial hiatus. *Neurology* 1992;42:1805–1807.

86. Pinto AN, Ferro FM, Canhao P, Campos J. How often is a perimesencephalic subarachnoid haemorrhage CT pattern caused by ruptured aneurysms? *Acta Neurochir (Wien)* 1993;124:79–81.

87. Marquardt G, Niebauer T, Schick U, Lorenz R. Long term follow up after perimesencephalic subarachnoid haemorrhage. *J Neurol Neurosurg Psychiatry* 2000;69:127–130.

88. Canhao P, Falcao F, Pinho, Ferro H, Ferro J. Vascular risk factors for perimesencephalic nonaneurysmal subarachnoid hemorrhage. *J Neurol* 1999;246:492–496.

89. Perex JJ, Arsura EL, Strategos S. Methamphetamine-related stroke: four cases. *J Emerg Med* 1999;17:469–471.

90. Karch SB, Stephens BG, Ho CH. Methamphetamine-related deaths in San Francisco: demographic, pathologic, and toxicologic profiles. *J Forensic Sci* 1999;44: 359–368.

91. Karch SB. Use of Ephedra-containing products and risk for hemorrhagic stroke. *Neurology* 2003;61:724–725.

92. Fessler RD, Esshaki CM, Stankewitz RC, Johnson RR, Diaz FG. The neurovascular complications of cocaine. *Surg Neurol* 1997;47:339–345.

93. Harrington H, Heller HA, Dawson D, Caplan L, Rumbaugh C. Intracerebral hemorrhage and oral amphetamine. *Arch Neurol* 1983;40:503.

94. Levine SR, Brust JC, Futrell N, et al. Cerebrovascular complications of the use of the "crack" form of alkaloidal cocaine. *N Engl J Med* 1990;323:699–704.

95. Morgenstern LB, Viscoli CM, Kernan WN, et al. Use of Ephedra-containing products and risk for hemorrhagic stroke. *Neurology* 2003;60:132–135.

96. Levine SR, Brust JC, Futrell N, et al. A comparative study of the cerebrovascular complications of cocaine: alkaloidal versus hydrochloride—a review. *Neurology* 1991; 41:1173–1177.

97. Aggarwal SK, Williams V, Levine SR, et al. Cocaine-associated intracranial hemorrhage: absence of vasculitis in 14 cases. *Neurology* 1996;46:1741–1743.

98. Kernan WN, Viscoli CM, Brass LM, et al. Phenylpropanolamine and the risk of hemorrhagic stroke. *N Engl J Med* 2000;343:1826–1832.

99. Nolte KB, Brass LM, Fletterick CF. Intracranial hemorrhage associated with cocaine abuse: a prospective autopsy study. *Neurology* 1996;46:1291–1296.

100. Oyesiku NM, Colohan ART, Barrow DL, et al. Cocaine-induced aneurysmal rupture: an emergent negative factor in the natural history of intracranial aneurysms. *Neurosurgery* 1993;32:518–526.

101. Nanda A, Vannemreddy PS, Polin RS, Willis BK. Intracranial aneurysms and cocaine abuse: analysis of prognostic indicators. *Neurosurgery* 2000;46:1063–1067.

102. Krendel DA, Ditter SM, Frankel MF, et al. Biopsy-proven cerebral vasculitis associated with cocaine abuse. *Neurology* 1990;40:1092–1094.

103. Storen EC, Wijdicks EF, Crum BA, Schultz G. Moyamoya-like vasculopathy from cocaine dependency. *AJNR Am J Neuroradiol* 2000;21:1008–1010.

104. Wen PY, Feske SK, Teoh SK, Stieg PE. Cerebral hemorrhage in a patient taking fenfluramine and phentermine for obesity. *Neurology* 1997;49:632–633.

105. Nighoghossian N, Derex L, Trouillas P. Multiple intracerebral hemorrhages and vasospasm following antimigrainous drug abuse. *Headache* 1998;38:478–480.

106. White H, Simes RJ, Anderson NE, et al. Pravastatin therapy and the risk of stroke. *N Engl J Med* 2000;343: 317–326.

107. Schwartz SM, Siscovick DS, Longstreth WT, Jr., et al. Use of low-dose oral contraceptives and stroke in young women. *Ann Intern Med* 1997;127:596–603.

108. Johnston SC, Colford JMJ, Gress DR. Oral contraceptives and the risk of subarachnoid hemorrhage: a meta-analysis. *Neurology* 1998;51:411–418.

109. Leppala JM, Paunio M, Virtamo J, et al. Alcohol consumption and stroke incidence in male smokers. *Circulation* 1999;100:1209–1214.

110. Berger K, Ajani UA, Kase CS, et al. Light-to-moderate alcohol consumption and the risk of stroke among U.S. male physicians. *N Engl J Med* 1999;341:1557–1564.

111. Solomon RA, Loftus CM, Quest DO, et al. Incidence and etiology of intracerebral hemorrhage following carotid endarterectomy. *J Neurosurg* 1986;64:29–34.

112. Piepgras DG, Morfan MK, Sundt TM, Jr., et al. Intracerebral hemorrhage after carotid endarterectomy. *J Neurosurg* 1988;68:532–536.

113. Ouriel K, Shortell CK, Illig KA, Greenberg RK, Green RM. Intracerebral hemorrhage after carotid endarterectomy: incidence, contribution to neurologic morbidity, and predictive factors. *J Vasc Surg* 1999;29:82–87.

114. Heros RC, Nelson PB. Intracerebral hemorrhage after microsurgical revascularization. *Neurosurgery* 1980;6: 371–375.

115. McCabe DJ, Brown MM, Clifton A. Fatal cerebral reperfusion hemorrhage after carotid stenting. *Stroke* 1999;30: 2483–2486.

116. Mori T, Fukuoka M, Kazita K, Mima T, Mori K. Intraventricular hemorrhage after carotid stenting. *J Endovasc Surg* 1999;6:337–341.

117. Snow RB, Zimmerman RD, Deviasky O. Delayed intracerebral hemorrhage after ventriuloperitoneal shunting. *Neurosurgery* 1986;19:305–307.

118. Kvam DA, Michelsen WJ, Quest DO. Intracerebral hemorrhage as a complication of artificial embolization. *Neurosurgery* 1980;7:491–494.

119. Modesti LM, Hodge CJ, Barnwell ML. Intracerebral hematoma after evacuation of chronic extracerebral fluid collection. *Neurosurgery* 1982;10:689–693.

120. D'Avella D, DeBlan F, Rotilio A, et al. Intracerebral hematoma following evacuation of chronic subdural hematomas. *J Neurosurg* 1986;65:710–712.

121. Humphreys RP, Hoffman HJ, Mustard WT, et al. Cerebral hemorrhage following heart surgery. *J Neurosurg* 1975;43: 671–675.

122. Onoyama K, Ibayashi S, Nahishi F, et al. Cerebral hemorrhage in patients on maintenance hemodialysis. *Eur Neurol* 1987;26:171–175.

123. Kawamura M, Fijimoto S, Hisanaga S, Yamamoto Y, Eto T. Incidence, outcome, and risk factors of cerebrovascular events in patients undergoing maintenance hemodialysis. *Am J Kidney Dis* 1998;31:991–996.

124. Caplan L. Intracerebral hemorrhage revisited. *Neurology* 1988;38:624–627.

125. Stanley LD, Suss RA. Intraverebral hematoma secondary to lightning strike: case report and review of the literature. *Neurosurgery* 1985;16:686–688.

126. Caplan LR, Neely S, Gorelick P. Cold-related intracerebral hemorrhage. *Arch Neurol* 1985;42:227–227.

127. Barbas N, Caplan LR, Baquis G, et al. Dental chair intracerebral hemorrhage. *Neurology* 1987;37:511–512.

128. Kasirajan V, Smedira N, McCarthy J, Casselman F, Boparai N, McCarthy P. Risk factors for intracranial hemorrhage in adults on extracorporeal membrane oxygenation. *Eur J Cardiothorac Surg* 1999;15:508–514.

129. Drislane FW, Wang AM. Multifocal cerebral hemorrhage in eclampsia and severe pre-eclampsia. *J Neurol* 1997; 244:194–198.

130. Qureshi AI, Frankel MR, Ottenlips JR, Stern BJ. Cerebral hemodynamics in preeclampsia and eclampsia. *Arch Neurol* 1996;53:1226–1231.

131. Qureshi AI, Giles WH, Croft JB, Stern BJ. Number of pregnancies and risk for stroke and stroke subtypes. *Arch Neurol* 1997;54:203–206.

132. Roh JK, Park KS. Postpartum cerebral angiopathy with intracerebral hemorrhage in a patient receiving lisuride. *Neurology* 1998;50:1152–1154.
133. Ursell MR, Marras CL, Farb R, Rowed DW, Black SE, Perry JR. Recurrent intracranial hemorrhage due to postpartum cerebral angiopathy: implications for management. *Stroke* 1998;29:1995–1998.
134. Singh S, Brensman MJ. Menkes' kinky hair syndrom (trichopoliodystrophy). *Am J Dis Child* 1973;39:773–775.
135. Casson IF, Cooke NT. Thyrotoxicosis and subarachnoid hemorrhage. *Br J Clin Pract* 1981;35:121–122.
136. Sterling GM. Conn's syndrome and subarachnoid hemorrhage. *Br Med J* 1965;1:839–840.
137. Boersma LV, Leyten QH, Meijer JW, Strubbe EJ, Bosch FH. Cerebral hemorrhage complicating exertional heat stroke. *Clin Neurol Neurosurg* 1998;100:112–115.
138. Chehrenama M, Zagardo MT, Koski CL. Subarachnoid hemorrhage in a patient with Lyme disease. *Neurology* 1997;48:520–523.
139. Vahedi K, Massin P, Guichard J-P, et al. Hereditary infantile hemiparesis, retinal arteriolar tortuosity, and leukoencephalopathy. *Neurology* 2003;60:57–63.

CHAPTER 17

Strokes in Children and Young Adults

While stroke usually is considered as a disease of older persons, vascular events of the nervous system are an important cause of death or disability in infants, children, and young adults. In developing countries, the impact of stroke in the young is especially high. For example, up to 30 percent of strokes in the Middle East and South Asia are diagnosed in persons younger than 45 (see Chapter 2).

Still, young persons with stroke differ from older individuals. A majority of cerebrovascular events in young adults are due to intracerebral hemorrhage or subarachnoid hemorrhage. This ratio differs markedly from older populations in which 80 percent of strokes are infarctions. Still, cerebral infarctions frequently occur in children and young adults. Unfortunately, stroke is among the leading causes of death in childhood.[1] Approximately 3 percent of ischemic strokes occur among persons aged 15–45.[2] The causes of ischemic stroke in teenagers and young adults differ from those seen in older persons. For example, atherosclerosis is a progressive vasculopathy that evolves over a lifetime. Thus, advanced atherosclerosis is a relatively uncommon cause of stroke among young people. Conversely, genetic or congenital diseases often lead to stroke in young persons. They become symptomatic early in life. The etiologies of intracranial hemorrhage among young persons also differ from those found among older persons. For example, the relative importance of a ruptured vascular malformation is high in young men and women. Conversely, chronic hypertension and amyloid angiopathy are rare causes of intracerebral hemorrhage in children and young adults.

Additional research on the causes and management of both hemorrhagic and ischemic strokes in young adults is needed. While the diagnosis, prognosis, and treatment of ischemic and hemorrhagic strokes in young adults have received considerable attention in the last two decades, information about vascular events in children has lagged. Much of pediatric stroke research has focused on treatment of children with sickle cell disease. This genetic disease, which is an important cause of stroke, merits this attention. However, the differential diagnosis of both hemorrhagic and ischemic stroke in infancy and childhood is broad and considerable additional research is needed. Other important causes of pediatric stroke need to be addressed. Research on the ways to manage stroke in children also is limited. While there are data about the safety and efficacy of blood transfusions in limited the cerebrovascular consequences of sickle cell disease, evidence about the utility of other therapies to prevent or treat stroke in the pediatric population is virtually nonexistent.[3] Additional epidemiological studies and research on the causes of and treatment of strokes in children and young adults are needed. Many of the causes of hemorrhagic or ischemic stroke in children and young adults are described in other chapters of this book. This chapter focuses on several of the etiologies of stroke that appear to occur primarily in younger persons.

▶ PERINATAL STROKE

Both cerebral infarction and hemorrhage occur in fetuses and infants (Table 17-1). Despite the potential for severe morbidity or mortality, the contribution of stroke to infantile neurological impairments does not receive much emphasis. The consequences of perinatal brain injury can lead to severe lifetime disability. Perinatal stroke also can lead to death. Many affected children also have residual mental retardation, behavioral problems, or seizures.[1,4,5] Neonatal strokes are one of the leading causes of cerebral palsy in children. In particular, those cases of cerebral palsy marked by spasticity, dystonia, or weakness of one side might be secondary to a brain hemorrhage or infarction. In addition, fetal intraventricular hemorrhage is a potential cause of congenital hydrocephalus. These events usually are not discussed in detail in neurological texts, even those that focusing on cerebrovascular diseases. Because many of the events occur in-utero or near the time of delivery, the strongest data are found in the obstetrical literature.

Hemorrhage

Periventricular (subependymal) and *intraventricular hemorrhage (germinal matrix hemorrhage)* are a leading cause of morbidity or mortality in premature infants. These hemorrhages are uncommon among term infants. Vergani et al.[6] reported that the incidence of intracranial bleeding is approximately 0.9/1000 pregnancies. They noted a very poor prognosis among affected babies. Many of these hemorrhages likely occur during the antepartum period and they can be diagnosed through prenatal sonography.[7] In addition, some hemorrhages might be secondary to the stresses and trauma of delivery. Babies with intraventricular or subependymal hemorrhages often need ventilatory assistance and appear in distress soon after birth. However, focal neurological impairments apparently are not obvious. Intrapartum fetal distress and possibly acidosis appear to predict which premature infants will have hemorrhagic complications.[8] No relationship to antepartum or intrapartum complications, type of delivery, duration of labor, or the presence of hyaline membrane disease has been found. Maternal factors that might be associated with fetal hemorrhages include thrombocytopenia, von Willebrand disease, drug abuse, and use of warfarin.[7,9]

Hyperhomocysteinemia is another potential cause of neonatal hemorrhage. In addition, genetic disorders of coagulation, such as factor V or factor X deficiency, affecting the fetus can induce major intracranial bleeding. For example, a European survey reported intracranial bleeding within 1 week of birth in 11 boys with *hemophilia*.[10] Hypoprothrombinemia is a cause of bleeding in newborns.[11] Congenital afibrinogenemia can be complicated by newborn bleeding.[12]

Infarction

Perinatal cerebral infarctions, which most commonly affect the territory of the middle cerebral artery, seem to occur primarily in full-term infants. The incidence of perinatal infarctions, which is approximately 25/100,000 births, appears to be higher than the risk of ischemic stroke in older children. Some of these strokes might not produce symptoms in the neonatal period and the vascular event is recognized only when the child is older and neurological deficits, such as cognitive impairments, are detected. Children can have seizures or respiratory distress as the only evidence of the acute brain event. Focal motor impairments, such as hemiparesis, usually are not obvious. The causes of perinatal ischemic stroke probably are diverse and include perinatal central nervous system infections, congenital cardiac disorders, severe anemia, prothrombotic coagulation disorders, hypoxia, asphyxia, and trauma. Stroke can be a presentation of *infantile AIDS*. Vahedi et al.[13] described infantile hemiparesis as a finding in *hereditary endotheliopathy* with *retinopathy, nephropathy,* and *stroke.* While severe anemia is included among the uncommon hematological disorders that can lead to stroke in older persons, the impact of iron deficiency anemia in leading to neonatal infarction might be considerable because many children, particularly those in underdeveloped countries, have *iron deficiency anemia.* The neonatal period is a

---

▶ **TABLE 17-1.** CAUSES OF PERINATAL HEMORRHAGE OR INFARCTION

Hemorrhage
  Subependymal and germinal matrix hemorrhage
    Hemorrhage in premature infarction
  Maternal factors associated with perinatal bleeding
    Thrombocytopenia
    Von Willebrand disease
    Drug abuse
    Use of oral anticoagulants
  Hyperhomocystinemia
  Factor V deficiency
  Hemophilia
  Hypoprothrombinemia
  Afibrinogenemia
Infarction
  Central nervous system infection
  Congenital heart disease
  Iron deficiency anemia
  Hypoxia
  Asphyxia
  Arterial trauma
  Neonatal purpura fulminans
  HERNS

---

time of particularly high risk for severe ischemic complications of some of the inherited disorders of coagulation, particularly those with homozygous inheritance; fulminant thromboembolic disease has been reported. For example, *neonatal purpura fulminans* can be secondary to an absence of protein C.[14] While children affected by neonatal/perinatal infarctions usually survive, many of them will have residual language, cognitive or motor impairments. No data exist to guide management of neonates with cerebral infarction. Recently, Crowther et al.[15] reported that administration of magnesium sulfate to women immediately before preterm birth was safe and that the medication might lower the risk for major neurological injuries in the child.

The risk of recurrent stroke appears to be relatively low. Kurnik et al.[16] followed 215 neonates with ischemic stroke and only 7 had recurrent events. Most of the children who had a second stroke had an underlying hypercoagulable disorder.

► ISCHEMIC STROKE IN CHILDREN

The incidence of infarctions in children older than 6 months of age is approximately 3–4/100,000 with higher rates in African-American children than in other ethnic groups.[1,17] The higher rate of stroke in African-Americans is largely secondary to *sickle cell disease*.[18] Most studies suggest that the frequencies of stroke suggest a slightly higher rate among boys than among girls; mortality from ischemic stroke also is higher among boys.[1] The mortality from childhood stroke has declined during the last 20 years.[1] Stroke remains an important cause of death in childhood.[19] In the past, the risk of recurrent infarction among children was thought to be relatively low, but this impression appears to be incorrect. The chances of recurrent events appear to be similar as to adults with an overall likelihood of a second stroke being approximately 10–30 percent in the subsequent 3–5 years.[1] On the other hand, Hurvitz et al.[20] found relatively good functional outcomes among adolescents and children who survived stroke. Those children with infarction secondary to embolism or heart disease and those with hemiparesis had poor outcomes. Girls and those with strokes at a young age had high rates of behavioral or cognitive impairments. Although no clinical trials have tested the utility of antithrombotic medications in treatment of children with stroke, these agents are prescribed to a broad spectrum of children.[21] In general, the guidelines for the use of these medications are similar to those for adults.

Clinical Findings

In general, the presentations of ischemic stroke in children mimic those found in adults. Ischemic stroke in children can result from a wide variety of arterial diseases, cardiac disorders, or diseases of coagulation[22,23] (Table 17-2). In many cases, multiple potential contributing causes or risk factors can be identified. Genetic diseases are a particularly important cause of stroke in children.[24] With an extensive evaluation, the likely cause of stroke can be determined in approximately 70 percent of children.

Arterial Causes

Atherosclerosis is not an important cause of infarctions in children. Exceptional cases of accelerated atherosclerosis might occur in teenagers who have an inherited disorder of lipid metabolism or another genetic disease that leads to early arterial occlusive disease. While most young men with arterial disease secondary to Fabry–Anderson disease usually do not develop ischemic neurological or cardiac symptoms until the third decade, some teenage boys could have stroke. Homocystinuria also could cause accelerated arterial disease in an adolescent. Patients with hyperhomocysteinemia or a deficiency of MTHFR also could have arterial stenoses or occlusions at a relatively young age.[25] In addition, the detection of risk factors for accelerated atherosclerosis in childhood does correlate with development of advanced disease in adulthood.[26–28]

Infections

Many strokes in children and adolescents are secondary to infectious or noninfectious, inflammatory vasculopathies.[22,29] In particular, infections seem to be key cause of major arterial occlusions in children. Stroke is a potential complication of *meningitis* secondary to streptococcus pneumoniae, haemophilus influenzae, or neisseria meningitides.[30] The inflammatory process in the meninges presumably leads to an arteritis. An inflammatory arteriopathy following *varicella* is a cause of stroke; the lag between the infection and the stroke can be several months. Askalan et al.[31] reported that 22 of 70 children with acute ischemic stroke had varicella in the previous year. The infarctions usually involve the basal ganglia in the distribution of the lenticulostriate arteries. Arteriography can demonstrate segmental areas of narrowing and irregularity. Chabrier et al.[32] described a transient arteriopathy that causes subcortical infarctions and that was characterized by multiple areas of narrowing of the basal arteries. It is unclear if this arteriopathy was infectious in origin. *Cysticercosis* can present as stroke in childhood.[33] This scenario is most likely among persons living in areas endemic for the parasite.

Occlusion of the internal carotid artery also can follow a *suppurative infection* of the *oropharynx* or *tonsillitis*. Severe dehydration and clotting derangements secondary to an infectious illness, which is complicated by vomiting and diarrhea, can also lead to arterial or

► **TABLE 17-2.** CAUSES OF ISCHEMIC STROKE IN CHILDREN

Noninflammatory Vasculopathies	Noninfectious Vasculitis
Arterial dissection	Systemic lupus erythematosus
Trauma	Kawasaki disease
Intraoral trauma	Takayasu disease
Moyamoya disease	Infectious Vasculopathies
Moyamoya syndrome	Bacterial meningitis
Migraine	Viral meningitis
Fibromuscular dysplasia	Lyme disease
Cardioembolism	Tuberculous meningitis
Pulmonary atresia	Fungal meningitis
Aortic stenosis	Varicella
Coarctation of the aorta	Parameningeal infection
Ventricular septal defect	AIDS
Atrial septal defect	Parasitic infection
Patent ductus arteriosus	Coagulopathy
Transposition of great vessels	Leukemia
Rheumatic fever	Thrombocytopenia
Prosthetic cardiac valve	Anemia
Endocarditis	Polycythemia
Cardiomyopathy	Sickle cell disease
Atrial myxoma	DIC
Rhabdomyoma	Hemophilia
Other causes of emboli	Prothrombin gene mutation
Air	Factor V Leiden
Fat	Protein C or S deficiency
Drugs or medications	Antithrombin deficiency
Chemotherapy	Fanconi anemia
Cocaine	
Methamphetamine	
Phencyclidine	

venous thrombosis. Noninfectious, autoimmune vascular diseases, such as Takayasu disease, Kawasaki disease, or systemic lupus erythematosus, are relatively uncommon causes of cerebral infarction in children.[34]

Dissection

Arterial dissection is a potential cause of stroke in children. In a review of the literature, Fullerton et al.[35] found 118 children. The actual number probably is much higher. Approximately 75 percent were boys and all had evidence of ischemia. Approximately 60 percent of the arterial dissections were intracranial were in location. Presumably most of these were spontaneous. In the series of Schievink et al.,[36] 18 of 263 persons with extracranial or intracranial dissections were younger than 18. Both carotid and vertebrobasilar dissections are found with most traumatic dissections being located extracranially.[37,38] The symptoms and signs in children are similar to those found in older persons. Both traumatic and spontaneous dissections can occur.[36] Among the latter, *Ehlers-Danlos syndrome* is one of the underlying arterial diseases.[18,30] Vertebral arterial dissection has complicated *Klippel-Feil syndrome*.[39] Trauma can cause extracranial dissection or occlusion of the vertebral or

internal carotid arteries. Because children are very physically active and involved in a large number of sports, which can be complicated by hyperrotation or hyperextension of the neck, secondary arterial injury is not surprising. The extracranial portion of the internal carotid artery, which lies behind in the tonsillar fossa, is vulnerable to *penetrating trauma*. The usual scenario is a child falling while having a foreign body such as a candy stick or ice cream stick in his mouth. The stick is forced into the posterior pharynx and either punctures the artery or cause an intramural hematoma ("popsicle stick palsy" or "lollypop palsy".) The prognosis of children with arterial dissections is similar to adults. The internal carotid artery also can be injured during *tonsillectomy*.

Moyamoya

Moyamoya disease is a genetic arteriopathy that is inherited in an autosomal dominant pattern.[40] The disease affects both children and young adults and is most common among persons of Northeast Asian ancestry. *Moyamoya syndrome* has been described as a vascular complication of *Down syndrome, neurofibromatosis, or sickle cell disease* (see Chapter 12). *Radiation-induced vasculopathy* can complicate radiation therapy for treatment of pediatric brain tumors such as *medulloblastoma*.[41] The radiation can cause vascular damage, a mineralizing microangiopathy, or moyamoya syndrome. Besides ischemic stroke, children with moyamoya disease or syndrome can initially have seizures or mental retardation.

Migraine

Pediatric migraine is a potential cause of stroke in children.[42] Because children often have prominent focal neurological symptoms with their migrainous attacks, an infarction must be differentiated from a complex migraine. In particular, most people affected by vertebrobasilar migraine are children or adolescents. These events can mimic a vertebrobasilar TIA or a brain stem stroke. The rules for diagnosing migrainous stroke in children should be the same as for young adults.

Cardioembolism

Approximately 15 percent of ischemic strokes in childhood are secondary to embolization from a cardiac lesion.[43] Most affected children have clinically overt heart disease. Many of the cardiac lesions are congenital and some are associated with cyanosis and right-to-left intracardiac shunts[22,44] (see Chapter 13). Besides stroke, *cyanotic congenital heart disease* in childhood also can be complicated by brain abscess. Presumably a septic embolus lodges in a cerebral artery and serves as a nidus for the bacterial infection. Children with congenital cardiac lesions also are at risk for infective endocarditis and warrant antibiotic prophylaxis during dental procedures and other operations. Acquired cardiac lesions include rheumatic heart disease and cardiomyopathies, some of which are secondary to genetic neuromuscular disorders including the muscular dystrophies. Children with severe heart disease often need major cardiovascular operations. Kirkham[45] has highlighted the relatively high risk of cognitive and other neurological sequelae of such surgery. Pua and Bissonnette[46] estimated that up to 30 percent of children might have postoperative ischemic brain injuries. The *Fontan procedure* appears to be particularly risky.[47]

Hypercoagulable Disorders

Inherited or acquired hypercoagulable states are an important cause of stroke in children.[43,48,49] Stroke is a leading neurological complication of childhood malignancies, including *acute lymphoblastic leukemia, acute myeloblastic leukemia,* and *neuroblastoma*.[50,51] Leukemia can lead to hyperviscosity and secondary thrombosis. In addition, stroke is a potential complication of chemotherapy including treatment with *methotrexate, asparaginase,* or *adrimycin*. Children also are risk for stroke secondary to thrombocytopenia, nonbacterial thrombotic

▶ **TABLE 17-3.** SICKLE CELL DISEASE AND STROKE

Children of African or Middle Eastern ancestry
Other evidence of disease
    Painful crises (hypoxia or infection)
    Severe anemia
    Cardiomegaly and heart failure
Neurological features
    Cerebral infarction
    Multiple lacunar infarctions
      Vascular dementia
    Moyamoya syndrome
    Intracranial hemorrhage—aneurysms

endocarditis, sepsis, or disseminated intravascular coagulation. Stroke can complicate *hemolytic-uremic syndrome* and *thrombotic thrombocytopenia purpura*[52](see Chapter 14). In addition, stroke has occurred among children having *bone marrow transplantation*. Dehydration complicating a severe systemic illness also can promote thrombosis through hyperviscosity. While polycythemia is uncommon among children, severe anemia, including iron deficiency anemia, is a potential etiology.

Sickle cell disease is a leading cause of stroke in children; the incidence of stroke among affected children is estimated as 1.29 per 100,000[53] (Table 17-3). The peak age for sickle cell disease induced cerebral infarction is approximately 4.[54] Because the childhood mortality from sickle cell disease is decreasing, the mean age of affected patients is increasing and the risk of stroke persists.[55] As children reach adulthood, the chances of cerebral infarction decline. Approximately 5–10 percent of children have clinically obvious strokes, while another 15 percent will have evidence of clinically silent infarctions found on brain imaging studies.[56–58] Sickle cell disease also can lead to progressive cognitive impairments secondary to recurrent ischemia.[59,60]

Affected children have other evidence of sickle cell disease including a history of painful crises. Attacks often are provoked by hypoxia or infections. In addition, children with severe anemia can have secondary cardiomegaly or congestive heart failure; cardioembolic stroke is a potential complication. Most strokes often are due to occlusion of small intracranial arteries. Such strokes usually are small and located in the basal ganglia or centrum semiovale. They often are aligned in a watershed pattern. Presumably the sickle cells adhere to the vascular endothelium and lead to inflammation and thickening of the vessel wall. In addition, larger vessels appear to be affected by changes in the vasa vasorum. Transcranial Doppler ultrasonography has become an important method of screening children with sickle cell disease. Detection of secondary changes in velocity (>200 cm/sec) can prompt transfusion of normal blood to lower the concentration of SS hemoglobin in the blood.[61,62] A systemic review of the available clinical trials suggests that regular blood transfusions can reduce the risk of stroke among children with sickle cell disease but there is risk from recurrent transfusions.[63] The benefit of the transfusions needs to be weighed against the potential for serious consequences from the repeated transfusions. Additional study about the potential efficacy of the intervention is needed.

Other inherited hypercoagulable disorders include either *Factor V Leiden* or the *prothrombin gene mutation*.[64] Both of these prothrombotic diseases have been described as a cause of stroke in infants and children. For example, Lynch et al.[65] described 128 children with stroke and Factor V Leiden. Other series have described similar data.[66,67] Infarctions secondary to arterial or venous occlusion have been described among children with decreased levels of proteins C or S, antithrombin, or plasminogen. Antiphospholipid antibodies also have been found in some children with stroke.[68] Management of children with hypercoagulable causes of ischemic stroke is similar to that given to adults.

Several of the inherited or acquired disorders of coagulation are described in more detail in Chapter 14. The inherited arterial causes of ischemic stroke, which lead to brain infarction, including the mitochondrial disorders, are reviewed in Chapter 12.

▶ HEMORRHAGIC STROKE IN CHILDREN

After excluding for germinal matrix and traumatic bleeding, Broderick et al.[17] found that the incidence of spontaneous intracerebral or subarachnoid hemorrhage was 1.5/100,000 children—a rate that exceeded that for infarction. A slightly higher rate was found among African-American children compared to whites.

Trauma

Trauma is the leading cause of intracranial hemorrhage in children. Intracranial bleeding can follow minor trauma in a child that has an inherited or acquired coagulopathy (Table 17-4). In some cases, the history of trauma, such as a fall from a swing or bicycle, is obvious. However, intracranial bleeding can be secondary to an *intentional injury*, especially when the child is younger than 3 and neurologists need to consider child abuse as a possible cause of bleeding. Wells et al.[69] noted that the imaging findings of a convexity subdural hematoma, interhemispheric subdural hematoma, subdural hygroma, or the absence of a skull fracture with an intracranial hemorrhage might be associated with an intentional injury.

▶ **TABLE 17-4.** CAUSES OF HEMORRHAGIC STROKE IN CHILDHOOD

Trauma
  Accidents
  Intentional (child abuse)
Vascular malformation
Aneurysm
  Saccular
  Dissection
  Infective
Moyamoya disease or syndrome
Coagulopathies
  Hemophilia
  Sickle cell disease
  Thrombocytopenia
  Leukemia
Medications
  Chemotherapy
  Antithrombotic medications
Alagille syndrome

Vascular Malformation

Hemorrhage in the brain, ventricles, or subarachnoid space can be secondary to rupture of a *vascular malformation*. Among the causes are arteriovenous malformations, arteriovenous fistulas, vein of Galen malformation, and aneurysms.[70] Vascular malformations are leading cause of subarachnoid hemorrhage in children and adolescents. The clinical findings of ruptured supratentorial or posterior fossa vascular malformations in childhood are similar to those found in adults. Besides hemorrhage, a large vein of Galen malformation also can cause compression of adjacent structures. In addition, the malformation can lead to a rapidly enlarging head or congestive heart failure in an infant. In general, the options for management of vascular malformations diagnosed in childhood are similar to those available for treatment of older persons. Although a leptomeningeal vascular anomaly (angiomatosis) is a key component of the *Sturge-Weber syndrome*, bleeding seems to be uncommon. Subarachnoid hemorrhage in a child has been attributed to a *dissecting aneurysm* that complicated fibromuscular dysplasia.[71] Bleeding also can be a complication of moyamoya disease and syndrome.[72–74]

Aneurysm

The frequency of bleeding secondary to aneurysms is relatively low in the pediatric population. The locations of the aneurysms generally are similar to those found in adults, although there is some suggestion that more of the lesions are located distally than in older persons. Occasionally, a large, intact aneurysm can produce compressive symptoms in a child. In general, the prognosis of children with ruptured aneurysms is poor.

Bleeding Diatheses

The frequency of intracranial hemorrhages complicating *hemophilia* has not changed in the last 20 years.[10,75–78] Intracranial bleeding usually is secondary to trauma. Affected children often have severe neurological sequelae including seizures, hemiparesis, or cognitive impairments. While infarction is an important cause of neurological morbidity among children with sickle cell disease, hemorrhage also occurs. Most hemorrhages are in adolescents.[79] A potential relationship between sickle cell disease and saccular aneurysms may exist.[79–81] Hemorrhages also can be secondary to *malignancies* or *chemotherapy*.[51,82] Thrombocytopenia secondary to chemotherapy is among the potential causes of pediatric intracranial hemorrhage. A potential scenario is bleeding in a child with leukemia who also has had a bone marrow transplant. The inherited and acquired disorders that promote bleeding are described in more detail in Chapter 14.

Intracranial hemorrhage is a cause of morbidity and mortality among children with *Alagille syndrome.* This autosomal dominant disorder presents with anomalies of the skeleton, face, eye, liver, and heart. Affected children can have major cardiac changes including tetralogy of Fallot or pulmonary atresia, which requires surgical correction. In addition, a coagulation disturbance causes a high risk of bleeding complications. Moyamoya syndrome also has been described as a finding in Alagille syndrome.

In general, the management of intracranial bleeding in childhood is similar to that recommended for treatment of adults. Based on a follow-up study involving 36 of 56 children with hemorrhagic stroke, Blom et al.[83] found cognitive impairments in 50 percent of children and motor impairments in almost as many. Only 25 percent of children did not have either cognitive or motor sequelae from the hemorrhage.

▶ STROKE IN YOUNG ADULTS

Stroke is an important health problem in young adults.[84] In stroke studies, the term, young adults, usually encompasses the age group of 15–45. While the patients aged 15–18 usually are included in a pediatric population, the types of vascular diseases of the brain begin to change at this age. For example, most serious congenital heart diseases that are associated with stroke already have been symptomatic by this time. Thus teenagers have diseases similar to persons who are slightly older.

Malm et al.[85] reported that approximately 6 percent of young adults with cerebral infarction died as a result of the stroke. Biller et al.[86] reported similar results. The mortality from hemorrhagic stroke is higher.[87] In addition, the societal consequences of stroke in the young are immense. Young adults are parents of small children, they are the persons who are active in the work force, and in some cases they are providing care for parents. As a result, their disability from stroke has a major economic impact. Virtually every young adult will comment on the adverse cognitive, physical, emotional, and societal sequelae of the stroke.[88] The stroke changed their lives and not for the better. While the stroke recurrence rate is not especially high, many young adults remain disabled and they are unable to return to work.[89] Musolino et al.[90] found that only 50 percent of young adults were fully independent, while 11 percent of were completely disabled. In their series, only 68 percent of stroke survivors were able to return to work but in many instances, major adjustments in employment were required.

The incidence of stroke in young adults might be increasing. In part, this rise might be secondary to improved recognition and detection. However, some of the high-risk behaviors associated with stroke also are increasing in this age group. For example, drug and alcohol abuse are important risk factors for stroke in young adults.[91] Some of the increase in hemorrhagic stroke is secondary to cocaine abuse. The list of causes of stroke in young adults is long. In some way, the listing represents a transition. Many of the congenital or inherited diseases that affect children also affect this age group. In addition, some of the acquired diseases that become more prevalent in the elderly begin to appear in young adults. Some researchers have divided this group into two subgroups: patients aged 15–35 and those aged 36–45. This division is based on the assumption that the majority of ischemic strokes in the younger subgroup are secondary to disorders of coagulation or heart disease, while some of the older patients start having strokes secondary to atherosclerotic vascular disease.

Many of the differences in stroke rates among the ethnic groups in the United States are most marked among young adults; in this age group the rates of stroke are three to four times higher in African-Americans and twice as high among Hispanics as than in whites[92,93] (see Chapter 2). The chances of subarachnoid and intracerebral hemorrhages also are considerably higher in young African-Americans compared to whites.[94,95] Qureshi et al.[96] found that the frequency of hypertensive intracerebral hemorrhage and lacunar infarctions, which probably are secondary to hypertensive disease of small arteries, were much more common in young African-Americans than in other ethnic groups. The likelihood of death from a stroke in African-American men and women is approximately twice that found in whites. Similar differences are noted among ethnic groups living in the United Kingdom. The explanations for the high incidence of stroke in young African-American men and women include high prevalences of heart disease, diabetes, hypertension, and obesity. Increased mortality from stroke in young adults also has been described in Asian/Pacific Islanders and Native Americans.[97] Much of the higher mortality is ascribed to subarachnoid hemorrhage. In several countries, increased mortality from stroke among young adults also has been correlated with a lower socioeconomic living environment.[98]

In addition, important differences in the causes of hemorrhagic and ischemic stroke are noted between young men and women.[99] In the general population, the incidence of stroke is higher in men than in women. Some of the high risk among men is attributed to the high prevalence of smoking and alcohol use (Table 17-5). The exception to the rule of higher rates of stroke among men is the age group of young adults. The relative frequency of both brain infarctions and hemorrhages is increased in young women, largely as the result of complications of pregnancy.[100,101] The important associations between stroke and pregnancy or the puerperium highlight the differences between sexes. Among women under the age of 45, cerebrovascular disease, in particular cerebral hemorrhage, is a more common cause of death than is ischemic heart disease.[102] The leading causes of stroke in young women are cardioembolism, nonatherosclerotic vasculopathies, hematological disorders, and migraine.[99] Reiner et al.[103] found that polymorphisms in Factor XIII are associated with an increased susceptibility to hemorrhagic stroke in women. In addition, the use of oral contraceptives is implicated as associated with an increased chance of stroke. Among young men, the importance of atherosclerosis as a cause of stroke increases after the age of 35. It can be a direct cause of cerebral infarction or an indirect cause via myocardial infarction with secondary cardioembolic stroke.

The differential diagnosis of causes of ischemic stroke in young adults is broad[84,104–106] (see Table 17-5). The etiologies are categorized as (1) atherosclerosis leading to large or small artery disease, (2) nonatherosclerotic vasculopathies, (3) cardiac sources of embolization, or (4) prothrombotic states. Despite an extensive evaluation, the etiology of cerebral infarction often is not determined. Stroke of undetermined etiology is diagnosed in approximately one-sixth to one-fourth of cases. The distribution of causes differs than in older individuals because atherosclerosis and ischemic heart disease with secondary atrial fibrillation are relatively uncommon among persons younger than 35. The causes of hemorrhage in young adults are similar to those occur in older adults. As with ischemic stroke, the ratio of the causes of hemorrhage in younger persons differs from older persons. Amyloid angiopathy and chronic hypertension are relatively uncommon, while aneurysms, vascular malformations, and acute hypertensive crises are important etiologies.

► ISCHEMIC STROKE IN YOUNG ADULTS

► ARTERIAL CAUSES

Atherosclerosis

Atherosclerosis is an important cause of cerebral infarction in young adults, especially among men older than 35 and its prevalence might be increasing (Table 17-6). Although estimates vary considerably between clinical series, approximately 10–25 percent of infarctions in young adults probably are secondary to atherosclerotic disease.[104] The disease can be either intracranial or

► **TABLE 17-5.** LEADING CAUSES OF ISCHEMIC STROKE IN YOUNG ADULTS

Large artery atherosclerosis	Small artery occlusive disease
Nonatherosclerotic vasculopathies	
Dissection	Cardioembolism
Trauma	Rheumatic mitral stenosis
Fibromuscular dysplasia	Prosthetic valve
Moyamoya disease	Patent foramen ovale
Moyamoya syndrome	Mitral valve prolapse
Susac syndrome	Myocardial infarction
Infectious vasculopathies	Cardiomyopathy
Herpes zoster	Migraine
Syphilis	Pregnancy
Meningitis	Eclampsia
AIDS	Postpartum vasculopathy
Aneurysms	Postpartum cardiomyopathy
CADASIL	Amniotic fluid embolism
Alcohol abuse	Air embolism
Drug abuse	Oral contraceptives
Cocaine	Homocystinuria
Methamphetamine	Fabry-Anderson disease
Heroin	Marfan syndrome

► **TABLE 17-6.** ATHEROSCLEROSIS IN YOUNG ADULTS

Frequency increases among men >35 years or women >45 years
Large artery intracranial or extracranial disease
Small artery occlusive disease
Familial or inherited risk factors for premature atherosclerosis
Hypercholesterolemia
Homocystinuria
Hyperhomocysteinemia
Fabry-Anderson disease
Other risk factors for premature atherosclerosis
Hypercholesterolemia
Hypertension
Diabetes mellitus
Smoking/tobacco abuse

extracranial in location. Infarctions also can be secondary to small vessel disease. A relatively young age should not automatically exclude the diagnosis of atherosclerotic cerebrovascular disease. Young persons at risk for premature atherosclerosis include those with a strong family history of premature atherosclerosis, hypertension, hypercholesterolemia, hyperhomocysteinemia, smoking, or diabetes mellitus.[107–110] For example, Tan et al.[111] found that hyperhomocysteinemia is an independent risk factor for stroke in young adults. In most instances, these young patients have a history of risk factors, which often are poorly controlled, for several years. Patients can have either intracranial or extracranial artery disease. Lacunar infarctions are particularly common in young African-Americans with chronic hypertension.[96] Young adults with juvenile onset diabetes mellitus also have a high risk for lacunar infarctions, which can be recurrent. Ischemic stroke presumably due to premature atherosclerosis in a young man can be secondary to *Fabry–Anderson disease.*[112] While this X-linked genetic disease is uncommon, most men affected with cerebral infarction or myocardial infarction are younger than 30 (see Chapter 12).

Many young adults (especially men) have a history of premature coronary artery disease and secondary embolization from an ischemic cardiac lesion is also a potential cause of infarction. Management of young adults with symptomatic atherosclerosis is similar to that recommended for evaluation and treatment of older persons. Aggressive treatment of diabetes mellitus, homocysteine, cholesterol, and hypertension are complemented by changes in lifestyle including avoidance of tobacco, drugs, and excessive alcohol use. In particular, a sizable majority of young adults who have atherosclerotic stroke have a history of heavy tobacco use. Both the duration of smoking and the daily consumption of cigarettes appear to be important.[109] Thus, efforts to stop smoking are a critical step in lowering the risk of atherosclerotic stroke in the young (see Chapter 4).

Nonatherosclerotic Vasculopathies

Nonatherosclerotic vasculopathies comprise a disproportionately large number of ischemic strokes in this population.

Dissection or Trauma

Arterial dissection accounts for approximately 10 percent of infarctions and the occasional hemorrhage.[104,113] Young adults are the most commonly affected age group (see Chapter 10). The classic clinical description of dissection is a cerebral infarction in a young adult, who does not have the traditional risk factors for stroke and who has pain or headache in association with the vascular event. When dissections involve the intracranial segment of the internal carotid artery, the middle

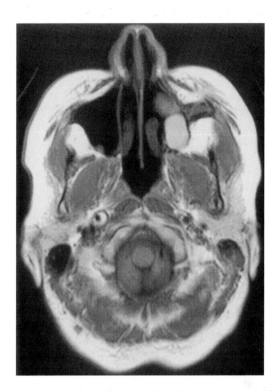

Figure 17-1. An axial view of a T-2 weighted MRI of the neck demonstrates a crescent sign with eccentric flow void in the right internal carotid artery. The results of this imaging study are consistent with the diagnosis of dissection of the internal carotid.

cerebral artery, or the basilar artery, most lesions affect the extracranial segment of the internal carotid artery or the distal vertebral artery (Fig. 17-1). Because many dissections are associated with sports or injuries, a majority of these arterial lesions are found in young men.[114–116] Dissection is a potential cause of stroke during labor and delivery. Some dissections are not associated with trauma and they are complications of an underlying arteriopathy (see Chapter 10).

Dissection of the aorta in a young adult can be secondary to *Marfan syndrome* or another inherited connective tissue disorder. A case of aortic dissection has been described with *Erdheim-Gsell cystic medial necrosis.*[117] The same pathological process also has been described in the extracranial arteries.

Arterial occlusion is a potential cause of neurological morbidity among young adults who have *craniocerebral trauma*[114] (see Chapter 10). The trauma can directly injure the artery without causing a dissection. *Posttraumatic vasospasm* can cause cerebral ischemia following a closed head injury with subarachnoid hemorrhage. Patients with multisystem trauma, including fracture of long bones, can have *fat embolization* (Table 17-7; Figs. 17-2 and 17-3). This scenario most commonly happens with fracture of the femur or tibia. Affected patients have sudden onset of

► **TABLE 17-7.** FAT EMBOLIZATION

Fracture of long bones—multisystem trauma
    Femur or tibia
Sudden respiratory distress or hypoxia
Multiple small lesions seen in lung
Neurological symptoms
    Decreased consciousness
    Seizures
    Multifocal neurological impairments
    Multiple lesions seen in brain imaging
Fat emboli found on ophthalmoscopy

respiratory distress, decreased consciousness, multifocal neurological impairments, and seizures. A chest X-ray usually shows multiple lesions in both lung fields. Examination of the ocular fundus can demonstrate the emboli.

Noninflammatory Vasculopathies

Moyamoya disease is not as important cause of infarction in young adults as it is in children. However, *moyamoya syndrome* is complicated by recurrent ischemic stroke in young adults, especially women (see Chapter 10). A strong relationship has been reported between the combination of smoking and use of oral contraceptives and the moyamoya syndrome in young women.[118,119] In the United States and most other western countries, women

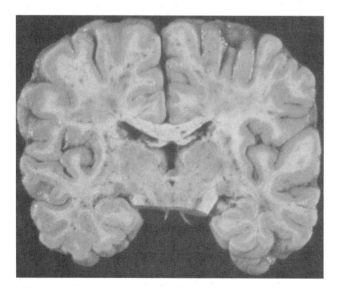

Figure 17-2. A coronal autopsy specimen demonstrates multiple small areas of hemorrhagic ischemia primarily located in the white matter in both cerebral hemispheres and the corpus callosum. The patient had been involved in a motor vehicle crash and had several injuries. The findings are those of fat embolization to the brain. (*Courtesy of S.S. Schochet, M.D., Department of Pathology, University of West Virginia, Morgantown WV.*)

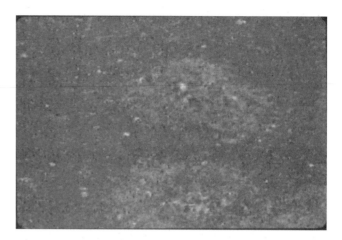

Figure 17-3. A microscopic examination of one of the lesions shown in Fig. 17-22 reveals multiple fat emboli within the arterioles. (*Courtesy of S.S. Schochet, M.D., Department of Pathology, University of West Virginia, Morgantown WV.*)

compromise the majority of young adults affected by moyamoya syndrome. *Fibromuscular dysplasia* is a relatively uncommon cause of stroke but it occurs primarily among young women.[120] The arteriopathy can be complicated by dissection or the presence of a saccular aneurysm. Ischemic stroke in a young adult can be a complication of a *giant intracranial aneurysm.*

Inflammatory or Infectious Vasculopathies

Infectious diseases that are associated with cerebral infarction include bacterial meningitis, fungal meningitis, tuberculous meningitis, malaria, or cysticercosis (see Chapter 11). *Herpes zoster ophthalmicus* occurs in young adults. A secondary arteritis of the internal carotid artery can lead to infarction of the ipsilateral cerebral hemisphere. The interval from the acute infection until the arterial occlusion can be up to several months. A zoster infection leading to a vasculitis can lead to hemorrhagic or ischemic stroke in an immunocompromised individual (see Chapter 11). *Meningovascular syphilis* is a potential cause of stroke in young adults. The arteritis, which generally occurs approximately 3–18 months following the primary exposure, usually affects medium-to-large caliber arteries. Strokes seem to occur primarily in the territory of the middle cerebral artery. Some of these young adults will have *AIDS* or other immune deficiency states associated with opportunistic infections that cause cerebral infarction. In addition, the shared risk factors mean that patients with AIDS also are at risk for meningovascular syphilis.

A variety of noninfectious inflammatory vasculopathies can cause neurological impairments in young adults (see Chapter 11). *Systemic lupus erythematosus* is common among young women. Neurological involvement usually causes psychiatric symptoms or an encephalopathy; these signs probably do not represent vascular disease but probably a direct autoimmune reaction. Ischemic strokes among young patients with systemic lupus erythematosus are due to thromboembolic events related to the presence of antiphospholipid antibodies, lupus anticoagulants, or Libman–Sacks endocarditis. Other multisystem rheumatological disorders occasionally complicated by brain ischemia include *rheumatoid arthritis, Churg–Strauss syndrome, periarteritis nodosa,* or *Wegener granulomatosis.* The group at highest risk for *Takayasu disease* is young women aged 20–40. Affected patients have headaches, visual loss, decreased pulses in the upper extremities, and recurrent stroke.

Inherited Vasculopathies

Cerebral autosomal dominant arteriopathy and *subcortical ischemic leukoencephalopathy* (CADASIL) is a leading genetic cause of recurrent stroke in young adults. Several other genetic diseases, including the *mitochondrial encephalopathies* or *homocystinuria,* also produce brain ischemia in young men and women.

▶ MIGRAINE AND STROKE

Approximately 10 percent of young men and 20 percent of young women in the United States have a history of migraine headaches[121] (Table 17-8). Most individuals have recurrent headache without other neurological findings (migraine without aura). However, some persons have neurological symptoms (migraine with aura) including visual disturbances, oculorotatory signs, hemiparesis,

▶ TABLE 17-8. MIGRAINE AND STROKE

Cause-and-effect relationship is difficult to establish
  Migraine is very common in population
  Migraine described as symptom of several diseases
  Headache common among patients with stroke
  Dissections often cause headache and stroke
  Thunderclap headache mimics subarachnoid hemorrhage
  Migraine a leading differential diagnosis for TIA
Risk of stroke probably higher among patients with migraine
  Particularly among young women
  Some strokes can are migrainous
  Risk increased in presence of other factors
  Risk increased with use of oral contraceptives
  Risk associated with antimigraine medications
  Risk increased among patients with migraine with aura
  Risk increased among patients with complex aura
    Hemiplegia
    Monocular visual loss (ocular)
    Ocular motility
    Vertebrobasilar

or language disturbances prior to, during, or following the headache. The binocular visual disturbances, usually with positive phenomena (scintillating scotoma or fortification spectra), are the most common neurological symptoms. Some patients have monocular visual symptoms (retinal migraine). Children and young adults have neurological symptoms, including prominent vertigo, which mimic the findings of vertebrobasilar ischemia (vertebrobasilar migraine). Because of the high prevalence of migraine and the prominent focal neurological symptoms, an interrelationship to ischemic stroke might exist.[122] Besides stroke, migraine also has been described as a risk factor for asymptomatic lesions found in the cerebral hemispheres.[123]

Migraine probably involves a process that affects cerebral blood flow and blood vessels. During the phase when the neurological signs are prominent, flow might be decreased.[124] The throbbing headache is speculated to be due to dilated intracranial vessels. The relationship between the neurological signs (brain dysfunction) and the vascular phenomena are not clear. An appealing theory is that the focal neurological signs are secondary to a progressive neuronal process. The vascular phenomena found in migraine might be the consequence of the neurological process rather than the cause. Still, a prolonged period of vasoconstriction could lead to an infarction. Some young adults with migraine are found to have cortical lesions found on brain imaging that appear to be stroke. In addition, stroke is a potential complication of medications used to treat migraine including the ergots and serotonin agonists. However, these interactions have not been established. Recently, Hall et al.[125] concluded that the use of triptans to treat migraine was not associated with an increased risk of vascular events, including stroke.

In some series, approximately 5–15 percent of strokes in young adults are attributed either directly or indirectly to migraine.[90] The upper figure seems too high. The potential interfaces are complex and diagnosing a cause-and-effect relationship is difficult. Chronic headache appears to be a marker for an increased risk for stroke (see Table 17-8). The age of the persons might be important. Although a history of migraine does not portend ischemic stroke in the elderly, it does identify a group of young adults at higher risk for stroke.[126–129] The person's sex also seems to affect risk. Migraine appears to increase the risk of ischemic stroke among men by a factor of approximately 2.[130] The relative risk appears to be approximately 3 among women.[129,131,132] Those persons with migraine accompanied by focal neurological symptoms appear to have a higher risk of stroke than do patients with migraine without aura. The presence of other risk factors or behaviors influences the interconnections between migraine and stroke. Among young women with migraine, the likelihood of stroke appears to be increased by the use of oral contraceptives, smoking, or arterial hypertension.[131] For example, Tzourio et al.[133] reported that the risk of stroke was increased by a factor of greater than 10 among women with migraine who also smoked more than 20 cigarettes/day. Silvestrini et al.[134] correlated an increased risk of ischemic events among persons with migraine who also had antiphospholipid antibodies. In addition, Tietjen et al.[135] reported that young women with migraine have an increased prevalence of livedo reticularis. This dermatological finding, which is often detected among persons with antiphospholipid antibodies, has been correlated with ischemic cardiac and cerebral events. Presumably, the migraine headaches are a symptom of an underlying prothrombotic disorder or vasculopathy. These data suggest that migraine is a contributing factor or marker for vascular diseases that lead to cerebral infarction. As such, young patients should be asked about a past history of headaches not necessarily to establish migraine as the cause of stroke but, rather, the history of headaches can serve as a maker for the disease that is leading to the cerebrovascular event.

Patients with several inherited disorders have had migraine as an important symptom. Complex (hemiparetic) migraine is one of the cardinal presenting features of CADASIL (see Chapter 12). This genetic disease is associated with a high risk for recurrent stroke and vascular dementia in young adults. *Familial hemiplegic migraine* also is associated with CADASIL.[136–138] Migraine also is feature of some mitochondrial disorders that also produce stroke. A potential relationship of migraine with a patent foramen ovale or atrial septal aneurysm also has been described. Presumably, these cardiac lesions would abet embolization of small thrombi that would serve as the precipitant of the migraines.

Migraine is an important alternative diagnosis to both hemorrhagic and ischemic stroke.[139] For example, *benign thunderclap headache,* which can be secondary to migraine, mimics the symptoms of aneurysmal subarachnoid hemorrhage. *Coital migraine* also can be associated with a sudden, severe headache and nausea, and vomiting, symptoms that imitate those occurring with a ruptured aneurysm. Unfortunately, too many patients with subarachnoid hemorrhage are misdiagnosed as having a migraine. Some of the persons with subarachnoid hemorrhage have a past history of migraine. If the patient relates that the new headache differs from the usual migraine, the prudent approach is to assume that the new symptoms are of a nonmigrainous origin.

Migraine is an alternative diagnosis for transient ischemic attacks. The focal neurological symptoms of a migrainous aura often mimic those occurring with a transient ischemic attack. On the other hand, transient ischemic attacks often are accompanied by headache, particularly when the events are in the posterior circulation.

The clinical clues to differentiate migraine and transient ischemic attacks are described in Chapter 5. Distinguishing a transient ischemic attack from migraine might be especially difficult when the patient does not have a concomitant headache. *Migraine equivalents* usually occur in older persons and involve the focal neurological symptoms of the aura.[140] However, the attacks are not associated with headache, nausea, vomiting, or malaise. In the absence of the development of other symptoms of migraine, the positive phenomena (scintillating scotoma or fortification spectra) or a march of symptoms supports the diagnosis of migraine equivalents. This distinction is important because migraine equivalents do not predict a high risk for a stroke that accompanies transient ischemic attacks. Rather than anticoagulants or antiplatelet aggregating agents, treatment focuses on prophylactic antimigraine agents such as beta-blocking or calcium channel-blocking medications.

Most migrainous aurae involve visual symptoms (Table 17-9). However, more complex migrainous attacks can produce other focal neurological symptoms including hemiparesis, aphasia, or cranial nerve palsies. In *ophthalmoplegic migraine*, the patient will have oculomotor nerve palsy that precedes, accompanies, or follows the headache. *Vertebrobasilar migraine* most commonly occurs in children and younger adults. Affected children often have prominent vertigo, ataxia, or bilateral motor or sensory symptoms with the headache. Patients with *hemiplegic migraine* have a contralateral hemiparesis often associated with a contralateral visual field disturbance. Aphasia can accompany a hemiplegic migrainous attack affecting the dominant hemisphere.

▶ **TABLE 17-9.** MIGRAINOUS AURA

Classic migraine
  Homonymous visual symptoms
    Scintillating scotoma
    Fortification spectra
    Visual loss
Ocular migraine
  Monocular sparkles and shimmers
  Evolving monocular visual loss
Ophthalmoplegic migraine
  Oculomotor paresis—diplopia
Hemiplegic migraine
  Contralateral hemiparesis
  Contralateral sensory loss
  Contralateral homonymous visual loss
  Aphasia (dominant hemisphere)
Vertebrobasilar migraine
  Vertigo
  Ataxia
  Bilateral motor weakness
  Bilateral sensory loss

A Danish epidemiological study found that women accounted for approximately 75 percent of the persons with hemiplegic migraine.[141] This research also found that familial and sporadic cases of hemiplegic migraine were roughly equal in number. Transient monocular visual disturbances in young adults secondary to *ocular migraine* can mimic amaurosis fugax. These attacks, which are vasospastic in origin, most commonly occur in persons younger than 45. Attacks of ocular migraine usually are associated with monocular positive visual phenomena (sparkles or shimmers) followed by gradually evolving visual loss. While most patients with ocular migraine have a periorbital or temporal headache, some patients may have only the ocular symptoms without the headache. In general, the chances of permanent residuals (migrainous stroke or migrainous retinal infarction) appear to be greater among patients with the more complex neurological auras than among patient with the classical visual disturbances.

Young persons with ischemic stroke often complain of headache and this symptom often prompts the diagnosis of migraine as the cause of the ischemia. This may be a misstep. Ferro et al.[142] found that headaches were prominent among patients with strokes of many causes that occur in the posterior circulation, especially in the distribution of the posterior cerebral artery. Headaches are relatively common among younger persons, women, and those with a past history of migraine.[143] The presence of a headache should not automatically lead to the diagnosis of migraine.[142,144] In fact, most young adults with stroke and headaches are not having a migrainous stroke. For example, a young person with stroke and severe headache or pain could have an arterial dissection. This scenario is supported by the observation of Tzourio et al.,[145] who found that migraine is a risk factor for cervical artery dissection. Because migraine is common among young adults with stroke secondary to arterial dissection, the association might be coincidence. Further research is needed to determine if migraine causes the arterial disease or whether the arterial disease presents symptoms that mimic migraine.

As a principle, a stroke should not be attributed to migraine until other etiologies have been excluded with a reasonable degree of certainty (Table 17-10). The diagnosis of migrainous stroke is particularly dangerous if the patient has not had prior migrainous attacks. A reasonable approach is to attribute stroke to migraine only when the patient has a stroke that mimics the aura of previous attacks.[146–148] The usual scenario of a migrainous stroke is a typical aura that persists with a resultant permanent neurological impairment. The most common permanent residual of a migrainous stroke is a homonymous hemianopia representing an infarction in the distribution of the posterior cerebral artery. The risk of recurrent migrainous stroke appears to be relatively

▶ **TABLE 17-10.** DIAGNOSIS OF MIGRAINOUS STROKE

The presence of headache is not sufficient for diagnosis
Most strokes are not due to migraine
Diagnosis of migrainous stroke should be a diagnosis of exclusion
Migrainous stroke
  Patient has prior attacks of migraine with aura
    Positive visual phenomena
    Focal neurological impairments
    March of symptoms
  Patient has a typical migrainous attack with aura
  Focal neurological symptoms of aura persist—stroke

low. Occasionally, patients have migraine as a consequence of stroke.

Stroke, including spinal cord infarction, has been attributed to complications of both prophylactic and abortive therapies prescribed to persons with migraine.[149] However, the risk of stroke from the use of these medications probably is low.[125] Because of the perceived high risk for stroke, triptans and ergots usually are not prescribed patients with complex neurological aura, such as hemiparesis, aphasia, or oculomotor nerve palsy or those who have had a previous stroke. Administration of the vasoconstrictive medications often is avoided to young patients that have other risk factors for stroke, including those with hypertension or diabetes. There are concerns that these agents can be associated with myocardial ischemia as well as stroke. Stroke also has been attributed to treatment of propranolol. Still, both beta-blockers and calcium channel-blockers are given to patients with migraine who also might be at risk for stroke. Patients treated with vasodilator medications including nitrates or dipyridamole can have a worsening of their migraines. Patients with a history of migraine should be warned about the possibility of an increase in the frequency of headaches if the combination of aspirin and extended release dipyridamole is administered following a TIA. While migraine was considered to be a contraindication for arteriography, data showing an increased risk of stroke with arteriography in migrainous patients are not available.

▶ CARDIOEMBOLIC CAUSES OF ISCHEMIC STROKE

The frequency of cardiac embolization as an etiology of stroke in young adults has varied between hospital-based studies but a reasonable estimate is that approximately 15–25 percent of all events are secondary to cardioembolism.[104,113] With the exception of patients with rheumatic mitral stenosis, the prevalence of atrial fibrillation in young persons is relatively low. Fortunately, improved management of acute rheumatic fever means that the frequency of *rheumatic mitral stenosis* in young persons has declined dramatically. However, rheumatic mitral stenosis, with or without atrial fibrillation, is a consideration if a patient has a loud cardiac murmur. In addition, rheumatic heart disease remains an important illness in countries with limited health care resources. The discovery of atrial fibrillation in a young adult with stroke should prompt a search for an underlying structural heart disease. The screening may be negative and the patient has lone atrial fibrillation, which has a relatively low risk of thromboembolism. Thus, stroke generally should not be attributed to cardioembolism if a young patient has lone atrial fibrillation. *Coronary artery disease* is increasingly diagnosed in young persons with multiple risk factors for atherosclerosis, embolic strokes can occur in this population secondary to a recent myocardial infarction or an ischemic cardiomyopathy. Some young patients with severe congenital or rheumatic heart disease have mechanical prostheses inserted. They are at risk for thromboembolism if their level of anticoagulation is not adequate. In addition, young patients with valvular heart disease are liable for infectious endocarditis. *Mitral valve prolapse* once was thought to be a leading cardiac cause of embolization in young adults (see Chapter 13). This association appears to be relatively weak. While most severe congenital cardiac abnormalities will have been identified in childhood, but a *patent foramen ovale* often is detected during the evaluation of a young adult with a cryptogenic stroke. The high prevalence of patent foramen ovale in the general population and the relatively common nature of stroke make the cause-and-effect relationship somewhat difficult to establish.

▶ PROTHROMBOTIC CAUSES OF ISCHEMIC STROKE

Most of the genetic or acquired hematological and coagulation disorders that lead to cerebral infarction in children also can occur in young adults (see Chapter 14). These prothrombotic disorders probably account for approximately 5–10 percent of ischemic strokes in this age group, a percentage that is much higher than in older persons.[104,150-152] The most common etiologies are the presence of *antiphospholipid antibodies* or *Factor V Leiden*. Deficiencies of protein C, protein S, antithrombin, or plasminogen also can be found. While many persons with sickle cell disease live to young adulthood, the frequency of ischemic stroke seems to be relatively low. Rather than infarction, young adults with sickle cell disease have subarachnoid hemorrhage, often due to the presence of an aneurysm.

▶ PREGNANCY AND STROKE

Stroke is among the leading causes of maternal morbidity or mortality. With the development of modern obstetrical care including the improved management of puerperal infections, the relative importance of vascular events of the brain as a cause of unfavorable outcomes after pregnancy has increased. Both hemorrhagic and ischemic stroke are complications (Table 17-11). Intracranial hemorrhage during pregnancy or the puerperium is associated with a maternal mortality as high as 35 percent and fetal mortality is approximately 25 percent.

In the United States and Western Europe, the frequency of cerebral infarction is estimated to be approximately 4–10/100,000 pregnancies and the rate

▶ TABLE 17-11. STROKE AND PREGNANCY

	Highest risk period
Hemorrhagic stroke	
Ruptured arteriovenous malformation	3rd trimester and delivery
Ruptured intracranial aneurysm	3rd trimester and delivery
Hypertensive hemorrhage	2nd and 3rd trimesters
Bleeding diathesis	Delivery
Metastatic choriocarcinoma	Puerperium
Ischemic stroke	
Eclampsia	2nd and 3rd trimesters, puerperium
Posterior reversible encephalopathy syndrome	same as eclampsia
Hypercoagulable state	2nd and 3rd trimesters, puerperium
Cardioembolism	
Paradoxical embolism	2nd and 3rd trimesters, delivery
Peripartum cardiomyopathy	Puerperium
Other causes	2nd and 3rd trimesters
Arterial dissection	Delivery
Air embolism	Delivery
Amniotic fluid embolism	Delivery

of hemorrhage is approximately the same.[153] In some series, the rates of hemorrhage appear to be higher than for ischemic stroke. Rates appear to be considerably higher in developing countries. The highest risk periods for cerebrovascular events are the third trimester, labor and delivery, and the first 6 weeks of the puerperium[154] (see Table 17-11). An increased risk for cerebrovascular events has been associated with eclampsia and cesarean section.[101,153,155–157] The latter might reflect the patient's condition rather than be a direct contributor to stroke. Both arterial and venous disease can lead to neurological impairments. In general, arterial occlusions leading to stroke and bleeding events are highest during the second and third trimesters and venous occlusions usually happen following delivery. Hemorrhages also occur primarily in the third trimester and during labor and delivery. *Venous thrombosis* is a particularly important cause of neurological dysfunction during the puerperium[158] (see Chapter 18). Lamy et al.[159] looked at the rates or recurrent among women who have had a stroke during pregnancy; they found a relatively low risk of a second stroke during a subsequent pregnancy. In general, the chances of another cerebrovascular event appear to be similar to the general population of women the same age.

Evaluation and treatment of a pregnant woman is similar to that recommended for other persons. The primary focus should be on the mother. MRI and radiological procedures including CT and angiography should be performed. However, special care should be implemented to protect the fetus. Because of the high teratogenic risk of warfarin, oral anticoagulants are not recommended (see Chapter 19). The risk is particularly high when the medication is used in the first trimester. In addition, the use of oral anticoagulants in the third trimester can be complicated by fetal vitamin K deficiency that leads to severe bleeding. A high-risk pregnant woman, for example, a woman with a prosthetic heart valve often is prescribed heparin or one of the low molecular weight agents. Aspirin has been used to prevent eclampsia and might be useful in forestalling stroke in high-risk patients. Aspirin also might be associated with bleeding complications. The safety of clopidogrel or dipyridamole is not known.

The differential diagnosis of the cause of stroke in a pregnant woman is similar to that entertained in other young women.[160] In addition, there are other causes of stroke that are directly associated with the pregnancy. Ischemic strokes complicating pregnancy often are attributed to disturbances in coagulation.[161,162] Increases in red blood cell mass and plasma volume lead to changes in hematocrit and viscosity. Hyperviscosity also results from dehydration (Table 17-12). Increases in platelet aggregation and levels of fibrinogen and factors II, VII, VIII, IX, and X occur especially during the third trimester. Declines in levels of proteins C and S also

▶ **TABLE 17-12.** HEMATOLOGICAL CHANGES IN PREGNANCY

Increased red blood cell mass
Increased plasma volume
Increased viscosity
Increased levels of fibrinogen
Increased levels of factors II, VII, VIII, IX, X
Increased platelet aggregation
Decreased levels of proteins C and S

occur. Nonbacterial thrombotic endocarditis also is a potential complication of pregnancy. The coagulation disturbances persist for a few weeks following delivery.

Nonatherosclerotic vasculopathies including arterial dissection, moyamoya, and fibromuscular dysplasia can be complicated by infarction. *Arterial dissection* has complicated hyperextension of the neck during delivery.[163,164] Pregnancy does increase the risk of ischemic stroke among women with moyamoya. However, special procedures to prevent complications from moyamoya including measures to control toxemia of pregnancy or hypertension have been recommended.[165] Noninfectious, inflammatory, or infectious arteritis has been implicated in exceptional cases of pregnancy-related stroke.

Peripartum vasculopathy can produce neurological symptoms through either ischemia or bleeding following delivery (Table 17-13). The vasculopathy also is associated with recurrent intracranial hemorrhage.[166] The woman develops focal neurological impairments, headache, seizures, nausea, and vomiting, which mimic migraine or subarachnoid hemorrhage.[163] The symptoms usually begin within a few days of delivery. This vasculopathy needs to be differentiated from vasospasm secondary to subarachnoid hemorrhage, drug-induced vasculitis, or an autoimmune vasculitis. The cause of the vasculopathy is not clear although the administration of bromocriptine, which is used to suppress lactation, has been implicated.[167–169] The cerebrospinal fluid usually shows an elevated protein and leucocytosis. Arteriography demonstrates areas of segmental arterial narrowing that appear similar to vasculitis or vasospasm. The arterial narrowing resolves during the subsequent days. While no specific

▶ **TABLE 17-13.** PERIPARTUM VASCULOPATHY

Begins within a few days of delivery
Causes either infarction or hemorrhage
Possibly related to the use of bromocriptine
Symptoms
   Headache, nausea, and vomiting
   Seizures
   Focal neurological signs
Elevated CSF protein and white blood cell count
Focal areas of arterial narrowing in multiple vessels

treatment has been established as effective, nimodipine often is prescribed. Angioplasty has been used to treat refractory arterial narrowing.

Women with congenital or acquired heart diseases are at risk for embolization during pregnancy. Among the potential cardiac sources of emboli are rheumatic valvular disease, a prosthetic cardiac valve, or a patent foramen ovale. In the latter situation, thrombi could arise in the pelvic veins and reach the brain via a patent foramen ovale or another right-to-left shunt. A *peripartum cardiomyopathy* is a potential cause of embolic stroke occurring during the first few weeks following delivery.[170,171] This cardiac complication is more commonly described in developing countries, African-American women and those who have a difficult or multiparous pregnancy. It should be considered as a potential cause of postpartum stroke, especially if the woman has evidence of congestive heart failure. Treatment of this dilated cardiomyopathy is challenging.

Less common causes of stroke include *air embolism* or *amniotic fluid embolism*.[161] A potential situation for air embolization is early termination of pregnancy, particularly criminal abortion. Air can enter the gravid uterus and traverse to the lung and brain. Amniotic fluid embolization usually within a few hours of delivery or dilatation and curettage performed in the second trimester.[172] Women with amniotic fluid embolism often have clotting and hematological studies compatible with a disseminated intravascular coagulation. Both air and amniotic fluid embolization present with decreased consciousness, seizures, and multiple focal neurological impairments. The air emboli can be detected readily by brain imaging, small bubbles usually lodge in terminal portions of cerebral arteries in a watershed pattern.

Eclampsia is an important alternative diagnosis to intracranial hemorrhage if a pregnant woman has a severe headache, seizures, or decreased consciousness (Table 17-14). Most eclamptic women have a history of hypertension, proteinuria, or edema. On occasion, a past history of pre-eclampsia might not be available. Most cases of eclampsia occur in the third trimester and distinguishing eclampsia from a subarachnoid hemorrhage or intracerebral hemorrhage is critical because bleeding might be secondary to a ruptured aneurysm or vascular malformation. Brain imaging usually shows bilateral abnormalities primarily located in the parieto-occipital region. Magnetic resonance imaging shows the changes of *posterior reversible encephalopathy syndrome* (PRES) that can be seen with eclampsia or any other hypertensive encephalopathy (Fig. 17-4). Servillo et al.[173] described four critically ill, pregnant women with PRES; two had seizures and the other two had cortical blindness and headache. They also noted that PRES occurs both during pregnancy and the puerperium. Transcranial Doppler ultrasonography can detect changes in flow

► **TABLE 17-14.** ECLAMPSIA

Usually develops in third trimester
  Can occur after delivery
History of hypertension, edema, and proteinuria
Symptoms
  Headache
  Seizures
  Cortical blindness
  Decreased consciousness
HELLP
  Hemolysis
  Abnormal liver function tests
  Thrombocytopenia
  Disseminated intravascular coagulation
MRI
  Posterior reversible encephalopathy syndrome
Transcranial Doppler ultrasonography
  Increased flow velocities in multiple vessels

velocities in the intracranial arteries, which point to an increased risk of neurological dysfunction. The *HELLP syndrome* is a potential complication of eclampsia. Besides stroke, other findings include hemolysis, abnormal liver function tests, and thrombocytopenia. Affected

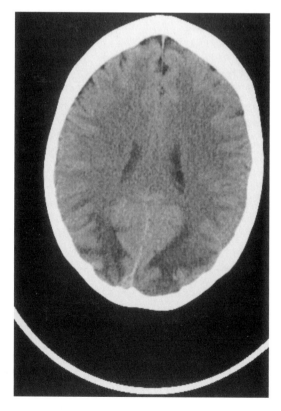

Figure 17-4. An unenhanced CT study in a young woman with pregnancy, elevated blood pressure, proteinuria, and headache. The CT shows changes in the white matter in the parieto-occipital regions bilaterally. The CT is suggestive of the diagnosis of eclampsia.

women can develop disseminated intravascular coagulation and severe bleeding.[174]

While a cerebral *arteriovenous malformation* is not a contraindication for pregnancy, concerns remain about the risk of bleeding. The chances of rupture seem to be increased among women who have had a previous hemorrhage. In particular, risks are greatest during the third trimester and during labor and delivery. Because of the potential for rupture during labor and delivery, Cesarean section sometimes is recommended. Management of a ruptured vascular malformation during pregnancy should be the same as when a woman is not pregnant. Surgical evacuation of the hematoma and resection of the malformation is the preferred management. The risk of bleeding from an *intracranial aneurysm* also reaches a peak during labor and delivery.[154] Management of aneurysmal subarachnoid hemorrhage with pregnancy is similar to other situations (see Chapter 23). While the management focuses on treatment of the intracranial lesion, decisions about vaginal delivery or Cesarean section depend upon the viability of the fetus and the mother's status. Recommendations about management of a pregnant woman with an unruptured aneurysm are not available. In general, plans should be similar to that for other persons. However, decisions about labor and delivery might be altered. For example, Cesarean section might be an option instead of vaginal delivery.

Intracranial hemorrhage can be the initial presentation of metastatic *choriocarcinoma*. Choriocarcinoma associated-bleeding usually occurs within 6 months of a normal pregnancy. The tumor also can occur with ectopic pregnancies or hydatiform moles. Most women will have pulmonary involvement (metastases) and many have hematological derangements that mimic disseminated intravascular coagulation. The presence of markedly elevated levels of beta-human chorionic gonadotropin points to the diagnosis. Besides treating the hemorrhage, management focuses on measure to treat the tumor.

▶ ORAL CONTRACEPTIVES AND STROKE

Shortly after the introduction of oral contraceptives in the 1960s, a possible relationship with an increased risk of stroke was found. Oral contraceptives are associated with increased chances of either hemorrhagic or ischemic stroke (Table 17-15). Cerebral venous thrombosis also is a potential complication. Although the data are conflicting, the relative increase in risk is estimated to be approximately 1.5–4.[132,175,176] The World Health Organization looked at the risk of hemorrhagic or ischemic stroke among women in Europe and several developing countries; the risk of stroke was increased by a factor of approximately 3.[177,178] The relative risk of hemorrhagic

▶ **TABLE 17-15.** ORAL CONTRACEPTIVES AND STROKE

Oral contraceptives modestly increase the risk of stroke
  Cerebral infarction
  Intracerebral hemorrhage
  Subarachnoid hemorrhage
  Venous thrombosis
  Moyamoya syndrome
In general, considered a contributing factor, rather than cause
Risk of vascular events reduced with 2nd and 3rd generation medications
  Lower dose of estrogen
  Lower dose of progesterone
Risk of vascular events increased among following groups of women
  Age >35
  Presence of following risk factors
    Hypertension
    Diabetes mellitus
    Smoking
    Migraine (especially with aura)
    Obesity
Risk of vascular events probably lower than that found with pregnancy

stroke, in particular subarachnoid hemorrhage, appears to be greater than for ischemic stroke. Although the risk of stroke is highest among women currently taking oral contraceptives, the chances of a cerebrovascular event also seem to be elevated among women who took the medications in the past.

In the last 40 years, the relative risk for stroke following use of oral contraceptives appears to have declined probably as a result in the reduction in doses of the medications. Risks probably are lowest among women taking the new low-dose oral contraceptives.[175] In fact, Schwartz et al.[179] concluded that the risk of stroke was not increased with the use of low-dose oral contraceptive medications. Lidegaard and Kreiner[180,181] evaluated the risks of stroke in relation to dosage of estrogen and the presence of progesterone in the oral contraceptive medications. In general, the risk of stroke is considerably lower with use of the second- and third-generation medications, which contain lower doses of estradiol. They found the odds ratio to decline from approximately 4.5 with 50 mcg preparations to 1 with 20 mcg dose formulations. The presence of the second-generation progestins seems to be associated with a higher risk of thromboembolic events compared to the third-generation progestins.

Most of the increase in the risk of ischemic stroke is attributed to changes in coagulation factors but no specific secondary hypercoagulable disorder has been identified. The increase in risk of subarachnoid hemorrhage has been attributed to secondary increases in blood pressure.

Some subgroups of young women appear to have a higher risk of stroke.[182] While the likelihood of cerebrovascular events increases among women older than 30, the chances seem greatest among women older than 35. One study found that the relative risk of stroke was increased by a factor of 16 among women older than 40.[183] In addition, smoking, obesity, and hypertension are correlated with an increased stroke risk. The risk of vascular events is significantly greater among young women who smoke than those who use oral contraceptives.[184] Based on these relationships, oral contraceptives should be prescribed with caution to any woman who has other risk factors for stroke. In particular, women older than 35 who have any of the above risk factors probably should not take the medication and other forms of birth control should be recommended. Although the data about the interactions between oral contraceptives and migraine leading to an increased risk of stroke are not clear, the combination probably is more dangerous than either factor alone. Thus, the use of oral contraceptives usually is discouraged if a young woman has a history of migraine with aura, particularly if the neurological symptoms involve nonvisual phenomena.[185,186] Oral contraceptives are avoided if a young woman has a coagulopathy such as antiphospholipid antibodies or heart disease associated with a high risk for embolism.

Because many women are taking oral contraceptives, finding a history of the use of the medications while assessing a young patient is not surprising. Undoubtedly, some strokes in young women are secondary to the use of oral contraceptives. However, in most cases, oral contraceptives probably are a contributing or aggravating factor rather than the direct cause. Most hemorrhagic or ischemic strokes in young women will be attributed to another etiology. Hemorrhages usually are due to an aneurysm, an arteriovenous malformation, or another vascular disease rather than the direct effects of oral contraceptives. Infarctions usually are secondary to arterial diseases, such as dissection, or cardioembolism. Thus, the diagnosis of stroke secondary to use of oral contraceptives should be one of exclusion.[104]

Although the risk of a second cerebrovascular event among women taking oral contraceptives is not known, women who have had a TIA, ischemic stroke, hemorrhagic stroke, or cerebral venous thrombosis should be advised to avoid continued use of the medication. Instead, another method of birth control should be advised.

Ovarian hyperstimulation syndrome can be complicated by cerebral infarction in young women.[187] The frequency of stroke, which presumably is secondary to changes in coagulation factors, among women with this relatively uncommon disorder is not known.

▶ SMOKING AND STROKE

Smoking is an important risk factor for cerebral infarction and myocardial infarction in persons of all ages.[188] The prevalence of smoking among young adults with stroke is extraordinarily high. The relationships are particularly obvious among young men.[107] Similar effects are seen among women.[184] The interactions between tobacco use and atherosclerosis or stroke are described in Chapter 4. A majority of young adults with stroke secondary to atherosclerosis are smokers. Both the duration of smoking and the number of cigarettes smoked per day have an effect on stroke risk.[109] Because smoking increases the risk of coronary artery disease, it can contribute to cerebral infarction through the mechanism of cardioembolism following an acute myocardial infarction or as the result of an ischemic cardiomyopathy. Such interactions are especially important among young adults. Smoking also is an important risk factor for hemorrhagic stroke in men. Kurth et al.[189] found that the risk of intracerebral hemorrhage was increased by a factor of 2 among smokers. The risk of subarachnoid hemorrhage was tripled among current smokers. While these effects are not directly related to atherosclerosis, presumably smoking increases blood pressure, which in turn promotes intracranial bleeding. Some persons who smoke also abuse alcohol or drugs and thus, the smoking may be a marker of other behaviors that place the patient at risk for cerebrovascular events. Regardless of the individual's age, they should be encouraged to stop smoking. This recommendation is especially important for young adults.

▶ ALCOHOL ABUSE AND STROKE

Light-to-moderate use (approximately 1 glass of wine, beer, or distilled spirits/mixed drink) of alcohol seems to slow the progression of atherosclerosis and lower the risk of coronary artery disease and cerebral infarction[190,191] (see Chapter 4). Alcohol use can lessen LDL cholesterol and increase HDL cholesterol concentrations. Modest levels of alcohol also can lower levels of platelet-derived thromboxane (Table 17-16). On the other hand, alcohol abuse (either chronic heavy use or binge drinking) is complicated by an increase in the risk of hemorrhagic or ischemic stroke.[192] The increase in risk for either hemorrhagic or ischemic stroke seems to be linear to the amount of alcohol consumed.[190] This association is present in men and women of all ethnic groups, but eems to be especially prominent among young adults.[132] Rodgers et al.[193] reported that weekly consumption of more than 180 gm of alcohol increases the risk of stroke by approximately 3. Kiechl et al.[194] found that daily consumption of >100 gm was correlated with increased progression of intimal-medial thickness and thus, atherosclerosis. Heavy alcohol

▶ **TABLE 17-16.** ALCOHOL AND STROKE

Moderate daily consumption of alcohol appears to lower risk
    Slows progression of atherosclerosis
        Decreases LDL cholesterol concentration
        Increases HDL cholesterol concentration
    Reduction in risk of myocardial infarction
Heavy alcohol consumption (daily or binge)
    Increased risk of hemorrhage or infarction in young adults
    Accelerates progression of atherosclerosis
    Increases blood pressure
        Subarachnoid hemorrhage
    Disturbances in clotting factors
        Hypercoagulable states—thrombosis
        Hemoconcentration—thrombosis
        Bleeding diathesis—hemorrhage
    Alcohol-induced cardiomyopathy

▶ **TABLE 17-17.** ISSUES IN MANAGEMENT OF ALCOHOLIC PATIENT WITH STROKE

Anticipate, prevent or treat
    Alcohol withdrawal syndrome
    Delirium tremens
    Seizures
Administer thiamine with intravenous fluids
    Wernicke–Korsakoff syndrome
Screen for hepatic dysfunction
    Bleeding risk
    Levels of clotting factors
    Interactions with medications
Screen for fall risk—affects mobilization or medications
    Acute intoxication
    Neuropathy
    Cerebellar disease
Compliance with treatment regimen
    Medications
    Rehabilitation
Social and economic issues
    Family or other support
    Return to society
    Violence

consumption also is associated with increases in blood pressure, heart rate, and cardiac output. The chronic hypertension can predispose to brain hemorrhage. Alcoholic persons also can have a dilated cardiomyopathy that is the source of emboli to the brain.

Haapaniemi et al.[195] reported that consumption of >40 gm of alcohol in the previous 24 hours was associated with increased risk of cerebral infarction. This relationship was much stronger for men than for women. The association with heavy alcohol consumption may explain the increased risk of stroke occurring on weekends and holidays that is noted in young adults.[195,196] The risk of cardioembolic stroke is particularly high in the hours following the heavy consumption of alcohol.[197] Because alcohol has a diuretic effect, heavy consumption can lead to hemoconcentration, changes in viscosity, or changes in clotting factors, which in turn promotes thrombosis. In addition, the changes in coagulation factors can promote bleeding. Thus, alcohol abuse in young patients can be complicated by intracerebral hemorrhage most commonly arising in lobar locations. However, the relative increase in bleeding risk with heavy alcohol use has not been established.[198] An increased risk of rupture of aneurysms or vascular malformations also is correlated with acute alcohol abuse. In addition, persons with acute alcohol intoxication can have falls that lead to either infarction or hemorrhage. Traumatic arterial injuries, including arterial dissection, can cause infarction in young adults.

Management of an acute stroke in a patient who chronically abused alcohol should include measures to prevent symptoms of *alcohol withdrawal* or to treat *delirium tremens* (Table 17-17). Because many alcoholic patients have poor diets, emergency treatment also should include administration of thiamine and other vitamins in order to avoid *Wernicke–Korsakoff syndrome*. Decisions about long-term management also are affected. Persons who abuse alcohol often are not compliant with their treatment regimens. Alcohol-induced hepatic disease can affect concentrations of coagulation factors that increase the risk for serious bleeding complications, particularly if oral anticoagulants are prescribed. In addition, patients may have secondary neuropathy or cerebellar degeneration, which increase the risk for falls with secondary traumatic intracranial bleeding. These factors often mean that most persons who abuse alcohol cannot be treated with long-term oral anticoagulants. Aspirin and the other antiplatelet agents are safer in this situation.

▶ DRUG ABUSE AND STROKE

Cerebral infarction, intracerebral hemorrhage and subarachnoid hemorrhage have been attributed to abuse of drugs. With the increasing use of illicit drugs, the frequency of complicating stroke likely will grow. Already, approximately 10 percent of strokes in young adults are attributed directly or indirectly to drug abuse[199,200] (Table 17-18). In one series of strokes in young adults, 73 of 214 patients had a history of drug abuse.[201] A study from Northern California reported that abuse of cocaine or amphetamine increased the risk of stroke among young women by a factor of approximately 7.[202] Most of the abused agents associated with stroke are vasoconstrictors. Abuse of *heroin, amphetamines* (including *methamphetamine*), *cocaine,* and other stimulants are most commonly implicated.[203] While stroke is a potential complication of the single use of one of these drugs, repeated or

▶ **TABLE 17-18.** STROKE AND DRUG ABUSE

Accounts for up to 10% of stroke in young adults
Both hemorrhages and infarctions
Drugs
    Heroin
    Cocaine (hydrochloride or alkaloid)
    Amphetamines
    Ephedra
    Ephedrine
    Phenylpropanolamine
    Marijuana
    Adulterants
Causes of stroke
    Hypertensive crisis
    Rupture of aneurysm or vascular malformation
    Arterial dissection—trauma
    Myocardial infarction with embolization
    Cardiac arrhythmias
    Endocarditis
    Coagulopathy
    Accelerated atherosclerosis
    Vasculitis

chronic use of cocaine or amphetamine is more commonly associated with an increased chance for cerebrovascular complications. Hemorrhages seem to be more common than ischemic events. The risk of ischemic stroke seems to be greater with the use of alkaloidal cocaine than with the hydrochloride form of the drug.[204] Hemorrhage seems to be greater among persons using hydrochloride form of cocaine than with the cocaine alkaloid (crack). Levine et al.[204] found a strong temporal relationship between the use of alkaloid cocaine and both hemorrhagic and ischemic stroke. However, Qureshi et al.[205] concluded that crack cocaine use was not a major cause of cerebral infarction in inner city populations of young adults. Cardiovascular complications of cocaine use include myocardial ischemia, hypertensive crises, cardiomyopathy, cardiac arrhythmias, aortic dissection and endocarditis.[206] Chronic cocaine use might be associated with accelerated atherosclerosis primarily by its effects on platelet function. In addition, stroke has been associated with use of *marijuana*. The strength of marijuana used today is greater than that consumed in the past, and the effects of the more-potent drug on the likelihood of vascular events are not known.

Cerebral infarction among persons abusing drugs can be secondary to infective endocarditis. Intravenous drug abuse is associated with acute infectious endocarditis that most commonly affects the right side of the heart. Fulminant cardiac failure can result. In addition, infectious endocarditis can lead to embolic events. Cardioembolism also can be secondary to drug-induced cardiomyopathy, cardiac arrhythmias, or coronary artery occlusion leading to myocardial infarction. The stimulants can cause

hypertensive crises, vasoconstriction, or vasculitis. The diagnosis of a drug-induced vasculitis has been debated. Data are inconclusive. Pathological confirmation of a vasculitis is not available. Many patients with cocaine or amphetamine-associated stroke do not have arterial narrowing. The arteriographic changes that mimic vasculitis might be secondary to drug-induced vasoconstriction.[207,208] Storen et al.[209] described two cases of a moyamoya-like vasculopathy in two patients who had chronically abused cocaine, one had a hemorrhage and the other had bilateral infarctions.

Intracranial hemorrhage can be secondary to a hypertensive crisis or vasculitis. The bleeding also can induce rupture of an intracranial aneurysm or a vascular malformation. A case of rapid growth of an aneurysm following abuse of amphetamine implies that the drug might cause hemorrhage via this mechanism.[210] Although most intracerebral hemorrhages are lobar in location, primary subarachnoid hemorrhage also occurs. Before the hemorrhage is attributed to drug abuse, a patient needs arterial imaging to eliminate an aneurysm or an arteriovenous malformation as the cause of the bleeding. In addition, bleeding can occur secondary to infective aneurysm found in association with infective endocarditis. Besides leading to rupture of an underlying vascular disease, drug abuse also affects prognosis. For example, Howington et al.[211] looked at the influence of cocaine use on the severity and prognosis of aneurysmal subarachnoid hemorrhage. In a series of 108 patients, 36 had used cocaine. Twenty of these patients had very severe hemorrhages (Hunt and Hess grades IV or V). The patients who had used cocaine had more vasospasm and their risk of unfavorable outcomes was increased by a factor of 3.

Perez et al.[212] described strokes secondary to methamphetamine abuse in four young adults. With the explosion of methamphetamine abuse in many parts of the United States, the rates of secondary stroke likely will increase in the years ahead. Presumably both hemorrhagic and ischemic stroke can be complications of methamphetamine abuse.

Stroke also complicates heroin abuse. Most strokes, which are in a watershed pattern, are ischemic and are secondary to hypotension. Heroin abuse can lead to respiratory depression and hypoxia. Trauma secondary to falls or a prolonged period of heroin-induced unresponsiveness can lead to arterial occlusions, including dissection. Because most heroin abusers take the drug intravenously, they also are at risk for secondary infective endocarditis. Inadvertent intra-arterial administration of heroin also can cause direct neurotoxicity. Stroke also can be secondary to adulterants, including talc, that lead to embolization to the brain.

Because of the widespread abuse of drugs, screening of the urine or blood for these is an important component of the evaluation of young adults with stroke. In addition, young adults with known drug abuse should have an evaluation for other causes of stroke, including brain, cardiac, and vascular imaging. Blood cultures should be done obtained if the patient has taken drugs intravenously and if the diagnosis of infective endocarditis is suspected. Patients with stroke secondary to drug abuse should be strongly advised to stop. Abstinence is a fundamental component of treatment to prevent recurrent stroke.

► HEMORRHAGIC STROKE IN YOUNG ADULTS

Several studies show that intracranial hemorrhages occur at a higher frequency than do infarctions among young adults.[213] In a population study in Italy, Nencini et al.[214] reported that the incidence of infarction was 3.4/100,000, while the rate of subarachnoid hemorrhage was 3.2 and for intracerebral hemorrhage, the rate was 1.9. Based on a mixed ethnic population in New York, Jacobs et al.[215] found that the annual rate of infarction was 10/100,000 young adults and the incidence of intracerebral hemorrhage was 7/100,000 and subarachnoid hemorrhage, it was 6/100,000. This ratio differs from that found in older persons in which subarachnoid hemorrhage seems to occur at a rate that is approximately one-half of that for primary bleeding within the brain. The 1-month mortality from intracranial hemorrhage among young adults is approximately 10–30 percent. The prognosis of young adults with intracerebral hemorrhage generally is better than for older patients. In part, the favorable prognosis is due to their better overall health and the lobar location for the bleeding is associated with a lower chance of death. Ogungbo et al.[216] reported that approximately 80 percent of young adults with subarachnoid hemorrhage had favorable outcomes. This figure seems high. Many young adults have subtle residual cognitive or behavioral impairments that limit their ability to return to society. The prognosis of patients with lobar hemorrhages is better than those with bleeding in the cerebellum or deep structures of the cerebral hemispheres.

Bleeding should be included in the differential diagnosis for the cause of the sudden onset of focal neurological impairments in any young adult. The likelihood of a hemorrhage increases if a young patient also has a severe headache, seizures, or alteration in consciousness. In many cases, hemorrhage occurs in vigorous exercise including sports and thus, young adults, especially men, should be considered as being at risk. Despite the rather stereotyped symptoms, the diagnosis of subarachnoid hemorrhage often is delayed. Mild subarachnoid hemorrhage is missed because the patient is complaining of primarily of headache. The young person also has nausea

► **TABLE 17-19.** CAUSES OF HEMORRHAGIC STROKE IN YOUNG ADULTS

Hypertension	Vascular malformation
Acute hypertension	Arteriovenous
Eclampsia	Cavernous
Chronic hypertension	Venous
Aneurysm	Telangiectasis
Saccular	Dural fistula
Infectious	Trauma
Neoplastic	Bleeding diathesis
Dissection	Sickle cell disease
Perimesencephalic	Leukemia
subarachnoid hemorrhage	Thrombocytopenia
Pregnancy	Medications
Autoimmune and Infectious	Antiplatelet agents
Periarteritis nodosa	Thrombolytic agents
Churg Strauss	Anticoagulants
Primary CNS vasculitis	Phenylpropanolamine
Surgical procedures	Cocaine
Craniocerebral trauma	Amphetamine
	Ephedra

and vomiting; the combination of symptoms often prompts the diagnosis of migraine. (Chapter 6)

Trauma is the leading cause of subarachnoid hemorrhage in young adults (Table 17-19). In most cases, the evidence for trauma is obvious. However, in some cases, particularly among those persons with decreased consciousness, the history of trauma might be lacking or the trauma will be relatively mild. A *spontaneous* or *post-traumatic dissection* of an intracranial artery can cause a subarachnoid hemorrhage. Still, the leading cause of spontaneous (nontraumatic) subarachnoid hemorrhage is rupture of an intracranial saccular aneurysm. While women account for the majority of persons with subarachnoid hemorrhage, more young men than young women have ruptured aneurysms. The high risk of aneurysmal rupture in young men is attributed to tobacco and alcohol abuse. A strong relationship exists between binge drinking on the weekends and aneurysmal rupture in the subsequent 24 hours. In addition, hypertensive effects from the abuse of stimulants also may induce subarachnoid hemorrhage. A potential association between aneurysmal subarachnoid hemorrhage and the inclusion of nicotine or caffeine in pharmaceutical products has been speculated.[217] A sizable percentage of young adults with hemorrhagic stroke will have a history of recent drug abuse.[218] The incidence of drug-associated hemorrhage, often from a ruptured arteriovenous malformation or aneurysm, likely will increase in the years ahead. Young women also have an increased likelihood of subarachnoid hemorrhage during pregnancy, especially at the time of labor and delivery. An interaction between the use of oral contraceptives and subarachnoid hemorrhage also is apparent. The increase in the relative risk for subarachnoid hemorrhage among women taking oral contraceptives is greater than is the chances of ischemic stroke. Other causes of subarachnoid bleeding in young adults include rupture of a *nonsaccular aneurysm*, rupture of a small *vascular malformation*, a *leptomeningeal tumor*, *bleeding diathesis*, or *perimesencephalic subarachnoid hemorrhage*. Hypertensive hemorrhages can occur with an acute elevation in blood pressure, such as that found with eclampsia, acute glomerulonephritis, or abuse of sympathomimetic agents.

Many intracerebral hemorrhages in young adults are lobar in location and most are secondary to rupture of a vascular malformation. Deep hemispheric hemorrhages secondary to hypertension are much less frequent in young persons than in the elderly. Ruiz-Sandoval et al.[219] found some disparities in etiologies among different ages of young persons. Almost all the hemorrhages among adults younger than 20 were due to rupture of an arteriovenous malformation while the majority of persons with hypertensive hemorrhages were older that 30. Toffol et al.[220] found that ruptured vascular malformations were the most common etiology of intracerebral hemorrhage in young adults. Other causes of intracerebral hemorrhage include bleeding diatheses, vasculitis, tumors, or venous thrombosis. Both moyamoya disease and sickle cell disease in young adults are complicated by subarachnoid or intracerebral hemorrhage. Intracerebral hemorrhage also has been described in young persons with AIDS. Roquer et al.[221] reported that intracranial bleeding occurs in approximately 1 percent of young persons with AIDS.

REFERENCES

1. American Heart Association. Heart disease and stroke statistics—2004 update. 2004. (Generic).
2. Adams HP, Jr., Butler MJ, Biller J, Toffol GJ. Nonhemorrhagic cerebral infarction in young adults. *Arch Neurol* 1986;43: 793–796.
3. Nowak-Gottl U, Straeter R, Sebire G, Kirkham F. Antithrombotic drug treatment of pediatric patients with ishemic stroke. *Paediatr Drugs* 2003;5:167–174.
4. Trauner DA, Nass R, Ballantyne A. Behavioural profiles of children and adolescents after pre- or perinatal unilateral brain damage. *Brain* 2001;124:995–1002.
5. Ramaswamy V, Miller SP, Barkovich AJ, Partridge JC, Ferriero DM. Perinatal stroke in term infants with neonatal encephalopathy. *Neurology* 2004;62:2088–2091.
6. Vergani P, Strobelt N, Locatelli A, et al. Clinical significance of fetal intracranial hemorrhage. *Am J Obstet Gynecol* 1996;175:536–543.
7. Sherer DM, Anyaegbunam A, Onyeije C. Antepartum fetal intracranial hemorrhage, predisposing factors and prenatal sonography: a review. *Am J Perinatol* 1998;15: 431–441.
8. Strauss A, Kirz D, Modanlou HD, Freeman RK. Perinatal events and intraventricular/subependymal hemorrhage in the very low-birth weight infant. *Am J Obstet Gynecol* 1985;151:1022–1027.
9. Zipursky A. Prevention of vitamin K deficiency bleeding in newborns. *British Journal of Haematology* 1999;104: 430–437.
10. Klinge J, Auberger K, Auerswald G, Brackmann HH, Mauz-Korholz C, Kreuz W. Prevalence and outcome of intracranial haemorrhage in haemophiliacs—a survey of the paediatric group of the German Society of Thrombosis and Haemostasis. *Eur J Pediatr* 1999;158:S162–S165
11. Sutherland J, Glucek H, Gleser G. Hemorrhagic disease of the newborn: breast feeding is a necessary factor in the pathogenesis. *Am J Dis Child* 1967;113:524–533.
12. Henselmans J, Meijer K, Haaxma R, Hew J, vanderMeer J. Recurrent spontaneous intracerebral hemorrhage in a congenitally afibrinogenemic patient: diagnostic pitfalls and therapeutic options. *Stroke* 1999;30:2479–2482.
13. Vahedi K, Massin P, Guichard J-P, et al. Hereditary infantile hemiparesis, retinal arteriolar tortuosity, and leukoencephalopathy. *Neurology* 2003;60:57–63.
14. Crowther MA, Kelton JG. Congenital thrombophilic states associated with venous thrombosis: a qualitative overview and proposed classification system. *Ann Intern Med* 2003; 138:128–134.
15. Crowther CA, Hiller JE, Doyle LW, Haslam RR, for the Australian Collaborative Trial of Magnesium Sulphate (ACTOMgSO4) Collaborative Group. Effect of magnesium sulfate given for neuroprotection before preterm birth. A randomized controlled trial. *JAMA* 2003;290:2669–2676.
16. Kurnik K, Kosch A, Strater R, et al. Recurrent thromboembolism in infants and children suffereing from symptomatic neonatal arterial stroke. A prospective follow-up study. *Stroke* 2003;34:2887–2893.
17. Broderick J, Talbot GT, Prenger E, Leach A, Brott T. Stroke in children within a major metropolitan area: the surprising importance of intracerebral hemorrhage. *J Child Neurol* 1993;8:250–255.
18. Earley CJ, Kittner SJ, Feeser BR, et al. Stroke in children and sickle-cell disease: Baltimore-Washington Cooperative Young Stroke Study. *Neurology* 1998;51:169–176.
19. Fullerton HJ, Chetkovich DM, Wu YW, Smith WS, Johnston SC. Deaths form stroke in US children, 1979 to 1998. *Neurology* 2002;59:34–39.
20. Hurvitz EA, Beale L, Ried S, Nelson VS. Functional outcome of paediatric stroke survivors. *Pediatr Rehabil* 1999; 3:43–51.
21. Nowak-Göttl U, Straeter R, Sebire G, Kirkham F. Antithrombotic drug treatment of pediatric patients with ischemic stroke. *Paediatr Drugs* 2003;5:167–175.
22. Giroud M, Lemesle M, Madinier G, Manceau E, Osseby GV, Dumas R. Stroke in children under 16 years of age. Clinical and etiological difference with adults. *Acta Neurol Scand* 1997;96:401–406.
23. deVeber G. Risk factors for childhood stroke: little folks have different strokes! *Ann Neurol* 2003;53:149–150.
24. Pavlakis SG, Kingsley PB, Bialer MG. Stroke in children: genetic and metabolic issues. *J Child Neurol* 2003;15: 308–315.

25. van Beynum I, Smeitink JA, den Heijer M, te Poele Pothoff MT, Blom HJ. Hyperhomocysteinemia: a risk factor for ischemic stroke in children. *Circulation* 1999;99:2070–2072.

26. Li S, Chen W, Srinivasan SR, et al. Childhood cardiovascular risk factors and carotid vascular changes in adulthood. The Bogalusa Heart Study. *JAMA* 2003;290:2271–2276.

27. Raitakari OT, Juonala M, Kähönen M, et al. Cardiovascular risk factors in childhood and carotid artery intima-media thickness in adulthood. The Cardiovascular Risk in Young Finns Study. *JAMA* 2003;290:2277–2283.

28. Ganesan V, Prengler M, McShane MA, Wade AM, Kirkham FJ. Investigation of risk factors in children with arterial ischemic stroke. *Ann Neurol* 2003;53:167–173.

29. Kerr LM, Anderson DM, Thompson JA, Lyver SM, Call GK. Ischemic stroke in the young: evaluation and age comparison of patients six months to thirty-nine years. *J Child Neurol* 1993;8:266–270.

30. Ferrera PC, Curran CB, Swanson H. Etiology of pediatric ischemic stroke. *Am J Emerg Med* 1997;15:671–679.

31. Askalan R, Laughlin S, Mayank S, et al. Chickenpox and stoke in childhood: a study of frequency and causation. *Stroke* 2001;32:1257–1262.

32. Chabrier S, Rodesch G, Lasjaunias P, Tardieu M, Landrieu P, Sebire G. Transient cerebral arteriopathy: a disorder recognized by serial angiograms in children with stroke. *J Child Neurol* 1998;13:27–32.

33. Cantu C, Barinagarrementeria F. Cerebrovascular complications of neurocysticercosis. Clinical and neuroimaging spectrum. *Arch Neurol* 1996;53:233–239.

34. Benseler SM, Silverman E, Aviv RI, et al. Primary central nervous system vasculitis in children. *Arthritis Rheum* 2006;54:1297–1297

35. Fullerton HJ, Johnston SC, Smith WS. Arterial dissection and stroke in children. *Neurology* 2001;57:1155–1160.

36. Schievink WI, Mokri B, Piepgras DG. Spontaneous dissections of cervicocephalic arteries in childhood and adolescence. *Neurology* 1994;44:1607–1612.

37. Cheon JE, Kim IO, Kim WS, Hwang YS, Wang KC, Yeon KM. MR diagnosis of cerebellar infarction due to vertebral artery dissection in children. *Pediatr Radiol* 2001;31:163–166.

38. Camacho A, Villarejo A, de Aragon AM, Simon R, Mateos F. Spontaneous carotid and vertebral artery dissection in children. *Pediatr Neurol* 2001;25:250–253.

39. Hasan I, Wapnick S, Kutscher ML, Couldwell WT. Vertebral arterial dissection associated with Klippel-Feil syndrome in a child. *Childs Nerv Syst* 2002;18:67–70.

40. Chiu D, Shedden P, Bratina P, Grotta JC. Clinical features of moyamoya disease in the United States. *Stroke* 1998;29:1347–1351.

41. Grenier Y, Tomita T, Marymont MH, Byrd S, Burrowes DM. Late postirradiation occlusive vasculopathy in childhood medulloblastoma. Report of two cases. *J Neurosurg* 1998;89:460–464.

42. Wober-Bingol C, Wober C, Karwautz A, Feucht M, Brandtner S, Scheidinger H. Migraine and stroke in childhood and adolescence. *Cephalalgia* 1995;15:26–30.

43. Williams LS, Garg BP, Cohen M, Fleck JD, Biller J. Subtypes of ischemic stroke in children and young adults. *Neurology* 1997;49:1541–1545.

44. Garcia JH, Pantoni L. Strokes in childhood. *Sem Pediatr Neurol* 1995;2:180–191.

45. Kirkham FJ. Recognition and prevention of neurological complications in pediatric cardiac surgery. *Pediatr Cardiol* 1998;19:331–345.

46. Pua HL, Bissonnette B. Cerebral physiology in paediatric cardiopulmonary bypass. *Can J Anaesth* 1998;45:960–978.

47. Quinones JA, Deleon SY, Bell TJ, et al. Fenestrated fontan procedure: evolution of technique and occurrence of paradoxical embolism. *Pediatr Cardiol* 1997;18:218–221.

48. Nestoridi E, Buonanno FS, Jones RM, et al. Arterial ischemic stroke in childhood: the role of plasma-phase risk factors. *Curr Opin Neurol* 2002;15:139–144.

49. deVeber G, Monagle P, Chan A, et al. Prothrombotic disorders in infants and children with cerebral thromboembolism. *Arch Neurol* 1998;55:1539–1543.

50. Gore RM, Weinberg PE, Anandappa E, Shkolnik A, White H. Intracranial complications of pediatric hematologic disorders: computed tomographic assessment. *Invest Radiol* 1981;16:175–180.

51. Priest JR, Ramsay NK, Latchaw RE, et al. Thrombotic and hemorrhagic strokes complicating early therapy for childhood acute lymphoblastic leukemia. *Cancer* 1980;46:1548–1554.

52. Mendoza PL, Conway EE, Jr. Cerebrovascular events in pediatric patients. *Pediatr Ann* 1998;27:665–674.

53. Adams RJ, McKie VC, Carl EM, et al. Long-term stroke risk in children with sickle cell disease screened with transcranial Doppler. *Ann Neurol* 1997;42:699–704.

54. Prengler M, Pavlakis SG, Prohovnik I, Adams RJ. Sickle cell disease: the neurological complications. *Ann Neurol* 2002;51:543–552.

55. Quinn CT, Rogers ZR, Buchanan GR. Survival of children with sickle cell disease. *Blood* 2004;103:4023–4027.

56. Liesner R, Mackie I, Cookson J, et al. Prothrombotic changes in children with sickle cell disease: relationships to cerebrovascular disease and transfusion. *Br J Haematol* 1998;103:1037–1044.

57. Ohene-Frempong K, Weiner SJ, Sleeper LA, et al. Cerebrovascular accidents in sickle cell disease: rates and risk factors. *Blood* 1998;91:288–294.

58. Kinney TR, Sleeper LA, Wang WC, et al. Silent cerebral infarcts in sickle cell anemia: a risk factor analysis. The Cooperative Study of Sickle Cell Disease. *Pediatrics* 1999;103:640–645.

59. Steen RG, Xiong X, Mulhern RK, Langston JW, Wang WC. Subtle brain abnormalities in children with sickle cell disease. Relationship to blood hematocrit. *Ann Neurol* 1999;45:279–286.

60. Steen RG, Xiong X, Langston JW, Helton KJ. Brain injury in children with sickle cell disease: prevalence and etiology. *Ann Neurol* 2003;54:564–572.

61. Adams RJ. Stroke prevention in sickle cell disease. *Curr Opin Hematol* 2000;7:101–105.

62. Adams RJ, Brambilla DJ, Granger S, et al. Stroke and conversion to high risk children screened with transcranial Doppler ultrasound during the STOP study. *Blood* 2004;103:3689–3694.

63. Riddington C, Wang W. Blood transfusion for preventing stroke in people with sickle cell disease. *Cochrane Database Syst Rev* 2002;CD003146.

64. Ganesan V, McShane MA, Liesner R, Cookson J, Hann I, Kirkham FJ. Inherited prothrombotic states and ischaemic stroke in childhood. *J Neurol Neurosurg Psychiatry* 1998; 65:508–511.

65. Lynch JK, Nelson KB, Curry CJ, Grether JK. Cerebrovascular disorders in children with the factor V Leiden mutation. *J Child Neurol* 2001;16:735–744.

66. Tosetto A, Ruggeri M, Castaman G, Rodeghiero F. Inherited abnormalities of blood coagulation in juvenile stroke. A case-control study. *Blood Coagul Fibrinolysis* 1997;8:397–402.

67. Kenet G, Sadetzki S, Murad H, et al. Factor V Leiden and antiphospholipid antibodies are significant risk factors for ischemic stroke in children. *Stroke* 2000;31:1283–1288.

68. Baca V, Garcia-Ramirez R, Ramirez-Lacayo M, Marquez-Enriquez L, Martinez I, Lavalle C. Cerebral infarction and antiphospholipid syndrome in children. *J Rheumatol* 1996; 23:1428–1431.

69. Wells RG, Vetter C, Laud P. Intracrainial hemorrhage in children younger than 3 years: prediction of intent. *Arch Pediatr Adolesc Med* 2002;156:252–257.

70. Chul Suh D, Alvarez H, Bhattacharya JJ, Rodesch G, Lasjaunias PL. Intracranial haemorrhage within the first two years of life. *Acta Neurochir* 2001;143:997–1004.

71. Nomura S, Yamashita K, Kato S, et al. Childhood subarachnoid hemorrhage associated with fibromuscular dysplasia. *Childs Nerv Syst* 2001;17:419–422.

72. Hamada JI, Hashimoto N, Tsukahara T. Moya-moya disease with repeated intraventricular hemorrhage due to aneurysm rupture. *J Neurosurg* 1994;80:328–331.

73. Yoshida Y, Yoshimoto T, Shirane R, Sakurai Y. Clinical course, surgical management, and long-term outcome of moyamoya patients with rebleeding after an episode of intracerebral hemorrhage: An extensive follow-Up study. *Stroke* 1999;30:2276.

74. Saeki N, Nakazaki S, Kubota M, et al. Hemorrhagic type moyamoya disease. *Clin Neurol Neurosurg* 1997;99(suppl 2):S196–S201.

75. Alaani WS, Awidi AS. Spontaneous intracranial bleeding in hemorrhagic diathesis. *Surg Neurol* 1982;17:137–140.

76. Papa ML, Schisano G, Franco A, et al. Congential deficiency of factor VII in subarachnoid hemorrhage. *Stroke* 1994;25:508–510.

77. Cahill MR, Colvin BT. Haemophilia. *Postgrad Med J* 1997; 73:201–206.

78. Arkin S, Cooper H, Hutter J, et al. Activated recombinant human coagulation factor VII therapy for intracranial hemorrhage in patients with himophilia A or B with inhibitors. Results of the novoseven emergency-use program. *Haemostasis* 1998;28:93–98.

79. Batjer HH, Adamson TE, Bowman GW. Sickle cell disease and aneurysmal subarachnoid hemorrhage. *Surg Neurol* 1991;36:145–149.

80. Oyesiku NM, Barrow DL, Eckman JR, et al. Intracranial aneurysms in sickle-cell anemia: Clinical features and pathogenesis. *J Neurosurg* 1991;75:356–363.

81. Preul MC, Cendes F, Just N, Mohr G. Intracranial aneurysms and sickle cell anemia: multiplicity and propensity for the vertebrobasilar territory. *Neurosurgery* 1998;42:971–977.

82. Graus F, Rogers LR, Posner JB. Cerebrovascular complications in patients with cancer. *Medicine* 1985;64:16–35.

83. Blom I, De Schryver EL, Kappelle LJ, Rinkel GJ, Jennekens-Schinkel A, Peters AC. Prognosis of haemorrhagic stroke in childhood: a long-term follow-up study. *Dev Med Child Neurol* 2003;45:233–239.

84. Rasura M, Spalloni A, Ferrari M, et al. A case series of young stroke in Rome. *Eur J Neurol* 2006;13:146–152.

85. Malm J, Kristensen B, Carlberg B, Fagerlund M, Olsson T. Clinical features and prognosis in young adults with infratentorial infarcts. *Cerebrovasc Dis* 1999;9:282–289.

86. Biller J, Adams HP, Jr., Bruno A, Love BB, Marsh EE. Mortality in acute cerebral infarction in young adults—a ten-year experience. *Angiology* 1991;42:224–230.

87. Biller J, Toffol GJ, Kassell NF, Adams HP, Jr., Beck DW, Boarini DJ. Spontaneous subarachnoid hemorrhage in young adults. *Neurosurgery* 1987;21:664–667.

88. Kappelle LJ, Adams HP, Jr., Heffner ML, Torner JC, Gomez F, Biller J. Prognosis of young adults with ischemic stroke. A long-term follow-up study assessing recurrent vascular events and functional outcome in the Iowa Registry of Stroke in Young Adults. *Stroke* 1994;25:1360–1365.

89. Adunsky A, Hershkowitz M, Rabbi R, Asher-Sivron L, Ohry A. Functional recovery in young stroke patients. *Arch Phys Med Rehabil* 1992;73:859–862.

90. Musolino R, La Spina P, Granata A, Gallitto G, Leggiadro N, Carerj S. Ischaemic stroke in young people: a prospective and long-term follow-up study. *Cerebrovasc Dis* 2003;15:121–128.

91. Martin PJ, Enevoldson TP, Humphrey PR. Causes of ischaemic stroke in the young. *Postgrad Med J* 1997;73:8–16.

92. Kittner SJ, McCarter RJ, Sherwin RW, et al. Black-white differences in stroke risk among young adults. *Stroke* 1993;I13–I15.

93. Kittner SJ, Stern BJ, Wozniak M, et al. Cerebral infarction in young adults: the Baltimore-Washington Cooperative Young Stroke Study. *Neurology* 1998;50:890–894.

94. Morgenstern LB, Spears WD. A triethnic comparison of intracerebral hemorrhage mortality in Texas. *Ann Neurol* 1997;42:919–923.

95. Broderick JP, Brott TG, Tomsick T. Intra-cerebral hemorrhage more than twice as common as subarachnoid hemorrhage. *J Neurosurg* 1993;78:188–191.

96. Qureshi AI, Safdar K, Patel M, Janssen RS, Frankel MR. Stroke in young black patients. Risk factors, subtypes, and prognosis. *Stroke* 1995;26:1995–1998.

97. Ayala C, Greenlund K, Croft JB, et al. Racial/ethnic disparities in mortality by stroke subtype in the United States. *Am J Epidemiol* 2001;154:1057–1063.

98. Jakovljevic D, Sivenius J, Sarti C, et al. Socioeconomic inequalities in the incidence, mortality and prognosis of subarachnoid hemorrhage: the FINMONICA Stroke Register. *Cerebrovasc Dis* 2001;12:7–13.

99. Barinagarrementeria F, Gonzalez-Duarte A, Miranda L, Cantu C. Cerebral infarction in young women: analysis of 130 cases. *Eur Neurol* 1998;40:228–233.

100. Knepper LE, Giuliani MJ. Cerebrovascular disease in women. *Cardiology* 1995;86:339–348.

101. Kittner SJ, Stern BJ, Feeser BR, et al. Pregnancy and the risk of stroke. *N Engl J Med* 1996;335:768–774.

102. Haddad N, Silva MB. Mortality due to cardiovascular disease in women during the reproductive age (15 to 49 years), in the State of Sao Paulo, Brazil from 1991 to 1995. *Arq Bras Cardiol* 2000;75:375–379.

103. Reiner AP, Schwartz SM, Frank MB, et al. Polymorphisms of coagulation factor XIII subunit A and risk of nonfatal hemorrhagic stroke in young white women. *Stroke* 2001;32:2580–2586.

104. Adams HP, Jr., Kappelle LJ, Biller J, Gordon DL, Love BB. Ischemic stroke in young adults. *Arch Neurol* 1995;52:491–495.

105. van den Berg JS, Limburg M. Ischemic stroke in the young: influence of diagnostic criteria. *Cerebrovasc Dis* 1993;3:227–230.

106. Chan MT, Nadareishvili ZG, Norris JW. Diagnostic strategies in young patients with ischemic stroke in Canada. *Can J Neurol Sci* 2000;27:120–124.

107. Haapaniemi H, Hillbom M, Juvela S. Lifestyle-associated risk factors for acute brain infarction among persons of working age. *Stroke* 1997;28:26–30.

108. You RX, McNeil JJ, O'Malley HM, Davis SM, Thrift AG, Donnan GA. Risk factors for stroke due to cerebral infarction in young adults. *Stroke* 1997;28:1913–1918.

109. Love BB, Biller J, Jones MP, Adams HP, Jr., Bruno A. Cigarette smoking. A risk factor for cerebral infarction in young adults. *Arch Neurol* 1990;47:693–698.

110. Carolei A, Marini C, Nencini P, et al. Prevalence and outcome of symptomatic carotid lesions in young adults. National Research Council Study Group. *Br Med J* 1995;310:1363–1366.

111. Tan NC, Venketasubramanian N, Saw S, Tjia HT. Hyperhomocyst(e)inemia and risk of ischemic stroke among young Asian adults. *Stroke* 2002;33:1956–1962.

112. Mitsias P, Levine SR. Cerebrovascular complications of Fabry's disease. *Ann Neurol* 1996;40:8–17.

113. Lisovoski F, Rousseaux P. Cerebral infarction in young people. A study of 148 patients with early cerebral angiography. *J Neurol Neurosurg Psychiatry* 1991;54:576–579.

114. Hilton-Jones D, Warlow CP. Non-penetrating arterial trauma and cerebral infarction in the young. *Lancet* 1985;1:1435–1438.

115. Thie A, Hellner D, Lachenmayer L, Janzen RWC, Kunze K. Bilateral blunt traumatic dissections of the extracranial internal carotid artery; report of eleven cases and review literature. *Cerebrovasc Dis* 1993;3:295–303.

116. Welling RE, Saul TG, Tew JMJ, Tomsick TA, Kremchek TE, Bellamy MJ. Management of blunt injury to the internal carotid artery. *J Trauma* 1987;27:1221–1226.

117. van Putten MJ, Bloem BR, Smit VT, Aarts NJ, Lammers GJ. An uncommon cause of stroke in young adults. *Arch Neurol* 1999;56:1018–1020.

118. Bruno A, Adams HP, Jr., Biller J, Rezai K, Cornell S, Aschenbrener CA. Cerebral infarction due to moyamoya disease in young adults. *Stroke* 1988;19:826–833.

119. Levine SR, Fagan SC, Pessin MS, et al. Accelerated intracranial occlusive disease, oral contraceptives, and cigarette use. *Neurology* 1991;41:1893–1901.

120. Wesen CA, Elliott BM. Fibromuscular dysplasia of the carotid arteries. *Am J Surg* 1986;151:448–451.

121. Launer LJ, Terwindt GM, Ferrari MD. The prevalence and characteristics of migraine in a population-based cohort. *Neurology* 1999;53:537–542.

122. Narbone MC, Leggiadro N, La Spina P, Rao R, Grugno R, Musolino R. Migraine stroke: a possible complication of both migraine with and without aura. *Headache* 1996;36:481–483.

123. Kruit MC, van Buchem MA, Hofman PAM, et al. Migraine as a risk factor for subclinical brain lesions. *JAMA* 2004;291:427–434.

124. Lance JW. The pathophysiology of migraine: a tentative synthesis. *Patholog Bio* 1992;40:355–360.

125. Hall GC, Brown MM, Mo J, MacRae KD. Triptans in migraine: the risks of stroke, cardiovascular disease, and death in practice. *Neurology* 2004;62:563–568.

126. Jousilahti P, Tuomilehto J, Rastenyte D, Vartiainen E. Headache and the risk of stroke: a prospective observational cohort study among 35,056 Finnish men and women. *Arch Intern Med* 2003;163:1058–1062.

127. Mosek A, Marom R, Korczyn AD, Bornstein N. A history of migraine is not a risk factor to develop an ischemic stroke in the elderly. *Headache* 2001;41:399–401.

128. Kurth T, Gaziano J, Cook NR, et al. Migraine and risk of cardiovascular disease in women. *JAMA* 2006;296:283–291.

129. Schwaag S, Nabavi DG, Frese A, Husstedt IW, Evers S. The association between migraine and jvenile stroke: a case-control study. *Headache* 2003;43:90–95.

130. Mitchell P, Wang JJ, Currie J, Cumming RG, Smith W. Prevalence and vascular associations with migraine in older Australians. *Aust N Z J Med* 1998;28:627–632.

131. Chang CL, Donaghy M, Poulter N. Migraine and stroke in young women: case-control study. The World Health Organisation Collaborative Study of Cardiovascular Disease and Steroid Hormone Contraception. *Br Med J* 1999;318:13–18.

132. Nightingale AL, Farmer RDT. Ischemic stroke in young women. A nested case-control study using the UK general practice research database. *Stoke* 2004;35:1574–1578.

133. Tzourio C, Iglesias S, Hubert JB, et al. Migraine and risk of ischaemic stroke: a case-control study. *Br Med J* 1993;307:289–292.

134. Silvestrini M, Cupini LM, Matteis M, De Simone R, Bernardi G. Migraine in patients with stroke and antiphospholipid antibodies. *Headache* 1993;33:421–426.

135. Tietjen GE, Gottwald L, Al-Qasmi MM, Gunda P, Khuder SA. Migraine is associated with livedo reticularis: a prospective study. *Headache* 2002;42:263–267.

136. Chabriat H, Tournier-Lasserve E, Vahedi K, et al. Autosomal dominant migraine with MRI white-matter abnormalities mapping to the CADASIL locus. *Neurology* 1995;45:1086–1091.

137. Hutchinson M, O'Riordan J, Javed M, et al. Familial hemiplegic migraine and autosomal dominant arteriopathy

with leukoencephalopathy (CADASIL). *Ann Neurol* 1995; 38:817–824.

138. Desmond DW, Moroney JT, Lynch T, Chan S, Chin SS, Mohr JP. The natural history of CADASIL: a pooled analysis of previously published cases. *Stroke* 1999;30:1230–1233.

139. Kowalski RG, Claassen J, Kreiter KT, et al. Initial misdiagnosis and outcome after subarachnoid hemorrhage. *JAMA* 2004;291:866–869.

140. Wijman CA, Wolf PA, Kase CS, Kelly-Hayes M, Beiser AS. Migrainous visual accompaniments are not rare in late life: the Framingham Study. *Stroke* 1998;29:1539–1543.

141. Thomsen LL, Eriksen MK, Roemer SF, Andersen I, Olesen J, Russell MB. A population-based study of familial hemiplegic migraine suggests revised diagnostic criteria. *Brain* 2002;125:1379–1391

142. Ferro JM, Melo TP, Oliveira V, et al. A multivariate study of headache associated with ischemic stroke. *Headache* 1995;35:315–319.

143. Jorgensen HS, Jespersen HF, Nakayama H, Raaschou HO, Olsen TS. Headache in stroke: the Copenhagen Stroke Study. *Neurology* 1994;44:1793–1797.

144. Gorelick PB, Hier DB, Caplan LR, Langenberg P. Headache in acute cerebrovascular disease. *Neurology* 1986;36:1445–1450.

145. Tzourio C, Benslamia L, Guillon B, et al. Migraine and the risk of cercial artery dissection: a case-control study. *Neurology* 2002;59:435–437.

146. Bogousslavsky J, Regli F, Van Melle G, Payot M, Uske A. Migraine stroke. *Neurology* 1988;38:223–227.

147. Broderick JP, Swanson JW. Migraine-related strokes. Clinical profile and prognosis in 20 patients. *Arch Neurol* 1987;44:868–871.

148. Hoekstra-van Dalen RA, Cillessen JP, Kappelle LJ, van Gijn J. Cerebral infarcts associated with migraine: clinical features, risk factors and follow-up. *J Neurol* 1996;243:511–515.

149. Meschia JF, Malkoff MD, Biller J. Reversible segmental cerebral arterial vasospasm and cerebral infarction: possible association with excessive use of sumatriptan and Midrin. *Arch Neurol* 1998;55:712–714.

150. Barinagarrementeria F, Cantu-Brito C, De La Pena A, Izaguirre R. Prothrombotic states in young people with idiopathic stroke. A prospective study. *Stroke* 1994;25:287–290.

151. Douay X, Lucas C, Caron C, Goudemand J, Leys D. Antithrombin, protein C and protein S levels in 127 consecutive young adults with ischemic stroke. *Acta Neurol Scand* 1998;98:124–127.

152. Munts AG, van Genderen PJ, Dippel DW, van Kooten F, Koudstaal PJ. Coagulation disorders in young adults with acute cerebral ischaemia. *J Neurol* 1998;245:21–25.

153. Lanska DJ, Kryscio RJ. Risk factors for peripartum and postpartum stroke and intracranialvenous thrombosis. *Stroke* 2000;31:1274–1282.

154. Salonen Ros H, Lichtenstein P, Bellocco R, Peterson G, Cnattinguis S. Increased risks of circulatory diseases in late pregnancy and puerperium. *Epidemiology* 2001;12:456–460.

155. Brown DW, Dueker N, Jamieson DJ, et al. Preeclampsia and risk of ischemic stroke among young women. Results from the Stroke Prevention in Young Women Study. *Stroke* 2006;37:1055–1059.

156. Kaplan PW. Neurologic issues in eclampsia. *Rev Neurol* 1999;155:335–341.

157. Qureshi AI, Giles WH, Croft JB, Stern BJ. Number of pregnancies and risk for stroke and stroke subtypes. *Arch Neurol* 1997;54:203–206.

158. Cantu C, Barinagarrementeria F. Cerebral venous thrombosis associated with pregnancy and puerperium. *Stroke* 1993;24:1880–1884.

159. Lamy C, Hamon JB, Coste J, Mas JL. Ischemic stroke in young women: risk of recurrence during subsequent pregnancies. French Study Group on Stroke Pregnancy. *Neurology* 2000;55:269–274.

160. Donaldson JO, Lee NS. Arterial and venous stroke associated with pregnancy. *Neurol Clin* 1994;12:583–599.

161. Wiebers DO. Ischemic cerebrovascular complications of pregnancy. *Arch Neurol* 1985;42:1106–1113.

162. Ballem P. Acquired thrombophilia in pregnancy. *Semin Thromb Hemost* 1998;24(suppl 1):41–47.

163. Calado S, Viana-Baptista M. Benign cerebral angiopathy; postpartum cerebral angiopathy. Characteristics and treatment. *Curr Treat Options Cardiovasc Med* 2006;8:201–212.

164. Van de Kelft E, Kunnen J, Truyen L, Heytens L. Postpartum dissecting aneurysm of the basilar artery. *Stroke* 1992;23:114–116.

165. Komiyama M, Yasui T, Kitano S, Sakamoto H, Fujitani K, Matsuo S. Moyamoya disease and pregnancy: case report and review of the literature. *Neurosurgery* 1998;43:360–368.

166. Geocadin RG, Razumovsky AY, Wityk RJ, Bhardwaj A, Ulatowski JA. Intracerebral hemorrhage and postpartum cerebral vasculopathy. *J Neurol Sci* 2002;205:29–34.

167. Raroque HGJ, Tesfa G, Purdy P. Postpartum cerebral angiopathy. Is there a role for sympathomimetic drugs? *Stroke* 1993;24:2108–2110.

168. Janssens E, Hommel M, Mounier-Vehier F, Leclerc X, Guerin dM, Leys D. Postpartum cerebral angiopathy possibly due to bromocriptine therapy. *Stroke* 1995;26:128–130.

169. Barinagarrementeria F, Cantu C, Balderrama J. Postpartum cerebral angiopathy with cerebral infarction due to ergonovine use. *Stroke* 1992;23:1364–1366.

170. Sharshar T, Lamy C, Mas JL. Incidence and causes of strokes associated with pregnancy and puerperium. A study in public hospitals of Ile de France. Stroke in Pregnancy Study Group. *Stroke* 1995;26:930–936.

171. Hodgman MT, Pessin MS, Homans DC, et al. Cerebral embolism as the initial manifestation of peripartum cardiomyopathy. *Neurology* 1982;32:668–671.

172. Mainprize TC, Maltby JR. Amniotic fluid embolism: a report of four probable cases. *Can Anaesth Soc J* 1986;33:382–387.

173. Servillo G, Striano P, Striano S, et al. Posterior reversible encephalopathy syndrome (PRES) in critically ill obstetric patients. *Inten Care Med* 2003;29:2323–2326.

174. Ertan AK, Wagner S, Hendrik HJ, Tanriverdi HA, Schmidt W. Clinical and biophysical aspects of HELLP-syndrome. *J Perinat Med* 2002;30:483–489.

175. Heinemann LA, Lewis MA, Thorogood M, Spitzer WO, Guggenmoos H, Bruppacher R. Case-control study of oral contraceptives and risk of thromboembolic stroke: results from International Study on Oral Contraceptives and Health of Young Women. *Br Med J* 1997;315:1502–1504.

176. Hannaford PC, Croft PR, Kay CR. Oral contraception and stroke. Evidence from the Royal College of General Practitioners' Oral Contraception Study. *Stroke* 1994;25:935–942.

177. WHO Collaborative Study of Cardiovascular Disease and Steroid Hormone Contraception. Ischaemic stroke and combined oral contraceptives: results of an international, multicentre, case-control study. *Lancet* 1996;348:498–505.

178. WHO Collaborative Study of Cardiovascular Disease and Steroid Hormone Contraception. Haemorrhagic stroke, overall stroke risk, and combined oral contraceptives: results of an international, multicentre, case-control study. *Lancet* 1996;348:505–510.

179. Schwartz SM, Petitti DB, Siscovick DS, et al. Stroke and use of low-dose oral contraceptives in young women: a pooled analysis of two US studies. *Stroke* 1998;29:2277–2284.

180. Lidegaard O, Kreiner S. Cerebral thrombosis and oral contraceptives. A case-control study. *Contraception* 1998;57:303–314.

181. Lidegaard O, Kreiner S. Contraceptives and cerebral thrombosis: a five-year national case-control study. *Contraception* 2002;65:197–205.

182. Chasan-Taber L, Stampfer MJ. Epidemiology of oral contraceptives and cardiovascular disease. *Ann Intern Med* 1998;128:467–477.

183. Thorogood M. Stroke and steroid hormonal contraception. *Contraception* 1998;57:157–167.

184. Vessey M, Painter R, Yeates D. Mortality in relation to oral contraceptive use cigarette smoking. *Lancet* 2003;362:185–191.

185. Becker WJ. Migraine and oral contraceptives. *Can J Neurol Sci* 1997;24:16–21.

186. Becker WJ. Use of oral contraceptives in patients with migraine. *Neurology* 1999;53:S19-S25

187. Yoshii F, Ooki N, Shinohara Y, Uehara K, Mochimaru F. Multiple Cerebral infarctions associated with ovarian hyperstimulation syndrome. *Neurology* 1999;53:225–227.

188. Boden-Albala B, Sacco RL. Lifestyle factors and stroke risk: exercise, alcohol, diet, obesity, smoking, drug use, and stress. *Curr Atheroscler Rep* 2000;2:160–166.

189. Kurth T, Kase CS, Berger K, Schaeffner ES, Buring JE, Gaziano JM. Smoking and the risk of hemorrhagic stroke in men. *Stroke* 2003;34:1151–1155.

190. Reynolds K, Lewis LB, NOlen JDL, Kinney GL, Sathya B, He J. Alcohol consumption and risk of stroke. A Meta-analysis. *JAMA* 2003;289:579–588.

191. Sacco RL, Eikind M, Boden-Albala B, et al. The potential effect of moderate alcohol consumption on ischemic stroke. *JAMA* 1999;281:53–60.

192. Gorelick PB. Stroke from alcohol and drug abuse. A current social peril. *Postgrad Med* 1990;88:171–174.

193. Rodgers H, Aitken PD, French JM, Curless RH, Bates D, James OF. Alcohol and stroke. A case-control study of drinking habits past and present. *Stroke* 1993;24:1473–1477.

194. Kiechl S, Willeit J, Rungger G, Egger G, Oberhollenzer F, Bonora E. Alcohol consumption and atherosclerosis: what is the relation? Prospective results from the Bruneck Study. *Stroke* 1998;29:900–907.

195. Haapaniemi H, Hillbom M, Juvela S. Weekend and holiday increase in the onset of ischemic stroke in young women. *Stroke* 1996;27:1023–1027.

196. Hillbom M, Numminen H, Juvela S. Recent heavy drinking of alcohol and embolic stroke. *Stroke* 1999;30:2307–2312.

197. Hillbom M, Haapaniemi H, Juvela S, Palomaki H, Numminen H, Kaste M. Recent alcohol consumption, cigarette smoking, and cerebral infarction in young adults. *Stroke* 1995;26:40–45.

198. Klatsky A, Armstrong M, Friedman G, Sidney S. Alcohol drinking and risk of hemorrhagic stroke. *Neuroepidemiology* 2002;21:115–122.

199. Sloan MA, Kittner SJ, Rigamonti D, Price TR. Occurrence of stroke associated with use/abuse of drugs. *Neurology* 1991;41:1358–1364.

200. Sloan MA, Kittner SJ, Feeser BR, Gardner J, Epstein A, Wozniak MA. illicit drug-associated ischemic stroke in the Baltimor-Washinton Stroke Study. *Neurology* 1998;50:1688–1693.

201. Kaku DA, Lowenstein DH. Emergence of recreational drug abuse as a major risk factor for stroke in young adults. *Ann Intern Med* 1990;113:821–827.

202. Petitti DB, Sidney S, Quesenberry C, Bernstein A. Stroke and cocaine or amphetamine use. *Epidemiology* 1998;9:596–600.

203. Nanda A, Vannemreddy P, Willis B, Kelley RL. Stroke in the young. Relationship of active cocaine use with stroke mechanisms and outcome. *Acta Neurochir Suppl* 2006;96:91–96.

204. Levine SR, Brust JC, Futrell N, et al. Cerebrovascular complications of the use of the "crack" form of alkaloidal cocaine. *N Engl J Med* 1990;323:699–704.

205. Qureshi AI, Akbar MS, Czander E, Safdar K, Janssen RS, Frankel MR. Crack cocaine use and stroke in young patients. *Neurology* 1997;48:341–345.

206. Lange R, Hillis L. Cardiovascular complications of cocaine use. *N Engl J Med* 2001;345:351–358.

207. Kokkinos J, Levine SR. Stroke. *Neurol Clin* 1993;11:577–590.

208. Wang AM, Suojanen JN, Colucci VM, Rumbaugh CL, Hollenberg NK. Cocaine- and methamphetamine-induced acute cerebral vasospasm: an angiographic study in rabbits. *Am J Neuroradiol* 1990;11:1141–1146.

209. Storen EC, Wijdicks EF, Crum BA, Schultz G. Moyamoya-like vasculopathy from cocaine dependency. *Am J Neuroradiol* 2000;21:1008–1010.

210. Chen HJ, Liang CL, Lu K, Lui CC. Rapidly growing internal carotid artery aneurysm after amphetamine abuse: case report. *Am J Forensic Med Pathol* 2003;24:32–34.

211. Howington JU, Kutz SC, Wilding GE, Awasthi D. Cocaine use as a predictor of outcome in aneurysmal subarachnoid hemorrhage. *J Neurosurg* 2003;99:271–275.

212. Perez JA, Jr., Arsura EL, Strategos S. Methamphetamine-related stroke: four cases. *J Emerg Med* 1999;17:469–471.

213. Marini C, Totaro R, De Santis F, Ciancarelli I, Baldassarre M, Carolei A. Stroke in young adults, in the community-based L'Aquila registry: incidence and prognosis. *Stroke* 2001;32:52–56.

214. Nencini P, Inzitari D, Baruffi MC, et al. Incidence of stroke in young adults in Florence, Italy. *Stroke* 1988;19: 977–981.

215. Jacobs BS, Boden-Albala B, Lin IF, Sacco RL. Stroke in the young in the northern Manhattan stroke study. *Stroke* 2002;33:2789–2793.

216. Ogungbo B, Gregson B, Blackburn A, et al. Aneurysmal subarchnoid hemorrhage in young adults. *J Neurosurg* 2003;98:43–49.

217. Broderick JP, Viscoli CM, Brott T, et al. Major risk factors for aneurysmal subarachnoid hemorrhage in the young are modifiable. *Stroke* 2003;34:1375–1381.

218. McEvoy AW, Kitchen ND, Thomas DG. Intracerebral haemorrhage and drug abuse in young adults. *Br J Neurosurg* 2000;14:449–454.

219. Ruiz-Sandoval JL, Cantu C, Barinagarrementeria F. Intracerebral hemorrhage in young people: analysis of risk factors, locations, causes, and prognosis. *Stroke* 1999;20: 537–541.

220. Toffol GJ, Biller J, Adams HP, Jr. Nontraumatic intracerebral hemorrhage in young adults. *Arch Neurol* 1987;44: 483–485.

221. Roquer J, Palomeras E, Knobel H, Pou A. Intracerebral haemorrhage in AIDS. *Cerebrovasc Dis* 1998;8:222–227.

CHAPTER 18

Venous Thrombosis, Pituitary Apoplexy, and Vascular Disease of the Spinal Cord

▶ VENOUS THROMBOSIS

Venous thrombosis of the brain occurs at a much lower frequency than does thromboembolic arterial occlusions. Still, cerebral venous thrombosis is not a rare illness and the estimates of this vascular disease partially reflect problems in diagnosis rather than the true incidence.[1] A sizable proportion of cases are probably not recognized. Because of the relative infrequency and variable presentations, the diagnosis of cerebral venous thrombosis is often difficult or delayed. Fortunately, with a reasonable index of suspicion and the availability of modern vascular imaging studies, in particular magnetic resonance venography (MRV), the recognition of cerebral venous thrombosis should improve. Early diagnosis is important because medical measures to halt propagation or speed lysis of the intravenous clot are available. Interventions help limit secondary neurological injury. In addition, prescription of anticoagulants to high-risk persons might prevent this serious illness.

Many patients have involvement of more than one cerebral venous sinus. In general, the most commonly involved veins are the superior sagittal sinus and the lateral sinus. Isolated venous thrombosis affecting the cavernous sinus, superior sagittal sinus, or lateral sinus also can occur. Less commonly, isolated cortical thrombophlebitis, deep venous sinus thrombosis, or cerebellar venous thrombosis develop.

Pathophysiology

The course of venous thrombosis is subacute. The time of onset of the thrombosis often is not known. Presumably, the intravenous occlusion gradually expands over several hours to possibly weeks. The severity of the neurological symptoms depends upon the size of the occluded venous structure, the location of the clot, and whether the thrombosis results in complete or partial obliteration of the vascular lumen.[2] The neurological signs are usually due to bleeding or brain edema that produces increased intracranial pressure. Still, because flow can proceed via collateral veins, secondary brain ischemia or major hemorrhage is often avoided. Venous occlusion (obstruction) leads to distension of the vessel and the swollen venous structures can compress adjacent neurological structures (Fig. 18-1). Venous occlusion locally or generally slows drainage of blood from the cranial vault. The vascular congestion also causes increases in intracranial pressure in part due to impaired absorption of cerebrospinal fluid. Depending upon the occluded vein, the brain edema can be unilateral or bilateral. The swelling can affect deep structures primarily or can be cortical in location. The vascular congestion also leads to capillary leakage and intracerebral bleeding (Fig. 18-2). Focal neurological signs might not be found with occlusions of larger venous structures (particularly the posterior venous sinuses) because the thrombus might not extend to cortical or deep veins.

A localized cortical thrombophlebitis or occlusion of a deep hemispheric vein can be complicated by a focal hemorrhage or ischemic brain injury, which produces discrete neurological impairments. The affected gray and white mater can be congested and associated with hemorrhage. The areas of bleeding can be solitary or multiple, and the severity ranges from small petechial areas to a large hematoma.

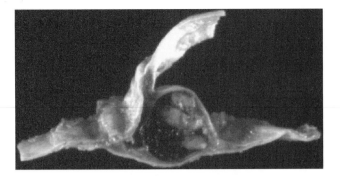

Figure 18-1. Cross section of the superior sagittal sinus illustrates a thrombus within the lumen of the venous structure. (*Courtesy of S.S. Schochet, M.D., Department of Pathology, University of West Virginia, Morgantown, WV*)

The course of venous thrombosis is variable. A majority of occluded veins have spontaneous recanalization.[3] Such recanalization usually occurs within the first 4 months. In some patients, alternative venous channels can be developed to maintain venous flow.

Epidemiology

Venous thrombosis is relatively uncommon in comparison to arterial occlusions. Estimates of its incidence are not very reliable because physicians often do not recognize cases of cerebral venous thrombosis. It affects men and women of all ages, although Breteau et al.[4] found that approximately 75 percent of affected patients were women. The marked predominance in women probably

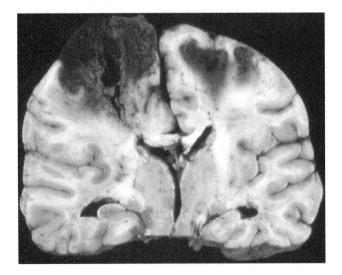

Figure 18-2. Coronal autopsy specimen reveals bilateral parasagittal hemorrhages in both cerebral hemispheres in a patient who died of thrombosis of the superior sagittal sinus. (*Courtesy of S.S. Schochet, M.D., Department of Pathology, University of West Virginia, Morgantown, WV*)

reflects the strong association of venous thrombosis to pregnancy or the puerperium. A Swedish study found that venous thrombosis was dramatically increased in the period around the time of delivery.[5] The incidence of puerperal cerebral venous thrombosis is estimated to be as high as 60 per 100,000 pregnancies in the United States. However, the incidence of venous thrombosis is considerably higher among pregnant women in developing countries. Venous thrombosis also occurs in children.[6] Neonates or infants might have involvement of the deep venous structures. Their symptoms are similar to those found in older persons. In addition, the number of cases of cerebral venous thrombosis diagnosed in childhood is increasing.[7] The explanation for this increase is not obvious. Data are not available to suggest any ethnic predisposition to this form of cerebrovascular disease.

Prognosis

The mortality of venous thrombosis is relatively low (10 percent).[8,9] Deaths are usually secondary to extensive brain edema and hemorrhage. Mortality is higher among patients with primary thrombosis of the deep veins than among those with cortical or sinus thrombosis. Patients with marked intracranial pressure, impaired consciousness, large hemorrhages, or diffuse brain edema have a poor prognosis.[9] In addition, mortality is related to the underlying etiology or factor that led to the thrombosis. Data about long-term prognosis are limited. The severity of the residual neurological impairments reflects the nature of the brain injury.[10] Patients with neurological worsening on admission or an encephalopathy have the highest risk for poor outcomes.[10] While most survivors have favorable outcomes, cognitive impairments and visual loss can occur.[4,11] Patients surviving cavernous sinus thrombosis usually have residual visual loss, disorders of ocular mobility, or pituitary insufficiency. The chances of recurrent cerebral venous thrombosis are relatively low. Ferro et al.[9] found that the rate of recurrent cerebral venous thrombosis was approximately 2 percent. Presumably, patients with some causes of venous thrombosis, such as an inherited or acquired hypercoagulable state, have a high risk for a second event.

Clinical Findings

The clinical manifestations and course of venous thrombosis differ from those found in patients with arterial occlusions (Table 18-1). Very few patients have the sudden onset of symptoms. Most patients have a course of gradually worsening or stepwise increase in symptoms over a few days to weeks. The most common symptoms are headache, nausea, vomiting, decreased consciousness, focal neurological complaints, and seizures.[1] The seizures can be focal or generalized.[12] While headache is the most common complaint, there is no particular

► **TABLE 18-1.** CLINICAL FEATURES OF CEREBRAL VENOUS THROMBOSIS

General symptoms
　Headache
　Focal or generalized seizures
　Focal neurological symptoms
　Papilledema
　Decreased consciousness
　Unilateral or bilateral abducens nerve palsies
Neurological symptoms—superior sagittal sinus
　Paraparesis
　Neurogenic bladder
　Encephalopathy or behavior disturbance
Neurological symptoms—cortical thrombophlebitis
　Unilateral motor or sensory impairments
　Visual impairments
　Cognitive impairments
Neurological symptoms—deep venous structures
　Coma
　Dystonia or movement disorder
Neurological symptoms—sigmoid or transverse sinus
　Headache
　Papilledema
　Decreased consciousness
　Cranial nerve palsies
Neurological symptoms—cavernous sinus (usually bilateral)
　Proptosis, chemosis
　Orbital edema
　Visual loss
　Oculomotor (III, IV, VI) nerve paralysis
　Trigeminal (V-1, and occasionally V-2) sensory loss
　Endocrine disturbances
　　Addisonian crisis
　　Diabetes insipidus

pattern or severity of the headache that is specific for venous thrombosis. A clinical presentation that mimics subarachnoid hemorrhage is a rare presentation.[13] The focal neurological symptoms depend upon the vein or venous sinus that is affected.

On examination, a disturbance in consciousness, which ranges from drowsiness or confusion to delirium or coma, is often found. Papilledema is found in approximately one-half of the cases. Although unilateral or bilateral abducens nerve palsies can be found, these false-localizing signs probably are secondary to the intracranial hypertension. Many patients have symptoms and signs of increased intracranial pressure only.[2] In such cases, the thrombosis usually involves the posterior venous sinuses (transverse, lateral, or sigmoid sinus). In the past, the term *otitic hydrocephalus* was used to describe venous thrombosis in these locations, which complicated serious otological infections. Affected patients usually have signs of intracranial hypertension only.

As implied by the term otitic hydrocephalus, venous thrombosis is one of the causes of a clinical syndrome

that mimics *pseudotumor cerebri*. Most patients are young women who are obese. Their complaints include headache and transient visual obscuration often associated with postural changes. Bilateral papilledema is the only abnormality found on examination. By definition, women with pseudotumor cerebri should have a normal evaluation except for increased cerebrospinal fluid pressure on lumbar puncture. However, magnetic resonance imaging (MRI) and MRV can detect an otherwise occult venous thrombus. There is some speculation that venous thrombosis might be a leading cause of pseudotumor cerebri. On the other hand, the increased intracranial pressure might lead to compression of the veins and create the false impression of a venous occlusion.

Depending upon the location of the clot, patients with *thrombosis of the superior sagittal sinus* have headache, decreased consciousness, focal or generalized seizures, and papilledema (Fig. 18-3). The neurological signs can be present unilaterally or bilaterally and, most commonly, involve the lower extremities. If the cortical veins (in particular the vein of Trolard) are secondary occluded, the patient can have a hemiparesis, aphasia, or focal cognitive impairments. Patients with *thrombosis of a lateral sinus* can have secondary congestion and hemorrhage involving the temporal lobe. *Thrombosis of the transverse sinus* or *sigmoid sinus* can

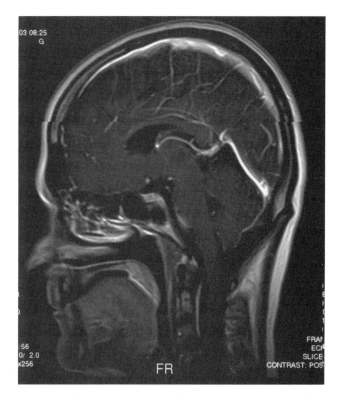

Figure 18-3. Midsagittal view of an enhanced T-1-weighted MRI study visualizes the major deep draining veins of the cerebral hemisphere, including the internal cerebral vein, the vein of Galen, and the straight sinus.

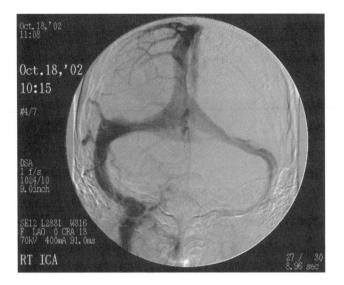

Figure 18-4. Anteroposterior view of a right carotid arteriogram shows the superior sagittal sinus, the torcula, the transverse sinuses, the sigmoid sinuses, and the internal jugular vein. The differences between the right and left sinuses are a normal variation.

cause isolated or multiple cranial nerves palsies[14] (Fig. 18-4). The most commonly affected nerves are III–VIII. An isolated cortical thrombophlebitis produces focal cognitive, sensory, motor, or visual impairments reflecting the area of secondary brain injury. Affected patients also have focal seizures. Patients with thrombosis of the deep venous structures (*vein of Galen* or *internal cerebral vein*) usually have the sudden onset of coma, extensor spasms, and hypertonia.

Cavernous sinus thrombosis has a rather distinct presentation (see Table 18-1). The course of the illness is usually acute with rapid evolution of symptoms over a few hours, particularly if the thrombosis is of infectious origin. Rarely, a subacute or chronic thrombosis develops. While the thrombosis initially involves one cavernous sinus, the abundant collateral vessels between the two cavernous sinuses mean that most patients develop bilateral involvement. In some cases, the spread evolves over a few hours. Patients have retro-orbital and frontal headache. They have prominent constitutional symptoms and can also have evidence of hypopituitarism, including diabetes insipidus, syndrome of inappropriate release of antidiuretic hormone, or an Addisonian crisis. Diplopia or unilateral or bilateral visual impairments also are prominent. On examination, patients have chemosis, proptosis, and ptosis. The face is often swollen. Unilateral or bilateral disk edema and visual loss, including an absent pupillary response to light, can be found. Additional signs include unilateral or bilateral involvement of the oculomotor, trochlear, abducens, and ophthalmic division of the trigeminal nerves. Less commonly, the maxillary division of the trigeminal nerve is affected.

▶ **TABLE 18-2.** IMAGING FINDINGS OF CEREBRAL VENOUS THROMBOSIS

MRI/CT
    Unilateral or bilateral hemispheric edema
    Unilateral or bilateral hemispheric hemorrhages
     (often multiple)
    Compression of sulci and ventricles
    Area of thrombosis in vein (cord sign)
    Empty-delta sign (CT)
    Hyperdensity in sinus (MRI)
    Absent flow void in sinus (MRI)
    Engorgement of sinus (MRI)
MRV
    Nonvisualization of deep or superficial venous structure
    Can demonstrate size and extent of thrombus
    Can be used to screen for recanalization

Diagnostic Studies

High-quality neuroimaging is key to diagnosis.[1,15] MRI is superior to computed tomography (CT) (Table 18-2). Direct evidence of venous involvement and indirect findings of the thrombosis are complemented by the secondary brain changes. The range of brain imaging findings is broad. Although some patients have normal studies, most have unilateral or bilateral areas of hemorrhage or brain swelling. Brain edema and intracranial hemorrhages that do not correspond to a specific arterial territory also point to venous thrombosis (see Fig. 18-5 and 18-6). The areas of hypodensity generally are more ill defined than those seen with arterial occlusions.

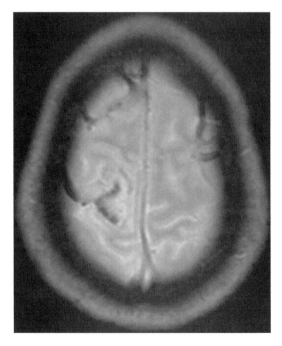

Figure 18-5. Gradient-echo MRI shows clots in multiple cortical veins in a patient with venous thrombosis.

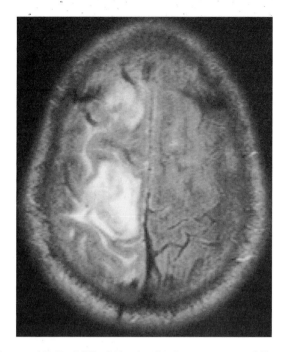

Figure 18-6. MRI of the brain demonstrates bilateral areas of edema and hemorrhage in a patient with sagittal sinus thrombosis.

Multiple areas of hypodensity, which are bilateral and primarily involving deep hemispheric structures or the white matter, are supportive of venous thrombosis. Thrombosis of the deep veins can produce bilateral changes in the thalamus, basal ganglia, rostral brain stem, and deep hemispheric white matter. Hemorrhagic changes range from petechiae to larger confluent areas of variable density. The hemorrhages often look less dense than that found with a primary brain hemorrhage. *Bilateral "thumbprint" hemorrhages* located parasagittally are highly suggestive of thrombosis of the superior sagittal sinus. Secondary changes include obliteration of the sulci and the compression of the ventricles. Hydrocephalus is rarely detected. The imaging might also demonstrate a local area of pathology, such as a tumor, which might be the underlying cause of the venous thrombus.

CT also detects more direct signs of the thrombus including the presence of increased density within a major vein, usually the superior sagittal sinus. The clot is usually adjacent to areas of hypodensity or bleeding within the brain. If the superior sagittal sinus is involved, the abnormality will be detected on multiple slices. If a vein that is aligned in the axial plane is affected, a long area of thrombosis (*cord sign*) can be found. The *empty-delta sign*, due to an absence of uniform enhancement of the sinus, can be detected with contrast-enhanced CT, most commonly with thrombosis of the superior sagittal sinus or one of the larger posterior fossa sinuses. A triangular-shaped area of enhancement occurs at the periphery of the vein with an absence of enhancement

in the center of the sinus, which represents the clot. Unfortunately, the finding lacks specificity and sensitivity. The finding of the empty-delta sign on one axial slice may be a false-positive change. Conversely, a large thrombus causing complete occlusion of the sinus might not permit enhancement of the periphery.

Swelling of the cavernous sinus on the basal CT slices can be found in cases of cavernous sinus thrombosis. In addition, imaging finds edema of the orbital contents. Obliteration of the sagittal or other bony sinuses consistent with an infectious process also can be found.

The imaging findings on MRI are influenced by the age of the thrombus (Fig. 18-7). The absence of the flow void within the vein can be seen. Sagittal slices can be used to detect hyperintensity within the superior sagittal sinus. Similar findings in the lateral or transverse sinus can be found on axial examinations of the posterior fossa (Fig. 18-7). Engorgement and slow flow also can be detected on evaluation of cortical or deep venous structures.

MRV, often with contrast enhancement, is a very useful imaging tool.[1] The sensitivity and specificity of MRV are very high. MRV can visualize both deep and superficial venous structures (Fig. 18-8). The size of the clot and extent of involvement of the thrombosis can be ascertained. Sequential studies can be used to assess the course of the thrombosis and to screen for recanalization of the vein. While MRV is highly useful, some caution should be exercised. Anatomic variations in the caliber of the veins, particularly those in the posterior fossa, might give the misleading impression of a thrombus.

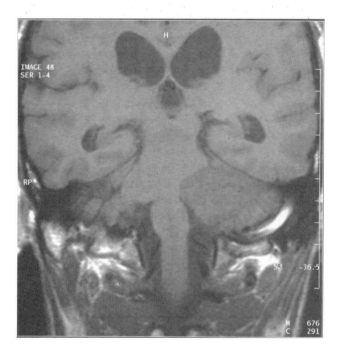

Figure 18-7. Coronal MRI study shows a thrombus in the left transverse sinus.

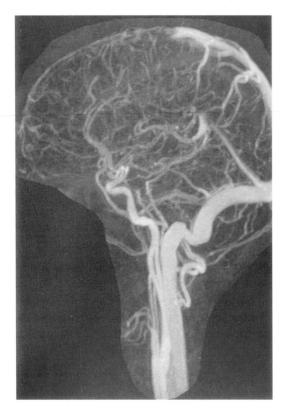

Figure 18-8. Sagittal view of an MRV reveals absence of filling of anterior half of the superior sagittal sinus in a patient with a thrombus.

External compression of the vein might be confused as a thrombus.

Until MRV became available, arteriography was the usual method for diagnosing venous thrombosis. However, the invasive study had limitations including the potential for side effects. The anatomic variations in venous drainage and issues in performing the test made interpretation of the results difficult. In addition, the yield of arteriography is probably lower than that of MRV. Thus, arteriography now is not recommended for evaluation of most patients with suspected venous thrombosis.

The results of examination of the cerebrospinal fluid usually are abnormal. Patients often have increased pressure. Other findings include an increased protein level and the presence of elevated counts of red blood cells and leukocytes. Other tests, such as assessments of coagulation factors, are aimed at looking at the cause of the venous thrombosis. Lalive et al.[16] recently reported measurement of D-dimer levels to be useful in screening for cerebral venous thrombosis. They found that patients with venous thrombosis generally have D-dimer levels greater than 500 ng/mL.

Causes

The causes of venous thrombosis can be categorized into (1) conditions that lead to a hypercoagulable state,

(2) factors that promote venous stasis or stagnation, or (3) diseases that cause direct invasion or involvement of the venous wall (Table 18-3). The latter causes usually are tumors or infections of the head, pharynx, or neck. In particular, lesions of the mastoid bone or the base of the skull can be complicated by venous thrombosis. Occasionally, a thrombus can develop adjacent to an inflammatory or neoplastic mass in a foramen or bony structure. Some tumors, particularly meningioma or otolaryngological malignancies, may invade the veins. Trauma or surgical procedures adjacent to a vein can prompt thrombosis. The most common are neurosurgical or otological operations. For example, surgery of the mastoid or inner ear can be complicated by a thrombus in the lateral sinus.

Cerebral venous thrombosis is a well-described vascular cause of neurological impairments in *pregnancy* and the *puerperium* (see Chapter 17). Peripartum venous thrombosis is an important cause of maternal morbidity and mortality. Most cases of venous thrombosis occur within 4–6 weeks of delivery. Because of the strong association of venous thrombosis to pregnancy, the condition needs to be a primary diagnostic consideration whenever a pregnant woman or a woman who recently delivered a child develops severe headache, especially if other neurological symptoms are present. No relationship to maternal age or parity has been found. Mehraein et al.[8] reported that the risk of recurrent venous thrombosis was low during subsequent pregnancies. However, the incidence of postpartum venous thrombosis is higher in developing countries than in the United States, Canada, or western Europe. Some of this association might be secondary to poor prenatal care or dehydration. Besides dehydration, venous thrombosis also might be secondary to changes in clotting factors that occur during pregnancy.

Cerebral venous thrombosis is often ascribed to *dehydration*. Presumably, the thrombus is the result of increased viscosity or stagnation of the blood. The dehydration can be secondary to serious systemic illnesses, fever, surgery, or prolonged vomiting. Depending upon the cause of the dehydration, changes in coagulation factors also can occur. The strong relationship between dehydration and venous thrombosis has an impact on the management of complicating increased intracranial pressure; for example, fluid restriction might not be a therapeutic option. Recently, sinus venous thrombosis was described as a complication of spontaneous intracranial hypotension.[17]

Venous thrombosis can complicate numerous systemic or cranial infections. Infection of the ear or mastoid sinus can lead to thrombosis of the transverse or lateral sinus. Cavernous sinus thrombosis is usually a complication of a facial, dental, or sinus infection. While most of the infections are bacterial, cavernous sinus thrombosis can occur with malignant *mucormycosis*.

▶ **TABLE 18-3.** CAUSES OR PREDISPOSING FACTORS OF CEREBRAL VENOUS THROMBOSIS

Craniocerebral trauma
Infection of head, face, or neck (most commonly bacterial or fungal)
  Orbital cellulitis
  Sinusitis or osteomyelitis
  Mastoiditis
  Dental infections (particularly maxillary)
  Otitis
  Facial or cutaneous cellulitis
  Tonsillitis
  Meningitis
  Encephalitis
  Brain abscess
  Subdural or epidural empyema
Other infections
  Septicemia
  Infectious endocarditis
  Typhoid
  Tuberculosis
  HIV
  Hepatitis
  Cytomegalovirus
  Malaria
  Trichinosis
  Aspergillosis
Neurosurgical, dental, or otolaryngological procedures
Tumors
  Meningioma
  Glomus jugulare tumor
  Carcinomatous meningitis
General surgery
Pregnancy and puerperium
Oral contraceptives
Hormonal replacement therapy
Ovarian hyperstimulation syndrome
Cancer
  Leukemia
  Hypereosinophilia
  Lymphoma
  Carcinoma, especially mucin producing
Vasculitis and inflammatory diseases
  Systemic lupus erythematosus
  Behçet disease
  Wegner disease
  Giant cell arteritis
  Sarcoidosis
  Inflammatory bowel disease
Nephrotic syndrome
Hepatic failure
Congestive heart failure
Congenital heart disease

Cerebral venous thrombosis in children can complicate systemic or head and neck infections.[7,18]

Cerebral venous thrombosis is a complication of a number of medications, including *oral contraceptives.* Venous thrombosis is a potential complication of *L-asparaginase* for the treatment of childhood leukemia.[19,20] Tamoxifen is a potential cause of cerebral venous sinus thrombosis.[21] Other systemic causes include inflammatory bowel disease (ulcerative colitis or regional arteritis), malignancies, Behçet disease, severe liver disease, severe heart disease, and autoimmune diseases.[22] Cerebral venous sinus thrombosis is a potential complication of infusions of intravenous immunoglobulin.[23] Among the potential scenarios would come administration of intravenous immunoglobulin for treatment of Guillain–Barré syndrome. Nephrotic syndrome has been complicated by cerebral venous thrombosis, presumably because of the loss of antithrombotic proteins.[15] AIDS-associated nephropathy has been complicated by venous thrombosis. Venous thrombosis can complicate craniocerebral trauma, affecting the head and neck.[18]

Venous thrombosis, particularly in children, is a potential complication of several inherited or acquired prothrombotic disorders, including factor V Leiden and the prothrombin G20210A mutation[6,24] (Table 18-4). Other causes include deficiencies of protein C, protein S, or antithrombin (see Chapters 14 and 17). An acquired prothrombotic condition, including the development of antiphospholipid antibodies or the lupus anticoagulant,

▶ **TABLE 18-4.** INHERITED OR ACQUIRED HYPERCOAGUABLE DISORDERS LEADING TO CEREBRAL VENOUS THROMBOSIS

Dehydration
Hyperviscosity syndrome
  Waldenstrom
  Monoclonal gammopathy
  Hyperfibrinogenemia
Polycythemia
Anemia
Sickle-cell disease
Thrombocytosis
Idiopathic thrombotic thrombocytopenia
Thrombotic thrombocytopenia purpura
Heparin-associated thrombocytopenia
Leukemia
Hypereosinophilia
Disseminated intravascular coagulation
Paroxysmal nocturnal hemoglobinuria
Protein C or S deficiency
Antithrombin deficiency
Factor V Leiden
Prothrombin G20210A gene mutation
Antiphospholipid antibodies
Dysfibrinogenemia
Cryofibrinogenemia
Plasminogen deficiency
Medications
  L-asparaginase
  Heparin-associated thrombocytopenia
  Epsilon-aminocaproic acid

is a leading cause of venous thrombosis in adults.[25] Venous thrombosis also has complicated disseminated intravascular coagulation, hyperfibrinogenemia, or disorders of plasminogen. Venous thrombosis is a potential complication of sickle-cell disease, polycythemia, thrombocytosis, heparin-induced thrombocytopenia, anemia, or hypereosinophilia.

Treatment

Management involves treatment of the underlying cause, therapy for brain edema and increased intracranial pressure, measures to halt propagation of thrombus, and interventions to speed lysis of the intravenous clot (Table 18-5). Depending upon the etiology, antibiotics, surgical interventions, rehydration, or anti-inflammatory therapies might be needed. Antibiotics are the key therapy for treatment of septic thrombophlebitis, in particular cavernous sinus thrombosis. Patients with cavernous sinus thrombosis often need corticosteroids or other hormone replacements to treat secondary endocrinopathies. Most patients with thrombosis of the major intracranial venous sinuses need measures to control brain edema and increased intracranial pressure. Choices include mannitol, steroids, furosemide, acetazolamide, repeated lumbar puncture, or drainage of cerebrospinal fluid (see Chapter 21). The latter interventions usually are recommended for treatment of long-term increased intracranial pressure following venous thrombosis, and the goal is to prevent visual loss.[26] Neurosurgical decompression of a vein by resection of a tumor or drainage of an abscess also might be indicated. Careful fluid management is indicated, with the goal of treating dehydration that has caused venous thrombosis.

▶ **TABLE 18-5.** TREATMENT OF VENOUS THROMBOSIS

Treat the underlying cause
   Rehydration
   Antibiotics
   Surgery
   Correct coagulopathy
Treat venous obstruction
   Anticoagulants
   Local intravenous infusion of thrombolytic agents
   Local intravenous mechanical thrombolysis
Treat seizures
Treat endocrinopathy (cavernous sinus thrombosis)
Treat increased intracranial pressure
   Osmotherapy
   Corticosteroids
   Furosemide
   Acetazolamide
   Repeated lumbar puncture
   Drainage of cerebrospinal fluid (shunt)

Although anticoagulants do not promote lysis of the intravascular clot, heparin remains the mainstay of treatment.[26] The rationale is that the anticoagulant halts propagation of the thrombus and helps maintain the patency of collateral veins. While uncertainty exists about the utility of anticoagulants in treatment of septic venous thrombosis, the medications are used to treat patients with occlusions secondary to other causes. The results of several studies demonstrate the potential utility of emergent anticoagulation, but the most important is a study performed by Einhäupl et al.[27] Brucker et al.[28] treated 42 patients with heparin followed by oral anticoagulants; 40 patients improved and 26 of these completely recovered. Based on the limited data available, a systemic review concluded that anticoagulants reduced the relative risk of death by 0.33 (95 percent CI 0.08–1.21) or death and disability by 0.46 (95 percent CI 0.16–1.31).[29] The usual regimen is a continuous intravenous infusion with adjustment of dosages in response to levels of activated partial thromboplastin time. Low-molecular-weight heparins or heparinoid are potential alternatives to unfractionated heparin. The goal is to start anticoagulation before the development of secondary hemorrhagic changes. Concerns that heparin might potentiate bleeding changes need to be weighed against their utility in halting propagation of the thrombus. Heparin is often delayed when the hemorrhagic infarctions are located in the temporal lobe, enlarging, or causing shift of midline structures. Still, other patients with minor hemorrhagic changes probably can receive heparin immediately after diagnosis. Careful monitoring of the level of anticoagulation is necessary and if appropriate, the medication can be discontinued. The use of the anticoagulants generally contraindicates the use of recurrent lumbar punctures or venous drainage to control the increased intracranial pressure. Most patients are treated subsequently with oral anticoagulants. The results of sequential MRV examinations can be used to guide long-term management. If the underlying cause has been successful treated or if the vein has recanalized, the oral anticoagulants are often discontinued after a few months, although there are no data to support any specific duration of treatment. On occasion, long-term administration of antiplatelet aggregating agents or anticoagulants is prescribed to treat an underlying hypercoagulable state.

With improvements in interventional neuroradiology and endovascular treatment, venous thrombosis now is treated with local infusions of thrombolytic agents, sometimes combined with mechanical measures. The goals are to promote lysis of the clot and to achieve recanalization. The catheter usually is inserted retrogradely into the cranial vault via the jugular vein. The thrombolytic agent is infused into the distal end of the thrombus and depending upon responses, the catheter can be advanced into the clot. Philips et al.[30] successfully treated six patients with either deep or superficial venous thrombosis. Mechanical devices, used to disrupt the clot, can be adjuncts to pharmacological thrombolysis. The thrombolytic agent could worsen bleeding complications and, in general, patients with major hemorrhages are not treated. Most patients treated with thrombolytic agents have worsened subsequently despite anticoagulant therapy. Because the intervention generally has been restricted to treatment of the most seriously affected patients, the role of thrombolytic therapy in management of less seriously ill patients has not been established. In addition, most patients are treated with anticoagulants following the thrombolytic intervention. The role of thrombolysis for treatment of cerebral sinus thrombosis remains to be established. A systemic review concluded that thrombolytics were safe but efficacy has not been determined.[31]

▶ PITUITARY APOPLEXY

Pituitary apoplexy can result from either a hemorrhage or an infarction of the gland, most often in the setting of a tumor.[32] It occurs among men and women of all ages. Most symptoms are secondary to the mass effects of the sudden enlargement of the intrasellar contents by the hematoma or edema secondary to the infarction. The symptoms are due to compression of the optic chiasm, adjacent oculomotor nerves, hypothalamus, or normal pituitary. Hemorrhage of the pituitary can extend into adjacent subcortical brain structures. In addition, patients often have evidence of acute endocrine failure. Most patients have a short history but a subacute course has also been described.

Clinical Findings

Patients with pituitary apoplexy usually have a sudden severe headache, nausea, and visual defects in one or both eyes[33,34] (Table 18-6). The headache can mimic migraine and it is usually retro-orbital or frontal and can be associated with nausea, vomiting, and constitutional

▶ **TABLE 18-6.** PRESENTATION OF PITUITARY APOPLEXY

Sudden onset of severe headache
Retro-orbital or frontal in location
Nausea, vomiting, prostration, and fever
Hypertension or hypotension
Addisonian crisis
Diabetes insipidus
Unilateral or bilateral visual loss
Orbital bruit
Unilateral or bilateral oculomotor nerve palsies
(III and VI nerves > IV nerve)

symptoms. The visual loss, which can be the result of injury to the optic nerve or chiasm, can be unilateral or bilateral and range from complete blindness to loss of a part of a visual field.

The mass also produces findings that mimic a cavernous sinus lesion. The most findings of parasellar involvement include unilateral or bilateral dysfunction of the oculomotor or abducens nerves, although trochlear nerve palsy can occur.[35,36] Milazzo et al.[37] found that oculomotor palsies were more common than were chiasmal or optic nerve impairments. An acute endocrinologic crisis (in particular an Addisonian crisis) or panhypopituitarism also happen. Other symptoms of signs include fever, arterial hypertension or hypotension, shock, or coma. The findings can mimic subarachnoid hemorrhage or aseptic meningitis. An orbital bruit occasionally can be auscultated.[38]

Causes

Most cases of pituitary apoplexy are secondary to a vascular event in either a functioning or nonfunctioning tumor (Table 18-7). Past reports suggest that hemorrhage or infarction of the pituitary could be found in 0.6–10.5 percent of persons with pituitary adenomas. However, a Polish series of patients with pituitary adenoma, hemorrhage, or ischemic necrosis of the adenoma was found in 14.4 percent of 783 patients treated surgically.[39] Presumably, the risk of vascular complications is related to the size and vascularity of the adenoma. Highly vascular tumors can lead to hemorrhage, while infarction can be secondary to the tumor outgrowing its blood supply. The tumor also could compress pituitary veins, which leads to secondary thrombosis.

Pituitary apoplexy is a well-described complication of pregnancy (*Sheehan syndrome*). Presumably, the enlargement of the pituitary during the pregnancy leads to

▶ **TABLE 18-7.** UNDERLYING PITUITARY DISEASES ASSOCIATED WITH APOPLEXY

Pituitary adenoma
Highly vascular—hemorrhage
Poor vasculature—infarction
Pregnancy (Sheehan syndrome)
Rathke's pouch cyst
Pituitary infection
Craniocerebral trauma
Irradiation to the pituitary
Strenuous coughing
Cardiovascular operations
Lumbar puncture
Use of anticoagulants or thrombolytic agents
Diabetic ketoacidosis
Hormone replacement therapy
Administration of bromocriptine

vascular compromise. Vascular events also have complicated Rathke's pouch cyst, tuberculosis, or lymphocytic hypophysitis. Rarely, a hemorrhage or infarction occurs in a normal pituitary gland. Pituitary apoplexy can occur spontaneously or be the result of craniocerebral trauma, pituitary irradiation, excessive coughing, radiological contrast procedures, cardiovascular procedures, or lumbar puncture.[40] Administration of anticoagulants or thrombolytic agents also has been complicated by pituitary hemorrhage. Vascular events also can complicate diabetic ketoacidosis or follow administration of estrogens, bromocriptine, or thyrotropin-releasing hormone.

Bleeding into the optic chiasm can mimic the symptoms of pituitary apoplexy. The usual cause of chiasmal apoplexy is rupture of a vascular malformation. Differentiating the source of the bleeding is important because surgical resection of the hematoma within the chiasm might preserve vision.[41]

Diagnostic Studies

A skull roentgenogram or CT can demonstrate enlargement or erosion of the sella. Both CT and MRI can demonstrate the intrasellar or suprasellar hematoma or mass. In general, the yield of MRI is better than CT.[33] If an aneurysm or vascular malformation is suspected as an alternative diagnosis, arteriography, magnetic resonance angiography (MRA), or computerized tomographic angiography (CTA) can be performed.

Treatment

Patients are usually treated with large doses of corticosteroids because of the potential of an Addisonian crisis (Table 18-8). Replacement of other hormones might be needed. The endocrine consequences of pituitary apoplexy also have been treated with bromocriptine.[42] Surgical resection of the pituitary mass usually is recommended. Surgery is often required to treat a patient with severe visual loss, impaired consciousness, or progressive neurological worsening.[33] Both intracranial and transsphenoidal approaches have been used. Postoperative radiation therapy also has been prescribed.

▶ **TABLE 18-8.** TREATMENT OF PITUITARY APOPLEXY

Treat acute endocrine emergency
   Steroid replacement
   Replace other hormones
   Pitressin for diabetes insipidus
Bromocriptine to shrink pituitary tumor
Surgical decompression (transsphenoidal or intracranial)
   Resect tumor
   Decompress optic nerves and optic chiasm

▶ SPINAL CORD INFARCTION

When compared to the frequency of vascular events affecting the brain, infarctions of the spinal cord are very uncommon. As a result, the incidence of spinal cord infarction is not known. In most years, a large medical center will not see a patient with spinal cord infarction not associated with trauma. Still, infarction is a relatively common cause of acute nontraumatic myelopathy.[43] In addition, spinal cord infarction as the result of secondary arterial injury is among the causes of neurological dysfunction following injuries to the neck or back. In such a situation, pathological findings include edema of the cord and occlusion of both anterior and posterior spinal arteries or cortical veins in addition to hemorrhage in the gray and white matter.[44] Presumably, much of the cord injury is secondary to injury to small penetrating and sulcal vessels, leading to infarctions.

Vascular Anatomy of the Cord

The abrupt time course and evolution of symptoms is similar to acute ischemic events of the brain. The clinical features of the infarction are dependent upon the vascular anatomy and the level of the cord injury (see Chapter 1). The anterior spinal artery is the most important source of blood supply to the cord. While the rostral portion of the anterior spinal artery is supplied via branches from the terminal portion of the vertebral arteries, radicular branches are the important source of blood at lower segments of the cord. These radicular arteries arise from the vertebral, deep cervical, intercostal, hypogastric, and sacral arteries. A large radicular branch (artery of Adamkiewicz) in the thoracolumbar region is a major source of blood to the caudal portions of the cord. The anatomic variations of these vessels are considerable and, in general, a watershed between more rostral and caudal arteries is located in the midthoracic cord. The anterior spinal artery supplies the anterior two-thirds of the cord. The paired posterior spinal arteries supply the dorsal portion of the spinal cord. The rostral portions are perfused via branches of the posteroinferior cerebellar artery or vertebral artery. Additional blood supply is achieved via radicular branches with caudal flow from higher branches and rostral flow from the lower arteries. An internal watershed between the anterior and posterior spinal arteries can be found in the central section of the cord.

Clinical Findings

Transient ischemia of the lumbosacral cord has been described in patients with severe arthritis (*spinal stenosis*) (Table 18-9). The symptoms of *intermittent claudication of the cord* can be provoked by exercise. Presumably, the arthritic process, which is compressing

▶ **TABLE 18-9.** CLINICAL PATTERNS OF SPINAL CORD ISCHEMIA

Intermittent claudication of the spinal cord
    Spinal stenosis (usually lumbar)
    Symptoms provoked by exercise
    Weakness leading to collapse
    Pain
Transverse spinal cord infarction
    Back, chest, abdominal, or radicular pain
    Flaccid paraplegia or quadriplegia
    Sensory loss below the level of infarction
    Acute areflexia (spinal shock)
    Subsequent hyperreflexia and spasticity
    Urinary incontinence or retention
    Ileus
    Impaired sweating or piloerection
    Impaired vasomotor control
Variations of spinal cord infarction
    Brown-Séquard syndrome
    Man-in-the-barrel syndrome
Centrospinal cord infarction
    Lower motor neuron signs at the level
    Dissociated sensory loss
Anterior spinal artery syndrome
    Flaccid paraplegia or quadriplegia
    Dissociated sensory loss below the level of lesion
        Preserved vibratory and position sense
        Loss of temperature and pain sense

radicular arteries, compromises the blood supply to the cord and as a result, blood flow is unable to meet the increased metabolic demands. Symptoms include pain and weakness of the lower extremities. The patient may collapse because of profound weakness. If transient ischemia affects the cervical cord, the patient may collapse with finding mimicking a drop attack. Spinal cord infarction is uncommon. Surgical treatment of the spine disease might lessen this ischemic symptom.

The features of spinal cord infarction depend upon the level of the affected cord, the size of the ischemic lesion, and the underlying cause. Most patients have pain at the segment of the cord, urinary incontinence or retention, and sensory loss and paralysis below the affected level of the cord.[45] With *transverse infarction of the cord*, the patient has a flaccid paraparesis or quadriparesis. Acutely, muscle stretch reflexes are lost and the plantar responses may be absent. As the course evolves, the signs of bilateral spastic paresis with hyperreflexia and Babinski signs appear. Beevor sign can be found with an infarction at the T-10 level. The patient has preserved motor function of the upper rectus abdominus muscles with flaccid muscles below the lesion. All sensory modalities are lost below the level of the lesion. The patient is aware of an area of hyperesthesia (tight band) at the level of the infarction. Besides causing a neuro-

genic bladder, other autonomic symptoms include ileus, unsettled sweating, impaired piloerection, orthostatic hypotension, reflex hypertension, or loss of vasomotor tone in the limbs. Many patients have back, chest, abdominal, or radicular pain. Sometimes the pain can be so severe that another diagnosis, including myocardial ischemia, is initially considered.[46] Most patients have bilateral impairments, although the *Brown-Séquard syndrome* has been described. The latter is due to the relative right-or-left pattern of penetrating sulcal branches of the anterior spinal artery.

Most strokes in the territory of the anterior spinal artery are located in the midthoracic cord. Thus, the *anterior spinal artery syndrome* usually produces a flaccid paraplegia or quadriplegia, loss to pain and temperature sensation below the level of the lesion, and early loss of sphincter function. Autonomic instability also can occur. Vibratory and position senses are relatively preserved (dissociated sensory loss) because the posterior columns usually are spared. Infarction in the rostral cervical cord can produce a quadriplegia. Infarction of the rostral cervical spinal cord can cause respiratory failure.[47] The usual level of the ischemia to compromise ventilation is C-3–C-4. Patients can have an absence of voluntary or automatic ventilatory movement and will require respiratory assistance. *Man-in-the-barrel syndrome*, which is usually found with bilateral watershed cerebral infarctions, has been described with an atypical infarction secondary to an occlusion of the anterior spinal artery.[48] Affected persons will have painful weakness of both upper extremities with normal lower extremity function.

Infarctions in the territory of the *posterior spinal artery* are relatively uncommon because of the extensive collateral circulation located on the dorsum of the cord. In addition, because of the collateral supply, the clinical findings of posterior spinal artery occlusion are highly variable. Patients usually have loss of vibration and position senses below the level of the lesion. Because the posterior horn can be affected, a segmental loss of all sensory modalities can be found. Rarely, weakness can be secondary to involvement of the lateral corticospinal tract.

A *centrospinal infarction* can complicate a hypoxic or hemodynamic event that produces ischemia to the gray matter regions of the cord. Patients have atrophy, lower motor neuron signs, and a dissociated sensory loss to pain and temperature in a segmental pattern. Infarction of the adjacent vertebral body can complicate ischemia to the spinal cord.[49] Infarction of the vertebral body is most commonly associated with ischemic lesions in the territory of the posterior spinal artery. Lacunar infarctions in the spinal cord also occur.

Venous infarction of the spinal cord usually produces severe pain, weakness and sensory loss of both lower extremities, and a neurogenic bladder. The

▶ **TABLE 18-10.** DIFFERENTIAL DIAGNOSIS OF SPINAL CORD INFARCTION OR HEMORRHAGE

Spinal cord infarction (for hemorrhage)
Spinal cord hemorrhage (for infarction)
   Intramedullary hemorrhage
   Extramedullary hemorrhage
Trauma
Mass (tumor or granuloma)
Infectious myelitis
Demyelinating diseases

patient's symptoms usually evolve over the first 48 h. A subacute necrosis of the spinal cord secondary to venous thrombosis also has been described (*Foix–Alajouanine syndrome*). The latter often is in the setting of a vascular malformation of the cord.

Differential Diagnosis

The differential diagnosis includes spinal cord hemorrhage, traumatic injury, cord compression by a mass, infectious myelitis, and an acute demyelinating disease (Table 18-10). The course and the pattern of the neurological impairments help distinguish the acute vascular event of the cord from the alternative diagnoses. Still, imaging of the cord is an important first step to look for a mass that might be surgically treated.

Prognosis and Complications

While spinal cord infarction usually is not a direct cause of death, most patients have permanent neurological sequelae that limit mobility and independence. A recent study of 57 patients with spinal cord infarctions reported that 41 percent had regained full mobility and 20 percent were wheelchair bound.[50] Younger patients seemed to have better outcomes than that of older adults. Most deaths are secondary to medical complications, including infections or pulmonary embolism. Because many patients are bedridden, they also have a high risk for pressure sores, pneumonia, and orthopedic complications. They usually need long-term indwelling catheters, which predispose to urinary tract infections and renal dysfunction. Autonomic instability, including reflex hypertensive crisis, can lead to cardiovascular complications, including intracranial hemorrhage.

Diagnostic Studies

MRI is the most useful way to assess the spinal cord in a patient with suspected vascular disease. The cord appears swollen on imaging (Figs. 18-9 and 18-10). The infarction is seen best on T-2-weighted images and diffu-

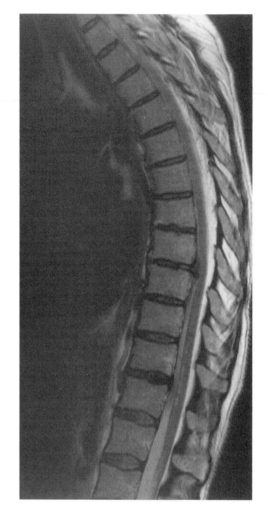

Figure 18-9. Sagittal view of a T-2-weighted MRI of the spinal cord demonstrates an infarction in the lower thoracic cord.

sion weighted imaging DWI. MRI changes in the adjacent vertebral body, which represents bony and bone marrow ischemia, can support the diagnosis of ischemia as the cause of an acute transverse myelitis.[51] Gadolinium enhancement can be used to assess the presence and age of an infarction. Subsequent imaging studies can demonstrate atrophy of the cord or the development of a syrinx. CT usually is not sufficiently sensitive to detect the ischemic lesion in the spinal cord. However, the test can be done in conjunction with myelography if the patient has a contraindication for MRI. CT has the advantages of detecting vertebral fractures and extramedullary hematomas. Occasionally, plain X-rays of the spine can demonstrate adjacent spinal or soft tissue pathology that might explain the infarction.

Arteriography of the spinal arteries can be done, but most patients do not have the test. Imaging of the

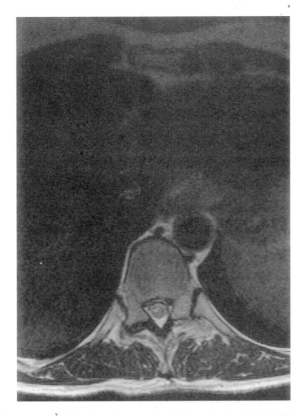

Figure 18-10. Axial view of a T-2-weighted MRI of the spinal cord shows an infarction in the lower thoracic cord.

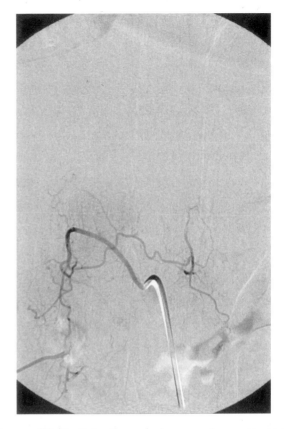

Figure 18-11. Selective arteriogram demonstrates a radicular artery supplying the cord.

vasculature is difficult because of the marked variations in the vascular anatomy and the small caliber of the arteries. Interpretation of an arterial occlusion must be made with caution because of these variables (Figs. 18-11 and 18-12). Arteriography also is time-consuming, expensive, and cumbersome. The procedure can be complicated by ischemia and the information gained from the arteriography might not change management. MRA also can provide information about the spinal cord vasculature.[52] The utility of MRA for examination of patients with suspected spinal cord infarction is not known.

Examination of the cerebrospinal fluid usually is not performed but a lumbar puncture can be done if an infectious or inflammatory process is an alternative diagnosis. Generally, the spinal fluid findings are normal. Spinal cord infarction also can produce abnormal response to somatosensory-evoked potentials. Changes in f-waves, H-reflexes, nerve conduction velocities, and compound muscle action potentials in the affected segments also can be found. A urological evaluation can demonstrate detrusor hyporeflexia or areflexia, abnormal bladder compliance, unstable detrusor contractions, or detrusor-external sphincter dyssynergia.[53]

Causes

Spinal cord infarction is due to vascular diseases of the aorta, vertebral artery, intercostal or other branch arteries, radicular arteries, or the anterior or posterior spinal arteries.[50] Thus, the list of causes of spinal cord infarction is extensive (Table 18-11). The aorta is the most common location for the underlying vascular pathology.

Infarction secondary to *dissection of the aorta* is a relatively common scenario. The patient has the sudden onset of severe back, chest, or abdominal pain associated with unstable vital signs. Spinal cord infarction results from the dissection tearing the orifices of the major intercostal or lumbar branches that are the origin of the radicular arteries that perfuse the cord. Most dissections are secondary to atherosclerosis but an arterial tear can be secondary to Marfan syndrome, collagen diseases, or syphilitic aortitis. The infarction usually involves several segments of the cord and produces complete dysfunction of the cord. Although the midthoracic cord is the most common site, cervical cord infarction also can happen. Patients have a flaccid paraplegia, loss of sensory modalities below the level of the lesion, and bladder and bowel dysfunction. In most cases, the pain is intense and prominent but painless

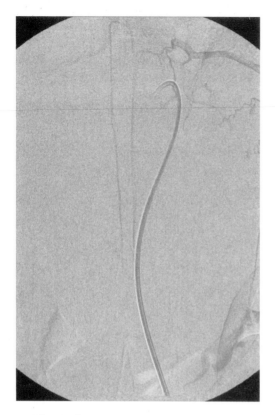

Figure 18-12. Selective arteriogram reveals a radicular artery perfusing the thoracic spinal cord.

▶ **TABLE 18-11.** CAUSES OF INFARCTION SPINAL CORD

Diseases of the aorta
  Atherosclerotic aneurysm
  Dissection of the aorta
    Atherosclerosis
    Marfan syndrome
    Syphilitic aortitis
  Coarctation of the aorta
  Surgical procedures
    Resection of aortic aneurysm
    Clamping of the aorta
    Extracorporeal cardiac-assist device
    Arteriography (aortography)
    Endovascular interventions
Diseases of the vertebral arteries
  Traumatic occlusion
  Dissection
Diseases of the intercostal, lumbar, or sacral arteries
  Pulmonary surgery
  Sympathectomy
Diseases of the spinal arteries or branches
  Meningovascular syphilis
  Bacterial meningitis
  Fungal meningitis
  Parasitic infections
  Sarcoidosis
  Lyme disease
  Giant cell arteritis
  Sickle-cell disease
  Atherosclerosis
  Periarteritis nodosa
  Systemic lupus erythematosus
  Sjögren syndrome
  Compression by subluxation of disk
  Compression by spondylosis/spurs
  Rheumatic subluxation
  Intrathecal injection
  Radiation therapy
  Compression by primary or metastatic tumor
  Trauma
  Osteoarthritis with kyphoscoliosis
  Hypercoagulable states
Hemodynamic events
  Cardiac arrest
  Shock
  Hemodialysis
Embolization
  Cardioembolism
  Cholesterol embolization
  Caisson disease
  Fibrocartilaginous emboli

aortic dissection can occur.[54] The prognosis of most patients with spinal cord injury secondary to aortic dissection is poor. The poor prognosis largely reflects the aortic lesion. Management focuses on limiting the arterial tear by measures such as reducing the blood pressure or surgical repair. Infarction also can result from aortic surgery, hemodialysis, placement of a central line, epidural anesthesia, spinal anesthesia, intrathecal administration of medications, endovascular treatment of aneurysms, ventricular-assist devices, arteriography, or repair of coarctation of aorta.[45,55]

Dissection of the vertebral artery as it ascends the neck can lead to spinal cord infarction.[56] On occasion, both vertebral arteries can be affected. The symptoms of brain stem ischemia secondary to vertebral artery dissection are described in Chapter 6. Ipsilateral nuchal and occipital pain can be prominent. The artery can also be injured acutely during blunt or penetrating trauma.[57] Dislocation or fracture-related stenosis of the transverse foramen secondarily impinges on the ascending vertebral arteries. Some of the neurological impairments following a cervical spine fracture probably are secondary to ischemia. Rather than directly injuring the cord, the fracture of dislocation impinges on the vertebral artery or radicular branches. Cervical spinal cord infarction also complicates atherosclerotic stenosis of the vertebral artery. Besides cervical cord dysfunction, vertebral lesions also can cause impairments, reflecting ischemia of the midline portion of the caudal medulla. Severe arthritis of the spine can secondarily compress the spinal cord and the arteries.

Diseases of smaller arteries including autoimmune or infectious vasculitides have been complicated by spinal cord infarction. Spinal cord infarction complicating AIDS can be secondary to a varicella-zoster-induced vasculitis.[58] Invasive aspergillosis or bacterial meningitis also has been complicated by spinal cord ischemia.[59,60] Other causes include steal by an extramedullary spinal cord vascular malformation, cocaine abuse, hypotension, hypercoagulable states, severe hypotension, disseminated intravascular coagulation, inflammatory vasculitis, or embolism.[61–64] Among the embolic causes are air (Caisson disease), cardioembolism, cholesterol emboli, or fibrocartilaginous emboli.

Treatment

Treatment generally focuses on symptomatic management, including treatment of pain, attention to the neurogenic bladder, and interventions to prevent acute or subacute complications. No studies have tested the utility of interventions aimed at limiting the ischemic consequences of the acute arterial or venous occlusions. Similar to management of patients with acute spinal cord injuries, large doses of corticosteroids are often administered, with the intention to limit cord edema. The efficacy of steroid treatment in this situation has not been tested. Neither anticoagulants nor neuroprotective agents are known to be effective. Acute treatment focuses on therapies aimed at the cause of the spinal cord ischemia. Rehabilitation is a key component of long-term management.

▶ SPINAL CORD HEMORRHAGE

Hemorrhages affecting the spinal cord include bleeding within the substance of the cord, or the subarachnoid space, subdural space, or epidural space. Hemorrhages occur at any segment of the cord, and spinal subarachnoid hemorrhage can mimic even an intracranial event.[65] Bleeding from a vascular malformation of the cord is a potential explanation for recurrent subarachnoid hemorrhage for which no intracranial pathology is found. Patients with recurrent subarachnoid hemorrhage and negative cerebral arteriography should be evaluated for a spinal source of bleeding. Spinal cord hemorrhages are uncommon but they can occur in men and women of any age. The causes of the bleeding are influenced by the location of the hemorrhage. Vascular malformations are the most common cause of intrathecal hemorrhages. Spinal cord vascular malformations have been described as a component of Cobb syndrome, Klippel–Trénaunay syndrome, and Rendu–Osler–Weber syndrome.[66] Bleeding also can occur within the substance of the spinal cord.[67] Epidural hemorrhages are more commonly related to trauma or a bleeding diathesis. These lesions are more common in young adults but they can affect children or men or women of any age.

Clinical Findings

A patient with a spinal hemorrhage usually complains of severe back or neck pain, often localized to the level of the bleeding[68,69] (Table 18-12). Radicular pain is prominent if the bleeding is primarily in the epidural or subdural space. If the bleeding has occurred in the neck, the patient may also have a severe headache that mimics the pain of aneurysmal subarachnoid hemorrhage. Other complaints include nausea and vomiting, photophobia, decreased consciousness, or seizures. Bleeding primarily into the cord might not produce prominent pain. Depending upon the location and extent of the hematoma, the patient can develop bilateral lower extremity weakness, sensory loss, and a neurogenic bladder. Nuchal rigidity or opisthotonos can be found. If the bleeding compresses the cauda equina, the neurological signs can be lateralized or involve primarily the bowel and bladder. Cobb syndrome involves a spinal arteriovenous malformation or arteriovenous fistula that is associated with changes in the extradural space. Recurrent hemorrhages also can occur.[65,70]

Patients with vascular malformations can also have a slowly progressive course, with intermittent neurological symptoms. The most common complaints are weakness of the lower extremities and difficulty in walking. In addition, pain, sensory loss, urinary or rectal incontinence, or impotence can occur. The symptoms often increase with standing, walking, or with Valsalva maneuver. Generally, the condition of patients gradually worsens over several years.

On neurological examination, the impairments reflect the area of injury to the spinal cord. The most common pattern is that of a transverse myelopathy. The Foix–Alajouanine syndrome also can be found. Occasionally, the impairments will reflect cord dysfunction that is several segments away from the vascular malformation. Rarely, a spinal bruit can be heard.

▶ **TABLE 18-12.** CLINICAL FINDINGS OF SPINAL CORD HEMORRHAGE

Severe neck, back, or radicular pain
Headache
Nausea, vomiting, or photophobia
Seizure
Decreased consciousness
Quadriplegia or paraplegia
Sensory loss below the level of the lesion
Acute areflexia (spinal shock)
Subsequently—hyperreflexia and spasticity
Urinary incontinence or retention

Differential Diagnosis

The differential diagnosis of an acute spontaneous spinal cord hemorrhage generally involves other mass lesions, including a traumatic fracture or dislocation, tumor, abscess, or granuloma. In addition, spinal cord infarction and an inflammatory transverse myelitis are alternative diagnoses.

Diagnostic Studies

MRI is the usual diagnostic procedure.[71] It can image the hemorrhagic lesion within the cord and demonstrate a vascular malformation within or adjacent to the cord. An extraspinal hematoma also can be found. Dilated vessels often can be seen on the surface of the cord. CT with myelography is an alternative diagnostic procedure for examination of patients who cannot have MRI. Multiple tortuous, snakelike, vessels are often seen on the surface of the cord, particularly on the dorsal aspect. MRA can be performed to help define the presence of a vascular malformation. Superselective arteriography remains the most definitive way to look for a vascular malformation. Multiple radicular arteries often are injected in order to define the extent of the lesion.

Causes

Vascular malformations are the most common cause of hemorrhage (Table 18-13). These lesions can occur anywhere in the spinal cord but are most frequent in thoracic segments. *Spinal cord arteriovenous malformations* consist of a nidus, arterial feeders, and draining veins. The nidus is most commonly located on the dorsal surface of the cord. One variety called an *angioma racemosum venosum* is usually found in the lower thoracic or lumbar cord. A single arterial feeder usually feeds the malformation and the multiple draining veins are enlarged. Another type labeled an *angioma racemosum arteriosum* usually is located in the cervical cord. It receives blood from several branches of the anterior spinal, vertebral, or posteroinferior cerebellar arteries. These lesions can produce subarachnoid or intramedullary hemorrhage. In addition, the mass of the malformation can cause compression of the cord or nerve roots. In addition, the lesion can steal blood from the cord and produce ischemia.[63] A *spinal (dural) arteriovenous fistula* is located on the surface of the cord and is in close proximity to the anterior or posterior spinal arteries. These lesions can cause subarachnoid hemorrhage, compression of the cord, or ischemia. The ischemia can be secondary to stealing of blood through the large fistula. Vascular malformations are relatively uncommon and account for approximately 5 percent of spinal cord masses. The intramedullary lesions are most commonly diagnosed in young adults, while the

▶ **TABLE 18-13.** CAUSES OF SPINAL CORD HEMORRHAGE

Vascular malformation
   Arteriovenous malformation
   Telangiectasis
   Venous malformation
Aneurysm of a spinal artery
Trauma
Lumbar puncture
Epidural anesthesia
Spinal surgery
Tumor
   Ependymoma
   Hemangioblastoma
   Neurofibroma
   Meningioma
   Metastases
Bleeding diathesis
   Anticoagulants
   Thrombolytic agents
   Hemophilia
   Thrombocytopenia
Hypertension
Autoimmune disease
   Polyarteritis nodosa
   Systemic lupus erythematosus
   Sjögren syndrome

---

spinal fistulas are more commonly recognized among older persons. Aneurysms can be found in association with vascular malformations of the spinal cord.[72,73]

Trauma can cause bleeding within the cord or lead to a hematoma that secondarily compresses the spinal cord. Bleeding is one of the leading causes of spinal cord dysfunction following fractures or penetrating injuries. Hemorrhages can be a complication of surgical procedures, including spinal operations. In addition, bleeding can complicate the use of oral anticoagulants or antiplatelet agents. For example, an acute epidural hematoma can complicate antithrombotic or thrombolytic medications.[74] Fortunately, spontaneous bleeding is relatively uncommon. Symptomatic hemorrhages can complicate lumbar puncture performed when a patient has been taking an anticoagulant. Lumbar puncture to assess a patient with a suspected stroke contraindicates the subsequent use of thrombolytic agents or anticoagulants to treat the stroke, primarily because of the potential for a spinal hemorrhage.

Treatment

Treatment of spinal cord hemorrhage is challenging. While an extramedullary hematoma can be evacuated operatively, an intramedullary lesion probably cannot be treated surgically. Corticosteroids can be administered to reduce the edema. In addition, the patient will need the rehabilitation efforts that are prescribed to other persons who have spinal cord injuries. Management of an underlying vascular malformation can include microsurgical neurosurgery and/or endovascular interventions. Patients often require both procedures. Eskandar et al.[75] treated 26 patients with dural arteriovenous malformations of the cord, 3 with surgery and 23 with endovascular interventions. Nine patients treated with endovascular balloon occlusion subsequently needed surgical resection.

REFERENCES

1. Fink JN, McAuley DL. Cerebral venous sinus thrombosis: a diagnostic challenge. *Intern Med J* 2001;31:384–390.

2. Bergui M, Bradac GB. Clinical picture of patients with cerebral venous thrombosis and patterns of dural sinus involvement. *Cerebrovasc Dis* 2003;16:211–216.

3. Baumgartner RW, Studer A, Arnold M, Georgiadis D. Recanalisation of cerebral venous thrombosis. *J Neurol Neurosurg Psychiatry* 2003;74:459–461.

4. Breteau G, Mounier-Vehier F, Godefroy O, et al. Cerebral venous thrombosis 3-year clinical outcome in 55 consecutive patients. *J Neurol* 2003;250:29–35.

5. Salonen Ros H, Lichtenstein P, Bellocco R, Peterson G, Cnattinguis S. Increased risks of circulatory diseases in late pregnancy and puerperium. *Epidemiology* 2001;12: 456–460.

6. Young G, Manco-Johnson M, Gill JC, et al. Clinical manifestations of the prothrombin G20210A mutation in children: a pediatric coagulation consortium study. *J Thromb Haemost* 2003;1:958–962.

7. Chan AK, deVeber G, Monagle P, Brooker LA, Massicotte PM. Venous thrombosis in children. *J Thromb Haemost* 2003;1:1443–1455.

8. Mehraein S, Ortwein H, Busch M, Weih M, Einhaupl K, Masuhr F. Risk of recurrence of cerebral venous and sinus thrombosis during subsequent pregnancy and puerperium. *J Neurol Neurosurg Psychiatry* 2003;74: 814–816.

9. Ferro JM, Canhão P, Stam J, Bousser M-G, Barinagarrementeria F, for the ISCVT Investigators. Prognosis of cerebral vein and dural sinus thrombosis. Results of the International Study on Cerebral Vein and Dural Sinus Thrombosis (ISCVT). *Stroke* 2004;35:664–670.

10. Ferro JM, Lopes MG, Rosas MJ, Ferro MA, Fontes J. Long-term prognosis of cerebral vein and dural sinus thrombosis. Results of the VENOPORT study. *Cerebrovasc Dis* 2002;13:272–278.

11. Buccino G, Scoditti U, Patteri I, Bertolino C, Mancia D. Neurological and cognitive long-term outcome in patients with cerebral venous sinus thrombosis. *Acta Neurol Scand* 2003;107:330–335.

12. Ferro JM, Correia M, Rosas MJ, Pinto AN, Neves G, for the Cerebral Venous Thrombosis Portuguese Collaborative Study Group. Seizures in cerebral vein and dural sinus thrombosis. *Cerebrovasc Dis* 2003;15:78–83.

13. Sztajzel R, Coeytaux A, Dehdashti AR, Delavelle J, Sinnreich M. Subarachnoid hemorrhage: a rare presentation of cerebral venous thrombosis. *Headache* 2001;41:889–892.

14. Kuehnen J, Schwartz A, Neff W, Hennerici M. Cranial nerve syndrome in thrombosis of the transverse/sigmoid sinuses. *Brain* 1998;121:381–388.

15. Lee SK, TerBrugge KG. Cerebral venous thrombosis in adults: the role of imaging evaluation and management. *Neuroimaging Clin N Am* 2003;13:139–152.

16. Lalive PH, de Moerloose P, Lovblad K, Sarasin FP, Mermillod B, Sztajzel R. Is measurement of D-dimer useful in the diagnosis of cerebral venous thrombosis? *Neurology* 2003;61:1057–1060.

17. Berroir S, Grabli D, Héran F, Bakouche P. Cerebral sinus venous thrombosis in two patients with spontaneous intracranial hypotension. *Cerebrovasc Dis* 2004;17:9–12.

18. Huisman TA, Holzmann D, Martin E, Willi UV. Cerebral venous thrombosis in childhood. *Eur Radiol* 2001;11: 1760–1765.

19. Kieslich M, Porto L, Lanfermann H, Jacobi G, Schwabe D, Bohles H. Cerebrovascular complications of L-asparaginase in the therapy of acute lymphoblastic leukemia. *J Pediatr Hematol Oncol* 2003;25:484–487.

20. Rogers LR. Cerebrovascular complications in cancer patients. *Neurol Clin* 1991;9:889–899.

21. Masjuan J, Pardo J, Callejo JM, Andrés MT, Álvarez-Cermeño JC. Tamoxifen: a new risk factor for cerebral sinus thrombosis. *Neurology* 2004;62:334–335.

22. Kawanishi M, Yoshida Y, Sakaguchi I, Nagano F, Kato K, Miyake H. Cerebral venous sinus thrombosis in a patient with ulcerative colitis. *J Stroke Cerebrovasc Dis* 2003;12: 271–275.

23. Evangelou N, Littlewood T, Anslow P, Chapel H. Transverse sinus thrombosis and IVIg treatment: a case report and discussion of risk-benefit assessment for immunoglobulin treatment. *J Clin Pathol* 2003;56:308–309.

24. Heckmann JG, Tomandl B, Erbguth F, Neidhardt B, Zingsem H, Neundörfer B. Cerebral vein thrombosis and prothrombin gene (G20210A) mutation. *Clin Neurol Neurosurg* 2001;103:191–193.

25. Christopher R, Nagaraja D, Dixit NS, Narayanan CP. Anticardiolipin antibodies: a study in cerebral venous thrombosis. *Acta Neurol Scand* 1999;99:121–124.

26. Biousse V, Tong F, Newman NJ. Cerebral venous thrombosis. *Curr Treat Options Cardiovasc Med* 2003;5:181–192.

27. Einhaupl KM, Villringer A, Meister W, et al. Heparin treatment in sinus venous thrombosis. *Lancet* 1991;338: 597–600.

28. Brucker AB, Vollert-Rogenhofer H, Wagner M, et al. Heparin treatment in acute cerebral sinus venous thrombosis: a retrospective clinical and MR analysis of 42 cases. *Cerebrovasc Dis* 1998;8:331–337.

29. Stam J, de Bruijn SFTM, deVeber G. Anticoagulation for cerebral sinus thrombosis. *Cochrane Database Syst Rev* 2002.

30. Philips MF, Bagley LJ, Sinson GP, et al. Endovascular thrombolysis for symptomatic cerebral venous thrombosis. *J Neurosurg* 1999;90:65–71.

31. Canhao P, Falcao F, Ferro JH. Thrombolytics for cerebral sinus thrombosis. *Cerebrovasc Dis* 2003;15:159–166.

32. Symon L, Mohanty S. Hemorrhage in pituitary tumors. *Acta Neurochir (Wien)* 1982;65:41–49.

33. Randeva HS, Schoebel J, Byrne J, Esiri M, Adams CB, Wass JA. Classical pituitary apoplexy: clinical features, management and outcome. *Clin Endocrinol (Oxf)* 1999;51: 181–188.

34. Masson EA, Atkin SL, Diver M, White MC. Pituitary apoplexy and sudden blindness following the administration of gonadotrophin releasing hormone. *Clin Endocrinol (Oxf)* 1993;38:109–110.

35. Riedl M, Clodi M, Kotzmann H, et al. Apoplexy of a pituitary macroadenoma with reversible third, fourth and sixth cranial nerve palsies following administration of hypothalamic releasing hormones: MR features. *Eur J Radiol* 2000; 36:1–4.

36. Famularo G, Pozzessere C, Piazza G, De Simone C. Abrupt-onset oculomotor paralysis: an endocrine emergency. *Eur J Emerg Med* 2001;8:233–236.

37. Milazzo S, Toussaint P, Proust F, Touzet G, Malthieu D. Ophthalmologic aspects of pituitary apoplexy. *Eur J Ophthalmol* 1996;6:69–73.

38. Watson SL, Francis IC, Coroneo MT. Pituitary apoplexy presenting with an orbital bruit. *Clin Experiment Ophthalmol* 2002;30:305–307.

39. Bonicki W, Kasperlik-Zaluska A, Koszewski W, Zgliczynski W, Wislawski J. Pituitary apoplexy: endocrine, surgical and oncological emergency. Incidence, clinical course and treatment with reference to 799 cases of pituitary adenomas. *Acta Neurochir* 1993;120:118–122.

40. Biousse V, Newman NJ, Oyesiku NM. Precipitating factors in pituitary apoplexy. *J Neurol Neurosurg Psychiatry* 2001; 71:542–545.

41. Pakzaban P, Westmark K, Westmark R. Chiasmal apoplexy due to hemorrhage from a pituitary adenoma into the optic chiasm: case report. *Neurosurgery* 2000;46:1511–1513.

42. Brisman MH, Katz G, Post KD. Symptoms of pituitary apoplexy rapidly reversed with bromocriptine. *J Neurosurg* 1996;85:1153–1155.

43. de Seze J, Stojkovic T, Breteau G, et al. Acute myelopathies: clinical, laboratory and outcome profiles in 79 cases. *Brain* 2001;124:1509–1521.

44. Tator CH, Koyanagi I. Vascular mechanisms in the pathophysiology of human spinal cord injury. *J Neurosurg* 1997; 86:483–492.

45. Castro-Vilanova MD, de Toledo M, Mateos F, Simon R. Spinal cord infarction/ischemia. *Rev Neurol* 1999;29: 977–980.

46. Cheshire WP, Jr. Spinal cord infarction mimicking angina pectoris. *Mayo Clin Proc* 2000;75:1197–1199.

47. Howard RS, Thorpe J, Barker R, et al. Respiratory insufficiency due to high anterior cervical cord infarction. *J Neurol Neurosurg Psychiatry* 1998;64:358–361.

48. Berg D, Mullges W, Koltzenburg M, Bendszus M, Reiners K. Man-in-the-barrel syndrome caused by cervical spinal cord infarction. *Acta Neurol Scand* 1998;97:417–419.

49. Suzuki T, Kawaguchi S, Takebayashi T, Yokogushi K, Takada J, Yamashita T. Vertebral body ischemia in the posterior spinal artery syndrome: case report and review of literature. *Spine* 2003;1:E260–E264.

50. Nedeltchev K, Loher TJ, Stepper F, et al. Long-term outcome of acute spinal cord ischemic syndrome. *Stroke* 2004;35:560–565.

51. Faig J, Busse O, Salbeck R. Vertebral body infarction as a confirmatory sign of spinal cord ischemic stroke: report of three cases and review of the literature. *Stroke* 1998;29: 239–243.

52. Bowen BC, Pattany PM. Contrast-enhanced MR angiography of spinal vessels. *Magn Reson Imaging Clin N Am* 2000;8:597–614.

53. Gomelsky A, Lemack GE, Weld KJ, Dmochowski RR. Urodynamic patterns following ischemic spinal cord events. *J Urol* 2003;170:122–125.

54. Inamasu J, Hori S, Yokoyama M, Funabiki T, Aoki K, Aikawa N. Paraplegia caused by painless acute aortic dissection. *Spinal Cord* 2000;38:702–704.

55. Pathak M, Kim RC, Pribram H. Spinal cord infarction following vertebral angiography: clinical and pathological findings. *J Spinal Cord Med* 2000;23:92–95.

56. Bergqvist CAG, Goldberg HI, Thorarensen O, Bird SJ. Posterior cervical spinal cord infarction following vertebral artery dissection. *Neurology* 1997;48:1112–1115.

57. Oliviero A, Insola A, Santilli V, et al. Concomitant post-traumatic craniocervical junction epidural hematoma and pontomedullary junction infarction: clinical, neurophysiologic, and neuroradiologic features. *Spine* 2000;25:888–890.

58. Kenyon LC, Dulaney E, Montone KT, Goldberg HI, Liu GT, Lavi E. Varicella-zoster ventriculo-encephalitis and spinal cord infarction in a patient with AIDS. *Acta Neuropathol* 1996;92:202–205.

59. O'Farrell R, Thornton J, Brennan P, Brett F, Cunningham AJ. Spinal cord infarction and tetraplegia—rare complications of meningococcal meningitis. *Br J Anaesth* 2000;84: 514–517.

60. Kastenbauer S, Winkler F, Fesl G, et al. Acute severe spinal cord dysfunction in bacterial meningitis in adults: MRI findings suggest extensive myelitis. *Arch Neurol* 2001;58: 806–810.

61. Di Lazzaro V, Restuccia D, Oliviero A, et al. Ischaemic myelopathy associated with cocaine: clinical, neurophysiological, and neuroradiological features. *J Neurol Neurosurg Psychiatry* 1997;63:531–533.

62. Galetta SL, Balcer LJ, Lieberman AP, Syed NA, Lee JM, Oberholtzer JC. Refractory giant cell arteritis with spinal cord infarction. *Neurology* 1997;49:1720–1723.

63. Bandyopadhyay S, Sheth RD. Acute spinal cord infarction: vascular steal in arteriovenous malformation. *J Child Neurol* 1999;14:685–687.

64. Young G, Krohn KA, Packer RJ. Prothrombin G20210A mutation in a child with spinal cord infarction. *J Pediatr* 1999;134:777–779.

65. Kim CH, Kim HJ. Cervical subarachnoid floating cavernous malformation presenting with recurrent subarachnoid haemorrhage. *J Neurol Neurosurg Psychiatry* 2002; 72:668.

66. Rodesch G, Hurth M, Alvarez H, Tadie M, Lasjaunias P. Classification of spinal cord arteriovenous shunts: proposal for a reappraisal—the Bicetre experience with 155 consecutive patients treated between 1981 and 1999. *Neurosurgery* 2002;51:374–379.

67. Sakamoto M, Watanabe T, Okamoto H. A case of ruptured aneurysm associated with spinal arteriovenous malformation presenting with hematomyelia: case report. *Surg Neurol* 2002;57:438–442.

68. Olivero WC, Hanigan WC, McCluney KW. Angiographic demonstration of a spinal epidural arteriovenous malformation. Case report. *J Neurosurg* 1993;79:119–120.

69. Acciarri N, Padovani R, Pozzati E, Gaist G, Manetto V. Spinal cavernous angioma: a rare cause of subarachnoid hemorrhage. *Surg Neurol* 1992;37:453–456.

70. Sharma RR, Selmi F, Cast IP, O'Brien C. Spinal extradural arteriovenous malformation presenting with recurrent hemorrhage and intermittent paraplegia: case report and review of the literature. *Surg Neurol* 1994;42:26–31.

71. D'Angelo V, Bizzozero L, Talamonti G, Ferrara M, Colombo N. Value of magnetic resonance imaging in spontaneous extradural spinal hematoma due to vascular malformation: case report. *Surg Neurol* 1990;34:343–344.

72. Konan AV, Raymond J, Roy D. Transarterial embolization of aneurysms associated with spinal cord arteriovenous malformations—report of four cases. *J Neurosurg* 1999;90:148–154.

73. Handa T, Suzuki Y, Saito K, Sugita K, Patel SJ. Isolated intramedullary spinal artery aneurysm presenting with quadriplegia. Case report. *J Neurosurg* 1992;77:148–150.

74. Clark MA, Paradis NA. Spinal epidural hematoma complicating thrombolytic therapy with tissue plasminogen activator—a case report. *J Emerg Med* 2002;23:247–251.

75. Eskandar EN, Borges LF, Budzik RF, Putman CM, Ogilvy CS. Spinal dural arteriovenous fistulas: experience with endovascular and surgical therapy. *J Neurosurg* 2002;96:162–167.

CHAPTER 19

Antithrombotic Medications to Prevent Cerebral Infarction

Prevention is the most cost-effective strategy in the management of patients with ischemic cerebrovascular disease. Prevention of a stroke avoids the costs of both acute hospital care and long-term rehabilitation. Thus, even an expensive therapy is very cost-effective if it is useful in preventing stroke. More importantly, prevention also avoids the consequences of disability or lost productivity of a patient or family members that might need to stop work in order to provide care. In addition, prevention of an ischemic stroke eliminates the tremendous human suffering that accompanies stroke. Although there is considerable room for improvement, physicians have ways to effectively lower the likelihood of an ischemic stroke. Although no intervention eliminates the problem, therapies can lower the risk considerably. Proper administration of these therapies to high-risk patients can prevent some strokes from happening.

Antithrombotic medications are a mainstay of management of patients at the highest risk for cerebral infarction (Table 19-1). These medications are also used for the primary prevention of asymptomatic patients who have risk factors for accelerated atherosclerosis or patients with atrial fibrillation. These medications are indicated for secondary prevention of ischemic vascular events among patients with previous ischemic stroke or TIA or symptomatic atherosclerotic disease in other vascular circulations (angina pectoris, myocardial infarction, or peripheral vascular disease). The goals of treatment are to prevent myocardial infarction, vascular death, or other ischemic events in addition to forestalling stroke. In addition, these medications are given to patients with nonatherosclerotic vasculopathies or disorders of coagulation that promote thromboembolism.

► FACTORS INFLUENCING DECISIONS ABOUT ANTITHROMBOTIC THERAPY

In general, prevention of stroke involves several interventions. Antithrombotic medications complement other treatment options including surgical procedures and management of those diseases and behaviors that promote atherosclerosis. The surgical procedures are discussed in Chapter 20. The behavioral and medical interventions to control the risk factors are described in Chapter 4. The choices for antithrombotic treatment include anticoagulants and antiplatelet aggregating agents (Table 19-2). Evidence about the safety and efficacy of these medications is robust. While several options currently are available, the list of medications that have antithrombotic effects and that could be used to prevent stroke likely will increase in the years ahead.

The choice of antithrombotic therapy is selected on a case-by-case basis. The factors that influence the decisions about treatment are listed in Table 19-3. The presumed cause of the ischemic neurological symptoms has a major impact on the selection of antithrombotic therapy. For

▶ **TABLE 19-1.** PERSONS AT HIGHEST RISK FOR ISCHEMIC STROKE

Clinical
  Previous ischemic stroke
  Transient ischemic attack
    Recent event
    Prolonged or severe event
    Crescendo
  Amaurosis fugax
  Atrial fibrillation
    Structural heart disease
    Lone atrial fibrillation
  Symptomatic atherosclerosis
    Coronary artery disease
      Myocardial infarction
      Angina pectoris
      Coronary artery surgery/endovascular therapy
    Peripheral artery disease
      Abdominal aortic aneurysm
      Intermittent claudication
      Digital ischemia
      Bowel ischemia
      Renal artery stenosis
      Arterial reconstruction operation
    Asymptomatic carotid bruit
    Asymptomatic retinal embolus
Imaging of the brain
  Clinically occult stroke
Imaging of vessel
  Intraluminal thrombus
  Severe stenosis or ulceration of artery
  Extensive aortic plaques
  Extensive atherosclerosis
Imaging of heart
  Intraventricular or intraatrial thrombus
  Valvular vegetations
  Dilated left ventricle or atrium
  Left atrial turbulence

▶ **TABLE 19-2.** ANTITHROMBOTIC MEDICATIONS TO PREVENT CEREBRAL INFARCTION

Anticoagulants
  Heparin
  Low-molecular-weight heparins
  Low-molecular-weight heparinoid
  Vitamin K antagonists (warfarin)
Direct thrombin inhibitor (ximelagatran, argatroban, napsagatran, inogatran, melagatran)
  Hirudin and Hirulog
  Factor Xa inhibitors (antistatin, tick anticoagulant peptide)
  Activated protein C
  Thrombomodulin
  Tissue factor inhibitors
  Factor VII inhibitors
Antiplatelet aggregating agents
  Aspirin
  Dipyridamole
  Thienopyridines (clopidogrel, ticlopidine)
  Glycoprotein IIb/IIIa receptor blockers

increased risk of bleeding complications from an oral anticoagulant. Patients with poorly controlled hypertension usually are not good candidates for anticoagulants. Symptomatic vascular disease in other territories, such as angina pectoris, might mandate the use of antiplatelet agents. A young woman who has a high-risk cardiac lesion and who is pregnant will likely need a parenteral anticoagulant instead of warfarin because of the potential teratogenic effects of the latter medication. Patients with neurological impairments that lead to poor compliance, poor balance, or a high risk for falls generally are not prescribed anticoagulants. Anticoagulants and some

▶ **TABLE 19-3.** FACTORS INFLUENCING DECISIONS FOR ANTITHROMBOTIC TREATMENT TO PREVENT STROKE

Presumed cause of stroke or transient ischemic attack
  Large artery atherosclerosis
  Small artery occlusion
  Nonatherosclerotic vasculopathy
  Cardioembolism
  Hypercoagulable disorder
  Undetermined cause
Overall health of the patient
  Age
  Concomitant medical diseases
  Concomitant neurological diseases
  Neurological impairments
Specific contraindications
  Allergic reactions
  Side effects of medications
  Ability to comply with treatment regimen
  Availability of necessary laboratory follow up
Previous antithrombotic treatment ("failure")
Wishes of the patient

example, non-antithrombotic medications, such as antibiotics or immunosuppressive agents, might be needed for treatment of a patient with an infectious vasculopathy or a noninfectious vasculitis that causes neurological symptoms. However, most other patients are administered either anticoagulants or antiplatelet agents. In general, anticoagulants are the preferred medical therapy for prevention of stroke among persons with high-risk cardiac lesions or those with several hypercoagulable disorders. Antiplatelet agents usually are the first choice for treatment of patients with stroke secondary to arterial diseases, including those for whom no specific underlying cause can be found. In some high-risk patients, a combination of an anticoagulant and an antiplatelet agent or the combination of two antiplatelet agents can be prescribed.

The overall health of the patient, including age and presence of risk factors also can affect decisions. For example, an advanced age might be associated with an antiplatelet agents are not given to patients who abuse alcohol or drugs or to persons who likely will not follow a treatment regimen. Specific contraindications such as an allergy to aspirin or a previous history of adverse experiences from a medication, such as erosive gastritis secondary to aspirin, also affects recommendations for treatment. Many patients previously were treated with one or more antithrombotic medications and despite their use, recurrent ischemic events have occurred. These "failures" of treatment, most commonly involving aspirin, often prompt treatment with another medication or the use of a combination of medications. Issues such as the cost of the medication or the necessity for follow-up laboratory studies might be crucial for some patients. For example, patients living in rural areas might not have the necessary laboratory monitoring readily available. Importantly, the patient's wishes need to be respected. Some patients might not want the inconvenience and hassle of the necessary laboratory studies or close follow-up that some of the medications require. Patients might reject the idea of a prolonged course of frequent parenteral injections of a medication, such as heparin.

When deciding about antithrombotic therapy, differentiating acute and long-term treatment is important. Patients seen within a few hours or days following a TIA or ischemic stroke have a considerably higher risk of a new, potentially serious, ischemic event than do those persons encountered several days later. Patients with a crescendo of ischemic events or those with a prolonged but reversible event appear to be at very high risk.[1,2] Such a high risk has prompted physicians to administer rapidly acting antithrombotic medications to these patients. The parenterally administered anticoagulants, in particular heparin, usually were recommended. More recently, the newer anticoagulants, aspirin, and clopidogrel have been used. Still, the data about the utility of these medications are limited. The short-term management with antithrombotic medications is described in more detail in Chapter 22. This chapter focuses on medications that are used on a long-term basis. Still, some of the shorter acting anticoagulants medications, such as heparin, are alternatives when a patient cannot tolerate an oral anticoagulant.

▶ ANTICOAGULANTS

Heparin, Low-Molecular-Weight Heparins, and Danaparoid

Heparin is the most commonly prescribed parenterally administered anticoagulant. Other options include the low-molecular-weight heparins or danaparoid. Some of the direct thrombin inhibitors, such as argatroban, can be given parenterally. These medications are discussed in more detail in Chapter 22.

Oral Anticoagulants

Since their development in the mid-twentieth century, oral anticoagulants have been a mainstay of medical treatment to avert thromboembolic disease including stroke. While the controversy about the use of these medications has been considerable, studies performed during the last two decades have greatly clarified their role. In addition, the development of increasingly effective methods to measure the biological responses to these agents has improved their safety. These medications are of established utility in preventing embolization among persons with high-risk cardiac lesions. The oral anticoagulants are the recommended therapy for treatment of patients with several hypercoagulable diseases. Still, these medications have important limitations. Patients need close observation and regular monitoring of the level of anticoagulation. Compliance with the treatment regimen is crucial. Interactions with medications are numerous. Concomitant diseases can affect the patient's responses to the medications. Many patients need frequent adjustments in the dosage of medication. The risk of serious bleeding complications, including intracranial hemorrhage, remains despite the improved methods of monitoring. As a result, there is a strong desire for better anticoagulant medications.

Pharmacology

The oral anticoagulants block hepatic vitamin K-reductases, which leads to a depletion of the levels of vitamin K and the vitamin K-dependent coagulation factors.[3,4] The levels of both the natural regulatory anticoagulant proteins (protein S and C) and several procoagulant factors (prothrombin {factor II}, factor VII, factor IX, and factor X) decline (Tables 19-3 and 19-4). Kamath et al.[5] found that adjusted dose warfarin reduced plasma levels of fibrin D-dimer, prothrombin fragment 1+2, and beta-thromboglobulin, factors that denote platelet aggregation. While several oral vitamin-K antagonists are available, warfarin is the medication that is most widely used in North America and Asia. Phenprocoumon is used in

▶ **TABLE 19-4.** EFFECTS OF ORAL ANTICOAGULANTS

Reduce levels of anticoagulant factors
Protein C
Protein S
Reduce levels of procoagulant factors
Factor II
Factor VII
Factor IX
Factor X
Reduce levels of D-dimer
Reduce levels of prothrombin fragment 1 + 2
Reduce levels of beta-thromboglobulin

Germany, The Netherlands, and Switzerland and aceno-coumarol usually is prescribed in Spain and Italy.[6] Most of the comments in this section are aimed at warfarin but they generally are applicable to the other agents, too. Warfarin is readily absorbed and maximal blood levels of the agent are achieved within 90 minutes. The half-life of warfarin is approximately 36–48 hours. While its actions are relatively predictable, patients' responses vary considerably. As a result, several different dosage formulations of warfarin are available to meet patients' needs. While a parenteral form of warfarin is available, it is of limited utility. The parenteral form does not act more rapidly than the oral medication. The primary indication would be for treatment of a patient with a major abdominal illness for whom no medications can be given orally or via a feeding tube. Presumably, some patients with recent cardiovascular operations might need parenteral warfarin.

The primary antithrombotic action of warfarin relates to its lowering of concentrations of prothrombin. The decline in the prothrombin level secondarily lowers concentrations of thrombin, which is the key for clot formation. Besides interacting with fibrin, the fibrin-bound thrombin stimulates thrombosis by affecting factor VII, tissue factors, platelets, leucocytes, and endothelial cell.[3,7] However, the antithrombotic effects of the oral anticoagulants are delayed by several days because it takes time for the stores of prothrombin to be depleted. This effect limits the utility of these medications in an acute setting. The delay in antithrombotic response probably reflects the 72-hour half-life of prothrombin. On the other hand, both proteins S and C have relatively short half-lives (approximately 6–24 hours) and thus, the pharmacological effects of warfarin on the levels of these anticoagulant proteins appear before the actions on thrombin. As a result, a transient prothrombotic state can occur during the initial administration of warfarin. This effect can lead to skin necrosis and the purple toe syndrome.[8,9] The ischemia is secondary to thrombi forming in small veins located in cutaneous tissue. Fortunately, these complications are rare and they are most commonly found among persons who have either an inherited or acquired deficiency of protein C or protein S.[10] Warfarin-induced skin necrosis also has occurred among patients with antiphospholipid antibodies or Factor V Leiden.[11,12] Most patients do not have any problems during the first days of treatment with oral anticoagulants. A short course of a parenteral anticoagulant, such as heparin, might be used to reduce this risk during the initiation of warfarin therapy. However, the utility of this strategy is not clear because heparin also can be complicated by prothrombotic side effects.[13] Because of concerns about potential drug interactions, Smythe et al.[14] recommend that warfarin anticoagulation be postponed among patients with heparin-induced thrombocytopenia until the platelet count has recovered. The strategy of starting a relatively low (maintenance) dose of warfarin has been used to initiate ther-

apy. Such an approach might slow/inhibit the levels of both the pro- and anticoagulant proteins while possibly avoiding the potential thrombotic complications.[15,16]

International Normalized Ratio

The biological effects of warfarin are measured by measuring the changes in the prothrombin time, which responds to declines in the concentrations of thrombin, factor VII, and Factor X. For many years, the ratio of the prothrombin time from the patient compared to control values was used to assess the therapeutic actions of the oral anticoagulants. Unfortunately, laboratories often used different thromboplastin reagents for doing the test and as a result prothrombin times and ratios varied considerably. Patients could be either overtreated or undertreated despite the "same" prothrombin time ratios. The overtreated patients would be at high risk for hemorrhage and the undertreated patients would remain at high risk for thromboembolism. Because of the potential for spurious laboratory values, some patients probably received excessive doses of warfarin with the resultant risk of major bleeding complications. Fortunately, the international normalized ratio (INR) was created to help resolve the confusion about the laboratory measurements.[17] The INR is based on a mathematical conversion of the ratio of the patient's and control prothrombin times as adjusted by thromboplastin reagent. Thus, the INR should allow for reliable assessment of the level of anticoagulation from any laboratory in the world. The INR now is the best way to describe a patient's level of anticoagulation. For most indications, the desired level of INR is approximately 2–3[18] (see Table 19-5).

Monitoring the level of anticoagulation is an integral component of management with anticoagulants (Table 19-5). Usually, the level of anticoagulation is monitored

▶ **TABLE 19-5.** DESIRED LEVELS OF ANTICOAGULATION INTERNATIONAL NORMALIZED RATION (INR)*

Indication	Desired INR
Nonvalvular atrial fibrillation	2–3
Rheumatic mitral stenosis with atrial fibrillation	2–3
Recent (<6 months) myocardial infarction	2–3
Dilated cardiomyopathy	2–3
Prosthetic cardiac valves	
Mechanical aortic or mitral valves	2.5–3.5
Bioprosthetic aortic or mitral valves	2–3
Mitral valve repair	2–3
Hypercoagulable disorder	2–3.5
Prevention or treatment of deep vein thrombosis	2–3
Cerebral venous thrombosis	2–3

*The course of anticoagulation might be short-term for some of these indications. Some of the indications might necessitate the addition of antiplatelet agents to the oral anticoagulants.
Adapted from Ref. 74.

every day during the initiation of treatment. The intense monitoring is performed when large daily doses of warfarin are used to start treatment. If a lower, maintenance, dose is given to begin treatment, the first assessment can be done after several days of therapy. Once the level is relatively stable, the interval between blood tests is expanded.[19] Most patients taking oral anticoagulants on a long-term basis need to have monitoring at least once a month. Follow-up laboratory tests are done after adjustments in dosage or if concomitant medications are administered. The effects of warfarin gradually abate over approximately 4 days after stopping the medication but phenocoumarol has a longer duration of effect.[6]

Initiation of Treatment

For many years, the usual method of starting anticoagulation was administration of warfarin in daily 10 mg doses for 2 or 3 days. The goal was to achieve suppression of prothrombin (and achieve anticoagulation) as rapidly as possible. However, this tactic often resulted in frequent dose adjustments during the first few days and many patients needed to remain in the hospital to assure safety. Another strategy can achieve effective levels of anticoagulation in a reasonable period of time and the medication can be started on an outpatient basis.[15,16,20,21] Patients would receive maintenance daily doses of warfarin, most commonly 5 mg, and the first dosage adjustment would be at approximately 1 week. This approach has worked very well for many patients. However, Kovacs et al.[22] reported that the older regimen of a daily 10 mg dose of warfarin was superior to initiating treatment with a 5 mg dose in rapidly achieving a therapeutic INR. Being able to rapidly reach a therapeutic INR might be more important for stroke prophylaxis than for prevention of deep vein thrombosis and thus the traditional strategy might be more useful. The overall risks of hemorrhage or recurrent stroke during the initiation of therapy need to be assessed. Further research on strategies to safely initiate warfarin therapy, hopefully on an outpatient basis, is needed.

Administration and Factors Affecting Responses to Treatment

Responses to oral anticoagulants vary greatly. Some patients achieve a therapeutic INR with as little as 1 mg of warfarin daily, other patients require much higher doses of the medication. No way of predicting individual patient responses is foolproof. As a rule of thumb, older patients (especially those >75 years) are more sensitive to the medication than are younger persons.[19,23] In order to compensate for advanced age, Roberts et al.[24] used a regimen that involved empiric dosage adjustments by physicians. They were able to rapidly achieve a stable INR and avoided excessive levels of anticoagulation. Children with high-risk cardiac lesions or procoagulant disorders can be treated with warfarin with a reasonable

degree of safety. Other factors that seem to affect patients' responses to warfarin include their weight, gender, serum albumin levels, and concomitant medications. A weight-based nomogram has been developed to help with adjustment of warfarin doses.[25] This nomogram seems to be most useful when initiating therapy but it has not been implemented widely. While a concern about differences in responses between proprietary and generic formulations of warfarin has been raised, this appears not to be a major problem. Monitoring of the INR can be done to assess for any changes in responses between different preparations.

Patients with polymorphisms of the cytochrome P450 gene (CYP2C9 or CYP2C19) have lower warfarin dose requirements to maintain therapeutic levels of anticoagulation than do other individuals.[26,27] These polymorphisms affect metabolic clearance of warfarin and affect management. The frequency of the genetic defects is not clear. It probably is relatively uncommon and screening patients for these abnormalities probably is not cost-effective. Conversely, Fregin et al.[28] reported a genetic disorder from combined deficiency of vitamin-K dependent clotting factors, which might affect warfarin resistance. Other cases of warfarin resistance are attributed to an inherited factor that causes an abnormal receptor or enzyme that has an increased affinity for vitamin K.[29]

A large number of medical conditions affect patients' responses to warfarin (Table 19-6). Both hepatic and bowel disease alter the affects of the oral anticoagulants by changing either the metabolism or absorption of vitamin K. Patients with inflammatory bowel diseases or

▶ **TABLE 19-6.** MEDICAL CONDITIONS THAT AFFECT RESPONSES TO ORAL ANTICOAGULANTS

Increase level of anticoagulation
Advanced age
Malignancy
Autoimmune diseases
Diarrhea
Malabsorption
Bowel disease
Hepatic disease
Hypoalbuminemia
Hyperthyroidism
Malnutrition
Vitamin K deficiency
Inherited deficiency of vitamin-K dependent clotting factors
Polymorphisms of cytochrome P450
Decrease level of anticoagulation
Inherited resistance to warfarin
Hyperlipidemia
Hypothyroidism
Nephrotic syndrome
Multiple vitamins containing vitamin K
Diet with foods high in vitamin K

chronic diarrhea have increased sensitivity to these medications. Dietary changes also affect the INR. While patients can eat foods high in vitamin K, they should have stable consumption so that the medication dose can be adjusted to achieve the desired INR. The foods high in vitamin K include green leafy vegetables, especially those in the cabbage family, peas, beans, tofu, soybean oil, and canola oil. The oils of some fish might potentiate the effects of warfarin. In addition, Japanese green tea, herbal products, ginseng, and garlic can affect the INR. Patients taking oral anticoagulants should be advised about potential interactions with herbal products such as gingko biloba.[6] While patients taking warfarin can consume modest amounts of alcohol, heavy alcohol use (either binge drinking or chronic abuse) can affect the INR.

Because many medications affect either hepatic metabolism or gastrointestinal function, the listing of potential drug interactions with oral anticoagulants is long.[4] Some medications prolong the INR and others have the opposite effect. The listings of medications in Tables 19-7 and 19-8 are not comprehensive. The data supporting the potential interactions between the medications and warfarin often are quite weak.[19] However, some important interactions with oral anticoagulants occur. For example, antibiotics can affect the absorption of vitamin K or warfarin and greatly alter the INR. The degrees of interactions vary; some medications might have a much greater impact than others. A few medications could either increase or decrease the INR in differing circumstances or patients. Physicians should not memorize which medications are most likely to increase or decrease the INR. Rather, an assumption should be

▶ **TABLE 19-7.** MEDICATIONS THAT CAN POTENTIATE THE EFFECTS OF ORAL ANTICOAGULANTS

Acetaminophen	Allopurinol
Amiodarone	Anabolic steroids
Chloral hydrate	Cimetidine
Cisapride	Clofibrate
Disulfiram	Erythromycin
Fluconazole	Fluorouracil
Fluoxetine	HMG coA reductase inhibitors
Isoniazid	Nalidixic acid
Propafenone	Propoxyphene
Propranolol	Quinidine
Sulfonamides	Tamoxifen
Tetracyclines	Thyroid replacement medications
Theophylline	Tricyclic antidepressants
Trimethoprim- sulphamethoxazole	
Amoxacillin	Gingko
Carbenicillin	Penicillin
Phenytoin	Statins
Sulfapyrazone	

▶ **TABLE 19-8.** MEDICATIONS THAT CAN LESSEN THE EFFECTS OF ORAL ANTICOAGULANTS

Azathioprine	Barbiturates
Benzodiazepines	Carbamazepine
Cholestyramine	Cyclosporine
Dicloxacillin	Griseofulvin
Nafcillin	Phenytoin
Propylthiouracil	Rifampin
Sucralfate	Garlic
Ginseng	St. John's wort

that any medication might have a potential interaction with warfarin. The prudent course is to monitor INR for potential changes in the level of anticoagulation if a new medication is prescribed. Besides being told about the interactions with prescription drugs, patients also should be informed about potential interactions with over-the-counter medications, particularly those that contain aspirin or other nonsteroidal anti-inflammatory agents.

Because of the high associated risk of bleeding, oral anticoagulants usually are temporarily discontinued before surgical procedures. However, stopping the medication can be associated with thromboembolic complications. This scenario does occur and patients need to be warned about the potential for such events. For example, a survey of dermatologic surgeons reported that patients had recurrent stroke or other major vascular events when anticoagulants were discontinued in preparation for a Mohs procedure.[30] This experience means that the decision to discontinue the antithrombotic therapy should be made with considerable thought. The duration of suspension before and after the operation depends upon the level of desired anticoagulation and the nature of the surgery. If the procedure is elective, the physicians and patient need to determine whether the risks of temporarily halting the oral anticoagulant are sufficiently high that the operation should be delayed. Patients with neurological events or ischemic symptoms who recently have become stable during warfarin therapy might need to have the operation postponed. For most elective operations, the medication is halted 3–4 days before the operation and an INR can be checked preoperatively.[19] In general, surgery can be done if the INR is < 1.4. If the patient's medical condition mandates urgent surgery, the anticoagulants need to be halted, and usually their effects reversed, even if the patient's neurological status is not completely stable. If the risks of recurrent thromboembolism would be very high when oral anticoagulants are halted, an interim course of heparin could be administered up to approximately 4–6 hours before surgery. For high-risk patients, either warfarin or heparin is restarted as soon as the surgeon believes it is safe to do so.

Because many patients are very sensitive to the medication, careful compliance with the treatment regimen is important. The patient should be advised not to make changes in their treatment regimen without the approval of their physician. The patient should not take additional (compensatory) doses of warfarin if one or two doses or medication are missed. Taking extra medication could lead to bleeding complications.

Safety

Oral anticoagulants are relatively safe. While their use requires precautions and close follow up, most patients can take these medications without a high likelihood of major complications (Tables 19-8 and 19-9). The initiation of warfarin can be complicated with skin necrosis and the *purple toe syndrome*.[4,11,12,14] Fortunately, these complications are uncommon. In addition, the administration of warfarin is a potential cause of digital (toe) ischemia among persons with a shagbark aorta. The cause-and-effect relationship is not clear, but it might relate to augmenting embolization of atherosclerotic (cholesterol) debris from mobile plaques within the aortic lumen. Vitamin K is important in the formation of bone matrix proteins and low levels of the vitamin can lead to decreased bone density, osteopenia, and possibly pathological fractures.[31] Although the risk is low, patients should be warned about the potential for these complications that accompany long-term administration of the medications. Patients can be given vitamin D or calcium supplements but the usefulness of these interventions is not clear.

Because of potential teratogenicity, the oral anticoagulants are not administered to women who are pregnant.[32,33] While the risk is relatively low, birth anomalies ascribed to warfarin use in the first trimester occur with sufficient frequency to mandate avoidance of the medication. Besides being teratogenic, these medications have other adverse effects during pregnancy. Most problems occur in the fetus. Cotrufo et al.[34] followed 71 pregnancies among women with mechanical valve prostheses who were treated with warfarin. The pregnancy was lost in 23 cases and 5 stillbirths occurred. Fetal embryopathy was found in 4 cases. They found that pregnancy-related complications were especially high among those women who required daily doses of warfarin, which exceeded 5 mg. Use of the these medications in the third trimester can be complicated by a vitamin K deficiency in the baby, which can cause severe bleeding after delivery. Because of these complications, pregnant women at high risk for thromboembolism often are treated with parenteral anticoagulants, either heparin or LMW heparin.[33]

Hemorrhage is the major safety issue associated with the use of oral anticoagulants.[4,35] While physicians are worried about the potential for bleeding complications, for patients, the fear of a stroke is a much higher concern.[36] Thus, the importance of the potential for bleeding complications needs to be emphasized to the patient. A relationship between bleeding and the use of anticoagulants is not surprising because the medications are given in an attempt to prevent thrombosis and these agents have potent antithrombotic effects. Bleeding can be secondary to excessive levels of anticoagulation or to some other pathology that is unmasked by the use of the medication; such a potential scenario would be detection of a gastrointestinal or urinary bladder tumor. Hemorrhages occur anywhere in the body including the brain and spinal cord. Oral anticoagulants are an important cause of hemorrhagic stroke. Intracranial hemorrhage is the most serious and potentially life-threatening complication of oral anticoagulant therapy (see Table 19-9). Patients with anticoagulant-associated intracerebral bleeding can have enlargement of the hematoma during the first 24 hours.[37] This may be one of the explanations for the high rate of poor outcomes. Usually, the risk of intracranial hemorrhage is correlated with the level of INR. While hemorrhage can complicate excessive levels of anticoagulation, the presence of the medication also can augment intracerebral bleeding from other causes including amyloid angiopathy or hypertension. Patients taking oral anticoagulants are at high risk for subdural bleeding that can follow rather trivial head trauma. In some cases the trauma is so minor that the patient does not remember the event. The frequency of subdural hemorrhage is similar to that bleeding that occurs within the brain. Bleeding in other intracranial sites is uncommon.

The risks of intracranial bleeding are highest among the elderly, persons with poor balance, or dementia (Table 19-10). Copland et al.[38] found that an advance age per-se is not a contraindication for use of oral anticoagulants. Still, decisions about antithrombotic therapy in elderly patients can be influenced by the age of the patient.[39] Patients with previous stroke have a high propensity for bleeding complications and physicians should use caution when prescribing oral anticoagulants to patients with cognitive or motor impairments. Persons with a history of stroke also have a high likelihood of intracranial bleeding. In addition, the findings on brain

▶ **TABLE 19-9.** COMPLICATIONS OF ORAL ANTICOAGULANTS

Transient prothrombotic state—purple toe syndrome
Teratogenicity
Osteopenia and pathological fractures
Bleeding
  Intracranial hemorrhage
    Intracerebral hemorrhage
    Subdural hematoma
  Spinal hemorrhage
  Gastrointestinal hemorrhage
  Urinary hemorrhage
  Retroperitoneal hemorrhage
  Intraocular hemorrhage
  Soft tissue hemorrhage
  Epistaxis

▶ **TABLE 19-10.** FACTORS ASSOCIATED WITH AN INCREASED RISK OF BLEEDING COMPLICATIONS WITH ORAL ANTICOAGULANTS

History of serious bleeding, in particular intracranial hemorrhage
History of previous bleeding when taking an anticoagulant
History of stroke, in particular causing motor or cognitive impairments
Advanced age (especially >75 years)
Poor balance or coordination or history of frequent falls
Dementia
History of poor compliance with medical treatment regimens
Alcohol or drug abuse
Serious medical illness
    Cancer   Peptic ulcer disease
    Hepatic failure   Renal failure
Nonavailability of close follow-up and laboratory monitoring

imaging help predict bleeding complications. For example, the presence of leukoaraiosis on brain imaging is associated with an increased risk of warfarin-related intracranial hemorrhage among persons who have had a stroke.[40] Serious bleeding also can occur in other parts of the body with gastrointestinal hemorrhage or urinary tract hemorrhage being the most common. The possibility of intraocular hemorrhage with resultant visual loss often limits the use of the medications among diabetic patients with retinopathy.

Estimates on the rates of serious bleeding complications vary considerably. Based on a population study in Minnesota, Petty et al.[41] found that the frequency of warfarin-related hemorrhages was 7.9/1000 patient-years. Another study reported that the chances of major bleeding complications were 2.7/100 patient-years.[42] The risk is greater than that associated with antiplatelet agents. A potential relationship is found with the duration of treatment. The risk of major hemorrhages is approximately 1.6 percent within 1 month of starting therapy, 3.3 percent during the first 3 months, 5.3 percent within 1 year, and 10.6 percent within 2 years.[43] A similar trend is seen for mortality. The frequency of anticoagulant-related deaths is estimated as approximately 1 percent within 6 months, 5 percent at 1 year, and 7 percent within 2–3 years.[44] Although these data are important, caution should be used because some of these figures represent data collected prior to the widespread use of the INR. The current chances of major bleeding complications probably are lower than these figures would imply.

Gullov et al.[45] reported that the 3-year risk of bleeding events was approximately 40 percent among patients receiving adjusted dose anticoagulation. The risk of bleeding appears to be lower with fixed low doses of warfarin than with adjusted dose regimens. The level of anticoagulation is a very strong predictor of serious bleeding complications, including intracranial hemorrhage. In general,

the risk of bleeding increases when the level of INR exceeds 3.[46] One clinical trial testing warfarin for prevention of stroke among patients with arterial disease was prematurely halted because of an unacceptably high rate of major bleeding complications.[47] The desired level of anticoagulation was an INR > 3. However, if care is used and the INR is kept within the range of 2–3, the risks of bleeding are low. For example, another trial testing the utility of anticoagulants in preventing recurrent stroke did not find an unacceptably high rate of bleeding.[48] This finding was confirmed by a recent analysis performed by the ESPRIT group.[49] With fixed low-dose warfarin, the INR usually is below 2 and the likelihood of an excessively high level of anticoagulation is low and as a result, bleeding complications are few.[46] Clinical trials testing different levels of anticoagulation report reduced rates of bleeding complications among patients given the lower doses of warfarin.[50] The chances of hemorrhage increase if the warfarin is supplemented with an antiplatelet agent. Bleeding risks remain high with the combination of low-dose warfarin with aspirin reported that bleeding risks remain high.[51] However, most bleeding is more commonly associated with adjusted dose regimens than with low-dose strategies.

Monitoring of INR levels in order to avoid excessive anticoagulation is a crucial component of management. Occasionally, a patient will not have bleeding despite an excessively prolonged INR. Levels of anticoagulation that are higher than those desired are relatively common and they occur most frequently among older patients.[23] Responses to a high INR vary depending upon the patient's clinical status and the INR level. A temporary interruption in treatment is the usual response to an INR of <6 detected in an asymptomatic patient. The level will drop after omitting one or two doses and the medication can be restarted at a slightly lower maintenance dose. Vitamin K can be given to an asymptomatic patient who has a markedly prolonged INR (>6). Patients with minor bleeding (skin ecchymoses) secondary to excessive anticoagulation probably can be managed similar to asymptomatic patients. However, serious bleeding mandates reversal of the effects of the medication. Vitamin K can be given either orally or intravenously in a dose of 1–10 mg.[19,52] Orally administered vitamin K is preferred. A recent study demonstrated that oral administered vitamin K was as effective when it is given subcutaneously.[53] When vitamin K is administered intravenously, it should be given slowly because rapid infusions have been complicated by anaphylaxis. Whenever vitamin K is administered, the physician should recognize that reinstitution of the oral anticoagulant might be difficult and achieving an adequate INR level can be delayed (warfarin resistance). In critical situations including cases of intracranial hemorrhage, the effects of the anticoagulant should be reversed aggressively (see Chapter 21). Intravenous administration of clotting factors is recommended. Among the choices are fresh frozen plasma or factor VII or IX concentrates[54,55] (see Chapter 21).

Potential Indications

Oral anticoagulants are used for treatment of patients with a wide variety of conditions. These medications are a mainstay in the treatment of patients at high risk for deep vein thrombosis and pulmonary embolism, including those persons immobilized following a stroke.[4,56,57] The timing of initiation of anticoagulant therapy depends upon the type and severity of stroke. For example, starting the medications might be delayed if the patient has an intracranial hemorrhage or a multilobar infarction. In some cases, the oral agents follow a parenteral anticoagulant. Specific trials of long-term anticoagulant therapy to prevent deep vein thrombosis among stroke survivors have not been done. However, Ridker et al.[58] reported that low-intensity (INR 1.5–2) warfarin therapy was effective in preventing venous thromboembolic events even when given for periods up to 4 years. Kearon et al.[59] found that a dosage-adjustment regimen of warfarin was superior to the low-dose approach for the long-term prevention of venous thromboembolism. While uncertainty exists about the type of anticoagulation program, consensus exists that anticoagulants are the mainstay for the prevention of deep vein thrombosis.

Oral anticoagulants often are given to prevent stroke among patients with cardiac lesions associated with a high risk of embolization or to those persons with an acquired or inherited hypercoagulable disorder[4,60] (Table 19-11). Evidence for the efficacy of anticoagulants is strongest for preventing cardioembolic stroke.[4,18,61] Most recent research has focused on the utility of anticoagulants in preventing embolization among persons with nonvalvular atrial fibrillation[62] (Fig. 19-1). Most trials tested oral anticoagulants for the primary prevention of stroke. A European study involved preventing recurrent ischemic symptoms among patients with atrial fibrilla-

▶ **TABLE 19-11.** POTENTIAL INDICATIONS FOR ORAL ANTICOAGULANTS PREVENTION OF ISCHEMIC STROKE

High-risk cardiac sources of embolization
    Atrial fibrillation-complicating structural heart disease
    Recent myocardial infarction
    Dilated cardiomyopathy
    Mechanical prosthetic valve (mitral position)
Intermediate-risk cardiac sources of embolization
    Patent foramen ovale
    Atrial septal aneurysm
Hypercoagulable disorders
    Antiphospholipid antibody syndrome
    Factor V Leiden
    Prothrombin gene mutation
Arterial diseases
    Aortic atherosclerosis
    High-grade extracranial or intracranial stenosis
    Posterior circulation disease
    Arterial dissection
Failure to respond to antiplatelet agents
Combination with antiplatelet agents

tion.[63] The trials have compared the utility of oral anticoagulants to either placebo (control) or aspirin (Fig. 19-2; Tables 19-12 to 19-14). The results of all the trials are similar; anticoagulants substantially reduce the risks of embolic stroke among high-risk patients with atrial fibrillation.[64–66] The factors that designate the highest risk patients are listed in Chapter 13 (Table 13-5). The overall relative reduction in the risk of stroke is approximately 60 percent. [62,67] Apparently, the benefit is primarily from preventing the development of thrombi in the left atrial appendage.[64] Not only are the oral anticoagulants superior to placebo, the medications are more effective than aspirin. Although some uncertainty exists, the adjusted dose regimen of oral anticoagulants seems to be superior to a low fixed dose of medication alone or when low-dose anticoagulation is combined with aspirin (Fig. 19-3). The

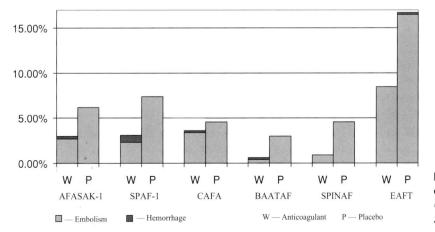

Figure 19-1. Placebo-controlled trials of anitcoagulations—atrial fibrillation. (*Adapted from Refs. 63, 228–231 and 233*).

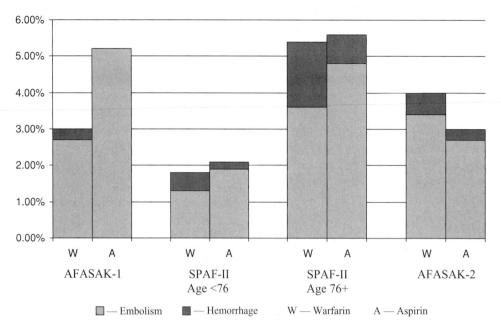

Figure 19-2. Comparison of oral anticoagulation or aspirin—atrial fibrillation. (*Adapted from Refs. 68, 228 and 234*).

lack of benefit of low-dose anticoagulation is demonstrated in the experience of SPAF-2, which could not show a therapeutic effect among persons younger than 76.[68] Edvardsson et al.[51] investigated the utility of low-dose oral anticoagulation combined with aspirin in a population of medium-risk patients with atrial fibrillation. While a reduction in embolic events was found when compared to control, the effects were not significant. However, in another study, Hylek et al.[69] found that anticoagulation that achieved an INR of 2 or greater was associated with a greater reduction in ischemic stroke,

severe stroke, or fatal stroke than when the medications were given at lower doses. These data support the use of adjusted dose warfarin as the desired treatment regimen for most patients with atrial fibrillation.

Anticoagulants are an important component of periprocedural management of patients having mechanical or electrical cardioversion for treatment of atrial fibrillation. Gallagher et al.[70] recommended that the INR be >2.5 at the time of conversion if the duration of atrial fibrillation is uncertain or if the arrhythmia had persistent for longer than 2 days. The medication is given for approximately

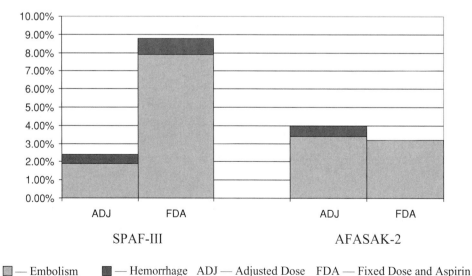

Figure 19-3. Comparison of adjusted dose anticoagulation to combined fixed dose anticoagulation and aspirin—atrial fibrillation. (*Adapted from Refs. 232 and 234*).

▶ **TABLE 19-12.** TRIALS OF ADJUSTED DOSE ORAL ANTICOAGULANTS PREVENTION OF EMBOLISM—ATRIAL FIBRILLATION

Trial	INR	Annual Rates of Embolic Events			
		OAC	Control	RRR	*P*-Value
AFASAK-1	2.8–4.2	2.7%	6.2%	56%	<0.05
SPAF-1	2.0–4.5	2.3%	7.4%	67%	0.01
BAATAF	1.5–2.7	0.4%	3.0%	86%	0.002
CAFA	2.0–3.0	3.4%	4.6%	26%	0.25
SPINAF	1.4–2.8	0.9%	4.3%	79%	0.001
EAFT	2.5–4.0	8.5%	16.5%	47%	0.001

INR = International normalized ratio, OAC = oral anticoagulant, RRR = relative risk reduction.
Adapted from Refs. 63, 228–231 and 233.

4 weeks before cardioversion and then continued for at least 2 weeks after treatment. Anticoagulants also are recommended for treating patients who will have cardioversion for treatment of atrial flutter.

Patients with the combination of atrial fibrillation and previous ischemic neurological symptoms are judged to have an especially high risk and, if possible, oral anticoagulants, with doses adjusted to maintain an INR of 2–3, are the preferred form of antithrombotic therapy[64] (see Table 19-15). Hart et al.[64] concluded that women with atrial fibrillation seem to benefit more from oral anticoagulants than do men. In part, this relationship may be ascribed to the age differences with women being older. Elderly women appear to have a very high risk for embolization. The other clinical variables that forecast a high embolic risk with atrial fibrillation and that mandate the use of anticoagulants are listed in Table 19-15. The utility of adjusted dose warfarin in prevention ischemic events among persons with lone atrial fibrillation and other lower risk situations is not established.[18] These patients have a low risk for thromboembolic events and thus it is hard to demonstrate a benefit of any intervention, in particular if important complications, such as bleeding, can occur. Most of these patients are prescribed aspirin.

Oral anticoagulants often are prescribed to patients with other cardiac lesions not associated with atrial fibrillation but that might be complicated embolization (Fig. 19-4). These conditions include sick sinus syndrome, a recent myocardial infarction, a patent foramen ovale (PFO), atrial septal aneurysm, left ventricular aneurysm or dysfunction, dilated cardiomyopathy, rheumatic mitral stenosis, and prosthetic heart valves.[18,71–74] Information about the utility of anticoagulants for treatment of these indications is limited. For example, Pullicino et al.[75] emphasized the importance of stroke as a complication of dilated cardiomyopathies, which can be of several etiologies, and the potential utility of oral anticoagulants. Still, data from controlled clinical trials are lacking and while anticoagulants usually are given to persons with dilated cardiomyopathies, additional data about their usefulness is needed.

For many patients, oral anticoagulants are the preferred treatment of patients with rheumatic mitral stenosis complicated by atrial fibrillation.[73] Although evidence about the usefulness of anticoagulants for this indication is limited, the success of the medications in preventing thromboembolic events among patients with nonvalvular atrial fibrillation buttresses this recommendation. In the modern antibiotic era, the frequency of

▶ **TABLE 19-13.** TRIALS OF ADJUSTED DOSE ORAL ANTICOAGULANTS IN COMPARISON TO ASPIRIN TO PREVENT EMBOLISM ATRIAL FIBRILLATION

Trial	INR	Annual Rates of Embolic Events			
		OAC	Control	RRR	*P*-Value
AFASAK-1	2.8–4.2	2.7%	5.2%	48%	<0.05
SPAF-2	2.0–4.5				
<76 years		1.3%	1.9%	33%	0.24
76+ years		3.6%	4.8%	27%	0.39
AFASAK-2	2.0–3.0	3.4%	2.7%	−21%	NS
Hellemons	2.5–3.5	2.5%	3.1%	19%	NS

INR = International normalized ratio, OAC = oral anticoagulant, RRR = relative risk reduction.
Adapted from Refs. 63, 68, 234 and 235.

▶ **TABLE 19-14.** TRIALS OF ADJUSTED DOSE ORAL ANTICOAGULANTS TO LOW, FIXED DOSE ANTICOAGULANTS WITH (#) OR WITHOUT ASPIRIN PREVENTION OF EMBOLIC EVENTS—ATRIAL FIBRILLATION

| Trial | INR | Annual Rates of Embolic Events | | | |
		ADJ Dose	Fixed	RRR	P-Value
AFASAK-2	2.0–3.0	3.4%	3.9%	13%	NS
			3.2%#	−6%	NS
SPAF-3	2.0–3.0	1.9%	7.9%#	74%	<0.0001
Hellemons	2.5–3.5	2.5%	2.2%	−14%	NS
Pengo		3.6%	6.2%	42%	0.29

INR = International normalized ratio, ADJ = adjusted dose, RRR = relative risk reduction.
Adapted from Refs. 46, 232, 234 and 235.

rheumatic heart disease should decline and hopefully this indication for anticoagulation will disappear.

Oral anticoagulants are the primary antithrombotic therapy for preventing embolic events among patients with prosthetic heart valves.[76] Because the risk of embolization from mechanical and bioprosthetic valves differs, the relative indications for antiplatelet agents or anticoagulants vary. The presence of atrial fibrillation, two prosthetic valves, left ventricular dysfunction, or a hypercoagulable state or a history of previous ischemic neurological symptoms supports the long-term use of oral anticoagulants. Although no clinical trials tested the efficacy of oral anticoagulants among patients with mechanical valves, particularly those in the mitral position, the very high rate of thromboembolic events, even with anticoagulant therapy implies the necessity for

▶ **TABLE 19-15.** INDICATIONS FOR ANTITHROMBOTIC TREATMENT SUBGROUPS OF PATIENTS WITH ATRIAL FIBRILLATION

Highest risk treatment with oral anticoagulants highly desirable
  Previous stroke or transient ischemic attack
High-risk treatment with oral anticoagulants desirable
  Patient's age >75 years
  Women (especially age >75 years)
  Presence of hypertension
    History of hypertension
    Systolic blood pressure >160 mm Hg
  Presence of diabetes mellitus
  History of coronary artery disease
  History of congestive heart failure
  Evidence of left ventricular dysfunction
  Detection of thrombus in left atrial appendage
  Detection of spontaneous contrast—left atrium
Intermediate risk treatment with either oral anticoagulants or aspirin
  Age >65 years but above factors absent
Lowest risk treatment with aspirin or no-specific antithrombotic agent
  Age <65 and above factors absent

treatment. Anticoagulants are the most important intervention for preventing stroke in this group of patients.[77] The desired level of anticoagulation (INR 2.5–4) is higher than for other indications largely because of the extraordinarily high embolic risk with these valves. Patients with mechanical valves should plan on taking anticoagulants for the remainder of their lives.

Oral anticoagulants usually are administered to patients with bioprosthetic valves during the first 3 months following surgery or if the patient has a history of previous thromboembolism.[76] In general, the level of anticoagulation is lower than that prescribed to patients with mechanical valves. After 3 months, aspirin usually is prescribed in lieu of the oral anticoagulants, particularly when if the patient has an aortic bioprosthetic valve.

Warfarin also is used to prevent recurrent myocardial ischemia or complicating embolic stroke following myocardial infarction (see Fig. 19-4). The selection for anticoagulants is made on a case-by-case basis. Most patients with a recent myocardial infarction do not have a high risk for embolic stroke and probably can be treated with antiplatelet agents. However, anticoagulants are administered to patients with a large anterior myocardial infarction in an attempt to prevent develop of an intraventricular thrombus.[78] Other factors that predict a high risk for thromboembolism are severe left ventricular dysfunction, congestive heart failure, or atrial fibrillation. Echocardiographic evidence of a mural thrombus or a history of complicating neurological symptoms also prompts initiation of anticoagulation. The results are impressive. Azar et al.[79] found that anticoagulants reduced the risk of stroke from 1.2/100 patient-years to 0.7/100 patient-years and that the risk of bleeding was low when the INR was maintained <3. The role of anticoagulation following a myocardial infarction appears to be growing. Van Es et al.[80] found that adjusted dose anticoagulants or the combination of low-dose anticoagulants and aspirin were superior to aspirin monotherapy. These results were buttressed by the findings of the study reported by Hurlen et al.[81] Rudnicka et al.[82] found that full compliance with adjusted dose oral anticoagulants

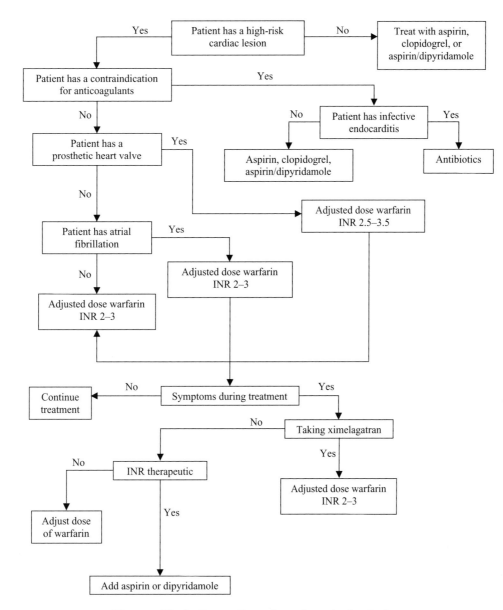

Figure 19-4. Prevention of cardioembolic stroke.

would lower the risk of fatal cardiac events by approximately 50 percent. While anticoagulants alone or in combination with aspirin were associated with more bleeding events following myocardial infarction, the reduction in new ischemic events more than compensated. In general, anticoagulants are administered for 3–6 months following the myocardial infarction. Long-term anticoagulation to prevent cardioembolic stroke is not needed because the cardiac disease usually stabilizes. No data are available to support the use of oral anticoagulants for treatment of patients with a ventricular aneurysm or akinetic ventricular segment. Most of the persons with these cardiac changes are treated with aspirin.

While anticoagulants often are administered to patients with cardiac diseases associated with a presumed lower risk for embolism, data about their usefulness are limited. Anticoagulants are recommended to many patients with PFO because the thrombi probably are of venous origin and because of the presence of a structural cardiac disease the venous thrombi can reach the brain. In a spin-off project of the Warfarin-Aspirin Recurrent Stroke Study (WARSS), Homma et al.[83] compared the utility of warfarin or aspirin in preventing stroke among patients with PFO. They found that patients with PFO did not have a significantly higher risk for recurrent ischemic events than did those patients without the cardiac change. In addition, no differences in rates of ischemic events were found between patients taking aspirin and those prescribed warfarin. No other data are available. At present, data are lacking about the usefulness

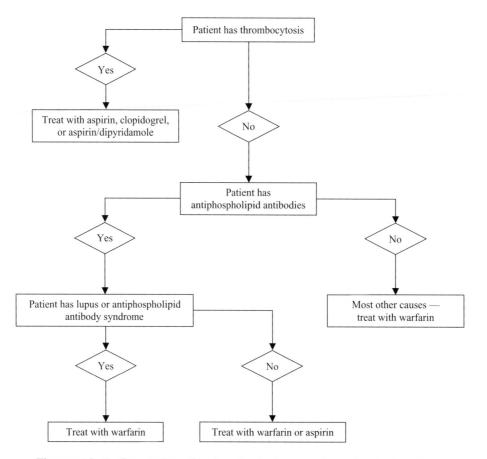

Figure 19-5. Prevention of ischemic stroke—prothrombotic disorders.

of anticoagulants in preventing thromboembolism among patients with PFO, atrial septal aneurysm, or other cardiac lesions of undeterminate risk. If the risks of embolization are low, demonstrating efficacy of anticoagulation will be a challenge.

Anticoagulants often are given to prevent stroke among patients with inherited or acquired hypercoagulable disorders[60,84] (see Chapter 14) (Fig. 19-5). In particular, patients with the antiphospholipid antibody syndrome usually are treated with anticoagulants. The goal often is to achieve an INR > 3.[85] In some instances, the INR will not be reliable among patients with antiphospholipid antibodies and measurement of factor II inhibition is required to monitor the level of anticoagulation. Until recently, data to support the use of anticoagulants or to recommend a specific INR level were not available. Crowther et al.[50] evaluated two doses of warfarin (INR 2–3 or 3.1–4) for treatment of patients with antiphospholipid antibody syndrome and recurrent thrombosis. They found that the two treatment regimens were equal in efficacy and that a goal INR of 2–3 was reasonable. Ruiz-Irastorza et al.[86] evaluated the safety and potential utility of several different doses of warfarin in treatment of patients with antiphospholipid syndrome. They found a high rate of recurrent

events (9.1/100 patient-years) regardless of the level of anticoagulation but that the rate of bleeding complications was not especially high among patients who had a target INR of 3.5. A spin-off project of WARSS compared the utility of warfarin (desired INR approximately 2) or aspirin in preventing recurrent ischemic events among persons with a previous stroke and antiphospholipid antibodies.[87] The results do not demonstrate the superiority for warfarin. These data imply that warfarin is not better than antiplatelet therapy for preventing recurrent stroke among most patients with antiphospholipid antibodies. Still, some patients with antiphospholipid antibodies, such as those with systemic lupus erythematosus or the clinical features of the antiphospholipid antibody syndrome, might benefit from anticoagulation. Research is needed to determine if these groups of patients are best treated with oral anticoagulants. Although warfarin often is prescribed to patients with Factor V Leiden, the prothrombin gene mutation and other inherited or acquired coagulopathies, data about efficacy of the intervention are lacking. The relatively low prevalence of these coagulopathies mean that the data needed to determine the utility of anticoagulants will be hard to achieve. Still, until such data are available, anticoagulants often are recommended.

Oral anticoagulants often are recommended for the treatment of patients with severe atherosclerotic disease of the aorta. In particular, patients with highly mobile or protruding plaques with secondary thrombus often are given anticoagulants. In a nonrandomized study, Dressler et al.[88] reported ischemic events in 27 percent of patients with severe aortic atherosclerosis who did not receive anticoagulants. No events occurred among the patients who were treated with the medication. Another study evaluated the utility of warfarin (INR 2–3) in treatment of patients with both advanced aortic plaques and atrial fibrillation.[89] The annual rate of recurrent events was 5.9 percent among patients treated with adjusted dose warfarin while it was 17.3 percent among patients who were treated with aspirin and low-dose warfarin. It is not clear if the emboli were arising from the heart or the aorta. In a nonrandomized study, Tunick et al.[90] could not demonstrate any benefit from warfarin in preventing thromboembolic events among patients with severe plaquing of the thoracic aorta found by transesophageal echocardiography. The risk of distal thromboembolism (purple toe syndrome) probably is not so high as to preclude anticoagulant therapy. The data do not provide guidance for the use of anticoagulants. Because many patients have symptomatic atherosclerosis in other vascular territories, antiplatelet agents might be the best choice.

Oral anticoagulants often are given to patients with stroke secondary to severely stenotic disease of intracranial arteries, in particular when the posterior circulation was involved. Information about the utility of anticoagulation is limited. A retrospective, nonrandomized study found the rates of recurrent strokes were 3.6/100 patient-years with warfarin and 10.4/100 patient-years with aspirin.[91] Another multicenter study reported that warfarin might be superior to aspirin in preventing recurrent stroke, especially among patients with disease in the vertebrobasilar circulation but this was not a randomized trial.[92] A randomized clinical trial testing the utility of either warfarin or aspirin in preventing strokes among patients with symptomatic severely stenotic atherosclerosis of intracranial arteries recently was halted because of a lack of a trend favoring the use of anticoagulants.[93] The potential utility of warfarin in treatment of patients with ischemic neurological symptoms not due to cardioembolic events was tested in two clinical trials. Most patients probably had larger artery atherosclerosis or small artery disease. One trial was prematurely halted because of the high rate of intracranial bleeding complications, which often were fatal, among the patients treated with the oral anticoagulant.[47] However, the level of anticoagulation probably was too high. WARSS compared the utility of warfarin (INR 1.4–2.8, preferred > 2) or aspirin 325 mg/day in preventing recurrent stroke among 2206 patients with noncardioembolic stroke.[48] The lower INR levels were associated with a low risk of

bleeding complications but no difference in the rates of ischemic events was noted between the two treatment groups. Subsequent analyses could not find a benefit from anticoagulation among subgroups of patients as influenced by either the INR level or presumed cause of stroke. A systemic review found that there was no evidence of benefit from long-term anticoagulant therapy for patients with stroke or transient ischemic attack presumably secondary to a noncardioembolic origin.[94] Another trial is comparing the utility of anticoagulation in preventing stroke among patients with arterial disease to either aspirin alone or aspirin and dipyridamole. To date, the investigators report that the anticoagulation regimen has been associated with an acceptable safety profile.[49]

Patients with cerebral ischemia secondary to an extracranial arterial dissection often are given anticoagulants but no data are available to support this recommendation. Patients with dissection generally have a favorable prognosis and a low risk for recurrent ischemia. A systemic review concluded that there were no data to support the use of anticoagulants or antiplatelet agents for treatment of patients with extracranial carotid dissections.[95] Because of the potential for transmural dissection leading to subarachnoid hemorrhage, anticoagulants are not given to patients with intracranial dissections. Thus, the rationale for long-term anticoagulation is not strong.

Oral anticoagulants often are prescribed to patients who have had recurrent ischemic symptoms despite treatment with antiplatelet agents, including combinations of medications. No clinical trials have evaluated the utility of anticoagulants in this situation. At present, data about the effectiveness of warfarin are insufficient to make any recommendation about the utility of anticoagulation among patients with arterial causes of stroke.

Oral anticoagulants are the mainstay of treatment to prevent recurrent or progression of cerebral venous thrombosis. Most patients are treated with agents following a course of heparin (see Chapter 18). Although clinical trials do not provide guidance about either the intensity or duration of treatment, a goal of an INR of 2–3 seems reasonable. Patients usually are treated for approximately 6 months unless an underlying hypercoagulable disorder mandates longer-term treatment.

Summary

Despite their utility, oral anticoagulants are underutilized partially because of concerns about safety. These agents can be administered with a reasonable degree of safety, even to elderly patients, if precautions are taken. For most indications, the desired INR is 2–3. Unfortunately, the possibility of major bleeding complications including intracranial or epidural spinal hemorrhage cannot be eliminated completely. The decision to administer oral anticoagulants must be made on a case-by-case basis. The potential benefit in lowering the risk of ischemic stroke must be weighed against the potential for major complications.

The data from clinical trials provide compelling data about the use of oral anticoagulants for the long-term prevention of cardioembolic stroke.[96] Oral anticoagulants are the medical therapy of choice for treatment of patients with atrial fibrillation complicating structural heart disease, prosthetic cardiac valves, dilated cardiomyopathies, rheumatic mitral stenosis, and a recent anterior myocardial infarction.[97] While several factors identify patients with heart disease who have a high risk for embolism, the occurrence of ischemic neurological symptoms denotes the highest risk for recurrent thromboembolism. The utility of these medications is not established in management of persons with other cardiac lesions, including a PFO. Many patients with low-risk cardiac lesions probably can be treated with aspirin. Oral anticoagulants are not established as useful alternative to antiplatelet agents for preventing thromboembolism secondary to intracranial or extracranial arterial disease.

Other Anticoagulants Including the Direct Thrombin Inhibitors

Several new antithrombotic agents have been developed.[98] *Argatroban* inhibits fibrin-clot activation of thrombin.[99] It is used to treat patients with heparin-associated thrombocytopenia and thrombosis.[100] Argatroban might be an effective alternative to heparin or other acutely administered anticoagulants, but it likely will not be used for long-term therapy. *Bivalirudin* is another direct thrombin inhibitor.[98] The data about the potential utility of bivalirudin are not available.

Hirudin or its derivative, *Hirulog*, was used to treat patients with unstable heart disease but the agents were associated with an unacceptably high rate of intracranial hemorrhages.[101,102] Because of the increased rates of major bleeding complications among patients with heart disease, these medications have not been tested for treatment of patients with cerebrovascular disease. These agents should not be used until there is evidence of their safety and efficacy.

The oral direct thrombin inhibitor, *ximelagatran*, is a potential therapy for prevention of venous thromboembolism and other ischemic events. The medication has potential advantages, including the lack of the requirement for adjustments in medication dosage in response to the level of anticoagulation.[103] Eriksson et al.[104] found that ximelagatran is as effective as the combination of dalteparin and warfarin in limiting venous thrombosis in the lower extremities. Francis et al.[105] found that ximelagatran was as effective as warfarin in preventing venous thromboembolism following knee surgery. A placebo-controlled trial found that ximelagatran effectively prevented deep vein thrombosis with no increase in bleeding.[106] Two large clinical trials compared ximelagatran to warfarin in preventing thromboembolism in patients with atrial fibrillation (Fig. 19-6).[107,108] In high-risk patients, fixed-dose ximelagatran was as effective as warfarin in preventing stroke or systemic embolism. The medication was generally well tolerated and the number of bleeding events was similar in the two treatment groups. Some patients can have secondary hepatic changes and monitoring the levels of hepatic enzymes appears to be part of the safe administration of ximelagatran. A potential disadvantage of ximelagatran is the absence of an antidote if severe

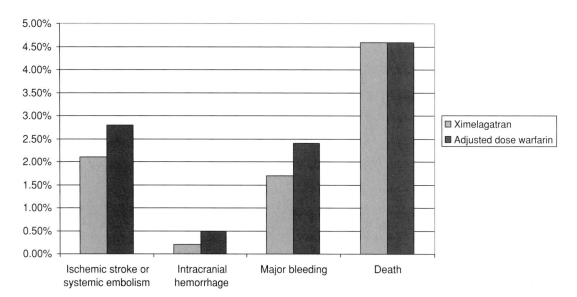

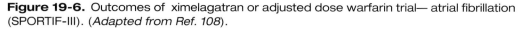

Figure 19-6. Outcomes of ximelagatran or adjusted dose warfarin trial— atrial fibrillation (SPORTIF-III). (*Adapted from Ref. 108*).

bleeding occurs. Treatment, including potentially surgical evacuation of a hematoma, will be delayed until the 12 hour duration of the effects of the medication are resolved. The role of this medication in preventing stroke will be defined during the next few years. It might become the primary alternative to warfarin for prevention of cardioembolic stroke.[109,110]

Other promising antithrombotic agents include activated protein C, tissue factor pathway inhibitor, and synthetic pentasaccharides.[98] Information about the utility of these medications in preventing stroke is not available.

▶ ANTIPLATELET AGENTS

Antiplatelet agents are the medications of choice for prevention of serious ischemic events secondary to arterial disease, including stroke and myocardial infarction. Antiplatelet agents are prescribed for the primary prevention of vascular events in asymptomatic patients who have factors associated with a high risk for atherosclerosis. Patients with symptomatic atherosclerotic disease also are prescribed these medications that can prevent ischemic events in several vascular territories. These medications are used alone or in combination with surgical interventions or oral anticoagulants. Data also support the efficacy of antiplatelet agents in the management of patients with peripheral artery disease.[111] Overall, the antiplatelet agents lowering the risk of major ischemic events (stroke, myocardial infarction, or vascular death) by approximately 25 percent.[112] These agents reduce the likelihood of major stroke by approximately 30 percent, the risk of nonfatal myocardial infarction by approximately 35 percent and vascular mortality by approximately 18 percent. On the other hand, an independent analysis looked at the utility of antiplatelet agents in treatment of patients with either TIA or stroke found that the medications lowered the chances of major vascular events by only approximately 16 percent.[113]

Systemic reviews show that these medications are equally effective in men and women.[112] The responses to antiplatelet agents also are not affected by the age of the patient, the presence or absence of hypertension, or the presence or absence of diabetes mellitus.[114–116] Although these medications are effective, the room for improvement is considerable; too many patients have stroke, myocardial infarction or a vascular death. The utility of the antiplatelet agents in preventing cardioembolic stroke is less impressive than for forestalling arterial thromboembolism. For example, antiplatelet agents have not achieved the reduction in risk of stroke complicating atrial fibrillation that is reported with the oral anticoagulants.

Besides being effective, antiplatelet agents generally have an acceptable safety profile (Table 19-16). The chances for major bleeding complications are lower than

▶ **TABLE 19-16.** MOST COMMON SIDE EFFECTS ANTIPLATELET AGGREGATING AGENTS

Aspirin
Bleeding, including intracranial hemorrhage
Gastritis, peptic ulcer, gastrointestinal bleeding
Allergic reactions including anaphylaxis
Ticlopidine or clopidogrel
Bleeding, including intracranial hemorrhage
Allergic reactions—skin rash, urticaria
Gastrointestinal distress or diarrhea
Hepatitis or jaundice
Pulmonary disease
Neutropenia or agranulocytosis
Thrombotic thrombocytopenia purpura
Aplastic anemia
Dipyridamole
Headache

those accompanying the use of the anticoagulants. Surgeons report an increased risk of perioperative bleeding complications but overall, the risk of major hemorrhage is small. Halting the use of the antiplatelet agents a few days prior to elective surgery can reduce the likelihood of perioperative bleeding complications. On the other hand, antiplatelet agents are an important component of perioperative care for patients have vascular procedures. For example, systemic reviews demonstrate that antiplatelet agents are effective in preventing vascular events, including stroke, among patients treated with carotid endarterectomy.[18,112,117,118] The other potential side effects are well known and other than for ticlopidine, laboratory monitoring for the development of complications is not needed. Still, despite their many attributes, the antiplatelet agents still are underused. Patients at high risk for either myocardial infarction or ischemic stroke often are not prescribed or are not taking these agents.[119] Obviously, with the low cost of aspirin, financial concerns are not a major reason for the nonuse of antiplatelet agents. Efforts to increase the utilization of antiplatelet medications need to be included in all components of health care.

Aspirin

Aspirin is the most extensively studied and the most widely used antiplatelet agent. It was the first medication found to be effective in lowering the risk of stroke among patients with arterial disease. Aspirin is easy to administer and it does not require laboratory monitoring. Aspirin is effective over a wide range of doses and it is relatively safe, especially at lower doses (Table 19-17). The side effects of aspirin are well known. The risk of gastrointestinal complications, which are the most common adverse experiences, can be lowered with the use of ancillary medications or enteric-coated preparations.

▶ **TABLE 19-17.** DOSAGES OF ANTIPLATELET AGENTS TO PREVENT CEREBRAL INFARCTION

Aspirin	30–1300 mg/day
Ticlopidine	500 mg/day
Clopidogrel	75 mg/day
Extended release dipyridamole	400 mg/ day

Because of its many advantages and strong track record, aspirin is the standard intervention to which other medications or surgical procedures to prevent stroke are compared. While aspirin is available as an over-the-counter medication is most countries, both physicians and patients need to remember that it is a potent medication. It has serious side effects. Patients need to follow their physician's recommendations about the use of aspirin.

Pharmacology and Dosages

Through its irreversible inhibition of prostaglandin function and cyclo-oxygenase activity, aspirin has potent effects on platelet aggregation.[118,120] In addition, aspirin also affects the activity of endothelial cells, which lowers levels of the vasodilator, prostacyclin. Aspirin also is a potent anti-inflammatory agent that influences the activity of white blood cells. Some of the utility of aspirin in preventing ischemic stroke probably is secondary to its anti-inflammatory actions, which could help stabilize the atherosclerotic plaques. Large doses of aspirin also might have some neuroprotective actions.[121]

Aspirin is rapidly absorbed from the gastrointestinal tract. Approximately 98 percent inhibition of thromboxane production can be achieved within 1 hour of taking a single 325 mg tablet.[122] The antithrombotic effects of aspirin increase more slowly with the administration of lower doses (81 mg) of the medication and a significant decline in platelet aggregation for several days. On the other hand, an initial (loading) dose of 325 mg of aspirin, which causes a rapid inhibition of platelet function, can be followed by lower daily doses of the medication to sustain the antithrombotic effects. Aspirin can be given as a rapid-release preparation, which can have a quicker effect on platelet aggregation than do conventional formulations.[123] However, this preparation probably is not necessary. On the other hand, the absorption of aspirin is slow with the use of an enteric-coated formulation and as a result, antiplatelet effects are delayed. While blood levels decline within a few hours, the antithrombotic effects persist for several days. Because of its irreversible effects on circulating platelets and megakaryocytes, the antithrombotic function of aspirin persists for 10 days. As a result, some antiplatelet actions will persist for approximately 1 week.

Aspirin's efficacy is demonstrated over doses ranging from 30 to 1300 mg/day[124] (see Table 19-17). In general, a daily dose of 40–160 mg/day causes greater than 80 percent inhibition of platelet cyclooxygenase activity.[125] The effects of aspirin on platelet function vary among individuals. Some patients may be relatively insensitive to the actions of aspirin and others might develop some degree of aspirin-resistance with prolonged use. The prevalence of persons who do not respond to aspirin is not known. Using a test of platelet function, Alberts et al.[126] found that normal platelet activity could be found in a sizable proportion of patients taking enteric-coated or low doses of aspirin. Based on the results of testing of platelet aggregation among patients taking aspirin, Helgason et al.[127,128] suggested that some patients might need an escalation in the dose in order to sustain adequate levels of platelet inhibition. This group of patients, sometimes called aspirin nonresponders, might have a high risk for ischemic events. Clinical evidence to support a high risk for stroke with development of aspirin nonresponsiveness has not been shown. The importance of acquired aspirin resistance is being investigated. Grundmann et al.[129] found that the return of normal platelet function was correlated with recurrent ischemic events in some patients taking aspirin. Aspirin resistance being an explanation for recurrent stroke despite the use of the medication is the subject of future bench and clinical research. Patients with aspirin resistance might be treated with increasing doses of the medication or the addition of other antiplatelet agents. This approach needs to be studied. At present, there is no evidence that increasing the dose of aspirin will efficacious when treating a patient who already has had an ischemic event while taking a lower dose of the medication. Currently, the usual dosage of aspirin for treatment of most patients with ischemic disease is 81–325 mg/day.

Safety

The side effects of aspirin are well known; the most common are gastritic irritation (gastritis), peptic ulcer disease, and gastrointestinal hemorrhage (see Table 19-16). Sze et al.[130] estimated that the regular use of aspirin increases the risk of peptic ulcer disease or gastric bleeding by approximately 350 percent. Rarely, patients can have serious, potentially life-threatening gastrointestinal hemorrhages. Severe erosive gastritis with multiple areas of superficial ulceration can be found during endoscopic evaluation. Some of the gastric side effects are related directly to aspirin's actions on prostaglandins and thus, the potential for gastrointestinal complications cannot be differentiated from the potential utility in suppressing platelet aggregation. A relationship between the dose of aspirin and gastric side effects is present. Patients generally tolerate lower daily doses (<325 mg/day) better than doses of 1300 mg/day or more.[131] Although gastric irritation and bleeding are reduced with lower daily doses (81–162 mg) than with higher doses, these adverse events occur. Patients should be warned about the potential for these side effects. Enteric-coated medications or ancillary treatment with antacids or other medications to protect the stomach can be used to further lower the frequency of side effects. However, some of the gastroprotective medications are expensive and the need for their use can negate the fiscal advantage of aspirin. Allergies to aspirin are relatively uncommon but are important contraindications to the use of the medication. Rarely, anaphylaxis can occur. Aspirin probably has some teratogenic effects but the absolute risk probably is small. Although the medication is avoided during the first few weeks, low-dose aspirin can be given safely after the first trimester of pregnancy.[132] Aspirin can be associated with an increased risk of maternal or neonatal bleeding.

The risk of any major bleeding complication from aspirin is approximately 3.5/100 patient-years.[41] Aspirin does not cause a generalized bleeding disorder unless a patient is also taking an anticoagulant or has an underlying coagulopathy. While gastrointestinal hemorrhage is the most frequent bleeding complication, hemorrhages in other locations, including inside the cranial vault can occur. Studies of the primary prevention of ischemic vascular disease in healthy persons noted that a slight increase in the risk of hemorrhagic stroke does occur with aspirin.[133] He et al.[134] reported that the risk of hemorrhagic stroke was 12/10,000. Although intracranial bleeding is a potential complication of aspirin, neither patients nor physicians should consider this risk to be so high as to preclude treatment. The risk of nongastrointestinal bleeding complications is not correlated with the dosage of aspirin. In particular, intracranial hemorrhage can complicate either high or low doses. Lower doses are not safer than the large amounts of aspirin. Such a lack of a dosage relationship should not be surprising because of the antiplatelet effects associated with a broad range of doses.

Potential Indications

Aspirin is effective for both primary and secondary prevention of major ischemic events including myocardial infarction[118,133](Table 19-18). It is used for primary prophylaxis of ischemic vascular events for both men and women, although the impact seems greater among men presumably because the lower risk for vascular events among women. The best dosage for prevention of myocardial infarction is 75–325 mg/day and presumably, the same doses should be effective for primary prevention of stroke.[135,136] Overall, the effect in primary prevention of ischemic stroke is less apparent than its utility in preventing myocardial ischemia. This situation is not surprising because coronary artery disease usually becomes symptomatic at a younger age than atherosclerotic cerebrovascular disease. Additional information about the utility of aspirin in primary stroke prevention is needed. However, until such data are available, aspirin

▶ **TABLE 19-18.** ASPIRIN IN PREVENTION OF STROKE

Easy to use
Good safety profile
Low economic costs
Can be started within 24–48 hours of stroke
Broad spectrum of vascular diseases
Alternative to anticoagulants
Low-risk cardiac lesions
High risk for bleeding
Combination with anticoagulants
Combination with other antiplatelet agents

should be prescribed to high-risk asymptomatic patients including the elderly and those with risk factors for premature atherosclerosis including hypertension, diabetes mellitus, and hypercholesterolemia. Still, the mechanisms of ischemic stroke and myocardial infarction are similar and the doses of aspirin to prevent the two vascular events are likely to be similar too.[135]

Aspirin is the primary medical therapy to prevent recurrent ischemic stroke. It is used to treat most patients with cerebral ischemia secondary to large artery atherosclerosis or small vessel occlusive disease.[18] This approach is supported by the clinical trials in stroke prevention, which enrolled patients with both lacunar strokes and those with symptoms secondary to intracranial or extracranial large artery atherosclerosis. The relative utility of aspirin in subgroups of patients with stroke is not known. While some physicians have assumed that patients with lacunar strokes should be given different medications that those with large artery atherosclerosis. Such an association is not established. The usefulness of aspirin among patients with large artery atherosclerosis may have been questioned; other antiplatelet agents might be superior but data to support that contention are not available. Aspirin often is prescribed to patients with nonatherosclerotic vasculopathies, such as arterial dissections, but the medication has not been tested in clinical trials.

The initial studies of aspirin tested a daily dosage that were >1000 mg although the reasons for selection of these relatively high doses were not obvious. These studies produced relatively positive results and aspirin was approved for prevention of stroke (Fig. 19-7). Subsequently, studies done primarily in Europe, tested lower daily doses of aspirin in part to improve its safety profile. These studies found that lower doses (30–300 mg/day) were effective in preventing ischemic stroke.[137–139] However, some experts were not convinced by the new data. The controversy about the dosage of aspirin was addressed in the Aspirin Carotid Endarterectomy study, which found that lower doses of aspirin (81–325 mg) were equal to or superior to higher dose

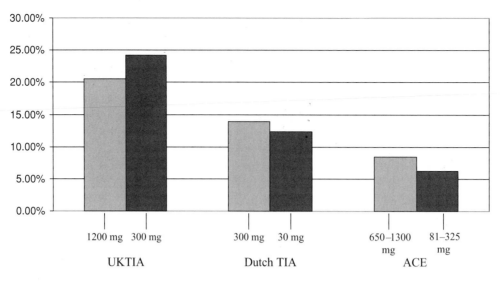

Figure 19-7. Rates of outcomes—trials comparing different doses of aspirin. (*Adapted from Refs. 137, 138 and 140*).

treatment (650–1300 mg) in reducing both cardiovascular and cerebrovascular events following carotid surgery.[140] The conclusion is that higher dose aspirin treatment is not better to lower dose regimens.[141] In addition, a meta-analysis found that the reduction in the risk of stroke was relatively uniform across doses that range from 50 to 1500 mg/day.[124]

The timing of starting of aspirin following cerebral infarction was tested in two large trials, when the medication when administered within 48 hours of onset of stroke.[142,143] Aspirin was associated with a modest increase in the risk of intracranial hemorrhage and a marginal, but statistically significant, improvement in outcomes probably because of prevention of subsequent stroke. A European trial found that the combination of aspirin and streptokinase given within the first hours after stroke was associated with an unacceptably high rate of serious, usually fatal, intracranial hemorrhages.[144]. Other trials testing

LMW heparin used aspirin as the control.[145,146] In general, aspirin was safer than the anticoagulants and the two medications were equally effective.

Aspirin has been given in conjunction with thrombolytic medications. The National Institute of Neurological Disorders and Stroke trial of rtPA prohibited initiation of aspirin therapy within 24 hours of treatment with the thrombolytic agent.[147] Based on the success of that trial, current guidelines advise that aspirin be withheld for 24 hours after rtPA treatment.[148] Most other patients can receive aspirin.

Based on analysis of the data available at the time, Algra and van Gijn[113] concluded that aspirin produced a modest benefit in prevention of stroke; they estimated that the risk of a major ischemic cerebrovascular event was reduced by approximately 16 percent. This assessment was buttressed by the results of the second European trial of aspirin and dipyridamole[149] (Fig. 19-8).

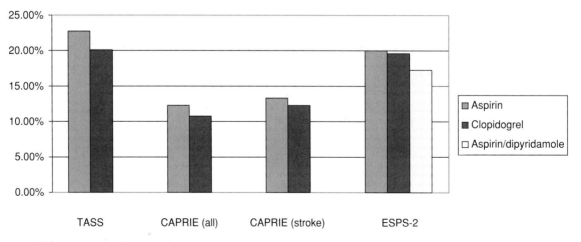

Figure 19-8. Rates of outcome events—comparisons of aspirin and other antiplatelet medications. (*Adapted from Refs. 149, 155 and 157*).

This large study found that aspirin (50 mg/day) reduced the risk of ischemic events by approximately 15 percent among a group of patients with TIA or stroke. Thus, the conclusion must be that while aspirin is effective, additional medical interventions or other strategies to prevent stroke are needed.

Despite treatment with aspirin, many patients have recurrent stroke that leads to moderate-to-severe disability. Some ischemic events likely are due to cardioembolism.[150] The data about the utility of aspirin in preventing strokes secondary to emboli arising in the heart are mixed. Aspirin is not effective in preventing the formation of a left ventricular mural thrombus following myocardial infarction.[78] Aspirin monotherapy is not effective in preventing embolization among patients with mechanical prosthetic cardiac valves.[151] Although aspirin often is prescribed to patients with bioprosthetic valves, it usually is not started until after a 3-month course of oral anticoagulant therapy following insertion of the prosthesis.[151] Low doses of aspirin are given as adjunctive agents to patients with mechanical valves who are also receiving oral anticoagulants. For example, the occurrence of a cerebral thromboembolic event in a patient with a prosthetic valve and who is receiving adequate levels of anticoagulation often prompts the addition of aspirin. Some very high-risk patients receive both aspirin and oral anticoagulants immediately following valve replacement.

Aspirin is an alternative therapy for management of patients with atrial fibrillation who cannot take warfarin (see Table 19-18). Aspirin reduces the risk of stroke among persons with atrial fibrillation by approximately 20–40 percent.[67,74] Still, it is not as effective as anticoagulants even when combined with clopidogrel.[152] Aspirin often is prescribed to patients with lone atrial fibrillation. Because the risk of embolization is low in this group of persons, aspirin has been recommended as the alternative therapy. A Norwegian demonstrated that aspirin was as effective as a low-molecular-weight heparin in preventing early recurrent embolism among patients with recent stroke and atrial fibrillation.[145] Subsequently, patients can be switched to long-term treatment with oral anticoagulants.

A French study evaluated the rates of recurrent events among patients with PFO alone, ASA alone, or the combination who were treated with aspirin[153] (see Table 19-18). Patients with PFO alone did not have a significantly higher rate of recurrent stroke than did those who did not have the cardiac lesion. Homma et al.[83] demonstrated that aspirin was equal to oral anticoagulants in preventing recurrent ischemic events among patients with PFO. By implication, aspirin might be a reasonable therapeutic option for treatment of patients with cardiac lesions associated with a low risk for embolization.

Although no clinical trials have tested the utility of aspirin in preventing stroke among patients with moyamoya syndrome, arterial dissections, or other noninflammatory vasculopathies, the medication often is prescribed. This seems to be a reasonable choice. In particular, the potential for intracranial hemorrhage favors aspirin instead of warfarin for prevention of recurrent infarction among patients with moyamoya. The relatively low risk of recurrent stroke among persons with arterial dissections supports the use of aspirin instead of warfarin.

Although the Antiplatelet Trialists Group[154] found that aspirin was effective in lowering the risk of deep vein thrombosis, the recommendation to use aspirin as an alternative to oral anticoagulants has not received considerable support. Presumably, the nature of peripheral venous thrombosis implies that anticoagulants or ximelgatran will remain superior to aspirin. Aspirin is not used to treat patients with cerebral venous thrombosis. However, aspirin replaces warfarin after of several months of treatment.

Summary

Aspirin remains a leading antithrombotic medication for prevention of stroke among high-risk persons.[18,74,96] The advantages of aspirin including ease of use, relatively good safety profile, and its low costs make it the first choice for treatment of most patients (see Table 19-18, Figs. 19-9 and 19-10). The medication can be safely started within the first 48 hours after stroke. Aspirin is not started within 24 hours of treatment of stroke with rtPA. Aspirin can be recommended for prevention of stroke among patients with large artery atherosclerosis, small artery occlusive disease, noninflammatory, nonatherosclerotic vasculopathies, and heart diseases associated with a low risk for embolism. Aspirin is an important adjunct to endovascular or surgical interventions to prevent stroke. Aspirin is a second-line therapy for treatment of high-risk patients with nonvalvular atrial fibrillation who cannot take oral anticoagulants. Aspirin also can be combined with other antiplatelet agents or oral anticoagulants. Therapy can be initiated with a 325 mg dose. Thereafter, patients can take 81–325 mg/day to maintain the antiplatelet effects. Increasing the dosage of aspirin after a patient has a new ischemic event does not seem to be necessary. Increasing the daily dose of aspirin does not appear to improve efficacy and the higher doses of the medication are complicated by increased chances of gastric side effects. In general, patients having recurrent events despite treatment with aspirin receive either another antiplatelet agent in addition to the aspirin or have the other medication as a substitute for the aspirin.

Ticlopidine and Clopidogrel

The thienopyridines, ticlopidine and clopidogrel, were developed specifically for their antiplatelet effects. Their chemical structures are similar. Ticlopidine was developed

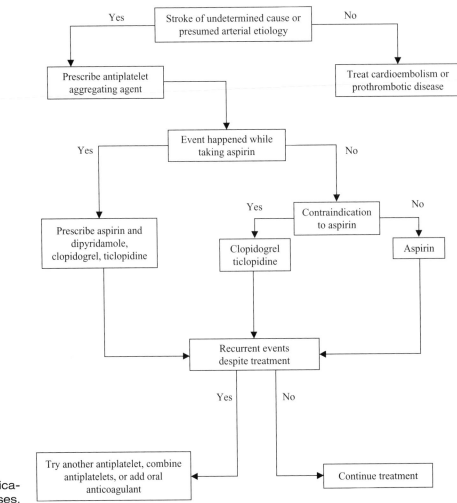

Figure 19-9. Selection of medication—patients with arterial diseases.

first and it was tested in two large clinical trials in the 1980s.[155,156] Subsequently, clopidogrel was tested in clinical studies in the mid-1990s.[157] Currently, clopidogrel is being tested in a number of clinical trials. The results of these trials might change the indications for this medication.

Pharmacology

These medications block platelet responses to adenosine diphosphate (ADP)-induced aggregation and signal transduction.[7,118,158] They do not inhibit platelet aggregation in in-vitro testing. This finding suggests that some transformation of the agents is required to achieve the antiplatelet effects. Clopidogrel also may reduce the number of ADP binding sites and both medications affect the glycoprotein IIb/IIIa receptors interactions with fibrinogen.[118] The changes in platelet function are irreversible and both medications prolong the bleeding time.

Both medications are administered orally. Approximately 90 percent of a single 250 mg dose of ticlopidine is rapidly absorbed. Plasma concentrations of ticlopidine reach a peak within 1–3 hours.[118] The usual dose of ticlopidine is 250 mg twice a day. Ticlopidine has a half-life of

approximately 24–36 hours (see Table 19-17). Inhibition of platelet aggregation is delayed by 24–48 hours after starting treatment.[158] The antiplatelet effects of ticlopidine increase slowly and maximal effects on platelet function are not achieved until 1–2 weeks following initiation of therapy. Therefore, ticlopidine is not useful for acute treatment of patients with vascular events. The pharmacokinetics of clopidogrel differ slightly.[118] The medication is rapidly absorbed and metabolized into a number of compounds. Within 2 hours of a loading dose of clopidogrel (400 mg), platelet aggregation can be reduced.[159] A dose of 300–600 mg of clopidogrel can be used when starting treatment in an acutely ill or unstable patient[160] (see Table 19-17). Thereafter, a daily dosage of 50–100 mg maintains the antiplatelet effects. The usual daily dosage of clopidogrel is 75 mg. The antiplatelet effects of clopidogrel gradually disappear within 1 week of stopping the treatment.[161]

Safety

While bleeding complications can occur with use of these medications, the chances of serious hemorrhage

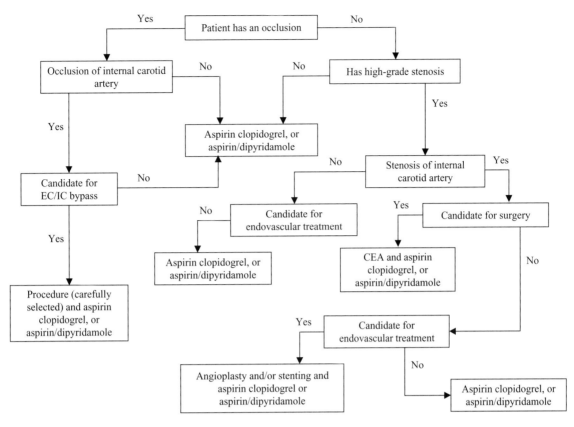

Figure 19-10. Prevention of stroke in large artery atherosclerosis.

are less than those found with oral anticoagulants (see Table 19-16). The frequency of gastrointestinal hemorrhage is lower with clopidogrel than with aspirin.[162] Gastrointestinal distress and diarrhea are the most common side effects (see Table 19-16). Unlike aspirin, these medications do not induce gastritis and gastrointestinal bleeding. Ticlopidine has been associated with rare cases of pulmonary disease, cholestatic hepatitis or jaundice.[163,164] Allergic reactions, which include urticaria or generalized skin eruptions, most commonly occur within the first 2 weeks of initiation of therapy. Ticlopidine is associated with important, potentially life-threatening, hematological reactions.[165] Cases of neutropenia, including agranulocytosis, occur in approximately 0.5 percent of patients. The decline in white blood cell count generally happens during the first 3–4 months of treatment. Thus, patients need to have hematological monitoring every 2 weeks during the first 4 months of treatment. The development of neutropenia should lead to discontinuance of ticlopidine. Seriously affected patients might need hospitalization or treatment with granulocyte colony stimulating factor because infectious complications can develop.[166] The risk of neutropenia is much less with clopidogrel and the hematological monitoring is not performed. The use of ticlopidine has dropped during the last 10 years largely because of the potential complication

of thrombotic thrombocytopenia purpura (TTP).[167] The frequency of TTP following treatment is estimated as 0.02 percent.[118,168] TTP can be associated with the hemolytic-uremic syndrome.[169] A few cases of TTP have been described among patients taking clopidogrel.[170] Overall, the risk of TTP is considerably less with clopidogrel than with ticlopidine.[162,171] Most cases of clopidogrel-associated TTP occur within 2 weeks of starting treatment. Patients with TTP usually are critically ill. They should be hospitalized and they often are treated with plasma exchange. Relapses of TTP can occur despite plasma exchange.[170] Fatal aplastic anemia has been described in patients taking clopidogrel.[172,173]

There was a concern about a potential interaction between clopidogrel and atorvastatin, lovastatin, simvastatin, or cerivastatin that might lessen the antiplatelet effects of the former medication. However, Saw et al.[174] looked at the rates of vascular events among patients taking the statins that effect CYP3A4 and clopidogrel and those patients taking the antiplatelet agents and either fluvastatin or pravastatin, which are not metabolized by the cytochrome P450 system. They could not find any effects on the rates of either bleeding or ischemic events. Angiotensin converting enzyme inhibitors, which might limit the effects of aspirin, appear not to have an interaction with clopidogrel.

Those patients requiring surgery should have the medications stopped approximately 1 week before the operation. The probability of bleeding complications, including intracranial hemorrhage, increases when a patient is prescribed the combination of aspirin and either ticlopidine or clopidogrel.

Potential Indications

Ticlopidine is effective in treatment of patients with angina pectoris, peripheral arterial disease, or diabetic retinopathy. A clinical trial enrolling patients with symptomatic peripheral vascular disease reported that ticlopidine reduced the risk of stroke or myocardial infarction by 11.4 percent.[175] Ticlopidine has been used effectively as a monotherapy or in combination with aspirin to treat patients with unstable coronary artery disease or those having cardiovascular interventions.[176,177] Another trial compared ticlopidine or aspirin treatment among patients with recent myocardial infarction, no major differences were noted between the two treatment groups.[178] Two large trials tested the usefulness of ticlopidine in preventing ischemic stroke. A placebo-controlled trial found that ticlopidine reduced the risk of recurrent stroke by approximately 30 percent.[156] The medication was effective in both men and women. Another trial showed that the use of ticlopidine was associated with an approximately 12–16 percent reduction in stroke in comparison to aspirin.[155] A post-hoc study suggested that ticlopidine was especially effective in African Americans.[179] This finding prompted the study of Gorelick et al.[180], which tested the relative usefulness of ticlopidine 500 mg/day or aspirin 650 mg/day in preventing recurrent stroke among African-American patients. Recurrent stroke, myocardial infarction or vascular death was diagnosed in 14.7 percent of patients treated with ticlopidine and 12.3 percent of patients administered aspirin. The investigators found a modest reduction in the risk of fatal or nonfatal stroke among patients given aspirin. In summary, ticlopidine was not superior among this group of high-risk patients.

A large international trial compared aspirin or clopidogrel for prevention of major vascular events among patients with peripheral vascular disease, coronary artery disease, or ischemic stroke.[157] The overall results of the trial showed that clopidogrel was superior to aspirin (5.32 percent vs. 5.83 percent rate of events) but the differences in favor of clopidogrel were detected primarily among persons with peripheral vascular disease (see Fig. 19-8). No significant difference in outcomes was noted among the patients who initially had TIA or ischemic stroke. In a subgroup analysis found that the superior of clopidogrel among patients who have previous ischemic symptoms before their qualifying events.[181] Subsequently, several clinical trials tested the efficacy of clopidogrel usually in combination with aspirin in comparison to aspirin monotherapy, oral anticoagulants, or ticlopidine and aspirin.[182,183] Most of these studies enrolled patients with unstable heart disease or those undergoing cardiac endovascular procedures. The combination of clopidogrel and aspirin was effective and relatively safe. The combination of aspirin and clopidogrel is used widely in interventional cardiology. Because of the utility of the combination of aspirin and clopidogrel in treatment of patients have coronary artery angioplasty and stenting; the combination of medications also has been used to treat patients with similar cerebrovascular procedures.[184–186] Additional trials comparing clopidogrel monotherapy to the combination of aspirin and clopidogrel or aspirin monotherapy in comparison to treatment with aspirin and clopidogrel showed no superiority of the combination. These studies are enrolling patients with stroke. Many patients with symptomatic ischemic cerebrovascular disease are being treated with clopidogrel and aspirin despite the lack of the data to support the use of the combination of medications.

Information is not available about the utility of ticlopidine or clopidogrel for prevention of embolic events among patients with cardiac sources of embolism. Although these medications often are prescribed to patients with nonatherosclerotic vasculopathies, data to support their use are lacking.

Summary

Ticlopidine and clopidogrel are important medical therapies for prevention of ischemic events among patients with arterial diseases[187] (see Figs. 19-9 and 19-10). A systemic review concluded that these medications are modestly but significantly more effective than aspirin in preventing serious vascular events among high-risk persons.[188] These medications can lower the risk of a serious vascular event (stroke, myocardial infarction or death) by approximately 9 percent and for any stroke by approximately 12 percent.[189] Clopidogrel is considered to be slightly more effective than aspirin.[96] Either ticlopidine or clopidogrel monotherapy is indicated for treatment of patients who cannot tolerate aspirin. While data about the relative efficacy of ticlopidine or clopidogrel are largely inferential, indirect comparisons of the two agents in reference to aspirin suggest that the ticlopidine is the more effective medication. The relative reduction of risk of vascular strokes is greater with ticlopidine than with clopidogrel. Unfortunately, the safety profile of ticlopidine has limited the use of the medication. In particular, concerns about the hematological reactions (neutropenia or TTP) have prompted many physicians to avoid prescribing the medication. Clopidogrel has a much better safety record and as a result it is the thienopyridine that is prescribed for stroke prophylaxis in most patients.[96,190] Still Gazpoz et al.[191] found that the economic costs of clopidogrel make it a less attractive medication for prevention of ischemic events than aspirin.

Dipyridamole

Dipyridamole is a potent vasodilator, which increases coronary artery blood flow. It also has reversible antiplatelet aggregating effects.[192] Because of its vasodilatory effects, dipyridamole often is prescribed as an adjunctive intervention to evaluate coronary artery blood flow. While dipyridamole has been evaluated in a series of studies over the last 25 years, its use remains controversial. For example, Gibbs and Lip[193] concluded that the data do not support the use of dipyridamole for treatment of patients with vascular disease. Based on a systemic review, De Schryver et al.[194] concluded that there was no evidence that dipyridamole reduced the risk of vascular death although it might lessen the number of further vascular events. Conversely, Albers et al.[18] and a Leys et al.[96] stated that dipyridamole was an effective adjunctive agent for prevention of stroke in high-risk patients.

Pharmacology

The mechanism of the antiplatelet actions of dipyridamole is uncertain. The medication inhibits cyclic nucleotide phosphodiesterase in the platelet.[118] As a result, cyclic adenosine monophosphate (AMP) accumulates within the platelet, which could inhibit aggregation. Dipyridamole also may block the uptake of adenosine within the platelet. Dipyridamole also may prolong platelet survival. The medication also can have some effect on prostaglandin synthesis.

The absorption of conventional formulations of dipyridamole is quite variable and as a result, systemic bioavailability can be low. A modified (sustained-release) formulation appears to increase the bioavailability of dipyridamole (see Table 19-17). The medication is hepatically metabolized. The half-life of the medication is approximately 10 hours, which means a twice-a-day regimen is needed to maintain therapeutic effects.

Safety

The safety profile of dipyridamole is good; the most common side effects are headache and gastrointestinal distress[122] (see Table 19-16). Patients with a history of migraine might not tolerate the medication. However, some patients with headaches can use dipyridamole if the medication is started as a once-a-day regimen and can be gradually escalated to a twice a day course of therapy.[195] Patients with headaches can develop tolerance to dipyridamole and the medication can be continued. Because dipyridamole is a coronary artery vasodilator, there have been concerns that the medication could worsen heart disease. However, Humphreys et al.[196] found no adverse cardiac effects from dipyridamole among patients with mild-to-moderate heart disease. The agent does not seem to lead to a permanent reduction in blood pressure.[197] Dipyridamole is not accompanied by a high risk of major bleeding complications. No special laboratory monitoring is required.

Potential Indications

Most studies evaluating dipyridamole focused on the utility of the medication in preventing stroke among high-risk patients. Studies tested dipyridamole monotherapy or the medication in combination with aspirin. Dipyridamole has been used as an adjunct to warfarin for prevention of embolic events among patients with prosthetic cardiac valves.[198] Early studies did not find any specific benefit in stroke prophylaxis from the addition of dipyridamole to aspirin.[199,200] Subsequently, a large European trial showed a reduction in the risk of stroke with the treatment with dipyridamole and aspirin but critics concluded that most of the benefit could be ascribed to aspirin.[201] Another European trial tested aspirin 50 mg/day, sustained release dipyridamole 400 mg/day, or the combination in comparison to placebo among patients with recent TIA or stroke[149] (see Fig. 19-8). An approximately 15 percent reduction in stroke risk was achieved with either aspirin or dipyridamole alone. With the combination, the stroke risk was reduced by approximately 24 percent. Another study found that the combination of aspirin and dipyridamole was superior to aspirin alone for prevention of stroke among patients with recent TIA or stroke.[202]

A meta-analysis of the studies testing dipyridamole in treatment of patients with vascular disease found that the medication was effective in reducing ischemic events, other than vascular death. Most of the benefit from dipyridamole was found when the medication was given with aspirin and the data are strongly influenced by the results of ESPS-2.[149] The combination of aspirin and dipyridamole is effective in reducing nonfatal strokes but it does not lessen the likelihood of myocardial infarction or fatal stroke.[122]

Summary

Dipyridamole is an important adjunctive medication for treatment of patients at high risk for stroke (see Figs. 19-9 and 19-10). The medication usually is administered in combination with aspirin, which appears to be superior to aspirin monotherapy[203,204] The sustained released formulation might improve the bioavailability and efficacy of the medication. Dipyridamole does not seem to lower the risk of noncerebrovascular ischemic events. The safety of dipyridamole is one of its major attributes. Side effects, such as headache, are self-limited. The combination of extended-release dipyridamole and aspirin appears to be cost-effective.[205,206]

Other Antiplatelet Agents

Sulfinpyrazone is a uricosuric agent that has antiplatelet effects. It was tested as a monotherapy or in combination with aspirin in comparison to aspirin monotherapy or placebo in a Canadian trial.[207] No benefit was found. Further study has not been done. *Indobufen* is a nonsteroidal anti-inflammatory agent that is a cyclooxygenase inhibitor. It was compared to ticlopidine for prevention of stroke but the frequency of bleeding complications was increased among the patients treated with indobufen.[208,209] *Ibuprofen* is a commonly used over-the-counter anti-inflammatory agent that also affects platelet function. While the medication is not used as an antithrombotic agent, administration of the medication can affect the platelet receptors and might limit the effectiveness of aspirin, when the latter is given in close proximity. It has not been tested for stroke prophylaxis.

The efficacy of *triflusal* for preventing vascular events was compared to aspirin in a trial that enrolled more than 2100 patients.[210] While triflusal was associated with a lower risk of bleeding than aspirin, the two medications were approximately equal in preventing ischemic events. In summary, no net benefit was found from treatment with triflusal.

The rapidly acting intravenously administered glycoprotein IIb/IIIa (GP IIa/IIIb) receptor blockers are potent inhibitors of platelet aggregation. These medications are used to treat patients with unstable coronary artery disease and coronary endovascular interventions.[211] Orally administered GP IIa/IIIb receptor blockers have been tested in clinical trials but these agents did not reduce the frequency of stroke and an increase in mortality was found among patients treated with the new agent.[212] A trial of *lotrafiban* in combination with aspirin in comparison to aspirin monotherapy was halted prematurely because of a high rate of adverse experiences with the combination of medications.[213] A large trial evaluated aspirin, low-dose *sibrafran,* or high-dose sibrafran to patients with recent coronary events.[214] Recurrent ischemic events were similar in all treatment groups but bleeding complications were more frequent among the patients treated with sibrafran. Mortality was increased among patients treated with *orbofiban* enrolled in another trial.[215] Unless strategies can improve the safety of the oral GP IIb/IIIa receptor blockers, this class of agents appears to have limited future for the long-term treatment of patients with ischemic vascular diseases.

Pentoxifylline affects the deformability of red blood cells, alters shear stress of blood and reduces platelet aggregation.[216] Pentoxifylline is used to treat patients with intermittent claudication and because of its effects on blood flow it might be used to treat patients with TIA. Limited data are available to provide evidence about the utility of pentoxifylline.[217] This medication usually is not used for treatment of patients with cerebrovascular disease.

▶ COMBINATIONS OF ANTITHROMBOTIC MEDICATIONS

Because the antiplatelet agents affect platelet aggregation by different mechanisms, they medications could be complementary.[218–221] Already, the combination of dipyridamole and aspirin is prescribed for treatment of patients at high risk for stroke because of strong evidence of efficacy. In a large clinical trial, the combination of dipyridamole and aspirin was more effective than either medication used alone.[149]

The combination of clopidogrel and aspirin has much more potent effects on platelet thrombus formation than does aspirin alone.[222] The combination of either ticlopidine or clopidogrel and aspirin has been tested primarily for treatment of patients with unstable cardiac disease. Trials testing clopidogrel (usually with an initial dose of 300 mg followed by 75 mg daily) and aspirin in treatment of patients found that the combination was superior to aspirin.[182,223] At 30 days, 5.4 percent of patients treated with aspirin and placebo had a cardiovascular death, myocardial infarction or stroke while 4.3 percent of patients with clopidogrel and aspirin had events.[183] However, the combination was associated with an increased risk of bleeding complications. A study enrolling patients undergoing coronary endovascular procedures found an approximately 25 percent reduction in the risk of stroke among patients who received the combination of aspirin and clopidogrel when compared to treatment with aspirin alone.[189] The combination of aspirin and clopidogrel might be useful in management of patients with extensive atherosclerotic disease of the aorta.[212] Additional studies are testing the combinations of antiplatelet agents to better define the use of multiple medications in high-risk patients. One can anticipate that the combination of antiplatelet agents is associated with a higher risk of bleeding complications than that accompanying the use of one medication. In a study looking at responses of coagulation markers, the combination of aspirin and clopidogrel was not as effective in warfarin in preventing either thrombogenesis or platelet activation in patients with atrial fibrillation.[5] Still, the combination of medications might be useful in preventing thromboembolism among patients with atrial fibrillation. Two trials testing the combination of clopidogrel and aspirin against either agent administered alone failed to demonstrate superiority of the combination of therapies.[224,225]

Aspirin has been used in conjunction with either fixed-dose or adjusted-dose oral anticoagulants. Data about the use of aspirin and warfarin are limited. One trial enrolling patients after myocardial infarction found that combination of 80 mg of aspirin and a small fixed dose of warfarin (1 mg/day) was not as effective as 160 mg of aspirin alone.[226] Despite the negative results of this trial, the combination of aspirin and warfarin often is prescribed to patients who have ischemic symptoms despite being treated with adequate levels of anticoagulation. A systemic analysis found that the addition of low-dose aspirin to warfarin decreases the risk of systemic embolism and death among persons with prosthetic heart valves.[227] The currently recommended dose is approximately 75–81 mg/day.

REFERENCES

1. Johnston SC, Gress DR, Browner WS, Sidney S. Short-term prognosis after emergency department diagnosis of TIA. *JAMA* 2000;284:2901–2906.
2. Johnston SC, Easton JD. Are patients with acutely recovered cerebral ischemia more unstable? *Stroke* 2003;34:2446–2450.
3. Hirsh J, Dalen JE, Anderson DR, et al. Oral anticoagulants: mechanism of action, clinical effectiveness, and optimal therapeutic range. *Chest* 2001;119:8S–21S.
4. Hirsh J, Fuster V, Ansell J, Halperin JL. American Heart Association/American College of Cardiology foundation guide to warfarin therapy. *Circulation* 2003;107:1692–1711.
5. Kamath S, Blann AD, Chin BS, Lip GY. A prospective randomized trial of aspirin-clopidogrel combination therapy and dose-adjusted warfarin on indices of thrombogenesis and platelet activation in atrial fibrillation. *J Am Coll Cardiol* 2002;40:484–490.
6. Chamorro A, Obach V. Anticoagulant therapy. *Cerebrovasc Dis* 2003;15:49–55.
7. Harker LA. Therapeutic inhibition of thrombin activities, receptors, and production. *Hematol Oncol Clin North Am* 1998;12:1211–1230.
8. Hyman BT, Landas SK, Ashman RF, Schelper RL, Robinson RA. Warfarin-related purple toes syndrome and cholesterol microembolization. *Am J Med* 1987;82:1233–1237.
9. Essex DW, Wynn SS, Jin DK. Late-onset warfarin-induced skin necrosis: case report and review of the literature. *Am J Hematol* 1998;57:233–237.
10. Sallah S, Abdallah JM, Gagnon GA. Recurrent warfarin-induced skin necrosis in kindreds with protein S deficiency. *Haemostasis* 1998;28:25–30.
11. Ng T, Tillyer ML. Warfarin-induced skin necrosis associated with Factor V Leiden and protein S deficiency. *Clin Lab Haematol* 2001;23:261–264.
12. Talmadge DB, Spyropoulos AC. Purple toes syndrome associated with warfarin therapy in a patient with antiphospholipid syndrome. *Pharmacotherapy* 2003;23:674–677.
13. Sallah S, Thomas DP, Roberts HR. Warfarin and heparin-induced skin necrosis and the purple toe syndrome: infrequent complications of anticoagulant treatment. *Thromb Haemost* 1997;78:785–790.
14. Smythe MA, Warkentin TE, Stephens JL, Zakalik D, Mattson JC. Venous limb gangrene during overlapping therapy with warfarin and a direct thrombin inhibitor for immune heparin-induced thrombocytopenia. *Am J Hematol* 2002;71:50–52.
15. Crowther MA, Ginsberg JB, Kearon C, et al. A randomized trial comparing 5-mg and 10-mg warfarin loading doses. *Arch Intern Med* 1999;159:46–48.
16. Harrison L, Johnston M, Massicotte MP, Crowther M, Moffat K, Hirsh J. Comparison of 5-mg and 10-mg loading doses in initiation of warfarin therapy. *Ann Intern Med* 1997;126:133–136.
17. Hirsh J, Poller L. The International Normalized Ratio. A guide to understanding and correcting its problems. *Arch Intern Med* 1994;154:282–288.
18. Albers GW, Amarenco P, Easton JD, Sacco RL, Teal P. Antithrombotic and thrombolytic therapy for ischemic stroke. *Chest* 2001;119:300S–320S.
19. Ansell J, Hirsh J, Dalen J, et al. Managing oral anticoagulant therapy. *Chest* 2001;119:22S–38S.
20. Oates A, Jackson PR, Austin CA, Channer KS. A new regimen for starting warfarin therapy in out-patients. *Br J Clin Pharmacol* 1998;46:157–161.
21. Shine D, Patel J, Kumar J, et al. A randomized trial of initial warfarin dosing based on simple clinical criteria. *Thromb Haemost* 2003;89:297–304.
22. Kovacs MJ, Rodger M, Anderson DR, et al. Comparison of 10-mg and 5-mg Warfarin initiation nomograms together with low-molecular-weight Heparin for outpatient treatment of acute venous thromboembolism. *Ann Intern Med* 2003;138:714–719.
23. Gladman JR, Dolan G. Effect of age upon the induction and maintenance of anticoagulation with warfarin. *Postgrad Med J* 1995;71:153–155.
24. Roberts GW, Helboe T, Nielsen CB, et al. Assessment of an age-adjusted warfarin initiation protocol. *Ann Pharmacother* 2003;37:799–803.
25. Dalere GM, Coleman RW, Lum BL. A graphic nomogram for warfarin dosage adjustment. *Pharmacotherapy* 1999;19:461–467.
26. Scordo MG, Pengo V, Spina E, Dahl ML, Gusella M, Padrini R. Influence of CYP2C9 and CYP2C19 genetic polymorphism on warfarin maintenance dose and metabolic clearance. *Clin Pharmacol Ther* 2002;72:702–710.
27. Linder MW, Looney S, Adams JE, III, et al. Warfarin dose adjustments based on CYP2C9 genetic polymorphisms. *J Thromb Thrombolysis* 2002;14:227–232.
28. Fregin A, Rost S, Wolz W, Krebsova A, Muller CR, Oldenburg J. Homozygosity mapping of a second gene locus for hereditary combined deficiency of vitamin K-dependent clotting factors to the centromeric region of chromosome 16. *Blood* 2002;100:3229–3232.
29. Hulse ML. Warfarin resistance: diagnosis and therapeutic alternatives. *Pharmacotherapy* 1996;16:1009–1017.
30. Kovich O, Otley CC. Thrombotic complications related to discontinuation of warfarin and aspirin therapy perioperatively for cutaneous operation. *J Am Acad Dermatol* 2003;48:233–237.
31. Sato Y, Honda Y, Kunoh H, Oizumi K. Long-term oral anticoagulation reduces bone mass in patients with previous hemispheric infarction and nonrheumatic atrial fibrillation. *Stroke* 1997;28:2390–2394.
32. Wehrmacher WH, Karlman RL, Scanlon P, Messmore HL, Jr. Anticoagulant therapy of thromboembolic disease during pregnancy. *Compr Ther* 1998;24:289–294.

33. Ginsberg JS, Greer I, Hirsh J. Use of antithrombotic agents during pregnancy. *Chest* 2001;119:122S-131S.

34. Cotrufo M, De Feo M, De Santo LS, et al. Risk of warfarin during pregnancy with mechanical valve protheses. *Obstet Gynecol* 2002;99:35–40.

35. Linkins LA, Choi PT, Douketis JD. Clinical impact of bleeding in patients taking oral anticoagulant therapy for venous thromboembolism. A meta-analysis. *Ann Intern Med* 2003;139:893–900.

36. Devereaux PJ, Anderson DR, Gardner MJ, et al. Differences between perspectives of physicians and patients on anticoagulation in patients with atrial fibrillation: observational study. *Br Med J* 2001;323:1218–1222.

37. Yasaka M, Minematsu K, Naritomi H, Sakata T, Yamaguchi T. Predisposing factors for enlargement of intracerebral hemorrhage in patients treated with warfarin. *Thromb Haemost* 2003;89:278–283.

38. Copland M, Walker ID, Tait RC. Oral anticoagulation and hemorrhagic complications in an elderly population with atrial fibrillation. *Arch Intern Med* 2001;161:2125–2128.

39. Man SH, Nichol G, Lau A, Laupacis A. Choosing antithrombotic therapy for elderly patients with atrial fibrillation who are at risk for falls. *Arch Intern Med* 1999;159:677–685.

40. Smith EE, Rosand J, Knudsen KA, Hylek EM, Greenberg SM. Leukoaraiosis is associated with warfarin-related hemorrhage following ischemic stroke. *Neurology* 2002;59:193–197.

41. Petty GW, Brown RD, Jr., Whisnant JP, Sicks JD, O'Fallon WM, Wiebers DO. Frequency of major complications of aspirin, warfarin, and intravenous heparin for secondary stroke prevention. *Ann Intern Med* 1999;130:14–22.

42. van der Meer FJ, Rosendaal FR, Vandenbroucke JP, Briet E. Bleeding complications in oral anticoagulant therapy. An analysis of risk factors. *Arch Intern Med* 1993;153:1557–1562.

43. Gitter MJ, Jaeger TM, Petterson TM, Gersh BJ, Silverstein MD. Bleeding and thromboembolism during anticoagulant therapy: a population-based study in Rochester, Minnesota. *Mayo Clin Proc* 1995;70:725–733.

44. Petty GW, Lennihan L, Mohr JP, et al. Complications of long-term anticoagulation. *Ann Neurol* 1988;23:570–574.

45. Gullov AL, Koefoed BG, Petersen P. Bleeding during warfarin and aspirin therapy in patients with atrial fibrillation: the AFASAK 2 study. Atrial Fibrillation Aspirin and Anticoagulation. *Arch Intern Med* 1999;159:1322–1328.

46. Pengo V, Zasso A, Barbero F, et al. Effectiveness of fixed minidose warfarin in the prevention of thromboembolism and vascular death in nonrheumatic atrial fibrillation. *Am J Cardio* 1998;82:433–437.

47. The Stroke Prevention in Reversible Ischemia Trial (SPIRIT) Study Group. A randomized trial of anticoagulants versus aspirin after cerebral ischemia of presumed arterial origin. *Ann Neurol* 1997;42:857–865.

48. Mohr JP, Thompson JLP, Lazar RM, et al. A comparison of warfarin and aspirin for the prevention of recurrent ischemic stroke. *N Engl J Med* 2001;345:1444–1451.

49. ESPRIT I. Oral anticoagulation in patients after cerebral ischemia of arterial origin and risk of intracranial hemorrhage. *Stroke* 2003;34:e45-e46

50. Crowther MA, Ginsberg JS, Julian J, et al. A comparison of two intensities of warfarin for the prevention of recurrent thrombosis in patients with the antiphospholipid antibody syndrome. *N Engl J Med* 2003;349:1133–1138.

51. Edvardsson N, Juul-Moller S, Omblus R, Pehrsson K. Effects of low-dose warfarin and aspirin versus no treatment on stroke in a medium-risk patient population with atrial fibrillation. *J Intern Med* 2003;254:95–101.

52. Weibert RT, Le DT, Kayser SR, Rapaport SI. Correction of excessive anticoagulation with low-dose oral vitamin K1. *Ann Intern Med* 1997;126:959–962.

53. Crowther MA, Douketis JD, Schnurr T, et al. Oral vitamin K lowers the international normalized ratio more rapidly than subcutaneous vitamin K in the treatment of warfarin-associated coagulapathy. A randomized, controlled trial. *Ann Intern Med* 2002;137:251–254.

54. Boulis NM, Bobek MP, Schmaier A, Hoff JT. Use of factor IX complex in warfarin-related intracranial hemorrhage. *Neurosurgery* 1999;45:1113–1119.

55. Deveras RA, Kessler CM. Reversal of warfarin-induced excessive anticoagulation with recombinant human factor VIIa concentrate. *Ann Intern Med* 2002;137:884–888.

56. Geerts WH, Heit JA, Clagett P, et al. Prevention of venous thromboembolism. *Chest* 2001;119:132S-175S.

57. Ginsberg JS, Bates SM, Oczkowski W, et al. Low-dose warfarin in rehabilitating stroke survivors. *Thromb Res* 2002;107:287–290.

58. Ridker PM, Goldhaber SZ, Danielson E, et al. Long-term, low-intensity warfarin therapy for the prevention of recurrent venous thromboembolism. *N Engl J Med* 2003;348:1425–1434.

59. Kearon C, Ginsberg JS, Kovacs MJ, et al. Comparison of low-intensity warfarin therapy with conventional-intensity warfarin therapy for long-term prevention of recurrent venous thromboembolism. *N Engl J Med* 2003;349:702–704.

60. Bauer KA. Management of thrombophilia. *J Thromb Haemost* 2003;1:1429–1434.

61. Gere J, Minier D, Osseby GV, Couvreur G, Moreau T, Giroud M. Indications for anticoagulant use in secondary prevention of strokes. *Presse Medicale* 2003;32:1175–1180.

62. Go AS, Hylek EM, Chang Y, et al. Anticoagulation therapy for stroke prevention in atrial fibrillation. How well do randomized trials translate into clinical practice? *JAMA* 2003;290:2685–2692.

63. EAFT (European Atrial Fibrillation Trial) Study Group. Secondary prevention in non-rheumatic atrial fibrillation after transient ischaemic attack or minor stroke. *Lancet* 1993;342:1255–1262.

64. Hart RG, Halperin JL, Pearce LA, et al. Lessons from the stroke prevention in atrial fibrillation trials. *Ann Intern Med* 2003;138:831–838.

65. Hart RG. Atrial fibrillation and stroke prevention. *N Engl J Med* 2003;349:1015–1016.

66. Hart RG, Palacio S, Pearce LA. Atrial fibrillation, stroke and acute antithrombotic therapy: analysis of randomzied clinical trials. *Stroke* 2002;33:2722–2727.

67. Mattle HP. Long-term outcome after stroke due to atrial fibrillation. *Cerebrovasc Dis* 2003;16(suppl):3–8.

68. Stroke Prevention in Atrial Fibrillation Investigators. Warfarin versus aspirin for prevention of thromboembolism in atrial fibrillation: Stroke Prevention in Atrial Fibrillation II Study. *Lancet* 1994;343:687–691.

69. Hylek EM, Go AS, Chang Y, et al. Effect of intensity of oral anticoagulation on stroke severity and mortality in atrial fibrillation. *N Engl J Med* 2003;349:1019–1026.

70. Gallagher MM, Hennessy BJ, Edvardsson N, et al. Embolic complications of direct current cardioversion of atrial arrhythmias: association with low intensity of anticoagulation at the time of cardioversion. *J Am Coll Cardiol* 2002; 40:926–933.

71. Hart RG. Oral anticoagulants for secondary prevention of stroke. *Cerebrovasc Dis* 1997;7(suppl 6):24–29.

72. Feinberg WM. Anticoagulation for prevention of stroke. *Neurology* 1998;51:S20-S22

73. Salem DN, Levine HJ, Pauker SG, Eckman MH, Daudelin DH. Antithrombotic therapy in valvular heart disease. *Chest* 1998;114:590S-601S.

74. Sacco RL, Adams R, Albers G, et al. Guidelines for prevention of stroke in patients with ischemic stroke or transient ischemic attack. A statement for healthcare professionals from the American Heart Association/American Stroke Association. *Stroke* 2006;37:577–617.

75. Pullicino PM, Halperin JL, Thompson JLP. Stroke in patients with heart failure and reduced left ventricular ejection fraction. *Neurology* 2000;54:288–294.

76. Tiede DJ, Nishimura RA, Gastineau DA, et al. Modern management of prosthetic valve anticoagulation. *Mayo Clin Proc* 1998;73:665–680.

77. Ezekowitz MD. Anticoagulation management of valve replacement patients. *J Heart Valve Dis* 2002;11(suppl 1): S56–S60

78. Vaitkus PT, Barnathan ES. Embolic potential, prevention and management of mural thrombus complicating anterior myocardial infarction: a meta-analysis. *J Am Coll Cardiol* 1993;22:1004–1009.

79. Azar AJ, Koudstaal PJ, Wintzen AR, et al. Risk of stroke during long-term anticoagulant therapy in patients after myocardial infarction. *Ann Neurol* 1996;39:301–307.

80. Van Es RF, Jonker JJ, Verheugt FW, Deckers JW, Grobbee DE. Aspirin and coumadin after acute coronary syndromes (the ASPECT-2 study): a randomized controlled trial. *Lancet* 2002;360:109–113.

81. Hurlen M, Abdelnoor M, Smith P, Erikssen J, Arnesen H. Warfarin, aspirin, or both after myocardial infarction. *N Engl J Med* 2002;347:969–974.

82. Rudnicka AR, Ashby D, Brennan P, Meade T. Thrombosis prevention trial: compliance with warfarin treatment and investigation of a retained effect. *Arch Intern Med* 2003;163:1454–1460.

83. Homma S, Sacco RL, Di Tullio MR, Sciacca RR, Mohr JP. Effect of medical treatment in stroke patients with patent foramen ovale: patent foramen ovale in cryptogenic stroke study. *Circulation* 2002;105:2625–2631.

84. Mannucci PM. Aspects of the clinical management of hereditary thrombophilia: a personal perspective. *Haemostasis* 2000;30(suppl):11–15.

85. Khamashta MA, Cuadrado MJ, Mujic F, Taub NA, Hunt BJ, Hughes GR. The management of thrombosis in the antiphospholipid-antibody syndrome. *N Engl J Med* 1995; 332:993–997.

86. Ruiz-Irastorza G, Khamashta MA, Hunt BJ, Escudero A, Cuadrado MJ, Hughes GR. Bleeding and recurrent thrombosis in definite antiphospholipid syndrome: analysis of a series of 66 patients treated with oral anticoagulation to a target international normalized ratio of 3.5. *Arch Intern Med* 2002;162:1164–1169.

87. The APASS Investigators. Antiphopholipid antibodies and subsequent thrombo-occlusive events in patients with ischemic stroke. *JAMA* 2004;291:576–584.

88. Dressler FA, Craig WR, Castello R, Labovitz AJ. Mobile aortic atheroma and systemic emboli: efficacy of anticoagulation and influence of plaque morphology on recurrent stroke. *J Am Coll Cardiol* 1998;31:134–138.

89. Blackshear JL, Zabalgoitia M, Pennock G, et al. Warfarin safety and efficacy in patients with thoracic aortic plaque and atrial fibrillation. SPAF TEE Investigators. Stroke Prevention and Atrial Fibrillation. Transesophageal Echocardiography. *Am J Cardiol* 1999;83:453–455.

90. Tunick PA, Nayar AC, Goodkin GM, et al. Effect of treatment on the incidence of stroke and other emboli in 519 patients with severe thoracic aortic plaque. *Am J Cardiol* 2002;90:1320–1325.

91. Chimowitz MI, Kokkinos J, Strong J, et al. The Warfarin-Aspirin Symptomatic Intracranial Disease Study. *Neurology* 1995;45:1488–1493.

92. The Warfarin-Aspirin Symptomatic Intracranial Disease (WASID) Study Group. Prognosis of patients with symptomatic vertebral or basilar artery stenosis. *Stroke* 1998; 29:1389–1392.

93. Chimowitz MI, Lynn MJ, Howlett-Smith H, et al. Comparison of warfarin and aspirin for symptomatic intracranial arterial stenosis. *N Engl J Med* 2005;353: 1305–1316.

94. Sandercock P, Mielke O, Liu M, Counsell C. Anticoagulants for preventing recurrence following presumed non-cardioembolic ischaemic stroke or transient ischaemic attack. Cochrane Database of Systematic Reviews 2003; CD000248.

95. Lyrer P, Engelter S. Antithrombotic drugs for carotid artery dissection. Cochrane Database of Systematic Reviews 2000;CD000255.

96. Goldstein LB, Adams R, Alberts MJ, et al. Primary prevention of ischemic stroke. A guideline from the American Heart Association, American Stroke Association Stroke Council. *Stroke* 2006;37:1583–1563.

97. Rubio F, Jato M. Usefulness of anticoagulants in the prevention of ischemic stroke. *Cerebrovasc Dis* 2004;17 (suppl 1):70–73.

98. Hirsh J. New anticoagulants. *Am Heart J* 2001;142:S3-S8

99. Lunven C, Gauffeny C, Lecoffre C, O'Brien DP, Roome NO, Berry CN. Inhibition by argatroban, a specific thrombin inhibitor, of platelet activation by fibrin clot-associated thrombin. *Thromb Haemost* 1996;75:154–160.

100. Lewis BE, Walenga JM, Wallis DE. Anticoagulation with Novastan (argatroban) in patients with heparin-induced thrombocytopenia and heparin-induced thrombocytopenia

and thrombosis syndrome. *Semin Thromb Hemost* 1997;23: 197–202.

101. Topol EJ, Fuster V, Harrington RA, et al. Recombinant hirudin for unstable angina pectoris. A multicenter, randomized angiographic trial. *Circulation* 1994;89:1557–1566.

102. The Global Use of Strategies to Open Occluded Coronary Arteries (GUSTO) IIa Investigators. Randomized trial of intravenous heparin versus recombinant hirudin for acute coronary syndromes. *Circulation* 1994;90:1631–1637.

103. Harenberg J, Ingrid J, Tivadar F. Treatment of venous thromboembolism with the oral thrombin inhibitor, ximelagatran. *Israel Med Assoc J* 2002;4:1003–1005.

104. Eriksson BI, Bergqvist D, Kalebo P, et al. Ximelagatran and melagatran compared with dalteparin for prevention of venous thromboembolism after total hip or knee replacemnt: the METHRO II randomised trial. *Lancet* 2002;360:1441–1447.

105. Francis CW, Davidson B, Berkowitz S, et al. Ximelgatran versus Warfarin for the prevention of venous thromboembolism after total knee arthroplasty. *Ann Intern Med* 2002;137:648–655.

106. Schulman S, Wåhlander K, Lundström T, Clason SB, Eriksson H, for the THRIVE III Investigators. Secondary prevention of venous thromboembolism with the oral direct thrombin inhibitor ximelagatran. *N Engl J Med* 2003;349:1713–1721.

107. Petersen P, Grind M, Adler J, SPORTIF II Invesitgators. Ximelagatran versus warfarin for stroke prevention in patients with nonvalvular atrial fibrillation. SPORTIF II: a dose-guiding tolerability, and safety study. *J Am Coll Cardiol* 2003;41:1445–1451.

108. Executive Steering Committe on behalf of the SPORTIF III Investigators. Stroke prevention with the oral direct thrombin inhibitor ximelagatran compared with warfarin in patients with non-valvular atrial fibrillation (SPORTIF III): randomised controlled trial. *Lancet* 2003;362:1691–1698.

109. Verheugt FWA. Can we pull the plug on warfarin in atrial fibrillation? *Lancet* 2003;362:1685–1687.

110. Hankey GJ, Klijn CJM, Eikelboom JW. Ximelagatran or warfarin for stroke prevention in patients with atrial fibrillation? *Stroke* 2004;35:389–391.

111. Peripheral Arterial Disease Antiplatelet Consensus Group. Antiplatelet therapy in peripheral arterial disease. Consensus statement. *Eur J Vasc Endovasc Surg* 2003;26: 1–16.

112. Antithrombotic Trialists' Collaboration. Collaborative meta-analysis of randomised trials of antiplatelet therapy for prevention of death, myocardial infarction, and stroke in high risk patients. *Br Med J* 2002;324:71–86.

113. Algra A, van Gijn J. Aspirin at any dose above 30 mg offers only modest protection after cerebral ischaemia. *J Neurol Neurosurg Psychiatry* 1996;60:197–199.

114. Sivenius J, Cunha L, Diener HC, et al. Second European Stroke Prevention Study: antiplatelet therapy is effective regardless of age. ESPS2 Working Group. *Acta Neurol Scand* 1999;99:54–60.

115. Puranen J, Laakso M, Riekkinen PJS, Sivenius J. Efficacy of antiplatelet treatment in hypertensive patients with TIA or stroke. *J Cardiovasc Pharmacol* 1998;32:291–294.

116. Puranen J, Laakso M, Riekkinen PS, Sivenius J. Risk factors and antiplatelet therapy in TIA and stroke patients. *J Neurol Sci* 1998;154:200–204.

117. Engelter S, Lyrer P. Antiplatelet therapy for preventing stroke and other vascular events after carotid endarterectomy. Cochrane Database of Systematic Reviews 2003; CD001458.

118. Patrono C, Coller B, Dalen JE, et al. Platelet-active drugs. *Chest* 2001;119:39S-63S.

119. Rojas-Fernandez CH, Kephart GC, Sketris IS, Kass K. Underuse of acetylsalicylic acid in individuals with myocardial infarction, ischemic heart disease or stroke: data from the 1995 population-based Nova Scotia Health Survey. *Can J Cardiol* 1999;15:291–296.

120. Awtry EH, Loscalzo J. Aspirin. *Circulation* 2000;101: 1206–1218.

121. Gomes I. Aspirin: a neuroprotective agent at high doses? *Natl Med J India* 1998;11:14–17.

122. Fleck JD, Biller J. Choices in medical management for prevention of acute ischemic stroke. *Curr Neurol Neurosci Rep* 2001;1:33–38.

123. Brandon RA, Eadie MJ. The basis for aspirin dosage in stroke prevention. *Clin Exp Neurol* 1987;23:47–54.

124. Johnson ES, Lanes SF, Wentworth CE, Satterfield MH, Abebe BL, Dicker LW. A metaregression analysis of the dose-response effect of aspirin on stroke. *Arch Intern Med* 1999;159:1248–1253.

125. Buchanan MR, Hirsh J. Effect of aspirin on hemostasis and thrombosis. *N Engl Reg Allergy Proc* 1986;7:26–31.

126. Alberts MJ, Bergman DL, Molner E, Jovanovic BD, Ushiwata I, Teruya J. Antiplatelet effect of aspirin in patients with cerebrovascular disease. *Stroke* 2004;35: 175–178.

127. Macchi L, Sorel N, Christiaens L. Aspirin resistance. Definitions, mechanisms, prevalence, and clinical significance. *Curr Pharm Des* 2006;12:252–258.

128. Helgason CM, Bolin KM, Hoff JA, et al. Development of aspirin resistance in persons with previous ischemic stroke. *Stroke* 1994;25:2331–2336.

129. Grundmann K, Jaschonek K, Kleine B, Dichgans J, Topka H. Aspirin non-responder status in patients with recurrent cerebral ischemic attacks. *J Neurol* 2003;250:63–66.

130. Sze PC, Reitman D, Pincus MM, Sacks HS, Chalmers TC. Antiplatelet agents in the secondary prevention of stroke: meta-analysis of the randomized control trials. *Stroke* 1988;19:436–442.

131. Adams HP, Jr., Bendixen BH. Low- versus high-dose aspirin in prevention of ischemic stroke. *Clin Neuropharmacol* 1993;16:485–500.

132. CLASP Collaborative Group. Low dose aspirin in pregnancy and early childhood development: follow up of the collaborative low dose aspririn study in pregnancy. *Br J Obstet Gynaecol* 1995;102:861–868.

133. Steering Committee of the Physicians' Health Study Research Group. Final report on the aspirin component of the ongoing Physicians' Health Study. *N Engl J Med* 1989;321:129–135.

134. He J, Whelton PK, Vu B. Aspirin and risk of hemorrhagic stroke. *JAMA* 1998;280:1930–1935.

135. Patrono C. Prevention of myocardial infarction and stroke by aspirin: different mechanisms? Different dosage? *Thromb Res* 1998;92:S7–12.

136. Hart R, Halperin J, McBride R. Aspirin for the primary prevention of stroke and other major vascular events. *Arch Neurol* 2000;57:326–332.

137. UK-TIA Study Group. United Kingdom transient ischaemic attack (UK-TIA) aspirin trial: interim results. *Br Med J* 1988;. 296:316–320.

138. The Dutch TIA Trial Study Group. A comparison of two doses of aspirin (30 mg vs. 283 mg a day) in patients after a transient ischemic attack or minor ischemic stroke. *N Engl J Med* 1991;325:1261–1266.

139. The SALT Collaborative Group. Swedish Aspirin Low-Dose Trial (SALT) of 75 mg aspirin as secondary prophylaxis after cerebrovascular ischaemic events. *Lancet* 1991;338:1345–1349.

140. Taylor DW, Barnett HJM, Haynes RB, et al. Low-dose and high-dose acetylsalicylic acid for patients undergoing carotid endarterectomy: a ransomised controlled trial. *Lancet* 1999;353:2179–2184.

141. van Gijn J. Low doses of aspirin in stroke prevention. *Lancet* 1999;353:2172–2173.

142. International Stroke Trial Collaborative Group. The International Stroke Trial (IST): a randomised trial of aspirin, subcutaneous heparin, both, or neither among 19435 patients with acute ischaemic stroke. *Lancet* 1997;349:1569–1581.

143. CAST (Chinese Acute Stroke Trial) Collaborative Group. CAST: randomised placebo-controlled trial of early aspirin use in 20,000 patients with acute ischaemic stroke. *Lancet* 1997;349:1641–1649.

144. Multicentre Acute Stroke Trial–Italy (MAST-I) Group. Randomised controlled trial of streptokinase, aspirin, and combination of both in treatment of acute ischaemic stroke. *Lancet* 1995;346:1509–1514.

145. Berge E, Abdelnoor M, Nakstad PH, Sandset PM, on behalf of the HAEST Study Group. Low molecular-weight heparin versus aspirin in patients with acute ischaemic stroke and atrial fibrillation: a double-blind randomised study. *Lancet* 2000;355:1205–1210.

146. Bath PM, Lindenstrom E, Boysen G, et al. Tinzaparin in acute ischaemic stroke (TAIST): a randomised aspirin-controlled trial. *Lancet* 2001;358:683–684.

147. The National Institute of Neurological Disorders and Stroke rt-PA Stroke Study Group. Tissue plasminogen activator for acute ischemic stroke. *N Engl J Med* 1995;333:1581–1587.

148. Adams HP, Adams RJ, Brott T, et al. Guidelines for the early management of patients with ischemic stroke. A scientific statement from the stroke council of the American Stroke Association. *Stroke* 2003;34:1056–1083.

149. Diener HC, Cunha L, Forbes C, Sivenius J, Smets P, Lowenthal A. European Stroke Prevention Study. 2. Dipyridamole and acetylsalicylic acid in the secondary prevention of stroke. *J Neurol Sci* 1996;143:1–13.

150. Chimowitz MI, Furlan AJ, Nayak S, Sila CA. Mechanism of stroke in patients taking aspirin. *Neurology* 1990;40:1682–1685.

151. Stein PD, Alpert JS, Dalen JE, Horstkotte D, Turpie AG. Antithrombotic therapy in patients with mechanical and biological prosthetic heart valves. *Chest* 1998;114:602S–610S.

152. ACTIVE Writing Group on behalf of the ACTIVE Investigators. Clopidogrel plus aspirin versus oral anticoagulation for atrial fibrillation in the Atrial Fibrillation Clopidogrel Trial with Irbesartan for prevention ov Vascular Events (ACTIVE W). A randomised controlled trial. *Lancet* 2006;367:1903–1912

153. Mas JL, Arquizan C, Lamy C, et al. Recurrent cerebrovascular events associated with patent foramen ovale, atrial septal aneurysm, or both. *N Engl J Med* 2001;345:1740–1746.

154. Antiplatelet Trialists' Collaboration. Collaborative overview of randomised trials of antiplatelet therapy - III: Reduction in venous thrombosis and pulmonary embolism by antiplatelet prophylaxis among surgical and medical patients. *Br Med J* 1994;308:235–246.

155. Hass WK, Easton JD, Adams HP, Jr., et al. A randomized trial comparing ticlopidine hydrochloride with aspirin for the prevention of stroke in high-risk patients. Ticlopidine Aspirin Stroke Study Group. *N Engl J Med* 1989;321:501–507.

156. Gent M, Blakely JA, Easton JD, et al. The Canadian American Ticlopidine Study (CATS) in thromboembolic stroke. *Lancet* 1989;1:1215–1220.

157. CAPRIE Steering Committee. A randomised, blinded, trial of clopidogrel versus aspirin in patients at risk of ischaemic events (CAPRIE). *Lancet* 1996;348:1329–1339.

158. Quinn MJ, Fitzgerald DJ. Ticlopidine and clopidogrel. *Circulation* 1999;100:1667–1672.

159. Helft G, Osende JI, Worthley SG, et al. Acute antithrombotic effect of a front-loaded regimen of clopidogrel in patients with atherosclerosis on aspirin. *Arterioscler Thromb Vasc Biol* 2000;20:2316–2321.

160. Pache J, Kastrati A, Mehilli J, et al. Clopidogrel therapy in patients undergoing coronary stenting: value of a high-loading-dose regimen. *Catheterizat Cardiovas Interven* 2002;55:436–441.

161. Weber AA, Braun M, Hohlfeld T, Schwippert B, Tschope D, Schror K. Recovery of platelet function after discontinuation of clopidogrel treatment in healthy volunteers. *Br J Clin Pharmacol* 2001;52:333–336.

162. Harker LA, Boissel JP, Pilgrim AJ, Gent M. Comparative safety and tolerability of clopidogrel and aspirin results from CAPRIE. CAPRIE Steering Committee and Investigators. Clopidogrel verus aspirin in patients at risk of ischaemic events. *Drug Saf* 1999;21:325–335.

163. Iqbal M, Goenka P, Young MF, Thomas E, Borthwick TR. Ticlopidine-induced cholestatic hepatitis: report of three cases and review of the literature. *Dig Dis Sci* 1998;43:2223–2226.

164. Persoz CF, Cornella F, Kaeser P, Rochat T. Ticlopidine-induced interstitial pulmonary disease: a case report. *Chest* 2001;119:1963–1965.

165. Love BB, Biller J, Gent M. Adverse haematological effects of ticlopidine. Prevention, recognition and management. *Drug Saf* 1998;19:89–98.

166. Hung MJ, Wang CH, Cherng WJ. Granulocyte colony stimulating factor treatment for delayed recovery of ticlopidine-related neutropenia. *Int J Clin Pract* 2002;56: 70–71.

167. Bennett CL, Weinberg PD, Rozenberg-Bendror K, Yarnold PR, Kwaan HC, Green D. Thrombotic thrombocytopenia purpura associated with ticlopidine. *Ann Intern Med* 1998;128:541–544.

168. Steinhubl SR, Tan WA, Foody JM, Topol EJ. Incidence and clinical course of thrombotic thrombocytopenic purpura due to ticlopidine following coronary stenting. EPISTENT Investigators. Evaluation of Platelet IIb/IIIa Inhibitor for Stenting. *JAMA* 1999;281:806–810.

169. Medina PJ, Sipols JM, George JN. Drug-associated thrombotic thrombocytopenic purpura-hemolytic uremic syndrome. *Curr Opin Hematol* 2001;8:286–293..

170. Zakarija A, Bandarenko N, Pandey DK, et al. Clopidogrel-associated TTP. An update of pharmacovigilance efforts conducted by independent researchers, pharmaceutical suppliers, and the Food and Drug Administration. *Stroke* 2004;35:533–538.

171. Nara W, Ashley I, Rosner F. Thrombotic thrombocytopenic purpura associated with clopidogrel administration: case report and brief review. *Am J Med Sci* 2001; 322:170–172.

172. Trivier JM, Caron J, Mahieu M, Cambier N, Rose C. Fatal aplastic anaemia associated with clopidogrel. *Lancet* 2001; 357:446

173. Meyer B, Staudinger T, Lechner K. Clopidogrel and aplastic anaemia. *Lancet* 2001;357:1446–1447.

174. Saw J, Steinhubl SR, Berger PB, et al. Lack of adverse clopidogrel-atorvastatin clinical interaction from secondary analysis of a randomized, placebo-controlled clopidogrel trial. *Circulation* 2003;108:921–924.

175. Janzon L. The STIMS trial: the ticlopidine experience and its clinical applications. Swedish Ticlopidine Multicenter Study. *Vasc Med* 1996;1:141–143.

176. van de Loo A, Nauck M, Noory E, Wollschlager H. Enhancement of platelet inhibition of ticlopidine plus aspirin vs aspirin alone given prior to elective PTCA. *Eur Heart J* 1998;19:96–102.

177. Goods CM, al-Shaibi KF, Liu MW, et al. Comparison of aspirin alone versus aspirin plus ticlopidine after coronary artery stenting. *Am J Cardio* 1996;78:1042–1044.

178. Scrutinio D, Cimminiello C, Marubini E, Pitzalis MV, Di Biase M, Rizzon P. Ticlopidine versus aspirin after myocardial infarction (STAMI) trial. *J Am Coll Cardiol* 2001;37: 1259–1265.

179. Weisberg LA. The efficacy and safety of ticlopidine and aspirin in non-whites: analysis of a patient subgroup from the Ticlopidine Aspirin Stroke Study. *Neurology* 1993;43:27–31.

180. Gorelick PB, Richardson D, Kelly M, et al. Aspirin and ticlopidine for prevention of recurrent stroke in black patients: a randomized trial. *JAMA* 2003;289:2947–2857.

181. Ringleb PA, Bhatt DL, Hirsch AT, Topol EJ, Hacke W, for the CAPRIE Investigators. Benefit of clopidogrel over aspirin is amplified in patients with a history of ischemic events. *Stroke* 2004;35:528–532.

182. Yusuf S, Zhao F, Mehta SR, et al. Effects of clopidogrel in addition to aspirin in patients with acute coronary syndromes without ST-segment elevation. *N Engl J Med* 2001; 345:494–502.

183. Yusuf S, Mehta SR, Zhao F, et al. Early and late effects of clopidogrel in patients with acute coronary syndromes. *Circulation* 2003;107:966–972.

184. Berger PB, Bell MR, Rihal CS, et al. Clopidogrel versus ticlopidine after intracoronary stent placement. *J Am Coll Cardiol* 1999;34:1891–1894.

185. Dangas G, Mehran R, Abizaid AS, et al. Combination therapy with aspirin plus clopidogrel versus aspirin plus ticlopidine for prevention of subacute thrombosis after successful native coronary stenting. *Am J Cardio* 1907;87:470–472.

186. Bhatt DL, Kapadia SR, Bajzer CT, et al. Dual antiplatelet therapy with clopidogrel and aspirin after carotid artery stenting. *J Invas Cardiol* 2001;13:767–771.

187. Jarvis B, Simpson K. Clopidogrel: a review of its use in the prevention of atherothrombosis. *Drugs* 2000;60:347–377.

188. Hankey GJ, Sudlow CLM, Dunbabin DW. Thienopyridine derivatives (ticlopidine, clopidogrel) versus aspirin for preventing stroke and other serious vascular events in high vascular risk patients. Cochrane Database of Systematic Reviews 2000;CD001246.

189. Easton JD. Evidence with antiplatelet therapy and ADP-receptor antagonists. *Cerebrovasc Dis* 2003;16:20–26.

190. Paciaroni M, Bogousslavsky J. Clopidogrel for cerebrovascular prevention. *Cerebrovasc Dis* 1999;9:253–260.

191. Gaspoz JM, Coxson PG, Goldman PA, et al. Cost effectiveness of aspirin, clopidogrel, or both for secondary prevention of coronary heart disease. *N Engl J Med* 2002;346: 1800–1806.

192. Rivey MP, Alexander MR, Taylor JW. Dipyridamole: a critical evaluation. *Drug Intell Clin Pharm* 1984;18:869–880.

193. Gibbs CR, Lip GY. Do we still need dipyridamole? *Br J Clin Pharmacol* 1998;45:323–328.

194. De Schryver ELLM, Algra A, van Gijn J. Dipyridamole for preventing stroke and other vascular events in patients with vascular disease. Cochrane Database of Systematic Reviews 2003;CD001820.

195. Theis JG, Deichsel G, Marshall S. Rapid development of tolerance to dipyridamole-associated headaches. *Br J Clin Pharmacol* 1999;48:750–755.

196. Humphreys DM, Street J, Schumacher H, Bertrand-Hardy JM, Palluk R. Dipyridamole may be used safely in patients with ischaemic heart disease. *Int J Clin Pract* 2002;56: 121–127.

197. De Schryver EL, ESPRIT Study Group. Dipyridamole in stroke prevention: effect of dipyridamole on blood pressure. *Stroke* 2003;34:2339–2342.

198. Sullivan JM, Harken DE, Gorlin R. Pharmacologic control of thromboembolic complications of cardiac-valve replacement. *N Engl J Med* 1971;284:1391–1394.

199. The Persantine-Aspirin Reinfarction Study (PARIS) Research Group. The Persantine-Aspirin Reinfarction Study. *Circulation* 1980;62:V85-V88.

200. The American-Canadian Co-Operative Study group. Persantine Aspirin Trial in cerebral ischemia. Part II: Endpoint results. *Stroke* 1985;16:406–415.

201. Sivenius J, Laakso M, Penttila IM. The European stroke prevention study: results according to sex. *Neurology* 1991;41:1189–1192.

202. ESPRIT Study Group. Aspirin plus dipyridamole versus aspirin alone after cerebral ischaemia of arterial origin (ESPRIT). Randomised controlled trial. *Lancet* 2006;367: 1665–1673.

203. Tijssen JG. Low-dose and high-dose acetylsalicylic acid, with and without dipyridamole: a review of clinical trial results. *Neurology* 1998;51:S15-S16

204. Wilterkink JL, Easton JD. Dipyridamole plus aspirin in cerebrovascular disease. *Arch Neurol* 1999;56:1087–1092.

205. Shah H, Gondek K. Aspirin plus extended-release dipyridamole or clopidogrel compared with aspirin monotherapy for the prevention of recurret ischemic stroke: a cost-effective analysis. *Clin Ther* 2000;22:362–370.

206. Chambers M, Hutton J, Gladman J. Cost-effectiveness analysis of antiplatelet therapy in the prevention of recurrent stroke in the UK. Aspirin, dipyridamole and aspirin-dipyridamole. *Pharmacoeconomics* 1999;16:577–593.

207. The Canadian Cooperative Study Group. A randomized trial of aspirin and sulfinpyrazone in threatened stroke. *N Engl J Med* 1978;299:53–59.

208. Bergamasco B, Benna P, Carolei A, Rasura M, Rudelli G, Fieschi C. A randomized trial comparing ticlopidine hydrochloride with indobufen for the prevention of stroke in high-risk patients (TISS Study). Ticlopidine Indobufen Stroke Study. *Funct Neurology* 1997;12:33–43.

209. Morocutti C, Amabile G, Fattapposta F, et al. Indobufen versus warfarin in the secondary prevention of major vascular events in nonrheumatic atrial fibrillation. SIFA (Studio Italiano Fibrillazione Atriale) Investigators. *Stroke* 1997;28:1015–1021.

210. Matias-Guiu J, Ferro JM, Alvarez-Sabín J, et al. Comparison of triflusal and aspirin for prevention of vascular events in patients after cerebral infarction: the TACIP Study: a randomized, double-blind, multicenter trial. *Stroke* 2003;34: 840–848.

211. Topol EJ. Prevention of cardiovascular ischemic complications with new platelet glycoprotein IIb/IIIa inhibitors. *Am Heart J* 1995;130:666–672.

212. Ringleb PA, Hacke W. Antiplatelet therapy in stroke prevention. *Cerebrovasc Dis* 2003;15:43–48.

213. Topol EJ, Easton JD, Amarenco P, et al. Design of the blockade of the glycoprotein IIb/IIIa receptor to avoid vascular occlusion (BRAVO) trial. *Am Heart J* 2000;139:927–933.

214. The SYMPHONY Investigators. Comparison of sibrafiban with aspirin for prevention of cardiovascular events after acute coronary syndromes: a randomised trial. *Lancet* 2000;355:337–345.

215. Cannon CP, McCabe CH, Wilcox RG, et al. Oral glycoprotein IIb/IIIa inhibition with orbofiban in patients with unstable coronary syndromes (OPUS-TIMI 16) trial. *Circulation* 2000;102:149–156.

216. Schneider R. Results of hemorheologically active treatment with pentoxifylline in patients with cerebrovascular disease. *Angiology* 1989;40:987–993.

217. Apollonio A, Castignani P, Magrini L, Angeletti R. Ticlopidine-pentoxifylline combination in the treatment of atherosclerosis and the prevention of cerebrovascular accidents. *J Int Med Res* 1989;17:28–35.

218. Bornstein NM. Antiplatelet drugs: how to select them and possibilities of combined treatment. *Cerebrovasc Dis* 2001;11:96–99.

219. Urbano LA, Bogousslavsky J. Antiplatelet drugs in ischemic stroke prevention: from monotherapy to combined treatment. *Cerebrovasc Dis* 2004;17(suppl 1):74–80.

220. Teal PA. Recent clinical trial results with antiplatelet therapy: implications in stroke prevention. *Cerebrovasc Dis* 2004;17(suppl 3):6–10.

221. Hankey GJ. Ongoing and planned trials of antiplatelet therapy in the acute and long-term management of patients with ischemic brain syndromes: setting a new standard of care. *Cerebrovasc Dis* 2004;17(suppl 3): 11–16.

222. Cadroy Y, Bossavy JP, Thalamas C, Sagnard L, Sakariassen K, Boneu B. Early potent antithrombotic effect with combined aspirin and a loading dose of clopidogrel on experimental arterial thrombogenesis in humans. *Circulation* 2000;101:2823–2828.

223. The Clopidogrel in Unstable Angina to Prevent Recurrent Events Trial Investigators. Effects of clopidogrel in addition to aspirin in patients with acute coronary syndromes without ST-segment elevation. *N Engl J Med* 2001;345: 494–502.

224. Diener HC, Bogousslavsky J, Brass LM, et al. Aspirin and clopidogrel compared to clopidogrel alone after recent ischemic stroke or transient ischemic attack in high-risk patients (MATCH). Randomised, double-blind, placebo-controlled trial. *Lancet* 2004;364:331–337.

225. Bhatt DL, Fox KA, Hacke W, et al. Clopidogrel and aspirin versus aspirin alone for prevention of atherothrombotic events. *N Engl J Med* 2006;354:1706–1717.

226. O'Connor CM, Gattis WA, Hellkamp AS, et al. Comparison of two aspirin doses on ischemic stroke in post-myocardial infarction patients in the warfarin (Coumadin) Aspirin Reinfarction Study (CARS). *Am J Cardio* 2001;88: 541–546.

227. Massel D, Little SH. Risks and benefits of adding antiplatelet therapy to warfarin among patients with prosthetic heart valves: a meta-analysis. *J Am Coll Cardiol* 2001;37:569–578.

228. Petersen P, Boysen G, Godtfredsen J, Andersen ED, Andersen B. Placebo-controlled, randomised trial of warfarin and aspirin for prevention of thromboembolic complications in chronic atrial fibrillation. The Copenhagen AFASAK study. *Lancet* 1989;1:175–179.

229. Stroke Prevention in Atrial Fibrillation Investigators. Stroke prevention in atrial fibrillation study. Final results. *Circulation* 1991;84:527–539.

230. Connolly SJ, Laupacis A, Gent M, Roberts RS, Cairns JA, Joyner C. Canadian Atrial Fibrillation Anticoagulation (CAFA) Study. *J Am Coll Cardiol* 1991;18:349–355.

231. Ezekowitz MD, Bridgers SL, James KE, et al. Warfarin in the prevention of stroke associated with nonrheumatic atrial fibrillation. Veterans Affairs Stroke Prevention in Nonrheumatic Atrial Fibrillation Investigators. *N Engl J Med* 1992;327:1406–1412.

232. The SPAF III Writing Committee for the Stroke Prevention in Atrial Fibrillation Investigators. Patients with non-valvular atrial fibrillation at low risk for stroke. Stroke Prevention in Atrial Fibrillation III Study. *JAMA* 1998;279:1273–1277.

233. The Boston Area Anticoagulation Trial for Atrial Fibrillation Investigators. The effect of low-dose warfarin on the risk of stroke in patients with non-rheumatic atrial fibrillation. *N Engl J Med* 1990;323:1505–1511.

234. Gullov AL, Koeford BG, Petersen P, et al. Fixed mini-dose warfarin and aspirin alone and in combination versus adjusted dose warfarin for stroke prevention in atrial fibrillation. Second Copenhagen Atrial Fibrillation, Aspirin, and Anticoagulation Study. *Arch Intern Med* 1998;158:1513–1521.

235. Hellemons BS, Langenberg M, Lodder J, et al. Primary prevention of arterial thromboembolism in non-rheumatic atrial fibrillation in primary care. Randomised, controlled trial comparing two intensities of coumarin with aspirin. *Br Med J* 1999;319:958–964.

CHAPTER 20

Surgical Interventions to Prevent Ischemic Stroke

Ever since the first carotid endarterectomy (CEA) was performed in the early 1950s, surgery has been an important aspect of strategies to lessen the risk of cerebral infarction among high-risk individuals. Several procedures have been developed to improve blood flow to the brain or to remove a source of emboli (Table 20-1). Operations have addressed both intracranial and extracranial arterial disease. More recently, cardiac procedures aimed at reducing the risk of embolism and endovascular procedures aimed at improving cerebral circulation have been introduced. Technical advances, particularly in endovascular interventions, portend dramatic changes in the surgical methods to prevent cerebral infarction. The operations are the subject of considerable controversy, which partially continues to this day. Still, modern clinical research provides important data about the safety and utility of the operations. Indications and contraindications for several of the procedures now are known. Both surgeons and physicians interested in prevention of stroke deserve credit for their support to these studies, which are the model for trials testing promising surgical interventions. Because some of the new surgical procedures will likely be shown to be successful, management to prevent stroke will likely differ radically in 10–20 years than what is recommended currently.

▶ CAROTID ENDARTERECTOMY

The rates of CEA in the United States have varied considerably during the last 30 years. Between 1971 and 1986, the annual frequency of CEA increased from 15,000 to more than 100,000 operations. It then declined to approximately 60,000 per year after neurologists expressed concerns about the overuse of the surgery.[1] After clinical trials demonstrated that surgery was effective in lowering the risk of stroke, especially among symptomatic patients, the frequency of CEA increased dramatically, and now approximately 128,000–140,000 operations are being done in the United States.[2,3] CEA now is one of the most commonly performed surgical procedures in the United States. Similar trends are reported in other countries. For example, the frequency of CEA in the United Kingdom has risen; still the number of operations is much lower in Britain than in the United States.[4] At present, CEA is the standard operation recommended for treatment of high-risk patients with atherosclerosis of the internal carotid artery. However, with the increasing popularity of angioplasty and stenting for treatment of extracranial arterial lesions, including stenoses at the origin of the internal carotid artery, the indications for CEA may change again. If endovascular procedures are found to be equal to or superior to CEA, the number of operations might decline dramatically in the future.

The rates of CEA in the United States vary with geographic location, age, sex, and ethnicity. The geographic variances have not been explained. The rate of CEA among men is approximately 1.9 times that of women.[5] This difference probably reflects the younger age of men

► **TABLE 20-1.** SURGICAL INTERVENTIONS TO PREVENT ISCHEMIC STROKE

Endarterectomy
    Internal carotid artery
    External carotid artery
    Middle cerebral artery
    Origin of vertebral artery
Bypass operations
    Superficial temporal artery-to-middle cerebral artery
    Branches of basilar artery
    Subclavian artery
    Innominate artery
    Vertebral artery
    Encephaloduroarteriomyosynangiosis
    Encephaloduromyosynangiosis
    Duroarteriosynangiosis
Other arterial operations
    Plication of the internal carotid artery—stump syndrome
    Resection of kink or loop of internal carotid artery
    Resection of arterial dissection
    Resection of a segment of the aorta
    Graded dilation of internal carotid artery—fibromuscular dysplasia
Cardiac operations to remove a source of embolization
    Valve replacement
    Cardioversion or pacemaker
    Resect atrial myxoma or other cardiac tumor
    Close PFO
        Surgery
        Endovascular insertion of device
    Obliteration of left atrial appendage
Endovascular arterial procedures
    Angioplasty and stenting
        Extracranial arteries
        Intracranial arteries
    Balloon occlusion or coiling

who develop severe atherosclerotic disease of the internal carotid artery. In the past, a difference in the rates of operations was noted between African American and white patients. This difference appears to be diminishing. Oddone et al.[6] found that the frequency of CEA was similar in black and white patients. Still, CEA is less commonly performed among persons of Asian ancestry, and the number of operations in eastern Asia is proportionally less than that in Europe or North America. These observations probably reflect differences in the location of atherosclerotic lesions in the intracranial or extracranial arteries among different ethnic groups.

Rationale

An advanced atherosclerotic plaque at the origin of the internal carotid artery can be the source of emboli that go to the eye or brain. Emboli can consist of atherosclerotic debris (cholesterol embolus) arising from an ulcerated plaque or of a piece of thrombus that develops at the site of a fractured plaque. The latter probably is the more common situation. The secondary thromboembolism can go to the eye, causing amaurosis fugax or retinal infarction, or it travels to the brain, most commonly to the territory of the middle cerebral artery, leading to transient ischemic attack (TIA) or cerebral infarction. In addition, a large thrombus at the site can occlude the internal carotid artery. A high-grade stenosis of the internal carotid artery also can reduce blood flow to the brain and hemodynamic insufficiency also can cause transient or permanent ischemic deficits (Fig. 20-1). Thus, the rationales for surgery are to (1) remove the plaque as a source for emboli and (2) restore or improve blood flow to the ipsilateral hemisphere and eye (Fig. 20-2). There is strong evidence of the effects of CEA on cerebral blood flow. Changes in blood flow, including collateral changes, can occur with CEA.[7] Among symptomatic patients, CEA improves mean transit time and increase cerebral blood flow in both white matter and watershed regions.[8,9] In addition, CEA improves cerebrovascular reactivity.[10] Even if the patient does not have symptoms secondary to hypoperfusion, improvement in blood flow might limit the ischemic symptoms due to small emboli. The improved flow may "wash" the emboli out of the small arterioles before they can cause ischemia.

Procedure

The operation is relatively straightforward[11] (Table 20-2). In some cases, the surgeon places a patch to increase the size of the lesion or to prevent recurrent arterial stenosis.[12] Both surgical and anesthesia techniques have evolved in an attempt to improve both the

► **TABLE 20-2.** PERIOPERATIVE PROCEDURES OF CEA

Anesthesia
    General
    Local or regional
Cardiac monitoring
Blood pressure monitoring
Neurological monitoring
    Electroencephalography
    Evoked potentials
Cerebrovascular monitoring
    Transcranial Doppler ultrasonography
    Measuring distal carotid artery pressure
Surgical techniques
    Use of a shunt
    Patch grafting
Prevent thromboembolism
    Heparin
    Aspirin
    Clopidogrel
Management of arterial hypertension

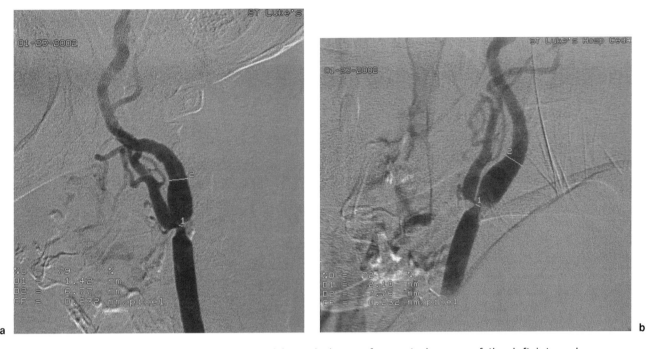

Figure 20-1. Anteroposterior and lateral views of an arteriogram of the left internal carotid artery demonstrate a high-grade stenosis of the origin of artery. The residual lumen at the stenosis (a) is compared to a normal distal segment of the vessel (b) to calculate the severity of the stenosis. A high-grade stenosis of the origin of the external carotid artery also is found.

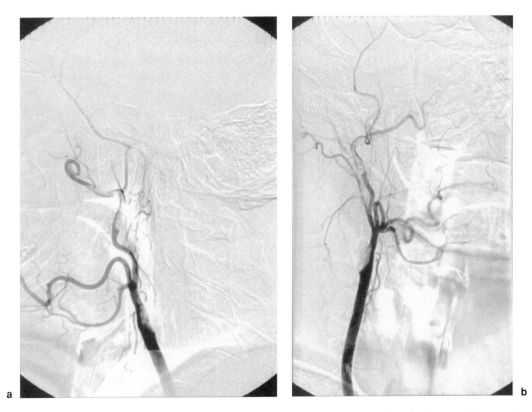

Figure 20-2. Two views of a left carotid arteriogram show intraluminal thrombi (a) just above the bifurcation and (b) in the intracavernous segment of the internal carotid artery.

safety and the efficacy of the operation. The use of synthetic or venous patches might lower the risk of perioperative stroke.[13] Patches generally are used when treating a female patient, largely because of the smaller caliber of the internal carotid artery among women. Limited data suggest that patches will lower the risk of recurrent arterial occlusion or recurrent stenosis, following carotid surgery.[14] However, the utility of this surgical adjunct in reducing the risk of stroke or death is not established.[14] Data about the relative usefulness of synthetic or venous patches in performing CEA also do not exist.[15] As such, the use of a patch remains at the discretion of the surgeon and the decision is made on a case-by-case basis. Intraoperative monitoring using the electroencephalography (EEG) or transcranial Doppler ultrasonography might permit detection of the early changes of hypoperfusion.[16] Shunts have been used to maintain flow around the arterial site. Some surgeons routinely place a shunt, while others use changes on EEG, transcranial Doppler flow measurements, or clinical status as a guide for use of this device. Still, the placement of shunt does involve additional arterial injuries that can be a source for thromboembolism. A systemic review of available data could find no information to support or refute the use of either routine or selective shunting as part of CEA.[17] Thus, as with the use of patches, shunting is decided on a case-by-case basis. Because the surgery involves exposure of the thrombogenic arterial wall tissue or residual plaque to the circulating blood and incites thrombosis, embolism is a potential complication. Intraoperative and postoperative use of heparin or antiplatelet agents might lessen the likelihood of intraluminal thrombosis. Although these medications are used regularly, no data are available to guide the selection of medications. In addition, these agents might be associated with an increased risk of perioperative bleeding.

While most operations are performed with the use of general anesthesia, some surgeons prefer local or regional anesthesia. As with most major operations, general anesthesia gives better control of the operative field. Some agents used for general anesthesia, such as barbiturates, might also have neuroprotective actions. Performing the operation under local or regional anesthesia allows the surgeon to monitor the patient's neurological status during the procedure.[18] Local or regional anesthesia can be performed if a patient has severe heart or pulmonary disease, which could increase operative risks if general anesthesia is used. One study found that regional or local anesthesia is associated with a reduced chance of major nonneurological complications following CEA.[19] Local or regional anesthesia also reduces length of stay in the hospital and hospital costs.[18,20] A systemic review of the available data does not provide information about the relative utility of either general or local anesthesia for patients undergoing carotid surgery.[21]

Thus, the surgeon will continue to decide about anesthesia on an individual patient basis.

In the clinical trials testing CEA, the findings of arteriography were used to select the patients to be treated surgically.[22–25] Unfortunately, arteriography is an invasive procedure that can be associated with serious complications, including stroke. In the trial of CEA for treatment of patients with an asymptomatic stenosis, the risks of arteriography were higher than those accompanying the operation.[23] As a result, surgeons are often using other vascular imaging studies to select patients for operation. The improvements in duplex imaging or contrast-enhanced magnetic resonance angiography are changing practice, and patients now are selected for CEA based on the results of these tests[26] (see Chapter 8). Arteriography, as a preoperative procedure, probably is limited to cases in which a high-grade stenosis (string sign) cannot be differentiated from an occlusion or if the noninvasive studies cannot determine the upper and lower limits of the plaque.[11]

CEA is relatively expensive and it involves a surgeon's fee, anesthesiologist's fee, operating room costs, costs of the baseline evaluation and monitoring, and hospitalization. With focused perioperative care, the length of hospitalization following CEA has been shortened. Hernandez et al.[27] reported that most patients might be discharged within 24 h of surgery. Patients who need longer hospitalizations usually have other serious comorbid diseases, including insulin-dependent diabetes mellitus, major cardiac diseases, or previous stroke. A strategy that involves no arteriography, regional anesthesia, avoidance of inpatient care in the intensive care unit, and early discharge of stable patients can reduce economic costs and yet maintains safety and efficacy of CEA.[28]

Safety

CEA usually is done as a prophylactic procedure for treatment of either symptomatic or asymptomatic patients. Because many operatively treated patients would never have stroke even without surgery, the operation must be extraordinarily safe. Even symptomatic patients with high-grade stenoses are not helped if the operation cannot be done with a reasonable degree of safety. The potential risk for serious side complications should be weighed in comparison to likely benefits before recommending surgery.[29] The serious complications include ischemic or hemorrhagic stroke, myocardial infarction or death, usually due to stroke or heart disease. Other less serious complications also occur (Table 20-3). Guidelines for the maximal rates of complications following CEA that can be accepted are available.[30] These statements provide guidance about the anticipated frequencies of serious adverse events as influenced by the patient's status and the indications for surgery. For example, the acceptable

▶ **TABLE 20-3.** COMPLICATIONS OF CEA

Cerebral infarction
   Arterial occlusion
   Thromboembolism
   Embolization of atherosclerotic debris
   Hypoperfusion
Recurrent arterial stenosis
Hyperperfusion syndrome
   Cerebral hemorrhage
   Seizures
   Headache
Cranial or cervical nerve palsy
   Hypoglossal nerve
   Facial nerve
   Vagus nerve
   Recurrent laryngeal nerve
Blood pressure disturbances
   Hypotension
   Hypertension
   Myocardial ischemia
Local complications
   Wound infection
   Perioperative hematoma
   Tracheal compression

rate of complications in an asymptomatic patient is much lower than that of a symptomatic patient having a second operation at the same site.

Even with the improvements in technique and perioperative care, the risks of CEA vary considerably. In a community study approximately 25 years ago, Easton and Sherman[31] found that almost 20 percent of patients had major complications. More recently, Chaturvedi et al.[32] reported a 30-day rate of stroke or death of approximately 11.4 percent. The North American Symptomatic Carotid Endarterectomy Trial (NASCET) investigators reported that the perioperative mortality of CEA was 1.1 percent and another 1.8 percent of patients had disabling strokes.[22] This trial involved participation of the surgeons who met specific standards for low perioperative morbidity and mortality. The rates among operatively treated patients in the Asymptomatic Carotid Atherosclerosis Study were very low.[23]

Overall, the rates of major complications in general practice are higher than those reported in clinical trials. In a large survey, Lanska and Kryscio[33] reported that in-hospital mortality was 1.2 percent following CEA; mortality was 0.9 percent among persons younger than 65 and 1.7 percent among persons older than 75. Still, age, per se, is not a contraindication for CEA. Surgery can be performed with a reasonable degree of safety in persons older than 80.[34] While there are concerns that the smaller caliber of the internal carotid artery in woman is associated with an increased risk of complications and might explain some of the lack of benefit of CEA in asymptomatic women, no major difference in perioperative morbidity was noted in women and men.[5,35] Women should be considered as reasonable candidates for CEA.[36,37] The rates of perioperative complications are similar among white and African-American patients.[38]

Several clinical or vascular imaging features predict the likelihood of major complications of CEA. The chances of stroke are highest among persons who are neurologically unstable.[29] However, such patients are at high risk for vascular events without surgery. Patients with crescendo TIA or recent stroke have a higher risk of neurological complications than do patients having CEA for treatment of an asymptomatic stenosis. In general, the risks are the same following a TIA or an ischemic stroke.[29] In the past, surgeons waited 6 or more weeks after stroke before performing CEA because of concerns that revascularization would lead to hemorrhage or worsening of brain edema. Several groups looked at the timing of surgery and concluded that CEA can be performed in neurologically unstable patients with a reasonable degree of safety.[39–42] Paty et al.[43] report that operative exploration and endarterectomy can be done safely and feasibly for acutely symptomatic occlusions of the internal carotid artery. Giordano[44] concluded that CEA can be performed within a few days of stroke if the computed tomography (CT) is normal. In a systematic review, no major difference was found between patients who had surgery within 3–6 weeks following stroke and those who had later operations.[29] Thus, minor stroke with minimal or no changes on CT does not preclude early CEA, but the operation should be delayed if the patient has major neurological impairments or a large infarction visualized by brain imaging.[45–48]

Other patient characteristics are associated with a high rate of operative complications. The presence of severe comorbid medical diseases increases the complexity of surgery, anesthesia, and perioperative medical management (Tables 20-4 and 20-5). While the rate of major complications is low among persons having CEA for treatment of asymptomatic carotid artery disease, the presence of severe comorbidity increases risks to approximately 5.56 percent.[49] Potential high-risk patients include those with congestive heart failure, recent myocardial infarction, oxygen-dependent pulmonary disease, renal disease, contralateral carotid occlusion, stenosis located above the second cervical vertebra, recurrent operation, recent coronary artery bypass graft (CABG), neurological symptoms of less than 6 weeks, or previous neck radiation.[50] Still, Gasparis et al.[50] found that CEA can be performed in high-risk patients with a reasonable degree of safety. However, the patients with another serious medical illnesses have a high likelihood of death or disability in the years following CEA. Most of the deaths are due to noncerebrovascular diseases, and thus overall medical management of the patients is as

▶ **TABLE 20-4.** RISK FACTORS FOR COMPLICATIONS OF CEA

Contraindications for surgery
    Recent myocardial infarction
    Unstable angina
    Recent major ipsilateral cerebral infarction
    Other life-threatening disease
Factors associated with increased risk for complications
    Neurologically unstable
        Recent TIA
        Crescendo TIA
        Acute ischemic stroke
        Events not responding to medical interventions
    Extensive vascular disease
        Occlusion of contralateral internal carotid artery
        Intracranial (tandem) atherosclerosis
        Intraluminal thrombus
        Previous CEA (recurrent stenosis)
        Radiation therapy—neck
    Clinical factors
        Advanced age
        History of coronary artery disease
        Chronic lung disease
        Hypertension
        Diabetes mellitus
        Obesity
    Surgeon's experience

important as CEA. The presence of more than two of the above-mentioned risk factors is associated with a reduced likelihood of a 5-year survival following CEA.[51] An Australian study found that approximately 20 percent of patients who have successful CEA are dead within 4 years and that most of the deaths are due to vascular disease.[52] Thus, most patients with a short life expectancy due to other serious diseases probably should not have CEA.

Many patients have severe coronary artery disease and carotid artery disease. Myocardial infarction is the most common cause of early or delayed death following CEA.[53] Patients having carotid surgery are at risk for myocardial infarction and stroke is a potential complica-

▶ **TABLE 20-5.** CLINICAL FACTORS THAT INCREASE THE RISK FOR CAROTID ENDARTERECTOMY

Asymptomatic stenosis 1.62 times greater than asymptomatic stenosis
Transient ischemic attack 2.31 times greater than ocular ischemia
Recurrent stenosis (previous surgery) 1.95 times greater than first operation
Urgent/evolving neurological symptoms 19.2 times greater than stable patients

Estimated increases in risk of surgery.

tion of CABG surgery. In some circumstances of treatment of patients with both diseases, CEA is performed first and in others CABG is done initially. In addition, a combined approach of treating severe coronary artery disease and carotid artery disease is widely used, but this strategy is controversial.[53] No data support the superiority of any strategy for doing the operations in any particular sequence. Blacker et al.[54] recently concluded that treatment of the symptomatic vessel should take precedence. A recent multistate study demonstrated that the combined stroke and death rate of patients having simultaneous CEA and CABG was 17.7 percent[55] In another study, Halm et al.[49] found that major complications occurred in 10.32 percent of patients having CEA and CABG. However, Vitali et al.[56] reported that combining CEA and CABG could be accomplished with reasonable safety. Evaluating another strategy, Naylor et al.[57] reported that 10–12 percent of patients having either staged or combined operative procedures had mortality or major morbidity within 30 days. Doing the coronary procedure first was associated with the highest risk of stroke. Conversely, myocardial infarction or death was increased among those patients who have CEA as the initial operative procedure. Prophylactic CEA prior to CABG probably is justified only in patients with stable coronary artery disease and good ejection fraction.[58] Patients with severe coronary artery disease should have local anesthesia for CEA.[58] The combination of off-pump concomitant CABG and CEA has been used because of the presumed lower risk for stroke.[59] This tactic likely will be evaluated further. Supplementing surgery (either CABG or CEA) with endovascular therapy also will likely be evaluated in the future. At present, no particular plan for treatment of severe or symptomatic carotid and coronary artery disease has been established as most useful.

The extent of the atherosclerotic cerebrovascular disease and the other findings detected by vascular imaging also affects decisions about surgery. The presence of an intraluminal thrombus is associated with a high risk of thromboembolism during CEA (see Fig. 20-2). Manipulation of the artery during surgery might promote release of pieces of thrombi. Intraluminal clots are most commonly associated with severe stenosis and most commonly, detected among symptomatic patients. The thrombus probably is secondary to fracturing and ulceration of the plaque. While surgery can be done in an emergency, the alternative approach is to give anticoagulants for a period of several weeks to allow for lysis of the clot prior to CEA. The presence of an occlusion of the contralateral internal carotid artery also is correlated with a high operative risk; the likelihood of perioperative mortality is approximately 5 percent.[60–62] Baker et al.[63] found no benefit from surgical treatment of a patient with an asymptomatic stenosis and contralateral internal carotid artery, but the lack of advantage of surgery probably is secondary to the generally low rate of strokes among asymptomatic patients. Reed et al.[51] found that contralateral occlusion was the only factor that predicted adverse events following CEA. However, the chances of death or stroke also are among medically treated patients. The risks of doing surgery must be compared to the chances of major morbidity or mortality if CEA is not done. Although the risks of surgery are increased, the long-term benefit in reducing stroke still supports operative treatment for most cases if the patient has no other contraindication.[64] The presence of a contralateral occlusion is not a contraindication for CEA. Intracranial atherosclerotic disease (siphon stenosis) or poor collateral circulation from the contralateral internal carotid artery or the posterior circulation also portend an increased risk of stroke. However, affected patients can have surgery.

Approximately 5–10 percent of patients have recurrent stenosis following CEA. Recurrent stenosis develops most commonly among women and persons with small carotid arteries.[65] Some cases of recurrent stenosis are associated with new neurological symptoms but most are asymptomatic and patients have the narrowing detected by follow-up vascular imaging. The new narrowing is often due to development of fibrosis and scar tissue rather than the formation of a new plaque. In addition, the soft tissues next to the carotid artery also will have postoperative changes. Thus, it is not surprising that the rate of perioperative complications is increased when the artery is operatively treated for a second time.[30] The risks may be particularly high if the contralateral internal carotid artery is occluded.[66] Rather than performing a second CEA, many physicians now are recommending angioplasty and stenting.[67] However, the utility of endovascular treatment in this situation has not been established. In addition, AbuRahma et al.[68] found that recurrent carotid stenosis generally can be treated with the same degree of safety as angioplasty and stenting, although patients having a second operation were at risk for complicating cranial nerve palsies. Surgery often is difficult if a patient has had prior radiation therapy to the neck. Besides inducing arterial changes that lead to a severe stenosis, the radiation also affects adjacent tissues. Both surgical dissection and postoperative healing can be hampered. In addition, baroreceptors in the carotid body can respond abnormally and blood pressure management can be challenging. While patients with radiation-induced carotid stenosis are being treated with endovascular interventions, surgery remains an option. Leseche et al.[69] reported that CEA could be done safely among patients who have had cervical radiation therapy.

A majority of complications of CEA are secondary to technical errors, and thus the skill of the surgeon is critical for success.[70,71] A surgeon with poor results should not perform the operation. Physicians and surgeons should know what are the surgeons' rates of complications. The operative success of the surgeon depends upon the type of practice. A surgeon who operates only on asymptomatic patients should have a much lower rate of complications than a colleague who treats neurologically unstable patients. Both the numbers of operations performed by the surgeons and the procedures done in an institution are important markers of the risk of complications.[72,73] Perioperative complications are lowest when surgeons who have done a large number of operations perform the operation. Such surgeons perform approximately half the operations in the United States.[74] Cowan et al.[74] found that perioperative mortality was 0.44 percent for high-volume surgeons, 0.63 percent for medium-volume surgeons, and 1.1 percent for low-volume surgeons. For same groups, the perioperative stroke rate was 1.14 percent for high-volume surgeons, 1.63 percent for medium-volume surgeons, and 2.03 percent for low-volume surgeons. Quality improvement measures can lower the rates of complications of CEA.[75] Both the surgeons and their institutions should implement them.

Ischemic stroke is the most common neurological complication of CEA. One report estimated the frequency as high as 7 percent.[76] Infarctions usually are the result of embolization of thrombi or pieces of atherosclerotic debris. Embolization usually occurs at the time of the initial manipulation of the artery or when the flow is restored to the brain at the end of surgery.[77] Strokes also can be secondary to hypoperfusion or acute thrombotic occlusion of the internal carotid artery. Most ischemic strokes are recognized as the patient is awakening from anesthesia. The discovery of new focal neurological deficits should lead to immediate reimaging of the brain and artery. Patients might need surgical reexploration with removal of the clot in order to restore flow. In order to lower the risk of ischemic stroke, surgeons often prescribe antiplatelet agents or anticoagulants in the perioperative period.

Besides cerebral infarction, hemorrhages that can be fatal or disabling are potential complications. The 30-day risk of ipsilateral hemorrhage in NASCET was 0.64 percent.[78,79] Presumably, the bleeding is secondary to a sudden increase of perfusion to a vulnerable area of brain. The perioperative use of anticoagulants might increase the chances of intracranial hemorrhage.

Cerebral hyperperfusion, which is an important cause of neurological impairments and which can lead to intracerebral hemorrhage, can follow CEA[76,80] (Table 20-6). Presumably, the increased perfusion to the brain is secondary to vascular changes that are secondary to impaired autoregulation distal to the original stenosis. Presumably, the sudden surge in flow overwhelms normal physiological responses and vascular congestion, brain edema, and bleeding results. In some ways, the changes mimic those found with hypertensive encephalopathy.

▶ **TABLE 20-6.** FEATURES OF HYPERPERFUSION SYNDROME

Treatment of high-grade stenosis of internal carotid artery
    Carotid endarterectomy
    Angioplasty and stenting
Develops within 1–8 days of procedure (peak 2–3 days)
Overwhelms cerebral autoregulation
    Develops brain edema
    Develops intracranial bleeding
    Occurs with volatile blood pressure
Symptoms
    Headache
    Seizures
    Focal neurological impairments
    Decreased consciousness
Prophylaxis aimed at controlling blood pressure

While this complication usually occurs among patients having CEA for treatment of a very severe stenosis, Ascher et al.[80] found no correlation between hyperperfusion syndrome and the presence of severe ipsilateral or contralateral carotid disease. In addition, the illness might occur more frequently among patients with a volatile blood pressure or severe hypertension following the operation.[80] Most cases of hyperperfusion syndrome occur within 1–8 days following surgery.[80] With the hyperperfusion syndrome, patients have increasingly severe headache, seizures, or progressively worsening focal neurological impairments. Some patients will have disturbances in consciousness. Careful control of blood pressure is the primary strategy to prevent hyperperfusion syndrome; the goal is to avoid postoperative hypertension. Hartsell et al.[81] concluded that the risk of hyperperfusion might be lowered if the operation is done under regional anesthesia rather than general anesthesia.

Seizures are a relatively uncommon complication; the frequency is estimated as approximately 0.8 percent.[82] Seizures are most common among patients with severe disease and might be related to severe hypertension or hyperperfusion following the surgery. Most seizures occur within the first few days following the operation.

Cranial neuropathies can be secondary to trauma in the operative field. The frequency and types of cranial and cervical nerve injuries complicating CEA were reviewed by Ballotta et al.[83] In the large international trial, Ferguson et al.[84] reported that approximately 8.6 percent have postoperative nerve palsies. The most commonly affected nerves are hypoglossal, recurrent laryngeal, superior laryngeal, marginal mandibular, and greater auricular. Injury to the vagal nerve or its branches can cause dysphagia or dysphonia. Trauma to the hypoglossal nerve causes paralysis of the ipsilateral side of the tongue. Stretching or traction on the nerve is the usual cause of the palsy. The nerves can also be compressed by a local hematoma.[85] The cranial and cervical nerve palsies are most commonly found among persons having a long plaque in the carotid artery, extensive dissection, or placement of a patch. Most cranial nerve palsies recover over several months. Dissection also can involve severing of small cutaneous nerves that can result in areas of anesthesia along the angle of the jaw. Men might note an area of numbness while shaving.

Other complications of CEA are relatively uncommon. Infections are potential complications and the risk might be increased if a patch is inserted.[86,87] Pseudoaneurysm formation can also complicate the use of patching of the internal carotid artery following CEA.[87] Postoperative bleeding can cause a cervical hematoma that can lead to compression of the trachea and compromise of the airway.

Potential Indications

Several studies, including clinical trials, evaluated the indications for carotid surgery (Table 20-7). When looking at the efficacy of the operation, the relative risk of the surgery causing early morbidity or mortality must be compared to the potential benefit of long-term reduction in stroke. Based on the results of the large clinical trials performed in Europe and North America in the late 1980s and early 1990s, one can conclude that CEA is effective. It does lower the risk of stroke among persons with high-grade stenosis and is especially helpful among persons who have had warning neurological symptoms. While the utility of the operation is influenced primarily by the severity of the stenosis, the presence of ulceration of the plaque also predicts a benefit from CEA. The indications for and the limitations of CEA are included in treatment guidelines[30]

The most robust evidence for utility of CEA is found for treatment of patients who have recent ischemic symptoms, as shown by large European and North

▶ **TABLE 20-7.** POTENTIAL INDICATIONS OF CEA

Symptomatic patients—desired maximal risk <3%
    Stenosis >50% (especially 70–90%)
    Presence of ulceration of plaque increases indication
    Reasonable surgical risk
        Neurological factors
        Extent of vascular disease
        Medical factors
    Availability of skilled surgeon
Asymptomatic patients—desired maximal risk <1.5%
    Stenosis >60% (especially 70–90%)
    Reasonable surgical risk
        Neurological factors
        Extent of vascular disease
        Medical factors
    Availability of skilled surgeon

American trials.[22,24,25] NASCET found that surgery resulted in dramatic lowering of the risk of stroke among persons with stenoses greater than 70 percent, a reduction in stroke among persons with stenoses of 50–70 percent, and no net benefit from surgery among persons with stenoses less than 50 percent.[22] The European trial found slightly different results but some of the discrepancies are due to differences in the measurement of the arterial narrowing.[25] Rothwell et al.[88] reanalyzed the data from the European Carotid Surgery Trials, using the criteria for stenosis similar to those used in NASCET. The new analyses found that surgery was highly beneficial for patients with stenoses of 70–99 percent and moderately beneficial for patients with stenoses of 50–69 percent. They found little benefit for surgical management of a near-total (>99 percent) stenosis of the internal carotid artery. Although the clinical trials did not demonstrate a benefit from CEA in the treatment of a near-occlusive lesion of the internal carotid artery, Morgenstern et al.[89] found that operation can be performed with reasonable safety and efficacy, among patients with very severe narrowing. The results of an analysis of pooled data from the trials of CEA for symptomatic patients are included in Table 20-8[90,91] (Fig. 20-3). Men and patients with hemispheric symptoms (minor stroke or TIA) had the greatest benefit from CEA. The advantage from surgery is less obvious among women and those with amaurosis fugax. The advantages of CEA are most obvious when the operation is performed within the first weeks after the last ischemic symptom.[91]

A major shift toward surgical management of asymptomatic patients has occurred.[49] Although a majority of patients having CEA do not have neurological symptoms, surgical treatment of an asymptomatic severe stenosis of

▶ **TABLE 20-8.** CHANGE IN THE RISK OF IPSILATERAL CEREBRAL INFARCTION WITHIN 5 YEARS OF CEA AS INFLUENCED BY SEVERITY OF STENOSIS

Degree of Stenosis	Absolute Change in Risk
<30%	Increase 2.2%
30–49%	Decrease 3.2%
50–69%	Decrease 4.6%
70–99%	Decrease 16.0%
Near occlusion	Increase 1.7%

Results of a meta-analysis of clinical trials
Endarterectomy for symptomatic narrowing
Adapted from Rothwell et al., *Lancet*, 2003;361:107–116.

the internal carotid artery remains controversial.[92,93] The criticism from these experts is particularly concerning because of their leadership in the trials testing CEA for treatment of symptomatic patients. Overall, the data from clinical trials testing CEA in asymptomatic persons are not as compelling as when the operation was tested in studies enrolling symptomatic patients. A systemic review of data concluded that evidence is meager for significant benefit of CEA in treatment of asymptomatic patients.[94] In large part, the lower risk of stroke among patients with asymptomatic stenoses makes demonstration of efficacy of a prophylactic operation more difficult to achieve. One large trial found that CEA reduced the projected 5-year risk of stroke from approximately 10 percent to 5 percent among persons who had a stenosis greater than 60 percent[23] (Fig. 20-4). The success was largely restricted to male patients. Other trials testing CEA in treatment of patients with asymptomatic narrowing have not been able to establish the success of the operation in preventing

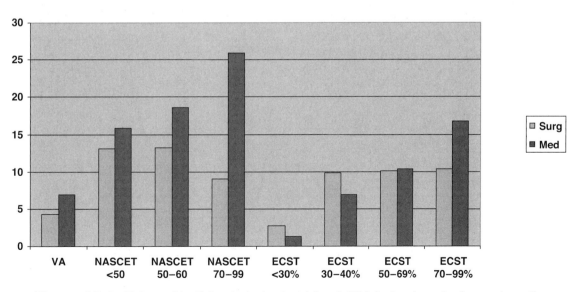

Figure 20-3. Rates of ipsilateral stroke in trials of CEA in treatment of symptomatic patients. (*Adapted from*[22,25,206]).

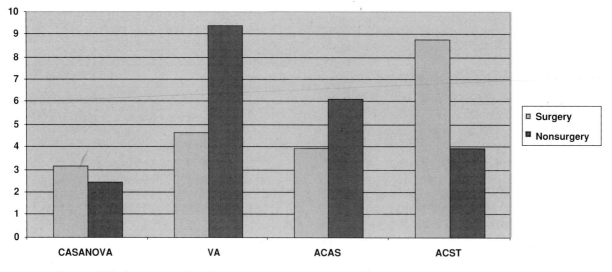

Figure 20-4. Rates of ipsilateral stroke in trials of CEA in treatment of asymptomatic patients. (*Adapted from*[23,95,208]).

stroke. A Veterans Administration Study found that the surgery was successful in lowering the risk of ipsilateral stroke or TIA.[95] However, most of the differences in outcome were attributed to a decline in the frequency of TIA. In a follow-up survey, European investigators reported that the risk of stroke ipsilateral to an asymptomatic stenosis was relatively low and did not justify the operation.[96] Critics of the operation for this indication have suggested that the surgery could be reserved until the patient develops ischemic symptoms, which suggests that the underlying arterial lesion has become unstable. Despite this criticism, CEA has become widely accepted as a therapy for good-condition patients with severe asymptomatic narrowing of the internal carotid artery.

While CEA is performed when a patient has a recurrent arterial stenosis, the risk of complications of the surgery appears to be higher than when the artery is operated for the first time. A patch is often placed in the arteriotomy in an effort to expand the caliber of the artery. In general, a second operation is done when a recurrent stenosis is found by imaging. Brown et al.[97] performed CEA for recurrent stenosis following angioplasty and stenting. With the increased use of angioplasty and stenting, such a situation might become more frequent. The treating physician will need to determine whether CEA or a second endovascular procedure is the best option. At present, no data are available to guide such a decision.

CEA has been done to treat patients with severe radiation-induced arterial narrowing. In one series, no major complications were noted with the surgery.[98] CEA can also be performed in a radiated field.[69] Still, the operation can be difficult and the role of CEA for this indication is not established.

While the success of CEA for reopening an occluded internal carotid artery is limited, some groups have reported that the operation can be done for this indication.[42,99] The most common scenario is emergency CEA to treat an acutely occluded artery—sometimes in the setting of occlusion immediately following surgery. CEA to reestablish perfusion in the setting of an acute ischemic stroke is not widely performed. Current guidelines do not recommend the use of CEA for treatment of most patients with acute ischemic stroke.[100]

Costa et al.[101] found that CEA could improve flow in the ophthalmic, retinal, and posterior ciliary arteries. Thus, it is done to improve perfusion to the eye among persons with severe ischemia and progressive visual loss. While no controlled trials have tested the operation for this indication, it should be considered as a treatment option for the patients with ischemic ophthalmopathy secondary to carotid artery disease. The goal is to preserve vision. CEA has been advocated as a therapy to improve cognitive functioning or lessen the risk of vascular dementia among persons with severe atherosclerotic disease. The rationale is that the operation would improve blood flow and lessen any cerebral ischemia. However, no data are available to establish the use of CEA in improving mental functioning among patients with severe carotid artery disease.[102] CEA is also used to treat patients with TIA or recurrent stroke in the vertebrobasilar circulation. The aim is to improve flow to the posterior circulation via the major intracranial branches of the internal carotid artery. To date, no data are available to show that CEA is useful for this indication.[103] Such findings are not surprising because most transient ischemic events are secondary embolization and surgery on the internal carotid artery does not remove the source of such emboli. In addition, the success of the operation in restoring perfusion in the vertebrobasilar circulation is not known.

Summary

Overall, many of the controversies about the utility of CEA are resolved. In particular, CEA is an established method to lower the risk of stroke among symptomatic patients.[104] When the operation can be performed with a reasonable safety, it is of proven efficacy in preventing stroke among patients with ischemic symptoms ipsilateral to a moderate-to-severe stenosis. A systemic review concluded that surgery reduces the relative risk of death or disabling stroke by approximately 48 percent among patients with severe narrowing.[105] The number of operations to prevent stroke over 2–6 years was 15. For patients with moderate narrowing, the operation reduced the risk of severe stroke or death by 27 percent.[105] The usefulness of CEA in preventing ipsilateral infarction among persons with asymptomatic narrowing is less apparent because the risk of a stroke is not as high as that among those with warning symptoms. A systemic review of the available data concluded that benefits of surgery were small.[94] Because the benefits of CEA are not apparent for several years, an asymptomatic patient should not have CEA if he/she has other severe diseases that will limit life expectancy. Still, the operation can be recommended for carefully selected patients with asymptomatic stenosis if the surgical morbidity is kept very low.[106] Recent guidelines recommend CEA, when a skilled surgeon is available, for the treatment of carefully selected asymptomatic patients who have severe narrowing.[30]

The decision to recommend CEA must be made on a case-by-case basis, using the following features: (1) the patient's neurological and general medical status, (2) the severity of the arterial pathology including collateral vessels, and (3) the availability of a skilled surgeon. The operation must be done with a low risk of major complications, in order for this prophylactic procedure to be efficacious.

▶ OTHER EXTRACRANIAL OPERATIONS

Several surgical procedures are done to treat atherosclerotic disease of the subclavian, common carotid, external carotid, or vertebral arteries. Because experience with these procedures is relatively limited, the indications and contraindications for these operations are not established with any certainty. No definitive data are available to provide guidance about recommending these revascularization procedures. On occasion, these operations are done in conjunction with surgical treatment of the internal carotid artery. In some cases, the external carotid artery could be the source of embolization. Endarterectomy of a stenotic external carotid artery can be performed to treat a patient with an occluded internal carotid artery and for whom prominent collateral flow is via the external carotid circulation. The goal is to improve flow and to eliminate another source of emboli.

Emboli can arise from the proximal (stump) segment of an occluded internal carotid artery[107] (Fig. 20-5). Blood would stagnate in the stump and secondary emboli can flow to the brain via branches of the external carotid artery.[108] Surgical plication of the stump could eliminate this source of embolization. The frequency of this clinical situation and the utility of surgical treatment of the stump have not been tested. Endovascular obliteration of the stump is another option. Grafting of vein or synthetic material can be used to develop a new arterial channel for treatment of severe disease of the proximal segments of cervical arteries. Reconstruction of a diseased common carotid artery can be performed using carotid–carotid artery crossover grafting.[109] Axillary-to-carotid bypass also can be used to treat severe disease of the common carotid artery.[110] Revascularization of the subclavian artery distal to a proximal occlusion can be done using a carotid-to-subclavian bypass.[111,112]

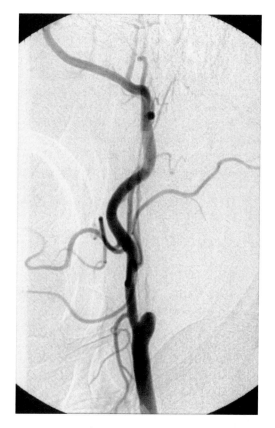

Figure 20-5. Lateral view of a left carotid arteriogram demonstrates a stump proximal to an occlusion of the internal carotid artery.

Surgeons have removed segments (kinks or loops) of the internal carotid artery, with the aim of improving perfusion and lessening turbulence of flow in the internal carotid artery.[113,114] However, the necessity for these operations is not clear. Most patients with tortuous extracranial arteries probably do not need to have resection of diseases segments. Surgical resection of an involved segment or ligation of the internal carotid or vertebral artery can be used to treat an arterial dissection with secondary aneurysmal formation.[115] The surgery is aimed at removing a source of emboli or preventing rupture. The location of the lesion, which is often at the base of the skull, makes surgery difficult. The benefit from surgical treatment of arterial dissections is not clear and because of advances in endovascular therapies, which can use coiling to obliterate the aneurysm, open surgical procedures will probably be indicated rarely. The generally benign prognosis of most patients with arterial dissections also weighs against surgical management.[116] Graded dilation or surgical resection can be used to treat fibromuscular dysplasia.[117] The segment of artery that is affected is long and deep, which makes surgery problematic. Because most affected patients have a good prognosis, the indications for these surgical procedures are not established. In addition, endovascular interventions will probably be the first treatment option.

Severe atherosclerotic disease of the aorta can be the source of emboli to either the anterior or posterior circulation. Clamping across these aortic plaques during cardiac surgery can produce massive embolization of debris. Surgical manipulation of the aorta also can be complicated by embolization. Replacement of a diseased segment of the aorta has been attempted, and localized endarterectomy, debridement, and surgical correction of the aortic lesions also can be performed. Experience is limited and results are mixed.[118,119] Because of the high risk for complications, surgical treatment of severe atherosclerosis of the arch of the aorta probably has limited utility. The primary reason probably is not for stroke prophylaxis.

▶ EXTRACRANIAL-TO-INTRACRANIAL ARTERIAL ANASTOMOSES

A variety of bypass procedures are used to restore or improve flow to the brain with severe occlusive disease of either the intracranial or extracranial vasculature. Among the possible indications are occlusion of the internal carotid artery or severe stenosis or occlusion of the major intracranial arteries in either the anterior or posterior circulation.

Rationale

These operations aim at restoring or improving perfusion distal to an occlusion or stenosis.[120] The most commonly performed anastomosis involves a connection of a branch of the superficial temporal artery to a branch of the middle cerebral artery. Less commonly, revascularization procedures involve attaching an extracranial branch of the external carotid artery to a major branch in the posterior circulation.[121] Unlike endarterectomy, the anastomosis procedures do not remove a source of embolization.

Procedures

The most common operation involves transposition of a cutaneous branch of the superficial temporal artery through a burr hole in the skull (Fig. 20-6). The vessel is attached to a branch of the middle cerebral artery. In addition, a long saphenous vein anastomosis can be attached to an artery of either the anterior or posterior circulation. Klijn et al.[122] modified the operation in an attempt to improve the technical success. Streefkerk et al.[123] used the excimer-laser-assisted nonocclusive anastomosis technique to improve vascularization. Still, the surgery is technically demanding because of the small caliber of both the donor and recipient arteries.

Extracranial-to-intracranial arterial anastomoses are most commonly done to treat patients with atherosclerotic cerebrovascular disease. The operation has been used as an adjunct to surgical procedures to treat tumors or other serious intracranial diseases.[124] In some instances, a parent artery is sacrificed during the surgery and the bypass is created to maintain adequate flow distally. Bypass operations have been performed to treat patients with intracranial arterial dissections or to improve flow to the eye among patients with ischemic oculopathy secondary to an occlusion of the internal carotid artery.[125,126] In addition, superficial temporal artery-to-middle cerebral artery bypass operations have been used to treat patients with moyamoya. Other operations have been used to improve perfusion among patients with moyamoya disease or syndrome, including encephaloduroarteriosynangiosis, encephalodurosynangiosis, and duroarteriosynangiosis.[127–129] Kim et al.[130,131] reported that encephaloduroarteriosynangiosis might be used successfully to treat patients with pediatric moyamoya disease. These procedures involve a craniotomy and placement of tissue (muscle, arteries, or meninges) on the surface of the ipsilateral cerebral hemisphere. Presumably, the operations stimulate angiogenesis to improve flow to the cerebral cortex.

Safety

Schmiedek et al.[132] reported that risk of major complications, including death, following bypass operations is approximately 14 percent. A similar rate was found in an international trial that tested the operation.[133] The rate of adverse experiences is higher among persons having posterior circulation anastomoses than that reported by superficial temporal artery-to-middle cerebral artery

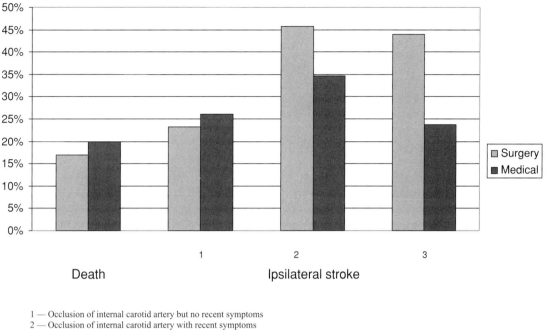

1 — Occlusion of internal carotid artery but no recent symptoms
2 — Occlusion of internal carotid artery with recent symptoms
3 — Stenosis of middle cerebral artery

Figure 20-6. Rates of death or ipsilateral stroke among subgroups of patients enrolled in the International Trial of Extracranial/intracranial Arterial Anastomosis. (*Adapted from[133]*).

bypass.[134] Because of the small caliber of the arteries involved in bypass procedures, the risk for occlusion of the anastomoses is high. The risk for occlusion of the bypass and result infarction is considerable. Because the operation involves a craniotomy, intracranial complications including bleeding, ischemia, seizures, edema, or infection can occur. The surgical procedure is not performed for several weeks following a stroke because of the high risk of neurological worsening. In part, this deterioration is because of a sudden increase in local perfusion pressure following creation of the bypass, which can lead to a hemorrhage. Infarction is the most common complication of extracranial-to-intracranial arterial bypass procedures.[135]

Potential Indications

Superficial temporal artery-to-middle cerebral artery bypass operations were tested in a large international trial.[133] The trial enrolled patients with symptomatic occlusions of the middle cerebral artery or internal carotid artery, or severe stenoses of the proximal segment of the middle cerebral artery or the distal portion of the internal carotid artery. Despite high success in maintaining patency of the bypass, the operation did not reduce the long-term risk of ipsilateral stroke. As a result of the trial and despite a number of severe criticisms of the conduct of the project, interest in the operation waned. Since then, additional research has focused on

those patients who have impaired vascular reserve. In addition, the development of endovascular techniques means that patients with stenotic lesions probably will not need bypass operations. Studies have identified a group of patients, with occlusion of the internal artery and an impaired collateral circulation, who have a high risk of recurrent stroke.[136,137] This group of patients might benefit from an operation to restore or improve flow. Research is ongoing.[120,138]

Summary

The status of extracranial-to-intracranial bypass operations remains unsettled. Until additional research negates the results of the large international trial, the role of bypass operations appears to be limited. This surgery can be an adjunct to major intracranial vascular operations that result in occlusion of major intracranial arteries. At present, treatment of moyamoya disease appears to be the most common indication. The other operations to improve perfusion among patients with moyamoya syndrome also are recommended, although definitive data about the utility of these procedures are lacking.

▶ INTRACRANIAL OPERATIONS

Endarterectomy of the middle cerebral artery can eliminate a stenosis of the first portion of the vessel. This operation is not performed widely and will likely be replaced by endovascular interventions. Resection of a fusiform (dolichoectatic) aneurysm has been attempted. The basilar artery is most commonly affected by this vascular pathology. Because of many small perforating arteries perfusing the brain stem from the basilar artery, resection of a segment of the basilar artery could be complicated by a major infarction. Thus, the utility of such surgery probably will be limited. Clipping of large intracranial aneurysms can lower the risk of embolization, leading to cerebral ischemia.[139–141] The number of cases of TIA or ischemic stroke secondary to a saccular aneurysm is relatively small, and thus the usefulness of surgical obliteration in prevention of stroke is unknown. Endovascular obliteration of the aneurysm by placing coils might be an alternative to operative clipping.

▶ ENDOVASCULAR PROCEDURES (ANGIOPLASTY AND STENTING)

Because of the success of endovascular interventions (angioplasty and stenting) in treatment of patients with coronary artery disease and severe atherosclerotic lesions in other vascular territories, interest about the potential use of these procedures for treating patients with cerebrovascular diseases has grown dramatically during the last few years. Severely stenotic lesions of either intracranial or extracranial arteries in either the carotid or vertebrobasilar circulations might be treated by angioplasty, with or without stenting. Research is ongoing. Technical advances including the use of protective devices are expanding the role for endovascular interventions.

Rationale

The goal for angioplasty and stenting is primarily for improving or restoring flow by increasing the diameter of the artery. In order to maintain the caliber of the artery and to prevent postprocedural recurrent stenosis, a stent often is placed. The stent usually consists of a fine mesh that lies on the endothelial surface of the vessel. Markus et al.[142] found that angioplasty can improve circulation to the ipsilateral hemisphere and that the effects are similar to those achieved with CEA. Transcranial Doppler ultrasonography also demonstrates increased flow velocities distal to angioplasty of the internal carotid artery.[143] The procedures do not remove an atherosclerotic lesion that can be a source of emboli. Angioplasty and stenting can be performed in locations that cannot be reached by conventional surgical procedures. Endovascular interventions can be performed in small caliber arteries. These procedures, which are less invasive than conventional vascular operations, can be done while the patient is awake.[144]

▶ **TABLE 20-9.** PERIPROCEDURAL CARE FOR ANGIOPLASTY AND STENTING

Performed under local or regional anesthesia
General anesthesia—intracranial disease
Stenting to prevent recurrent stenosis
Balloon-mounted stent
Self-expanding stent
Distal protective device to trap released emboli
Prevent thrombosis at the arterial site
Aspirin and clopidogrel
Glycoprotein IIb/IIIa antagonists
Treat fluctuations in blood pressure

Procedure

The procedure is invasive and involves placing a microcatheter into the lumen of the stenotic artery. Once the catheter is located over the stenotic lesion, a small balloon is inflated to dilate the artery (Table 20-9). The balloon fractures the underlying atherosclerotic plaque, compresses the connective tissue, and stretches the internal elastic lamina and intramural smooth muscle. The stent is placed to maintain the arterial patency (Fig. 20-7). Both balloon-mounted and self-expanding stents have been used. No differences have been noted between the types of stents used.[145] A protective device (filter or balloon) is inserted distally to protect the brain from debris and thromboembolism. At the completion of the procedure, the device is removed. Based on their experience in treating more than 400 patients, Cremonesi et al.[146] found that stenting of the carotid artery with the use of a cerebral protection device was feasible and not associated with a high risk of complications. Their experience was buttressed by the report by McKevitt et al.[147] In a series of 333 procedures including 97 with distal protection devices, they found that the 30-day risk for serious stroke or death was 2.1 percent. Antiplatelet agents (most commonly, aspirin and clopidogrel) are prescribed prior to and after the endovascular procedure, in an effort to reduce thromboembolism. Administration of glycoprotein IIb/IIIa receptor blockers also can prevent early thrombosis following angioplasty and stenting.[148–150]

Safety

Endovascular procedures are often recommended instead of CEA to patients with severe heart disease because of the lack of a requirement for anesthesia. On the other hand, endovascular procedures can be complicated by serious morbidity, including stroke (Table 20-10). Tearing of the arterial wall can lead to the formation of an intramural hematoma or a dissection. Vasospasm also can occur. Intracranial endovascular procedures can be complicated by subarachnoid

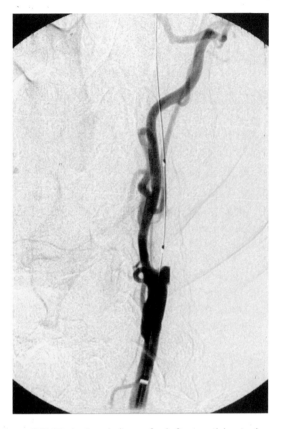

Figure 20-7. Lateral view of a left carotid arteriogram shows the placement of catheter across a high-grade stenosis.

hemorrhage. Injury to the artery can lead to thrombotic occlusion of the artery. In addition, the fracturing of the plaque can cause embolization of atherosclerotic debris. The placement of a distal protection device could prevent embolization of thrombi or debris to the brain. Castriota et al.[151] concluded that the use of the device

could reduce the risk of cerebral embolism by approximately 80 percent. McKevitt et al.[147] found that placement of a cerebral protection device reduced the risk of complications during carotid angioplasty and stenting from approximately 4–2.1 percent. Albuquerque et al.[152] found that angioplasty without stenting can be associated with a high rate of moderate-to-severe restenosis. In addition, the blood pressure can be volatile after endovascular treatment of a severe stenosis of the internal carotid artery.

The frequency of serious complications following angioplasty and stenting varies considerably among institutions.[153–155] In a single-center study, Kastrup et al.[156] found that the rates of complications were similar among patients treated with CEA or angioplasty and stenting.

Potential Indications

Several groups report the potential utility of angioplasty and stenting in treatment of patients with stenosis of the extracranial segment of the internal carotid artery[157–163] (Table 20-11). In a multicenter study, Qureshi et al.[164] found that placement of stent was feasible for treatment of patients with stenosis of the internal carotid artery. Hayashi et al.[165] used endovascular therapy to treat patients with severe stenosis of the extracranial segment of the internal carotid artery and progressing stroke. Carotid angioplasty prior to CABG can be recommended for treatment of carotid artery disease in high-risk patients when the center has sufficient expertise.[58] Angioplasty and stenting has become an important treatment option

▶ **TABLE 20-10.** POTENTIAL COMPLICATIONS OF ANGIOPLASTY AND STENTING

Infarction
    Embolization of atherosclerotic debris
    Thrombotic occlusion
    Thromboembolism
Hyperperfusion syndrome
Arterial vasospasm
Arterial rupture
    Subarachnoid hemorrhage
Local bleeding
Recurrent stenosis of artery
Cardiovascular events
    Volatile blood pressure
    Cardiac arrhythmias
    Myocardial ischemia
Death

▶ **TABLE 20-11.** POTENTIAL INDICATIONS OF CEREBROVASCULAR ANGIOPLASTY AND STENTING

Extracranial segment of internal carotid artery—stenosis
    Not a good candidate for CEA
        Neurological factors
        Extensive vascular disease
        Medical factors—heart disease in particular
        Stenosis not easily approached by surgery
    Recurrent stenosis following CEA
    Presence of tandem or intracranial stenoses
    Radiation-induced arterial narrowing
    Dissection or fibromuscular disease
    Aneurysm
Intracranial segment of internal carotid artery—stenosis
    Siphon
    Distal internal carotid artery
Middle cerebral artery stenosis
Basilar artery stenosis
Vertebral artery stenosis
    Extracranial segment
    Intracranial segment
Subclavian artery stenosis

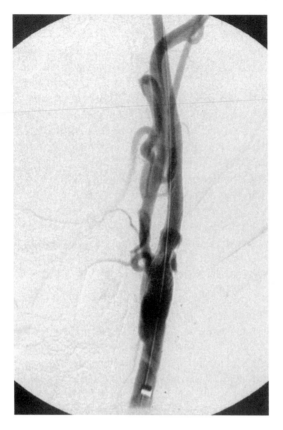

Figure 20-8. Lateral view of a left carotid arteriogram demonstrates the presence of a stent in the artery.

for management of patients at high risk for complications from CEA[166,167] (Fig. 20-8). One of the indications for angioplasty and stenting has been treatment of a recurrent carotid stenosis following a CEA. Recently, AbuRahma et al.[64] found that endovascular treatment was not safer than a second CEA. Bowser et al.[168] found that the rates of complications were similar among patients having a second CEA or angioplasty and stenting. On the other hand, Fox et al.[169] reported that angioplasty and stenting was safe and potentially effective for management of patients, with high-grade symptomatic carotid stenosis, who were not good surgical candidates.

A European trial compared angioplasty and stenting or CEA in treatment of patients with carotid artery disease.[170] The rates of most complications of the two procedures were similar, although endovascular treatment is associated with a much lower rate of cranial nerve palsies than was found with CEA. While the trial found a higher rate of recurrent stenosis among patients having endovascular treatment than with CEA, most patients did not have stents inserted. Overall, the rates of recurrent cerebrovascular ischemic events were similar in the two treatment groups. Another study compared CEA with angioplasty and stenting in high risk patients, the endovascular intervention appeared superior.[171] Additional trials are underway.[172]

Angioplasty has been used to treat stenoses of the cervical portion of the vertebral artery, including its origin from the subclavian artery[111,152] (Fig. 20-9). These procedures are used to treat lesions of the cavernous segment of the internal carotid artery, the distal segment of the extracranial internal carotid artery, and the brachiocephalic artery. Angioplasty and stenting have been done in conjunction with CEA or coronary angioplasty.[173-176] Angioplasty has also been used to treat severe stenoses of the middle cerebral artery or the basilar artery.[177-179] Based on a series of 10 patients, Lee et al.[180] found that angioplasty could be performed with a reasonable degree of safety, although recurrent stenosis does occur. Angioplasty has also been used to treat stenoses of major branches of the basilar artery.[181]

Angioplasty and stenting have been used to treat patients with fibromuscular dysplasia.[182] These procedures have also been used to treat patients with radiation-induced arteriopathy, vasculitis, or arterial dissections, including those with false aneurysms.[183-187]

Summary

The utility of angioplasty and stenting in treatment of patients with ischemic cerebrovascular disease has not been established.[104,188,189] Experience with these procedures is relatively limited. Systemic reviews of the usefulness of angioplasty in the treatment of extracranial carotid artery stenosis or vertebral artery stenosis concluded that the data are insufficient to make any recommendations.[190,191] However, the promise for these procedures seems very bright. Improvements in technique and technology are rapidly improving the safety of endovascular interventions and broadening their indications. These procedures will likely be the best way to locally treat severe atherosclerotic disease of the posterior circulation and intracranial arteries. Angioplasty and stenting might replace CEA for treatment of patients with severe atherosclerosis of the extracranial segment of the internal carotid artery.

▶ CARDIAC OPERATIONS

Prevention of embolization is one of the indications for several cardiac operations or endovascular procedures. With improvements in endovascular techniques, the spectrum of structural lesions of the heart, which can be treated, likely will grow in the future. Surgical procedures include valve replacement operations. Replacement of a rheumatic mitral or aortic valve is often performed to improve cardiac function and to lessen the formation of emboli on the diseased valves. Vikram et al.[192] demonstrated that surgical replacement of infected left-sided native valves was associated with a reduction in 6-month

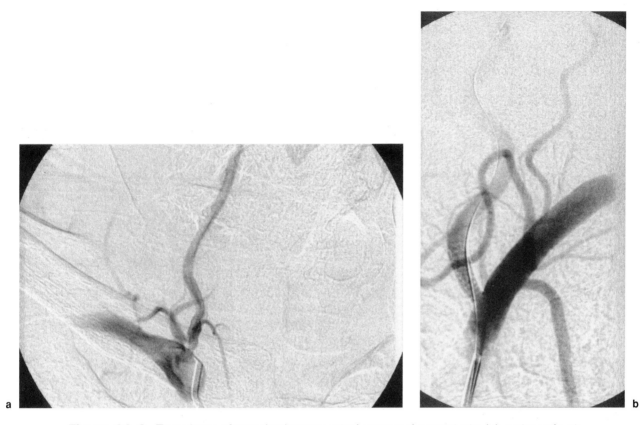

Figure 20-9. Two views of vertebral artery arteriograms demonstrate (a) a stenosis at the origin of the vessel and (b) subsequent enlargement of ortium after angioplasty.

mortality following endocarditis. Surgical resection of an atrial myxoma also will eliminate embolization. Cardioversion, interruption of the bundle of His, a pacemaker, or an external defibrillator have been used to improve cardiac function and lower the formation of thrombi.

Open surgical procedures have been used to occlude a patent foramen ovale (PFO).[193,194] However, the risk of recurrent embolization among patients with a patent foramen ovale appears to be relatively low, and the risk of the operation needs to be compared to the potential efficacy in preventing stroke.[195,196] Operative repair of a patent foramen ovale will likely be replaced by endovascular placement of occlusive devices or filters.[197–200] Du et al.[201] found that endovascular closure could be performed safely and successfully among patients with PFO. Khositseth et al.[202] found that transcatheter device closure of a PFO could be done safely. While they presume that the procedure is effective, they also concluded that recurrent ischemic events could occur even in the absence of a residual shunt. While these devices are being placed in a large number of persons, particularly young adults with cryptogenic stroke, their utility is not established.[194,203] Clinical trials are ongoing. Endovascular obliteration of the left atrial appendage

has been used to lower the risk of thromboembolism among persons with nonvalvular atrial fibrillation.[204,205] While this intervention shows promise, additional research is needed to determine if this therapy is superior to medical management.

REFERENCES

1. Pokras R, Dyken ML. Dramatic changes in the performance of endarterectomy for diseases of the extracranial arteries of the head. *Stroke* 1988;19:1289–1290.
2. Chassin MR. Appropriate use of carotid endarterectomy. *N Engl J Med* 1998;339:1468–1471.
3. American Heart Association. Heart disease and stroke statistics—2004 update. 2004.
4. Brittenden J, Murie JA, Jenkins AM, Ruckley CV, Bradbury AW. Carotid endarterectomy before and after publication of randomized controlled trials. *Br J Surg* 1999;86:206–210.
5. Sheikh K, Bullock C. Sex differences in carotid endarterectomy utilization and 30-day postoperative mortality. *Neurology* 2003;60:471–476.
6. Oddone EZ, Horner RD, Johnston D, et al. Carotid endarterectomy and race: do clinical indications and patient preferences account for differences? *Stroke* 2002; 33:2936–2943.

7. Hendrikse J, Eikelboom BC, van der Grond J. Magnetic resonance angiography of collateral compensation in asymptomatic and symptomatic internal carotid artery stenosis. *J Vasc Surg* 2002;36:799–805.

8. Soinne L, Helenius J, Saimanen E, et al. Brain diffusion changes in carotid occlusive disease treated with endarterectomy. *Neurology* 2003;61:1061–1065.

9. Soinne L, Helenius J, Tatlisumak T, et al. Cerebral hemodynamics in asymptomatic and symptomatic patients with high-grade carotid stenosis undergoing carotid endarterectomy. *Stroke* 2003;34:1655–1661.

10. D'Angelo V, Catapano G, Bozzini V, et al. Cerebrovascular reactivity before and after carotid endarterectomy. *Surg Neurol* 1999;51:321–326.

11. Loftus CM. Carotid endarterectomy: how the operation is done. *Clin Neurosurg* 1997;44:243–265.

12. Shi Q, Wu MH, Sauvage LR. Clinical and experimental demonstration of complete healing of porous Dacron patch grafts used for closure of the arteriotomy after carotid endarterectomy. *Ann Vasc Surg* 1999;13:313–317.

13. AbuRahma AF, Robinson PA, Stickler DL. Analysis of regression of postoperative carotid stenosis from prospective randomized trial of carotid endarterectomy comparing primary closure versus patching. *Ann Surg* 1999;229:767–772.

14. Counsell C, Salinas R, Warlow C, Naylor R. CD000160. *Cochrane Database Syst Rev* 2000;CD000160.

15. Counsell C, Warlow C, Naylor R. Patches of different types for carotid patch angioplasty. *Cochrane Database Syst Rev* 2000;CD000071.

16. Pinkerton JA. EEG as a criterion for shunt need in carotid endarterectomy. *Ann Vasc Surg* 2002.

17. Bond R, Rerkasem K, Rothwell PM. Routine or selective carotid artery shunting for carotid endarterectomy (and different methods of monitoring in selective shunting). *Cochrane Database Syst Rev* 2002;CD000190.

18. Gurer O, Yapici F, Enc Y, Cinar B, Ketenci B, Ozler A. Local versus general anesthesia for carotid endarterectomy: report of 329 cases. *Vasc Endovascular Surg* 2003;37:171–177.

19. Papavasiliou AK, Magnadottir HB, Gonda T, Franz D, Harbaugh RE. Clinical outcomes after carotid endarterectomy: comparison of the use of regional and general anesthetics. *J Neurosurg* 2000;92:291–296.

20. Nuri M, Barbaccia JJ, Schunn CD. Effect of anesthetic management on resource utilization and outcome in carotid endarterectomy patients. *W V Med J* 2003;99:100–104.

21. Tangkanakul C, Counsell C, Warlow C. Local versus general anaesthesia for carotid endarterectomy. *Cochrane Database Syst Rev* 2000;CD000126.

22. North American Symptomatic Carotid Endarterectomy Trial Collaborators. Beneficial effect of carotid endarterectomy in symptomatic patients with high-grade carotid stenosis. *N Engl J Med* 1991;325:445–453.

23. Executive Committee for the Asymptomatic Carotid Atherosclerosis Study. Endarterectomy for asymptomatic carotid artery stenosis. *JAMA* 1995;273:1421–1428.

24. European Carotid Surgery Trialists' Collaborative Group. MRC European Carotid Surgery Trial: interim results for symptomatic patients with severe (70–99%) or with mild (0–29%) carotid stenosis. *Lancet* 1991;337:1235–1243.

25. European Carotid Surgery Trialists' Collaborative Group. Randomised trial of endarterectomy for recently symptomatic carotid stenosis: final results of the MRC European Carotid Surgery Trial (ECST). *Lancet* 1998;351:1379–1387.

26. Johnston D, Eastwood JD, Nguyen T, Goldstein LB. Contrast-enhanced magnetic resonance angioplasty of carotid arteries: utility in routine clinical practice. *Stroke* 2002;33:2834–2838.

27. Hernandez N, Salles-Cunha SX, Daoud YA, et al. Factors related to short length of stay after carotid endarterectomy. *Vasc Endovascular Surg* 2002;36:425–437.

28. Back MR, Harward TR, Huber TS, Carlton LM, Flynn TC, Seeger JM. Improving the cost-effectiveness of carotid endarterectomy. *J Vasc Surg* 1997;26:456–462.

29. Bond R, Rerkasem K, Rothwell PM. Systematic review of the risks of carotid endarterectomy in relation to the clinical indication for the timing of surgery. *Stroke* 2003;34:2290–2301.

30. Biller J, Feinberg WM, Castaldo JE, et al. Guidelines for carotid endarterectomy: a statement for healthcare professionals from a Special Writing Group of the Stroke Council, American Heart Association. *Circulation* 1998;97:501–509.

31. Easton JD, Sherman DG. Stroke and mortality rate in carotid endarterectomy: 228 consecutive operations. *Stroke* 1977;8:565–568.

32. Chaturvedi S, Aggarwal A, Murugappan A. Results of carotid endarterectomy with prospective neurologist follow-up. *Neurology* 2000;55:769–772.

33. Lanska DJ, Kryscio RJ. In-hospital mortality following carotid endarterectomy. *Neurology* 1998;51:440–447.

34. Pruner G, Castellano R, Jannello AM, et al. Carotid endarterectomy in the octogenarian: outcomes of 345 procedures performed from 1995–2000. *Cardiovasc Surg* 2003;11:105–112.

35. Kapral MK, Wang H, Austin PC, et al. Sex differences in carotid endarterectomy outcomes: results from the Ontario Carotid Endarterectomy Registry. *Stroke* 2003;34:1120–1125.

36. Rockman CB, Castillo J, Adelman MA, et al. Carotid endarterectomy in female patients: are the concerns of the Asymptomatic Carotid Atherosclerosis Study valid? *J Vasc Surg* 2001;33:240–241.

37. Akbari CM, Pulling MC, Pomposelli FB, Jr., Gibbons GW, Campbell DR, Logerfo FW. Gender and carotid endarterectomy: does it matter? *J Vasc Surg* 2000;31:1103–1108.

38. Conrad MF, Shepard AD, Pandurangi K, et al. Outcome of carotid endarterectomy in African Americans: is race a factor? *J Vasc Surg* 2003;38:129–137.

39. Gay J, Curtil A, Buffliere S, Favre J, Barral X. Urgent carotid artery repair: retrospective study of 21 cases. *Ann Vasc Surg* 2002;16:401–406.

40. Huber R, Muller BT, Seitz RJ, Siebler M, Modder U, Sandmann W. Carotid surgery in acute symptomatic patients. *Eur J Vasc Endovasc Surg* 2003;25:60–67.

41. Schneider C, Johansen K, Konigstein R. Emergency carotid thromboendarterectomy: safe and effective. *World J Surg* 1999;23:1163–1167.

42. Eckstein HH, Schumacher H, Klemm K, et al. Emergency carotid endarterectomy. *Cerebrovasc Dis* 1999;9:270–281.

43. Paty PS, Darling RC, Woratyla S, et al. Timing of carotid endarterectomy in patients with recent stroke. *Surgery* 1997;122:850–854.

44. Giordano JM. The timing of carotid endarterectomy after acute stroke. *Semin Vasc Surg* 1998;11:19–23.

45. Hoffmann M, Robbs J. Carotid endarterectomy after recent cerebral infarction. *Eur J Vasc Endovasc Surg* 1999; 18:6–10.

46. Parrino PE, Lovelock M, Shockey KS, King C, Tribble CG, Kron IL. Early carotid endarterectomy after stroke. *Cardiovasc Surg* 2000;8:116–120.

47. Eckstein HH, Ringleb P, Dorfler A, et al. The Carotid Surgery for Ischemic Stroke Trial: a prospective observational study on carotid endarterectomy in the early period after ischemic stroke. *J Vasc Surg* 2002;36:997–1004.

48. Ballotta E, Da Giau G, Baracchini C, Abbruzzese E, Saladini M, Meneghetti G. Early versus delayed carotid endarterectomy after a nondisabling ischemic stroke: a prospective randomized study. *Surgery* 2002;131:287–293.

49. Halm EA, Chassin MR, Tuhrim S, et al. Revisiting the appropriateness of carotid endarterectomy. *Stroke* 2003; 34:1464–1472.

50. Gasparis A, Ricotta L, Cuadra S, Char D, Purtill W, Van Bemmelen P. High-risk carotid endarterectomy: fact or fiction. *J Vasc Surg* 2003;37:40–46.

51. Reed AB, Gaccione P, Belkin M, et al. Preoperative risk factors for carotid endarterectomy: defining the patient at high risk. *J Vasc Surg* 2003;37:1191–1199.

52. Middleton S, Donnelly N, Harris J, Lusby R, Ward J. Audit of long-term mortality and morbidity outcomes for carotid endarterectomy. *Aust Health Rev* 2002;25: 81–91.

53. Brown KR. Treatment of concomitant carotid and coronary artery disease. Decision-making regarding surgical options. *J Cardiovasc Surg* 2003;44:395–399.

54. Blacker DJ, Flemming KD, Link MJ, Brown RD, Jr. The preoperative cerebrovascular consultation: common cerebrovascular questions before general or cardiac surgery. *Mayo Clin Proc* 2004;79:223–229.

55. Brown K, Kresowik TF, Chin M, Kresowik RA, Grund SL, Hendel ME. Multistate population-based outcomes of combined carotid endarterectomy and coronary artery bypass. *J Vasc Surg* 2003;37:32–39.

56. Vitali E, Lanfranconi M, Bruschi G, Colombo T, Russo C. Combined surgical approach to coexistent carotid and coronary artery disease: early and late results. *Cardiovasc Surg* 2003;11:113–119.

57. Naylor AR, Cuffe RL, Rothwell PM, Bell PR. A systematic review of outcomes following staged and synchronous carotid endarterectomy and coronary artery bypass. *Eur J Vasc Endovasc Surg* 2003;25:380–389.

58. Bandyk DF, Back MR, Johnson BL, Shames ML. Carotid intervention prior to or during coronary artery bypass grafting. When is it necessary? *J Cardiovasc Surg* 2003;44: 401–405.

59. Beauford RB, Saunders CR, Goldstein DJ. Off pump concomitant coronary revascularization and carotid endarterectomy. *J Cardiovasc Surg* 2003;44:407–415.

60. Gasecki AP, Eliasziw M, Ferguson GG, Hachinski V, Barnett HJM. Long-term prognosis and effect of endarterectomy in patients with symptomatic severe carotid stenosis and contralateral carotid stenosis or occlusion: results from NASCET. North American Symptomatic Carotid Endarterectomy Trial (NASCET) Group. *J Neurosurg* 1995;83:778–782.

61. Aungst M, Gahtan V, Berkowitz H, Roberts AB, Kerstein MD. Carotid endarterectomy outcome is not affected in patients with a contralateral carotid artery occlusion. *Am J Surg* 1998;176:30–33.

62. Klijn CJM, van Buren PA, Kappelle LJ, et al. Outcome in patients with symptomatic occlusion of the internal carotid artery. *Eur J Vasc Endovasc Surg* 2003;19:579–586.

63. Baker WH, Howard VJ, Howard G, Toole JF. Effect of contralateral occlusion on long-term efficacy of endarterectomy in the Asymptomatic Carotid Atherosclerosis Study (ACAS). *Stroke* 2000;31:2330–2334.

64. AbuRahma AF, Robinson P, Holt SM, Herzog TA, Mowery NT. Perioperative and late stroke rates of carotid endarterectomy contralateral to carotid artery occlusion: results from a randomized trial. *Stroke* 2000;31:1566–1571.

65. Johnson CA, Tollefson DF, Olsen SB, Andersen CA, McKee-Johnson J. The natural history of early recurrent carotid artery stenosis. *Am J Surg* 1999;177:433–436.

66. Domenig C, Hamdan AD, Belfield AK, et al. Recurrent stenosis and contralateral occlusion: high-risk situations in carotid endarterectomy? *Ann Vasc Surg* 2003;17:622–628.

67. Hobson RW, Goldstein JE, Jamil Z, et al. Carotid restenosis: operative and endovascular management. *J Vasc Surg* 1999;29:228–235.

68. AbuRahma AF, Bates MC, Wulu JT, Stone PA. Early post-surgical carotid restenosis: redo surgery versus angioplasty/stenting. *J Endovasc Ther* 2002;9:566–572.

69. Leseche G, Castier Y, Chataigner O, et al. Carotid artery revascularization through radiated field. *J Vasc Surg* 2003; 38:244–250.

70. Hamdan AD, Pomposelli FBJ, Gibbons GW, Campbell DR, LoGerfo FW. Perioperative strokes after 1001 consecutive carotid endarterectomy procedures without an electroencephalogram: incidence, mechanism, and recovery. *Arch Surg* 1999;134:412–415.

71. Gorelick PB. Carotid endarterectomy. Where do we draw the line? *Stroke* 1999;30:1745–1750.

72. Hannan EL, Popp AJ, Feustel P, et al. Association of surgical specialty and processes of care with patient outcomes for carotid endarterectomy. *Stroke* 2001;32: 2890–2897.

73. Kucey DS, Bowyer B, Iron K, Austin P, Anderson G, Tu JV. Determinants of outcome after carotid endarterectomy. *J Vasc Surg* 1998;28:1051–1058.

74. Cowan JA, Jr., Dimick JB, Thompson BG, Stanley JC, Upchurch GR, Jr. Surgeon volume as an indicator of outcomes after carotid endarterectomy: an effect independent of specialty practice and hospital volume. *J Am Coll Surg* 2002;195:814–821.

75. Kresowik TF, Hemann RA, Grund SL, et al. Improving the outcomes of carotid endarterectomy: results of a statewide quality improvement project. *J Vasc Surg* 2000;31:918–926.

76. Hingorani A, Ascher E, Tsemekhim B, et al. Causes of early post carotid endarterectomy stroke in a recent series: the

increasing importance of hyperperfusion syndrome. *Acta Chir Belg* 2002;102:435–438.

77. Riles TS, Imparato AM, Jacobowitz GR, et al. The cause of perioperative stroke after carotid endarterectomy. *J Vasc Surg* 1994;19:206–214.

78. Cheung RTF, Eliasziw M, Meldrum HE, Fox AJ, Barnett HJM, for the North American Symptomatic Carotid Endarterectomy Trial (NASCET) Group. Risk, types, and severity of intracranial hemorrhage in patients with symptomatic carotid artery stenosis. *Stroke* 2003;34:1847–1851.

79. Wilson PV, Ammar AD. The incidence of ischemic stroke versus intracerebral hemorrhage after carotid endarterectomy. A review of 2452 cases. *Ann Vasc Surg* 2005;19:1–4.

80. Ascher E, Markevich N, Schutzer RW, Kallakuri S, Jacob T, Hingorani AP. Cerebral hyperperfusion syndrome after carotid endarterectomy: predictive factors and hemodynamic changes. *J Vasc Surg* 2003;37:769–777.

81. Hartsell PA, Calligaro KD, Syrek JR, Dougherty MJ, Raviola CA. Postoperative blood pressure changes associated with cervical block versus general anesthesia following carotid endarterectomy. *Ann Vasc Surg* 1999;13:104–108.

82. Naylor AR, Evans J, Thompson MM, et al. Seizures after carotid endarterectomy: hyperperfusion, dysautoregulation or hypertensive encephalopathy? *Eur J Vasc Endovasc Surg* 2003;26:39–44.

83. Ballotta E, Da Giau G, Renon L, et al. Cranial and cervical nerve injuries after carotid endarterectomy: a prospective study. *Surgery* 1999;125:85–91.

84. Ferguson GG, Eliasziw M, Barr HW, et al. The North American Symptomatic Carotid Endarterectomy Trial. Surgical results in 1415 patients. *Stroke* 1999;30:1751–1758.

85. Zannetti S, Parente B, De Rango P, et al. Role of surgical techniques and operative findings in cranial and cervical nerve injuries during carotid endarterectomy. *Eur J Vasc Endovasc Surg* 1998;15:528–531.

86. Rockman CB, Su WT, Domenig C, et al. Postoperative infection associated with polyester patch angioplasty after carotid endarterectomy. *J Vasc Surg* 2003;38:251–256.

87. Borazjani BH, Wilson SE, Fujitani RM, Gordon I, Mueller M, Williams RA. Postoperative complications of carotid patching: pseudoaneurysm and infection. *Ann Vasc Surg* 2003;17:156–161.

88. Rothwell PM, Gutnikov SA, Warlow CP, for the European Carotid Surgery Trialists' Collaboration. Reanalysis of the final results of the European Carotid Surgery Trial. *Stroke* 2003;34:514–523.

89. Morgenstern LB, Fox AJ, Sharpe BL, Eliasziw M, Barnett HJM, Grotta JC. The risks and benefits of carotid endarterectomy in patients with near occlusion of the carotid artery. North American Symptomatic Carotid Endarterectomy Trial (NASCET) Group. *Neurology* 1997;48:911–915.

90. Rothwell PM, Eliasziw M, Gutnikov SA, et al. Analysis of pooled data from the randomised controlled trials of endarterectomy for symptomatic carotid stenosis. *Lancet* 2003;361:107–116.

91. Rothwell PM, Eliasziw M, Gutnikov SA, Warlow CP, Barnett HJM, for the Carotid Endarterectomy Trialists' Collaboration. Endarterectomy for symptomatic carotid stenosis in relation to clinical subgroups and timing of surgery. *Lancet* 2004;363:915–924.

92. Barnett HJM, Eliasziw M, Meldrum HE, Taylor DW. Do the facts and figures warrant a 10-fold increase in the performance of carotid endarterectomy on asymptomatic patients? *Neurology* 1996;46:603–608.

93. Warlow C. Carotid endarterectomy for asymptomatic carotid stenosis. Better data, but the case is still not convincing. *BMJ* 1998;317:1468.

94. Chambers BR, You RX, Donnan GA. Carotid endarterectomy for asymptomatic carotid stenosis. *Cochrane Database Syst Rev* 2000;CD001923.

95. Hobson RW, Weiss DG, Fields WS, et al. Efficacy of carotid endarterectomy for asymptomatic carotid stenosis. The Veterans Affairs Cooperative Study Group. *N Engl J Med* 1993;328:221–227.

96. The European Carotid Surgery Trialists' Collaborative Group. Risk of stroke in the distribution of an asymptomatic carotid artery. *Lancet* 1995;345:209–212.

97. Brown KR, Desai TR, Schwartz LB, Gewertz BL. Operative intervention for recurrent stenosis after carotid stent angioplasty: a report. *Ann Vasc Surg* 2002;16:575–578.

98. Kashyap VS, Moore WS, Quinones-Baldrich WJ. Carotid artery repair for radiation-associated atherosclerosis is a safe and durable procedure. *J Vasc Surg* 1999;29:90–96.

99. McCormick PW, Spetzler RF, Bailes JE, Zabramski JM, Frey JL. Thromboendarterectomy of the symptomatic occluded internal carotid artery. *J Neurosurg* 1992;76:752–758.

100. Adams HP, Adams RJ, Brott T, et al. Guidelines for the early management of patients with ischemic stroke. A scientific statement from the stroke council of the American Stroke Association. *Stroke* 2003;34:1056–1083.

101. Costa VP, Kuzniec S, Molnar LJ, Cerri GG, Puech-Leao P, Carvalho CA. The effects of carotid endarterectomy on the retrobulbar circulation of patients with severe occlusive carotid artery disease. An investigation by color Doppler imaging. *Ophthalmology* 1999;106:306–310.

102. Irvine CD, Gardner FV, Davies AH, Lamont PM. Cognitive testing in patients undergoing carotid endarterectomy. *Eur J Vasc Endovasc Surg* 1998;15:195–204.

103. McNamara JO, Heyman A, Silver D, Mandel ME. The value of carotid endarterectomy in treating transient cerebral ischemia of the posterior circulation. *Neurology* 1977;27:682–684.

104. Sacco RL, Adams R, Albers G, et al. Guidelines for prevention of stroke in patients with ischemic stroke or transient ischemic attack. A statement for healthcare professionals from the American Heart Association/American Stroke Association Council on Stroke. *Stroke* 2006;37:577–617.

105. Cina CS, Clase CM, Haynes RB. Carotid endarterectomy for symptomatic carotid stenosis. *Cochrane Database Syst Rev* 2000;CD001081.

106. Castaldo J. Is carotid endarterectomy appropriate for asymptomatic stenosis? Yes. *Arch Neurol* 1999;56:877–879.

107. Hankey GJ, Warlow CP. Prognosis of symptomatic carotid artery occlusion. *Cerebrovasc Dis* 1991;1:245–256.

108. Ryan PG, Day AL. Stump embolization from an occluded internal carotid artery. Case report. *J Neurosurg* 1987;67:609–611.

109. Ozsvath KJ, Roddy SP, Darling RC, III, et al. Carotid–carotid crossover bypass: is it a durable procedure? *J Vasc Surg* 2003;37:582–585.

110. Archie JP, Jr. Axillary-to-carotid artery bypass grafting for symptomatic severe common carotid artery occlusive disease. *J Vasc Surg* 1999;30:1106–1112.

111. Molnar RG, Naslund TC. Vertebral artery surgery. *Surg Clin N Am* 1998;78:901–913.

112. Law MM, Colburn MD, Moore WS, Quinones-Baldrich WJ, Machleder HI, Gelabert HA. Carotid-subclavian bypass for brachiocephalic occlusive disease. Choice of conduit and long-term follow-up. *Stroke* 1995;26:1565–1571.

113. Radonic V, Baric D, Giunio L, Buca A, Sapunar D, Marovic A. Surgical treatment of kinked internal carotid artery. *J Cardiovasc Surg* 1998;39:557–563.

114. Grego F, Lepidi S, Cognolato D, Frigatti P, Morelli I, Deriu GP. Rationale of the surgical treatment of carotid kinking. *J Cardiovasc Surg* 2003;44:79–85.

115. Schievink WI, Piepgras DG, McCaffrey TV, Mokri B. Surgical treatment of extracranial internal carotid artery dissecting aneurysms. *Neurosurgery* 1994;35:809–815.

116. Touze E, Gauvrit JY, Moulin T, Meder JF, Bracard S, Mas JL. Risk of stroke and recurrent dissection after a cervical artery dissection: a multicenter study. *Neurology* 2003;61:1347–1351.

117. Chiche L, Bahnini A, Koskas F, Kieffer E. Occlusive fibromuscular disease of arteries supplying the brain: results of surgical treatment. *Ann Vasc Surg* 1997;11:496–504.

118. Bojar RM, Payne DD, Murphy RE, et al. Surgical treatment of systemic atheroembolism from the thoracic aorta. *Ann Thorac Surg* 1996;61:1389–1393.

119. King RC, Kanithanon RC, Shockey KS, Spotnitz WD, Tribble CG, Kron IL. Replacing the atherosclerotic ascending aorta is a high-risk procedure. *Ann Thorac Surg* 1998;66:396–401.

120. Grubb RL, Jr. Extracranial–intracranial arterial bypass for treatment of occlusion of the internal carotid artery. *Curr Neurol Neurosci Rep* 2004;4:23–30.

121. Ausman JI, Diaz FG, Vacca DF, Sadasivan B. Superficial temporal and occipital artery bypass pedicles to superior, anterior inferior, and posterior inferior cerebellar arteries for vertebrobasilar insufficiency. *J Neurosurg* 1990;72:554–558.

122. Klijn CJ, Kappelle J, van der Zwan A, van Gijn J, Tulleken CA. Excimer lasar-assisted high-flow extracranial/intracranial bypass in patients with symptomatic carotid artery occlusion at high risk of recurrent cerebral ischemia: safety and long-term outcome. *Stroke* 2002;33:2451–2458.

123. Streefkerk HJ, van der Zwan A, Verdaasdonk RM, Beck HJ, Tulleken CA. Cerebral revascularization. *Adv Tech Stand Neurosurg* 2003;28:145–225.

124. Sekhar LN, Kalavakonda C. Cerebral revascularization for aneurysms and tumors. *Neurosurgery* 2002;50:321–331.

125. Vishteh AG, Marciano FF, David CA, Schievink WI, Zabramski JM, Spetzler RF. Long-term graft patency rates and clinical outcomes after revascularization for symptomatic traumatic internal carotid artery dissection. *Neurosurgery* 1998;43:761–768.

126. Kawaguchi S, Sakaki T, Kamada K, Iwanaga H, Nishikawa N. Effects of superficial temporal to middle cerebral artery bypass for ischaemic retinopathy due to internal carotid artery occlusion/stenosis. *Acta Neurochir (Wien)* 1994;129:166–170.

127. Kawaguchi T, Fujita S, Hosoda K, et al. Multiple burr-hole operation for adult moyamoya disease. *J Neurosurg* 1996;84:468–476.

128. Iwama T, Hashimoto N, Miyake H, Yonekawa Y. Direct revascularization to the anterior cerebral artery territory in patients with moyamoya disease: report of five cases. *Neurosurgery* 1998;42:1157–1161.

129. Sehgal M, Swanson JW, DeRemee RA, Colby TV. Neurologic manifestations of Churg–Strauss syndrome. *Mayo Clin Proc* 1995;70:337–341.

130. Kim SK, Wang KC, Kim IO, Lee DS, Cho BK. Combined encephaloduroarteriosynangiosis and bifrontal encephalogaleo(periosteal) synangiosis in pediatric moyamoya disease. *Neurosurgery* 2002;50:88–96.

131. Kim CY, Wang KC, Kim SK, Chung YN, Kim HS, Cho BK. Encephaloduroarteriosynangiosis with bifrontal encephalogaleo(periosteal)synangiosis in the pediatric moyamoya disease: the surgical technique and its outcomes. *Childs Nerv Syst* 2003;19:316–324.

132. Schmiedek P, Piepgras A, Leinsinger G, Kirsch CM, Einhupl K. Improvement of cerebrovascular reserve capacity by EC-IC arterial bypass surgery in patients with ICA occlusion and hemodynamic cerebral ischemia. *J Neurosurg* 1994;81:236–244.

133. The EC/IC Bypass Study Group. Failure of extracranial–intracranial arterial bypass to reduce the risk of ischemic stroke. Results of an international randomized trial. *N Engl J Med* 1985;313:1191–1200.

134. Hopkins LN, Budny JL. Complications of intracranial bypass for vertebrobasilar insufficiency. *J Neurosurg* 1989;70:207–211.

135. Sundt TMJ, Whisnant JP, Fode NC, Piepgras DG, Houser OW. Results, complications, and follow-up of 415 bypass operations for occlusive disease of the carotid system. *Mayo Clin Proc* 1985;60:230–240.

136. Vorstrup S, Haase J, Waldemar G, Andersen A, Schmidt J, Paulson OB. EC-IC bypass in patients with chronic hemodynamic insufficiency. *Acta Neurol Scand* 1996;(suppl 166):79–81.

137. Grubb RL, Jr., Derdeyn CP, Fritsch SM, et al. Importance of hemodynamic factors in the prognosis of symptomatic carotid occlusion. *JAMA* 1998;280:1055–1060.

138. Adams HP, Jr., Powers WJ, Grubb RLJ, Clarke WR, Woolson RF. Preview of a new trial of extracranial-to-intracranial arterial anastomosis: the carotid occlusion surgery study. *Neurosurg Clin N Am* 2000;12:613–624.

139. Qureshi AI, Mohammad Y, Yahia AM, et al. Ischemic events associated with unruptured intracranial aneurysms: multicenter clinical study and review of the literature. *Neurosurgery* 2000;46:282–289.

140. Carvi y Nievas MN, Haas E, Hollerhage HG. Unruptured large intracranial aneurysms in patients with transient cerebral ischemic episodes. *Neurosurg Rev* 2003;26:215–220.

141. Carvi y Nievas MN. Unruptured intracranial aneurysms in patients with transient cerebral ischemic episodes. Optional managements and literature review. *Neurol Res* 2003;25:217–221.

142. Markus HS, Clifton A, Buckenham T, Taylor R, Brown MM. Improvement in cerebral hemodynamics after carotid angioplasty. *Stroke* 1996;27:612–616.

143. Schoser BG, Heesen C, Eckert B, Thie A. Cerebral hyperperfusion injury after percutaneous transluminal angioplasty of extracranial arteries. *J Neurol* 1997;244:101–104.

144. Chaturvedi S. Medical, surgical, and interventional treatment for carotid artery disease. *Clin Neuropharmacol* 1998;21:205–214.

145. Wholey MH, Tan WA, Eles G, Jarmolowski C, Cho S. A comparison of balloon-mounted and self-expanding stents in the carotid arteries: immediate and long-term results of more than 500 patients. *J Endovasc Ther* 2003; 10:171–181.

146. Cremonesi A, Manetti R, Setacci F, Setacci C, Castriota F. Protected carotid stenting. Clinical advantages and complications of embolic protection devices in 442 consecutive patients. *Stroke* 2003;34:1936–1943.

147. McKevitt FM, Macdonald S, Venables GS, Cleveland TJ. Complications following carotid angioplasty and carotid stenting in patients with symptomatic carotid artery disease. *Cerebrovasc Dis* 2004;17:28–34.

148. Qureshi AI, Suri FK, Khan J, Fessler RD, Guterman LR, Hopkins LN. Abciximab as an adjunct to high-risk carotid or vertebrobasilar angioplasty: preliminary experience. *Neurosurgery* 2000;46:1316–1325.

149. Wholey MH, Eles G, Toursakissian B, Bailey S, Jarmolowski C, Tan WA. Evaluation of glycoprotein IIb/IIIa inhibitors in carotid angioplasty and stenting. *J Endovasc Ther* 2003;10:33–41.

150. Kopp CW, Steiner S, Nasel C, et al. Abciximab reduces monocyte tissue factor in carotid angioplasty and stenting. *Stroke* 2003;34:2560–2567.

151. Castriota F, Cremonesi A, Manetti R, et al. Impact of cerebral protection devices on early outcome of carotid stenting. *J Endovasc Ther* 2002;9:786–792.

152. Albuquerque FC, Fiorella D, Han P, Spetzler RF, McDougall CG. A reappraisal of angioplasty and stenting for the treatment of vertebral origin stenosis. *Neurosurgery* 2003;53: 607–614.

153. Golledge J, Mitchell A, Greenhalgh RM, Davies AH. Systematic comparison of the early outcome of angioplasty and endarterectomy for symptomatic carodis artery disease. *Neurology* 2000;31:1439–1443.

154. Qureshi AI, Luft AR, Sharma M, Guterman LR, Hopkins LN. Prevention and treatment of thromboembolic and ischemic complications associated with endovascular procedures: part I—pathophysiological and pharmacological features. *Neurosurgery* 2000;46:1344–1359.

155. Qureshi AI, Luft AR, Sharma M, Guterman LR, Hopkins LN. Prevention and treatment of thromboembolic and ischemic complications associated with endovascular procedures: part II—clinical aspects and recommendations. *Neurosurgery* 2000;46:1360–1376.

156. Kastrup A, Skalej M, Krapf H, Nagele T, Dichgans J, Schulz J. Early outcome of carotid angioplasty and stenting versus carotid endarterectomy in a single academic center. *Cerebrovasc Dis* 2003;15:84–89.

157. Yadav JS, Roubin GS, King P, Iyer S, Vitek J. Angioplasty and stenting for restenosis after carotid endarterectomy. Initial experience. *Stroke* 1996;27:2075–2079.

158. Yadav JS, Roubin GS, Iyer S, et al. Elective stenting of the extracranial carotid arteries. *Circulation* 1997;95:376–381.

159. Wholey MH, Jarmolowski CR, Eles G, Levy D, Buecthel J. Endovascular stents for carotid artery occlusive disease. *J Endovasc Surg* 1997;4:326–338.

160. Wholey MH, Wholey M, Bergeron P, et al. Current global status of carotid artery stent placement. *Cathet Cardiovasc Diagn* 1998;44:1–6.

161. Lanzino G, Mericle RA, Lopes DK, Wakhloo AK, Guterman LR, Hopkins LN. Percutaneous transluminal angioplasty and stent placement for recurrent carotid artery stenosis. *J Neurosurg* 1999;90:688–694.

162. Pucillo AL, Mateo RB, Aronow WS. Effect of carotid angioplasty-stenting on short-term mortality and stroke. *Heart Dis* 2003;5:378–379.

163. Chaloupka JC, Weigele JB, Mangla S, Lesley WS. Cerebrovascular angioplasty and stenting for the prevention of stroke. *Curr Neurol Neurosci Rep* 2001;1:39–53.

164. Qureshi AI, Knape C, Maroney J, Suri MFK, Hopkins LN. Multicenter clinical trial of the NexStent coiled sheet stent in the treatment of extracranial carotid artery stenosis: immediate results and late clinical outcomes. *J Neurosurg* 2003;99:264–270.

165. Hayashi K, Kitagawa N, Takahata H, et al. Endovascular treatment for cervical carotid artery stenosis presenting with progressing stroke: three case reports. *Surg Neurol* 2002;58:148–154.

166. Hanel RA, Xavier AR, Kirmani JF, Yahia AM, Qureshi AI. Management of carotid artery stenosis: comparing endarterectomy and stenting. *Curr Cardiol Rep* 2003;5: 153–159.

167. Ouriel K, Yadav JS. The role of stents in patients with carotid disease. *Rev Cardiovasc Med* 2003;4:61–67.

168. Bowser AN, Bandyk DF, Evans A, et al. Outcome of carotid stent-assisted angioplasty versus open surgical repair of recurrent carotid stenosis. *J Vasc Surg* 2003;38: 432–438.

169. Fox D, Moran CJ, Cross DT, et al. Long-term outcome after angioplasty for symptomatic extracranial stenosis in poor surgical candidates. *Stroke* 2002;33:2877–2880.

170. CAVATAS Investigators. Endovascular versus surgical treatment in patients with carotid stenosis in the Carotid and Vertebral Artery Transluminal Angioplasty Study (CAVATAS). A randomized trial. *Lancet* 2001;357:1729–1737.

171. Yadav JS, Wholey MH, Kurtz RE, et al. Protected carotid artery stenting versus endarterectomy in high-risk patients. *N Engl J Med* 2004;351:1493–1501.

172. Roubin GS, Hobson RW, White R, et al. CREST and CARESS to evaluate carotid stenting: time to get to work! *J Endovasc Ther* 2001;8:107–110.

173. Levien LJ, Benn CA, Veller MG, Fritz VU. Retrograde balloon angioplasty of brachiocephalic or common carotid artery stenoses at the time of carotid endarterectomy. *Eur J Vasc Endovasc Surg* 1998;15:521–527.

174. Widenka DC, Spuler A, Steiger H. Treatment of carotid tandem stenosis by combined carotid endarterectomy and balloon angioplasty: technical case report. *Neurosurgery* 1999;45:179–182.

175. Mathur A, Roubin GS, Yadav JS, Iyer SS, Vitek J. Combined coronary and bilateral carotid stenting: a case report. *Cathet Cardiovasc Diagn* 1997;40:202–206.

176. Hofmann R, Kerschner K, Kypta A, Steinwender C, Bibl D, Leisch F. Simultaneous stenting of the carotid artery and other coronary or extracoronary arteries: does a combined procedure increase the risk of interventional therapy? *Catheter Cardiovasc Interv* 2003;60:314–319.

177. Marks MP, Wojack JC, Al-Ali F, et al. Angioplasty for symptomatic intracranial stenosis. Clinical outcome. *Stroke* 2006;37:1016–1020.

178. Callahan AS, III, Berger BL. Balloon angioplasty of intracranial arteries for stroke prevention. *J Neuroimaging* 1997;7:232–235.

179. Higashida RT. Intracranial stenting: which patients and when? *Cleve Clin J Med* 2004;71(suppl 1):S50–S51.

180. Lee JH, Kwon SU, Suh DC, Kim JS. Percutaneous transluminal angioplasty for symptomatic middle cerebral artery stenosis: long-term follow-up. *Cerebrovasc Dis* 2003;15: 90–97.

181. Koenigsberg RA, McCormick D, Thomas C, Yee M, Williams N. Vertigo secondary to isolated PICA insufficiency: successful treatment with balloon angioplasty. *Surg Neurol* 2003;60:306–310.

182. Kellogg JX, Nesbit GM, Clark WM, Barnwell SL. The role of angioplasty in the treatment of cerebrovascular disease. *Neurosurgery* 1998;43:549–555.

183. Hurst RW, Haskal ZJ, Zager E, Bagley LJ, Flamm ES. Endovascular stent treatment of cervical internal carotid artery aneurysms with parent vessel preservation. *Surg Neurol* 1998;50:313–317.

184. Gomez CR. The role of carotid angioplasty and stenting. *Semin Neurol* 1998;18:501–511.

185. Hacein-Bey L, Koennecke HC, Pile-Spellman J, et al. Pilot study for cerebral balloon angioplasty: design considerations and case-control methods. *Cerebrovasc Dis* 1998; 8:354–357.

186. Ahuja A, Blatt GL, Guterman LR, Hopkins LN. Angioplasty for symptomatic radiation-induced extracranial carotid artery stenosis: case report. *Neurosurgery* 1995;36:399–403.

187. Rabinov JD, Hellinger FR, Morris PP, Ogilvy CS, Putman CM. Endovascular management of vertebrobasilar dissecting aneurysms. *AJNR Am J Neuroradiol* 2003;24:1421–1428.

188. Bettmann MA, Katzen BT, Whisnant J, et al. Carotid stenting and angioplasty: a statement for healthcare professionals from the Councils on Cardiovascular Radiology, Stroke, Cardio-Thoracic and Vascular Surgery, Epidemiology, and Prevention, and Clinical Cardiology, American Heart Association. *Circulation* 1998;97:121–123.

189. Joint Officers of the Congress of Neurological Surgeons and the American Association of Neurological Surgeons. Carotid angioplasty and stent: an alternative to carotid endarterectomy. *Neurosurgery* 1997;40:344–345.

190. Crawley F, Brown MM. Percutaneous transluminal angioplasty and stenting for vertebral artery stenosis. *Cochrane Database Syst Rev* 2000;CD000516.

191. Crawley F, Brown MM. Percutaneous transluminal angioplasty and stenting for carotid artery stenosis. *Cochrane Database Syst Rev* 2000;CD000515.

192. Vikram HR, Buenconsejo J, Hasbun R, Quagliarello VJ. Impact of valve surgery on 6-month mortality in adults with complicated, left-sided native valve endocarditis. A propensity analysis. *JAMA* 2003;290:3207–3214.

193. Giroud M, Tatou E, Steinmetz E, et al. The interest of surgical closure of patent foramen ovale after stroke: a preliminary open study of 8 cases. *Neurol Res* 1998;20:297–301.

194. Rodriguez CJ, Homma S. Management of patients with stroke and a patent foramen ovale. *Curr Neurol Neurosci Rep* 2004;4:19–22.

195. Mas JL, Arquizan C, Lamy C, et al. Recurrent cerebrovascular events associated with patent foramen ovale, atrial septal aneurysm, or both. *N Engl J Med* 2001;345:1740–1746.

196. Mas JL. Specifics of patent formane ovale. *Adv Neurol* 2003;92:197–202.

197. Onorato E, Melzi G, Casilli F, et al. Patent foramen ovale with paradoxical embolism: mid-term results of transcatheter closure in 256 patients. *J Interv Cardiol* 2003; 16:43–50.

198. Sievert H, Horvath K, Zadan E, et al. Patent foramen ovale closure in patients with transient ischemia attack/ stroke. *J Interv Cardiol* 2001;14:261–266.

199. Martin F, Sanchez P, Doherty E, et al. Precutaneous transcatheter closure of patent foramen ovale in patients with paradoxical embolism. *Circulation* 2002;106:1121–1126.

200. Braun MU, Fassbender D, Schoen SP, et al. Transcatheter closure of patent foramen ovale in patients with cerebral ischemia. *J Am Coll Cardiol* 2002;39:2019–2025.

201. Du ZD, Cao QL, Joseph A, et al. Transcatheter closure of patent foramen ovale in patients with paradoxical embolism: intermediate-term risk of recurrent neurological events. *Catheter Cardiovasc Interv* 2002;55:189–194.

202. Khositseth A, Cabalka AK, Sweeney JP, et al. Transcatheter amplatzer device closure of atrial septal defect and patent foramen ovale in patients with presumed paradoxical embolism. *Mayo Clin Proc* 2004;79:35–41.

203. Adams HP, Jr. Patent foramen ovale: paradoxical embolism and paradoxical data. *Mayo Clin Proc* 2004;79:15–20.

204. Sievert H, Lesh MD, Trepels T, et al. Percutaneous left atrial appendage transcatheter occlusion to prevent stroke in high-risk patients with atrial fibrillation: early clinical experience. *Circulation* 2002;105:1887–1889.

205. Blackshear JL, Johnson WD, Odell JA, et al. Thoracoscopic extracardiac obliteration of the left atrial appendage for stroke risk reduction in atrial fibrillation. *J Am Coll Cardiol* 2003;42:1249–1252.

206. Mayberg MR, Wilson JE, Yatsu F, et al. Carotid endarterectomy and prevention of cerebral ischemia in symptomatic carotid stenosis. VA Cooperative Study Program 309 Trialists group. *JAMA* 1991;266:3289–3294.

207. The CASANOVA Study Group. Carotid surgery versus medical therapy in asymptomatic carotid stenosis. *Stroke* 1991;22:2179–2184.

208. MRC Asymptomatic Carotid Surgery Trial (ACST) Collaborative Group. Prevention of disabling and fatal stroke by successful carotid endarterectomy in patients without recent neurological symptoms. Randomised, controlled trial. *Lancet* 2004;363:1491–502.

CHAPTER 21

Emergency Management of Patients with Suspected Stroke

The management of patients with acute stroke involves general emergency treatment measures in addition to specific interventions aimed at treating the acute brain hemorrhage or infarction itself. The emergency department is the usual location for initial management of most patients. In the future, certification organizations and governmental bodies likely will designate regional centers that will specialize in the treatment of patients with acute stroke. The personnel and other requirements for an emergency department and hospital are outlined in Chapter 3. Among the components will be an acute stroke team that is directed by a physician, most commonly a neurologist or emergency medicine specialist, who has expertise in the evaluation and treatment of patients with stroke. Depending upon the type of stroke (infarction or hemorrhage) and the severity of the neu-

rological injury, a neurosurgeon often needs to be involved early in treatment. The aims of the acute stroke care team are to rapidly evaluate and treat the patient. Organizations have developed a series of time goals for the initial evaluation and treatment of patients with suspected stroke (Table 21-1). Although these goals are focused on expediting thrombolytic treatment, the same actions are appropriate for management of all patients with stroke. Similar steps should be undertaken for evaluation and treatment of patients with acute spinal cord lesions, including spinal cord infarction or hemorrhage. Overall, much of the initial evaluation and treatment of patients with stroke is similar whether the patient has an infarction or a hemorrhage. Each institution should develop protocols and care maps to meet these goals (see Chapter 3).

▶ EMERGENCY DIAGNOSTIC STUDIES

The necessary baseline diagnostic tests should be obtained quickly. A list of needed studies can be included in preprinted orders[1,2] (Table 21-2). Blood samples should be forwarded to the laboratory immediately and the brain imaging tests should be readily available. Fortunately, several diagnostic tests may be done simultaneously (see Chapter 8). CT is the single most important diagnostic study because of its ability to differentiate hemorrhagic from ischemic stroke (Figs. 21-1 and 21-2).

Examination of the CSF is usually reserved for those patients with suspected subarachnoid hemorrhage and who have a normal CT examination. Depending upon the results of CT, other studies including vascular imaging, are ordered on a case-by-case basis. For example, arteriographic screening for a saccular aneurysm might be required in the emergency treatment of a patient with a subarachnoid hemorrhage. Blood samples should be sent to the institution's blood bank for typing and matching for possible need of blood transfusions during a surgical intervention.

▶ **TABLE 21-1.** TIMELINE FOR INITIAL EVALUATION AND TREATMENT OF
A PATIENT WITH STROKE

Action	Time from Arrival in Emergency Department
Seen by a physician	10 minutes
Seen by a physician from stroke team	15 minutes
Completion of brain imaging study (CT)	25 minutes
Interpretation of brain imaging study and other tests	45 minutes
Initiation of treatment for stroke	60 minutes

▶ INITIAL EVALUATION AND DIAGNOSIS

Several key questions are critical in the initial evaluation
of a patient with a suspected stroke. The sequence of
questions outlined in Table 21-3 is critical because they
influence decisions about acutely used therapies. For
example, intravenous thrombolysis is not administered
if the patient is first assessed more than 3 hours following onset of symptoms. These questions are addressed
as the patient is undergoing the initial clinical evaluation
and emergency treatment.

Upon arrival in the emergency department, physicians and other medical personnel should urgently assess
the patient's overall status (see Chapter 3). Although the
history and physical examination are described sepa-
rately in this chapter, in fact, both components of the clinical evaluation are performed simultaneously. Some components of the history influence the differential diagnosis
and emergency treatment. Still, the emergency assessment first focuses on examination. Simultaneously, management of critical aspects of care, including the ABC's of
life support should be done. Several neurological and
medical complications of stroke occur within the first
hours after the ictus and plans to address these problems
must be part of initial care.[3,4] In addition, the interval
from stroke, the severity of the neurological injury, the
patient's premorbid status, the presence of concomitant
diseases, and the patient's and family's wishes effect decisions about management.

▶ **TABLE 21-2.** GENERAL EMERGENCY
DEPARTMENT ORDERS
PATIENT WITH SUSPECTED STROKE

Nursing assessments
  Pulse, respiratory rate, and blood pressure checked
    every 15 minutes
  Temperature checked every 4 hours
  Neurological assessments every 15 minutes
  Cardiac monitoring
  Pulse oximetry
General management
  Bed rest
  Nothing given by mouth
  Intravenous access with normal saline rate approximately
    100 mL/hour
  Supplemental oxygen if patient is hypoxic
  Treat elevated temperature with antipyretic
Diagnostic studies
  Computed tomography of brain without contrast
  Electrocardiogram
  Complete blood count and platelet count
  Prothrombin time (INR) and activated partial
    thromboplastin time
  Blood glucose
  Serum electrolytes
  Blood for typing and crossing (if transfusion planned)
  If febrile, cultures of blood, urine, and sputum
  Examination of CSF if subarachnoid hemorrhage
    suspected and CT is negative

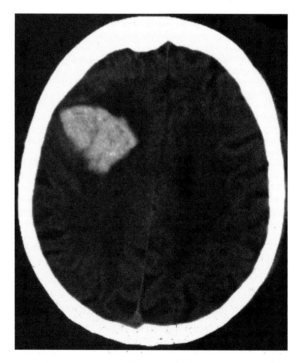

Figure 21-1. An unenhanced CT scan demonstrates
a right frontral hemorrhage in a patient presenting with
an acute onset of left hemiparesis.

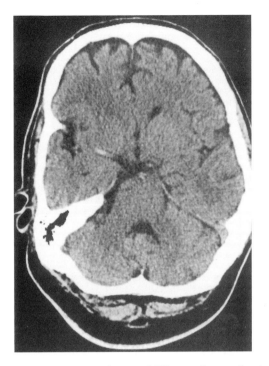

Figure 21-2. An unenhanced CT scan in a patient with an acute onset of left hemispheresis shows an embolus in the in the right middle cerebral artery (dense artery sign). No area of the brain ischemia is detected.

► EMERGENCY ASSESSMENT AND MANAGEMENT

Level of Consciousness

The patient's level of consciousness is a vital sign and often is disturbed following a stroke. The initial level of consciousness is a strong predictor of outcome.[5] The

► TABLE 21-3. CRITICAL QUESTIONS EVALUATION OF PATIENT WITH SUSPECTED STROKE

When did the symptoms of stroke begin?
  Any neurological worsening or improvement?
  Any warning events during the preceding days?
  Was recovery from warning events complete?
What are the symptoms of the new stroke?
Any recent (previous 6 weeks) medical problems?
  Previous stroke—ischemic or hemorrhagic?
  Other neurological illness?
  Myocardial infarction or other cardiac event?
  Major bleeding events?
  Major operation?
  Major injury, including at time of possible stroke?
What medications are being taken?
  Anticoagulants?
  Antiplatelet aggregating events?
  Cardiac medications?
  Insulin?

spectrum of impairments in consciousness ranges from drowsiness to deep coma. In an elegant neuroanatomic-clinical study, Parvizi and Damasio[6] found that coma most commonly results from discrete vascular lesions of the pons and midbrain. These lesions usually are large and affect the tegmentum. Generally, patients with ischemic stroke do not develop stupor or coma during the first few hours; most will be alert, drowsy, or stunned. Although many patients with major hemispheric infarctions have profound cognitive impairments, their awareness of the environment and their responses to stimuli are not impaired. Cucchiara et al.[7] found no association between the involved hemisphere and the subsequent development of impairments in consciousness among patients with major infarctions. Patients with bilateral hemispheric ischemic events might be unconscious but these events are relatively uncommon. Coma commonly accompanies a major intracranial hemorrhage. In general, impaired consciousness is secondary to increased intracranial pressure that results from mass effect of a hematoma or the development of acute hydrocephalus. Some of the alternative diagnoses to stroke, including hypoglycemia, also are associated with a depressed level of alertness.

Some strokes are complicated by seizures, which also may impair consciousness. Patients with hemorrhagic stroke, in particular those with severe headache after subarachnoid hemorrhage, may have a delirium. A delirious patient can be agitated and require restraints in order to be protected from serious injury. Delirium is uncommon in most patients with ischemic stroke although it may be found in elderly patients, those with preexisting dementia, or patients with infectious or metabolic complications of the stroke.[8,9] A delirium also might be secondary to severe headache or nausea and vomiting.

The cause of impaired consciousness should be sought. Because such a patient is unable to relate the details of the event, family members or other observers should be asked about the course of the illness and any complicating diseases or trauma. The diagnostic battery of tests listed in Table 8-1 in Chapter 8 addresses the most common causes of coma. Other potential causes of delirium or coma, such as alcohol or drug overdose and an infectious disease, also can be evaluated. If a seizure is suspected by the history or examination, an EEG should be obtained. Patients with seizures should receive anticonvulsants (see below). Treating any metabolic of infectious disease that complicates stroke is part of the management of the coma. In addition, patients with a depressed level of consciousness need protection of the airway and other urgent management prior to evaluation and treatment of the stroke. Unconscious patients are at risk for orthopedic, dermatologic, muscular, or peripheral nerve trauma, and care should include measures to avoid such injuries. If a patient might have fallen at the time of the stroke or loss of consciousness, a secondary cervical spine injury should

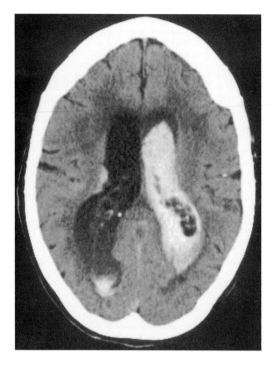

Figure 21-3. An unenhanced CT scan in a patient with a massive intraventricular hemorrhage. Hydrocephalus with dilation of the contralateral lateral ventricle also is present.

be considered. In such a situation, protection of the neck and screening for a fracture should be included in the emergent evaluation.

Nurses should repeatedly assess the patient's level of consciousness during the first few hours after stroke. Any deterioration in consciousness suggests worsening of the stroke or the development of acute complications, such as hemorrhagic transformation of the infarction, hydrocephalus, or malignant brain edema that warrants emergency treatment (Fig. 21-3). In addition, deterioration in alertness also may accompany acute medical complications including hypoglycemia, hyponatremia, or hypoxia. A decline in consciousness mandates reevaluation of the patient to screen for the cause and emergency treatment.

Airway and Breathing

Unconscious patients should have their airway protected to avoid obstruction, aspiration, hypoventilation, and cardiovascular complications (Table 21-4). Hypoventilation can lead to increased concentrations of pCO2, which in turn leads to cerebral vasodilation and increased intracranial pressure. Hypoxia and respiratory acidosis also depress consciousness. Patients with intracranial hemorrhage often have vomiting and protection of the airway is critical to avoid aspiration pneumonia and subsequent hypoxia.[10] Patients with severe paralysis of the oropha-

ryngeal muscles or loss of protective reflexes also must have the airway secured.[11] Patients lying in the supine position and those with typical risk factors for obstructive sleep apnea, such as obesity or large neck circumference, have a high risk for upper airway obstruction.[12]

Although no clinical trial has tested the usefulness of endotracheal intubation in the emergent treatment of patients with stroke, there is general agreement that an endotracheal tube should be placed if the airway is threatened.[1,2] Intubation is critical because it helps prevent obstruction, atelectasis, aspiration, and pneumonia. Impaired consciousness is the primary indication for endotracheal intubation. While patients with hemorrhage requiring endotracheal intubation usually have a Glasgow Coma Scale score of 10 or less, the procedure often is indicated by evidence of imminent respiratory failure rather than a specific score on the Glasgow Coma Scale.[13] The prognosis of patients who require endotracheal intubation generally is poor; approximately 50 percent are dead at 30 days.[14–16] On the other hand, Roch et al.[17] found that many patients with intracerebral hemorrhage who require ventilatory assistance will survive the illness and some will have favorable outcomes. Thus, there is a reason to be aggressive. In addition to protecting the airway, elective intubation can assist in the management of increased intracranial pressure or brain edema.[15] Emergency intubation expedites all subsequent components of care. Placement of an oral or nasal airway is not a sufficient substitute of endotracheal intubation.

Intubation should be performed with care with maximal preoxygenation. Medications such as atropine, thiopental, propofol, and succinylcholine may be needed

▶ **TABLE 21-4.** ABC'S OF LIFE SUPPORT ACUTE STROKE

Protect airway—endotracheal intubation
    Decreased consciousness
    Bulbar dysfunction
    Screen for possible cervical spine fracture
Breathing
    Treat hypoxia
    Avoid hypercarbia
    Treat increased intracranial pressure
    Supplemental oxygen
Circulation
    Treat acute cardiac arrhythmias
    Treat acute myocardial ischemia
    Treat arterial hypertension
    Treat arterial hypotension
Glucose
    Treat hyperglycemia
    Treat hypoglycemia
Temperature
    Treat fever

to ease intubation and in order to avoid secondary hypertensive crises or cardiac arrhythmias.[13] Similarly, measures to avoid vomiting and aspiration are included. If complicating craniocerebral trauma and cervical spine injury are suspected, screening for a neck injury must be done prior to elective intubation. Pulmonary suctioning often is needed to help maintain patency of the airway.

Many patients with stroke have preexisting cardiovascular or pulmonary diseases that may affect oxygenation and ventilation. Secondary hypoxia is reversed by supplemental oxygenation.[18] However, many patients with intracerebral hemorrhages or brainstem hemorrhages or infarctions also have abnormalities in breathing.[19] Lesions of the distal medulla and rostral spinal cord may lead to Ondine curse.[20] Paralysis of the intercostal muscles or diaphragm secondary to spinal cord infarction or hemorrhage may impair breathing.[21] Subarachnoid hemorrhage may lead to secondary lung injury and respiratory failure.[22,23] Disturbances in breathing may be secondary to metabolic disorders, especially hyperglycemia and acidosis.

Abnormal ventilatory patterns are of particular importance among comatose patients. Ventilatory failure is a leading cause of sudden death among persons with acute neurological events. Ventilatory assistance is indicated if the arterial blood gases demonstrate a pO2 < 60 mm Hg or pCO2 > 50 mm Hg.[13] In addition to protecting the airway, ventilatory assistance is a critical step in saving a patient's life. While most patients are initially treated with an external ventilator, noninvasive positive pressure ventilation might be used in a few patients with spinal cord vascular events who have intercostal and diaphragmatic paralysis but preserved central respiratory drive.[21] Hyperventilation often is needed as a temporary emergency measure to help control increased intracranial pressure. This indication for intubation and ventilatory assistance is discussed below.

Supplemental Oxygen

Most patients do not require supplemental oxygen. Measuring oxygen saturation concentrations with a pulse oximeter is often sufficient to guide decisions about oxygenation assistance. The goal is to maintain oxygen saturation levels of 95 percent or greater.[24] Hypoxic patients or those with blood oxygen desaturation should receive oxygen either via nasal prongs or a facemask.[1,25,26] A recent controlled study found that the use of supplemental oxygen (3 L/minute) did not improve outcomes following stroke.[27] Subsequent assessments of arterial blood gases may affect subsequent management. In particular, patients with preexisting lung disease may need supplemental oxygen on a long-term basis. While hyperbaric oxygen therapy might be useful in treatment of patients with acute neurological symptoms secondary to air embolization or Caisson disease, evidence to support its use in treatment of acute ischemic stroke is lacking.[28–30]

Fever

Most patients with acute cerebrovascular events are not febrile. However, among patients with hemorrhages or major infarctions, the body temperature usually begins to rise in the first 4–6 hours.[31] Fever is commonly detected among patients hospitalized for treatment of stroke.[32] The presence of fever, particularly at 10–12 hours after onset, is a poor prognostic sign.[29] A temperature > 37°C on admission to the hospital is associated with more severe strokes, diabetes mellitus, and poor outcomes.[33] Elevation of body temperature is associated with increased metabolic demands, free-radical production, and release of neurotransmitters.[34,35] All of these factors have a negative effect on an acutely ill brain. In a meta-analysis of the clinical reports of the influence of fever on outcomes, Hajat et al.[36] concluded that pyrexia after stroke was associated with marked increases in morbidity and mortality. Regardless of the severity of bleeding or the presence of infectious complications, the development of fever after subarachnoid hemorrhage is independently predictive of vasospasm or a poor outcome.[37]

Therefore, the source of any fever should be sought. Grau et al.[38] found that most fevers following stroke are secondary to complicating infections, most commonly pneumonia. Patients with decreased consciousness or paralysis of bulbar muscles have a potential for aspiration and secondary pneumonia. Other potential sources of fever include urinary tract infection or sepsis. The latter might be associated with infective endocarditis, which could explain a cardioembolic stroke or an unusual intracranial hemorrhage (ruptured infective aneurysm). The infectious source for a fever should be treated. Blood in the subarachnoid space and ventricles also might incite an inflammatory reaction and fever and may require neurosurgical management.

A central (neurogenic) fever should not be diagnosed unless other explanations for the elevated temperature are excluded. A neurogenic cause of fever is most commonly detected among patients with a subarachnoid hemorrhage. Presumably central fever is due to a disturbance in hypothalamic thermoregulatory centers, although the release of endogenous pyrogens also has been implicated.[39] Central fever, which most commonly occurs soon after the vascular event, does not respond well to antipyretic medications.[39] The levels of temperature vary widely with central fever. Among patients with severe intracranial bleeding, both brain and core body temperatures are elevated and these elevations are associated closely with elevated intracranial pressure readings.[40] Neurogenic fever is uncommon following a cerebral infarction.

Febrile patients should have their temperature lowered.[1] Lowering an elevated body temperature may improve prognosis.[41] Although antipyretic agents are prescribed, data about their utility are limited. Clinical trials have tested the utility of oral medications for lowering body temperatures in improving outcomes following stroke.[42–44] Acetaminophen produces a modest reduction in core body temperature. Early administration of aspirin or other nonsteroid anti-inflammatory agents also might lower body temperatures. Although these agents may be used to lower temperature, their effects on platelet function restrict their use following the administration of rt-PA. Cormio et al.[45] administered continuous low-dose diclofenac infusions to patients with acute brain injuries, including those with subarachnoid hemorrhage. They found that normalizing the temperature was associated with improved intracranial pressure. Still, Sulter et al.[46] concluded that neither aspirin or acetaminophen would lower temperatures sufficiently to be neuroprotective. Sustained fevers may be treated with other measures including internal or external cooling devices. Hypothermia has been shown to be effective in protecting the brain in the setting of acute ischemia.[46] The use of hypothermia, which is an emerging therapy to treat acute ischemic stroke, is discussed in Chapter 22.

Cardiac Complications Including Arrhythmias

The interactions between heart disease and stroke are numerous. Patients with preexisting heart disease can have secondary cardioembolic stroke (see Chapter 13). Stroke may be the initial manifestation of an underlying acute cardiac event, such as a clinically occult myocardial infarction or infective endocarditis. Stroke may be the result of treatment of the acute coronary occlusions, such as an intracranial hemorrhage following administration of thrombolytic agents, anticoagulants, and antiplatelet medications. Cardiac complications of stroke are not uncommon. They include myocardial ischemia and cardiac arrhythmias.

Myocardial Ischemia

Myocardial ischemia can occur among patients without known coronary artery disease. Presumably ischemia is due to high levels of catecholamines from hypothalamic and autonomic nervous system dysfunction. Myocardial infarction is a cause of death among patients with intracranial vascular events, especially those with hemorrhage.[4,48,49] In patients with subarachnoid hemorrhage, myocardial injury is seen primarily among persons with severe bleeding. Among patients with cerebral infarction, cardiac changes were most commonly found among patients with lesions affecting the insular cortex.[50] Thus, while silent coronary artery disease may preexist the

stroke, the stress of the cerebrovascular event also may lead to secondary cardiac ischemia. Myocardial ischemia can occur among patients without known coronary artery disease.

On examination of the heart among patients dying of acute cerebrovascular events, subendocardial ischemic lesions, small hemorrhages, or focal areas of myocardial necrosis may be found.[51] Electrocardiographic changes suggestive of myocardial ischemia include ST depression and pathological Q waves[52] (Table 21-5). The frequency of serious secondary electrocardiographic changes following subarachnoid hemorrhage can exceed 50 percent.[53] The presence of Q waves in more than two cardiac leads is predictive of death from cerebral infarction.[54] McDermott et al.[55] found ST wave changes consistent with acute myocardial ischemia within 5 days of stroke in approximately 20 percent of patients. The presence of ST changes is associated with an increased risk of severe cardiovascular complications of stroke.[56] Macmillan et al.[57] reported that increased QT dispersion was associated with cardiorespiratory failure among patients with severe subarachnoid hemorrhage. QT prolongation following subarachnoid hemorrhage is more common in women and those with hypokaliemia.[58] Other cardiac effects include abnormalities in left ventricular wall motion, presumably due to myocardial damage. In addition, patients

▶ **TABLE 21-5.** CARDIOVASCULAR COMPLICATIONS OF STROKE

Myocardial ischemia
  Acute subendocardial myocardial infarction
  Abnormal electrocardiogram
    Changes in ST segment—depression, elevation, inversion
    Inverted T waves
    Pathological Q waves
    QT wave dispersion or prolongation
    U waves
  Elevated levels of MB component of creatine kinase
  Elevated levels of troponin
Cardiac arrhythmias
  Atrial or blocks
    Sinus bradycardia
    Atrial fibrillation
    Sinoatrial block
    Atrioventricular block
    Asystolic intervals
  Ventricular
    Unifocal premature ventricular contractions
    Multifocal premature ventricular contractions
    Bigeminy or trigeminy
    Ventricular tachycardia
    Torsades de pointes
    Ventricular fibrillation
  Congestive heart failure—neurogenic pulmonary edema

can have elevated levels of enzymes suggesting myocardial damage including increases in troponin and the MB band of creatine kinase.[48,59] Treatment of myocardial ischemia should be part of emergency management. In most circumstances, the urgent advice of a cardiologist should be sought. Cardiac measures such as thrombolytic agents, antiplatelet agents, and anticoagulants might not be appropriate in the setting of stroke but other interventions might be helpful. For example, medications such as beta-blockers could be prescribed to protect the heart.[60] A pacemaker also might be required.

Cardiac Arrhythmias

Cardiac arrhythmias, including potentially life-threatening disturbances, are more common among persons with intracranial hemorrhage than with cerebral infarctions. Cardiac arrhythmias are a leading cause of sudden death among patients with stroke. Impaired autonomic regulation of heart rate leading to changes in cardiac instability is strongly associated with an increased risk of death following stroke.[61] Serious arrhythmias are less common among patients with cerebral infarction than among those with bleeding.[62] In particular, subarachnoid hemorrhage is complicated by cardiac disturbances[63] (see Table 21-5). Arrhythmias may be secondary to myocardial ischemia, which is secondary to excessive levels of catecholamines leading to vasospasm of coronary arteries or to the direct neurotoxic effects of catecholamines.[50,64–67] Cardiac rhythm disturbances are common in the elderly and among those with a history of heart disease.[50] Cardiac arrhythmias are correlated with lesions of the medulla or the cerebral hemispheres.[68] In particular, ischemic and hemorrhagic lesions of the insular cortex have a rate of cardiac arrhythmias. Some reports suggest that infarction of the right insular cortex is strongly associated with cardiac conduction disturbances, while others correlate arrhythmias with strokes affecting the left insular region.[69–71] Presumably, insular lesions lead to parasympathetic or sympathetic nervous system dysfunction. Changes in circadian control of the heart rate also may lead to cardiac arrhythmias within the first days following stroke.[72] Cardiac arrhythmias often are secondary to hypoxia or metabolic disturbances, in particular electrolyte disorders.

Ventricular arrhythmias, including torsades de pointes, or conduction defects are potential complications of stroke. Fortunately, these events are relatively uncommon. Following stroke, atrial fibrillation is the most commonly detected arrhythmia. It often is preexisting and, in some cases, may be markers for the cause of stroke. While atrial fibrillation is the leading marker of cardioembolic stroke, it also may represent a complication of the vascular event. In particular, atrial fibrillation is described as a complication of intracranial hemorrhage. Monitoring of cardiac rate and rhythm should be performed during the first hours after the stroke. If serious arrhythmias are detected, medical interventions should be prescribed as directed by a cardiologist.

Neurogenic Pulmonary Edema

Congestive heart failure is a relatively uncommon complication of stroke. Still, this cardiac complication greatly affects acute management. In one series, severe congestive heart failure with pulmonary edema was one of the leading indications for emergency ventilatory assistance.[73] Congestive heart failure may be secondary to neurogenic factors that cause decreased myocardial contractility. The resultant pulmonary edema leads to increased hypoxia and hypercarbia. These factors, in turn, worsen brain edema and increase intracranial pressure. Neurogenic pulmonary edema is a rare but life-threatening complication of serious intracranial hemorrhages, particularly among patients with ruptured aneurysms.[23] It is characterized by the presence of acute accumulation of protein-rich fluid within the lungs. This complication is correlated with hypothalamic injury or dysfunction. Neurogenic pulmonary edema is most commonly found among patients with other evidence of acute cardiac dysfunction, including QT dispersion and large negative T waves found on electrocardiography.[57,74] Presumably, pulmonary edema is due to acute left ventricular dysfunction. A sudden increase in pulmonary pressure may be secondary to vasoconstriction of pulmonary arteries due to sympathetic hyperactivity, increased capillary permeability and hydrostatic mechanisms.[75] Patients require intense cardiovascular monitoring. Ventilatory support and oxygen supplementation is fundamental. Fletcher and Atkinson[76] found that placing a patient in the prone position improved oxygenation. Infusions of dobutamine also may be administered.[77] Overall, patients with pulmonary edema have a poor prognosis.

Arterial Hypertension

Frequent blood pressure measurements are a component of emergency care. Physicians should be prepared to respond to changes in blood pressure readings. Either a sudden increase or decrease in blood pressure may occur with acute neurological or medical complications of the stroke.

An elevated blood pressure is detected commonly within the first few hours of hemorrhagic and ischemic stroke.[10,78] Broderick et al.[79] found elevated blood pressures (systolic > 160 mm Hg) within 90 minutes of onset of stroke in approximately 40 percent of patients. In a series of 624 patients, Brott et al.[80] found elevated blood pressures in 60 percent within the first 24 hours of ischemic stroke. Subsequently, most patients had a spontaneous decline of 20 percent or 25 percent or greater during the first 24 hours following stroke.[81] Aslanyan et al.[82]

found that while an acutely elevated blood pressure is not associated with poor outcomes, subsequent increases are correlated with unfavorable results. Other evidence exists that early hypertension or stability in blood pressure is a predictor of unfavorable outcomes, including death.[83–85] Elevated blood pressures are associated with a high rate of neurological worsening. Markedly elevated blood pressures may aggravate brain edema, potentiate continued bleeding from a ruptured intracranial vessel, lead to growth of an intracerebral hematoma, promote recurrent rupture of an aneurysm, or lead to hemorrhagic transformation of an infarction.[86,87] Such relationships may not be surprising since those patients with the most severe strokes have the highest levels of blood pressure.

There are several causes of elevated blood pressure (Table 21-6). It may represent preexisting arterial hypertension or may be a response to pain, nausea, vomiting, agitation or the stress of the neurological event. Arterial hypertension also might be a natural compensatory mechanism to maintain blood flow via collaterals in acute ischemic stroke or to maintain perfusion to the brain in a patient with increased intracranial pressure.[81] Despite its high prevalence in acutely ill patients, the optimal management of arterial hypertension is not established.[88] Moderate lowering of blood pressure might improve outcomes.[84,89]

Cerebral autoregulation is dysfunctional in the setting of an acute cerebrovascular event and cerebral blood flow becomes pressure-dependent.[88] Thus, there is concern that mitigates overly aggressive treatment of blood pressure; a decrease in blood pressure may reduce cerebral perfusion pressure and thereby worsen the ischemic injury.[1,2,13,88] However, another review found that lowering of blood pressure did not have a negative effect on outcomes among the most seriously ill patients.[90]

Treatment of agitation, headache, nausea, and vomiting may have a secondary effect in lowering blood pressure. Management of cardiopulmonary disease and elimination of an airway obstruction also can lessen

▶ **TABLE 21-6.** CAUSES OF INCREASED BLOOD PRESSURE FOLLOWING STROKE

Preexisting arterial hypertension
  Chronic hypertension
  Acute hypertensive crisis
Consequences of acute stroke
  Increased intracranial pressure—perfusion pressure
  Autonomic (sympathetic nervous system) disturbances
Symptomatic hypertension
  Headache
  Seizures
  Agitation
  Stress
  Nausea and vomiting

▶ **TABLE 21-7.** INDICATIONS FOR TREATMENT OF ELEVATED BLOOD PRESSURE

To lower markedly high levels—hemorrhagic stroke
  Slow continued bleeding
  Prevent recurrent arterial rupture
To treat hypertensive encephalopathy
To allow administration of thrombolytic agents—ischemic stroke
To treat other acute vascular or medical diseases
  Acute myocardial ischemia
  Acute heart failure—pulmonary edema
  Arterial (aortic) dissection
  Acute renal failure

arterial hypertension. Management of increased intracranial pressure, including the avoidance of hypercarbia, may secondarily lower blood pressure. As a result, many patients have spontaneous and dramatic declines in blood pressure levels without the institution of antihypertensive agents. However, even without these other factors, the natural history of blood pressure after acute stroke appears to be a reduction to prestroke levels during a course of several weeks.

Several factors influence decisions in the management of arterial hypertension following stroke (Table 21-7). Patients with concomitant myocardial ischemia, pulmonary edema, renal failure, or arterial dissection likely need emergent treatment. In addition, the urgency of lowering blood pressure is influenced by plans to treat the stroke. Most notably, sustained hypertension (systolic blood pressure > 185 mm Hg or diastolic blood pressure > 110 mm Hg) disqualifies a patient for treatment with intravenous rt-PA.[1] Although severe arterial hypertension is of concern, no data define the levels of blood pressure that mandate emergent management in other circumstances.

Current guidelines generally are based on consensus and the recommendations regarding blood pressure are quite broad.[1,2,13,91] In general, management of arterial hypertension is more aggressive among patients with intracranial bleeding than among persons with ischemic stroke[10,87] (Table 21-8). Among patients with ischemic stroke, antihypertensive medications are withheld unless the systolic blood pressure is > 220 mm Hg or diastolic blood pressure is > 120 mm Hg.[1] A mean blood pressure > 130 mm Hg has been the threshold for administering antihypertensive medications to patients with intracranial hemorrhage.[13] These guidelines may need further revision as additional data related to outcome measures and blood pressure, such as those described above, become available in the future.

Patients with simultaneous arterial hypertension and increased intracranial pressure pose a special problem. The difficult goal is to lower the blood pressure

▶ **TABLE 21-8.** MANAGEMENT OF ARTERIAL HYPERTENSION IN ACUTE ISCHEMIC STROKE

General principles
  Blood pressure often declines as patient's status stabilizes
    Response to treatment of increased intracranial pressure
    Response to treatment of hypoxia or hypercarbia
  Blood pressure often declines as other symptoms are treated
  Blood pressure should be reduced cautiously
  Monitor blood pressure carefully
  Medications with short duration of actions preferred
  Parenteral medications preferred initially
  Titrate medications in response to blood pressure declines
  Halt medications if blood pressure declines too rapidly
General blood pressure values that prompt treatment
  Mean blood pressure >130 mm Hg
  Systolic blood pressure >220 mm Hg
Blood pressure goals that permit treatment with rt-PA
  Diastolic blood pressure <110 mm Hg
  Systolic blood pressure <185 mm Hg

without compromising cerebral perfusion pressure. Cerebral perfusion pressure can be calculated among patients with increased intracranial pressure. Low levels of cerebral perfusion pressure can aggravate ischemia and if the cerebral perfusion pressure is less than 70 mm Hg, antihypertensive medications should be withheld.[13]

In general, blood pressure is lowered cautiously. A reasonable goal is to drop the blood pressure by approximately 15 percent per day until the patient has achieved desired levels. Medications may be given orally, transdermally, or parenterally. Transdermal glyceryl trinitrate can lower blood pressure but maintain cerebral blood flow after stroke.[92] Intravenously administered medications act the most rapidly and may be indicated for some of the above management indications (Table 21-9). In general, desirable medications should lower blood pressure promptly but the duration of action should be relatively brief. Potent antihypertensive agents that produce a sustained lowering of blood pressure should be avoided in the acute setting. For example, sublingual administration of nifedipine is problematic due to its long half-life.[93] Current guidelines recommend the use of intravenous labetalol or transdermal nitropaste to lower the blood pressure prior to administration of rt-PA.[1] Other choices for early antihypertensive management include captopril and nicardipine. Some patients may require an intravenous infusion of sodium nitroprusside or nitroglycerine. These medications might lead to vasodilation of intracranial arteries that may promote increases in intracranial pressure. Thus, they are prescribed to patients with malignant elevations of blood pressure. Some of the angiotensin converting enzyme inhibitors and calcium channel blockers also affect intracranial pressure. However, there is no clinical evidence that antihypertensive medications cause increased neurological impairments by an adverse effect on intracranial pressure. Still, if these medications lower blood pressure too rapidly or dramatically, the infusion should be slowed or discontinued. Then, a medication could be restarted at a reduced rate or concentration to maintain the desired level of blood pressure.

Some specific pharmacological effects influence the choice of other medications to treat arterial hypertension. For example, captopril should be avoided if concomitant renal artery stenosis is suspected.[94] Nifedipine and similar agents may increase heart rate while clonidine and the beta-blockers slow the pulse and may lower cardiac output.[94] Because many patients are dehydrated, the use of diuretics solely as an antihypertensive agent in the acute setting generally is avoided. Maintenance antihypertensive therapy usually is begun as soon as the patient is stable. This component of management generally will occur in the days after the patient is admitted to the hospital.

Arterial Hypotension

A low blood pressure following stroke is uncommon. Most hypotensive patients have a serious underlying disease that mandates emergency attention and, as a result, a low blood pressure is a poor prognostic sign.[83,85] A secondary drop in perfusion pressure may lead to impaired alertness or a worsening of focal neurological impairments. Potential causes are aortic dissection, blood loss, dehydration, side effects of medications, and decreased cardiac output secondary to myocardial ischemia or cardiac

▶ **TABLE 21-9.** MEDICATIONS TO LOWER BLOOD PRESSURE TREATMENT OF ACUTE STROKE

Intravenous administration of labetalol
  Initial dose of 10–20 mg
  Subsequent doses of 20–80 mg every 10–15 minutes OR
    Infuse 2–8 mg/minute and adjust dose
  Stop if no response after 150 mg
Intravenous administration of sodium nitroprusside
  Initial dose of 0.5 μg/kg/minute
  Adjust treatment in response to blood pressure
  Dose range 0.5–10 μg/kg/minute
Intravenous administration of nicardipine
  Initial dose 5 mg/hour
  Titrate up by 0.25 mg/hour at 5–15 minute intervals if blood pressure is elevated
  Maximum dose 15 mg/hour
  When desired blood pressure reached reduce dose to 3 mg/hour
Alternative medications
  Transdermal nitropaste
  Captopril

▶ **TABLE 21-10.** CAUSES OF HYPOTENSION IN PATIENTS WITH ACUTE STROKE

Cardiovascular causes
    Myocardial ischemia
    Cardiac arrhythmias
    Aortic or arterial dissection
    Decreased cardiac output
Side effects of medications
Decreased volume
    Blood loss
    Dehydration
    Syndrome of inappropriate antidiuretic hormone
    Release of brain natruretic peptide

arrhythmia (Table 21-10). Low circulating blood volume may be secondary to bleeding or dehydration. While the volume of intracranial hemorrhage is relatively small, a patient with a coagulopathy also may have bleeding elsewhere in the body. Patients with intracranial hemorrhage may have acute erosive gastritis and gastrointestinal bleeding.[60] A disturbance in baroreceptor activity, such as that following surgery or angioplasty and stenting of the origin of the internal carotid artery, also may lead to hypotension.

Treatment usually involves restoration of the circulating volume with infusions of saline or colloids, including blood among patients who are anemic. Vasopressors, such as dopamine, also may be needed. Drug-induced hypertension has been used to treat ischemic symptoms secondary to vasospasm following subarachnoid hemorrhage. Induced elevations of blood pressure also have been used to treat acute stroke.[91,95,96] While preliminary data are promising, additional research is needed (see Chapter 22). Urgent medical treatment of hypotension following internal carotid artery angioplasty and stenting may require anticholinergic agents, such as atropine or glycopyrrolate, to treat concurrent bradycardia.

Hyperglycemia

Hyperglycemia is associated with an increased likelihood of an unfavorable outcome following stroke.[97–100] One study found that a blood glucose concentration greater than 8 mmol/L was associated with a poor outcome following stroke even when the data were corrected for the patient's age, the severity of stroke, and the likely cause.[101] The volumes of infarctions among patients with hyperglycemia also are larger than those noted among patients with normal blood glucose concentrations. Baird et al.[102] found that persistent hyperglycemia is associated with expansion of the volume of cerebral infarction during the first hours after stroke. In addition, the presence of hyperglycemia is associated with an increased risk of neurological worsening in the first few hours following stroke among patients with nonlacunar infarctions.[97] Hyperglycemia also might be a marker of increased risk

of hemorrhagic transformation of an infarction, particularly after reperfusion.[97,103] Hyperglycemia also increases the development of brain edema and perihematomal cell death after intracerebral hemorrhage.[104]

There is a strong scientific explanation for the negative effects of hyperglycemia in the presence of acute stroke. Hyperglycemia in the presence of hypoxia (the situation in acute cerebral ischemia) stimulates anaerobic glycolysis and lactic acidosis; this may worsen the neurological injury. It also can affect blood–brain barrier permeability. Still, the interactions between hyperglycemia and stroke outcome appear to be more complex. Blood glucose levels increase during the first hours following a severe stroke.[105] An elevation of the blood glucose concentration is a potential stress response to a severe stroke and hyperglycemia might primarily be a marker of a serious brain event.[106,107] In general, the level of glucose on admission is correlated with the severity of neurological impairments.[108] The finding that neither outcomes nor severity of stroke are correlated with levels of glycosylated hemoglobin (an indicator of preexisting hyperglycemia) supports the concept that hyperglycemia may represent a stress response to a severe stroke.[109]

Unfortunately, considerable uncertainty remains about optimal management of hyperglycemia. Current guidelines advocate efforts to reduce markedly elevated glucose concentrations but the data to support this recommendation are lacking.[1] Efforts to lower a markedly elevated blood glucose concentration seem prudent but the level that prompts initiation of insulin is not clear. Similarly, the rapidity of lowering blood glucose concentrations and desired level of glucose are not known. Baird et al.[102] recommended that normalization of blood glucose concentrations. A small trial demonstrated that an infusion containing both insulin and glucose could be given safely to patients with mild-to-moderate hyperglycemia following stroke.[110] Another series found that intravenous insulin could be given safely during treatment of acute stroke.[111] A trial testing intensive insulin therapy among critically ill patients (not necessarily with stroke) found that maintaining a blood glucose concentration under 110 mg/dL reduces morbidity and mortality.[112] Gray et al.[113] found that infusions of glucose, potassium, and insulin rapidly achieved euglycemia following stroke. While this regimen appears to be safe, additional research is needed to demonstrate efficacy. Trials are testing the utility of aggressive management of hyperglycemia on outcomes of patients with stroke.

Hypoglycemia

Hypoglycemia is included in the differential diagnosis of acute stroke because low glucose concentrations can produce focal neurological impairments that mimic acute stroke. In addition, hypoglycemia may exacerbate the acute effects of a stroke. Most affected patients have a history of diabetes mellitus and are taking insulin or an oral hypoglycemic agent. Still, the history of diabetes mellitus might not be available readily. Rapid screening of the blood glucose level should be followed by intravenous administration of glucose-containing fluids (most commonly an ampule of 50 percent dextrose in water). Many patients with hypoglycemia also have impaired consciousness that may result in a poor history regarding prior alcohol abuse. In theory, glucose administration may exacerbate the effects of thiamine deficiency and cause Wernicke–Korsakoff syndrome, so the simultaneous administration of thiamine should be given in conjunction with dextrose.

Fluid and Electrolyte Balance

Evaluation of the patient's fluid and electrolyte status should be part of the baseline evaluation in the emergency department. Patients with intracranial hemorrhages or infarctions involving the brainstem may have severe nausea and vomiting, which can lead to dehydration or electrolyte disturbances. Some patients, especially the elderly and those who are febrile, might have preexisting dehydration. The presence of hypotension is a clue that the patient likely has hypovolemia.

Expanding the vascular compartment may improve the neurological status of the patient by augmenting cerebral perfusion.[114] In general, the goal is to maintain a euvolemic state. Although many patients with stroke have a history of heart disease and congestive heart failure, the administration of fluids usually can be done safely. If there is a concern about cardiac failure or pulmonary edema, monitoring of pulmonary arterial wedge pressure or central venous pressure may be helpful. Typically normal saline is sufficient to normalize hydration status, although in some cases, blood products or colloids are needed. Hypo-osmolar fluids, such as 5 percent dextrose in water, are not given for rehydration purposes because of the associated risk of increasing brain edema. Serum electrolytes should be checked at regular intervals so that additional therapy can be given to maintain a normal electrolyte status.

Hypovolemia and hyponatremia are frequently found in the first hours after subarachnoid hemorrhage, especially among those patients with major bleeding.[60,115] These findings are secondary to disturbances in the release of brain natruretic peptides or antidiuretic hormone presumably secondary to hypothalamic dysfunction.[116,117] The low sodium is partially due to the loss of the kidney's ability to conserve sodium and water.[116] Often, patients have decreased circulating blood volume in addition to hyponatremia.[118] While patients with hyponatremia often are treated with fluid restriction, the presence of a low sodium concentration following subarachnoid hemorrhage should not prompt this response.

Restricting fluids can lead to an additional decline in blood volume, increased blood viscosity, and hemoconcentration.[119] This contraction in intravascular volume is particularly critical among patients with aneurysmal subarachnoid hemorrhage because of their high risk for ischemia secondary to vasospasm.[119] Rather, patients are given adequate amounts of fluids (approximately 2–3 L/day) and hypertonic saline can be used to correct the hyponatremia.

Hypervolemic hemodilution, which has been used to treat ischemia in patients with acute infarctions and to prevent ischemia among patients with vasospasm following subarachnoid hemorrhage, is reviewed in Chapters 22 and 23.

▶ SPECIFIC EMERGENCY INTERVENTIONS

Treatment of a Coagulopathy

Spinal or intracranial hemorrhages may be serious complications of a congenital or acquired disorder of coagulation (Table 21-11). Patients with intracranial hemorrhage associated with a coagulopathy have a much poorer prognosis than do such patients without a disturbance of coagulation. Sjoblom et al.[120] found that the 30-day mortality among patients with anticoagulant-associated hemorrhage was greater than 50 percent. The coagulation defect facilitates enlargement of the hematoma and neurological worsening.[121] The resultant large hematoma leads to additional brain damage and increases in intracranial pressure.

▶ TABLE 21-11. ACUTE TREATMENT OF COAGULATION DEFECTS IN PATIENTS WITH INTRACRANIAL HEMORRHAGE

Coagulation screening
Platelet count
Prothrombin time/ International Normalized Ratio (INR)
Activated partial thromboplastin time (aPTT)
Bleeding secondary to hemophilia
    Administer concentrates of factor VII or VIII
Bleeding secondary to anticoagulants
    Vitamin K—oral, subcutaneous, intravenous
    Fresh frozen plasma
    Concentrates of factors VII, VIII, or IX
Bleeding secondary to heparin
    Protamine sulfate
Bleeding secondary to rt-PA
    Cryoprecipitate
    Fresh frozen plasma
    Aminocaproic acid
    Platelets
Bleeding secondary to thrombocytopenia or antiplatelet agents
    Platelets

Yasaka et al.[122] found enlargement of an intracerebral hematoma within 24 hours of onset in approximately one-third of cases of bleeding secondary to medications. Abnormalities in coagulation factors also are associated with an increased risk of brain edema.[123] A coagulopathy should be suspected if a patient has other evidence of bleeding or a history of medications that affect coagulation. Screening for a coagulopathy is part of the initial evaluation of all patients with stroke. A disturbance in platelet count, prothrombin time/INR, or activated partial thromboplastin time provides strong evidence for a bleeding disorder. Additional coagulation tests also might be needed.

Patients with a coagulopathy need rapid correction of the defect.[121] The goal is to halt continued bleeding and thereby possibly avoid the necessity of surgical evacuation. In addition, the coagulation defect must be corrected prior to a neurosurgical intervention. The selection of therapies to reverse the coagulation defect is based on the type of coagulopathy. Choices for treatment of bleeding associated with oral anticoagulants include vitamin K, fresh frozen plasma, and coagulation factor concentrates. Vitamin K can be administered orally, intravenously or subcutaneously; the usual doses are 10–20 mg[124] (see Chapter 19). Oral vitamin K lowers the INR more rapidly than subcutaneously administered medication.[125] If an intravenous route is used, it should be infused over 30–60 minutes in order to avoid an allergic reaction. Cartmill et al.[126] found that prothrombin complex concentrate is superior to vitamin K for reversing the effects of anticoagulants. Boulis et al.[127] reported that Factor IX concentrate was superior to fresh frozen plasma for treatment of anticoagulant medication-associated intracranial hemorrhage. Administration of recombinant activated factor VII also can rapidly lower a prolonged INR.[128] The goal is to have the INR under 1.4 before surgical evacuation of the hematoma. Recombinant activated Factor VII or Factor VIII has been used to treat bleeding in patients with hemophilia.[121,129] A recent study reported that early administration of activated Factor VII would slow progression of hematoma growth and would improve neurological outcomes. While the details of this report are not available because the study has not been published, the results appear very promising.[130] A pilot study did not demonstrate benefit of emergency administration of aminocaproic acid for halting progression of intracerebral bleeding.[131] Patients with bleeding secondary to heparin usually are prescribed protamine sulfate (see Chapters 19 and 22). However, protamine sulfate does not reverse the antithrombotic effects of the low molecular weight heparins or danaparoid. Patients with intracranial bleeding secondary to these agents need replacement with clotting factors. Bleeding secondary to thrombolytic therapy often requires administration of cryoprecipitate, fresh frozen plasma or aminocaproic acid. Patients with

bleeding secondary to thrombocytopenia or the effects of glycoprotein IIb/IIIa receptor blocking agents need an infusion of platelets.

Patients with suspected acute ischemic stroke also are screened for a coagulation defect that could influence decisions about prescribing intravenous thrombolysis or other therapies that affect coagulation. A prolongation of the INR greater than 1.8 or a prolonged activated partial thromboplastin time or thrombocytopenia precludes intravenous administration of rt-PA. However, there is little reason to try an antidote such as vitamin K or protamine sulfate to reverse the effects of anticoagulants in order to then give rt-PA.

Some patients could be candidates for treatment with antithrombotic medications to prevent complications of the stroke or to prevent recurrent stroke. A systemic review concluded that antithrombotic medications should be avoided whenever possible among patients with acute intracranial bleeding.[132] In particular, heparin doubled the risk of early recurrent hemorrhage. Antiplatelet agents might be safer because they seem not to increase either mortality or the risk of recurrent bleeding.

Seizures

Seizures are a complication of either hemorrhagic or ischemic stroke. Several groups have looked at the frequency of seizures following stroke and their impact on neurological outcomes.[133,134] Although estimates vary widely (2–33 percent), a reasonable assumption is that approximately 5–10 percent of patients have early seizures, which typically occur at the time of the vascular event or within the first 24 hours.[135] Davalos et al.[136] found that seizures occurred at the time of ischemic stroke in approximately 5 percent of patients. Seizures more commonly occur with thrombotic or embolic occlusions that lead to ischemia of the cerebral cortex than with subcortical or brain stem ischemic events.[137] Seizures also occur with both intracerebral and subarachnoid hemorrhage.[10,138] Dennis[139] noted that seizures are more common among patients with hemorrhages than among those with infarctions.

Seizures are one of the potential explanations for a delirium or coma following a stroke.[140] Postictal focal neurological impairments also can give a false impression about the severity of the neurological event. Nonconvulsive status epilepticus can occur among seriously ill patients, especially older persons and those with cerebral edema.[141] In general, patients with seizures are more seriously ill, probably as a result of the underlying stroke. Seizures also could be secondary to hypoxia or another metabolic disturbance. Approximately 20–80 percent of patients with seizures will have recurrent events. Fortunately, the presence of intermittent seizures does not negatively alter the prognosis of patients with cerebral infarction. Physiological stresses associated with recurrent seizures could adversely affect a patient with a recently ruptured aneurysm. Status epilepticus, which may occur in up to one-fourth of patients with seizures, is a rare complication associated with an increased likelihood of disability following stroke.[137,142,143]

Patients with cerebral infarction are not treated with prophylactic anticonvulsants because the risk of seizures is low.[1] On the other hand, patients with intracranial hemorrhage often are prescribed anticonvulsants.[13,91,138] However, patients who have had seizures as part of a stroke should receive anticonvulsants. Most commonly these medications are administered parenterally. If a patient is having seizures, intravenous administration of a short-acting anticonvulsant (diazepam or lorazepam) usually is followed by phenytoin or fosphenytoin (Table 21-12). Phenobarbital can be administered but it usually is avoided because of its sedating side effects. Patients with recurrent seizures despite the administration of phenytoin likely will need intubation and treatment with a medication such as thiopental, midazolam, or propofol.[144] Oral medications may be given to less seriously ill patients who had a seizure at the time of stroke but who are not actively seizing during the evaluation. Prophylactic anticonvulsants usually are discontinued after 1 month of treatment.[13]

Increased Intracranial Pressure

While intracranial pressure is defined as elevated when the value is measured as greater than 20 mm Hg for a

▶ **TABLE 21-12.** TREATMENT OF SEIZURES AND STATUS EPILEPTICUS

Patient has had seizures but is not having seizures
Administer anticonvulsant
Parenteral
Phenytoin
Phenobarbital
Orally or via nasogastric tube
Phenytoin
Valproate
Carbamazepine
Patient is having frequent seizures or status epilepticus
Initial intravenous therapy
Lorazepam (0.1 mg/kg; usual dose 2 mg)
Diazepam (0.15–0.25 mg/kg; usual dose 5–10 mg)
Subsequent intravenous administration
Phenytoin (15–20 mg/kg; usual dose 1000 mg)
Fosphenytoin (15–20 mg/kg; usual dose 1000 mg)
Phenobarbital (up to 20 mg/kg)
If status epilepticus—uncontrolled
Thiopental
Midazolam
Propofol
Start maintenance anticonvulsant therapy

▶ **TABLE 21-13.** PATIENTS AT GREATEST RISK FOR MALIGNANT BRAIN EDEMA OR INCREASED INTRACRANIAL PRESSURE

Clinical findings—neurological
Decreased consciousness
Low Glasgow Coma Scale score
High National Institutes of Health Stroke Scale score
Combination of major motor, sensory, visual, and behavioral signs
Seizures
Clinical findings—medical
Abnormal vital signs
Fever
Hypercarbia
Hypoxia
Hyperglycemia
Patients with hemorrhage
Large hematoma
2.5 cm in cerebellum
3.0 cm in hemisphere
Intraventricular hemorrhage
Diffuse or thick subarachnoid hemorrhage
Acute hydrocephalus
Patients with infarction
Multilobar infarction in cerebral hemisphere
Occlusion of internal carotid artery
Occlusion of proximal segment of middle cerebral artery
Large cerebellar infarction
Patients with infarction—brain imaging findings
Hypodensity involving > one-third of cerebral hemisphere
Early sulcal effacement
Early loss of corticomedullary contrast
Dense artery sign

period greater than 5 minutes, most symptomatic patients have much higher values[13] (Table 21-13). Increased intracranial pressure is a leading cause of neurological deterioration, including declines in consciousness with serious brain illnesses including stroke.[10,46,145] Increased intracranial pressure may be secondary to expansion in the volume of the intracranial vasculature (blood volume), cerebrospinal fluid (most commonly hydrocephalus), or brain (hematoma or brain edema). Because the cranial vault is a closed compartment, the increase in volume leads to an increase in pressure. With a slow enlargement of a space-occupying mass, compensatory mechanisms, such as reduction of the cerebrospinal fluid compartment, may initially compensate for mass effect to maintain normal intracranial pressure. However, such compensation might not occur during a rapidly evolving illness, such as a hemorrhage. The short time course is one explanation that increased intracranial pressure is such an important problem with stroke. In addition, a mass that obstructs the normal egress of cerebrospinal fluid from the ventricles also may elevate intracranial pressure. Thus, a large hematoma or infarction in the cerebellum can compress

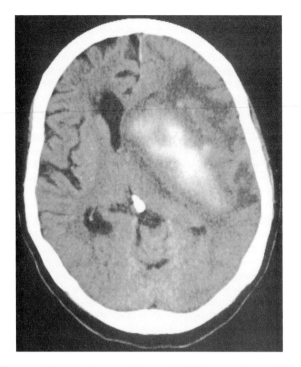

Figure 21-4. An unenhanced CT scan ina patient with a multilobar infarction of the left hemisphere with secondary brain edema, hemorrhagic transformation of the infarction, dilation of the right lateral ventricle and shift of midline structure.

the fourth ventricle or aqueduct of Sylvius and lead to neurological deterioration secondary to increased intracranial pressure and hydrocephalus. Blood in the subarachnoid space also interferes with absorption of cerebrospinal fluid along the arachnoid villi, which predisposes to hydrocephalus. The increase in intracranial pressure is directly tied to venous pressure and if venous obstruction occurs, intracranial pressure rises.[146] As a result, the signs and symptoms of increased intracranial pressure are commonly found among patients with thrombosis of the major venous sinuses.

The increase in intracranial pressure adversely affects cerebral perfusion pressure. Marked increases in intracranial pressure may lead to generalized brain ischemia. A sudden marked increase in intracranial pressure at the time of aneurysmal rupture, which transiently causes a dramatic decline in perfusion pressure, might explain the sudden loss of consciousness often described among patients with subarachnoid hemorrhage. An intracranial pressure that exceeds mean arterial pressure leads to a lack of perfusion to the brain and brain death. A decline of perfusion pressure also can promote local ischemia in a penumbral region around a cerebral infarction or hematoma and the focal signs and symptoms of a stroke then can progress.

In addition, the cranial vault is divided into three subunits by the falx cerebri and the tentorium. As a con-

sequence, pressure gradients can develop within the cranial vault. Differences in pressure in these three subunits (right hemisphere, left hemisphere, posterior fossa) can lead to shift of structures from the region of higher pressure to one with lower pressure. This shift, called herniation, is a leading neurological cause of death following stroke.

Brain edema can result from vasogenic and cellular changes (Fig. 21-4).[147] In stroke, edema may be the result of vasogenic, cytotoxic, neurotoxic, or interstitial factors that lead to accumulation of water in the brain (see Chapter 24). Brain edema and increased intracranial pressure account for more than three-fourths of the deaths that occur within the first week following of stroke.[134] Malignant brain edema that leads to neurological worsening or death usually peaks at 2–5 days[148,149] (Fig. 21-5). Edema and increased intracranial pressure develop more rapidly among patients with hemorrhages than with infarctions, largely because the hematoma itself is a mass while the mass-effects of infarction are secondary to brain edema that evolves over the first few days following stroke (Fig. 21-6). Successful management of patients with stroke should include measures to prevent or treat increased intracranial pressure. These measures should be started in the emergency department. Early interventions to treat increased intracranial pressure are especially urgent among patients with intracranial hemorrhage.

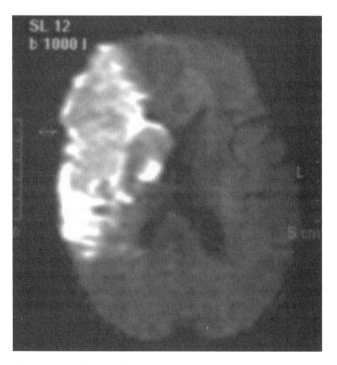

Figure 21-5. A diffusion-weighted MRI study shows a large infarction in the distribution of the right middle cerebral artery. A patient with this size of ischemic lesion would be at high risk for secondary brain edema and increased intracranial pressure.

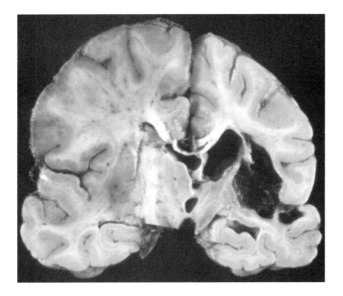

Figure 21-6. A coronal autopsy specimen through both cerebral hemispheres reveals an old infarction in the right hemisphere. An acute infarction is seen to involve most of the left hemisphere. The left hemisphere is edematous and midline structures are displaced to the left (herniation). In addition, areas of hemorrhage are found in the corpus callosum and the rostral brainstem, representing areas of brain injury secondary to herniation. (*Courtesy of S.S. Schochet, M.D., Department of Pathology, University of West Virginia.*)

The clinical examination and the results of imaging obtained in the emergency department provide clues as to which patients are at high risk for serious elevations of intracranial pressure (see Table 21-13). Patients with impaired consciousness or evidence of a major brain injury (high NIH Stroke Scale score) are at the greatest risk for malignant brain edema and increased intracranial pressure.[150] Imaging findings of a multilobar infarction, extensive subarachnoid blood, hydrocephalus, or a large intracerebral hematoma also forecast problems of increased intracranial pressure[150] (Figs. 21-7 and 21-8). Patients with lacunar infarctions or small deep hematomas in the deep hemispheric structures or brain stem do not have a high risk of increased intracranial pressure because the volume of the lesion is not sufficiently large to have significant secondary mass effects. Most patients with small (<3 cm) lobar cerebral infarctions or hemorrhages are not at risk for malignant brain edema. However, patients with similar sized infarctions or hematomas located in the posterior fossa do have a high risk for increased intracranial pressure and neurological worsening, in part because mass effects that lead to compression of the brainstem or secondary obliteration of the fourth ventricle or aqueduct of Sylvius cause acute obstructive hydrocephalus.[151,152] Other factors predicting malignant brain edema or increased intracranial pressure include hypoxia, hypercarbia, and hyperglycemia.

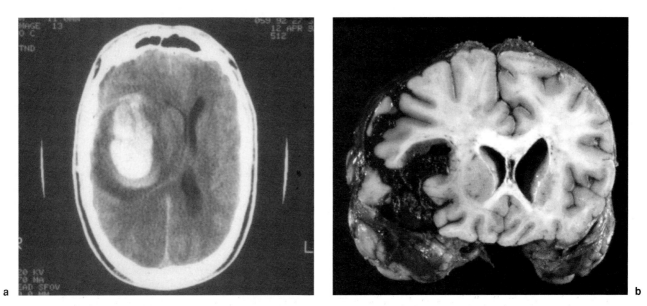

a   b

Figure 21-7. (a) An unenhanced CT scan obtained shortly before death in a patient with a massive right hemisphere hemorrhage with secondary edema reveals a marked displacement of midline structures to the left. (b) A coronal autopsy specimen from the same patient shows a large hematoma in the sylvian fissure and temporal lobe secondary to the ruptured aneurysm of the middle cerebral artery. The midline structures are displaced to the left and the right cingulated gyrus has herniated under the flax cerebri. (*Courtesy of S.S. Schochet, M.D., Department of Pathology, University of West Virginia.*)

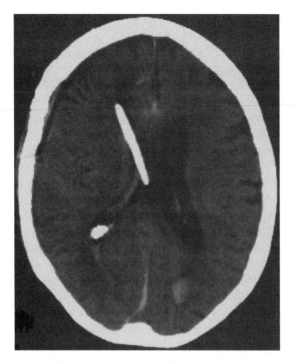

Figure 21-8. An uenhanced CT scan shows an intraventricular catheter inserted into the right lateral ventricle to treat acute hydrocephalus in a patient with an acute hemorrhage. Blood is present in the occipital horns of both lateral ventricles.

A progressive decline in consciousness is the earliest clinical warning of increased intracranial pressure (Table 21-14). Patients with a mass-producing intracerebral hemorrhage may have bradycardia and hypertension (Cushing response) in addition to impaired consciousness but these signs are not very common. The course of the illness generally is too brief for the finding of papilledema on ophthalmoscopic examination. However, patients with major intracranial hemorrhages might have intraocular hemorrhages found on visualization of the ocular fundus. Signs of herniation, most commonly an ipsilateral oculomotor nerve paresis, presenting with pupillary dilation or an ipsilateral hemiparesis (Kernohan notch—secondary to compression of the contralateral cerebral peduncle) appear relatively late in the course of increased intracranial pressure. Rarely cardiovascular or respiratory arrest also occurs.

A major emphasis of the frequent neurological assessment of patients during the first hours after stroke is to screen for signs of increased intracranial pressure. Follow-up brain imaging studies can be done to look for worsening brain edema, mass effect including shift of midline structures or compression of the ventricles, growth of the hematoma, or increasing hydrocephalus.[10] Either imaging or clinical deterioration stimulates additional measures to treat the brain edema and increased intracranial pressure.

▶ TABLE 21-14. CLINICAL FEATURES OF INCREASED INTRACRANIAL PRESSURE

Decrease in level of consciousness
   Waxing and waning in consciousness
   Progression to coma
Papilledema appears late
Increase in blood pressure
Decrease in heart rate
Herniation (uncal)
   Ipsilateral pupillary dilation (III nerve palsy)
   Periodic breathing
   New ipsilateral hemiparesis (Kernohan notch)

Valentin et al.[153] found that measuring intracranial pressure helped guide management of acutely ill patients and lowering of mortality resulted. Catheters, which can be inserted into the subdural space, ventricle, or brain parenchyma to monitor intracranial pressure, expedite management.[153-155] Measurement of intracranial pressure permits rapid calculation of cerebral perfusion pressure when the values are compared to arterial pressure readings. The cerebral perfusion pressure is estimated as mean arterial pressure minus intracranial pressure, which approximates mean venous pressure. A reasonable goal is to maintain a cerebral perfusion pressure greater than 70 mm Hg. Broderick et al.[13] recommend placement of a pressure monitor following hemorrhages when the patient's condition is worsening or when the patient is stuporous or comatose. The selection of the monitoring device depends upon the experience of the neurosurgeon and the patient's status. Intraventricular devices usually are indicated when the patient has hydrocephalus.[10] The ventricular drain and monitor may be placed by the neurosurgeon via a burr hole. The advantage of an intraventricular catheter is that cerebrospinal fluid can be drained if the pressure rises. This tactic is an effective method of lowering intracranial pressure. Other pressure monitors that do not have drainage capabilities may affect the use of medications or other interventions to lower intracranial pressure. In general, the goal is to keep the drain or monitor in place for less than 1 week. If intracranial pressure monitoring is used, the patient must be assessed regularly for signs of a complicating infection.[156]

Medical Management

Patients at high risk for brain edema who do not have signs of neurological worsening or increased intracranial pressure often are treated with prophylactic measures, which should be started in the emergency department. While many individual components have not been tested in clinical trials, there is general consensus that such interventions should be used. The earliest and easiest interventions are those aimed at treating factors that might aggravate intracranial pressure or brain edema such as hypoxia, hypercarbia, or hyperglycemia.[157] In addition, controlling fever, pain, nausea, vomiting, agitation, or seizures may be helpful. Postures that hamper venous drainage, such as hyperextension or rotation of the neck are avoided (Table 21-15). Modest elevation of the head of the bed (20–30°) can expedite venous drainage. However, Schwarz et al.[158] concluded that while elevation of the head can reduce intracranial pressure, cerebral perfusion pressure also drops. If cerebral perfusion pressure declines, keeping the patient flat is preferred. Reinprecht et al.[159] found that the prone posture may improve oxygenation, in turn counteracting some of the adverse effects on intracranial pressure. Potentially hypo-osmolar fluids, such as 5 percent dextrose in water, are avoided. Modest restriction of fluids also is recommended.

Most patients who have malignant increases in intracranial pressure require intubation and ventilatory assistance. Elective intubation before the patient decompensates is preferred. Neuromuscular blocking agents or sedation can help lower intrathoracic pressure during intubation. These are advised because elevated intrathoracic pressure hampers venous return, which further increases intracranial pressure. Ketamine and volatile anesthetics are avoided because they might increase intracranial pressure.[47] Positive end-expiratory pressure as part of respiratory management appears not to have a major effect on either intracranial pressure or cerebral perfusion pressure.[160]

Hyperventilation is recommended as an emergency intervention.[1,13] Hyperventilation reduces pCO2 levels and thereby causes constriction of intracranial vessels and contraction of the vascular compartment.[161] Cerebral vasoconstriction results in a decrease in cerebral blood volume and an almost instantaneous decline in intracranial pressure. A reduction of pCO2 of only 5–10 mm Hg can lower intracranial pressure by approximately 25–30 percent.[16,162] The main drawback to hyperventilation is the reduction in cerebral blood flow, an issue that is of concern for patients with cerebrovascular disease, especially those with acute ischemia.[157,161] The pCO2 level should not be lowered to below 30 mm Hg because more intensive lowering could lead to insufficient cerebral blood flow and increased ischemia.[47] Unfortunately, the effects of hyperventilation are time limited and it should be considered as an adjunct to other interventions.[161]

Although corticosteroids are used to treat the edema that accompanies brain tumors and to reduce the swelling of the spinal cord following trauma, their utility in treatment of acute cerebrovascular disease is not established. Studies of conventional or large doses of corticosteroids for treating brain edema following either hemorrhagic or ischemic stroke found no benefit in improving neurological outcomes.[163,164] Conversely, one study of corticosteroids found an increase in the frequency of infectious complications with their use.[10,165] A systemic review did not demonstrate any evidence for efficacy of corticosteroid treatment of patients with presumed ischemic stroke.[166] As a result, guidelines for treatment of hemorrhagic and ischemic stroke advise against the use of steroids.[1,13,167,168] However, uncertainty about the role of corticosteroids still exists and some experts propose additional research on the utility of these agents.[169–171] Other effects of acutely administered steroids also might be helpful. For instance, these medications might reduce the meningeal inflammatory reaction to subarachnoid hemorrhage. Although no trials have tested the utility of steroids as an ancillary treatment of patients with acute vascular events of the spinal cord, the efficacy of steroids in treating patients with traumatic spinal cord injuries provides a rationale for investigation.

An intravenous 40 mg bolus of furosemide often is given to patients who are rapidly deteriorating.[1] Presumably the diuretic effect of furosemide causes a loss of water, thereby reducing edema, and it also might slow production of cerebrospinal fluid. No trials have tested the efficacy of furosemide in the emergency management of patients with acute stroke.

While osmotherapy is recommended for treatment of patients with malignant brain edema and increased intracranial pressure, data about the utility of this intervention are limited.[1,13] The rationale for the interventions

▶ **TABLE 21-15.** PREVENTION OR TREATMENT OF BRAIN EDEMA AND INCREASED INTRACRANIAL PRESSURE

General preventive measures
  Avoid hypoxia
  Avoid hypercarbia
  Treat hyperthermia
  Avoid administration of hypo-osmolar fluids
  Elevate head of bed—improve venous drainage
Medical measures
  Osmotherapy
    Glycerol
    Mannitol
    Hypertonic saline
  Diuretics
    Furosemide
    Acetazolamide
  Steroids
Ventilatory assistance and hyperventilation
Intraventricular drainage of cerebrospinal fluid
Hypothermia
Barbiturates
Surgical interventions
  Evacuation of hematoma
  Surgical resection
  Surgical decompression

is that increasing the osmolarity of the circulating blood achieved by the administration of hypertonic solutions, serves as a stimulus for the movement of water out of the brain.[172–175] However, the blood–brain barrier must be intact for this therapy to be effective. Improvement of cerebral blood flow to an ischemic area may follow administration of such therapy.[176] Indications include worsening brain edema as detected by clinical examination or brain imaging or elevations of intracranial pressure as detected by monitoring.

Choices for treatment include hypertonic saline, urea, glycerol, and mannitol. Several studies evaluated glycerol.[177,178] Glycerol does not worsen mass effects among patients with large hemispheric infarctions.[179] A systemic review found that glycerol is associated with a favorable impact on short-term survival but it appears not to improve long-term outcomes.[180] Glycerol is sweet and not well tolerated when taken orally and intravenous infusions of glycerol may cause hemolysis. Hypervolemia, lactic acidosis and electrolyte disturbances also may occur with intravenous administration of glycerol.[47] As a result, glycerol is not used widely in North America. Urea is another hypertonic agent, but it has not been tested in treatment of stroke.

Intravenous infusions of 20 percent mannitol are the most widely used osmotherapy. Mannitol usually is given in a dose of 0.25–0.5 g/kg over 20 minutes.[181] The effects of mannitol are seen within a few minutes and the pressure can remain low for up to 6 hours.[182] The medication can be repeated every 4–6 hours as needed. The usual maximal daily dose is 2 g/kg. Patients receiving recurrent doses of mannitol should have careful fluid management. In general, the goal is to replace urinary losses every 6 hours. In addition, assessments of serum osmolarity should be done regularly. The aim is to avoid a serum osmolarity >330 mmol/L.[47] Mannitol also can affect renal function.[183] In addition, prolonged osmotherapy can result in an increase in osmolarity in the brain, which draws water into the brain (rebound phenomenon). The goal is to limit the use of mannitol to a maximum of 5 days.[13] Cruz et al.[184] found that early administration of high doses of mannitol (in the emergency room) improves outcomes among comatose patients with hemorrhage causing early signs of herniation. A randomized trial tested early administration of mannitol for treatment of patients with temporal lobe hematomas who had signs of herniation.[184] The mannitol, which was given in a dose of 1.4 g/kg, was associated with improved clinical outcomes and better postoperative control of increased intracranial pressure. Conversely, a recent report found no net benefit from the use of mannitol in reducing mortality after stroke.[185] A systemic review of available data concluded that there was no evidence that the routine use of mannitol following stroke would result in any benefit or harm.[186] Additional research of the utility of mannitol is needed.

At present, the use of mannitol is reserved for treatment of patients who are deteriorating from brain edema despite less aggressive medical interventions.

Administration of hypertonic saline leads to development of an osmotic gradient that draws water from the brain, increases cardiac output, promotes absorption of cerebrospinal fluid, decreases viscosity, and increases blood pressure.[175] These features could be particularly advantageous in treating patients with acute cerebrovascular events. One study found that a 75 ml infusion of 10 percent saline could reduce intracranial pressure and improve cerebral perfusion pressure among patients who were not responding to mannitol.[187] Infusions of hypertonic saline have been shown to increase cerebral blood flow in seriously ill patients with subarachnoid hemorrhage.[188] Presumably, the infusions improve the rheology of the blood by reducing concentrations of hemoglobin. Qureshi et al.[189] reported that infusions of 3 percent saline/acetate were promising for the treatment of patients with brain edema. While hypertonic saline was effective in reducing intracranial pressure some patients had serious side effects such as diabetes insipidus or pulmonary edema. The rebound phenomenon also can occur.[190] Other potential complications include decreased consciousness secondary to hypernatremia, central pontine myelinolysis, congestive heart failure, hypokalemia, blood pressure disturbances, and a coagulopathy.[175] Additional research on the use of hypertonic saline as an alternative to mannitol is indicated.

Even with these measures, a sizable proportion of patients with malignant strokes continue to deteriorate. The risk of death is extraordinarily high. Berrouschot et al.[191] evaluated a series of 53 patients with malignant brain infarctions managed with osmotherapy and mild hyperventilation and all became comatose despite treatment and 37 were dead within 4 days. Additional interventions to treat brain edema and increased intracranial pressure are needed. Barbiturate-induced coma, which suppresses brain metabolic activity, has been prescribed. However, it requires electroencephalographic monitoring with the goal of reaching a burst-suppression pattern.[47] This regimen is rigorous and includes intensive cardiovascular support.[192,193] No net benefit from barbiturate-induced coma has been found. Hypothermia also is used and appears promising.[194–196] Both external and internal cooling regimens are used. Besides reducing intracranial pressure, hypothermia also might be neuroprotective in the setting of an acute ischemic insult. While hypothermia cannot be recommended for management of most patients with increased intracranial pressure, it is being tested in clinical trials.[197]

Surgical Management

Approximately 20 percent of patients with intracranial bleeding have acute hydrocephalus, a complication that is more common among elderly patients.[198–200] Drainage of cerebrospinal fluid via an intraventricular catheter can be used to treat increased intracranial pressure in a patient with acute hydrocephalus.[10,155] Instillation of a thrombolytic agent via a catheter can expedite resolution of an intraventricular clot and improve drainage of the cerebrospinal fluid.[10,201] Kumar et al.[202] successfully treated intraventricular hemorrhage secondary to a ruptured vascular malformation prior to surgical resection of the vascular lesion. They concluded that the therapy reduced the volume of intraventricular blood, helped control hydrocephalus, and lowered intracranial pressure. Still, a systemic review of available data concluded that most of the evidence about the utility of intraventricular fibrinolytic therapy is anecdotal and additional research is needed.[203] Because acute obstructive hydrocephalus is most commonly found among patients with major intraventricular or subarachnoid bleeding, mass-producing hematomas, or large infarctions, ventricular drainage is an option for a limited number of patients with stroke. Ventriculostomy often is recommended to improve consciousness as part of early treatment of patients with ruptured intracranial aneurysms.[204] However, a sudden decline in intracranial pressure might lower transmural pressure and predispose to a recurrent rupture of the aneurysm. The frequency of this complication probably is relatively low and the potential for rebleeding should not be a reason for avoiding placement of a ventricular drain in a critically ill patient.

► EMERGENCY SURGICAL MEASURES TO TREAT A MASS-PRODUCING STROKE

Because of the slow evolution of complicating brain edema, decisions about potential surgical treatment of mass-producing infarction usually are made after the patient is admitted to the hospital (see Chapter 24). A possible exception is the patient with a large cerebellar infarction that is causing compression of the brain stem or leading to acute obstructive hydrocephalus secondary to obliteration of the fourth ventricle or the aqueduct of Sylvius[205] (Table 21-16; Fig. 21-9). In general, cerebellar infarctions that prompt consideration of surgical resection are larger than 3 cm in diameter.[206] Placement of a ventricular catheter to drain cerebrospinal fluid and suboccipital craniectomy, in combination with medical interventions, can relieve the hydrocephalus and brainstem compression.[205,207,208] Mortality among comatose patients with a mass-producing cerebellar infarction is approximately 80 percent, which is lowered to 30 percent if surgery is performed.[47] Although the data supporting surgical treatment of large cerebellar infarctions are not extensive, decompression is recommended for treatment of a deteriorating patient.[1,10,157]

Patients with large cerebellar hematomas have a more rapid course of neurological worsening than

► **TABLE 21-16.** SIGNS OF MASS EFFECT LARGE CEREBELLAR HEMORRHAGE OR INFARCTION

Early signs of cerebellar hemorrhage or infarction
  Headache
  Vertigo, nausea, and vomiting
  Ipsilateral limb ataxia
  Nystagmus
  Dysarthria
  Nuchal stiffness
Signs of secondary dysfunction (compression) of brain stem
  Ipsilateral trigeminal nerve dysfunction
  Ipsilateral facial nerve dysfunction
  Oculorotatory impairments
    Ipsilateral or bilateral abducens nerve dysfunction
    Ocular bobbing
  Quadriparesis
  Bilateral Babinski signs
  Small pupils
Signs of increased intracranial pressure
  Decreased consciousness
Late signs of brain stem dysfunction
  Pinpoint, unreactive pupils
Ataxic or agonal respiratory pattern

patients with similar sized infarctions. As a result, surgery is recommended for treatment of patients with large (>3 cm diameter) hemorrhages of the cerebellar hemispheres[10,13,47,209–211] (Fig. 21-10). Smaller hemorrhagic lesions of the vermis (25 mm × 35 mm) also often require

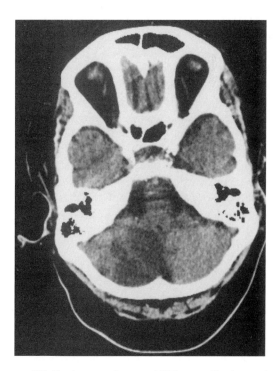

Figure 21-9. An unenhanced CT scan displays a large infarction in the right cerebellar hemisphere in the territory of the posterior inferior cerebellar artery.

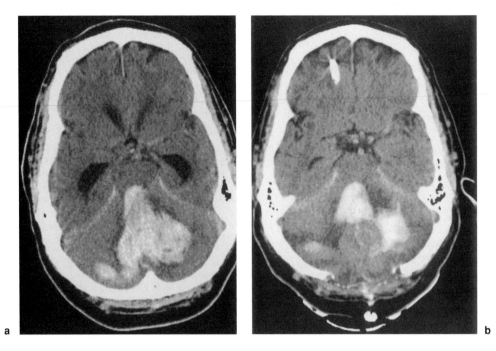

a   b

Figure 21-10. Two unenhanced CT scans from a patient with a large cerebellar hemor-rhage. (a) The first scan was performed before surgery. A large hematoma compressing the brainstem and fourth ventricle is present. Acute hydrocephalus with dilation of both temporal horns also is seen. The cisterns in the posterior fossa are obliterated. (b) The second scan done after surgical evacuation demonstrates a craniectomy defect as well as reduction in the volume of the hematoma.

surgery.[212] Early detection of secondary brainstem injury can prompt early surgical treatment of the cerebellar clot.[213] Imaging indicating obliteration of the posterior fossa cisterns usually predicts a high risk for brainstem compression. The decision for early ventriculostomy and suboccipital craniectomy often is made while the patient is in an emergency department. Patients with smaller cerebellar hematomas may be observed closely or treated only with ventricular drainage. Although Pollak et al.[214] found that results were poorer among patients with hemorrhage than those with infarction, patients who have surgical treatment have the greatest potential for favorable outcomes.

Surgery also is a treatment option for management of large hematomas in other brain locations.[10] Rabinstein et al.[215] treated 26 comatose or stuporous patients with expanding cerebral hemisphere hematomas, who also had signs of secondary midbrain dysfunction and imaging evidence of a shift of midline structures. Despite surgery, 56 percent died and 22 percent had severe disability. They concluded that craniotomy for treatment of deteriorating patients with evidence of brainstem dysfunction secondary to a cerebral hemorrhage usually is not successful. Still, advances in anesthesia and neurosurgical techniques permit more patients to be treated. The basic principle of surgery is to remove as much of the hematoma as possible

without injuring normal brain tissue. The goal is to remove a clot that is producing mass symptoms and increased intracranial pressure. Concomitant treatment of a ruptured aneurysm or vascular malformation also can be done. In addition, histological examination of the hematoma might permit pathological confirmation of another cause of the bleeding. However emergency evacuation of the hematoma is aimed primarily at stabilizing the patient's neurological condition. Craniotomy is the traditional surgical approach.[13] This procedure allows for good visualization of the hematoma but it can lead to additional brain injury, particularly if the hemorrhage is located in deep structures. Recurrent bleeding can accompany the operation. Because surgeons are not satisfied with conventional operations, other approaches including stereotactic evacuation are being developed.[216] Ancillary techniques, such as installation of a thrombolytic agent within the hematoma, have been used to ease surgical evacuation of the clot.[217,218] Naff et al.[219] reported that intraventricular administration of urokinase to patients with intraventricular hemorrhage could lower mortality. Similar results were reported by Lee et al.[220] Several studies describe the results of surgical evacuation of the hematoma.[221–225] The trials compared surgical drainage (either direct or endoscopic) with conventional medical therapy. Unfortunately, the results do not provide compelling evidence for surgical treatment.[13] A recent trial did not demonstrate the superiority of surgery in improving outcomes among patients with hematomas.[226]

These trials enrolled critically ill or deteriorating patients who already have a poor prognosis. The chances for a favorable outcome were low regardless of treatment. As a result surgery might not have been tested adequately. Most trials suggest that early surgery can be performed with reasonable safety. For example, Murthy et al.[225] found that surgery done within 8 hours of onset of hemorrhage is associated with a trend toward an increased likelihood of favorable outcomes. This approach involves surgery within a few hours of arrival in an emergency department. Marquardt et al.[227] concluded that early stereotactic aspiration of basal ganglia hematomas might improve consciousness and reduce the risk of major complications. Further study of the potential usefulness of emergency surgical evacuation of the hematoma is indicated.[228] Factors that influence responses to surgery include the patient's age, the presence of comorbid diseases, the volume of the hematoma, the location of the hematoma including whether the bleeding is affecting the dominant or nondominant hemisphere, severity of neurological impairments, the interval from hemorrhage until surgery, and the type of required surgical intervention.[228] A systemic review of surgical options concluded that there was no strong evidence to support the use of craniotomy, stereotactic surgery, or endoscopic evacuation of hemispheric hematomas.[224]

Surgical options also include emergency craniectomy.[229] While this approach has been used most frequency for surgical management of intractable brain edema complicating hemispheric infarctions, Smith et al.[230] did prophylactic decompressive craniectomy for treatment of poor condition patients with ruptured middle cerebral artery aneurysms. They noted prompt improvement in intracranial pressure readings and some patients did well. Ziai et al.[231] did hemicraniectomy for treatment of severe brain edema following a major hemorrhage. Outcomes among patients with subarachnoid hemorrhage generally were poor but the authors suggested that early surgical treatment (before signs of herniation) might be successful. Jaeger et al.[232] found that decompressive craniectomy reduces intracranial pressure and improves oxygenation among patients with severe subarachnoid hemorrhage but outcomes still were poor.

The decision to perform emergency surgery remains controversial. Current guidelines provide recommendations based on limited data.[13] The indications for treatment of cerebellar hematomas, described previously, are the most commonly accepted. The decision to recommend surgery is based on the patient's overall health, the neurological status, the location and size of the hematoma, and the presence of a source of bleeding that

can be cured if surgery is performed rapidly. Deteriorating patients with hematomas larger than 50 cm³ can be treated with surgical evacuation. Patients with lobar hemorrhages, especially those close to the cortical surface, can be more easily treated than those located in the thalamus or basal ganglia. Patients with small clots (volume < 10 cm³) within the brain usually do not need surgical evacuation because their prognosis generally is good and drainage of the hematoma probably will not improve outcomes.[13] Conversely, surgery is unlikely to help patients with profound neurological impairments. For example, an operation is not recommended for treatment of patients with a Glasgow Coma Scale score less than 5.[13] Surgical evacuation of a large hematoma arising within the brainstem usually is not recommended.

► EARLY SYMPTOMATIC TREATMENT

While much of the initial management of patients with stroke focuses on basic life support and prevention or treatment of serious complications, patients also have nonlife threatening complaints that need to be treated. Patients with intracranial hemorrhage, particularly those with subarachnoid bleeding, have severe headaches that should be treated aggressively, most commonly with parenteral opiates. Besides relieving the pain, effective analgesics also help lower blood pressure and lessen agitation. Morphine is typically used in this setting; its administration can be titrated to the patient's pain. Agitated or delirious patients also might need sedating medications to protect them from injury. However, medications should not be given unless absolutely necessary because pharmacological sedation may mask neurological worsening from other causes. Occasionally physical restraints might be needed. Patients with intense nausea and vomiting should receive antiemetic medications such as ondansetron. Patients should not receive food or fluid by mouth until their neurological status is stable and their ability to swallow safely has been assessed. Intermittent catheterization or placement of an indwelling bladder catheter can relieve the pain of a full bladder.

► PALLIATIVE CARE

Unfortunately some patients have a fatal brain injury. Such critically ill patients have extensive hemorrhages or infarctions demonstrated on brain imaging studies. They usually have profound neurological impairments, including deep coma and signs of brainstem dysfunction. They often have unstable vital signs including irregular breathing patterns. Despite the measures previously described in this chapter, their prognosis remains dismal. Many people do not wish to survive if devastating brain injuries would result in a prolonged coma or state of permanent incapacity. Some people have advanced directive documents that provide physicians with guidance about emergency treatment in situations such as a profound stroke. For example, the document might include a prohibition against intubation, mechanical ventilation, or other forms of aggressive life support. Physicians should honor those directives. In other circumstances, advanced directives are not available and the physician should involve family members (spouse, adult child, parent, or other next-of-kin) in decision making. A frank discussion of the nature of the brain illness, the prognosis, and the treatment options is critical. After the discussion, the family might elect to forgo aggressive therapy. They also may opt to employ all potential interventions. Alternatively, they may decide for an initial period of intensive care with the option to withdraw such therapy in subsequent days. Both physicians and families should be aware that in-hospital mortality is increased among patients who have do-not-resuscitate orders written.[233]

Patients with stroke often have severe preexisting neurological or medical diseases that cause severe impairments. For example, an elderly patient with advanced Alzheimer disease causing severe incapacity may be seen for a brain hemorrhage secondary to amyloid angiopathy. The new cerebrovascular event likely will add more disability to the brain disease. In such circumstances, the patient's guardian (often an adult child with a medical power-of-attorney) makes decisions about treatment of the stroke. The option to forego aggressive medical measures to prolong an otherwise terrible illness, now complicated by stroke, often is selected. This decision often is humane and kind and medical personnel should support it.

Some patients with devastating cerebrovascular events who are not likely to survive, such as subarachnoid hemorrhage, could be organ donors. With the pressing need for organs, the physician and the patient's family should consider this option. In many circumstances, family members find organ donation as a positive consequence of an otherwise horrendous experience.

REFERENCES

1. Adams HP, Adams RJ, Brott T, et al. Guidelines for the early management of patients with ischemic stroke. A scientific statement from the stroke council of the American Stroke Association. *Stroke* 2003;34:1056–1083.
2. Brainin M, Olsen TS, Chamorro A, et al. Organization of stroke care: education, referral, emergency management and imaging, stroke units and rehabilitation. *Cerebrovasc Dis* 2004;17(suppl 2):1–14.
3. Gebel JM, Broderick JP. Intracerebral hemorrhage. *Neurol Clin* 2000;18:419–438.
4. Solenski NJ, Haley ECJr, Kassell NF. Medical complication of aneurysmal subarachnoid hemorrhage: A report of the multicenter, cooperative aneurysm study. *Crit Care Med* 1995;23:1007–1017.
5. Gladman JR, Harwood DM, Barer DH. Predicting the outcome of acute stroke: prospective evaluation of five multivariate models and comparison with simple methods. *J Neurol Neurosurg Psychiatry* 1992;55:347–351.
6. Parvizi J, Damasio AR. Neuroanatomical correlates of brainstem coma. *Brain* 2003;126:1524–1536.
7. Cucchiara B, Kasner SE, Wolk DA, et al. Lack of hemispheric dominance for consciousness in acute ischaemic stroke. *J Neurol Neurosurg Psychiatry* 2003;74:889–892.
8. Ferro JM, Caeiro L, Verdelho A. Delirium in acute stroke. *Curr Opin Neurol* 2002;15:51–55.
9. Sandberg O, Franklin KA, Bucht G, Gustafson Y. Sleep apnea, delirium, depressed mood, cognition, and ADL ability after stroke. *J Am Geriat Soc* 2001;49:391–397.
10. Qureshi AI, Tuhrim S, Broderick JP. Spontaneous intracerebral hemorrhage. *N Engl J Med* 2001;344:1450–1460.
11. Hacke W, Krieger D, Hirschberg M. General principles in the treatment of acute ischemic stroke. *Cerebrovasc Dis* 1991;1(suppl 1):93–99.
12. Turkington PM, Bamford J, Wanklyn P, Iliott MW. Prevalence and predictors of upper airway obstruction in the first 24 hours after acute stroke. *Stroke* 2002;33:2037–2042.
13. Broderick JP, Adams HP, Jr., Barsan W, et al. Guidelines for the management of spontaneous intracerebral hemorrhage: A statement for healthcare professionals from a special writing group of the Stroke Council, American Heart Association. *Stroke* 1999;30:905–915.
14. Grotta J, Pasteur W, Khwaja G, Hamel T, Fisher M, Ramirez A. Elective intubation for neurologic deterioration after stroke. *Neurology* 1995;45:640–644.
15. Bushnell CD, Phillips-Bute BG, Laskowitz DT, Lynch JR, Chilukuri V, Borel CO. Survival and outcome after endotracheal intubation for acute stroke. *Neurology* 1999;52:1374–1381.
16. Gujjar AR, Deibert E, Manno EM, Duff S, Diringer MN. Mechanical ventilation for ischemic stroke and intracerebral hemorrhage: indications, timing, and outcome. *Neurology* 1998;51:447–451.
17. Roch A, Michelet P, Jullien AC, et al. Long-term outcome in intensive care unit survivors after mechanical ventilation for intracerebral hemorrhage. *Crit Care Med* 2003;31:2651–2656.
18. Nachtmann A, Siebler M, Rose G, Sitzer M, Steinmetz H. Cheyne-strokes respiration in ischemic stroke. *Neurology* 1995;45 (4):820–821.
19. Vingerhoets F, Bogousslavsky J. Respiratory dysfunction in stroke. *Clin Chest Med* 1994;15:729–737.
20. Oya S, Tsutsumi K, Yonekura I, Inoue T. Delayed central respiratory dysfunction after Wallenberg's syndrome—case report. *Neurol Med Chir* 2001;41:502–504.
21. Rabinstein AA, Wijdicks EF. Warning signs of imminent respiratory failure in neurological patients. *Sem Neurology* 2003;23:97–104.
22. Gruber A, Reinprecht A, Gorzer H, et al. Pulmonary function and radiographic abnormalities related to neurological

outcome after aneurysmal subarachnoid hemorrhage. *J Neurosurg* 1998;88:28–37.

23. Friedman JA, Pichelmann MA, Piepgras DG, McIver JI, Toussaint LG, McClelland RL. Pulmonary complications of aneurysmal subarachnoid hemorrhage. *Neurosurgery* 2003;52:1025–1031.

24. Treib J, Grauer MT, Woessner R, Morgenthaler M. Treatment of stroke on an intensive storke unit: a novel concept. *Intensive Care Med* 2000;26 (11):1598–1611.

25. The European Ad Hoc Consensus Group. Optimizing intensive care in stroke. A European perspective. *Cerebrovasc Dis* 1997;7:113–128.

26. Chiu EH, Liu CS, Tan TY, Chang KC. Venturi mask adjuvant oxygen therapy in severe acute ischemic stroke. *Arch Neurol* 2006;63:741–744.

27. Ronning OM, Guldvog B. Should stroke victims routinely receive supplemental oxygen? A quasi-randomized controlled trial. *Stroke* 1999;30:2033–2037.

28. Rockswold GL, Ford SE, Anderson DC, Bergman TA, Sherman RE. Results of a prospective randomized trial for treatment of severely brain-injured patients with hyperbaric oxygen. *J Neurosurg* 1992;76:929–934.

29. Nighoghossian N, Trouillas P, Adeleine P, Salord F. Hyperbaric oxygen in the treatment of acute ischemic stroke. A double-blind pilot study. *Stroke* 1995;26:1369–1372.

30. Rusyniak DE, Kirk MA, May JD, et al. Hyperbaric oxygen therapy in acute ischemic stroke: results of the hyperbaric oxygen in acute ischemic stroke trial pilot study. *Stroke* 2003;34:571–574.

31. Boysen G, Christensen H. Stroke severity determines body temperature in acute stroke. *Stroke* 2001;32:413–417.

32. Albrecht RF, II, Wass CT, Lanier WL. Occurrence of potentially detrimental temperature alterations in hospitalized patients at risk for brain injury. *Mayo Clin Proc* 1998;73:629–635.

33. Kammersgaard LP, Jorgensen HS, Rungger G, et al. Admission body temperature predicts long-term mortality after acute stroke. The Copenhagen stroke study. *Stroke* 2002;33:1759–1762.

34. Castillo J, Davalos A, Marrugat J, Noya M. Timing for fever-related brain damage in acute ischemic stroke. *Stroke* 1998;29:2455–2460.

35. Ginsberg M, Busto R. Combating hyperthermia in acute stroke: a significant clinical concern. *Stroke* 1998;29:529–534.

36. Hajat C, Hajat S, Sharma P. Effects of poststroke pyrexia on stroke outcome. A meta-analysis of studies in patients. *Stroke* 2000;31:410–414.

37. Oliveira-Filho J, Ezzeddine MA, Segal AZ, et al. Fever in subarachnoid hemorrhage: Relationship to vasospasm and outcome. *Neurology* 2001;56:1299–1304.

38. Grau AJ, Buggle F, Schnitzler P, Spiel M, Lichy C, Hacke W. Fever and infection early after ischemic stroke. *J Neurol Sci* 1999;171:115–120.

39. Morales-Ortiz A, Jimenez-Pascual M, Perez-Vicente JA, Monge-Arguiles A, Bautista-Prados J. Fever of central origin during stroke. *Rev Neurol* 2001;32:1111–1114.

40. Rossi S, Zanier ER, Mauri I, Columbo A, Stocchetti N. Brain temperature, body core temperature, and intracranial pressure in acute cerebral damage. *J Neurol Neurosurg Psychiatry* 2001;71:448–454.

41. Jorgensen HS, Reith J, Nakayama H, Kammersgaard LP, Raaschou HO, Olsen TS. What determines good recovery in patients with the most severe strokes? The Copenhagen Stroke Study. *Stroke* 1999;30:2008–2012.

42. Dippel DWJ, van Breda EJ, van Gemert HMA, et al. Effect of Paracetamol (acetaminophen) on body temperature in acute ischemic stroke. A double-blind, randomized phase II clinical trial. *Stroke* 2001;32:1607–1612.

43. Kasner SE, Wein T, Piriyawat P, et al. Acetaminophen for altering body temperature in acute stroke: a randomized clinical trial. *Stroke* 2002;33:130–134.

44. Dippel DWJ, van Breda EJ, van der Worp HB, et al. Timing of the effect of acetaminophen on body temperature in patients with acute ischemic stroke. *Neurology* 2003;61:677–679.

45. Mattioli C, Beretta L, Gerevini S, et al. Traumatic subarachnoid hemorrhage on the computerized tomography scan obtained at admission: a multicenter assessment of the accuracy of diagnosis and the potential impact on patient outcome. *J Neurosurg* 2003;98:37–42.

46. Sulter G, Elting JW, Maurits N, Luyckx GJ, De Keyser J. Acetylsalicylic acid and acetaminophen to combat elevated body temperature in acute ischemic stroke. *Cerebrovasc Dis* 2004;17:118–122.

47. Broderick JP, Hacke W. Treatment of acute ischemic stroke. Part II: neuroprotection and medical management. *Circulation* 2002;106:1736–1740.

48. Ay H, Koroshetz W, Benner T, et al. Neuroanatomic correlates of stroke-related myocardial injury. *Neurology* 2006;66:1325–1329.

49. Hays A, Diringer MN. Elevated troponin levels are associated with higher mortality following subarachnoid hemorrhage. *Neurology* 2006;66:1330–1334.

50. Abboud H, Berroir S, Labreuche, et al. Insular involvement in brain infarction increases risk for cardiac arrhythmia and stroke. *Ann Neurol* 2006;59:691–699.

51. Todd GL, Baroldi G, Pieper GM, Clayton F, Eliot RS. Experimental catecholamine induced myocardial necrosis. I. Morphology, quantification and regional distribution of acute contraction band lesions. *J Mol Cell Cardiol* 1985;17:317–338.

52. Anderson GB, Ashforth R, Steinke DE, Findlay JM. CT angiography for the detection of cerebral vasospasm in patients with acute subarachnoid hemorrhage. *AJNR Am J Neuroradiol* 2000;21:1011–1015.

53. Manninen PH, Ayra B, Gelb AW. Association between electrocardiographic abnormalities and intracranial blood in patient with acute subarachnoid hemorrhage. *J Neurosurg Anesthesiol* 1995;7:12–16.

54. Tanaka M, Nakayama Y, Maeda Y, Nishioka T, Shirakawa M, Tsumura K. Electrocardiographic Q-waves as a predictor of mortality in patients with cerebral infarction. *Neurology* 2004;62:1818–1821.

55. McDermott MM, Lefevre F, Arron M, Martin GJ, Biller J. ST segment depression detected by continuous electrocardiography in patients with acute ischemic stroke or transient ischemic attack. *Stroke* 1994;25:1820–1824.

56. Chua HC, Sen S, Cosgriff RF, Gerstenblith G, Beauchamp NJ, Jr., Oppenheimer SM. Neurogenic ST depression in stroke. *Clin Neurol Neurosurg* 1999;101:44–48.

57. Macmillan CS, Andrews PJ, Struthers AD. QTc dispersion as a marker for medical complications after severe subarachnoid haemorrhage. *Eur J Anaesthesiol* 2003;20:537–542.

58. Fukui S, Katoh H, Tsuzuki N, et al. Multivariate analysis of risk factors for QT prolongation following subarachnoid hemorrhage. *Crit Care* 2003;7:R7–R12.

59. Sato K, Masuda T, Izumi T. Subarachnoid hemorrhage and myocardial damage clinical and experimental studies. *Japan Heart J* 1999;40:683–701.

60. Wijdicks EFM. Worst case scenario: Management in poor-grade aneurysmal subarachnoid hemorrhage. *Cerebrovasc Dis* 1995;5:163–169.

61. Mäkikallio AM, Mäkiallio TH, Korpelainen JT, Sotaniemi KA, Huikuri HV, Myllylä VV. Heart rate dynamics predict poststroke mortality. *Neurology* 2004;62:1822–1826.

62. Britton M, de Faire U, Helmers C, Miah K, Ryding C, Wester PO. Arrhythmias in patients with acute cerebrovascular disease. *Acta Med Scand* 1979;205:425–428.

63. Sakr YL, Ghosn I, Vincent JL. Cardiac manifestations after subarachnoid heomrrhage: a systematic review of the literature. *Progress Cardiovas Dis* 2002;45:67–80.

64. Brouwers PJAM, Wijdicks EFM, Hasan D, et al. Serial electrocardiographic recording in aneurysmal subarachnoid hemorrhage. *Stroke* 1989;20:1162–1167.

65. Cruickshank JM, Neil-Dwyer G, Brice J. Electrocardiographic changes and their prognostic significance in subarachnoid hemorrhage. *J Neurol Neurosurg Psychiatry* 1974;37:755–759.

66. Grad A, Kiauta T, Osredkar J. Effect of elevated plasma norepinephrine on electrocardiographic changes in subarachnoid hemorrhage. *Stroke* 1991;22:746–749.

67. Tung P, Kopelnik A, Banki N, et al. Predictors of neurocardiogenic injury after subarachnoid hemorrhage. *Stroke* 2004;35:548–553.

68. Korpelainen JT, Sotaniemi KA, Makikallio A, Huikuri HV, Myllyla VV. Dynamic behavior of heart rate in ischemic stroke. *Stroke*. 1999;30:1008–1013.

69. Oppenheimer SM. Neurogenic cardiac effects of cerebrovascular disease. *Curr Opin Neurol* 1994;7:20–24.

70. Lane RD, Wallace JD, Petrosky PP, Schwartz GE, Gradman AH. Supraventricular tachycardia in patients with right hemisphere strokes. *Stroke* 1992;23:362–366.

71. Tokgozoglu SL, Batur MK, Topcuoglu MA, Saribas O, Kes S, Oto A. Effects of stroke localization on cardiac autonomic balance and sudden death. *Stroke* 1999;30:1307–1311.

72. Korpelainen JT, Sotaniemi KA, Huikuri HV, Myllyla VV. Circadian rhythm of heart rate variability is reversibly abolished in ischemic stroke. *Stroke* 1997;28:2150–2154.

73. Wijdicks EF, Scott JP. Causes and outcome of mechanical ventilation in patients with hemispheric ischemic stroke. *Mayo Clin Proc* 1997;72:210–213.

74. Takahashi M, Mitsuhashi T, Katsuki T, et al. Neurogenic pulmonary edema and large negative T waves associated with subarachnoid hemorrhage. *Intern Med* 2001;40:826–828.

75. Smith WS, Matthay MA. Evidence for a hydrostatic mechanism in human neurogenic pulmonary edema. *Chest* 1997;111:1326–1333.

76. Fletcher SJ, Atkinson JD. Use of prone ventilation in neurogenic pulmonary edema. *Br J Anaesth* 2003;90:238–240.

77. Deehan SC, Grant IS. Haemodynamic changes in neurogenic pulmonary edema: effect of dobutamine. *Intensive Care Med* 1996;22:672–676.

78. Morfis L, Schwartz RS, Poulos R, Howes LG. Blood pressure changes in acute cerebral infarction and hemorrhage. *Stroke* 1997;28:1401–1405.

79. Broderick J, Brott T, Barsan W, et al. Blood pressure during the first minutes of focal cerebral ischemia. *Ann Emerg Med* 1993;22:1438–1443.

80. Brott T, Lu M, Kothari R, et al. Hypertension and its treatment in the NINDS rt-PA Stroke Trial. *Stroke* 1998;29:1504–1509.

81. Phillips SJ. Pathophysiology and management of hypertension in acute ischemic stroke. *Hypertension* 1994;23:131–136.

82. Aslanyan S, Fazekas F, Weir CJ, Horner S, Lees KR, for the GAIN International Steering Committee and Investigators. Effect of blood pressure during the acute period of ischemic stroke on stroke outcome. A tertiary analysis of the GAIN International Trial. *Stroke* 2003;34:2420–2425.

83. Stead LG, Gilmore RM, Vedula KC, et al. Impact of acute blood pressure variability on ischemic stroke outcome. *Neurology* 2006;66:1878–1881.

84. Willmot M, Leonardi-Bee J, Bath PMW. High blood pressure in acute stroke and subsequent outcome. A systematic review. *Hypertension* 2004;43:1–7.

85. Castillo J, Leira R, García MM, Serena J, Blanco M, Dávalos A. Blood pressure decrease during the acute phase of ischemic stroke is associated with brain injury and poor stroke outcome. *Stroke* 2004;35:520–527.

86. Rasool AH, Rahman AR, Choudhury SR, Singh RB. Blood pressure in acute intracerebral haemorrhage. *J Hum Hypertens* 2004;18:187–192.

87. Ohwaki K, Yano E, Nagashima H, Hirata M, Nakagomi T, Tamura A. Blood pressure management in acute intracerebral hemorrhage. Relationship between elevated blood pressue and hematoma enlargement. *Stroke* 2004;35:1364–1367.

88. Powers WJ. Acute hypertension after stroke: the scientific basis for treatment decisions. *Neurology* 1993;43:461–467.

89. Lawes CMM, Bennett DA, Feigin VL, Rodgers A. Blood pressure and stroke. An overview of published reviews. *Stroke* 2004;35:776–785.

90. Ahmed N, Wahlgren NG. Effects of blood pressure lowering in the acute phase of total anterior circulation infarcts and other stroke subtypes. *Cerebrovasc Dis* 2003;15:235–243.

91. Mayberg MR, Batjer HH, Dacey R, et al. Guidelines for the management of aneurysmal subarachnoid hemorrhage. A statement for healthcare professionals from a special writing group of the Stroke Council, American Heart Association. *Stroke* 1994;25:2315–2328.

92. Willmot M, Ghadami A, Whysall B, et al. Transdermal glyceryl trinitrate lowers blood pressure and maintains cerebral blood flow in recent stroke. *Hypertension* 2006;47:1209–1215.

93. Grossman E, Messerli FH, Grodzicki T, Kowey P. Should a moratorium be placed on sublingual nifedipine capsules

given for hypertensive emergencies and pseudoemergencies? *JAMA* 1996;276:1328–1331.

94. Grossman E, Ironi AN, Messerli FH. Comparative tolerability profile of hypertensive crisis treatments. *Drug Saf* 1998;19:99–122.

95. Rordorf G, Cramer SC, Efird JT, Schwamm LH, Buonanno F, Koroshetz WJ. Pharmacological elevation of blood pressure in acute stroke. Clinical effects and safety. *Stroke* 1997;28:2133–2138.

96. Rordorf G, Koroshetz WJ, Ezzeddine MA, Segal AZ, Buonanna FS. A pilot study of drug-induced hypertension for treatment of acute stroke. *Neurology* 2001;56:1210–1213.

97. Bruno A, Biller J, Adams HP, Jr., et al. Acute blood glucose level and outcome from ischemic stroke. Trial of Org 10172 in Acute Stroke Treatment (TOAST) Investigators. *Neurology* 1999;52:280–284.

98. Bruno A, Levine SR, Frankel M, et al. Admission glucose level and clinical outcomes in the NINDS rt-PA Stroke Trial. *Neurology* 2002;59:669–674.

99. Kagnasky N, Levy S, Knobler H. The role of hyperglycemia in acute stroke. *Arch Neurol* 2001;58:1209–1212.

100. Parsons MW, Barber A, Desmond PM, et al. Acute hyperglycemia adversely affects stroke outcome: a magnetic resonance imaging and spectroscopy study. *Ann Neurol* 2002;52:20–28.

101. Weir CJ, Murray GD, Dyker AG, Lees KR. Is hyperglycaemia an independent predictor of poor outcome after acute stroke? Results of a long-term follow up study. *Br Med J* 1997;314:1303–1306.

102. Baird TA, Parsons MW, Phanh T, et al. Persistent poststroke hyperglycemia is independently associated with infarct expansion and worse clinical outcome. *Stroke* 2003;34:2208–2214.

103. Broderick JP, Hagen T, Brott T, Tomsick T. Hyperglycemia and hemorrhagic transformation of cerebral infarcts. *Stroke* 1995;26:484–487.

104. Song EC, Chu K, Jeong SW, et al. Hyperglycemia exacerbates brain edema and perihematomal cell death after intracerebral hemorrhage. *Stroke* 2003;34:2215–2220.

105. Christensen H, Boysen G. Blood glucose increases early after stroke onset: a study on serial measurements of blood glucose in acute stroke. *Eur J Neurology* 2002;9:297–301.

106. Candelise L, Landi G, Orazio EN, Boccardi E. Prognostic significance of hyperglycemia in acute stroke. *Arch Neurol* 1985;42:661–663.

107. Capes SE, Hunt D, Malmberg K, Pathak P, Gerstein HC. Stress hyperglycemia dn prognosis of stroke in nondiabetic and diabetic patients: a systematic overview. *Stroke* 2001;32:2426–2432.

108. Adams HP, Jr., Olinger CP, Marler JR, et al. Comparison of admission serum glucose concentration with neurologic outcome in acute cerebral infarction. A study in patients given naloxone. *Stroke* 1988;19:455–458.

109. Murros K, Fogelholm R, Kettunen S, Vuorela AL, Valve J. Blood glucose, glycosylated haemoglobin, and outcome of ischemic brain infarction. *J Neurol Sci* 1992;111:59–64.

110. Scott JF, Robinson GM, French JM, O'Connell JE, Alberti KG, Gray CS. Glucose potassium insulin infusions in the treatment of acute stroke patients with mild to moderate hyperglycemia: the Glucose Insulin in Stroke Trial (GIST). *Stroke* 1999;30(4):793–799.

111. Bruno A, Saha C, Williams LS, Shankar R. IV insulin during acute cerebral infarction in diabetic patients. *Neurology* 2004;62:1441.

112. Van den Berghe G, Wouters P, Weekers F, et al. Intensive insulin therapy in critically ill patients. *N Engl J Med* 2001;345:1359–1367.

113. Gray CS, Hildreth AJ, Alberti GKMM, O'Connell JE, on behalf of the GIST Collaboration. Poststroke hyperglycemia. Natural history and immediate management. *Stroke* 2004;35:122–126.

114. Lyden PD, Marler JR. Acute Medical Therapy. J Stroke *Cerebrovasc Dis* 1999;8:139–145.

115. Wijdicks EF. Neurologic complications in critically ill patients. *Anesth Analg* 1996;83:411–419.

116. Diringer MN, Wu KC, Verbalis VG, Hanley D. Hypervolemic therapy prevents volume contraction but not hyponatremia following subarachnoid hemorrhage. *Ann Neurol* 1992;31:543

117. Berendes E, Walter M, Cullen P, et al. Secretion of brain natriuretic peptide in patients with aneurysmal subarachnoid haemorrhage. *Lancet* 1997;349:245–249.

118. Sato K, Karibe H, Yoshimoto T. Circulating blood volume in patients with subarachnoid haemorrhage. *Acta Neurochir* 1999;141:1069–1073.

119. Wijdicks EFM, Vermuelen M, Hijdra A. Hyponatremia and cerebral infarction in patients with ruptured intracranial aneurysms: Is fluid restriciton harmful? *Ann Neurol* 1985;17:137–140.

120. Sjoblom L, Hardemark HG, Lindgren A, et al. Management and prognostic features of intracerebral hemorrhage during anticoagulant therapy: a Swedish multicenter study. *Stroke* 2001;32:2567–2574.

121. Mayer SA. Ultra-early hemostatic therapy for intracerebral hemorrhage. *Stroke* 2003;34:224–229.

122. Yasaka M, Minematsu K, Naritomi H, Sakata T, Yamaguchi T. Predisposing factors for enlargement of intracerebral hemorrhage in patients treated with warfarin. *Thromb Haemost* 2003;89:278–283.

123. Sansing LH, Kaznatcheeva EL, Perkins CJ, Komaroff E, Gutman FB, Newman GC. Edema after intracerebral hemorrhage: correlations with coagulation parameters and treatment. *J Neurosurg* 2003;98:985–992.

124. Butler AC, Tait RC. Management of oral anticoagulant-induced intracranial haemorrhage. *Blood Rev* 1998;12:35–44.

125. Crowther MA, Douketis JD, Schnurr T, et al. Oral vitamin K lowers the international normalized ratio more rapidly than subcutaneous vitamin K in the treatment of warfarin-associated coagulopathy. *Ann Intern Med* 2002;137:251–254.

126. Cartmill M, Dolan G, Byrne JL, Byrne PO. Prothrombin complex concentrate for oral anticoagulant reversal in neurosurgical emergencies. *Br J Neurosurg* 2000;14:458–461.

127. Boulis NM, Bobek MP, Schmaier A, Hoff JT. Use of factor IX complex in warfarin-related intracranial hemorrhage. *Neurosurgery* 1999;45:1113–1119.

128. Deveras RA, Kessler CM. Reversal of warfarin-induced excessive anticoagulation with recombinant human factor VIIa concentrate. *Ann Intern Med* 2002;137:884–888.

129. Morenski JD, Tobias JD, Jimenez DF. Recombinant activated factor VII for cerebral injury-induced coagulopathy in pediatric patients. Report of three cases and review of the literature. *J Neurosurg* 2003;98:611–616.

130. Mayer, S. A., Brun, N., Broderick, J., and et al. Recombinant factor VIIa for acute intracerebral hemorrhage. 2004. (Generic).

131. Piriyawat P, Morgenstern LB, Yawn DH, Hall CE, Grotta JC. Treatment of acute intracerebral hemorrhage with epsilon-aminocaproic acid: a pilot study. *Neurocrit Care* 2004;1:47–52.

132. Keir SL, Wardlaw J, Sandercock P, Chen Z. Antithrombotic therapy in patients with any form of intracranial haemorrhage: a systematic review of the available controlled studies. *Cerebrovasc Dis* 2002;14:197–206.

133. Bladin CF, Alexandrov AV, Bellavance A, et al. Seizures Stroke Study Group: Seizures after stroke - A prospective multicenter study. *Arch Neurol* 2000;57:1617–1622.

134. van der Worp HB, Kappelle LJ. Complications of acute ischaemic stroke. *Cerebrovasc Dis* 1998;8:124–132.

135. Camilo O, Goldstein LB. Seizures and epilepsy after ischemic stroke. *Stroke* 2004;35:1769–1775.

136. Davalos A, de Cendra E, Molins A, Ferrandiz M, Lopez-Pousa S, Genis D. Epileptic seizures at the onset of stroke. *Cerebrovasc Dis* 1992;2:327–331.

137. DeReuck J, Claeys I, Martens S, et al. Computed tomographic changes of the brain and clinical outcome of patients with seizures and epilepsy after an ischemic hemispheric stroke. *Eur J Neurol* 2006;13:402–407.

138. Passero S, Rocchi R, Rossi S, Ulivelli M, Vatti G. Seizures after spontaneous supratentorial intracerebral hemorrhage. *Epilepsia* 2002;43:1175–1180.

139. Dennis MS. Outcome after brain haemorrhage. *Cerebrovasc Dis* 2003;16(suppl 1):9–13.

140. Towne AR, Waterhouse EJ, Boggs JG, et al. Prevalence of nonconvulsive status epilepticus in comatose patients. *Neurology* 2000;54:340–345.

141. Dennis LJ, Claassen J, Hirsch LJ, Emerson RG, Connally ES, Mayer SA. Nonconclusive status epilepticus after subarachnoid hemorrhage. *Neurosurgery* 2002;51:1136–1143.

142. Rumbach L, Sablot D, Berger E, Tatu L, Vuillier F, Moulin T. Status epilepticus in stroke. Report on a hospital-based stroke cohort. *Neurology* 2000;54:350–354.

143. Velioglu SK, Ozmenoglu M, Boz C, Alioglu Z. Satus epilepticus after stroke. *Stroke* 2001;32:1169–1172.

144. Prasad A, Worrall BB, Bertram EH, Bleck TP. Propofol and midazolam in the treatment of refractory status epilepticus. *Epilepsia* 2001;42:380–386.

145. Zazulia AR, Diringer MN, Derdeyn CP, Powers WJ. Progression of mass effect after intracerebral hemorrhage. *Stroke* 1999;30:1167–1173.

146. Nemoto EM. Dynamics of cerebral venous and intracranial pressures. *Acta Neurochir Suppl* 2006;96:435–437.

147. Mamarou A. The pathophysiology of brain edema and elevated intracranial pressure. *Cleve Clin J Med* 2004;71 (suppl 1):S6–S8.

148. Hacke W, Schwab S, Horn M, Spranger M, De Georgia M, von Kummer R. 'Malignant' middle cerebral artery territory infarction: clinical course and prognostic signs. *Arch Neurol* 1996;53:309–315.

149. Wijdicks EF, Diringer MN. Middle cerebral artery territory infarction and early brain swelling: progression and effect of age on outcome. *Mayo Clin Proc* 1998;73:829–836.

150. Krieger DW, Demchuk AW, Kasner SE, Jauss M, Hantson L. Early clinical and radiological predictors of fatal brain swelling in ischemic stroke. *Stroke* 1999;30:287–292.

151. Horwitz NH, Ludolph C. Acute obstructive hydrocephalus caused by cerebellar infarction. Treatment alternatives. *Surg Neurol* 1983;20:13–19.

152. Greenberg J, Skubick D, Shenkin H. Acute hydrocephalus in cerebellar infarct and hemorrhage. *Neurology* 1979;29: 409–413.

153. Valentin A, Lang T, Karnik R, Ammerer HP, Ploder J, Slany J. Intracranial pressure monitoring and case mix-adjusted mortality in intracranial hemorrhage. *Crit Care Med* 2003; 31:1539–1542.

154. Fernandes HM, Gregson B, Siddique S, Mendelow AD. Surgery in intracerebral hemorrhage: the uncertainty continues. *Stroke* 2000;31:2511–2416.

155. Hamani C, Zanetti MV, Pinto FC, Andrade AF, Ciquini O, Jr., Marino R, Jr. Intraventricular pressure monitoring in patients with thalamic and ganlionic hemorrhages. *Arquivos de Neuro-Psiquiatria* 2003;61:376–380.

156. Guyot LL, Dowling C, Diaz FG, Michael DB. Cerebral monitoring devices: analysis of complications. *Acta Neurochir* 1998;71:47–49.

157. Kappelle LJ, van der Worp HB. Treatment or prevention of complications of acute ischemic stroke. *Curr Neurol Neurosci Rep* 2004;4:36–41.

158. Schwarz S, Georgiadis D, Aschoff A, Schwab S. Effects of body position on intracranial pressure and cerebral perfusion in patients with large hemispheric stroke. *Stroke* 2002;33:497–501.

159. Reinprecht A, Greger M, Wolfsberger S, Diterich W, Illievich UM, Gruber A. Prone position in subarachnoid hemorrhage patients with acute respiratory distress syndrome: effects on cerebral tissue oxygenation and intracranial pressure. *Crit Care Med* 2003;31:1831–1838.

160. Georgiadis D, Schwarz S, Baumgartner RW, Veltkamp R, Schwab S. Influence of positive end-expiratory pressure on intracranial pressure and cerebral perfusion pressure in patients with acute stroke. *Stroke* 2001;32: 2088–2092.

161. Robertson C. Every breath you take: hyperventilation and intracranial pressure. *Cleve Clin J Med* 2004;71(suppl 1): S14–S15.

162. Crockard HA, Copper DL, Morrow WFK. Evaluation of hyperventilation in treatment of head injuries. *Br Med J* 1973;4:634–640.

163. Bauer RB, Tellez H. Dexamethasone as treatment in cerebrovascular disease. 2. A controlled study in acute cerebral infarction. *Stroke* 1973;4:547–555.

164. Norris JW, Hachinski VC. High dose steroid treatment in cerebral infarction. *Br Med J* 1986;292:21–23.

165. Pugvarin N, Bhodpat W, Viriyajakul A. Effects of dexamethasone in primary supratentorial intracerebral hemorrhage. *N Engl J Med* 1987;316:1229–1233.

166. Qizilbash N, Lewington SL, Lopez-Arrieta JM. Corticosteroids for acute ischaemic stroke. Cochrane Database of Systematic Reviews 2002; CD000064.

167. Mayberg MR, Batjer HH, Dacey R. Guidelines for the management of aneurysmal subarachnoid hemorrhage. *Circulation* 1994;90:2592–2605.

168. Stead LG, Rowe BH, EBEM Commentators. Corticosteroid treatment for acute ischemic stroke. *Ann Emerg Med* 2003;42:150–152.

169. Norris JW. Steroids may have a role in stroke therapy. *Stroke* 2004;35:228–229.

170. Poungvarin N. Steroids have no role in stroke therapy. *Stroke* 2004;35:229–230.

171. Davis SM, Donnan GA. Steroids for stroke: another potential therapy discarded prematurely? *Stroke* 2004;35:230–231.

172. Pullicino PM, Alexandrov AV, Shelton JA, Alexandrova NA, Smurawska LT, Norris JW. Mass effect and death from severe acute stroke. *Neurology* 1997;49:1090–1095.

173. Qureshi AI, Suarez JI, Bhardwaj A. Malignant cerebral edema in patients with hypertensive intracerebral hemorrhage associated with hypertonic saline infusion: a rebound phenomenon? *J Neurosurg Anesthesiol* 1998;10:188–192.

174. Qureshi AI, Wilson DA, Traystman RJ. Treatment of elevated intracranial pressure in experimental intracerebral hemorrhage: comparison between mannitol and hypertonic saline. *Neurosurgery* 1999;44:1055–1064.

175. Suarez JI. Hypertonic saline for cerebral edema and elevated intracranial pressure. *Cleve Clin J Med* 2004;71 (suppl 1):S9–S13.

176. Stoll M, Hagen T, Bartylla K, Weber M, Jost V, Treib J. Changes of cerebral perfusion after osmotherapy in acute cerebral edema assessed with perfusion weighted MRI. *Neurol Res* 1998;20:474–478.

177. Mathew NT, Rivera VM, Meyer JS, Charney JZ, Hartmann A. Double-blind evaluation of glycerol therapy in acute cerebral infarction. *Lancet* 1972;2:1327–1329.

178. Bayer AJ, Pathy MS, Newcombe R. Double-blind randomised trial of intravenous glycerol in acute stroke. *Lancet* 1987;1:405–408.

179. Sakamaki M, Igarashi H, Nishiyama Y, et al. Effect of glycerol on ischemic cerebral edema assessed by magnetic resonance imaging. *J Neurol Sci* 2003;209:69–74.

180. Righetti E, Celani MG, Cantisani TA, Sterzi R, Boysen G, Ricci S. Glycerol for acute stroke: a Cochrane systematic review. *J Neurol* 2002;249:445–451.

181. Marshall LF, Smith RW, Rauscher LA, Shapiro HM. Mannitol dose requirements in brain-injured patients. *J Neurosurg* 1978;48:169–172.

182. Manno EM, Adams RE, Derdeyn CP, Powers WJ, Diringer MN. The effects of mannitol on cerebral edema after large hemispheric cerebral infarct. *Neurology* 1999;52:583–587.

183. Dziedzic T, Szczudlik A, Klimkowicz A, Rog TM, Slowik A. Is mannitol safe for patients with intracerebral hemorrhages? Renal considerations. *Clin Neurol Neurosurg* 2003;105:87–89.

184. Cruz J, Minoja G, Okuchi K. Major clinical and physiological benefits of early high doses of mannitol for intraparenchymal temporal lobe hemorrhages with abnormal pupillary widening: a randomized trial. *Neurosurgery* 2002;51:628–637.

185. Bereczki D, Mihalka L, Szatmari S, et al. Mannitol use in acute stroke: case fatality at 30 days and 1 year. *Stroke* 2003;34:1730–1735.

186. Bereczki D, Liu M, do Prado GF, Fekete I. Mannitol for acute stroke. Cochrane Database of Systematic Reviews 2001; CD001153.

187. Schwarz S, Georgiadis D, Aschoff A, Schwab S. Effects of hypertonic (10%) saline in patients with raised intracranial pressure after stroke. *Stroke* 2002;33:136–140.

188. Tseng M-Y, Al-Rawi PG, Pickard JD, Rasulo FA, Kirkpatrick PJ. Effect of hypertonic saline on cerebral blood flow in poor-grade patients with subarchnoid hemorrhage. *Stroke* 2003;34:1389–1397.

189. Qureshi AI, Suarez JI, Bhardwaj A, et al. Use of hypertonic (3%) saline/acetate infusion in the treatment of cerebral edema: Effect on intracranial pressure and lateral displacement of the brain. *Crit Care Med* 1998;26:440–446.

190. Qureshi AI, Suarez JI. Use of hypertonic saline solutions in treatment of cerebral edema and intracranial hypertension. *Crit Care Med* 2000;28:3301–3313.

191. Berrouschot J, Sterker M, Bettin S, Koster J, Schneider D. Mortality of space-occupying ('malignant') middle cerebral artery infarction under conservative intensive care. *Intensive Care Med* 1998;24:620–623.

192. Woodcock J, Ropper AH, Kennedy SK. High dose barbiturates in non-traumatic brain swelling: ICP reduction and effect on outcome. *Stroke* 1982;13:785–787.

193. Schwab S, Spranger M, Schwarz S, Hacke W. Barbiturate coma in severe hemispheric stroke: useful or obsolete? *Neurology* 1997;48:1608–1613.

194. Schwab S, Schwarz S, Spranger M, Keller E, Bertram M, Hacke W. Moderate hypothermia in the treatment of patients with severe middle cerebral artery infarction. *Stroke* 1998;29:2461–2466.

195. Schwab S, Spranger M, Aschoff A, Steiner T, Hacke W. Brain temperature monitoring and modulation in patients with severe MCA infarction. *Neurology* 1997;48:762–767.

196. Schwab S, Schwarz S, Aschoff A, Keller E, Hacke W. Moderate hypothermia and brain temperature in patients with severe middle cerebral artery infarction. *Acta Neurochir* 1998;71:131–134.

197. McDonald C, Carter BS. Medical management of increased intracranial pressure after spontaneous intracerebral hemorrhage. *Neurosurg Clin N Am* 2002;13:335–338.

198. Graff-Radford NR, Torner J, Adams HP, Jr. Factors associated with hydrocephalus after subarachnoid hemorrhage: A report of the Cooperative Aneurysm Study. *Arch Neurol* 1989;46:744–752.

199. Sheehan JP, Polin RS, Sheehan JM, Baskaya MK, Kassell NF, and Participants. Factors associated with hydrocephalus after aneurysmal subarachnoid hemorrhage. *Neurosurgery* 1999;45:1120–1128.

200. Yoshioka H, Inagawa T, Tokuda Y, Inokuchi F. Chronic hydrocephalus in elderly patients following subarachnoid hemorrhage. *Surg Neurol* 2000;53:119–124.

201. Engelhard HH, Andrews CO, Slavin KV, Charbel FT. Current management of intraventricular hemorrhage. *Surg Neurol* 2003;60:15–21.

202. Kumar K, Demeria DD, Verma A. Recombinant tissue plasminogen activator in the treatment of intraventricular

hemorrhage secondary to periventricular arteriovenous malformation before surgery: case report. *Neurosurgery* 2003;52:964–968.

203. Lapointe M, Haines S. Fibrinolytic therapy for intraventricular hemorrhage in adults. Cochrane Database of Systematic Reviews 2002; CD003692.

204. Suzuki M, Otawara Y, Doi M, Ogasawara K, Ogawa A. Neurological grades of patients with poor-grade subarachnoid hemorrhage improve after short-term pretreatment. *Neurosurgery* 2000;47:1098–1104.

205. Mathew P, Teasdale G, Bannan A, Oluoch-Olunya D. Neurosurgical management of cerebellar haematoma and infarct. *J Neurol Neurosurg Psychiatry* 1995;59:287–292.

206. Brandt T, Grau AJ, Hacke W. Severe stroke. *Baillieres Clin Neurol* 1996;5:515–541.

207. Rieke K, Krieger D, Aschoff A, Meyding-Lamade V, Hacke W. Therapeutic strategies in in space-occupying cerebellar infarction based on clinical, neuroradiological, and neurophysical logical data. *Cerebrovasc Dis* 1993;3:45–55.

208. Chen HJ, Lee TC, Wei CP. Treatment of cerebellar infarction by decompressive suboccipital craniectomy. *Stroke* 1992;23:957–961.

209. St.Louis EK, Wijdicks EF, Li H. Predicting neurologic deterioration in patients with cerebellar hematomas. *Neurology* 1998;51:1364–1369.

210. Wijdicks EF, St Louis EK, Atkinson JD, Li H. Clinician's biases toward surgery in cerebellar hematomas: an analysis of decision-making in 94 patients. *Cerebrovasc Dis* 2000;10:93–96.

211. Cohen ZR, Ram Z, Knoller N, Peles E, Hadani M. Management and outcome of non-traumatic cerebellar haemorrhage. *Cerebrovasc Dis* 2002;14:207–213.

212. Salvati M, Cervoni L, Raco A, Delfini R. Spontaneous cerebellar hemorrhage: clinical remarks on 50 cases. *Surg Neurol* 2001;55:156–161.

213. Yanaka K, Matsumaru Y, Nose T. Management of spontaneous cerebellar hematomas: a prospective treatment protocol. *Neurosurgery* 2002;51:524–525.

214. Pollak L, Rabey JM, Gur R, Schiffer J. Indication to surgical management of cerebellar hemorrhage. *Clin Neurol Neurosurg* 1998;100:99–103.

215. Rabinstein A, Atkinson JL, Wijdicks FM. Emergency craniotomy in patients worsening due to expanded cerebral hematoma. To what purpose? *Neurology* 2002;58:1367–1372.

216. Montes J, Wong J, Fayad P, Awad IA. Stereotactic computed tomographic-guided aspiration and thrombolysis of intracerebral hematoma: protocol and preliminary experience. *Stroke* 2000;31:834–840.

217. Naff N, Carhuapoma J, Williams M, et al. Treatment of intraventricular hemorrhage with urokinase: effects on 30-day survival. *Stroke* 2000;31:841–847.

218. Nieuwkamp DJ, De Gans K, Rinkel GJ, Algra A. Treatment and outcome of severe intraventricular extension in patients with subarachnoid or intracerebral hemorrhage: a systematic review of the literature. *J Neurol* 2000;247:117–121.

219. Naff NJ, Hanley DF, Keyl PM, et al. Intraventricular urokinase speeds clot resolution: results of a pilot, prospective, randomized, double blind, controlled trial. *Neurosurgery* 2004;54:1–7.

220. Lee MW, Pang KY, Ho W, Wong CK. Outcome analysis of intraventricular thrombolytic therapy for intraventricular hemorrhage. *Hong Kong Med J* 2003;9:335–340.

221. Marchuk G, Kaufmann AM. Spontaneous supratentorial intracerebral hemorrhage. The role of surgical management. *Can J Neurol Sci* 2005;32(suppl 2):S22–S30.

222. D'Ambrosio AL, Sughrue ME, Yorgason JG, et al. Decompressive hemicraniectomy for poor-grade aneurysmal subarachnoid hemorrhage patients with associated intracerebral hemorrhage. Clinical outcome and quality of life assessment. *Neurosurgery* 2005;56:12–19.

223. Morgenstern LB, Demchuk AM, Kim DH, Frankowski RF, Grotta JC. Rebleeding leads ot poor outcome in ultra-early craniotomy for intracerebral hemorrhage. *Neurology* 2001;56:1294–1299.

224. Morioka J, Fujii M, Kato S, et al. Surgery for spontaneous intracerebral hemorrhage has greater remedial value than conservative therapy. *Surg Neurol* 2006;65:67–72.

225. Murthy JM, Chowdary GV, Murthy TV, Bhasha PS, Naryanan TJ. Decompressive craniectomy with clot evacuation in large hemispheric hypertensive intracerebral hemorrhage. *Neurocrit Care* 2005;2:258–262.

226. Mendelow AD, Investigators and Steering Committee. The international surgical trial in intracerebral hemorrhage (ISTICH). *Acta Neurochir* 2003;86:441–443.

227. Marquardt G, Wolff R, Sager A, Janzen RW, Seifert V. Subacute stereotactic aspiration of haematomas within the basal ganglia reduces occurrence of complications in the course of haemorrhagic stroke in non-comatose patients. *Cerebrovasc Dis* 2003;15:252–257.

228. Little KM, Alexander MJ. Medical versus surgical therapy for spontaneous intracranial heomrrhage. *Neurosurg Clin N Am* 2002;13:339–347.

229. Foroohar M, Macdonald RL, Roth S, Stoodley M, Weir B. Intraoperative variables and early outcome after aneurysm surgery. *Surg Neurol* 2000;54:304–315.

230. Smith ER, Carter BS, Ogilvy CS. Proposed use of prophylactic decompressive craniectomy in poor-grade aneurysmal subarachnoid hemorrhage patients presenting with associated large sylvian hematomas. *Neurosurgery* 2002;51:117–124.

231. Ziai WC, Port JD, Cowan JA, Garonzik IM, Bhardwaj A, Rigamonti D. Decompressive craniectomy for intractable cerebral edema: experience of a single center. *J Neurosurg Anesthesiol* 2003;15:25–32.

232. Jaeger M, Soehle M, Meixensberger J. Effects of decompressive craniectomy on brain tissue oxygen in patients with intracranial hypertension. *J Neurol Neurosurg Psychiatry* 2003;74:513–515.

233. Hemphill JC, III, Newman J, Zhao S, Johnston SC. Hospital usage of early do-not-resuscitate orders and outcome after intracerebral hemorrhage. *Stroke* 2004;35:1130–1134.

CHAPTER 22

Treatment of Acute Ischemic Stroke

Until 1995, treatment of acute ischemic stroke focused on general management to control or prevent complications of the vascular event (see Chapter 21). While these therapies are crucial for achieving favorable outcomes, they are not aimed at lessening the acute neurological injury. With the announcement of the results of trials testing intravenous recombinant tissue plasminogen activator (rtPA) in late 1995 and the approval of the agent by the Food and Drug Administration approximately 6 months later, the entire approach to treatment of patients with acute ischemic stroke changed.[1] Since then intravenous rtPA has been approved for treatment of patients in several other countries, including Canada. At last, a therapy of proven utility was available to limit the neurological consequences of acute thromboembolic occlusions. Statements to guide decisions about treatment with rtPA and other therapies have been authored by groups in the United States and other countries.[2–7] The success of rtPA has stimulated a large number of trials testing other promising interventions to treat acute ischemic stroke (Table 22-1). To date, none of the other therapies has demonstrated the efficacy and safety achieved with rtPA. Additional therapies currently are being tested and one or more will likely be shown as useful. Indeed, one of the stimuli for additional research is the limited usefulness of intravenous rtPA. Because of the short time window (less than 3 h from onset of stroke) and the perceived high risk for bleeding complications, the majority of patients are not treated with thrombolysis.

▶ STRATEGIES TO TREAT ACUTE ISCHEMIC STROKE

In general, potential therapies involve interventions that restore or improve blood flow to the region of ischemia and those that halt the cellular and metabolic consequences of stroke (neuroprotection) (Figs. 22-1 to 22-4). Surgical interventions include emergency carotid endarterectomy or endovascular procedures that remove or destroy an intra-arterial thrombus. Endovascular interventions can be combined with intra-arterial administration of thrombolytic or antithrombotic agents. Thrombolytic agents promote lysis of the clot, and antiplatelet or anticoagulant medications may halt propagation of a thrombus, forestall early recurrent embolization, or improve collateral flow. Cerebral blood flow also can be augmented by the use of agents that alter vascular diameter, increase blood pressure, or alter the rheological characteristics of blood. Neuroprotective agents may ultimately prove to be beneficial in protecting the brain from the effects of anaerobic glycolysis, membrane depolarization, apoptosis, inflammation, or release of excitatory amino acids.

▶ PHARMACOLOGICAL THROMBOLYSIS

Rationale

The endogenous thrombolysin, plasminogen, is converted to plasmin at the time of an acute thromboembolic occlusion.[8] Plasmin helps halt the propagation of a

▶ **TABLE 22-1.** INTERVENTIONS TO TREAT ACUTE ISCHEMIC STROKE

Restore or improve blood flow and perfusion
    Pharmacological thrombolysis
        Intravenous administration
        Intra-arterial administration
        Combined intravenous and intra-arterial administration
        Combined with mechanical or other medical therapies
    Mechanical thrombolysis—endovascular procedures
        Clot-removal devices
        Ultrasound
        Angioplasty and stenting
    Surgical interventions
        Carotid endarterectomy
        Embolectomy
    Fibrinogen depleting agents
    Anticoagulants
    Antiplatelet aggregating agents
    Volume expansion and hemodilution
    Induced hypertension
Neuroprotection therapies
    Antagonists to excitatory amino acids
    Calcium-channel-blocking agents
    Free-radical antagonists
    Metabolic depressants, including hypothermia
    Antiapoptotic medications
    Membrane stabilizing agents
    Anti-inflammatory agents
    Hyperbaric oxygen

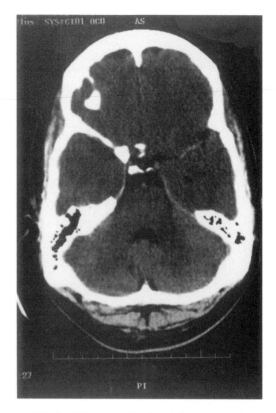

Figure 22-1. CT scan obtained from a patient seen within 3 h of the onset of aphasia and right hemiparesis. The study demonstrates a thrombus in the left middle cerebral artery (dense artery sign).

thrombus, speeds lysis of a formed clot, and helps maintain normal hemostasis. These effects help restore patency of an occluded artery. Unfortunately, natural recanalization does not happen with sufficient rapidity to restore circulation and prevent infarction of ischemic tissue. Several pharmacological therapies have been developed to speed the conversion of plasminogen to plasmin, with the goal of achieving recanalization and reperfusion as quickly as possible[8–10] (Table 22-2).

Pharmacology

The first thrombolytic agents were streptokinase and urokinase. Subsequently developed thrombolytic agents

▶ **TABLE 22-2.** THROMBOLYTIC AGENTS

Streptokinase
Urokinase
Alteplase (recombinant tissue plasminogen activator/rtPA)
Reteplase
Tenectoplase
Prourokinase
Antistreplase (anisoylated plasminogen streptokinase
    activator complex)
Staphylokinase

include rtPA (alteplase), reteplase, prourokinase, antistreplase, staphylokinase, and tenectoplase.[9] These agents have differences in pharmacological action, duration of effect, and risk of bleeding. For example, the third-generation thrombolytic agents have longer half-lives and greater penetration into the thrombus matrix than the initial agents and may prove faster and more efficacious than other thrombolytic agents. Streptokinase is produced by group A beta-hemolytic streptococci. Urokinase is secreted from human renal cells and is a direct plasminogen activator. Prourokinase, which is a single-chain urokinase plasminogen activator, is a precursor or urokinase.[10,11] While it has higher specificity for a thrombus, its thrombolytic effects are similar to urokinase. Alteplase (rtPA) is a recombinant double-chain thrombolytic agent that affects the lysine sites of plasminogen.[12,13] It increases plasminogen binding to fibrin and controls the inhibition of plasmin by alpha-2-antiplasmin. For treatment of acute ischemia, rtPA is usually given as a bolus followed by a 1-h infusion. Reteplase is a single-chain tissue plasminogen activator, including the kringle 2-protease domains of tissue plasminogen activator.[14] Reteplase has a longer half-life than rtPA. Twenty units of reteplase are approximately equal to 100 mg of rtPA. In

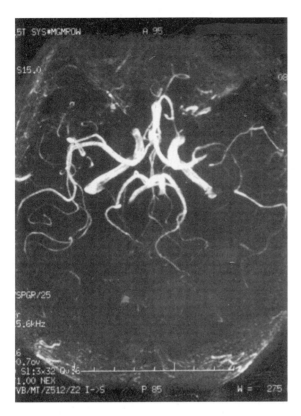

Figure 22-2. Basal view of an emergency MRA performed within 3 h of onset of stroke shows an embolic occlusion of the left middle cerebral artery.

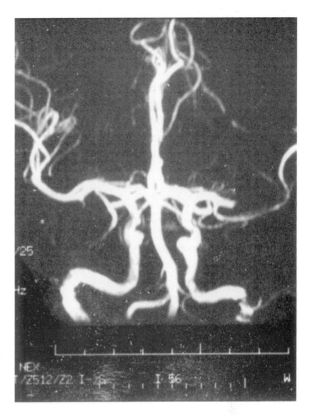

Figure 22-3. Anteroposterior view of an emergency MRA shows an embolic occlusion of the upper division of the left middle cerebral artery.

treatment of myocardial infarction, reteplase is given in two doses approximately 30 min apart. Both rtPA and reteplase are given intravenously or intra-arterially. Following administration of thrombolytic agents, levels of fibrin degradation products, D-dimer, and plasmin inhibitor complex are elevated.[15] The effects are measured by declines in the alpha-2-plasmin level. They may activate coagulation and the formation of fibrin. Streptokinase and rtPA can increase prothrombin fragments 1 + 2 through their stimulation of thrombin.[16–18] They also affect platelet aggregation by altering von Willebrand factor and binding at the platelet glycoprotein IIb/IIIa receptor. Staphylokinase has a high affinity for fibrin but it does not prolong the bleeding time to the same degree as rtPA. Ancrod is a defibrinogenating enzyme derived from snake venom.[19] It rapidly lowers blood levels of fibrinogen, halts propagation of thrombi, and results in increased levels of fibrin degradation products and D-dimer.

Experimental models of stroke demonstrate that thrombolytic agents can improve blood flow, decrease infarction volume, decrease brain edema, and increase neurological recovery. Metabolic studies also show recovery of brain activity, with restoration of blood flow. Based on changes in diffusion and perfusion magnetic resonance imaging (MRI) studies, Marks et al.[20] demonstrated

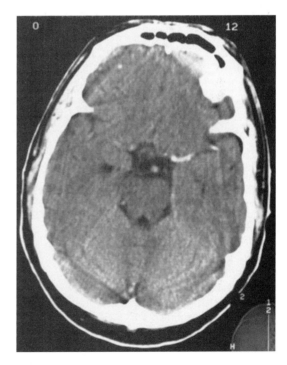

Figure 22-4. CT scan obtained within a few hours of an acute ischemic stroke shows a dense artery sign (embolus in the proximal segment) and dot sign (embolus in second segment) in the left middle cerebral artery.

early reperfusion with the use of thrombolytics. Heiss et al.[21] found that early thrombolysis protected ischemic brain tissue. Administration of these medications achieves recanalization of occluded arteries in patients with acute stroke, which can be detected by transcranial Doppler ultrasonography, arteriography, magnetic resonance angiography (MRA), or cerebral flow studies. Using transcranial Doppler ultrasonographic monitoring, Christou et al.[22] found that recanalization within 5 h of onset of stroke was associated with neurological recovery. Doppler ultrasonography is also used to monitor for recurrent thrombotic occlusion of the artery. Persistent occlusion or reocclusion following rtPA is associated with a lack of neurological improvement.[23] Alexandrov and Grotta[24] found that early reocclusion occurs in approximately one-third of patients treated with intravenous thrombolysis. Reocclusion usually develops in patients who have only partial recanalization. It is associated with an increased likelihood of neurological worsening after initial improvement, and outcomes are generally worse.

Safety

Bleeding is the main complication of thrombolytic agents (Table 22-3). While intracranial hemorrhage is the most serious and feared complication, hemorrhages also occur in other locations. Therefore, the potential for bleeding affects decisions about prescribing thrombolytic agents. For example, recent trauma or surgery usually precludes the thrombolytic treatment of acute myocardial or cerebral ischemia.

The frequency of serious intracranial bleeding is approximately 0.5–0.8 percent of patients receiving thrombolytic medications for treatment of acute myocardial ischemia.[25,26] The relative risk of serious intracranial bleeding following myocardial infarction is increased by a factor of approximately 3.5, with the use of thrombolytic medications. Bleeding may be intracerebral, intra-

▶ **TABLE 22-3.** COMPLICATIONS OF THROMBOLYSIS

Intracranial bleeding
  Hemorrhagic transformation of infarction
    Symptomatic
    Asymptomatic
  Intracerebral hemorrhage
  Intraventricular hemorrhage
  Subarachnoid hemorrhage
Bleeding in other locations
Myocardial rupture (patient with recent myocardial
  infarction)
Allergic idiosyncratic reactions
  Urticaria
  Angioedema of throat, mouth and tongue
  Anaphylaxis

---

ventricular, subdural, or subarachnoid in location. Among patients receiving thrombolytic agents for treatment of acute myocardial ischemia, the risk of hemorrhage is highest among persons older than 65 years (especially those older than 80 years), women, African Americans, persons weighing less than 70 kg, and those with diabetes or hypertension.[26,27] A past history of stroke is associated with a high risk of complicating intracranial hemorrhage following thrombolytic treatment of acute myocardial ischemia. The concomitant use of antiplatelet or anticoagulant medications also increase the likelihood of intracranial bleeding.

The likelihood of intracranial hemorrhage is increased considerably when thrombolytic agents are given to persons with acute stroke.[28] This risk is a major limitation of thrombolytic therapy. The rate of symptomatic (including fatal) intracranial hemorrhage was so high in the trials testing streptokinase that the trials were halted prematurely due to safety concerns.[29–32] The risk of bleeding following streptokinase was increased among patients with elevated levels of blood pressure.[33] Administration of rtPA increases the risk of symptomatic hemorrhagic transformation of an infarction by a factor of approximately 10.[1] A recent analysis of pooled data from several trials of rtPA found that the risk of hemorrhage was approximately 5.9 percent.[34] Bleeding risks are increased among older persons, those with severe neurological impairments (often measured as high National Institute of Health Stroke Scale (NIHSS) score), profound declines in pretreatment blood flow, occlusion of major intracranial arteries, and extensive changes on brain imaging.[35,36] Bleeding risk may also be increased with delayed administration of the thrombolytic agent, elevated fibrin degradation products, and an elevated blood glucose concentrations. In particular, hemorrhagic complications are highest among patients with a baseline NIHSS score greater than 20.[36] In this group, the risk of symptomatic hemorrhage following intravenous rtPA is approximately 16 percent. The chance of bleeding complications is also increased among patients with baseline hyperglycemia.[37] Trouillas et al.[38] found that the risk of symptomatic intracranial hemorrhage also was higher among persons with elevated levels of fibrin degradation products. Prior treatment with aspirin does not increase the risk of bleeding from rtPA.[39]

Since the approval of rtPA for treatment of stroke, several groups have reported that the rate of bleeding complications was similar to that found in the National Institutes of Neurological Disorders and Stroke (NINDS) trials.[1,40–43] An exception was the study reported by Katzan et al.[44]; in this community-based review in Cleveland, OH, the bleeding rate was 15.7 percent and mortality was increased with treatment. However, violations of the protocol for administration of rtPA were noted in many of the patients with hemorrhagic complications.

This experience is buttressed by the observation of Lopez-Yunez et al.,[45] who found that violations of the thrombolytic protocols are relatively common and these breaches are associated with an increased rate of hemorrhagic complications.

Cardiac rupture is a potential complication of thrombolytic therapy given for treatment of myocardial infarction, especially among women older than 70 years.[46] This complication is most likely to occur when the treatment is given for more than 12 h following a myocardial infarction.[47] Such a scenario could occur if thrombolytics are given to treat a stroke that follows a myocardial infarction. Kasner et al.[48] reported three cases of hemopericardium and cardiac tamponade, following use of rtPA for treatment of stroke. The potential for this fatal complication precludes the use of rtPA for treatment of stroke among patients with recent (within 6 weeks) myocardial infarction.

A recent operation is a relative contraindication. In particular, bleeding in a site that might not be easily treated is a potential concern. Despite the prohibition against giving thrombolytic therapy following surgery, Katzan et al.[49] safely administered rtPA to treat patients within 2-13 days following cardiac operations. In a series of 36 patients having stroke following surgery at an average interval of 21 h, intra-arterial thrombolysis was found to be relatively safe.[50] Therefore, the risk of bleeding must be weighed against the potential utility of limiting a serious brain injury. If the surgeon agrees to help manage bleeding related to the operative site, rtPA could be given during the perioperative period. A recent injury, including a fall at the time of stroke that leads to a fracture, also is a relative contraindication to thrombolysis because of the potential for serious bleeding at that site.

Idiosyncratic reactions may accompany the use of rtPA in treatment of stroke.[51–53] Patients may develop anaphylaxis including marked edema of the tongue and mouth, and the airway could become compromised. In that setting, the edema usually is worse on the side of the hemiparesis and seems to be more severe among persons who are also receiving angiotensin converting enzyme inhibitors. Severe allergic reactions also can complicate the administration of streptokinase.[54]

Intravenous Thrombolysis

Intravenous thrombolysis has several advantages. It can be administered in a community hospital and therefore greatly expands the number of patients who could be treated. It requires a minimal number of pretreatment diagnostic studies. It requires neither the technology nor the physician expertise required to administer the medication intra-arterially. Intravenous therapy may be given more quickly than intra-arterial therapy because additional time is required to transfer a patient to a large hospital, mobilize physicians and other personnel, and activate the necessary interventional facility.

Clinical trials tested the potential utility of thrombolytic medications in the late 1960s and early 1970s.[55] These trials, which were performed before the implementation of computed tomography (CT), enrolled patients up to 24 h, following onset of stroke. Because these trials showed an unacceptably high rate of hemorrhagic complications, including fatal intracranial bleeding, pharmacological thrombolysis was abandoned. Subsequently, cardiologists found that thrombolytic agents could substantially increase survival when administered within a few hours of myocardial infarction.[56] In addition, new, more selective thrombolytic medications were introduced. Advances in endovascular medicine permitted the use of intra-arterial thrombolysis. Based on a meta-analysis of several preliminary, uncontrolled studies reported prior to 1992, Wardlaw and Warlow[57] concluded that intravenous thrombolysis could improve outcomes after stroke, without causing an increased risk of intracranial bleeding. This analysis correctly predicted that thrombolysis would improve outcomes but incorrectly concluded that these medications did not increase bleeding risks.

Three trials tested *streptokinase* in a dose of 1.5 million units administered up to 6 h following stroke.[29–32] This time window and dose are similar to that used to treat patients with acute myocardial ischemia. The trials also enrolled seriously ill patients, those at highest risk for intracranial bleeding. In the Multicenter Acute Stroke Trial, Europe, the risk of symptomatic hemorrhage was 21.2 percent among 156 patients treated with streptokinase and 2.6 percent among 154 patients given placebo.[32] The trial was halted prematurely because of an unacceptably high rate of early deaths, largely due to bleeding, among the patients treated with streptokinase.[30] The Multicentre Acute Stroke Trial, Italy, also was stopped prematurely because of a high rate of fatal or symptomatic intracranial hemorrhages among patients treated with streptokinase and aspirin[31] (Figs. 22-5 to 22-8). Based on these results, Motto et al.[58] concluded that bleeding following streptokinase therapy was associated with a markedly increased risk of unfavorable outcomes following stroke. An Australian trial found a high rate of intracranial bleeding and mortality when streptokinase therapy was initiated more than 3 h after onset of stroke.[29] However, earlier administration of streptokinase was not associated with a significant increase in mortality. While these trials may be criticized, they demonstrate that streptokinase has not passed the test for safety. At present, no evidence exists to support the use of intravenous streptokinase for treatment of patients with stroke. Additional research, including preliminary studies that determine the optimal safe dose, is needed before streptokinase could be used to treat patients with stroke.

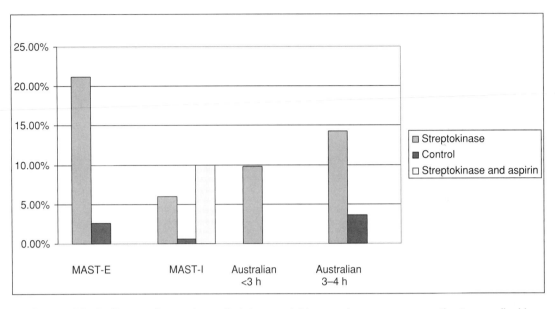

Figure 22-5. Rates of symptomatic intracranial hemorrhage among patients enrolled in the trials of streptokinase for treatment of acute ischemic stroke. (*Adapted from Refs. 29, 31, and 32*).

Streptokinase cannot be used as a substitute for management of patients with stroke.

Six phase III trials tested rtPA when administered up to 6 h after the onset of stroke.[1,59–63] In a placebo-controlled, randomized trial, Hacke et al.[59] enrolled 620 patients; half received rtPA 1.1 mg/kg up to 100 mg (Figs. 22-9 and 22-10). Based on a retrospective review of baseline CT criteria, approximately one-sixth of the patients were judged ineligible because they had large, multilobar infarctions. No net improvement of outcomes was noted in this study but the patients with large

infarctions had an increased rate of intracranial hemorrhages. A post hoc review of the data from patients treated within 3 h of onset of stroke showed a trend of increased likelihood of favorable outcomes with rtPA treatment.[65]

The investigators of the NINDS trials performed two back-to-back studies, which were published in a single report.[1] Patients were treated within 3 h of onset of stroke and one-half of these were enrolled within 90 min. The dose of rtPA (0.9 mg/kg–maximum of 90 mg) was selected on the basis of previously performed

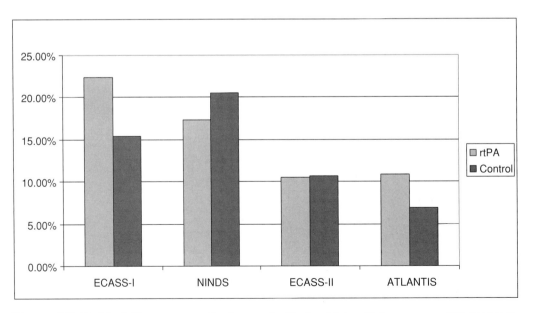

Figure 22-6. Mortality among patients enrolled in the trials of intravenous rtPA for treatment of acute ischemic stroke. (*Adapted from Refs. 1, 34, 58 and 59*).

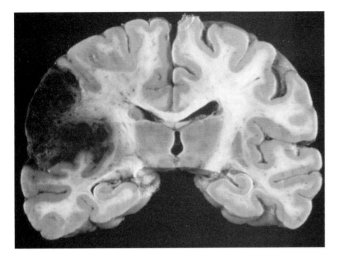

Figure 22-7. Coronal autopsy specimen shows a large area of hemorrhage within an infarction that followed an embolic occlusion of the middle cerebral artery. *(Courtesy of S.S. Schochet, M.D., Department of Pathology, University of West Virginia, Morgantown, WV)*

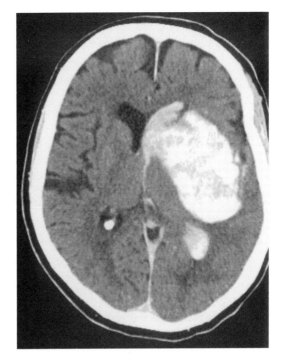

dose-escalation/safety studies.[66–68] Despite the very short interval from treatment, very few patients with suspected transient ischemic attack (TIA) were enrolled; only 2 percent of placebo-treated patients had complete recovery by 24 h following stroke. Favorable outcomes, as judged by complete or nearly complete recovery as rated on several outcome measures, were found in 31–50 percent of patients treated with rtPA compared to 20–38 percent of

Figure 22-8. CT scan of a brain obtained in a patient who deteriorated suddenly following intravenous administration of a thrombolytic agent for treatment of an acute right hemisphere infarction. A fluid level is seen within the hematoma.

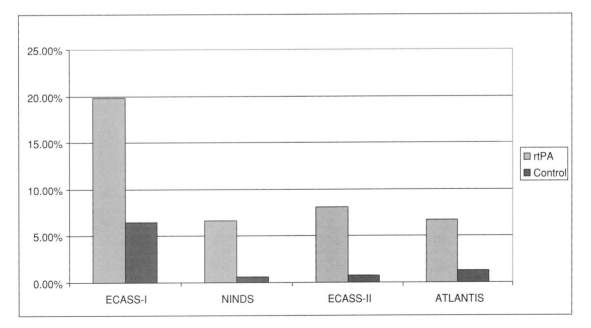

Figure 22-9. Frequency of symptomatic hemorrhage among patients enrolled in trials testing intravenously administered rtPA. In all four trials, the trials reported higher rates of symptomatic intracranial hemorrhage among patients given rtPA than among those in the control group. *(Adapted from Refs. 1, 34, 58 and 59).*

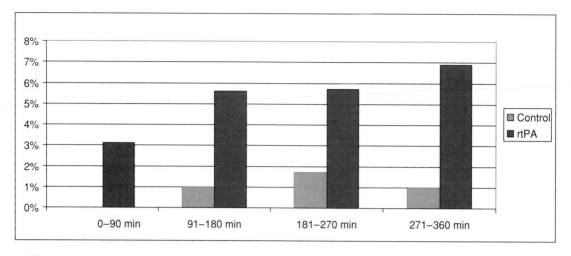

Figure 22-10. Frequency of symptomatic hemorrhage among patient enrolled in trials testing intravenously administered rtPA. The aggregate data are from randomized trials and report the rate of bleeding as influenced from the interval from onset of stroke until administration of medication. The frequency of hemorrhage is higher among patients treated more than 90 min after stroke. (*Adapted from Ref. 64*).

placebo-treated patients. Outcomes were similar among the patients treated within 90 min to those treated within 91–180 min. Patients with mild to moderately severe strokes (NIHSS score <20) and younger patients had the best response to treatment.[69] Because of concerns raised about the results of the trial, another panel reevaluated the data and concluded that the rtPA was effective.[70] The data have been validated by this independent review.

Another placebo-controlled, randomized trial of rtPA, using the dose and entry criteria included in the NINDS trials, enrolled 800 patients treated within 6 h of onset of stroke.[60] They used very strict criteria for CT screening and as a result, most patients with very large infarctions were not enrolled. Favorable outcomes were noted in 40.3 percent of patients treated with rtPA and 36.6 percent of those given placebo, a difference that was not statistically significant. Clark et al.[61] could not demonstrate a benefit from rtPA when the agent was administered up to 6 h after stroke. Another American trial looked at the potential utility of rtPA administered within 3–5 h following stroke.[63] Excellent outcomes were recorded in approximately one-third of the patients in each treatment group. In general, the responses to treatment are correlated with the baseline severity of neurological impairments as documented by the score on the NIHSS.[64] Recently, a pooled analysis of several trials testing rtPA showed that a benefit of thrombolysis was strongly associated with the interval from onset of stroke until treatment; earlier treatment was associated with the best chances of favorable outcomes.[34] A similar study found that the beneficial effects of treatment with rtPA were especially prominent when the medication was

▶ **TABLE 22-4.** KEY DECISIONS ABOUT INTRAVENOUS ADMINISTRATION OF rtPA

Interval from onset of stroke to treatment <3 h
  Time of onset must be known
  Most patients with stroke upon awakening cannot be
    treated
  Onset must be <3 h, even with subsequent worsening
  If previous TIA, signs must have cleared completely
High risk for bleeding complications
  History of recent serious trauma, fracture
  History of recent illness
    Myocardial infarction
    Ischemic stroke
    Serious bleeding
  History of recent major surgery
  Elevated blood pressure
    Systolic >185 mm Hg
    Diastolic >110 mm Hg
  Abnormal baseline coagulation tests
Neurological status
  Very severe stroke (NIHSS score >20 points)
  Very mild stroke (NIHSS score <4 points)
  Rapidly clearing neurological impairments
Brain imaging
  Age of new infarction
  Presence of multilobar infarction
    Hypodensity greater than one-third of hemisphere
    Early hypodensity—basal ganglia
    Early hypodensity—insular cortex
    Hyperdense artery sign
Patient and family informed of potential benefits and
  risks

started within 90 min of onset of stroke[71] (see Fig. 22-9). A pooled analysis of the data from several trials of rtPA suggest that women appeared to benefit more from rtPA than did men; this finding differs from those noted in most other experiences in management of cerebrovascular disease.[72]

The results of the NINDS trials led to the approval of rtPA for treatment of stroke. At present, it is indicated for treatment of carefully selected patients within 3 h of onset of symptoms (Table 22-4; Fig. 22-11). However, based on the review of the several trials of rtPA, Ringleb et al.[71] suggested that rtPA could be used successfully up to 6 h after onset of stroke. On the other hand, some physicians have not accepted the conclusion that intravenous rtPA is useful for treatment of patients with

stroke.[73,74] Some experts concluded that the magnitude of risks and benefits of intravenous rtPA are imprecise.[75] A systemic review of thrombolysis for management of patients with acute ischemic stroke concluded that the intervention results in a reduction in the patients who are dead or disabled at a cost of an increased number of deaths due to hemorrhage.[76] These conclusions seem valid and much more reliable than those made in 1992.[57] Still, combining the data from the trials testing streptokinase with those that evaluated rtPA can be questioned. While there are limited data that any particular thrombolytic agent is significantly safer than the others for treatment of ischemic stroke, the only trials that demonstrated a reasonable safety profile are those that tested rtPA.[77] Clinical trials of intravenous administration of new

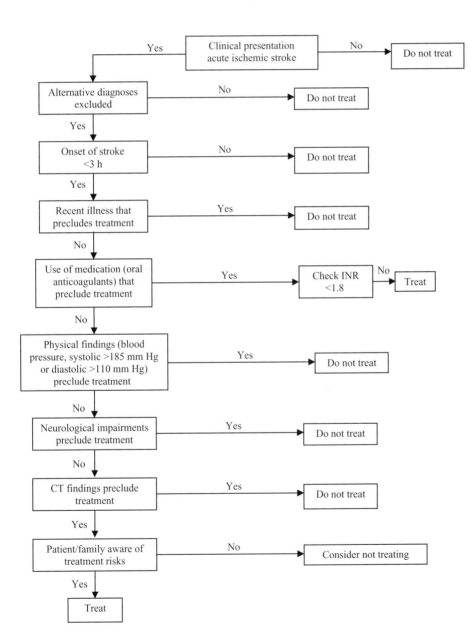

Figure 22-11. Algorithm used in decision making when considering intravenous administration of rtPA for treatment of patients with acute ischemic stroke.

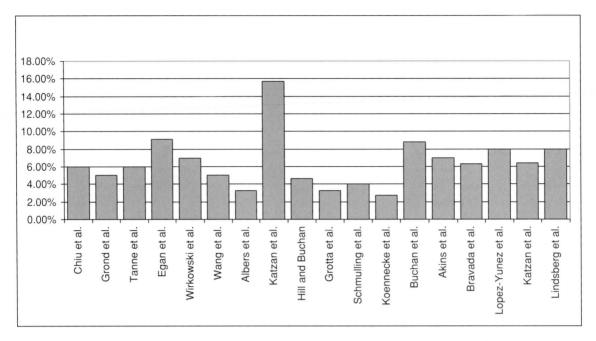

Figure 22-12. Rates of symptomatic hemorrhage among patients receiving intravenous administration of rtPA for treatment of acute ischemic stroke are reported from several population or community studies. (*Adapted from Refs. 37–41, 44, 45, 75, 79, 82, 83, and 87–92*).

thrombolytic agents are under way but data about safety and efficacy are limited.

Following approval of rtPA, several groups evaluated its utility in the treatment of stroke[40–42,44,78–86] (Figs. 22-12 and 22-13). These reports provide important information about the utility of intravenous thrombolysis outside the setting of a clinical trial. Grond et al.[84] found that intravenous thrombolysis could be used to effectively treat patients with acute strokes in the vertebrobasilar circulation. Felberg et al.[85] described dramatic recovery within 24 h of treatment, with rtPA in 22 percent of patients with occlusions of the middle cerebral artery.

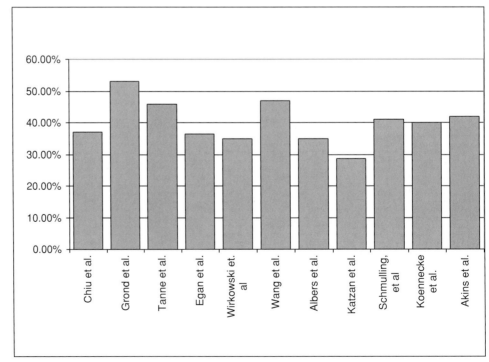

Figure 22-13. Rates of favorable outcomes among patient receiving intravenous administration of rtPA for treatment of acute ischemic stroke are reported from several population or community studies. (*Adapted from Refs. 40–42, 75, 79, 82, 83 and new references 87–92*).

Smith et al.[86] noted that physicians carefully adhering to the protocols could administer rtPA successfully in an emergency department setting. Wang et al.[42] reported that rtPA could be given in community hospitals, with reasonable safety and efficacy. Rudolf et al.[93] gave IV rtPA to 15 patients with strokes secondary to occlusions of the internal carotid artery, including 6 with dissections. No hemorrhages were diagnosed, and four deaths and four poor outcomes were attributed to the stroke. A French study reported that intravenous rtPA could be given with a reasonable chance of success for treatment up to 7 h, following onset of stroke in the vertebrobasilar circulation.[94] Despite the small numbers, this experience is important because it showed that patients with acute arterial dissections could receive rtPA with a reasonable expectation for safety. Ribo et al.[95] used the combination of MRI and transcranial Doppler ultrasonongraphy to select patients to treat, within 3–6 h following stroke. They found acceptable degrees of safety and potential efficacy. Although the utility of rtPA for treatment of children has not been tested, it is prescribed to children with acute ischemic stroke.[96]

Overall, these trials show a rate of bleeding complications that are similar to that found in the NINDS trials. They also show that neurological worsening following thrombolysis, possibly due to recurrent occlusion, most commonly occurs among patients with severe strokes. Still, these trials show that rtPA has limited utility. Despite ongoing efforts to increase the number of patients that are treated, a minority (approximately 3–5 percent) is treated. With aggressive community and professional efforts, the number of patients that can be treated should grow. For example, a project in Houston showed that approximately 15 percent of patients with acute stroke could reach the hospital in time for treatment with rtPA.[83] Grotta et al.[83]

found an acceptably low rate of bleeding when rtPA was administered in a general clinical setting.

Pilot studies testing the utility of tenecteplase and desmotoplase have been reported.[97–99] The preliminary data of these dose-escalation studies suggest that these agents might be useful as an alternative to rtPA. Further research is likely to be forthcoming. Yamaguchi et al.[100] report that lower dose rtPA (0.6 mg/kg-up to 60 mg) might be safe and useful when given more than 3 h after stroke to carefully selected patients.

Intra-Arterial Thrombolysis

Intra-arterial thrombolysis has several advantages.[101] It permits administration of larger doses of thrombolytic agent directly at the site of the occlusion. The amount of agent that reaches systemic tissues likely is lower than the amount given intravenously, which may improve safety in situations such as stroke shortly after a surgical procedure. Intra-arterial thrombolysis may be given alone or in conjunction with other endovascular interventions.[102,103] Intra-arterial administration of thrombolytic agents appears to achieve a higher rate of recanalization than does intravenous therapy (Fig. 22-14). However, it has the disadvantage of requiring a specialized facility and personnel, and therefore additioinal costs.

The relative utility of either intravenous or intra-arterial thrombolysis is not established.[3] Several small clinical series of intra-arterial thrombolysis using rtPA, urokinase, or streptokinase were published prior to the treatment guidelines written in 1996.[2] At that time, the conclusion was that intra-arterial therapy was promising but that it was not established as effective for improving outcomes. Since then, several series and one clinical trial testing different thrombolytic medications have been

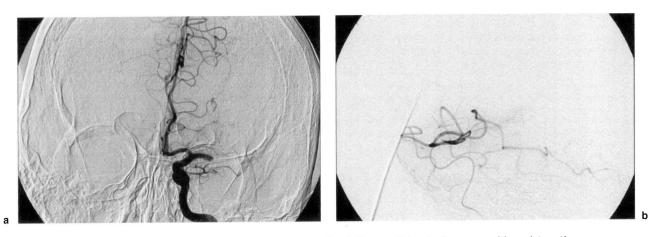

Figure 22-14. Anteroposterior view (a) of a left carotid arteriogram with subtraction technique demonstrates an occlusion of the first segment of the middle cerebral artery in a patient with an acute ischemic stroke. A selective catheterization of the artery (b) shows filling of the branches of the middle cerebral artery distal to the occlusion.

reported. Updated evidence suggests that intra-arterial administration of rtPA or another thrombolytic agent might become a useful form of treatment of patients with acute stroke.[3]

Most research focuses on patients with thromboembolic events in the anterior circulation. Results are mixed. Intra-arterial administration of rtPA up to 40 mg is relatively safe.[104] Urbach et al.[105] gave urokinase to 12 patients with embolic occlusions of the distal internal carotid artery or the proximal portions of the anterior or middle cerebral arteries. Few patients had recanalization and only four patients had good outcomes. A subsequent report by the same group emphasized the influence of the type of embolism on the rate of recanalization.[106] Endo et al.[107] treated 33 patients with severe strokes and occlusion of the cervical portion of the internal carotid artery. Recanalization was achieved in eight patients and good outcomes were noted in four. Gonner et al.[108] reported good or excellent responses in 26 of 43 patients who had occlusions in the anterior circulation. Jahan et al.[109] gave urokinase within 6 h of onset of stroke to 26 patients. Recanalization was achieved in 11 patients and 7 of these had favorable outcomes. They noted that success was greater if the occlusion was in the middle cerebral artery or one of its branches rather than in the distal segment of the internal carotid artery. This experience was similar to that described by other investigators. In general, patients with occlusions of the middle cerebral artery do better with thrombolytic therapy than do those with occlusions of the internal carotid artery.[110] Eckert et al.[111] looked at the rates of recanalization among patients given intra-arterial thrombolysis. No difference in responses was noted among the type of thrombolytic medication. However, recanalization was more likely among patients with either proximal or distal occlusions of the middle cerebral artery than with distal occlusions of the internal carotid artery. They noted that favorable outcomes were most likely among patients with early recanalization. Intra-arterial thrombolysis given to 54 patients within 6 h of stroke was evaluated by Suarez et al.[112] Mortality was 24 percent, and 17 percent had CT evidence of hemorrhage. Recanalization occurred with occlusions of the horizontal segment of middle cerebral artery but not with occlusion of distal internal carotid artery. Arnold et al.[113] administered urokinase via an intra-arterial approach to 100 patients. Symptomatic hemorrhages occurred in seven cases and complete recanalization was achieved in 20 patients. Excellent outcomes were associated with complete recanalization. In another study, these investigators noted that intra-arterial thrombolysis could be given effectively and safely for treatment of patients with arterial dissections.[114] Based on a review of the published trials of intra-arterial thrombolysis, Lisboa et al.[115] also concluded that intra-arterial thrombolysis increased the likelihood of favorable outcomes with lower mortality. They reported that mortality was reduced from 40 to 27.2 percent ($p = 0.004$) and favorable outcomes increased from 23 to 41.5 percent ($p = 0.002$). Intra-arterial thrombolysis increased the risk of symptomatic hemorrhage from 3 to 9.5 percent ($p = 0.046$). Using a case-control paradigm, Inoue et al.[116] reported that intra-arterial administration of urokinase could improve outcomes among critically ill patients with cardioembolic stroke.

Several investigators described the potential utility of intra-arterial thrombolysis in treatment of patients with stroke secondary to occlusion of the basilar artery.[117–123] These reports imply that the intervention lowers mortality among patients with this highly fatal form of ischemic cerebrovascular disease.

A series of studies evaluated the potential utility of prourokinase.[124–126] A phase II trial tested the combination of intra-arterial prourokinase with two different doses of heparin. The rates of both recanalization and bleeding complications were higher among patients receiving the larger of the two doses of heparin.[124] These results prompted a phase III trial that evaluated the utility of prourokinase among patients, with middle cerebral artery occlusions, who could be treated within 6 h of stroke.[126] Recanalization was achieved in 66 percent of 121 patients treated with prourokinase and 18 percent of the control group. Favorable outcomes at 3 months were recorded in 40 percent of the patients in the prourokinase group and in 25 percent of the patients in the control group. However, prourokinase was associated with a 10 percent rate of symptomatic hemorrhage compared to a 2 percent rate for placebo. Hemorrhage complicating intra-arterial administration of prourokinase usually occurred soon after treatment and it was associated with high mortality and poor outcomes.[127] It is not yet available for general clinical use. However, the results of this trial have been the stimulus for intra-arterial administration of rtPA and other agents.[128] Current guidelines conclude that intra-arterial thrombolysis is an option for the treatment of patients with occlusions of the middle cerebral artery if the medication can be administered within 6 h of onset of stroke.[3] At present, the potential availability of intra-arterial thrombolysis should not be a reason to forego treatment with intravenous thrombolysis.[3]

Intravenous Followed by Intra-Arterial Thrombolysis

Thrombolytic agents may be given intravenously on an urgent basis while the patient is being prepared for intra-arterial therapy.[129–135] The goal is to improve blood flow and neurological status, and then locally administer a thrombolytic agent to augment recanalization. The

Emergency Stroke Management Bridging Trial showed that such an approach was feasible.[129,130] Ernst et al.[131] combined intravenous rtPA (0.6 mg/kg—15 percent in bolus and remainder over 30 min) with intra-arterial rtPA (maximum dose of 24 mg) to 20 patients with a mean NIHSS score of 20 and found that 10 patients made very good outcomes. Suarez et al.[132] treated 45 patients with the combination of intravenous rtPA (0.6 mg/kg) followed by intra-arterial rtPA or urokinase. A majority of survivors had good outcomes and symptomatic hemorrhage occurred in 4.4 percent of cases. Keris et al.[133] found that the combination of intravenous followed by intra-arterial thrombolysis could be given safely and effectively within 6 h of stroke. However, Zaidat et al.[134] did not find a difference in outcomes among patients given combined intra-arterial and intravenous thrombolysis when compared to patients receiving intra-arterial treatment alone. Still, based on community experience, Hill et al.[135] concluded that intravenous thrombolysis followed by intra-arterial treatment is a promising strategy for treatment of patients with severe stroke and that early neurovascular and neurometabolic imaging helps select patients. Based on the available data, Lisboa et al.[115] concluded that the combination of intravenous and intra-arterial treatment may be superior to intra-arterial therapy alone.

▶ ANCROD

Experience with ancrod is limited. A placebo-controlled trial tested the utility of this defibrinogenating agent in the treatment of patients with acute ischemic stroke.[136] Patients were treated within 3 h of onset of stroke and received continuous infusions for 72 h. The goal was to reduce plasma fibrinogen levels. While mortality was not different between the two treatment groups, favorable outcomes were more frequent among the patients treated with ancrod. Both symptomatic and asymptomatic intracranial hemorrhages were detected more commonly among patients treated with ancrod. An analysis demonstrated that ancrod started within 3 h was associated with an increased likelihood of favorable outcomes. A European trial apparently did not show a benefit from ancrod. Unfortunately, the results of this study are not yet published. One disadvantage of this therapy is the requirement for frequent monitoring and adjustment of doses or infusions in responses to fibrinogen concentrations. The prolonged course of treatment (72 h) also is a potential disadvantage. A systemic review found that defibrinogenating enzymes were not associated with a significant reduction in either death or disability.[137] A nonsignificant increase in bleeding also was found. Further research is needed to determine if ancrod has a role in the management of patients with acute stroke.[138]

▶ HEPARIN, LOW-MOLECULAR-WEIGHT HEPARINS, AND DANAPAROID

Anticoagulants are a crucial component of long-term management to prevent ischemic stroke (see Chapter 19). However, the usefulness of anticoagulants is not established for the urgent treatment of patients with acute ischemic stroke.[3,139,140] The most commonly prescribed rapidly acting anticoagulants are heparin, low-molecular-weight (LMW) heparins, and danaparoid. Because the biological actions of warfarin are delayed, it does not have a role in emergency management.

Rationale

Anticoagulants are administered in an attempt to halt neurological worsening by limiting the propagation of a thrombus, limiting the neurologic injury by helping maintain collateral flow to the ischemic locus, preventing early recurrent thromboembolic events, especially among patients with cardiac lesions, and forestalling venous thromboembolism and pulmonary embolism (Fig. 22-15). Despite the lack of strong data about their usefulness, anticoagulants are widely administered agents for treatment of patients with recent stroke.[141–143] Their use is controversial.[139,144–151] In 1994, the panel writing the guidelines for management of patients with acute ischemic stroke concluded that there were insufficient data to make a recommendation about the use of heparin.[55] Since then, several of these agents have been tested in clinical trials and the results of these studies provide

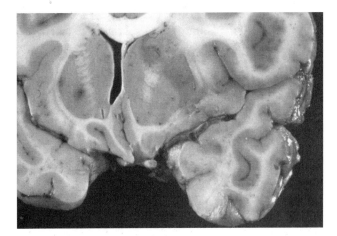

Figure 22-15. Coronal autopsy specimen reveals an acute infarction in the distribution of the left middle cerebral artery. An embolus, which was attributed to a recent anterior wall myocardial infarction, is present with the artery. (*Courtesy of S.S. Schochet, M.D., Department of Pathology, University of West Virginia, Morgantown, WV*)

information about the role of anticoagulants in treatment of patients with ischemic stroke.[139,140]

Pharmacology

Heparin is a mixture of glycosaminoglycans of biological origin that cannot be given orally.[152] The preferred routes of administration are subcutaneous or intravenous injections. Adequate anticoagulation is achieved with either route, although therapeutic levels usually are not reached until 24 h after starting subcutaneous injections. If immediate anticoagulation is needed, heparin is given intravenously in a bolus dose followed by an infusion. A continuous infusion is preferred to intermittent intravenous injections because of the stability of the level of anticoagulation. Variations in concentrations of plasma proteins that bind heparin partially explain the marked differences in anticoagulant effects among patients.[152] The antithrombotic effect of heparin is mediated through its binding with antithrombin III, which in turn inhibits thrombin, activated factor X, and activated factor IX.[152,153] Thus, the inactivation of thrombin is the primary anticoagulant action of heparin. Heparin also inactivates thrombin through its effects on heparin cofactor II. Heparin also affects endothelial cell function and alters platelet activity via an interaction with platelet factor IV. Chamorro et al.[154] speculated that unfractionated heparin has some anti-inflammatory actions that could improve recovery if it is given soon after stroke. The anti-inflammatory effects of heparin appear to be differentiated from its anticoagulant actions.[155] The activated partial thromboplastin time (aPTT) is the most widely used test to assess the anticoagulant effects of heparin. The usual therapeutic level of aPTT is assumed to be approximately 1.5 times of control levels. Unfortunately, data to support this level of anticoagulation are not available. An alternative method to examine the level of anticoagulation is to measure the level of inhibition of activated factor X, with desired levels being 0.3–0.5 units/mL.[156]

While most patients are treated with daily doses of approximately 24,000–30,000 units, the range of doses is broad. Traditionally, patients were treated with a bolus of 5000 units of heparin followed by an hourly infusion of 1000 units. Subsequently, the infusion would be adjusted in response to the aPTT levels. Unfortunately, this strategy does not account for the wide variation among patients. Some patients achieve excessive levels of anticoagulation with a resultant risk of bleeding, while others have inadequate levels with a potential for a subtherapeutic effect. The patient's weight is an important variable in affecting responses to heparin and to compensate, weight-based nomograms for the administration of heparin are available[157–159] (Table 22-5). This approach allows for more accurate administration of heparin. In addition, such a weight-based nomogram might improve

▶ **TABLE 22-5.** WEIGHT-BASED NOMOGRAM—INTRAVENOUS ADMINISTRATION OF HEPARIN

Initial loading (bolus) dose	80 U/kg
Initial intravenous infusion	18 U/kg/h
Check aPTT at 6 h	
Adjust heparin therapy in response to level of aPTT	
If aPTT is <35 s (<1.2 × control)	
Give another bolus of heparin	80 U/kg
Increase infusion dose	22 U/kg/h
If aPTT is 35–45 s (1.2 – 1.5 × control)	
Give another bolus of heparin	40 U/kg
Increase infusion dose	20 U/kg/h
If aPTT is 46–70 s (1.5 – 2.3 × control)	
Continue infusion	18 U/Kg/h
If aPTT is 71–90 s (2.3 – 3 × control)	
Decrease infusion dose	16 U/Kg/h
If aPTT is >91 s (>3 × control)	
Halt infusion for 1 h	
Restart infusion with dose	15 U/Kg/h
Recheck aPTT at 6 h	
Readjust regimen in response to aPTT	

Adapted from Refs. 157–159.

the usefulness of heparin in treatment of patients with recent ischemic neurological symptoms.[159]

Many of the antithrombotic effects of heparin are reversed by the administration of protamine sulfate. Approximately 1 mg of protamine counteracts the effects of 100 units of heparin.[152] In an emergency, protamine can be given. However, intravenous protamine should be administered slowly because it may induce hypotension. Anaphylaxis also is a potential complication of protamine.

The LMW heparins and danaparoid also are of biological origin. They are created by chemical or enzymatic depolarization of conventional heparin.[160–162] The several LMW heparins have slightly different effects but they act primarily through inhibition of factor X activity (Table 22-6). The ratio of inhibition of thrombin and activated factor X varies considerably among compounds. As such, the safety and efficacy profiles of one LMW heparin cannot be assumed to be true for another agent. Although danaparoid differs from the other LMW heparins because it consists primarily of heparan sulfate, its actions are similar to those of the other LMW compounds.[164] The smaller size of the LMW compounds results in reduced binding to plasma proteins, endothelial cells, macrophages, and platelets. These agents have more stable pharmacological effects and a longer half-life than that of conventional heparin. LMW heparins also may have some neuroprotective effects.[165] These agents usually do not alter the aPTT, and monitoring of pharmacological effects is performed via measurement of inhibition of activated factor X. The desired level of anticoagulation is 0.3-0.5 μ/mL of inhibition of activated factor X.[166] A prolonged aPTT happens when excessive doses are prescribed. Based on

▶ **TABLE 22-6.** ADVANTAGES AND DISADVANTAGES OF LMW HEPARINS AND DANAPAROID IN COMPARISON TO UNFRACTIONATED HEPARIN

Advantages
    Longer duration of anticoagulation
        More predictable response to injections
        Fewer injections
    Selective antithrombotic effects
        Less inhibition of thrombin
        Focused effects on activated factor X
        Little effects on platelets or endothelium
    Lower risk of bleeding
    Less antigenic—lower risk of thrombocytopenia
Disadvantages
    No specific antidote—no effect from protamine sulfate
    Expensive

their pharmacological effects, LMW heparins appear to be superior to conventional heparin for treatment of patients with arterial occlusions.[163]

Safety

Bleeding is the most common side effect (Table 22-7). Among patients with TIA, Petty et al.[167] estimated that the risk of hemorrhage with heparin is 0.3 per 100 patient-days, a rate that is considerably higher than that associated with either aspirin or oral anticoagulants. Even higher rates happen in the setting of acute stroke. The chances of bleeding seem to be very similar regardless of the route of administration (intravenous or subcutaneous). A continuous intravenous infusion appears to be safer than intermittent intravenous bolus doses. In general, the risk of hemorrhage increases with marked

▶ **TABLE 22-7.** COMPLICATIONS OF HEPARIN

Intracranial hemorrhage
    Hemorrhagic transformation of infarction
        Symptomatic
        Asymptomatic
    Hemorrhage
        Intracerebral hemorrhage
        Subdural hematoma
Other serious hemorrhage
    Retroperitoneal
    Gastrointestinal
    Genitourinary
Thrombocytopenia
Autoimmune thrombocytopenia—white clot syndrome
    Cerebral infarction
    Myocardial infarction
    Peripheral artery occlusion
Digital ischemia—purple toe syndrome
Osteoporosis

prolongation of the aPTT levels.[168] Bleeding also is the primary complication of administration of the LMW heparins and danaparoid.

Minor bleeding includes epistaxis, ecchymoses, and microscopic hematuria. Serious hemorrhages including gastrointestinal, genitourinary, intra-articular, or retroperitoneal bleeding also complicate the use of these medications. In the recent stroke trials, the frequency of serious nonneurological hemorrhage was as high as symptomatic hemorrhagic transformation.[169–172] These hemorrhages were an important cause of morbidity and unfavorable outcomes. In general, the risk of bleeding is approximately same for all the anticoagulants.[139]

Intracranial hemorrhage is the primary life-threatening bleeding complication of heparin for treatment of patients with stroke.[139] The risk of serious bleeding is lower than that accompanying administration of thrombolytic agents, but it is higher than that associated with use of antiplatelet agents. Jaillard et al.[173] and Chamorro et al.[169] examined the safety of emergency anticoagulation in treatment of recent stroke. Bleeding complications were highest among patients with severe neurological impairments, reflecting a multilobar infarction, and those with the highest levels of anticoagulation. Bleeding was thought to be more likely associated with embolic events than with thrombotic infarctions. Based on limited data, the Cerebral Embolism Study Group speculated that the administration of a bolus dose of heparin was associated with an increased risk of hemorrhage.[174]

Several clinical trials demonstrate that these agents increase the risk of both hemorrhagic transformation of the infarction and symptomatic intracranial bleeding.[151,170–172,175–177] One trial found that the risk of symptomatic intracranial bleeding was highest among patients with an NIHSS score greater than 15.[172] Most trials administered the anticoagulant subcutaneously and without a bolus dose. The exception is the trial of danaparoid, which gave the agent intravenously, included an adjusted the infusion in response to the level of inhibition of factor Xa.[172] Some trials found a dose-response association with bleeding; the rate of hemorrhage was highest among patients receiving larger doses of medication.[151,170,171,175,177]

Differences in the rate of bleeding reported in clinical trials cannot be attributed to different agents. For example, heparin is neither safer nor more dangerous than the other anticoagulants. These trials do not show that subcutaneously administered anticoagulants are either safer or more dangerous than intravenously given medications. No data demonstrate that the use of a bolus dose to start anticoagulation is particularly dangerous. Rather, differences in populations, ancillary care, and the level of monitoring probably are the key factors to explain the discrepancies in the data. In summary, recent trials show that early anticoagulation is accompanied with an increased

▶ **TABLE 22-8.** MAJOR ADVERSE EVENTS OF INTERNATIONAL STROKE TRIAL

Event	Treatment Group					
	Control	Aspirin	Aspirin LD Heparin	Aspirin HD Heparin	LD Heparin	HD Heparin
	N	N	N	N	N	N
	4859	4858	2431	2430	2429	2426
	N(%)	N(%)	N(%)	N(%)	N(%)	N(%)
Recurrent Stroke	214(4.4)	156(3.2)	50(2.1)	60(2.8)	78(3.2)	86(3.5)
Pulmonary Embolus	45(0.9)	36(0.7)	13(0.5)	8(0.3)	20(0.8)	12(0.5)
Intracranial Hemorrhage	15(0.3)	26(0.5)	19(0.8)	42(1.7)	16(0.7)	43(1.8)
Other serious Bleeding	14(0.3)	23(0.5)	20(0.8)	66(2.7)	10(0.4)	33(1.4)

Adapted from International Stroke Trial Collaborative Group.[177]

risk of intracranial hemorrhage, especially among patients with moderate-to-severe stroke.[3,139,140,147]

Some agents are complicated by thrombocytopenia. A benign decline in platelet count occurs in many patients given heparin.[178] While the risk of thrombocytopenia is highest with unfractionated heparin, it may also occur with the LMW heparins. A more serious autoimmune thrombocytopenia may appear after several days of treatment with heparin. It can lead to the so-called white clot syndrome and arterial thrombosis, which causes myocardial or cerebral ischemia.[179,180] The development of ischemia with heparin-associated thrombocytopenia presents a serious problem in the management of these patients. The LMW heparins should not be used; the usual choices are argatroban or danaparoid.

Heparin

In a small trial, Duke et al.[181] tested intravenous infusions of heparin in treatment of patients with stroke. No significant differences in outcomes were noted, although mortality was higher at 1 year among the heparin-treated group. The Cerebral Embolism Study Group speculated that heparin may be effective in reducing the risk of early recurrent embolic stroke.[174,182,183] They estimated that the risk of early recurrent embolization was approximately 12 percent, a figure that now appears to be too high. While the study of Berge et al.[176] found that recurrent embolic events were approximately 8 percent among persons with atrial fibrillation and stroke, most other recent studies show much lower rates of early recurrent embolization.[172,177,184] If the risks of early recurrent stroke were approximately 0.3–0.5 percent per day as shown in the control/placebo groups in several recent trials, then the urgency for administration of a potentially dangerous medication, such as heparin, is low.

A large international trial studied two doses of subcutaneously administered heparin alone or in combination with aspirin.[177] Patients were enrolled within 48 h of onset of stroke and they were treated for 14 days. This trial has several limitations, including the lack of a requirement for a brain imaging study before entry, no monitoring of the level of anticoagulation, no dosage adjustments, and no follow-up brain imaging tests. However, the trial found that heparin was associated with a dose-related increase in the risk of both intracranial and extracranial bleeding (Table 22-8). A modest reduction in early recurrent stroke was noted with heparin but this benefit was counterbalanced by the bleeding complications. As a result, no improvement in outcomes was found (Figs. 22-16 to 22-18). In a subgroup analysis of the International Stroke Trial, Saxena et al.[185] studied the impact of heparin therapy among patients with atrial fibrillation and stroke. While heparin was associated with a lower rate of recurrent stroke during the first 14 days, this benefit also was negated by a higher rate of intracranial hemorrhage. Despite the serious problems in the design of the International Stroke Trial, it provided evidence that heparin is not dramatically effective, at least in the regimen used in the study. A Swedish study could not demonstrate any benefit from heparin in halting neurological worsening or improving outcomes among persons with stroke-in-evolution.[186] A systemic review could not demonstrate any net benefit from treatment with heparin.[187] The current evidence shows that heparin does not improve clinical outcomes after stroke.[139,188] Despite the negative results, some physicians continue to prescribe intravenous heparin.[143] A sizable proportion of physicians reported that they would give heparin to patients with stroke-in-evolution and many physicians cited medicolegal reasons for this decision.[143] The International Stroke Trial does not provide conclusive data that heparin is not useful in any situation even if

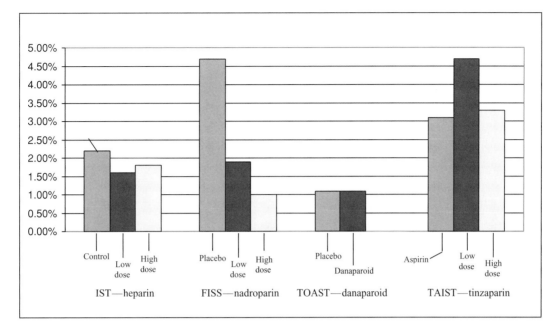

Figure 22-16. The effects of early parenteral administration of anticoagulants (LMW heparin, or danaparoid) on the rates of early recurrent stroke among patients with recent stroke enrolled in clinical trials. (*Adapted from Refs. 171, 172, 175 and 177*).

administered using a different strategy (intravenous bolus and frequent dose adjustments) to carefully selected patients. Indeed, heparin may be considered for treating patients at especially high risk for early recurrent stroke.[189] Other physicians advocate a new approach to test heparin, including the use of intravenous doses of heparin following the use of vascular imaging, to select patients to treat.[190]

Current guidelines prohibit the use of heparin during the first 24 h following administration of rtPA.[3] However, interest persists regarding the use of heparin as an adjunct to thrombolysis. Two trials of intra-arterial prourokinase included heparin as part of the treatment regimen.[124–126] del Zoppo et al.[124] found that the larger dose of heparin was associated with increased recanalization, but that it

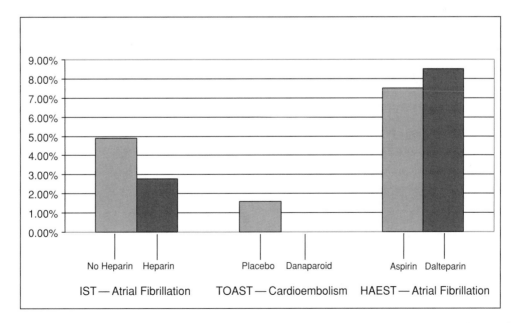

Figure 22-17. Effects of early parenteral administration of heparin, danaparoid, or dalteparin on the risk of early recurrent stroke among patients with recent stroke an atrial fibrillation enrolled in clinical trials. (*Adapted from Refs. 172, 176 and 177*).

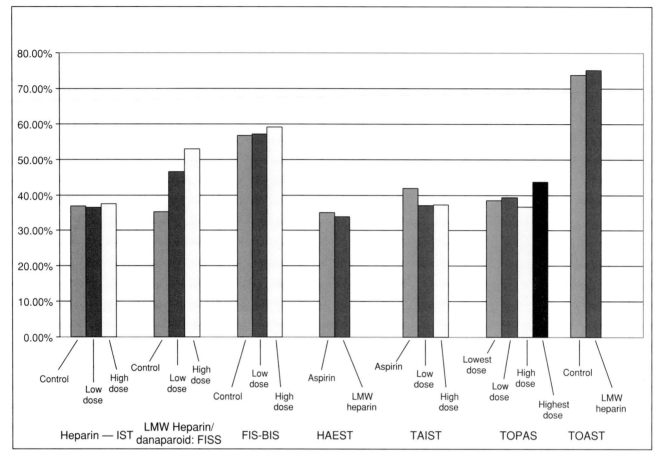

Figure 22-18. Effects of early parenteral administration of anticoagulants (LMW heparin or danaparoid) on outcomes following acute ischemic stroke among patient enrolled in clinical trials. (*Adapted from Refs. 150, 170–172, 175 and 177*).

was also accompanied by an increased risk of serious bleeding. Grond et al.[84] and Trouillas et al.[38] gave heparin shortly after administering rtPA; no increase in bleeding complications was noted. Schmulling et al.[39] also reported that heparin could be given following thrombolytic treatment. The utility of heparin as an adjunctive therapy following pharmacological thrombolysis has not been established and the current prohibition against the use of heparin should be honored until further data become available.

LMW Heparins and Danaparoid

Results of the trials testing different LMW heparins and danaparoid are mixed. In a placebo-controlled trial, Kay et al.[175] subcutaneously administered two doses of nadroparin to patients within 48 h of onset of stroke. The rates of recurrent embolism and bleeding were low in this study. No difference in outcomes was noted at 3 months but at 6 months, the group that received the large dose of nadroparin had a higher rate of favorable outcome. The success of this project prompted another trial

of nadroparin.[150] Unfortunately, no improvements in outcome were found, and patients given the largest dose of the LMW heparin had a 6.1 percent rate of intracranial hemorrhage, approximately twice that found with placebo (2.8 percent). A German trial tested four different doses of the LMW heparin, certoparin, given subcutaneously in treatment of acute stroke.[170] No difference in outcomes was noted among the four groups. Berge et al.[176] tested the ability of either dalteparin or aspirin to reduce recurrent thromboembolic events among patients with atrial fibrillation who had a recent stroke. Modest increases in the frequency of bleeding and recurrent ischemic events were found with dalteparin. No difference in halting neurological worsening or in improving outcomes was noted between the two groups. Two doses of subcutaneously administered tinzaparin were tested in another aspirin-controlled trial.[171] No difference in the rate of recurrent stroke, neurological worsening, bleeding complications, or outcomes was noted among the three treatment groups (see Figs. 22-16 and 22-17). In a placebo-controlled trial of danaparoid administered intravenously within 24 h of onset of stroke, investigators reported that it was associated with an increased risk of bleeding complications, especially among patients with severe infarctions.[172] This anticoagulant did not reduce the chance of recurrent embolization within the first week following stroke, including patients with presumed cardioembolic events. Overall, the trial did not demonstrate any effect from danaparoid in improving outcomes following stroke. A post hoc analysis examined patients whose stroke was ipsilateral to a high-grade stenosis or occlusion of the internal carotid artery.[191] The data suggested that danaparoid might improve outcomes in this subgroup of patients. Recently, Lovett et al.[192] reported that the risk of early recurrent stroke is highest among patients with large-artery atherosclerosis. However, these patients often have major hemispheric infarctions that could be accompanied by an increased risk of bleeding complications. Further research on the utility of anticoagulants in this subgroup of patients would be valuable.

In a meta-analysis, Bath et al.[193] found that the LMW heparins and danaparoid are effective in preventing venous thromboembolic events but at an increased risk of bleeding. A trend for increased intracranial bleeding complications also was found. A nonsignificant reduction in death and disability was observed. They concluded that LMW heparins should not be used in the routine management of patients with ischemic stroke.

A systemic review of the clinical trials testing anticoagulants concluded that immediate anticoagulant therapy is not associated with any net short-term or long-term benefit.[194] A similar review could not find any difference between conventional heparin and the newer antithrombotic agents. Based on a review of the recent trials of anticoagulation in treatment of patients with recent stroke, Adams[139] concluded that most patients with stroke should not be treated with unfractionated heparin or other rapidly acting anticoagulant medications. The only established indication is prevention of deep vein thrombosis among bedridden patients. A panel jointly sponsored by the American Stroke Association and the American Academy of Neurology found that the use of anticoagulants was not associated with improved outcomes.[140] The current guidelines for stroke care do not recommend the use of conventional heparin or any of the LMW anticoagulants for treatment of patients with acute ischemic stroke.[3]

► ARGATROBAN AND OTHER DIRECT THROMBIN INHIBITORS

Argatroban inhibits platelet activation of fibrin-clot-associated thrombin and it is used to treat heparin-associated thrombocytopenia.[195–197] In an experimental model, Morris et al.[198] concluded that the combination of argatroban and rtPA might prolong the time period for effective treatment of stroke. A pilot study of argatroban demonstrated a modest increase in bleeding risk but no major difference in outcomes.[199] The administration of direct thrombin inhibitors, including hirudin, has been associated with a high risk for intracranial bleeding, so these agents have not been evaluated in the setting of acute ischemic stroke.

► ANTIPLATELET AGENTS

Rationale

Platelet activation, adhesion, and aggregation are key components of arterial thromboembolism and ischemic stroke; therefore, interest in the use of these medications in the treatment of acute stroke is considerable.[200] Aspirin is a component of the emergency management of patients with acute myocardial ischemia; patients are advised to self-medicate with aspirin en route to an emergency department. Aspirin and other acutely acting antiplatelet agents are given in conjunction with anticoagulants and either mechanical or pharmacological thrombolysis. However, data about the usefulness of antiplatelet agents in the treatment of acute ischemic stroke are less conclusive than those for treatment of myocardial infarction.

Pharmacology

Aspirin inhibits platelet function within a few minutes of administration (see Chapter 19). A large loading dose of clopidogrel (in most cases 300 mg) also rapidly inhibits platelet activity. Data from clinical trials of patients with unstable heart disease show that the combination of aspirin and clopidogrel effectively improves outcomes.[201–204] Ridogrel also has potent antiplatelet effects through its inhibition of thromboxane synthase. While this agent has been used in treating patients with myocardial ischemia, it has not been tested in the setting of acute cerebral ischemia.[205]

The glycoprotein IIb/IIIa receptor is a central mediator of platelet-mediated thrombosis.[206] Antagonists to the glycoprotein IIb/IIIa receptor block the fibrinogen-binding sites of the platelet.[207,208] Schwarz et al.[209] reported that the glycoprotein IIb/IIIa blocker, abciximab, binds the leukocyte integrin Mac-1, fibrinogen, and factor X. Abciximab also limits thrombus formation by reducing monocyte tissue factor.[210] In experimental models, these medications halt the accumulation of platelets and fibrin in microvascular thrombosis.[211–213] A systemic review of the utility of intravenous glycoprotein IIb/IIIa receptor blocking agents found that these medications reduce mortality at 30 days and 6 months after myocardial infarction with a moderate increased risk of bleeding.[214] Recently, Kastrati et al.[215] reported that abciximab alone was as effective as abciximab combined with reteplase in limiting the extent of myocardial injury in the setting of acute myocardial infarction. These agents have been given safely in conjunction with thrombolytic agents in treatment of myocardial infarction and, in some cases, stroke. For example, a glycoprotein IIb/IIIa receptor blocker could be administered to prevent recurrent arterial occlusion after successful recanalization with rtPA. Adjunctive treatment with glycoprotein IIb/IIIa receptor inhibitors may increase the therapeutic window and reduce the dose of rtPA needed for recanalization.[215]

Safety

The safety profile of antiplatelet agents is superior to both anticoagulants and thrombolytic agents. Still, bleeding is a potential complication as these agents do have antithrombotic effects. Two large trials tested the potential utility of aspirin when administered within 48 h of onset of stroke.[177,184] In the International Stroke Trial, aspirin (300 mg/day) was given as a monotherapy or in conjunction with heparin.[171] Both studies showed a modest increase in bleeding complications. Chen et al.[216] concluded that the risk of hemorrhage secondary to aspirin was increased by a rate of 2 per 1000. Another trial gave aspirin alone or in combination with streptokinase for treatment of patients with acute ischemic stroke.[31] While the frequency of bleeding with aspirin was not significantly increased in comparison to placebo, the combination of aspirin and streptokinase was associated with an unacceptably high rate of serious, often fatal, hemorrhagic complications. Indeed, the combination was much more dangerous than streptokinase given alone. No data

are available about the risks of bleeding following the administration of large doses of clopidogrel for treatment of patients with stroke.

Bleeding is a potential complication of the glycoprotein IIb/IIIa receptor blockers. A dose-escalation study of abciximab as monotherapy found that it could be given safely.[217] While no case of symptomatic hemorrhage was reported among patients given abciximab, the frequency of asymptomatic hemorrhage detected by brain imaging was increased. A subsequent study, which was presented at meetings but not yet published, demonstrated a modest increase in symptomatic bleeding with abciximab when it was administered within 6 h of onset of stroke.[218] While bleeding is a potential complication of other glycoprotein IIb/IIIa receptor blocking agents, the degree of risk among patients with stroke is not clear. Morris et al.[219] gave a half-dose of rtPA and abciximab to five patients; one had an asymptomatic hemorrhagic transformation. Abciximab may also induce thrombocytopenia. Overall, the data suggest that antiplatelet agents may be given within the first hours of stroke, with a reasonable degree of safety.

Aspirin

The data from each of two large trials failed to establish the efficacy of the early use of aspirin[177,184] (Fig. 22-19). However, an analysis that combined the data from these studies showed that aspirin administered within 48 h of onset of stroke reduced the risk of recurrent ischemic events by approximately 7 per 1000.[216] A systemic review concluded that aspirin, given orally or per rectum, started within 48 h of stroke reduces the risk of early recurrent

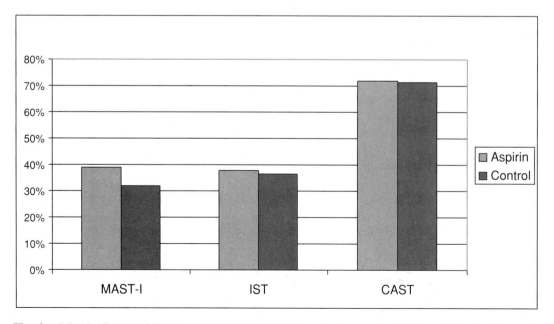

Figure 22-19. Rates of favorable outcomes among patients enrolled in three trials testing early administration of aspirin following acute ischemic stroke. (*Adapted from Refs. 31, 177 and 184*).

stroke.[220] However, it is not clear if aspirin improves outcomes following stroke by limiting the effects of the acute ischemic event. In fact, the degree of improvement in outcomes with aspirin is so small that it should not be considered as a definitive treatment for acute stroke.[221] Recently, a clinical trial failed to demonstrate any efficacy of aspirin in preventing progression of neurological signs in acute stroke.[222] A small study examined the safety and potential efficacy of aspirin combined with an LMW heparin.[223] No difference in the rate of bleeding was noted with that combination compared to treatment with aspirin alone. Current guidelines recommend that aspirin be started within 48 h of onset of stroke.[3] However, the guidelines also conclude that aspirin should not be considered an alternative to rtPA or other acute interventions to treat stroke. On the other hand, aspirin may be an effective adjunctive therapy for overall management of patients with recent stroke.

Other Antiplatelet Agents

Information about the potential efficacy of clopidogrel, alone or in combination with aspirin, in improving outcomes following stroke is not available.

Experience with the glycoprotein IIb/IIIa receptor blockers is limited. Seitz et al.[224] gave tirofiban and low-dose rtPA to 37 patients. When compared to another group treated with rtPA alone at another hospital, outcomes were similar. Intravenous tirofiban also was used to treat patients with an occlusion in the vertebrobasilar circulation.[225] In a pilot study, Junghans et al.[226] found that tirofiban could be given safely. Staub et al.[227] successfully administered a reduced intravenous dose of rtPA in combination with tirofiban. No hemorrhage occurred and patients who had recanalization of the middle cerebral artery showed improvement. Ho et al.[228] gave abciximab to three patients with acute ischemic stroke, and found that they all did well. Lee et al.[229] gave a reduced dose of intra-arterial urokinase and intravenous abciximab to 10 patients and were able to achieve recanalization. While they noted an improvement in outcomes, no reduction in bleeding was found. Kwon et al.[230] found that intra-arterially administered abciximab was an effective adjunct to thrombolytic agents for treatment of patients with acute stroke. Abciximab also has been used as an adjunct for carotid angioplasty and stenting.[231] A dose-escalation study of abciximab administered within 24 h of symptom onset found it to be safe and that it may improve outcomes.[217] The results of the study prompted other clinical trials that emphasized treatment within 6 h of onset of cerebral ischemia.[218] A subsequent larger trial enrolling patients within 5 h did not demonstrate safety or efficacy of abciximab. Trials testing the combination of rtPA and abciximab also are in progress. Although several glycoprotein IIb/IIIa receptor blocking agents are prescribed in clinical practice, their use in the management of stroke is not yet established.[232] They should not be prescribed as an alternative to other acute interventions to restore or improve blood flow to the brain.

▶ OTHER MEASURES TO IMPROVE BLOOD FLOW

Vasoconstrictors and Induced Hypertension

Cerebral blood flow to the brain becomes pressure dependent (linear) in the setting of acute stroke. Induced hypertension through the use of vasopressors could improve blood flow to the ischemic locus.[233,234] Already, Drug-induced hypertension is used to reverse ischemic symptoms among patients with vasospasm, complicating subarachnoid hemorrhage.[235,236] Thus far, the results of studies testing induced hypertension for treatment of patients with other forms of stroke are inconclusive. In a pilot study, Hillis et al.[237] showed some improvement in neurological outcomes among patients with induced hypertensive therapy. Marzan et al.[238] found that infusions of norepinephrine could be given with reasonable safety to patients with acute ischemic stroke. However, this therapy has potential limitations. The elevation of blood pressure may at the same time increase the likelihood of symptomatic hemorrhagic transformation of the infarction or aggravation of brain edema. In addition, vasopressors also may induce cardiac arrhythmias or myocardial ischemia. Hypertensive encephalopathy is another potential complication. At present, drug-induced hypertension is not indicated for treatment of most patients with stroke and further research is needed to determine its utility in the setting of acute ischemic stroke.

Theophylline, aminophylline, and caffeine cause constriction in vessels in nonischemic locations in the brain. As a result of the diversion of blood flow, these medications could increase flow to the area of the brain surrounding the ischemic locus. Based on limited data, there is insufficient evidence to know whether these medications improve outcomes.[239] A dose-escalation study of the combination of caffeine and ethanol (caffeinol) found it to be relatively safe.[240] Further research is planned. Until such data become available, vasoconstrictors should not be used as part of the management of acute ischemic stroke.

Vasodilators

Vasodilators increase blood flow in normal cerebral vessels. However, their usefulness in treating patients with acute ischemic stroke is not clear. Presumably, vasodilation could lead to increased intracranial pressure by expanding the vascular compartment. In addition, they could possibly "steal" blood from the ischemic locus to areas of normal brain. Vinpocetine, a vinca alkaloid vasodilator, failed to improve outcomes.[241]

Pentoxifylline, propentofylline, and pentifylline are vasodilators that also inhibit platelet function and decrease the release of free radicals. Pentoxifylline also prevents the deformability of red blood cells. In theory, these effects could improve blood flow to ischemic areas.[242] A review of the small trials testing these medications found that current evidence is insufficient to state whether these medications have an impact on outcomes following stroke.[243] Prostacyclin, another vasodilator, also has effects on platelets and blood vessels. It also could have neuroprotective actions. Limited clinical data are available to provide information about the utility of this medication in stroke.[244] Until more compelling positive data are available, vasodilators should not be used to treat acute ischemic stroke.

Volume Expansion and Hemodilution

The viscosity of blood has a major effect on flow in the microvasculature of the brain, and therefore increases in hematocrit or red blood cell mass, the major determinants of viscosity, may slow blood flow. On the other hand, a reduction in blood viscosity by volume expansion and hemodilution may improve blood flow to the brain.[245] Treatment involves changes in viscosity through the infusion of fluids (crystalloids or colloids) and, on occasion, venesection. Volume expansion is used successfully as an adjunct to carotid endarterectomy and to prevent ischemia secondary to vasospasm complicating subarachnoid hemorrhage.[235,236,246] Potential complications of volume expansion and hemodilution include aggravation of brain edema, worsening of heart failure, and worsening of myocardial ischemia. It may require intensive cardiovascular monitoring and support. Because patients with ischemic stroke are often elderly and have heart disease, volume expansion should be administered with care. LMW dextran may be used but it also may be complicated by allergic reactions, including anaphylaxis.

Trials testing LMW dextran, pentoxifylline, diaspirin (a cross-linked hemoglobin oxygen carrier), albumin, and hydroxyethyl starch have not demonstrated efficacy.[247–252] Two large trials of hemodilution found no evidence that the intervention improved outcomes after stroke.[253,254] In a review of the trials that included various combinations of interventions to reduce viscosity and expand volume, Asplund[255] found that hemodilution had no effect on outcomes. In a subsequent systemic review, he[256] concluded that the trials do not demonstrate efficacy for volume expansion interventions.

Extracorporeal membrane filtration has been used to treat patients with stroke.[257] The goal of this intervention is to improve the rheological characteristics of the blood by reducing fibrinogen and macroglobulins. A preliminary study of extracorporeal rheopheresis found that it may improve outcomes.[258] Rossler et al.[259] treated 17 patients with extracorporeal rheopheresis within 12 h of stroke. The results in treated patients were compared with 16 controls. While treatment resulted in an 18 percent reduction in blood viscosity, no differences in clinical outcomes were noted. Retrograde transvenous administration of fluids has been used to improve blood flow to the brain via the venous system among patients with major arterial occlusions. Clinical experience with this invasive procedure, which involves placement of catheters in the major intracranial venous sinuses and the recirculation of oxygenated blood, is limited and no conclusions about its efficacy may yet be drawn.[260]

Additional trials of albumin and other volume-expansion interventions are currently under way. However based on the current data, hemodilution should not be used to treat patients outside the setting of a clinical trial. Current guidelines recommend that hemodilution and volume expansion should not be prescribed.[3]

Surgical and Endovascular Interventions

Surgical or endovascular procedures to remove an intraluminal thrombus or to create collateral channels might improve flow in sufficient time to reverse the effects of acute ischemic stroke. Choices include carotid endarterectomy, bypass operations, angioplasty and stenting, and the use of endovascular devices to promote lysis of the thrombus. While none of these interventions is established as effective, interest in the use of these therapies alone or in combination with pharmacological thrombolysis is considerable. In particular, some endovascular interventions might be combined with intra-arterial administration of a thrombolytic agent.

Carotid Endarterectomy

Experience with emergency carotid endarterectomy is limited. No controlled trials are available. Meyer et al.[261] were able to reestablish patency in 94 percent of 34 patients having surgery, and while most patients had severe neurological residuals, nine patients had excellent outcomes. Walters et al.[262] did emergency carotid endarterectomy in 64 patients with a wide variety of acute neurological impairments; 10 of 13 patients with severe strokes remained stable or improved following surgery. Eckstein et al.[263] performed emergency carotid endarterectomy and found favorable outcomes in 9 of 16 patients with acute stroke and 26 of 34 patients with stroke-in-evolution. Eckstein et al.[264] combined carotid endarterectomy with intra-arterial thrombolysis for lysis of a distal embolus in 14 patients; 4 patients completely recovered, while 6 others had minor residuals. In another report, emergency carotid endarterectomy was performed in 43 patients with acute stroke.[265] Patients in coma or with major infarction on imaging were excluded. No complications or deaths related to surgery were reported. Gay et al.[266] looked at the effectiveness of urgent carotid endarterectomy in 21 high-risk patients with acute cerebral ischemia and concluded that the operation might be indicated in some patients. Huber et al.[267] performed surgery in 67 patients (58 percent with stroke) with occlusion of the internal carotid artery but with normal blood flow in the middle cerebral artery by ultrasonography. Flow was restored in all but five cases. A recent report suggested that the presence of a diffusion/perfusion mismatch on MRI could be used to select patients for emergency carotid endarterectomy.[268] Patients with severe neurological impairments but without large areas of brain injury might be helped by surgery. Due to very limited data, current guidelines do not make a specific recommendation for carotid endarterectomy for treatment of acute ischemic stroke.[3]

Other Surgical Procedures

Other surgical procedures include embolectomy to remove a clot in the first segment of the middle cerebral artery. Only a few patients have been treated.[269,270] Endovascular procedures to remove the thrombus in the middle cerebral artery likely will replace this operation.

Emergency revascularization operations (superficial temporal artery-to-middle cerebral artery bypass/extracranial-to-intracranial arterial anastomosis) are not recommended for treatment of patients with acute or progressing cerebral infarction, largely because of a concern or reperfusion injury, edema, and hemorrhage in the ischemic region.

Endovascular Procedures

Mechanical endovascular interventions include lasers, ultrasonography, angioplasty, microsnares, and clot-retrieval devices.[271-274] Advantages include early recanalization, a longer treatment window, and the use of reduced doses or no thrombolytic agents (Fig. 22-20). Mechanical disruption of a clot in conjunction with intra-arterial rtPA may be associated with recanalization, good outcomes, and a low risk of bleeding.[272] Ringer et al.[275] found that balloon angioplasty is an effective adjunct for treatment of patients who are also receiving intra-arterial thrombolysis. It might help prevent occlusion of the stenotic artery and permit distal infusion of thrombolytic medications.[275] Qureshi et al.[276] found that up to eight units of reteplase combined with or without angioplasty achieved recanalization. They proposed this as an alternative intervention for patients considered poor candidates for intravenous thrombolytic treatment. A small trial has demonstrated the potential utility of a clot extraction

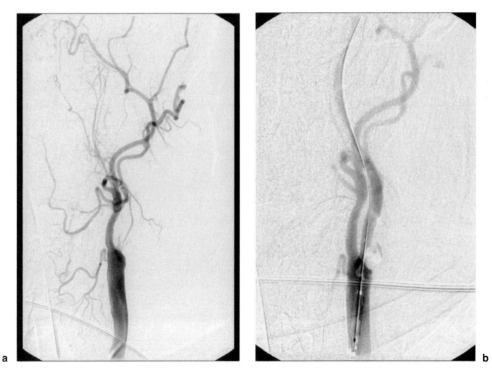

a b

Figure 22-20. Two lateral views of a left carotid arteriogram obtained in a patient with an acute ischemic stroke. The left internal carotid artery is occluded (a). Following mechanical measures, flow is restored in the vessel (b). Residual thrombus is seen in the artery.

device.[273] Experimental evidence shows that therapeutic ultrasonography may break fibrin monomers, increase clot lysis, and improve recanalization. Ultrasonography also could be used to enhance the effects of thrombolytic agents and speed recanalization.[277] Behrens et al.[278] examined the utility of transcranial ultrasonography (185 kHz or 1 MHz) in an experimental model of middle cerebral artery thrombosis and found that the device could speed lysis. Clinical experience is limited. These mechanical interventions hold promise but they are not established as effective in treatment of acute ischemic stroke. Current guidelines do not recommend the routine use of endovascular procedures.

▶ NEUROPROTECTIVE INTERVENTIONS

Neuroprotective interventions may protect ischemic neurons from metabolic effects or reperfusion-related injury.[279] These medications could be given alone or in combination with other neuroprotective therapies or interventions to restore or improve blood flow to the brain. These therapies have widely varying neuroprotective properties (Table 22-9). While the focus has been to protect ischemic neurons, therapies aimed at defending the white matter, oligodendroglia, astrocytes, and axons also are critical. Protection of the endothelial cells and the blood–brain barrier also is important.

Several neuroprotective strategies have been tested. Some therapies could limit the metabolic or biochemical consequences of ischemia. Others may stabilize membranes, slow the effects of apoptosis, or limit reperfusion injury. Strategies include limiting the effects of the excitotoxic glutamate cascade, entry of calcium, intracellular protease activation, free-radical damage, inflammatory responses, and membrane repair. Several variables affect responses to neuroprotective therapy and some interventions have issues related to side effects or tolerability. In a review of the trials of neuroprotection, Lees[280] concluded that, while results were disappointing, new medications and new clinical trial designs might result in one or more medications being shown as effective. Some neuroprotective agents, including N-methyl-D-aspartate (NMDA) receptor antagonists and antileukocyte adhesion molecules, were associated with serious side effects or drug reactions that limit their use.[281] Other neuroprotective agents, including citicoline, clomethiazole, and nalmefene, might be effective in some subgroups of patients with stroke.[282]

Antagonists to Excitatory Amino Acids

Acute brain ischemia induces the release of excitatory amino acids, including glutamate, in toxic levels. Antagonists to the release of glutamate or its effects could protect brain tissue from having been used in several stroke trials. None of these trials testing NMDA glutamate antagonists had positive results.[283]

The first NMDA antagonist, dizocilpine, was not tested in humans because of serious side effects.[284] A pilot study concluded that the competitive NMDA antagonist, selfotel, improved outcomes.[285] However, subsequent trials of this agent were stopped because of an increased rate of unfavorable outcomes, which raised the possibility of neurotoxicity from the medication.[286,287] Aptiganel, a noncompetitive NMDA channel blocker, was tested in a clinical trial. It was not efficacious and may be harmful in patients with stroke.[288] Aptiganel was accompanied by side effects, such as confusion, agitation, sedation, or hallucinations.[289] While dextromethorphan was found to be safe in a pilot study, it has not been tested for efficacy.[290] Dextrophan, a noncompetitive NMDA blocker, also was complicated by a high rate of adverse effects.[291] While memantine appeared efficacious in experimental models, it has not been tested in clinical studies.[284] Remacemide is a low-affinity NMDA receptor antagonist that affects sodium channels. A study suggested that remacemide might lower the frequency of neurological side effects of cardiac surgery.[292] A subsequent dose-escalation study evaluated this medication but additional reports about its efficacy have not been published.[293] Orgogozo et al.[294] then used remacemide to treat patients with mild-to-moderate dementia. Its future use is unclear. Diener et al.[295] tested another low-affinity NMDA antagonist in a randomized multicenter trial in Germany, France, and the Netherlands. Pharmacokinetic data showed that this agent (AR-R15896AR) achieved therapeutic levels but was, unfortunately, associated with

▶ **TABLE 22-9.** NEUROPROTECTIVE AGENTS TESTED IN TREATMENT OF PATIENTS WITH ISCHEMIC STROKE

Citicoline	Clomethiazole
Nalmefene	Selfotel
Aptiganel	Dextromethorphan
Dextrophan	Memantine
Remacemide	Gavestinel
CV 150526	Licostinel
Eliprodil	Lubeluzole
Magnesium	Nicardipine
Nimodipine	Flunarizine
Isradipine	Darodipine
Tirilazad	Edaravone
Diazepam	Naloxone
GM1 ganglioside	Ebselen
Piracetam	Repinotan
Fosphenytoin	Sipatrigine
L-arginine	Enlimomab
Recombinant erythropoietin	Hypothermia
Hyperbaric oxygen	

psychiatric symptoms and other side effects that made it intolerable.

Gavestinel, a glycine antagonist at the NMDA receptor complex, was found to be relatively well tolerated and, although the trial had imbalances, further testing for efficacy was planned.[296] In a parallel trial, Sacco et al.[297] enrolled 1369 patients (701 active) in a placebo-controlled trial. No significant improvement in the rate of favorable outcomes was found. Another glycine antagonist, GV 150526, was associated with hepatotoxicity and likely will not be tested further.[298] Licostinel is a competitive antagonist of glycine at the NMDA receptor. High doses were associated with numerous side effects.[299] A trial of eliprodil, a polyamine glutamate antagonist, was halted prematurely due to toxicity and side effects.[300] Weiser[301] proposed that the AMPA receptor antagonists might be a new approach to neuroprotective therapy. A systemic review of excitatory amino acid antagonists involving data from 36 trials enrolling more than 11,000 participants found no differences in death or disability, although there were differences among the agents.[302] Trends for increased mortality were seen with selfotel, aptiganel, and gavestinel. Aptiganel was associated with more neurological worsening. No major differences between calcium-channel-blocking agents and NMDA blockers were demonstrated.

Sodium Ion Channel Blocker

Lubeluzole, a sodium ion channel and nitric oxide blocker, was tested in a series of clinical trials. A pilot study found it to be safe in a daily dose of 10 mg and that it may reduce mortality.[303] Grotta[304] found no improvements in neurological outcomes with lubeluzole treatment. These findings were supported by those from a double-blind clinical trial that tested lubeluzole (10 mg/day for 5 days).[305] No significant differences in mortality or favorable outcomes were found. The combination of rtPA and lubeluzole could be administered feasibly and with a reasonable degree of safety.[306] Because the other trials were negative, this combination of medications was not tested further. Gandolfo et al.[307] also evaluated the data from the clinical trials of lubeluzole and concluded that evidence for efficacy was lacking.

Magnesium

Magnesium has several actions, including voltage gating the NMDA receptor, thereby preventing the ingress of calcium, and stimulating the production of adenosine triphosphate.[308-310] Preliminary studies of magnesium revealed that it was well tolerated.[311,312] A small study conducted in Israel found that intravenous magnesium sulfate could be given safely to patients with acute stroke, and outcomes were improved.[313] Because magnesium is relatively safe and easy to administer, it has several

advantages. It could be given by emergency medical personnel in the field, in an attempt to stabilize a patient prior to treatment with other interventions. Based on the evaluation of experimental and small clinical studies, Muir[312] concluded that there was solid evidence that magnesium may improve outcomes after stroke. Recently, a large clinical trial of magnesium was administered within 12 h of onset of stroke.[314] Magnesium did not improve outcomes and mortality was slightly increased among patients treated with the agent.

Calcium Antagonists

Transmembrane calcium flux is a critical step in excitoxic cell death, and thus agents that limit movement of calcium into the cell have the potential for treating stroke. Besides affecting the membranes of ischemic neurons, these medications also have vasodilator effects.[315] The calcium channel blocker, nimodipine, is recommended for prevention of brain ischemia among patients with vasospasm following subarachnoid hemorrhage.[235] Nimodipine was tested in 15 clinical trials in acute ischemic stroke, with generally negative results.[316-318] In the Intravenous Nimodipine West European Stroke Trial, outcomes were worse among patients treated with nimodipine than among controls.[318] A randomized trial of nimodipine started within 6 h of stroke failed to demonstrate any benefit from the calcium-channel-blocking agent; poor outcomes were found in 71 of 225 patients administered the medication and 62 of 229 placebo-treated patients.[319] Rosenbaum et al.[320] tested nicardipine in a dose-escalation study but no subsequent studies were conducted. Flunarizine was tested in a European trial but no improvement in outcomes was noted.[321] Other studies evaluated isradipine and darodipine; likewise, no benefit was observed from treatment.[322,323] A systemic review of the calcium-channel-blocking agents found no effect of these medications in reducing death or unfavorable outcomes among patients with ischemic stroke.[324] Intravenous treatment may be complicated by an increased number of unfavorable outcomes related to a decline in blood pressure. Starting the medication more than 12 h after onset of stroke also is associated with an increased risk of unfavorable outcomes. A membrane-activated calcium chelator may reduce intracellular levels of free calcium and is currently under investigation.

Antioxidants

Tirilazad, a 21-aminosteroid that has antioxidant properties, was tested in several studies in patients with subarachnoid hemorrhage and acute ischemic stroke. One study was halted prematurely when interim results demonstrated that the medication was not likely to be useful.[325] A systemic review of all clinical trials testing tirilazad concluded that it did not alter mortality (OR 1.12,

CI 0.88–1.44) but it did increase the likelihood of being dead or disabled (OR 1.23, CI 1.01–1.51).[326] Further studies of tirilazad probably are not warranted. Another free-radical scavenger, edaravone, was tested in a small clinical trial and it seemed to improve outcomes.[327] NKY 059 has been demonstrated as effective in a recent trial.[328]

GABA Agonists

Clomethiazole may have a neuroprotective effect by increasing concentrations of gamma-aminobutyric acid (GABA). In a pilot study, Lyden et al.[329] found that the combination of rtPA and clomethiazole could be given safely and feasibly. Preliminary results suggested that it could be given to patients with intracerebral hemorrhage and that it may improve outcomes among patients with a major stroke.[330,331] Unfortunately, subsequent clinical trials failed to demonstrate improved long-term outcomes.[332–334] Diazepam is a GABA agonist currently under investigation for use in acute stroke.

Opiate Antagonists

Pilot studies of the opiate antagonist, naloxone, did not find a net benefit from treatment.[335,336] Nalmefene (cervene), another opioid antagonist that selectively blocks κ-opioid receptors, was tested in clinical trials but no significant benefit was found with treatment.[337,338]

Membrane Stabilizers

Several studies tested citicoline, a medication that appears to stabilize membranes. A small placebo-controlled trial suggested that citicoline in doses of 500 or 2000 mg was associated with favorable outcomes, although an intermediate dose did have such an effect.[339] Subsequent studies did not demonstrate a benefit from treatment.[340,341] Although the individual trials gave inconclusive results, a meta-analysis concluded that it may improve outcomes among patients with moderate-to-severe stroke when started within 24 h.[342] The authors found good recovery at 3 months in 25.2 percent of patients treated with citicoline and 20.2 percent of placebo-treated patients. The treatment effect was greatest at the 2000-mg dose. Citicoline might have some efficacy in certain subgroups of patients with stroke.[343]

Trials of GM1 gangliosides, which may serve to stabilize membranes, found no net improvement in outcomes after stroke.[343–348] A systemic review of the available clinical data failed to demonstrate a benefit from treatment with gangliosides.[348] Further research testing with these agents is unlikely at this time.

Anti-Inflammatory Agents

Ebselen, which has glutathione peroxidase and anti-inflammatory properties, was tested in combination with rtPA in an animal model. It was found to have a narrow therapeutic window, particularly when given in combination with rtPA.[349] A small study tested ebselen in patients with stroke.[350] Later, Martinez-Vila and Sieira[343] concluded that ebselen may have some efficacy in certain subgroups of patients with stroke.

Other Neuroprotective Agents

Piracetam affects the phospholipid layer of membranes. It was tested in patients with stroke but mortality at 3 months was 23.9 percent among patients given piracetam and 19.2 percent among patients administered placebo.[351] Other studies demonstrated safety and suggested that it also may be effective.[352–354] One review concluded that piracetam may be effective in some patients with acute stroke.[354] However, in a systemic analysis, Ricci et al.[355] noted a trend for an increased risk of early mortality among patients treated with piracetam. Repinotan is a serotonin agonist that has been tested in clinical trials and early results are promising.[356] Fosphenytoin, an anticonvulsant that blocks sodium channels, and sipatrigine, the sodium channel antagonist, were shown to be ineffective.

Increases in nitric oxide concentrations could treat stroke via antiplatelet, antiatherosclerotic, hemodynamic, and neuroprotective properties. Increased nitric oxide synthase also might limit brain injury. Based on a review of available data, Bath et al.[357] concluded that clinical data were insufficient to make any conclusions about the utility of nitric oxide donor, L-arginine, or nitric oxide synthase inhibitors in treatment of patients with stroke. Stimulation of adenosine A-1 receptors by agonists appears to reduce ischemic injury in animal models of stroke but clinical trials are not yet done.[358]

Hyperbaric Oxygen

Hyperbaric oxygen is used to treat patients with carbon monoxide poisoning, Caisson disease, and air embolization.[359] Clinical studies of hyperbaric oxygen for treatment of patients with ischemic stroke provide inconclusive or conflicting data. Most studies are small and uncontrolled, and thus even seemingly beneficial results should be viewed with caution.[360,361] Rusyniak et al.[362] tested hyperbaric oxygen (2.5 atmosphere vs 1.4 atmosphere) in 33 patients with stroke. Patients treated with higher pressures had poorer outcomes. Until more positive data become available, hyperbaric oxygen therapy should not be considered useful for treatment of acute ischemic stroke.

Hypothermia

Hypothermia is a very potent neuroprotective intervention.[363–367] Lowering of the body temperature slows the cerebral metabolism and protects neurons in an ischemic environment. It also might enhance reperfusion. Hypothermia is used to treat patients following cardiac arrest.[367] In an Australian trial,[368] patients were treated with hypothermia (33°C core temperature) or normothermia within 2 h of cardiac arrest. In many cases, paramedics started treatment in the field. The odds ratio for a good outcome increased by a factor of 5.25 in the hypothermic group. Hypothermia has been used to treat patients with malignant brain edema.[369] The combination of hypothermia and medications also holds promise.[370] Therapeutic hypothermia is feasible but it does have serious side effects, including hypotension, cardiac arrhythmias, and pneumonia.[371] One important issue is the time required to lower body temperature. Endovascular cooling appears to be an option.[372,373] Endovascular cooling mechanisms provide rapid induction in hypothermia and maintain stable temperatures.[374] In a pilot study, Krieger et al.[375] tested the feasibility of endovascular cooling in patients with acute stroke. The treated patients generally did well. However, a systemic review found no convincing evidence for the routine use of physical or chemical cooling for the treatment of acute ischemic stroke.[376] Because hypothermia holds promise, future research is under way.[377]

Medications That Affect White Blood Cells

Reperfusion may induce inflammation that leads to additional neuronal injury following stroke. Medications that reduce white blood cell adhesion might limit the size of an infarction. Accumulation of inflammatory cells following stroke may contribute to the evolution of tissue injury through the generation of toxic substances. A randomized trial of enlimomab (a murine intercellular adhesion molecule—1 {ICAM-1}) found poorer outcomes, including increased mortality, among patients receiving the medication.[378] Another inhibitor of white blood cells was tested in a clinical trial and it was not associated with serious side effects; it did not improve outcomes following stroke.[379] In general, these agents appear not to be effective in improving outcomes after stroke. Because interferon-β has anti-inflammatory properties as well as possible role in stimulating antiapoptotic genes, it could be useful in treating patients with stroke.

Other Interventions

Erythropoietin appears to protect neurons from hypoxic/ischemic injury. Recombinant erythropoietin has anti-apoptotic, anti-inflammatory, and neurotrophic properties that increase within the brain after ischemic insults.[380] Intravenous recombinant erythropoietin is well tolerated among patients with stroke.

Therapies that could limit brain injury from cerebral infarction and that could be administered several days after the onset of the neurological symptoms include growth factors, medications that stimulate release of neurotransmitters, or transplants. At present, data are limited.

The pharmacological effects of some medications, including anticonvulsants, sedatives, and major tranquilizers, may hamper recovery from a stroke.[381,382] Conversely, some medications, including the amphetamines, may speed recovery[383] (see Chapter 25).

► TRANSPLANTATION

Transplantation of neural tissue into the area of brain injury was recently attempted.[384,385] A larger number of patients could be treated with administration of growth factors or stem cell transplants if they are useful in improving recovery.[386,387] Among the options for transplantation are fetal cells, neuroprogenitor cells, bone marrow stromal cells, multipotential cells isolated from umbilical cord blood, and immortalized cell lines.[384] Future strategies for transplantation would include a combination of interventions to replace lost neurons and glia, attract new blood supply, and enhance intrinsic plasticity and repair mechanisms.[387] Chopp and Li[388] concluded that implantation of stroma cells may be an effective strategy to treat patients with stroke. Modo et al.[389] tested transplantation of neural stem cells in a rat model of stroke, using a conditionally immortalized murine neuroepithelial stem cell line. Immune reactions were minimal. Experimental implantation of stem cell grafts showed some improvement in cognitive and sensorimotor deficits. Human bone marrow stem cells can be stimulated to exhibit a neural phenotype; they might lessen neurological impairments. In an experimental model, Li[390] administered marrow stromal cells intra-arterially, with the goal of improving neurological outcomes after cerebral infarction, and found positive results.

Gunnett and Heistad[391] proposed that gene transfer therapy could lead to production of functional proteins in brain parenchyma and cerebral blood vessels, but this work is limited. Gene therapy using recombinant adeno-associated virus vectors showed success in treatment of experimental stroke models. Yenari et al.[392] used the neurotropic herpes simplex viral vector system to transfer protective genes to neurons and concluded that they could enhance neuronal survival after ischemia.

Nerve growth factors or other proteins also might be used for treating patients with stroke. For example, the antiapoptotic protein BCL-2 appears to protect cells from apoptotic death by preventing release of cytochrome c from mitochondria and reducing caspase activation.[392] Trafermin (basic fibroblast growth factor) can reduce infarct volume in acute stroke models. A clinical trial of trafermin found that it was well tolerated.[393]

There was a trend that the medication could improve outcomes; however, another trial found higher mortality among patients treated with trafermin than among those given placebo.

These areas of experimental and clinical research hold great promise. While none has yet been established as effective, they do provide new approaches to treatment of cerebral infarction. If these interventions were effective, even when given several hours or days following stroke, they would greatly expand the number of patients who could be helped.

► COMBINATIONS OF INTERVENTIONS

At present, most interventions for treatment of stroke are being tested as monotherapy. Because of the complex metabolic and vascular effects of stroke, the use of combinations of interventions makes a great deal of sense. For example, agents that reduce the risk of hemorrhagic transformation after rtPA might be useful for concomitant therapy, including the spin-trap agents that scavenge free radicals, matrix metalloproteinase inhibitors that prevent membrane and vessel remodeling, and glycoprotein IIb/IIIa receptor antagonists. Some studies have already looked at the combination of rtPA and neuroprotective agents.[394] While these studies are small and do not establish the utility of such an approach, they do predict that future trials will examine the usefulness of several therapies aimed at restoring and maintaining circulation as well as protecting neurons from the consequences of acute ischemia. In the future, acute stroke care might mimic the approach used to treat acute myocardial ischemia, in which pharmacological and mechanical interventions are used.

► REFERENCES

1. The National Institute of Neurological Disorders and Stroke rt-PA Stroke Study Group. Tissue plasminogen activator for acute ischemic stroke. *N Engl J Med* 1995; 333:1581–1587.
2. Adams HP, Jr., Brott TG, Furlan AJ, et al. Guidelines for thrombolytic therapy for acute stroke: a supplement to the guidelines for the management of patients with acute ischemic stroke. A statement for healthcare professionals from a Special Writing Group of the Stroke Council, American Heart Association. *Circulation* 1996;94:1167–1174.
3. Adams HP, Adams RJ, Brott T, et al. Guidelines for the early management of patients with ischemic stroke. A scientific statement from the stroke council of the American Stroke Association. *Stroke* 2003;34:1056–1083.
4. Norris JW, Buchan A, Cote R, et al. Canadian guidelines for intravenous thrombolytic treatment in acute stroke. A consensus statement of the Canadian Stroke Consortium. *Can J Neurol Sci* 1998;25:257–259.
5. European Stroke Initiative. European stroke initiative recommendations for stroke management. *Cerebrovasc Dis* 2000;10:335–351.
6. ECC Guidelines. Part 7: the era of reperfusion, section 2: stroke. *Circulation* 2003;102(suppl 1):I204–I216.
7. Broderick JP, Hacke W. Treatment of acute ischemic stroke: part 1: recanalization strategies. *Circulation* 2002; 106:1563–1569.
8. Bell WR, Jr. Evaluation of thrombolytic agents. *Drugs* 1997;54(suppl 3):11–16.
9. Lijnen HR, Collen D. Fibrinolytic agents: mechanisms of activity and pharmacology. *Thromb Haemost* 1995;74: 387–390.
10. Fox D, Ouriel K, Green RM, Stoughton J, Riggs P, Cimino C. Thrombolysis with prourokinase versus urokinase: an in vitro comparison. *J Vasc Surg* 1996;23:657–666.
11. Credo RB, Burke SE. Fibrinolytic mechanism, biochemistry, and preclinical pharmacology of recombinant prourokinase. *J Vasc Interv Radiol* 1995;6:8S–18S.
12. Collen D, Lijnen HR. Molecular basis of fibrinolysis, as relevant for thrombolytic therapy. *Thromb Haemost* 1995; 74:167–171.
13. Koster RW, Cohen AF, Kluft C, et al. The pharmacokinetics of recombinant double-chain t-PA (duteplase): effects of bolus injection, infusions, and administration by weight in patients with myocardial infarction. *Clin Pharmacol Ther* 1991;50:267–277.
14. Martin U, Kaufmann B, Neugebauer G. Current clinical use of reteplase for thrombolysis. A pharmacokinetic-pharmacodynamic perspective. *Clin Pharmacokinet* 1999; 36:265–276.
15. Ueda T, Hatakeyama T, Sakaki S, Ohta S, Kumon Y, Uraoka T. Changes in coagulation and fibrinolytic system after local intra-arterial thrombolysis for acute ischemic stroke. *Neurol Med Chir (Tokyo)* 1995;35:136–143.
16. Figueroa BE, Keep RF, Betz AL, Hoff JT. Plasminogen activators potentiate thrombin-induced brain injury. *Stroke* 1998;29:1202–1207.
17. Chen H, Wu YI, Hsieh YL, et al. Perturbation of platelet adhesion to endothelial cells by plasminogen activation in vitro. *Thromb Haemost* 1997;78:934–938.
18. Lijnen HR, Stassen JM, Collen D. Differential inhibition with antifibrinolytic agents of staphylokinase and streptokinase induced clot lysis. *Thromb Haemost* 1995;73: 845–849.
19. Bell WR, Jr. Defibrinogenating enzymes. *Drugs* 1997; 54(suppl 3):18–30.
20. Marks MP, Tong DC, Beauliew TC, Albers GW, de Crespigny A, Moseley ME. Early reperfusion and IV tPA therapy using diffusion- and perfusion-weighed MRI. *Neurology* 1999;52:1792–1798.
21. Heiss WD, Graf R, Grond M, Rudolf J. Quantitative neuroimaging for the evaluation of the effect of stroke treatment. *Cerebrovasc Dis* 1998;8(suppl 2):23–29.
22. Christou I, Alexandrov AV, Burgin WS, et al. Timing of recanalization after tissue plasminogen activator therapy determined by transcranial Doppler correlates with

clinical recovery from ischemic stroke. *Stroke* 2000;31: 1812–1816.

23. Alexandrov AV, Demchuk AM, Felberg RA, et al. High rate of complete recanalization and dramatic clinical recovery during tPA infusion when continuously monitored with 2-MHz transcranial Doppler monitoring. *Stroke* 2000;31: 610–614.

24. Alexandrov AV, Grotta JC. Arterial reocclusion in stroke patients treated with intravenous tissue plasminogen activator. *Neurology* 2002;59:862–867.

25. Hillegass WB, Jollis JG, Granger CB, Ohman EM, Califf RM, Mark DB. Intracranial hemorrhage risk and new thrombolytic therapies in acute myocardial infarction. *Am J Cardiol* 1994;73:444–449.

26. Gurwitz JH, Gore JM, Goldberg RJ, et al. Risk for intracranial hemorrhage after tissue plasminogen activator treatment for acute myocardial infarction. Participants in the National Registry of Myocardial Infarction 2. *Ann Intern Med* 1998;129:597–604.

27. Alpert JS. Intracranial hemorrhage after thrombolytic therapy: a therapeutic conflict. *J Am Coll Cardiol* 1992;19: 295–296.

28. Larrue V, von Kummer R, del Zoppo G, Bluhmki E. Hemorrhagic transformation in acute ischemic stroke. Potential contributing factors in the European Cooperative Acute Stroke Study. *Stroke* 1997;28:957–960.

29. Donnan GA, Davis SM, Chambers BR, et al. Streptokinase for acute ischemic stroke with relationship to time of administration: Australian Streptokinase (ASK) Trial Study Group. *JAMA* 1996;276:961–966.

30. Hommel M, Boissel JP, Cornu C, et al. Termination of trial of streptokinase in severe acute ischaemic stroke. MAST Study Group. *Lancet* 1995;345:57.

31. Multicentre Acute Stroke Trial–Italy (MAST-I) Group. Randomised controlled trial of streptokinase, aspirin, and combination of both in treatment of acute ischaemic stroke. *Lancet* 1995;346:1509–1514.

32. Multicenter Acute Stroke Trial–Europe Study Group. Thrombolytic therapy with streptokinase in acute ischemic stroke. *N Engl J Med* 1996;335:145–150.

33. Gilligan AK, Markus R, Read S, et al. Baseline blood pressure but not early computed tomography changes predicts major hemorrhage after streptokinase in acute ischemic stroke. *Stroke* 2002;33:2236–2242.

34. The ATLANTIS ECASS, and NINDS rt-PA study group Investigaters. Association of outcome with early stroke treatment: pooled analysis of ATLANTIS, ECASS, and NINDS rt-PA stroke trials. *Lancet* 2004;363:768–774.

35. Levy DE, Brott TG, Haley EC, Jr., et al. Factors related to intracranial hematoma formation in patients receiving tissue-type plasminogen activator for acute ischemic stroke. *Stroke* 1994;25:291–297.

36. The NINDS t-PA Stroke Study Group. Intracerebral hemorrhage after intravenous t-PA therapy for ischemic stroke. *Stroke* 1997;28:2109–2118.

37. Demchuk AM, Morgenstern LB, Krieger DW, et al. Serum glucose level and diabetes predict tissue plasminogen activator-related intracerebral hemorrhage in acute ischemic stroke. *Stroke* 1999;30:34–39.

38. Trouillas P, Nighoghossian N, Derex L, et al. Thrombolysis with intravenous rtPA in a series of 100 cases of acute carotid territory stroke: determination of etiological, topographic, and radiological outcome factors. *Stroke* 1998;29: 2529–2540.

39. Schmulling S, Rudolf J, Strotmann-Tack T, et al. Acetylsalicylic acid pretreatment, concomitant heparin therapy and the risk of early intracranial hemorrhage following systemic thrombolysis for acute ischemic stroke. *Cerebrovasc Dis* 2003;16:183–190.

40. Grond M, Stenzel C, Schmulling S, et al. Early intravenous thrombolysis for acute ischemic stroke in a community-based approach. *Stroke* 1998;29:1544–1549.

41. Tanne D, Bates VE, Verro P, et al. Initial clinical experience with IV tissue plasminogen activator for acute ischemic stroke: a multicenter survey. The t-PA Stroke Survey Group. *Neurology* 1999;53:424–427.

42. Wang DZ, Rose JA, Honings DS, Garwacki DJ, Milbrandt JC, for the OSF Stroke Team. Treating acute stroke patients with intravenous tPA. *Stroke* 2000;31:77–81.

43. Alberts MJ. Hyperacute stroke therapy with tissue plasminogen activator. *Am J Cardiol* 1997;80:29D–34D.

44. Katzan IL, Furlan AJ, Lloyd LE, et al. Use of tissue-type plasminogen activator for acute ischemic stroke: the Cleveland area experience. *JAMA* 2000;283:1151–1158.

45. Lopez-Yunez AM, Bruno A, Williams LS, Yilmaz E, Zurru C, Biller J. Protocol violations in community-based rtPA stroke treatment are associated with symptomatic intracerebral hemorrhage. *Stroke* 2001;32:12–16.

46. Becker RC, Hochman JS, Cannon CP, et al. Fatal cardiac rupture among patients treated with thrombolytic agents and adjunctive thrombin antagonists: observations from the Thrombolysis and Thrombin Inhibition in Myocardial Infarction 9 Study. *J Am Coll Cardiol* 1999;33:479–487.

47. Becker RC, Charlesworth A, Wilcox RG, et al. Cardiac rupture associated with thrombolytic therapy: impact of time to treatment in the Late Assessment of Thrombolytic Efficacy (LATE) study. *J Am Coll Cardiol* 1995;25:1063–1068.

48. Kasner SE, Villar-Cordova CE, Tong D, Grotta JC. Hemopericardium and cardiac tamponade after thrombolysis for acute ischemic stroke. *Neurology* 1998;50:1857–1859.

49. Katzan IL, Masaryk TJ, Furlan AJ, et al. Intra-arterial thrombolysis for perioperative stroke after open heart surgery. *Neurology* 1999;52:1081–1084.

50. Chalela JA, Katzan I, Liebeskind DS, et al. Safety of intra-arterial thrombolysis in the postoperative period. *Stroke* 2001;32:1365–1369.

51. Rudolf J, Grond M, Prince WS, Schmulling S, Heiss WD. Evidence of anaphylaxy after alteplase infusion. *Stroke* 1999;30:1142–1143.

52. Rudolf J, Grond M, Schmulling S, Neveling M, Heiss WD. Orolingual angioneurotic edema following therapy of acute ischemic stroke with alteplase. *Neurology* 2000;55: 599–600.

53. Pancioli A, Brott T, Donaldson V, Miller R. Asymmetric angioneurotic edema associated with thrombolysis for acute stroke. *Ann Emerg Med* 1997;30:227–229.

54. Stephens MB, Pepper PV. Streptokinase therapy. Recognizing and treating allergic reactions. *Postgrad Med* 1998;103:89–90.

55. Adams HP, Jr., Brott TG, Crowell RM, et al. Guidelines for the management of patients with acute ischemic stroke. A statement for healthcare professionals from a special writing group of the Stroke Council, American Heart Association. *Circulation* 1994;90:1588–1601.

56. Boersma E, Maas AC, Deckers JW, Simoons ML. Early thrombolytic treatment in acute myocardial infarction: reappraisal of the golden hour. *Lancet* 1996;348:771–775.

57. Wardlaw JM, Warlow CP. Thrombolysis in acute ischemic stroke: does it work? *Stroke* 1992;23:1826–1839.

58. Motto C, Ciccone A, Aritzu E, et al. Hemorrhage after an acute ischemic stroke. *Stroke* 1999;30:761–769.

59. Hacke W, Kaste M, Fieschi C, et al. Intravenous thrombolysis with recombinant tissue plasminogen activator for acute hemispheric stroke. The European Cooperative Acute Stroke Study (ECASS). *JAMA* 1995;274:1017–1025.

60. Hacke W, Kaste M, Fieschi C, et al. Randomised double-blind placebo-controlled trial of thrombolytic therapy with intravenous alteplase in acute ischaemic stroke (ECASS II). Second European–Australasian Acute Stroke Study Investigators. *Lancet* 1998;352:1245–1251.

61. Clark WM, Albers GW, for the ATLANTIS Stroke Study Investigators. The ATLANTIS rt-PA (alteplase) Acute Stroke Trial. Final results. *Stroke* 1999;30:234.

62. Clark WM, Albers GW, Madden KP, Hamilton S, for the Thrombolytic Therapy in Acute Ischemic Stroke Study Investigators. The rtPA (alteplase) 0- to 6-hour acute stroke trial, part A (A0276g). Results of a double-blind, placebo-controlled, multicenter study. *Stroke* 2000;31:811–816.

63. Clark WM, Wissman S, Albers GW, et al. Recombinant tissue-type plasminogen activator (alteplase) for ischemic stroke 3 to 5 hours after symptom onset. The ATLANTIS Study: a randomized controlled trial. *JAMA* 1999;282:2019–2026.

64. Hacke W, Donnan G, Fieschi C, et al. Association of outcome with early stroke treatment: pooled analysis of ATLANTIS, ECASS, and NINDS rt-PA stroke trials. *Lancet* 2004;363:768–774.

65. Steiner T, Bluhmki E, Kaste M, et al. The ECASS 3-hour cohort. *Cerebrovasc Dis* 1998;8:198–203.

66. Brott TG, Haley EC, Jr., Levy DE, et al. Urgent therapy for stroke. Part I. Pilot study of tissue plasminogen activator administered within 90 minutes. *Stroke* 1992;23:632–640.

67. Haley EC, Jr., Levy DE, Brott TG, et al. Urgent therapy for stroke. Part II. Pilot study of tissue plasminogen activator administered 91–180 minutes from onset. *Stroke* 1992;23:641–645.

68. Haley EC, Jr. Thrombolytic therapy for acute ischemic stroke. *Clin Neuropharmacol* 1993;16:179–194.

69. The NINDS t-PA Stroke Study Group. Generalized efficacy of t-PA for acute stroke. Subgroup analysis of the NINDS t-PA Stroke Trial. *Stroke* 1997;28:2119–2125.

70. Schlegel DJ, Tanne D, Demchuk AM, Levine SR, Kasner SE, for the Multicenter rt-PA Stroke Survey Group. Prediction of hospital disposition after thrombolysis for acute ischemic stroke using the National Institutes of Health Stroke Scale. *Arch Neurol* 2004;61:1061–1064.

71. Ringleb PA, Schellinger PD, Schranz C, Hacke W. Thrombolytic therapy within 3 to 6 hours after onset of ischemic stroke: useful or harmful? *Stroke* 2002;33:1437–1441.

72. Bath P. Alteplase not yet proven for acute ischaemic stroke. *Lancet* 1998;352:1238–1239.

73. Hankey GJ. Thrombolytic therapy in acute ischaemic stroke: the jury needs more evidence. *Med J Aust* 1997;166:419–422.

74. Wardlaw JM, Sandercock PAG, Berge E. Thrombolytic therapy with recombinant tissue plasminogen activator for acute ischemic stroke. Where do we go from here? A cumulative meta-analysis. *Stroke* 2003;34:1437–1442.

75. Buchan AM, Barber PA, Newcommon N, et al. Effectiveness of t-PA in acute ischemic stroke. Outcome relates to appropriateness. *Neurology* 2000;54:679–684.

76. Wardlaw JM, del Zoppo G, Yamaguchi T, Berge E. Thrombolysis for acute ischaemic stroke. *Cochrane Database Syst Rev* 2003;CD000213.

77. Liu M, Wardlaw J. Thrombolysis (different doses, routes of administration and agents) for acute ischaemic stroke. *Cochrane Database Syst Rev* 2000;CD000514.

78. Chiu D, Krieger D, Villar-Cordova C, et al. Intravenous tissue plasminogen activator for acute ischemic stroke: feasibility, safety, and efficacy in the first year of clinical practice. *Stroke* 1998;29:18–22.

79. Egan R, Lutsep HL, Clark WM, et al. Open label tissue plasminogen activator for stroke: the Oregon experience. *J Stroke Cerebrovasc Dis* 1999;8:287–290.

80. Wirkowski E, Gottesman MH, Mazer C, Brody GM, Manzella SM. Tissue plasminogen activator for acute stroke in everyday clinical practice. *J Stroke Cerebrovasc Dis* 1999;8:291–294.

81. Katzan IL, Graber TM, Furlan AJ, et al. Cuyahoga County operation stroke speed of emergency department evaluation and compliance with National Institutes of Neurological Disorders and Stroke time targets. *Stroke* 2003;34:799–800.

82. Katzan IL, Hammer MD, Furlan AJ, Hixson ED, Nadzam DM. Quality improvement and tissue-type plasminogen activator for acute ischemic stroke: a Cleveland update. *Stroke* 2003;34:799–800.

83. Grotta JC, Burgin WS, El-Mitwalli A, et al. Intravenous tissue-type plasminogen activator therapy for ischemic stroke: Houston experience 1996 to 2000. *Arch Neurol* 2001;58:2009–2013.

84. Grond M, Rudolf J, Neveling M, Stenzel C, Heiss WD. Risk of immediate heparin after rt-PA therapy in acute ischemic stroke. *Cerebrovasc Dis* 1997;7:318–323.

85. Felberg RA, Okon NJ, El-Mitwalli A, Burgin WS, Grotta JC, Alexandrov AV. Early dramatic recovery during intravenous tissue plasminogen activator infusion: clinical pattern and outcome in acute middle cerebral artery stroke. *Stroke* 2002;33:1301–1307.

86. Smith RW, Scott PA, Grant RJ, Chudnofsky CR, Frederiksen SM. Emergency physician treatment of acute stroke with recombinant tissue plasminogen activator: a retrospective analysis. *Acad Emerg Med* 1999;6:618–625.

87. Akin PT, Delemos C, Wentworth D, et al. Can emergency department physicians safely and effectively initiate

thrombolysis for acute ischemic stroke. *Neurology* 2000; 55:1801–1805.

88. Bravada DM, Kim N, Concato J, Krumholz HM, Brass LM. Thrombolysis for acute stroke in routine clinical practice. *Arch intern Med* 2002;162:1994–2001.

89. Albers GW, Bates VE, Clark WM, et al. Intravenous tissue type plasminogen activator for treatment of acute stroke. The Standard Treatment with Alteplase to Reverse Stroke (STARS) study. *JAMA* 2000;283:1154–1150.

90. Chiu D, Krieger D, Villar-Cordova C, et al. Intravenous tissue plasminogen activitor for acute ischemic stroke. Feasibility, safety, and efficacy in the first year of clinical practice. *Stroke* 1998;29:18–22.

91. Koennecke H, Nohr S, Leistner S, Marx P. Intravenous tPA for ischemic stroke team performance over time, safety, and efficacy in single-center, 2-year experience. *Stroke* 2001;32:1074–1078.

92. Lindsberg PJ, Soinne L, Roine O, et al. Community-based thrombolytic therapy for acute ischemic stroke in Helsinki. *Stroke* 2003;34:1443–1449.

93. Rudolf J, Neveling M, Grond M, Schmülling S, Stenzel C, Heiss W-D. Stroke following internal carotid artery occlusion—contra-indication for intravenous thrombolysis? *Eur J Neurol* 1999;6:51–55.

94. Montavont A, Nighoghossian N, Derex L, et al. Intravenous r-TPA in vertebrobasilar acute infarcts. *Neurology* 2004;62: 1854–1856.

95. Ribo M, Molina CA, Rovina A, et al. Safety and efficacy of intravenous tissue plasminogen activator stroke treatment in the 3- to 6- hour window using multimodal transcranial Doppler, MRI selection protocol. *Stroke* 2005;36:602–606.

96. Nowak-Göttl U, Straeter R, Sebire G, Kirkham F. Antithrombotic drug treatment of pediatric patients with ischemic stroke. *Paediatr Drugs* 2003;5:167–175.

97. Hacke W, Albers G, Bogousslavsky A, et al. The desmoteplase in acute ischemic stroke trial (DIAS). A phase II MRI-based 9-hour window acute stroke thrombolysis trial with intravenous desmoteplase. *Stroke* 2005;36:66–75.

98. Haley EC, Lyden PD, Johnston KC, et al. A pilot dose escalation study of tenecteplase in acute ischemic stroke. *Stroke* 2005;36:607–612.

99. Furlan AJ, Eyding D, Albers GW, et al. Dose escalation study of desmoteplase for acute ischemic stroke (DEDAS). Evidence of safety and efficacy 3 to 9 hours after stroke onset. *Stroke* 2006;37:1227–1231.

100. Yamaguchi T, Mori E, Minematsu K, et al. Alteplase at 0.6 mg/kg for acute ischemic stroke within 3 hours of onset. Japan Alteplase Clinical Trial (J-ACT). *Stroke* 2006;37: 1810–1815.

101. Furlan A. Intra-arterial thrombolysis for acute stroke. *Cleve Clin J Med* 2004;71(suppl 1):S31–S38.

102. Saver JL. Intra-arterial thrombolysis. *Neurology* 2001;57: S58–S60.

103. Bourekas EC, Slivka AP, Shah R, Sunshine J, Suarez JI. Intraarterial thrombolytic therapy within 3 hours of the onset of stroke. *Neurosurgery* 2004;54:39–46.

104. Qureshi AI, Suri MFK, Shatla AA, et al. Intraarterial recombinant tissue plasminogen activator for ischemic stroke: an accelerating dosing regimen. *Neurosurgery* 2000;47:473–479.

105. Urbach H, Ries F, Ostertun B, Solymosi L. Local intra-arterial fibrinolysis in thromboembolic "T" occlusions of the internal carotid artery. *Neuroradiology* 1997;39: 105–110.

106. Urbach H, Hartmann A, Pohl C, Omran H, Wilhelm H, Flacke S. Local intra-arterial thrombolysis in the carotid territory: does recanalization depend on the thromboembolus type? *Neuroradiology* 2002;44:695–699.

107. Endo S, Kuwayama N, Hirashima Y, Akai T, Nishijima M, Takaku A. Results of urgent thrombolysis in patients with major stroke and atherothrombotic occlusion of the cervical internal carotid artery. *AJNR Am J Neuroradiol* 1998; 19:1169–1175.

108. Gonner F, Remonda L, Mattle H, et al. Local intra-arterial thrombolysis in acute ischemic stroke. *Stroke* 1998;29: 1894–1900.

109. Jahan R, Duckwiler GR, Kidwell CS, et al. Intraarterial thrombolysis for treatment of acute stroke: experience in 26 patients with long-term follow-up. *AJNR Am J Neuroradiol* 1999;20:1291–1299.

110. Linfante I, Llinas RH, Selim M, et al. Clinical and vascular outcome in internal carotid artery versus middle cerebral artery occlusions after intravenous tissue plasminogen activator. *Stroke* 2002;33:2066–2071.

111. Eckert B, Kucinski T, Neumaier-Probst E, Fiehler J, Röther J, Zeumer H. Local intra-arterial fibrinolysis in acute hemispheric stroke: effect of occlusion type and fibrinolytic agent on recanalization success and neurological outcome. *Cerebrovasc Dis* 2003;15:258–263.

112. Suarez JI, Sunshine JL, Tarr R, et al. Predictors of clinical improvement, angiographic recanalization, and intracranial hemorrhage after intra-arterial thrombolysis for acute ischemic stroke. *Stroke* 1999;30:2094–2100.

113. Arnold M, Schroth G, Nedeltchev K, et al. Intra-arterial thrombolysis in 100 patients with acute stroke due to middle cerebral artery occlusion. *Stroke* 2002;33:1828–1833.

114. Arnold M, Nedeltchev K, Sturzenegger M, et al. Thrombolysis in patients with acute stroke caused by cervical artery dissection: analysis of 9 patients and review of the literature. *Arch Neurol* 2002;59:549–553.

115. Lisboa R, Jovanovic B, Alberts MJ. Analysis of the safety and efficacy of intra-arterial thrombolytic therapy in ischemic stroke. *Stroke* 2002;33:2866–2871.

116. Inove T, Kimura K, Minematsu K, et al. A case-control analysis of intra-arterial urokinase thrombolysis in acute cardioembolic stroke. *Cerebrovasc Dis* 2005;19:225–228.

117. Becker KJ, Monsein LH, Ulatowski J, Mirski M, Williams M, Hanley DF. Intraarterial thrombolysis in vertebrobasilar occlusion. *AJNR Am J Neuroradiol* 1996;17:255–262.

118. Becker KJ, Purcell LL, Hacke W, Hanley DF. Vertebrobasilar thrombosis: diagnosis, management, and the use of intra-arterial thrombolytics. *Crit Care Med* 1996;24:1729–1742.

119. Brandt T, von Kummer R, Muller-Kuppers M, Hacke W. Thrombolytic therapy of acute basilar artery occlusion. Variables affecting recanalization and outcome. *Stroke* 1996;27:875–881.

120. Wijdicks EF, Nichols DA, Thielen KR, et al. Intra-arterial thrombolysis in acute basilar artery thromboembolism: the initial Mayo Clinic experience. *Mayo Clin Proc* 1997; 72:1005–1013.

121. Levy EI, Firlik AD, Wisniewski S, et al. Factors affecting survival rates for acute vertebrobasilar artery occlusions treated with intra-arterial thrombolytic therapy: a meta-analytical approach. *Neurosurgery* 1999;45:539–548.

122. Qureshi AI. Endovascular treatment of cerebrovascular diseases and intracranial neoplasms. *Lancet* 2004;363: 804–813.

123. Sasahara AA, Barker WM, Weaver WD, et al. Clinical studies with the new glycosylated recombinant prourokinase. *J Vasc Interv Radiol* 1995;6:84S–93S.

124. del Zoppo GJ, Higashida RT, Furlan AJ, Pessin MS, Rowley HA, Gent M. PROACT: a phase II randomized trial of recombinant pro-urokinase by direct arterial delivery in acute middle cerebral artery stroke. PROACT Investigators. Prolyse in acute cerebral thromboembolism. *Stroke* 1998; 29:4–11.

125. Furlan AJ, Higashida R, Wechsler L, Schultz G, PROACT II Investigators. PROACT II. Recombinant prourokinase (r-ProUK) in acute cerebral thromboembolism. Initial trial results. *Stroke* 1999;30:234.

126. Furlan A, Higashida R, Wechsler L, et al. Intra-arterial prourokinase for acute ischemic stroke. The PROACT II Study: a randomized controlled trial. *JAMA* 1999;282: 2003–2011.

127. Kase CS, Furlan AJ, Wechsler LR, et al. Cerebral hemorrhage after intra-arterial thrombolysis for ischemic stroke: the PROACT II trial. *Neurology* 2001;57:1603–1610.

128. Higashida RT, Furlan AJ, for the Technology Assessment Committees of the American Society of Interventional and Therapeutic Neuroradiology and the Society of Interventional Radiology. Trial design and reporting standards for intra-arterial cerebral thrombolysis for acute ischemic stroke. *Stroke* 2003;34:1923–1924.

129. The IMS Study Investigators. Combined intravenous and intra-arterial recanalization for acute ischemic stroke: The International Management of Stroke Study. *Stroke* 2004;35:904–912.

130. Lewandowski CA, Frankel M, Tomsick TA, et al. Combined intravenous and intra-arterial r-TPA versus intra-arterial therapy of acute ischemic stroke: emergency management of stroke (EMS) trial. *Stroke* 1999;30: 2598–2605.

131. Ernst R, Pancioli A, Tomsick T, et al. Combined intravenous and intra-arterial recombinant tissue plasminogen activator in acute ischemic stroke. *Stroke* 2000;31:2552–2557.

132. Suarez JI, Zaidat OO, Sunshine JL, Tarr R, Selman WR, Landis DM. Endovascular administration after intravenous infusion of thrombolytic agents for the treatment of patients with acute ischemic strokes. *Neurosurgery* 2002;50:251–260.

133. Keris V, Rudnicka S, Vorona V, Enina G, Tilgale B, Fricbergs J. Combined intraarterial/intravenous thrombolysis for acute ischemic stroke. *AJNR Am J Neuroradiol* 2001;22:352–358.

134. Zaidat OO, Suarez JI, Santillan C, et al. Response to intra-arterial and combined intravenous and intra-arterial therapy in patients with distal internal carotid artery occlusion. *Stroke* 2002;33:1821–1827.

135. Hill MD, Barber PA, Demchuk AM, et al. Acute intravenous-intra-arterial revascularization therapy for severe ischemic stroke. *Stroke* 2002;33:279–282.

136. Sherman DG, Atkinson RP, Cheppendale T, et al. Intravenous ancrod for treatment of acute ischemic stroke: the STAT study: a randomized controlled trial. Stroke Treatment with Ancrod Trial. *JAMA* 2000;283: 2395–2403.

137. Liu M, Counsell C, Zhao XL, Wardlaw J. Fibrinogen depleting agents for acute ischaemic stroke. *Cochrane Database Syst Rev* 2003;CD000091.

138. Sherman DG. Antithrombotic and hypofibrinogenetic therapy in acute ischemic stroke: what is the next step? *Cerebrovasc Dis* 2004;17(suppl 1):138–143.

139. Adams HP, Jr. Emergent use of anticoagulation for treatment of patients with ischemic stroke. *Stroke* 2002;33: 856–861.

140. Coull BM, Williams LS, Goldstein LB, et al. Anticoagulants and antiplatelet agents in acute ischemic stroke. Report of the Joint Stroke Guideline Development Committee of the American Academy of Neurology and the American Stroke Association (a division of the American Heart Association). *Neurology* 2002;59:13–22.

141. Marsh EE, Adams HP, Jr., Biller J, et al. Use of antithrombotic drugs in the treatment of acute ischemic stroke: a survey of neurologists in practice in the United States. *Neurology* 1989;39:1631–1634.

142. Anderson DC. How Twin Cities neurologists treat ischemic stroke. Policies and trends. *Arch Neurol* 1993;50:1098–1103.

143. Al-Sadat A, Sunbulli M, Chaturvedi S. Use of the intravenous heparin by North American neurologists: do the data matter? *Stroke* 2002;33:1574–1577.

144. Grau AJ, Hacke W. Is there still a role for intravenous heparin in acute stroke? Yes. *Arch Neurol* 1999;56:1159–1160.

145. Sandercock P. Is there still a role for intravenous heparin in acute stroke? No. *Arch Neurol* 1999;56:1160–1161.

146. Sandercock P. Full heparin anticoagulation should not be used in acute ischemic stroke. *Stroke* 2003;34:231–232.

147. Albers GW, Amarenco P, Easton JD, Sacco RL, Teal P. Antithrombotic and thrombolytic therapy for ischemic stroke. *Chest* 2001;119:300S–20S.

148. Caplan LR. Resolved: heparin may be useful in selected patients with brain ischemia. *Stroke* 2003;34:230–231.

149. Donnan GA, Davis SM. Heparin in stroke: not for most, but the controversy lingers. *Stroke* 2003;34:232–233.

150. Chamorro A. Heparin in acute ischemic stroke: the case for a new clinical trial. *Cerebrovasc Dis* 1999;9(suppl 3): 16–23.

151. Chamorro A, Obach V. Anticoagulant therapy. *Cerebrovasc Dis* 2003;15:49–55.

152. Hirsh J, Anand SS, Halperin JL, Fuster V. Guide to anticoagulant therapy: heparin. *Circulation* 2001;103:2994–3018.

153. Fareed J, Callas D, Hoppensteadt DA, Walenga JM, Bick RL. Antithrombin agents as anticoagulants and antithrombotics. Implications in drug development. *Med Clin N Am* 1998;82:569–586.

154. Chamorro A, Cervera A, Castillo J, Davalos A, Aponte JJ, Planas AM. Unfractionated heparin is associated with a lower rise of serum vascular cell adhesion molecule-1 in acute ischemic stroke patients. *Neurosci Lett* 2002;328: 299–232.

155. Lever R, Page C. Glycosaminoglycans, airways inflammation and bronchial hyperresponsiveness. *Pulm Pharmacol Ther* 2001;14:249–254.

156. Becker RC, Ansell J. Antithrombotic therapy. An abbreviated reference for clinicians. *Arch Intern Med* 1995;155:149–161.

157. Raschke RA, Reilly BM, Guidry JR, Fontana JR, Srinivas S. The weight-based heparin dosing nomogram compared with a "standard care" nomogram. A randomized controlled trial. *Ann Intern Med* 1993;119:874–881.

158. Raschke R, Hirsh J, Guidry JR. Suboptimal monitoring and dosing of unfractionated heparin in comparative studies with low-molecular-weight heparin. *Ann Intern Med* 2003;138:720–723.

159. Toth C, Voll C. Validation of a weight-based nomogram for the use of intravenous heparin in transient ischemic attack or stroke. *Stroke* 2002;33:670–674.

160. Hirsh J. New anticoagulants. *Am Heart J* 2001;142:S3–S8.

161. Hirsh J, Warkentin TE, Shaughnessy SG, et al. Heparin and low-molecular-weight heparin. Mechanisms of action, pharmacokinetics, dosing, monitoring, efficacy, and safety. *Chest* 2001;119:64S–94S.

162. Hirsh J, Weitz JI. New antithrombotic agents. *Lancet* 1999;353:1431–1436.

163. Nenci GG, Minciotti A. Low molecular weight heparins for arterial thrombosis. *Vasc Med* 2000;5:251–258.

164. Magnani HN. Heparin-induced thrombocytopenia (HIT): an overview of 230 patients treated with orgaran (Org 10172). *Thromb Haemost* 1993;70:554–561.

165. Mary V, Wahl F, Uzan A, Stutzmann JM. Enoxaparin in experimental stroke: neuroprotection and therapeutic window of opportunity. *Stroke* 2001;32:993–999.

166. Laposata M, Green D, Van Cott EM, Barrowcliffe TW, Goodnight SH, Sosolik RC. College of American Pathologists Conference XXXI on laboratory monitoring of anticoagulant therapy: the clinical use and laboratory monitoring of low-molecular-weight heparin, danaparoid, hirudin and related compounds, and argatroban. *Arch Pathol Lab Med* 1998;122:799–807.

167. Petty GW, Brown RD, Jr., Whisnant JP, Sicks JD, O'Fallon WM, Wiebers DO. Frequency of major complications of aspirin, warfarin, and intravenous heparin for secondary stroke prevention. *Ann Intern Med* 1999;130:14–22.

168. Levine MN, Raskob G, Landefeld S, Kearon C. Hemorrhagic complications of anticoagulant treatment. *Chest* 1998;114:511S–523S.

169. Chamorro A, Vila N, Saiz A, Alday M, Tolosa E. Early anticoagulation after large cerebral embolic infarction: a safety study. *Neurology* 1995;45:861–865.

170. Diener HC, Ringelstein EB, von Kummer R, et al. Treatment of acute ischemic stroke with the low-molecular-weight heparin certoparin. *Stroke* 2001;32:22–29.

171. Bath PM, Lindenstrom E, Boysen G, et al. Tinzaparin in acute ischaemic stroke (TAIST): a randomised aspirin-controlled trial. *Lancet* 2001;358:683–684.

172. The Publications Committee for the Trial of ORG 10172 in Acute Stroke Treatment (TOAST) Investigators. Low molecular weight heparanoid, ORG 10172 (danaparoid), and outcome after acute ischemic stroke: a randomized controlled trial. *JAMA* 1998;279:1265–1272.

173. Jaillard A, Cornu C, Durieux A, et al. Hemorrhagic transformation in acute ischemic stroke. *Stroke* 1999;30:1326–1332.

174. Cerebral Embolism Study Group. Immediate anticoagulation of embolic stroke: brain hemorrhage and management options. *Stroke* 1984;15:779–789.

175. Kay R, Wong KS, Yu YL, et al. Low-molecular-weight heparin for the treatment of acute ischemic stroke. *N Engl J Med* 1995;333:1588–1593.

176. Berge E, Abdelnoor M, Nakstad PH, Sandset PM, on behalf of the HAEST Study Group. Low molecular-weight heparin versus aspirin in patients with acute ischaemic stroke and atrial fibrillation: a double-blind randomised study. *Lancet* 2000;355:1205–1210.

177. International Stroke Trial Collaborative Group. The International Stroke Trial (IST): a randomised trial of aspirin, subcutaneous heparin, both, or neither among 19435 patients with acute ischaemic stroke. *Lancet* 1997;349:1569–1581.

178. Ramirez-Lassepas M, Cipolle RJ, Rodvold KA, et al. Heparin induced thrombocytopenia in patients with cerebrovascular ischemic disease. *Neurology* 1986;34:736–740.

179. Atkinson JL, Sundt TMJ, Kazmier FJ, Bowie EJ, Whisnant JP. Heparin-induced thrombocytopenia and thrombosis in ischemic stroke. *Mayo Clin Proc* 1988;63:353–361.

180. Becker PS, Miller VT. Heparin-induced thrombocytopenia. *Stroke* 1989;20:1449–1459.

181. Duke RJ, Bloch RF, Turpie AG, Trebilcock R, Bayer N. Intravenous heparin for the prevention of stroke progression in acute partial stable stroke. *Ann Intern Med* 1986;105:825–828.

182. Cerebral Embolism Study Group. Immediate anticoagulation and embolic stroke. A randomized trial. *Stroke* 1983;14:668–676.

183. Cerebral Embolism Study Group. Cardioembolic stroke, early anticoagulation, and brain hemorrhage. *Arch Intern Med* 1987;147:636–640.

184. CAST (Chinese Acute Stroke Trial) Collaborative Group. CAST: randomised placebo-controlled trial of early aspirin use in 20,000 patients with acute ischaemic stroke. *Lancet* 1997;349:1641–1649.

185. Saxena R, Lewis S, Berge E, Sandercock PA, Koudstaal PJ. Risk of early death and recurrent stroke and effect of heparin in 3169 patients with acute ischemic stroke and atrial fibrillation in the International Stroke Trial. *Stroke* 2001;32:2333–2337.

186. Roden-Jullig A, Britton M. Effectiveness of heparin treatment for progressing ischaemic stroke: before and after study. *J Intern Med* 2001;248:287–291.

187. Gubitz G, Counsell C, Sandercock P, Signorini D. Anticoagulants for acute ischaemic stroke. *Cochrane Database Syst Rev* 2000;CD000024.

188. Pereira AC, Brown MM. Aspirin or heparin in acute stroke. *Br Med Bull* 2000;56:413–421.

189. Moonis M, Fisher M. Considering the role of heparin and low-molecular-weight heparins in acute ischemic stroke. *Stroke* 2002;33:1927–1933.

190. Daffertshofer M, Grips E, Dempfle CE, Hennerici M. Heparin during acute ischemic stroke. Present data and clinical situation. *Nervenarzt* 2003;74:307–319.

191. Adams HP, Jr., Bendixen BH, Leira E, Chang KC, Davis PH, Woolson RF. Treatment of ischemic stroke in patients with occlusion or stenosis of the internal carotid artery. *Neurology* 1999;53:122–125.

192. Lovett JK, Coull AJ, Rothwell PM. Early risk of recurrence by subtype of ischemic stroke in population-based incidence studies. *Neurology* 2004;62:569–573.

193. Bath PM, Iddenden R, Bath FJ. Low-molecular-weight heparins and heparanoids in acute ischemic stroke. A meta-analysis of randomized controlled trials. *Stroke* 2000;31:1770–1778.

194. Counsell C, Sandercock P. CD000480. *Cochrane Database Syst Rev* 2001;CD000119.

195. Lunven C, Gauffeny C, Lecoffre C, O'Brien DP, Roome NO, Berry CN. Inhibition by argatroban, a specific thrombin inhibitor, of platelet activation by fibrin clot-associated thrombin. *Thromb Haemost* 1996;75:154–160.

196. Lewis BE, Walenga JM, Wallis DE. Anticoagulation with novastan (argatroban) in patients with heparin-induced thrombocytopenia and heparin-induced thrombocytopenia and thrombosis syndrome. *Semin Thromb Hemost* 1997;23:197–202.

197. Imiya M, Matsuo T. Inhibition of collagen-induced platelet aggregation by argatroban in patients with acute cerebral infarction. *Thromb Res* 1997;88:245–250.

198. Morris DC, Silver B, Mitsias P, et al. Treatment of acute stroke with recombinant tissue plasminogen activator and abciximab. *Acad Emerg Med* 2003;10:1396–1399.

199. LaMonte MP, Nash ML, Wang DZ, et al. Argatroban anticoagulation in patients with acute ischemic stroke (ARGIS-1). A randomized, placebo-controlled safety study. *Stroke* 2004;35:1677–1682.

200. del Zoppo GJ. The role of platelets in ischemic stroke. *Neurology* 1998;51:S9–S14.

201. The Clopidogrel in Unstable Angina to Prevent Recurrent Events Trial Investigators. Effects of clopidogrel in addition to aspirin in patients with acute coronary syndromes without ST-segment elevation. *N Engl J Med* 2001;345:494–502.

202. Yusuf S, Zhao F, Mehta SR, et al. Effects of clopidogrel in addition to aspirin in patients with acute coronary syndromes without ST-segment elevation. *N Engl J Med* 2001;345:494–502.

203. Steinhubl SR, Ellis SG, Wolski K, Lincoff AM, Topol EJ. Ticlopidine pretreatment before coronary stenting is associated with sustained decrease in adverse cardiac events: data from the Evaluation of Platelet IIb/IIIa Inhibitor for Stenting (EPISTENT) Trial. *Circulation* 2001;103:1403–1409.

204. Gerschutz GP, Bhatt DL, Clopidogrel in Unstable Angina to Prevent Recurrent Events Study. The Clopidogrel in Unstable Angina to Prevent Recurrent Events (CURE) study: to what extent should the results be generalized? *Am Heart J* 2003;145:595–601.

205. The Ridogrel Versus Aspirin Patency Trial (RAPT). Randomized trial of ridogrel, a combined thromboxane A2 synthase inhibitor and thromboxane A2/prostaglandin endoperoxide receptor antagonist, versus aspirin as adjunct to thrombolysis in patients with acute myocardial infarction. *Circulation* 1994;89:588–595.

206. Fintel DJ. From bench to bedside: GP IIb-IIIa inhibitors. *Neurology* 2001;57:S12–S19.

207. Bednar MM, Gross CE. Antiplatelet therapy in acute cerebral ischemia. *Stroke* 1999;30:887–893.

208. Ferguson JJ, Waly HM, Wilson JM. Fundamentals of coagulation and glycoprotein IIb/IIIa receptor inhibition. *Eur Heart J* 1998;19(suppl D):D3–D9.

209. Schwarz M, Nordt T, Bode C, Peter K. The GP IIb/IIIa inhibitor abciximab (c7E3) inhibits the binding of various ligands to the leukocyte integrin Mac-1 (CD11b/CD18). *Thromb Res* 2002;107:121–128.

210. Kopp CW, Steiner S, Nasel C, et al. Abciximab reduces monocyte tissue factor in carotid angioplasty and stenting. *Stroke* 2003;34:2560–2567.

211. Choudhri TF, Hoh BL, Zerwes HG, et al. Reduced microvascular thrombosis and improved outcome in acute murine stroke by inhibiting GP IIb/IIIa receptor-mediated platelet aggregation. *J Clin Invest* 1998;102:1301–1310.

212. Zhang L, Zhang ZG, Zhang R, et al. Adjuvant treatment with a glycoprotein IIb/IIIa receptor inhibitor increases the therapeutic window for low-dose tissue plasminogen administration in a rat model of embolic stroke. *Circulation* 2003;107:2837–2843.

213. Zhang L, Shang ZG, Zhang RL, et al. Postischemic (6-hour) treatment with recombinant human tissue plasminogen activator and proteasome inhibitor PS-519 reduces infarction in a rat model of embolic focal cerebral ischemia. *Stroke* 2001;32:2926–2931.

214. Bosch X, Marrugat J. Platelet glycoprotein IIb/IIIa blockers for percutaneous coronary revascularization, and unstable angina and non-ST-segment elevation myocardial infarction. *Cochrane Database Syst Rev* 2001;CD002130.

215. Kastrati A, Mehilli J, Schlotterbeck K, et al. Early administration of reteplase plus abciximab vs. abciximab alone in patients with acute myocardial infarction referred for percutaneous coronary intervention. A randomized controlled trial. *JAMA* 2004;291:947–954.

216. Chen ZM, Sandercock P, Pan HC, et al. Indications for early aspirin use in acute ischemic stroke: a combined analysis of 40 000 randomized patients from the Chinese acute stroke trial and the international stroke trial. On behalf of the CAST and IST collaborative groups. *Stroke* 2000;31:1240–1249.

217. The Abciximab in Ischemic Stroke Investigators. Abciximab in acute ischemic stroke. A randomized, double-blind, placebo-controlled, dose-escalation study. *Stroke* 2000;31:601–609.

218. Abciximab Emergent Stroke Treatment Trial (AbESTT) Investigators. Emergency administration of abciximab for treatment of patients with acute ischemic stroke. Results of a randomized, phase 2 trial. *Stroke* 2005;36:880–890.

219. Morris DC, Silver B, Mitsias P, et al. Treatment of acute stroke with recombinant tissue plasminogen activator and abciximab. *Acad Emerg Med* 2003;10:1396–1399.

220. Sandercock P, Gubitz G, Foley P, Counsell C. Antiplatelet therapy for acute ischaemic stroke. *Cochrane Database Syst Rev* 2003;CD000029.

221. Read SJ, Hirano T, Davis SM, Donnan GA. Limiting neurological damage after stroke: a review of pharmacological treatment options. *Drugs Aging* 1999;14:11–39.

222. Roden-Jullig A, Britton M, Malmkvist K, Leijd B. Aspirin in the prevention of progressing stroke: a randomized controlled study. *J Intern Med* 2003;254:584–590.

223. Sarma GR, Roy AK. Nadroparin plus aspirin versus aspirin alone in the treatment of acute ischemic stroke. *Neurol India* 2003;51:208–210.

224. Seitz RJ, Hamzavi M, Junghans U, Ringleb PA, Schranz C, Siebler M. Thrombolysis with recombinant tissue plasminogen activator and tirofiban in stroke. Preliminary observations. *Stroke* 2003;34:1932–1935.

225. Liebeskind DS, Pollard JR, Schwartz ED, Cucchiara BL, McGarvey ML, Hurst RW. Verterbrobasilar thrombolysis with intravenous tirofiban: case report. *J Thromb Thrombolysis* 2002;13:84–91.

226. Junghans U, Seitz RJ, Aulich A, Freund H-J, Siebler M. Bleeding risk of tirofiban, a nonpeptide GPIIb/IIIa platelet receptor antagonist in progressive stroke: an open pilot study. *Cerebrovasc Dis* 2001;12:308–312.

227. Staub S, Junghans U, Jovanovic V, Wittsack HJ, Seitz RJ, Siebler M. Systematic thrombolysis with recombinant tissue plasminogen activator and tirofiban in acute middle cerebral artery occlusion. *Stroke* 2004;35:705–709.

228. Ho DS, Wang Y, Chui M, Ho SL, Cheung RT. Intracarotid abciximab injection to abort impending ischemic stroke during carotid angioplasty. *Cerebrovasc Dis* 2001;11:300–304.

229. Lee DH, Jo KD, Kim HG, et al. Local intra-arterial urokinase thrombolysis of acute ischemic stroke with or without intravenous abciximab: a pilot study. *J Vasc Interv Radiol* 2002;13:769–773.

230. Kwon O-K, Lee KJ, Han MH, Oh C-W, Han DH, Koh YC. Intra-arterially administered abciximab as an adjuvant thrombolytic therapy: report of three cases. *AJNR Am J Neuroradiol* 2002;23:447–451.

231. Kapadia SR, Bajzer CT, Ziada KM, et al. Initial experience of platelet glycoprotein IIb/IIIa inhibition with abciximab during carotid stenting: a safe and effective adjunctive therapy. *Stroke* 2001;32:2328–2332.

232. Fisher M, Davalos A. Emerging therapies for cerebrovascular disorders. *Stroke* 2004;35:367–379.

233. Rordorf G, Koroshetz WJ, Ezzeddine MA, Segal AZ, Buonanna FS. A pilot study of drug-induced hypertension for treatment of acute stroke. *Neurology* 2001;56:1210–1213.

234. Mistri AK, Robinson TG, Potter JF. Pressor therapy in acute ischemic stroke. Systematic review. *Stroke* 2006;37:1565–1571.

235. Mayberg MR, Batjer HH, Dacey R, et al. Guidelines for the management of aneurysmal subarachnoid hemorrhage. A statement for healthcare professionals from a special writing group of the Stroke Council, American Heart Association. *Stroke* 1994;25:2315–2328.

236. Kassell NF, Peerless SJ, Durward QJ, Beck DW, Drake CG, Adams HP, Jr. Treatment of ischemic deficits from vasospasm with intravascular volume expansion and induced arterial hypertension. *Neurosurgery* 1982;11:337–343.

237. Hillis AE, Ulatowski JA, Barker PB, et al. A pilot randomized trial of induced blood pressure elevation: effects on function and focal perfusion in acute and subacute stroke. *Cerebrovasc Dis* 2003;16:236–246.

238. Marzan AS, Hungerbühler H-J, Studer A, Baumgartner RW, Georgiadis D. Feasibility and safety of norepinephrine-induced arterial hypertension in acute ischemic stroke. *Neurology* 2004;62:1193–1195.

239. Mohiuddin AA, Bath FJ, Bath PMW. Theophylline, aminophylline, caffeine and analogues for acute ischaemic stroke. *Cochrane Database Syst Rev* 2000;CD000211.

240. Piriyawat P, Labiche LA, Burgin WS, Aronowski JA, Grotta JC. Pilot dose-escalation study of caffeine plus ethanol (caffeinol) in acute ischemic stroke. *Stroke* 2003;34:1242–1245.

241. Bereczki D, Fekete I. Vinpocetine for acute ischaemic stroke. *Cochrane Database Syst Rev* 2000;CD000480.

242. Schneider R. Results of hemorheologically active treatment with pentoxifylline in patients with cerebrovascular disease. *Angiology* 1989;40:987–993.

243. Bath PMW, Bath FJ, Asplund K. Pentoxifylline, propentofylline and pentifylline for acute ischaemic stroke. *Cochrane Database Syst Rev* 2000;CD000162.

244. Bath PMW, Bath FJ. Prostacyclin and analogues for acute ischaemic stroke. *Cochrane Database Syst Rev* 2000; CD000177.

245. Walzl M, Schied G, Walzl B. Effects of ameliorated haemorheology on clinical symptoms in cerebrovascular disease. *Atherosclerosis* 1998;139:385–389.

246. Gross CE, Bednar MM, Lew SM, Florman JE, Kohut JJ. Preoperative volume expansion improves tolerance to carotid artery cross-clamping during endarterectomy. *Neurosurgery* 1998;43:222–226.

247. Matthews WB, Oxbury JM, Grainger KM, Greenhall RC. A blind controlled trial of dextran 40 in the treatment of ischaemic stroke. *Brain* 1976;99:193–206.

248. Saxena R, Wijnhoud AD, Carton H, et al. Controlled safety study of hemoglobin-based oxygen carrier, DCLHb, in acute ischemic stroke. *Stroke* 1999;30:993–996.

249. The Hemodilution in Stroke Study Group. Hypervolemic hemodilution treatment of acute stroke. Results of a randomized multicenter trial using pentastarch. *Stroke* 1989; 20:317–323.

250. Kaste M, Fogelholm R, Waltimo O. Combined dexamethasone and low-molecular-weight dextran in acute brain infarction: double-blind study. *Br Med J* 1976;2:1409–1410.

251. Strand T. Evaluation of long-term outcome and safety after hemodilution therapy in acute ischemic stroke. *Stroke* 1992;23:657–662.

252. Hsu CY, Norris JW, Hogan EL, et al. Pentoxifylline in acute nonhemorrhagic stroke. A randomized, placebo-controlled double-blind trial. *Stroke* 1988;19:716–722.

253. Italian Acute Stroke Study Group. Haemodilution in acute stroke: results of the Italian haemodilution trial. *Lancet* 1988;1:318–321.

254. Scandinavian Stroke Study Group. Multicenter trial of hemodilution in acute ischemic stroke. Results of subgroup analyses. *Stroke* 1988;19:464–471.

255. Asplund K. Hemodilution in acute stroke. *Cerebrovasc Dis* 1991;1(suppl 1):129–138.

256. Asplund K. Haemodilution for acute ischaemic stroke. *Cochrane Database Syst Rev* 2002;CD000103.

257. Berrouschot J, Barthel H, Scheel C, Koster J, Schneider D. Extracorporeal membrane differential filtration—a new

and safe method to optimize hemorheology in acute ischemic stroke. *Acta Neurol Scand* 1998;97:126–130.

258. Berrouschot J, Barthel H, Koster J, et al. Extracorporeal rheopheresis in the treatment of acute ischemic stroke: a randomized pilot study. *Stroke* 1999;30:787–792.

259. Rossler A, Berrouschot J, Barthel H, Hesse S, Koster J, Schneider D. Potential of rheopheresis for the treatment of acute ischemic stroke when initiated between 6 and 12 hours. *Ther Apher* 2000;4:358–362.

260. Frazee JG, Luo X, Luan G, et al. Retrograde transvenous neuroperfusion: a back door treatment for stroke. *Stroke* 1998;29:1912–1916.

261. Meyer FB, Piepgras DG, Sundt TMJ. Emergency embolectomy for acute occlusion of the middle cerebral artery. *J Neurosurg* 1985;62:639–647.

262. Walters BB, Ojemann RG, Heros RC. Emergency carotid endarterectomy. *J Neurosurg* 1987;66:817–823.

263. Eckstein HH, Schumacher H, Klemm K, et al. Emergency carotid endarterectomy. *Cerebrovasc Dis* 1999;9:270–281.

264. Eckstein HH, Schumacher H, Dorfler A, et al. Carotid endarterectomy and intracranial thrombolysis: simultaneous and staged procedures in ischemic stroke. *J Vasc Surg* 1999;29:459–471.

265. Schneider C, Johansen K, Konigstein R. Emergency carotid thromboendarterectomy: safe and effective. *World J Surg* 1999;23:1163–1167.

266. Gay J, Curtil A, Buffliere S, Favre J, Barral X. Urgent carotid artery repair: retrospective study of 21 cases. *Ann Vasc Surg* 2002;16:401–406.

267. Huber R, Muller BT, Seitz RJ, Siebler M, Modder U, Sandmann W. Carotid surgery in acute symptomatic patients. *Eur J Vasc Endovasc Surg* 2003;25:60–67.

268. Krishnamurthy S, Tong D, McNamara KP, Steinberg GK, Cockroft KM. Early carotid endarterectomy after ischemic stroke improves diffusion/perfusion mismatch resonance imaging: report of two cases. *Neurosurgery* 2003;52:238–242.

269. Linskey ME, Sekhar LN, Hecht ST. Emergency embolectomy for embolic occlusion of the middle cerebral artery after internal carotid artery balloon test occlusion. Case report. *J Neurosurg* 1992;77:134–138.

270. Kakinuma K, Ezuka I, Takai N, Yamamoto K, Sasaki O. The simple indicator for revascularization of acute middle cerebral artery occlusion using angiogram and ultraearly embolectomy. *Surg Neurol* 1999;51:332–341.

271. Leary MC, Saver JL, Gobin YP, et al. Beyond tissue plasminogen activator: mechanical intervention in acute stroke. *Ann Emerg Med* 2003;41:838–846.

272. Qureshi AI, Siddiqui AM, Suri MFK, et al. Aggressive mechanical clot disruption and low-dose intra-arterial third-generation thrombolytic agent for ischemic stroke: a prospective study. *Neurosurgery* 2002;51:1319–1329.

273. Smith WS, Sung G, Starkman S, et al. Safety and efficacy of mechanical embolectomy in acute ischemic stroke. Results of the MERCI Trial. *Stroke* 2005;36:1432–1438.

274. Choi JH, Bateman BT, Mangla S, et al. Endovascular recanalization therapy in acute ischemic stroke. *Stroke* 2006;37:419–424.

275. Ringer AJ, Qureshi AI, Fessler RD, Guterman LR, Hopkins LN. Angioplasty of intracranial occlusion resistant to thrombolysis in acute ischemic stroke. *Neurosurgery* 2001; 48:1282–1288.

276. Qureshi AI, Ali Z, Suri MFK, et al. Intra-arterial third-generation recombinant tissue plasminogen activator (reteplase) for acute ischemic stroke. *Neurosurgery* 2001; 49:41–50.

277. Alexandrov AV, Molina CA, Grotta JC, et al. Ultrasound enhanced systemic thrombolysis for acute ischemic stroke. *N Engl J Med* 2004;351:2170–2178.

278. Behrens S, Spengos K, Daffertshofer M, Schroeck H, Dempfle CE, Hennerici M. Transcranial ultrasound-improved thrombolysis: diagnostic vs. therapeutic ultrasound. *Ultrasound Med Biol* 2002;27:1683–1689.

279. Albers GW. Rationale for early intervention in acute stroke. *Am J Cardiol* 1997;80:4D–10D.

280. Lees KR. Neuroprotection. *Br Med Bull* 2000;56:401–412.

281. Lutsep HL, Clark WM. Neuroprotection in acute ischaemic stroke. Current status and future potential. *Drugs R D* 2002;1:3–8.

282. Wahlgren NG, Ahmed N. Neuroprotection in cerebral ischaemia: facts and fancies—the need for new approaches. *Cerebrovasc Dis* 2004;17(suppl 1):153–166.

283. Muir KW, Lees KR. Excitatory amino acid antagonists for acute stroke. *Cochrane Database Syst Rev* 2003; CD001244.

284. Stieg PE, Sathi S, Warach S, Le DA, Lipton SA. Neuroprotection by the NMDA receptor-associated open-channel blocker memantine in a photothrombotic model of cerebral focal ischemia in neonatal rat. *Eur J Pharmacol* 1999;375:115–120.

285. Grotta J, Clark W, Coull B, et al. Safety and tolerability of the glutamate antagonist CGS 19755 (selfotel) in patients with acute ischemic stroke: results of a phase IIa randomized trial. *Stroke* 1995;26:602–605.

286. Morris GF, Bullock R, Marshall SB, et al. Failure of the competitive *N*-methyl-D-aspartate antagonist selfotel (CGS 19755) in the treatment of severe head injury: results of two phase III clinical trials. *J Neurosurg* 1999; 91:737–743.

287. Davis SM, Lees KR, Albers GW, et al. Selfotel in acute ischemic stroke. Possible neurotoxic effects of an NMDA antagonist. *Stroke* 2000;31:347–354.

288. Albers GW, Goldstein LB, Hall D, Lesko LM. Aptiganel hydrochloride in acute ischemic stroke: a randomized controlled trial. *JAMA* 2001;286:2673–2682.

289. Dyker AG, Edwards KR, Fayad PB, Hormes JT, Lees KR. Safety and tolerability study of aptiganel hydrochloride in patients with an acute ischemic stroke. *Stroke* 1999;30: 2038–2042.

290. Albers GW, Saenz RE, Moses JAJ, Choi DW. Safety and tolerance of oral dextromethorphan in patients at risk for brain ischemia. *Stroke* 1991;22:1075–1077.

291. Albers GW, Atkinson RP, Kelley RE, Rosenbaum DM. Safety, tolerability, and pharmacokinetics of the N-methyl-D-aspartate antagonist dextrophan in patients with acute stroke. Dextrophan Study Group. *Stroke* 1995; 26:254–258.

292. Arrowsmith JE, Harrison MJ, Newman SP, Stygall J, Timberlake N, Pugsley WB. Neuroprotection of the brain during cardiopulmonary bypass: a randomized trial of

remacemide during coronary artery bypass in 171 patients. *Stroke* 1998;29:2357–2362.

293. Dyker AG, Lees KR. Remacemide hydrochloride: a double-blind, placebo-controlled, safety and tolerability study in patients with acute ischemic stroke. *Stroke* 1999; 30:1796–1801.

294. Orgogozo J, Rigaud A, Stoffler A, Mobius H, Forette F. Efficacy and safety of memantine in patients with mild moderate vascular dementia. A randomized, placebo-controlled trial (MMM 300). *Stroke* 2002;33:1834–1839.

295. Diener HC, Alkhedr A, Busse O, et al. Treatment of acute ischemic stroke with the low-affinity, use-dependent NMDA antagonist AR-R15896AR: a safety and tolerability study. *J Neurol* 2002;249:518–528.

296. Lees KR, Lavelle JF, Cunha L, et al. Glycine antagonist (GV1505526) in acute stroke: a multicentre, double-blind placebo-controlled phase II trial. *Cerebrovasc Dis* 2001; 11:20–29.

297. Sacco RL, DeRosa JT, Haley EC, Jr., et al. Glycine antagonist in neuroprotection for patients with acute stroke: GAIN Americas: a randomized controlled trial. *JAMA* 2001;285:1719–1728.

298. Dyker AG, Lees KR. Safety and tolerability of GV150526 (a glycine site antagonist at the N-methyl-D-aspartate receptor) in patients with acute stroke. *Stroke* 1999;30:986–992.

299. Albers GW, Clark WM, Atkinson RP, Madden K, Data JL, Whitehouse MJ. Dose escalation study of the NMDA glycine-site antagonist licostinel in acute ischemic stroke. *Stroke* 1999;30:508–513.

300. Lees KR. Cerestat and other NMDA antagonists in ischemic stroke. *Neurology* 1997;49(suppl 4):S66–S69.

301. Weiser T. AMPA receptor antagonists with additional mechanisms of action: new opportunities for neuroprotective drugs? *Curr Pharm Des* 2002;8:941–951.

302. Muir KW, Lees KR. Clinical experience with excitatory amino acid antagonist drugs. *Stroke* 1995;26:503–513.

303. Diener HC, Hacke W, Hennerici M, Radberg J, Hantson L, De Keyser J. Lubeluzole in acute ischemic stroke. A double-blind, placebo-controlled phase II trial. Lubeluzole International Study Group. *Stroke* 1996;27:76–81.

304. Grotta J. Lubeluzole treatment of acute ischemic stroke. The US and Canadian Lubeluzole Ischemic Stroke Study Group. *Stroke* 1997;28:2338–2246.

305. Diener HC, Cortens M, Ford G, et al. Lubeluzole in acute ischemic stroke treatment: a double-blind study with an 8-hour inclusion window comparing a 10-mg daily dose of lubeluzole with placebo. *Stroke* 2000;31:2543–2351.

306. Grotta J, The Combination Therapy Stroke Trial Investigators. Combination Therapy Stroke Trial: recombinant tissue-type plasminogen activator with/without lubeluzole. *Cerebrovasc Dis* 2001;12:258–263.

307. Gandolfo C, Sandercock P, Conti M. Lubeluzole for acute ischaemic stroke. *Cochrane Database Syst Rev* 2002; CD001924.

308. Muir KW. New experimental and clinical data on the efficacy of pharmacological magnesium infusions in cerebral infarcts. *Magnes Res* 1998;11:43–56.

309. Muir KW. Magnesium for neuroprotection in ischaemic stroke: rationale for use and evidence of effectiveness. *CNS Drugs* 2001;15:921–930.

310. Muir KW. Magnesium in stroke treatment. *Postgrad Med J* 2002;78:641–645.

311. Muir KW, Lees KR. Dose optimization of intravenous magnesium sulfate after acute stroke. *Stroke* 1998;29:918–923.

312. Muir KW, Lees KR. A randomized, double-blind, placebo-controlled pilot trial of intravenous magnesium sulfate in acute stroke. *Stroke* 1995;26:1183–1188.

313. Lampl Y, Gilad R, Geva D, Eshel Y, Sadeh M. Intravenous administration of magnesium sulfate in acute stroke: a randomized double-blind study. *Clin Neuropharmacol* 2001;24:11–15.

314. Muir KW, Lees KR, Ford I, Davis S, Intravenous Magnesium Efficacy in Stroke (IMAGES) Study Investigators. Magnesium for acute stroke (Intravenous Magnesium Efficacy in Stroke Trial): randomised controlled trial. *Lancet* 2004;363:439–445.

315. Kobayashi T, Mori Y. Ca2+ channel antagonists and neuroprotection from cerebral ischemia. *Eur J Pharmacol* 1998;363:1–15.

316. Kaste M, Fogelholm R, Erila T, et al. A randomized, double-blind, placebo-controlled trial of nimodipine in acute ischemic hemispheric stroke. *Stroke* 1994;25:1348–1353.

317. Bogousslavsky J, Regli F, Zumstein V, Kobberling W. Double-blind study of nimodipine in non-severe stroke. *Eur Neurol* 1990;30:23–26.

318. Wahlgren NG, MacMahon DG, DeKeyser J, Indredavik B, Ryman T. Intravenous Nimodipine West European Stroke Trial (INWEST) of nimodipine in the treatment of acute ischaemic stroke. *Cerebrovasc Dis* 1994;4:204–210.

319. Horn J, de Haan RJ, Vermeulen M, Limburg M. Very early nimodipine use in stroke (VENUS): a randomized, double-blind, placebo-controlled trial. *Stroke* 2001;32:461–465.

320. Rosenbaum D, Zabramski J, Frey J, et al. Early treatment of ischemic stroke with a calcium antagonist *Stroke* 1991;22:437–441.

321. Franke CL, Palm R, Dalby M, et al. Flunarizine in stroke treatment (FIST): a double-blind, placebo-controlled trial in Scandinavia and the Netherlands. *Acta Neurol Scand* 1996;93:56–60.

322. Azcona A, Lataste X. Isradipine in patients with acute ischaemic cerebral infarction: an overview of ASCLEPIOS programme. *Drugs* 1990;40(suppl 2):52–57.

323. Oczkowski WJ, Hachinski VC, Bogousslavsky J, Barnett HJ, Carruthers SG. A double-blind, randomized trial of PY 108-068 in acute ischemic cerebral infarction. *Stroke* 1989;20:604–608.

324. Horn, Limburg M. Calcium antagonists for acute ischemic stroke. *Cochrane Database Syst Rev* 2000;CD001928.

325. The RANTTAS Investigators. A randomized trial of tirilazad mesylate in patients with acute stroke (RANTTAS). *Stroke* 1996;27:1453–1458.

326. Bath PM, Iddenden R, Bath FJ, Orgogozo JM, The Tirilazad International Steering Committee. Tirilazad for acute ischaemic stroke. *Cochrane Database Syst Rev* 2001; CD002087.

327. Endaravone Acute Infarction Study Group. Effect of a novel free radical scavenger, edaravone (MCI-186), on acute brain infarction. Randomized, placebo-controlled, double-blind study at multicenters. *Cerebrovasc Dis* 2003; 15:222–229.

328. Lees KR, Zivin JR, Ashwood T, et al. NKY-059 for acute ischemic stroke. *N Engl J Med* 2006;354:588–600.

329. Lyden P, Jacoby M, Schim J, et al. The Clomethiazole Acute Stroke Study in tissue-type plaminogen activator-treated stroke (CLASS-T): final results. *Neurology* 2001;57:1199–1205.

330. Wahlgren NG, Diez-Tejedor E, Teitelbaum JK. Results in 95 hemorrhagic stroke patients included in CLASS, a controlled trial of clomethiazole versus placebo in acute stroke patients. *Stroke* 2000;31:82–85.

331. Wahlgren NG, Bornhov S, Sharma A, et al. The Clomethiazole Acute Stroke Study (CLASS): efficacy results in 545 patients classified as total anterior circulation syndrome (TACS). *Cerebrovasc Dis* 1999;8:231–239.

332. Wahlgren NG, Ranasinha KW, Rosolacci T, et al. Clomethiazole acute stroke study (CLASS): results of a randomized, controlled trial of clomethiazole versus placebo in 1,360 acute stroke patients. *Stroke* 1999;30:21–28.

333. Wahlgren NG, The Clomethiazole Acute Stroke Study Collaborative Group. The clomethiazole acute stroke study (CLASS): results of a randomised controlled study of clomethiazole versus placebo in 1360 acute stroke patients. *Cerebrovasc Dis* 1997;7(suppl 4):24–30.

334. Wester P, Strand T, Wahlgren NG, Ashwood T, Osswald G. An open study of clomethiazole in patients with acute cerebral infarction. *Cerebrovasc Dis* 1998;8:188–190.

335. Barsan WG, Olinger CP, Adams HP, Jr., et al. Use of high dose naloxone in acute stroke: possible side-effects. *Crit Care Med* 1989;17:762–727.

336. Olinger CP, Adams HP, Jr., Brott TG, et al. High-dose intravenous naloxone for the treatment of acute ischemic stroke. *Stroke* 1990;21:721–725.

337. Clark WM, Raps EC, Tong DC, Kelly RE, for the Cervene Stroke Study Investigators. Cervene (Nalmefene) in acute ischemic stroke. Final results of a phase III efficacy study. *Stroke* 2000;31:1234–1239.

338. Clark W, Ertag W, Orecchio E, Raps E. Cervene in acute ischemic stroke: results of a double-blind, placebo-controlled, dose-comparison study. *J Stroke Cerebrovasc Dis* 1999;8:224–230.

339. Clark WM, Warach SJ, Pettigrew LC, Gammans RE, Sabounjian LA. A randomized dose-response trial of citicoline in acute ischemic stroke patients. Citicoline Stroke Study Group. *Neurology* 1997;49:671–678.

340. Clark WM, Williams BJ, Selzer KA, et al. A randomized efficacy trial of citicoline in patients with acute ischemic stroke. *Stroke* 1999;30:2592–2597.

341. Clark WM, Wechsler LR, Sabounjian LA, Schwiderski UE, Citicoline Stroke Study Group. A phase III randomized efficacy trial of 2000 mg citicoline in acute ischemic stroke patients. *Neurology* 2001;57:1595–1602.

342. Davalos A, Castillo J, Alvarez-Sabín J, et al. Oral citicoline in acute ischemic stroke: an individual patient data pooling analysis of clinical trials. *Stroke* 2002;33:2850–2857.

343. Martinez-Vila E, Sieira PI. Current status and perspectives of neuroprotection in ischemic stroke treatment. *Cerebrovasc Dis* 2001;11:60–70.

344. Lenzi GL, Grigoletto F, Gent M, et al. Early treatment of stroke with monosialoganglioside GM-1. Efficacy and safety results of the Early Stroke Trial. *Stroke* 1994;25:1552–1558.

345. The SASS Trial. Ganglioside GM1 in acute ischemic stroke. *Stroke* 1994;25:1141–1148.

346. Bassi S, Albizzati MG, Sbacchi M, Frattola L, Massarotti M. Double-blind evaluation of monosialoganglioside (GM1) therapy in stroke. *J Neurosci Res* 1984;12:493–498.

347. Argentino C, Sacchetti ML, Toni D, et al. GM1 ganglioside therapy in acute ischemic stroke. *Stroke* 1989;20:1143–1149.

348. Candelise L, Ciccone A. Gangliosides for acute ischaemic stroke. *Cochrane Database Syst Rev* 2001;CD000094.

349. Lapchak PA, Zivin JA. Ebselen, a seleno-organic antioxidant, is neuroprotective after embolic strokes in rabbits. Synergism with low-dose tissue plasminogen activator. *Stroke* 2003;34:2013–2038.

350. Ogawa A, Yoshimoto T, Kikuchi H, et al. Ebselen in acute middle cerebral artery occlusion: a placebo-controlled, double-blind clinical trial. *Cerebrovasc Dis* 1999;9:112–118.

351. De Deyn PP, Reuck JD, Deberdt W, Vlietinck R, Orgogozo JM. Treatment of acute ischemic stroke with piracetam. Members of the Piracetam in Acute Stroke Study (PASS) Group. *Stroke* 1997;28:2347–2352.

352. De Reuck J, Van Vleymen B. The clinical safety of high-dose piracetam—its use in the treatment of acute stroke. *Pharmacopsychiatry* 1999;32(suppl 1):33–37.

353. Huber W. The role of piracetam in the treatment of acute and chronic aphasia. *Pharmacopsychiatry* 1999;32(suppl 1):38–43.

354. Orgogozo JM. Piracetam in the treatment of acute stroke. *Pharmacopsychiatry* 1999;32(suppl 1):25–32.

355. Ricci S, Celani MG, Cantisani AT, Righetti E. Piracetam for acute ischaemic stroke. *Cochrane Database Syst Rev* 2002;CD000419.

356. Lutsep HL. Repinotan Bayer. *Curr Opin Investig Drugs* 2002;3:924–927.

357. Bath PMW, Willmot M, Leonardi-Bee J, Bath FJ. Nitric oxide donors (nitrates), L-arginine, or nitric oxide synthase inhibitors for acute stroke. *Cochrane Database Syst Rev* 2002;CD000398.

358. von Lubitz DK. Adenosine in the treatment of stoke: yes, maybe or absolutely not? *Expert Opin Investig Drugs* 2001;10:619–632.

359. Bitterman H, Melamed Y. Delayed hyperbaric treatment of cerebral air embolism. *Isr J Med Sci* 1993;29:22–26.

360. Nighoghossian N, Trouillas P, Adeleine P, Salord F. Hyperbaric oxygen in the treatment of acute ischemic stroke. A double-blind pilot study. *Stroke* 1995;26:1369–1372.

361. Nighoghossian N, Trouillas P. Hyperbaric oxygen in the treatment of acute ischemic stroke: an unsettled issue. *J Neurol Sci* 1997;150:27–31.

362. Rusyniak DE, Kirk MA, May JD, et al. Hyperbaric oxygen therapy in acute ischemic stroke: results of the hyperbaric oxygen in acute ischemic stroke trial pilot study. *Stroke* 2003;34:571–574.

363. Berger C, Schwab S, Georgiadis D, Steiner T, Aschoff A. Effects of hypothermia on excitatory amino acids and metabolism in stroke patients: a microdialysis study. *Stroke* 2002;33:519–524.

364. Kollmar R, Schabitz WR, Heiland S, et al. Neuroprotective effect of delayed moderate hypothermia after focal cerebral ischemia. An MRI study. *Stroke* 2002;33:1899–1904.

365. Krieger DW. Therapeutic hypothermia may enhance reperfusion in acute ischemic stroke. *Cleve Clin J Med* 2004;71(suppl 1):S39.

366. Jian S, Yongming Q, Zhihua C, Yan C. Feasibility and safety of moderate hypothermia after acute ischemic stroke. *Int J Dev Neurosci* 2003;21:353–356.

367. Krieger DW, Yenari MA. Therapeutic hypothermia for acute ischemic stroke. What do laboratory studies teach us? *Stroke* 2004;35:1482–1489.

368. Bernard SA, Gray TW, Buist M, et al. Treatment of comatose survivors of out-of-hospital cardiac arrest with induced hypothermia. *N Engl J Med* 2002;346:557–563.

369. Georgiadis D, Schwarz S, Aschoff A, Schwab S. Hemicraniectomy and moderate hypothermia in patients with severe ischemic stoke. *Stroke* 2002;33:1568–1573.

370. Schmid-Elsaesser R, Hungerhuber E, Zausinger S, Baethmann A, Reulen HJ. Combination drug therapy and mild hypothermia. A promising treatment strategy for reversible, focal cerebral ischemia. *Stroke* 1999;30:1891–1899.

371. Olsen TS, Weber UJ, Kammersgaard LP. Therapeutic hypothermia for acute stroke. *Lancet Neurol* 2003;2:410–416.

372. Feigin VL, Anderson CS, Rodgers A, Anderson NE, Gunn AJ. The emerging role of induced hypothermia in the management of acute stroke. *J Clin Neurosci* 2002;9:502–507.

373. Schwab S, Schwarz S, Aschoff A, Keller E, Hacke W. Moderate hypothermia and brain temperature in patients with severe middle cerebral artery infarction. *Acta Neurochir Suppl (Wien)* 1998;71:131–134.

374. Keller E, Imhof HG, Gasser S, Terzic A, Yonekawa Y. Endovascular cooling with heat exchange catheters: a new method to induce and maintain hypothermia. *Intensive Care Med* 2003;29:939–943.

375. Krieger D, De Georgia M, Abou-Chebl A, et al. Cooling for acute ischemic brain damage (cool aid): an open pilot study of induced hypothermia in acute ischemic stroke. *Stroke* 2002;32:1847–1854.

376. Correia M, Silva M, Veloso M. Cooling therapy for acute stroke. *Cochrane Database Syst Rev* 2000;CD001247.

377. Hammer MD, Krieger DW. Hypothermia for acute ischemic stroke: not just another neuroprotectant. *Neurology* 2003;9:280–289.

378. Enlimomab Acute Stroke Trial Investigators. Use of anti-ICAM-1 therapy in ischemic stroke: results of the Enlimomab Acute Stroke Trial. *Neurology* 2001;57:1428–1434.

379. Krams M, Lees KR, Hacke W, et al. Acute stroke therapy by inhibition of neutrophils (ASTIN). An adaptive dose-response study of UK-279,276 in acute ischemic stroke. *Stroke* 2003;34:2543–2548.

380. Eid T, Brines M. Recombinant human erythropoietin for neuroprotection: what is the evidence? *Clin Breast Cancer* 2002;3(suppl 3):S109–S115.

381. Goldstein LB. Potential effects of common drugs on stroke recovery. *Arch Neurol* 1998;55:454–456.

382. Goldstein LB. Common drugs may influence motor recovery after stroke. The Sygen in Acute Stroke Study Investigators. *Neurology* 1995;45:865–871.

383. Goldstein LB, Davis JN. Restorative neurology. Drugs and recovery following stroke. *Stroke* 1990;21:1636–1640.

384. Wechsler LR. Stem cell transplantation for stroke. *Cleve Clin J Med* 2004;71(suppl 1):S40–S41.

385. Savitz SI, Rosenbaum D, Dinsmore JH, Wechsler LR, Caplan LR. Cell transplantation for stroke. *Ann Neurol* 2002;266:275.

386. Cairns K, Finklestein SP. Growth factors and stem cells as treatments for stroke recovery. *Phys Med Rehabil Clin N Am* 2003;14(suppl 1):S135–S142.

387. Roitberg B. Transplantation for stroke. *Neurol Res* 2004;26:256–264.

388. Chopp M, Li Y. Treatment of neural injury with marrow stromal cells. *Lancet Neurol* 2002;1:92–100.

389. Modo M, Stroemer P, Tang E, Patel S, Hodges H. Effects of implantation site of stem cell grafts on behavioral recovery from stroke damage. *Stroke* 2002;33:2270–2278.

390. Li Y, Chen J, Wang L, Lu M, Chopp M. Treatment of stroke in rat with intracarotid administration of marrow stromal cells. *Neurology* 2001;566:1666–1672.

391. Gunnett CA, Heistad DD. The future of gene therapy for stroke. *Curr Hypertens Rep* 2001;3:36–40.

392. Yenari MA, Zhao H, Giffard RG, Sobel RA, Sapolsky RM, Steinberg GK. Gene therapy and hypothermia for stroke treatment. *Ann N Y Acad Sci* 2003;993:54–68.

393. Bogousslavsky J, Victor SJ, Salinas EO, et al. Fiblast (trafermin) in acute stroke: results of the European–Australian phase II/III safety and efficacy trial. *Cerebrovasc Dis* 2002;14:239–251.

394. Lapchak PA. Hemorrhagic transformation following ischemic stroke: significance, causes, and relationship to therapy and treatment. *Curr Neurol Neurosci Rep* 2002;2:38–43.

CHAPTER 23
Treatment of Hemorrhagic Stroke

In comparison to management of acute ischemic stroke, research has lagged on the medical and surgical therapies to limit the neurological injuries secondary to hemorrhagic stroke. Despite this difference, oral nimodipine was the first agent approved for treatment of patients with any form of acute cerebrovascular disease—those with recent aneurysmal subarachnoid hemorrhage. Much of the management of intracranial hemorrhages is focused on interventions that are specifically aimed at treating the underlying cause. In particular, treatment of patients with ruptured intracranial aneurysms or vascular malformations has been emphasized.

Management of patients with hemorrhage involves both medical and surgical interventions (Table 23-1). Because of the very acute nature of the disease, many decisions about management of hemorrhage are made when the patient is first seen in an emergency department (see Chapter 21). Issues such as treating acute hypertension or an underlying coagulopathy are addressed within the first few hours after hemorrhage. Plans to evacuate a mass-producing intracranial hematoma or surgically decompress acute hydrocephalus also are made during this time (see Chapter 21). Still, the utility of emergency operations for treatment of patients with large cerebral hemorrhages has not been established.[1]

Evaluation for the cause of hemorrhage, which greatly affects subsequent treatment, is performed when the patient's condition has been stabilized. Much of the subsequent management is aimed at preventing or controlling medical or neurological complications of the bleeding (Table 23-2).

▶ GENERAL MANAGEMENT

Most patients with intracranial hemorrhage are admitted to an intensive care unit or stroke unit because treatment in such a nursing facility is associated with reduced mortality.[2–4] The utility of specialized management of patients with hemorrhage is confirmed by regional and statewide surveys. For example, in New York, Berman et al.[5] looked at the results of treatment of intracranial aneurysms. They found that those hospitals that are treating the largest number of patients had the best results. They concluded that the development of regional referral programs to transfer patients to specialized centers could improve outcomes after subarachnoid hemorrhage.

The components of acute care started in the emergency department usually are continued (see Chapter 21). Patients should have monitoring of vital signs and neurological assessments. Management should emphasize controlling intracranial pressure, brain edema, hydrocephalus, seizures, and medical complications.[2,6]

▶ HYPERTENSIVE HEMORRHAGE

Most hemorrhages secondary to hypertension occur deep in the cerebral hemispheres (basal ganglia, thalamus, and lobar white matter) (see Chapter 16). Other common locations are the brain stem and deep portions of the

▶ **TABLE 23-1.** TREATMENT OF PATIENTS
 HOSPITALIZED WITH INTRACRANIAL
 HEMORRHAGE

Continue monitoring
  Clinical observations
  Cardiovascular status
  Oxygen saturation
Intubation and ventilation
  Selective cases
  Early
 Blood pressure management
  Avoid high blood pressure
    Prevent recurrent bleeding
    Keep mean pressure ≤130 mm Hg
    Keep systolic pressure <180 mm Hg
  Avoid low blood pressure
    Prevent cerebral ischemia
    Keep systolic pressure >140 mm Hg
Keep normothermia
  Treat fever
Maintain hydration and nutrition
Give anticonvulsants only if seizures occur

cerebellum. Despite the typical location and the frequency of hypertensive hemorrhage, alternative causes for the intracranial bleeding should be sought, especially if the patient does not have other evidence for chronically elevated blood pressure. Usually the impairments secondary to a hypertensive hemorrhage are at maximal severity within a few hours of the ictus. Still, expansion probably secondary to continued bleeding from the primary ruptured artery or from disruption of surrounding blood vessels can occur.[2] The neurological impairments are secondary to both the mass effect of the hematoma and the destruction or compression of adjacent areas of

▶ **TABLE 23-2.** COMPLICATIONS OF
 HEMORRHAGIC STROKE

Recurrent hemorrhage	Hydrocephalus
Brain edema	Increased intracranial pressure
Convulsions	Vasospasm
Cerebral infarction	Neurogenic pulmonary edema
Cardiac arrhythmias	Myocardial infarction
Arterial hypertension	Pneumonia
Airway obstruction	Respiratory failure
Atelectasis	Hypoxia
Aspiration	Stress ulcers
Vomiting	Erosive gastritis
Gastrointestinal bleeding	Diabetes insipidus
Inappropriate secretion antidiuretic hormone	Dehydration
Cerebral salt wasting	Urinary tract infection
Pressure sores	Contractures
Pituitary dysfunction	

the brain. The secondary development of brain edema also leads to neurological worsening during the first days after hemorrhage. Management of arterial hypertension, which was often started in the emergency department, should continue. Lowering the blood pressure is particularly important among patients with bleeding secondary to an acute hypertensive crisis. In these situations, the elevated blood pressure might require frequent adjustments in medications or the use of multiple or parenteral agents (see Chapter 21).

Surgical Management

The main decision for subsequent treatment of the hematoma relates to whether surgical removal or aspiration of the blood should be attempted. Because the utility of surgery, including imaging-guided aspiration techniques, is not established, current guidelines provide general recommendations[6] (see Chapter 21). In general, surgery is reserved for patients who are deteriorating. However, patients with massive hypertensive hemorrhages who are in coma likely will not survive even with surgery, and palliative care may be the most appropriate response. Patients with small hemorrhages and those with bleeding causing minor neurological impairments generally are treated medically. Measures to prevent complications and rehabilitation should be recommended on a case-by-case basis (see Chapters 24 and 25). The risk of a second episode of bleeding occurring within the first few days is relatively low. The overall risk of a second hemorrhage within 2 years of the ictus is estimated as 2–5 percent.[7–10] Delayed recurrent hemorrhage is possible if the blood pressure is not adequately treated.[10–12] Long-term management should emphasize treatment of hypertension.[6]

▶ COAGULATION DISORDERS

Anticoagulant-related hemorrhage has a 30-day mortality of more than 50 percent.[13] Approximately 90 percent of patients with secondary intracranial bleeding who arrive in coma are dead within 1 month. Those with large hematomas or extension of bleeding within the ventricles also had a high mortality. Much of the management of bleeding secondary to a coagulation defect usually is performed in the emergency department. Early correction of the coagulopathy is important in minimizing growth of the hematoma.[14] Enlargement of the hematoma is common among patients whose international normalized ratio (INR) is greater than 2 at 24 h after hemorrhage.[15] Administration of antidotes such as protamine sulfate, vitamin K, platelets, or clotting factors is given to reverse the effects of antithrombotic medications or clotting disorders. Correction of the INR is important among patients with hemorrhage secondary to oral anticoagulants. Among patients with intracranial hemorrhage secondary to oral anticoagulants, vitamin K is supplemented by replacement with clotting factors. Mortality is lower among patients given fresh frozen plasma than among those treated with vitamin K or clotting factors.[13] However, the use of fresh frozen plasma requires time to type, cross match, thaw, and administer.[16] More rapid reversal of the anticoagulant effects is achieved with the use of recombinant activated factor VII. Besides treating hemophilia, Morenski et al.[16] also used recombinant activated factor VII to treat bleeding secondary to closed head injury. A trial testing the utility of recombinant activated factor VII in the early treatment of intracranial hemorrhage is planned.[17]

Some patients with bleeding were taking antithrombotic agents to prevent recurrent thromboembolic events. A potential scenario is the patient who has a high-risk cardiac lesion and a hemorrhage and is taking oral anticoagulants to prevent recurrent embolism. This patient likely will need to receive oral anticoagulants again but the primary question is when to reinitiate treatment. No data are available to guide this decision. Pessin et al.[18] found that anticoagulants could be continued safely among some patients despite the presence of a hemorrhagic infarction. While this experience implies that oral anticoagulants can be continued in exceptional cases, the most prudent course is to wait several days before starting the anticoagulants.[19] An interim course of heparin could be given as an initial step because its effects could be promptly reversed if bleeding recurs. Still, Keir et al.[19] found a high rate of recurrent bleeding with the use of heparin. On the other hand, restarting the oral anticoagulant at maintenance doses gradually achieves the desired level of antithrombotic effects and might be complicated by bleeding. Broderick et al.[6] recommended careful control of anticoagulation in order to reduce the risk of recurrent hemorrhage. In most instances, the desired INR is less than 3.

The risk of recurrent bleeding is probably less among patients taking antiplatelet agents. These medications, in particular aspirin, probably can be started when the patient is stable neurologically. Information about the safety of clopidogrel, combinations of antiplatelet agents, or the combination of antiplatelet agent and oral anticoagulant when started shortly after a brain hemorrhage is not available.

Presumably, the risk of bleeding is increased with the use of a combination of medications. There are no specific antidotes for the effects of antiplatelet agents. Platelet transfusions can be given.

Patients with inherited or other acquired disorders of coagulation, including hemophilia, leukemia, or thrombocytopenia, have a persisting risk for recurrent intracranial bleeding. Many of the affected patients are children. In general, management focuses on continued administration of factors to treat the underlying coagulopathy (see Chapter 14).

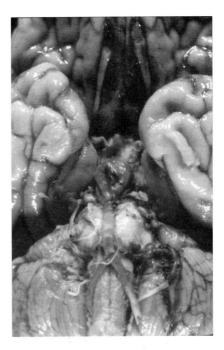

Figure 23-1. Basal view of the brain shows a large ruptured aneurysm arising at the distal portion (bifurcation) of the basilar artery.

► SACCULAR ANEURYSMS

Patients with ruptured saccular aneurysms are critically ill (Fig. 23-1). Approximately 50 percent of patients die as a consequence of the hemorrhage and one-third of the survivors have severe neurological sequelae.[20–22] Deaths and disability are the consequences of the initial hemorrhage, recurrent hemorrhage, vasospasm leading to cerebral infarction, or complications of medical or surgical procedures (Table 23-3). Acute effects of the subarachnoid hemorrhage include cardiac arrhythmias, electrolyte disturbances, seizures, hydrocephalus, and increased intracranial pressure (see Chapter 21). Elderly patients with ruptured aneurysms had higher rates of intraventricular hemorrhage, early hydrocephalus requiring drainage, and medical complications than do younger persons.[23]

► **TABLE 23-3.** LEADING CAUSES OF POOR OUTCOME OF ANEURYSMAL SUBARACHNOID HEMORRHAGE

Direct effects of initial hemorrhage
   Mass effect and increased intracranial pressure
   Brain injury
   Medical complications
Recurrent hemorrhage
Vasospasm and secondary ischemic stroke
Hydrocephalus
Complications of surgical interventions
Complications of medical interventions

▶ **TABLE 23-4.** COMPONENTS OF TREATMENT IN PATIENTS WITH RECENTLY RUPTURED ANEURYSMS

Close observation
Bed rest with restricted activity
    Assistance with self-care
    Gentle physical therapy—range of motion
    External pneumatic calf compression stockings
    Maintain hydration with intravenous saline
    Maintain nutrition
        Alert patients—soft, high-fiber diet
        Other patients—nasogastric feedings
    Stool softeners
    Antacids
Symptomatic treatment
    Analgesics—usually require narcotics
    Antiemetics—ondansetron
    Sedatives—short acting barbiturates or benzodiazepine
Anticonvulsant prophylaxis—phenytoin
Continue measures to treat cardiac arrhythmias or
    hypertension
Treat hyponatremia
    Administration of fluids—normal saline, hyperosmolar
        saline
    Generally avoid fluid restriction
    Avoid diuretics
Treat increased intracranial pressure
Prevent or treat vasospasm and secondary ischemia
    Avoid dehydration or arterial hypotension
    Treat increased intracranial pressure
    Nimodipine
    Hypervolemic hemodilution and drug-induced
        hypertension
    Intravenous administration of papaverine
    Angioplasty and stenting
Prevent rebleeding
    Antihypertensive agents
    Aminocaproic acid or tranexamic acid
    Surgical clipping
    Endovascular obliteration

Approximately 20–40 percent of patients with ruptured aneurysms have intracerebral hematomas.[20,24,25] Surgical evacuation of the hematoma may be necessary to treat mass effects and increased intracranial pressure (Table 23-4). Treatment of the hematoma and the aneurysm could be done simultaneously. For example, Su et al.[26] found that ultraearly surgical treatment of a ruptured aneurysm could be combined with aggressive medical treatment and ventriculostomy to manage patients with massive intrasylvian hematomas. Evacuation of a secondary subdural hematoma also can be done.[27]

Increased intracranial pressure secondary to acute hydrocephalus can be relieved, with the insertion of an intraventricular catheter. This interim measure might allow the patient to stabilize so that surgery can be performed.

Concerns have been expressed about the potential danger of placing an intraventricular catheter to lower intracranial pressure in a patient with a recently ruptured aneurysm. The sudden change in transmural pressure might promote recurrent bleeding. However, McIver et al.[28] reported that perioperative ventriculostomy was not accompanied by an increased risk of early recurrent hemorrhage.

Recurrent Hemorrhage

Rebleeding within the first few hours occurs in up to 15 percent of patients[29] (Fig. 23-2). The subsequent risk of rebleeding during the first 2 weeks is approximately 2 percent per day.[30,31] Overall, approximately 20 percent of patients have a recurrent hemorrhage within the first 10 days.[30] Thereafter, the likelihood of recurrent hemorrhage declines. At, 6 months, the risk of rebleeding drops to approximately 2.2 percent per year among patients whose aneurysms have not been treated surgically. The risk of early recurrent hemorrhage, which is often fatal, lends urgency to the accurate diagnosis of a ruptured aneurysm.[32] Although recurrent hemorrhage is most likely to occur among those patients who are already seriously ill from the initial bleeding event, all patients are at risk. Women and those who have severe hypertension also have a high risk of bleeding. No imaging factors predict rebleeding.

Presumably, the second hemorrhage occurs via the previous tear in the wall of the aneurysm. The

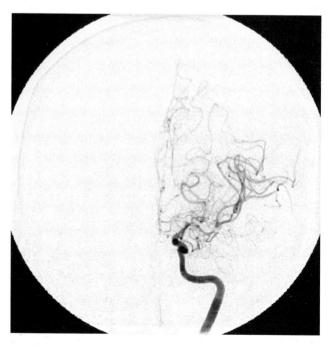

Figure 23-2. Anteroposterior view of a left carotid arteriogram shows narrowing (vasospasm) of the proximal segment of the middle cerebral artery.

perianeurysmal clot lyses through the effects of natural lysins, and thus the thrombus that could be buttressing the aneurysm wall is lost. Among the factors that promote rebleeding is a sudden surge in blood pressure or a seizure. Rebleeding is suspected if the patient has the sudden onset of a new, severe headache.[33] Other findings include a change in vital signs or worsening of the neurological status, including a decline in consciousness. However, recurrent hemorrhage can be missed if a patient already has depressed consciousness. Because new areas of blood can be detected on computed tomograhy (CT), it is the most useful diagnostic test. Examination of the cerebrospinal fluid is not particularly helpful in distinguishing a new hemorrhage from the previous one.[34] The differential diagnosis of rebleeding includes cerebral ischemia from vasospasm, brain edema, seizures, hydrocephalus, electrolyte disturbances, or complications from medications[33] (Table 23-5).

Medical Management

Several interventions have been used to lower the risk of rebleeding.[20] The most conservative measures include bed rest and close observation with the administration of sedatives, analgesics, and antihypertensive medications. The rationale for the use of antihypertensive agents is to lower transmural pressure. The results of these therapies have been unsatisfactory. In addition, the aggressive use of antihypertensive medications might increase the risk of ischemia secondary to vasospasm.

Antifibrinolytic medications (tranexamic acid and aminocaproic acid) have been used to lower the risk of recurrent hemorrhage[35] (Fig. 23-3). The rationale for these agents is that they would slow natural lysis of the

▶ **TABLE 23-5.** DIFFERENTIAL DIAGNOSIS OF NEUROLOGICAL WORSENING OF ANEURYSMAL SUBARACHNOID HEMORRHAGE

Recurrent aneurysmal rupture—rebleeding
Vasospasm—cerebral ischemia
Increased intracranial pressure
    Brain edema
    Subacute hydrocephalus
Seizures
Metabolic disturbance
    Hyponatremia
    Hypocalcemia
    Hypoxia
    Hypoglycemia
    Hyperglycemia
Medical complications
    Pneumonia
    Renal failure
    Hypotension
    Infections
Complications of medical interventions
Complications of surgical interventions

perianeurysmal thrombus and allow the patient to stabilize before other interventions are used to occlude the aneurysmal sac. These medications do lower the risk of rebleeding but neither mortality nor outcomes are improved.[36–39] Roos et al.[39] found that the combination of tranexamic acid and nimodipine was not effective. The benefit in prevention of recurrent hemorrhage is negated by an increased risk of ischemic stroke. Presumably, these agents promoted factors that augmented the development of vasospasm or secondary cerebral ischemia.

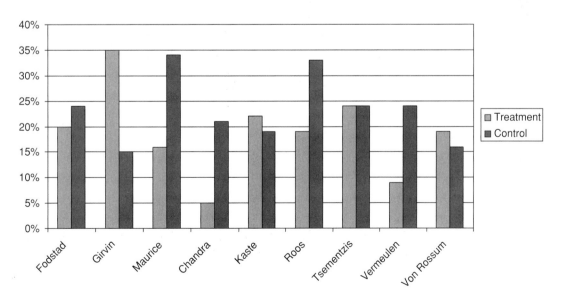

Figure 23-3. Rates of rebleeding—trials of antifibrinolytic therapy for aneurysmal subarachnoid hemorrhage. Adapted from references: 36, 39, 231–236.

Systemic reviews do not demonstrate utility of the administration of either tranexamic acid or aminocaproic acid for treatment of patients with aneurysmal subarachnoid hemorrhage.[40,41] Besides the risk of ischemia, these medications are associated with an increased risk of hydrocephalus or a fulminant myopathy. However, a very short course of antifibrinolytic therapy during the first hours following hemorrhage might help prevent early rebleeding while surgery or endovascular treatment is being arranged. Hillman et al.[42] reported that a short course of tranexamic acid might lower the likelihood of very early rebleeding (within 12 h) prior to surgical clipping of the aneurysm. They found no increase in ischemic symptoms secondary to the use of the medication. Additional research on such a tactic is needed.

Surgical Management

Direct surgical obliteration of the aneurysm (clipping) has been the mainstay of management to prevent recurrent rupture[20,43–46] (Fig. 23-4). Up until the mid-1980s, the usual approach was to allow the patient to recover from the effects of the initial hemorrhage before performing surgery. This delay, which was approximately of 2 weeks, was favored because the risks of early operation were considered unacceptably high. However, patients died of rebleeding while waiting for surgery. In addition, the development of vasospasm and cerebral ischemia occurred during the first 2 weeks compounded medical management. Efforts to prevent ischemia by expanding volume or increasing blood pressure could be accompanied by recurrent rupture of an untreated aneurysm. In addition, early surgery might be the setting for evacuation of the subarachnoid space with removal of clot, thus effectively reducing the risk of subsequent vasospasm. Although a large international study did not demonstrate the superiority of early surgery (usually more than 3 days

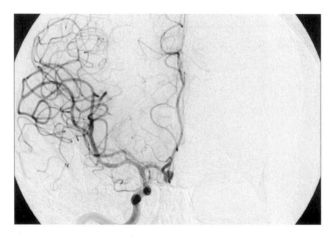

Figure 23-4. Anteroposterior view of a carotid arteriogram shows an acomm aneurysm of the anterior communicating artery.

of subarachnoid hemorrhage), many neurosurgeons advocate early operative treatment.[47,48] In a small, randomized trial, patients treated with early surgery (<3 days) seemed to have better outcomes than those who have operations at later intervals.[49] In an observational, nonrandomized study, Ross et al.[50] concluded that patients with subarachnoid hemorrhage secondary to rupture of an anterior circulation aneurysm could have early operation regardless of age. The primary reasons for doing early surgery are to avoid the risk of early rebleeding and to shorten the length of hospitalization. Still, a systemic review could not demonstrate superiority of early intracranial operation over delayed surgery in treating patients with ruptured aneurysms.[51] However, despite the lack of strong data, most physicians and neurosurgeons favor early operative treatment of the procedure.

Nonsaccular aneurysms also can be treated surgically. Nussbaum et al.[52] successfully treated fusiform aneurysms of the peripheral portion of the posteroinferior cerebellar artery. All patients had resection of the aneurysm with establishment of an anastomosis to maintain blood flow to the inferior portion of the cerebellum. Leibowitz et al.[53] found that occlusion of the patent vessel can be used to treat fusiform aneurysms. While these reports are promising, additional research is needed. Fusiform and dissecting aneurysms often involve major vessels and surgical management can be complicated by ischemia if penetrating arteries are sacrificed.

The combination of occlusion of the parent artery of an aneurysm with creation of an extracranial-to-intracranial bypass operation using a saphenous vein graft also has been used.[54]

Despite advances in anesthesia and neurosurgical technique, operative clipping of the aneurysm remains a dangerous procedure. Complex aneurysms and those located in remote sites, such as the posterior circulation, are often difficult to treat. Complications include premature recurrent rupture of the aneurysm secondary to manipulation inadvertent occlusion of proximal or adjacent vessels, trauma to adjacent neurological structure, and increased intracranial pressure secondary to postoperative brain. Both hemorrhages and infarctions are complications of aneurysm surgery. In some cases, the aneurysm might not be completely occluded. Fracturing or slipping of the aneurysm clip can occur. In some cases, the surgeon cannot clip the aneurysm and wrapping of the aneurysm is tried.

Endovascular Management

A major change in management of ruptured intracranial aneurysms is under way, with increased endovascular placement of detachable platinum coils (Guglielmi coils) within the sac. The coils become a nidus for thrombosis and occlusion of the aneurysm[44,55–59] (Fig. 23-5). Aneurysms that are not easily approachable by direct

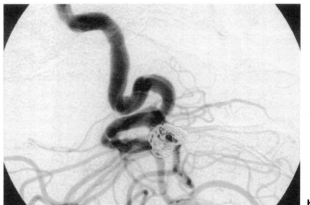

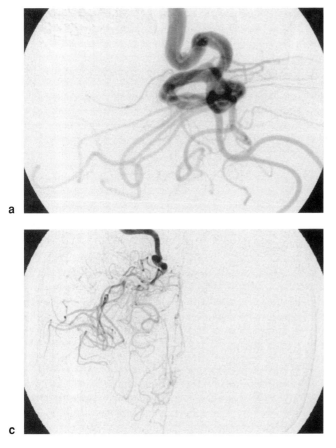

Figure 23-5. Lateral views of a carotid arteriogram show a large aneurysm of the internal carotid artery prior to (a) and following (b) placement of coils.

surgical dissection, such as those located on the internal carotid artery within the cavernous sinus, or that have been difficult to clip, such as aneurysms located in the posterior circulation, can be approached using endovascular techniques.[60–64] In particular, endovascular treatment of posterior circulation aneurysms avoids manipulation of the brain stem and cranial nerves.[65] Experiences from individual institutions and case series support the potential efficacy of endovascular therapy. Based on a series of 73 cases, Park et al.[66] found that endovascular interventions could treat paraclinoid saccular aneurysms. Groden et al.[67] treated 110 patients with vertebrobasilar aneurysms with coils. They did not achieve complete occlusion of the aneurysm in 23 cases. The other patients generally did well. In a series of 79 patients with aneurysmal subarachnoid hemorrhage, Kremer et al.[68] found two episodes of rebleeding following endovascular treatment. Based on a series of 818 patients with 916 aneurysms treated with endovascular placement of coils, Murayama et al.[69] showed that the overall morbidity and mortality of the procedure was approximately 9 percent. Delayed rupture of the aneurysms was found in 1.6 percent of cases. Weir et al.[70] treated 27 patients with severe subarachnoid hemorrhage with endovascular coiling of the aneurysm. Successful occlusion of the aneurysm was achieved in 13 cases. No cases of rebleeding were

reported. Wide-necked aneurysms can be treated with a self-expanding stent system.[71] The use of the stent can expedite embolization or coiling of the aneurysmal sac. Han et al.[72] treated 10 patients with broad-based aneurysms with the combination of coiling and stenting. The stents proved useful in improving the hemodynamic and mechanical aspects of these complex aneurysms. One of the advantages of endovascular treatment is that it might be associated with a lower risk of vasospasm than that associated with surgery. For example, Rabinstein et al.[73] concluded that patients with better clinical grades were less likely to have symptomatic vasospasm when they were treated with endovascular therapy than with surgical clipping.

While endovascular therapy avoids a major operation, patients usually need general anesthesia for the procedure, although a regimen of conscious sedation also is used. Critically ill patients with a recent subarachnoid hemorrhage likely will need anesthesia and anesthesia-related complications are possible. In addition, other potential complications of coiling include rupture of the aneurysm during the procedure, inadvertent occlusion of the parent artery, delayed occlusion of the aneurysm leaving the patient at risk for early recurrent bleeding, or delayed rebleeding.[74,75] Transcranial color-coded duplex ultrasonography can be used to monitor the status of coiled intracranial aneurysms.[76] Friedman et al.[77] reported no cases of rebleeding in 83 patients treated with coiling. Three patients needed surgery because of incomplete occlusion of the aneurysm. Cases of recurrent rupture of aneurysm or failure of coiling might mandate surgical treatment of patients with previously managed endovascular interventions.[78] Based on the available data, Brilstra et al.[79] and Johnston et al.[80] concluded that endovascular therapy had not been established as equal to or superior to operatively clipping. Johnston et al.[80] in another systemic review noted that endovascular embolization is moderately effective in completely occluding aneurysms of the posterior circulation, including those at the basilar apex, and that the intervention was effective in preventing early recurrent hemorrhage.[81]

Endovascular interventions have been used to treat nonsaccular aneurysms or aneurysms complicating other cerebrovascular diseases. Endovascular treatment was used for management of a posterior circulation aneurysm in a patient with moyamoya.[82] Endovascular treatment for dissecting aneurysms of the vertebrobasilar circulation includes trapping or proximal occlusion.[83–85] The selection of endovascular interventions is based on aneurysm location, configuration, collateral circulation, and time of presentation. Parent vessel occlusion can be used to treat dissecting aneurysms in the vertebrobasilar circulation.[53] Rabinov et al.[83] treated 26 cases with dissecting aneurysms of the vertebral artery; 14 were above the origin of the posteroinferior cerebellar artery. Recurrent hemorrhages occurred in two cases and overall mortality was 20 percent. In another study of 12 patients with intracranial dissections with hemorrhages, 6 were treated with coils and 6 with balloon occlusion.[84] Four of the patients had ischemic complications but none had rebleeding.

A small trial comparing endovascular or direct surgical clipping performed by Koivisto et al.[86] was inconclusive. Subsequently, the results of a large international trial became available. The study enrolled 2143 patients with ruptured intracranial aneurysms into a randomized trial comparing surgical or endovascular treatment; 1070 patients were assigned clipping and 1073 patients were treated with detachable platinum coils.[87,88] At 1 year, death or dependency was described in 190 of 801 patients (23.7 percent) assigned endovascular treatment and 243 of 793 patients (30.6 percent) assigned neurosurgical clipping (6.9 percent absolute risk reduction and 22.6 percent relative risk reduction) (see Fig. 23-3). The risk of rebleeding after 1 year with endovascular treatment was 2 per 1276 patient-years. The results of this study are impressive. However, patients were followed for only 1 year and the risk of delayed (very late) rebleeding among the patients treated with coiling is not known. In addition, some potential bias in selection of patients might have occurred. Patients with aneurysms of the middle cerebral artery were excluded because of

the perception that they might best respond to surgical clipping. Conversely, patients with ruptured aneurysms in the posterior circulation also were not enrolled because of the assumption that endovascular therapy already was known to be superior.[64] Thus, most of the patients had ruptured aneurysms of either the internal carotid or anterior communicating arteries. Still, this trial is a landmark and its results will change management dramatically. The role of endovascular coiling for treatment of patients with recently ruptured aneurysms likely will grow and the use of conventional surgical procedures probably will decline in the years ahead.[89]

At present, management to lower the risk of recurrent hemorrhage in patients with recently ruptured aneurysms is made on a case-by-case basis. Medical therapy, including the use of antifibrinolytic agents, remains adjunctive to surgical procedures. Operative clipping of the neck of the aneurysm and endovascular insertion of coils into the aneurismal sac are among the preferred methods. The selection of treatment is made on the basis of several variables, including the patient's overall condition, the severity of the hemorrhage, and the characteristics of the aneurysm. Patients with large aneurysms in difficult locations, such as the posterior circulation, are usually treated with coiling. Patients with aneurysms that can easily be approached by surgery are often advised to have operative clipping. Some patients might be treated with a combination of interventions. For example, Lawton et al.[90] treated patients with a multimodality approach, including microvascular surgical management, selective revascularization, and coiling. They reported that the combination of interventions might be used to treat complex aneurysms.

Vasospasm and Ischemic Stroke

Cerebral infarction secondary to hypoperfusion resulting from localized or generalized vasospasm is a leading cause of morbidity and mortality, following aneurysmal subarachnoid hemorrhage.[20,91] Thus, management includes therapies to prevent or reverse vasospasm, or to prevent or reverse the ischemic consequences of the arterial narrowing.[43,92,93] While the pathogenesis of vasospasm is not established with certainty, it is secondary to active contraction of smooth muscles and proliferation of cellular elements within the intracranial arteries.[94–97] Although vasospasm can accompany other types of subarachnoid hemorrhage, such as that found with trauma, it primarily occurs among patients with ruptured aneurysms. It is not seen with primary intraventricular or intracerebral hemorrhage. Vasospasm rarely occurs following a rupture of a vascular malformation or with perimesencephalic subarachnoid hemorrhage.[98] Generally, vasospasm develops in the presence of a thick area of blood in the subarachnoid space, and it might involve arterial or other factors in its pathogenesis. Vasospasm can rarely be detected in less than 48 h of subarachnoid hemorrhage.[99] However, vasospasm usually peaks at approximately 6–10 days after the hemorrhage and persists up to 2–3 weeks.[100] Thereafter, the arterial narrowing gradually resolves.

Presumably, red blood cells within the subarachnoid clot release a factor or combination of spasmogenic factors that promote the arterial narrowing. The formation of oxyhemoglobin may activate lipid peroxidation, decrease production of high-energy phosphates, or decrease arterial nourishments.[92,96,101] Potential mediators of vasospasm following subarachnoid hemorrhage include superoxide free radicals, ferrous hemoglobin that acts as a nitric oxide scavenger, endothelins, protein kinase C, and rho kinase.[102] Microvascular dysfunction and autoregulatory failure also may occur.[102] Dumont et al.[103] proposed that inflammation is critical in the development of vasospasm. Possible inflammation in the pathogenesis of vasospasm include adhesion molecules, cytokines, white blood cells, immunoglobulins, and complement.[103]

Vasospasm is most commonly diagnosed among seriously ill patients. Women and those with prominent meningeal signs, dehydration, hyponatremia, or hydrocephalus also have a high risk. The results of initial CT forecast the risk of vasospasm.[104–107] Patients with either local or diffuse thick collections of blood in the subarachnoid space are most likely to develop vasospasm. Early operative clipping might be associated with a higher risk of vasospasm than that accompanied by endovascular therapy.[31] This association has been disputed. Charpentier et al.[104] concluded that there was no difference between neurosurgical or endovascular interventions and the likelihood of vasospasm. Evacuation of the subarachnoid hematoma, possibly including lavage of the subarachnoid space using adjunctive instillation of thrombolytic agents, has been proposed as a way to avoid vasospasm.[108–110] The utility of this approach has not been established. A small, randomized trial did not show efficacy of intraoperative administration of thrombolytic agents in preventing ischemia.[110] A major limitation of antifibrinolytic agents to prevent recurrent hemorrhage is the association of increased risk of ischemia.[36,37] In part, this association may be secondary to the agents' effects on delaying lysis of the subarachnoid thrombus. Drug-induced hypotension and dehydration also promote the development of ischemic symptoms secondary to vasospasm.

Arteriography is the traditional way to diagnose vasospasm (see Fig. 23-2). At approximately 1 week following the hemorrhage, the arterial narrowing can be detected in up to 70 percent of patients.[94,95] The severity of the narrowing varies. Arterial changes are often generalized and affect multiple intracranial arteries or be localized—most commonly in the arteries adjacent to the

ruptured aneurysm. Vasospasm affects the distal portion of the internal carotid artery and the proximal segments of the anterior and middle cerebral arteries. The arterial narrowing reduces cerebral flood flow in the involved arteries. Transcranial Doppler ultrasonography (TCD) also detects changes in velocities in the affected vessels.[111–114] An increase in flow velocity is correlated with arteriographic narrowing. Sequential TCD studies can be used to monitor for increases in flow velocity, which are the first marker of impending ischemia. In general, flow velocities above 200 mL/min are predictive of severe arterial narrowing. Because the sensitivity and specificity of TCD changes are high, it has largely replaced arteriography for diagnosis of vasospasm.

The clinical features of vasospasm are secondary to ischemia and course usually is less precipitous than that occurring with recurrent hemorrhage.[94,95] Patients develop increasingly severe headache, confusion, decreased alertness, or focal neurological symptoms, such as hemiparesis, paraparesis, dysarthria, or aphasia. The focal signs reflect the affected brain areas. Neurological signs fluctuate but as the course of the illness evolves, the patient may develop coma or persisting focal neurological deficits. Brain imaging studies demonstrate areas of infarction. The differential diagnosis of vasospasm-induced ischemia includes recurrent hemorrhage, hydrocephalus, seizures, electrolyte disturbances, or complications of medical or surgical interventions (see Table 23-5).

Medical Management

Several interventions have been used to treat patients with vasospasm and secondary cerebral ischemia. Maintaining adequate hydration helps. Because the vascular compartment is contracted and many patients have a negative sodium balance, patients are at risk for hypoperfusion secondary to changes in viscosity or impaired flow.[115] In general, patients should receive approximately 3 L of saline, unless they have signs of cardiac failure. Data about the utility of adequate hydration or prophylactic expansion of circulating blood volume are mixed in preventing ischemia following subarachnoid hemorrhage.[116–118] Avoiding dehydration and use of intravenous fluids that maintain adequate circulating volume while preventing hyponatremia are part of initial management. Infusions of hypertonic saline have been shown to increase cerebral blood flow in seriously ill patients with subarachnoid hemorrhage.[119] Presumably, the infusions improve the rheology of circulating blood by reducing hemoglobin concentrations.

The adjunctive administration of the calcium-channel-blocking agent, nimodipine, is a standard part of management.[43] The medication presumably counteracts the effects of calcium on the vascular smooth muscle, and thus has an antivasospasm effect. In addition, it might have some prophylactic neuroprotective actions. Several studies have tested nimodipine.[120–122] In a systemic review of available data, Rinkel et al.[123] found that the calcium-channel-blocking agents reduce the proportion of patients with poor outcomes or ischemic strokes following subarachnoid hemorrhage. The risk of poor outcomes was 0.82 (95 percent CI 0.72–0.93). The medication was associated with a reduction in mortality—odds ratio 0.94 (0.80–1.10). More importantly, the odds of ischemic stroke were 0.67 (0.59 – 0.76), with the use of the medication. The use of the calcium channel blocker was associated with a reduction of CT evidence of infarction—an odds ratio of 0.80 (0.71 – 0.89). The results are largely influenced by the British trial of nimodipine.[120] Nimodipine (60 mg every 4 h) is recommended for treatment of patients with aneurysmal subarachnoid hemorrhage. Nimodipine is given orally but if the patient cannot take the medication by mouth, capsules can be crushed and given via a nasogastric tube. Nimodipine is relatively safe. Hypotension is the primary complication. In some cases, the agent might need to be discontinued in order to elevate a patient's blood pressure.

Nicardipine is another calcium-channel-blocking agent that has an advantage of the medication in which it can be given intravenously. Kasuya et al.[124] inserted prolonged-release implants of nicardipine into subarachnoid clots in dogs and showed that the intervention was successful in preventing vasospasm. A randomized trial of nicardipine demonstrated a reduction in the frequency of vasospasm but outcomes were not improved with treatment, largely because patients in the control group received rescue therapies, including drug-induced hypertension and volume expansion when patients developed ischemic complications.[125] Because of the negative results of the trial, nicardipine has not replaced nimodipine for treatment of patients with recently ruptured aneurysms.

Hypervolemic hemodilution and drug-induced hypertension (triple-H therapy) is used to treat patients with ischemic symptoms from vasospasm[43] (see Table 23-4). The rationale is that because autoregulation is lost, blood flow becomes pressure-dependent and increasing blood pressure will increase perfusion to areas of the brain distal to the vasospastic arteries. In addition, lowering the viscosity of the blood by hemodilution also improves blood flow.[122,126] Most of the evidence for efficacy of triple-H therapy is from anecdotal studies.[126–128] Sen et al.[129] concluded that triple-H therapy is effective in improving outcomes. Still, no randomized trial of triple-H therapy has been attempted.[129] A systemic review of hemodilution in preventing ischemic deficits following subarachnoid hemorrhage concluded that the intervention has not been properly studied.[117] The triple-H regimen is vigorous, and complications including recurrent rupture of an untreated aneurysm, hypertensive encephalopathy, increased cerebral edema, hemorrhagic transformation of the infarction, myocardial infarction, pulmonary edema,

and congestive heart failure have been reported.[130,131] In addition, elevation of the blood pressure can be difficult if the patient is also receiving nimodipine.

Several other agents have been tested, including tirilazad, ebselen, papaverine, and calcitonin-gene-related peptide.[132–140] In general, these medications have not been demonstrated as effective. The potential efficacy of tirilazad was seen only among women receiving the higher dose of the medication.[133–136] The other studies were negative.

Andaluz et al.[141] concluded that a single-dose infusion of papaverine can be done if angioplasty is not possible. Other uncontrolled studies have suggested that superselective administration of papaverine might improve outcomes.[142–145] Additional data are needed to determine the role of this intervention as a monotherapy or as an adjunct to angioplasty. Chia et al.[146] suggested that magnesium would limit ischemic symptoms from vasospasm following subarachnoid hemorrhage. A study demonstrated that infusions of magnesium are well tolerated among patients with subarachnoid hemorrhage and that the medication might be useful for preventing ischemia from vasospasm.[147] Other promising new treatments include fasudil hydrochloride, erythropoietin, and induced hypothermia.[102] Intermittent intrathecal injections of sodium nitroprusside and thiosulfate also have been used to treat symptomatic vasospasm following aneurysmal subarachnoid hemorrhage.[148] Transdermal nitroglycerin ointment can be used to treat cerebral vasospasm following subarachnoid hemorrhage.[149] Patients with mild-to-moderate ischemic symptoms secondary to vasospasm might benefit from ipsilateral cervical sympathetic block.[150] Juvela[151] speculated that patients taking aspirin prior to subarachnoid hemorrhage have a reduced risk of ischemic complications, presumably because of the medication's antithrombotic effects. However, the use of the antiplatelet agent might increase the risk of early rebleeding. A small study of aspirin administered to patients after surgical treatment found that aspirin was safe.[152] Additional study about the potential utility of aspirin or other antiplatelet agents is needed.

Endovascular Management

Dilation of the vasospastic arteries by angioplasty has been used to treat patients with intractable arterial narrowing or severe ischemia. Anecdotal reports suggest that the risk of complications of angioplasty is relatively low and that ischemic symptoms can be reversed.[122,153–156] Murayama et al.[157] combined endovascular coiling of the aneurysm with angioplasty for treatment of symptomatic vasospasm in 12 seriously ill patients with ruptured aneurysms; 8 patients had complete occlusion of the aneurysm. Favorable outcomes were found in six cases. In a series of 62 patients with intractable vasospasm not responding to measures including drug-induced hypertension and hemodilution, angioplasty, and intra-arterial administration of papaverine was attempted.[141] Single or multiple vascular territories were treated. In another recent report, balloon angioplasty also has been used to treat patients with ischemia secondary to persistent vasospasm.[102] Hoelper et al.[158] found that angioplasty for treatment of severe vasospasm is associated with improved biochemical parameters. Angioplasty might be used as a prophylactic intervention.[102,159] The procedure would be performed before ischemic symptoms appear. Complications of angioplasty include rupture of the intracranial vessel or hyperperfusion syndrome.[160,161]

Future management of patients with symptomatic vasospasm likely will change. Several treatment options are already available. The initial efforts involve avoiding hydration and hyponatremia. Nimodipine is started as soon as the diagnosis of aneurysmal subarachnoid hemorrhage is made. Patients who have ischemic symptoms receive aggressive medical measures, including triple-H therapy. Patients not responding to other interventions can be treated with angioplasty or other intra-arterial therapies.

Other Aspects of Management

Pituitary failure, with impaired release of adrenocorticotropic hormone (ACTH), is a potential complication of subarachnoid hemorrhage.[162] Steroid replacement might be needed in such exceptional cases. Patients with infective aneurysms are treated with intensive antibiotic therapy and local interventions (surgical or endovascular obliteration).[163,164]

▶ VASCULAR MALFORMATIONS

Vascular malformations are a leading cause of intracerebral hemorrhage and primary intraventricular hemor-

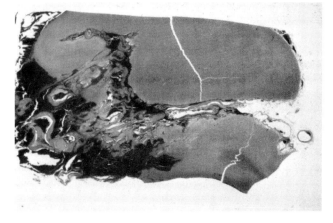

Figure 23-6. A microscopic section of a cerebral arteriovenous malformation shows dilated vessels and adjacent areas of hemorrhage. Courtesy of S.S. Schochet, M.D. Department of Pathology, University of West Virginia, Morgantown, WV.

rhage[165] (Figs. 23-6 and 23-7). Intracranial hemorrhage is the initial presentation of approximately one-half of all cases of cerebral vascular malformations.[166] The annual risk of bleeding from a vascular malformation is estimated to be 1–3 percent.[167,168] Eventually, approximately 60 percent of all patients with vascular malformations have hemorrhages. Fleetwood et al.[169] showed that the risk of bleeding with vascular malformations of the basal ganglia or thalamus is much higher than that associated with lesions in other locations. Bleeding is most likely to occur among smaller malformations with deep venous drainage.[170,171] Vascular malformations in the borderzone locations in the hemisphere have the lowest risk for hemorrhage.[172] Because of the risk of bleeding, most patients with arteriovenous malformations receive some treatment to lower the likelihood of a major hemorrhage.[173]

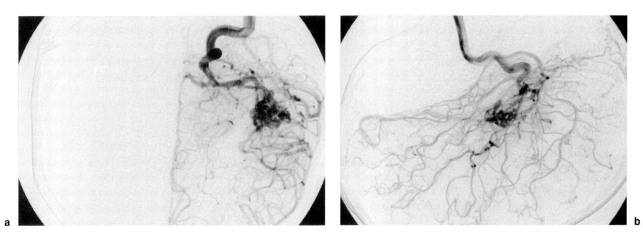

a   b

Figure 23-7. Anteroposterior and lateral views of a right arteriogram show a temporal arteriovenous malformation.

Overall, the prognosis of hemorrhage from vascular malformations is better than that of bleeding from other causes.[165] Rather than causing death, rupture of a vascular malformation usually leads to neurological disability because of intracerebral bleeding.[165,174] Thus, the consequences of bleeding from a vascular malformation are as ominous as the risks of hemorrhage from ruptured aneurysms.[174] While the risk of early recurrent hemorrhage is relatively low, such chances are increased among patients who already have had an episode of bleeding when compared to those who have symptomatic but intact vascular malformations.[168] The frequency of a second hemorrhage is approximately 6–10 percent during the first year.[168] Thereafter, the risk of bleeding is estimated as 3–4 percent per year.[175] The combined rate of major morbidity or mortality following recurrent rupture of a cerebral arteriovenous malformation is approximately 2.7 percent per year.[175]

Aneurysms can be detected in association with a vascular malformation in approximately 10–25 percent of patients.[176,177] The presence of the aneurysm complicates management because changes in hemodynamics secondary to treatment of the vascular malformation might promote rupture of the aneurysm. Stapf et al.[177] concluded that the risk of hemorrhage from an aneurysm on a feeding artery might be as high as 6 percent. The presence of an aneurysm on a feeding artery is an independent predictor of intracranial hemorrhage. While the urgency of treating a ruptured vascular malformation is not as great as that of obliterating a ruptured saccular aneurysm, the risk of another bleeding event is sufficiently high that some treatment to eradicate the vascular lesion is justified. Much of the management of acute intracranial hemorrhage that is started in an emergency setting (see Chapter 21) is continued. The options for management of the vascular malformation include surgical resection, endovascular obliteration, and focused irradiation therapy.[178] Clinical studies on management of vascular malformations involve treatment of patients with intact lesions as well as those with hemorrhages. Because vascular malformations often produce neurological symptoms other than hemorrhage, decisions about treatment often is in other settings. As a result, the number of studies that report the results of management of the vascular lesions following intracranial hemorrhage is relatively small. In addition, studies have not compared the safety and efficacy of the several interventions. As a result, all recommendations are based on the results of clinical series. Trials to compare the utility of surgery, endovascular therapy, and stereotactic radiotherapy are being planned. Hopefully, these studies' results will provide the information to guide physicians and surgeons. Such information is important because the costs of management of vascular malformations are high.[179] Patients with large vascular malformations utilize a large number of hospital resources because of poor neurological outcomes and a relatively high rate of neurological deficits following surgical interventions.

Surgical Management

Surgical resection has been the traditional treatment.[178,180] While surgery often is needed to aspirate a large intracerebral hemorrhage, the desired situation is for the surgical resection to be done as an elective procedure. In order to ease resection of the malformation, surgery often is delayed for at least several days following the hemorrhage. The goal of the operation is to completely remove the vascular lesion, including the nidus and the draining veins. Surgical ligation of one or more feeding arteries is not effective unless the nidus of the malformation is removed. The operation usually involves microsurgical techniques. Arteriography usually is performed at the end of the operation to assess whether the resection has completely removed the lesion. Still, Ali et al.[181] recently reported that recurrence of the vascular malformation might recur even after presumed complete surgical excision.

In order to guide decisions about operative resections, Spetzler and Martin[182] developed a system to estimate the risk of serious neurological consequences of the surgical procedure (see Chapter 15). The system is based on the location of the vascular malformation, the size of the lesion, and the number of feeding arteries. Malformations with multiple feeding vessels, large lesions, and those located in eloquent areas of the brain might not be treatable with surgery. Eloquent regions would be areas of brain, such as primary motor cortices or language cortices. Deep vascular malformations usually are not as easily treated surgically as those lesions that are located near the surface. Cortical arteriovenous malformations with a nidus smaller than 10 mL in volume can be treated surgically.[183]

Favorable outcomes of surgery can be anticipated in more than 90 percent of patients with the lowest risk malformations.[184] Among patients with more advanced and complicated vascular malformations, the chances of success drop. Lawton et al.[185] reported that some of the intermediate-grade vascular malformations might be treated with the same chances of success as that with the smaller lesions. Vascular malformations of the brain stem, thalamus, or basal ganglia also can be resected with a reasonable chance for success.[186] Huh et al.[187] concluded that microsurgery was the preferred treatment for lesions associated with a high risk of hemorrhage, including those with previous bleeding. However, Soderman et al.[183] concluded that deep vascular malformations with a nidus greater than 20 mL in volume should not be treated surgically. Ferch and Morgan[188] reported that surgical management of patients with deep complex vascular malformations was associated with a high rate of neurological deterioration due to hemorrhage, ischemia, and seizures. They concluded that large, complex malformations with feeding vessels from the lenticulostriate, choroidal, and deep thalamic perforating arteries and those with deep meningeal arterial involvement should be treated conservatively. Han et al.[189] found that treatment of some of the very complex vascular malformations was associated with considerable risk and that partial treatment of the lesions might be worse than the natural history for bleeding. In another report of 110 patients with small arteriovenous malformations, success was achieved in most patients; only 1 of 64 patients with surgical treatment of a lesion in a noneloquent area was neurologically worse, following operation.[190] In another report of outcomes of microsurgical treatment of arteriovenous malformations, neurological sequelae were more common among women, those with large lesions, and those with drainage to the deep venous system.[191] Currently, surgical excision of those lesions considered a low risk for operative complications, as defined by preoperative scales such as those rated as grade I or II on the Spetzler–Martin scale.[178] Zimmerman et al.[192] found that small cavernous malformations of the brain stem could be performed with reasonable safety and that the surgical excision could be curative.

A postoperative hyperperfusion syndrome can complicate resection of a large, high-flow, vascular malformation.[193] The cerebral circulation has adapted to the high-flow state and the sudden removal of the fistula can cause excessive blood flow to adjacent brain areas. The long-standing preoperative venous hypertension probably makes areas of the brain hypoxic or ischemic.[193] These areas might be vulnerable to the sudden changes in perfusion. Seizures, brain edema, and hemorrhage can result.[194] Morgan et al.[194] concluded that blood pressure be strictly controlled in order to limit effects on reperfusion. Patients with high-flow malformations often have staged procedures with several segmental resections or endovascular obliteration of feeding vessels combined with surgical resection.[178,183,195–198] The preoperative endovascular therapy can shorten the operation and limit blood loss. In addition, the endovascular treatment allows the surgeon to focus on the nidus of the malformation but help occlude deep, surgically inaccessible arteries.[199]

Deep vascular malformations with a nidus volume greater than 10 mL could benefit from targeted endovascular treatment followed by either conventional resection or radiosurgery.[183] Kinouchi et al.[198] successfully used the combination of endovascular embolization followed by surgery and noted that the surgery could be performed safely and successfully as soon as possible after hemodynamic changes were observed following the embolization. Chang et al.[200] reported that the combination of endovascular therapy, radiotherapy, and surgical resection could be used successfully to treat patients with giant arteriovenous malformations. Friedman et al.[201] reported that the combination of staged arterial embolization and radiotherapy could be used to treat low-flow dural arteriovenous fistulas. These procedures often are performed sequentially over several weeks. Still, there is considerable uncertainty about the utility of staged procedures for treatment of patients with large vascular malformations.[178]

Endovascular Management

Endovascular modalities include injection of sclerosing agents, therapeutic embolization, or insertion of coils. The sclerosing agents include I-butyl cyanoacrylate, *n*-butyl cyanoacrylate (NCBA), and ethylene vinyl alcohol copolymer (Figs. 23-8 and 23-9). The Food and Drug Administration approved the use of NCBA for treatment of cerebral arteriovenous malformations.[178] Solid polyvinyl alcohol particles, microcoils, and microballoons also have been used. The treated lesions have prominent feeding and draining vessels that can be canalized, such as arteriovenous malformations or fistulas. Slow-flow vascular malformations, such as venous or cavernous malformations, cannot be treated. These modalities can be used as an adjunct to surgical resection or as the primary intervention for treatment of nonresectable malformations.[178] Vinuela et al.[202] found that endovascular treatment alone was curative in 9.9 percent of 405 patients. Success was achieved primarily in treatment of small lesions that did not have a large number of feeding vessels. However, the success of endovascular occlusion of feeding vessels often is temporary. Obliteration of the nidus is critical, or otherwise new feeding collaterals appear to develop. Patients having only endovascular treatment need to be followed closely the appearance of new feeding vessels. For example, Gobin et al.[203] reported revascularization of the vascular malformation in approximately 12 percent of patients treated with embolization, and they concluded that the risk of bleeding among such patients is similar to patient's natural history. They also recommended radiosurgery to treat patients with residual vascular malformation. Liu et al.[204] successfully used endovascular interventions to treat vascular malformations of the brain stem. Endovascular interventions can be used to treat patients with deep vascular malformations located in the cerebral hemispheres.[205]

Endovascular interventions are associated with a procedural mortality of approximately 1 percent and a neurological morbidity of 2–5 percent.[59,178,202,206,207] The relatively high rate of complications should not be surprising, because patients treated with embolization are those who are at the highest risk for neurological sequelae.[208] Still, no specific feature portends a high risk of complications from endovascular management.[207] Hemorrhages are a potential complication. Keller et al.[209] described management of

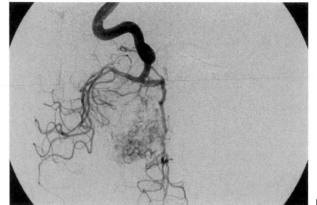

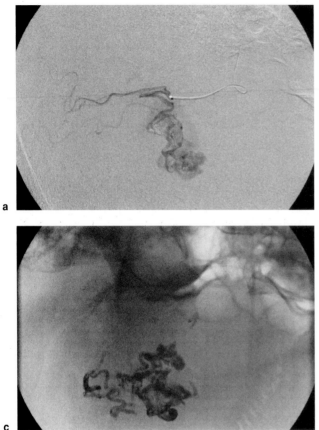

Figure 23-8. Three views of endovascular treatment of a vascular malformation (a) selective catheterization of the lesion, (b) partial occlusion, and (c) lateral view show occlusive material.

18 patients with severe bleeding following endovascular treatment of vascular malformations. Sources of bleeding include arterial perforation, rupture of an artery, or sudden occlusion of a vein. Hartmann et al.[207] reported the results of 233 patients treated with 545 endovascular treat-

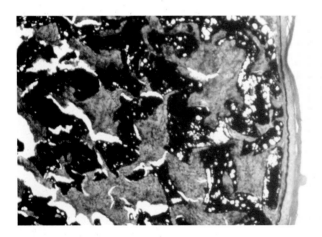

Figure 23-9. Elastic stained surgical specimen of an arteriovenous malformation that was treated previously with embolization shows the polymerization material within the lumen of the vessels. (*Courtesy of S.S. Schochet, M.D., Department of Pathology, University of West Virginia, Morgantown, WV*)

ments; 33 patients had some treatment-related neurological deficits. Complications were found among older patients and those who required multiple treatments. They concluded that the factors predicting a high risk for endovascular interventions differed from those for complications of microsurgery.

Currently, endovascular embolization or obliteration of feeding vessels should not be considered as curative. Embolization may be recommended for adjunctive treatment of patients with large, inoperable cortical and subcortical arteriovenous malformations.[178,206,210] Current guidelines recommend endovascular treatment as an adjunct to either surgical resection or radiosurgery for moderately complex vascular malformations.[178] The procedure should be performed for those patients who have larger arteriovenous malformations if the goal is to reduce flow or edema in association with another therapy.[178]

Radiation Therapy

Holocranial, focused, or stereotactic irradiation has become an important intervention for treatment of patients whose lesions cannot be treated surgically. In general, focused, stereotactic radiosurgery is most commonly recommended, because it can be performed to give high amounts of radiation to a discrete area of the brain.[211,212] The aim of radiosurgery is to cause progressive obliteration of the blood vessels of the malformation. The radiation exposure causes inflammation and involution of the nidus and the feeding and draining vessels. This process does take time. In general, the vascular malformation gradually shrinks during the first 2 years after treatment. Best suited for focused irradiation are malformations that are less than 3 cm in diameter or less than 10 cm^3 in volume.[183,213–216] Radiosurgery leads to eradication of the arteriovenous malformation in approximately 80 percent of cases within 2–3 years. Firlik et al.[217] suggested that microsurgical resection of the nidus of the residual vascular malformation could follow radiosurgery.

Flickinger et al.[218] found that success is greatest for small lesions. Pollock and Flickinger[219] proposed a system to predict responses to radiation therapy; the scores were based on the volume and location of the lesion and the patient's age. In general, obliteration of a cerebral arteriovenous malformation is most likely to be achieved when the lesion is small.[220] Success is greatest when treating smaller malformations in the lobar white matter, corpus callosum, or cerebellar treated than with larger arteriovenous lesions located in the basal ganglia, diencephalon, or brain stem. All types of vascular malformations have been treated. However, one report noted that complications might be greater among patients with cavernous malformations than for persons with other types of vascular malformation.[221] The success of radiosurgery seems greater when larger doses of radiation are used.[222]

In general, the results of the uncontrolled studies of therapy are positive. Based on treatment of 144 patients, Pollock et al.[223] reported excellent outcomes (obliteration of the lesion and no neurological impairment) in 96 patients. Huh et al.[187] concluded that radiosurgery was an effective treatment option for management of small vascular malformations located in eloquent regions. However, the risk of bleeding remains for several months after the intervention. Hasegawa et al.[224] reported that radiosurgery was helpful in reducing the risk of hemorrhage among patients with high-risk cavernous malformations. Most of their treated patients had lesions in the brain stem or diencephalon. Smyth et al.[225] reported that stereotactic radiosurgery could be done safely in children.

Radiosurgery can be complicated by hemorrhage or radiation-induced neurological injury. Karlsson et al.[226] reported 56 cases of hemorrhage within 2 years of treatment among 1593 patients having gamma knife radiosurgery. Hemorrhage following treatment was related to the older age of the patient, a larger volume vascular lesion, and if high doses of radiation were found. Twenty patients had major neurological impairments following treatment. In another study, recurrent posttreatment hemorrhage was detected in 10 percent of cases.[222] Kim et al.[227] treated 22 patients with cavernous malformations with linear accelerator or gamma knife radiosurgery. One patient had a hemorrhage during the follow-up period.

However, six patients had neurological worsening, which might be secondary to the radiation. In another study, hemorrhages occurred up to 42 months following gamma knife radiation therapy in 7 percent of 115 treated patients.[228] Malformations with multiple draining veins and those located in deep hemispheric structures had the highest risk for bleeding. Protection against bleeding is not achieved if the nidus is not obliterated following radiation therapy.[229] Other complications of radiosurgery include seizures, cranial nerve palsies, and radiation-induced parenchymal changes.[230] However, the risk of permanent radiation-induced complications seems to be relatively low.[222]

Radiosurgery is recommended for treatment of patients who are considered to be at too high risk for conventional surgery or endovascular therapy.[178] Current guidelines recommend that the procedure be primarily used to treat small lesions, especially those that are not easily approachable by direct surgical exploration.

REFERENCES

1. Prasad K, Shrivastava A. Surgery for primary supratentorial intracerebral haemorrhage. *Cochrane Database Syst Rev* 2000.
2. Qureshi AI, Tuhrim S, Broderick JP. Spontaneous intracerebral hemorrhage. *N Engl J Med* 2001;344:1450–1460.
3. Brainin M, Olsen TS, Chamorro A, et al. Organization of stroke care: education, referral, emergency management and imaging, stroke units and rehabilitation. *Cerebrovasc Dis* 2004;17(suppl 2):1–14.
4. Diringer MN, Edwards DF. Admission to a neurologic/neursurgical intensive care unit is associated with reduced mortality rate after intracerebral hemorrhage. *Crit Care Med* 2001;29:635–640.
5. Berman MF, Solomon RA, Mayer SA, Johnston SC, Yung PP. Impact of hospital-related factors on outcome after treatment of cerebral aneurysms. *Stroke* 2003;34:2200–2205.
6. Broderick JP, Adams HP, Jr., Barsan W, et al. Guidelines for the management of spontaneous intracerebral hemorrhage: a statement for healthcare professionals from a special writing group of the Stroke Council, American Heart Association. *Stroke* 1999;30:905–915.
7. Bae H, Jeong D, Doh J, Lee K, Yun I, Byun B. Recurrence of bleeding in patients with hypertensive intracerebral hemorrhage. *Cerebrovasc Dis* 1999;9:102–108.
8. Hill MD, Silver FL, Austin PC, Tu JV. Rate of stroke recurrence in patients with primary intracerebral hemorrhage. *Stroke* 2000;31:123–127.
9. Gonzalez-Duarte A, Cantu C, Ruiz-Sandoval JL, Barinagarrementeria F. Recurrent primary cerebral hemorrhage: frequency, mechanisms, and prognosis. *Stroke* 1998;29:1802–1805.
10. Arakawa S, Saku Y, Ibayashi S, Nagao T, Fujishima M. Blood pressure control and recurrence of hypertensive brain hemorrhage. *Stroke* 1998;29:1806–1809.

11. Passero S, Burgalassi L, D'Andrea P. Recurrence of bleeding in patients with primary intracerebral hemorrhage. *Stroke* 1995;26:1189–1192.

12. Chen ST, Chiang CY, Hsu CY. Recurrent hypertensive intracerebral hemorrhage. *Acta Neurol Scand* 1995;91: 128–132.

13. Sjoblom L, Hardemark HG, Lindgren A, et al. Management and prognostic features of intracerebral hemorrhage during anticoagulant therapy: a Swedish multicenter study. *Stroke* 2001;32:2567–2574.

14. Mayer SA. Ultra-early hemostatic therapy for intracerebral hemorrhage. *Stroke* 2003;34:224–229.

15. Yasaka M, Minematsu K, Naritomi H, Sakata T, Yamaguchi T. Predisposing factors for enlargement of intracerebral hemorrhage in patients treated with warfarin. *Thromb Haemost* 2003;89:278–283.

16. Morenski JD, Tobias JD, Jimenez DF. Recombinant activated factor VII for cerebral injury-induced coagulopathy in pediatric patients. Report of three cases and review of the literature. *J Neurosurg* 2003;98:611–616.

17. Mayer SA. Intracerebral hemorrhage: natural history and rationale of ultra early hemostatic therapy. *Intensive Care Med* 2002;28(suppl 2):S235–S240.

18. Pessin MS, Estol CJ, Lafranchise F, Caplan LR. Safety of anticoagulation after hemorrhagic infarction. *Neurology* 1993;43:1298–1303.

19. Keir SL, Wardlaw J, Sandercock P, Chen Z. Antithrombotic therapy in patients with any form of intracranial haemorrhage: a systematic review of the available controlled studies. *Cerebrovasc Dis* 2002;14:197–206.

20. Suarez JI, Tarr RW, Selman WR. Aneurysmal subarachnoid hemorrhage. *N Eng J Med*, 2006;354:387–396.

21. Hop JW, Rinkel GJE, Algra A, van Gijn J. Quality of life in patients and partners after aneurysmal subarachnoid hemorrhage. *Stroke* 1998;29:798–804.

22. Hop JW, Rinkel GJE, Algra A, van Gijn J. Changes in functional outcome and quality of life in patients and caregivers after aneurysmal subarachnoid hemorrhage. *J Neurosurg* 2001;95:957–963.

23. Ferch R, Pasqualin A, Barone G, Pinna G, Bricolo A. Surgical management of ruptured aneurysms in the eighth and ninth decades. *Acta Neurochir (Wien)* 2003;145: 439–445.

24. Adams HP, Jr., Kassell NF, Torner JC. CT and clinical correlations in recent aneurysmal subarachnoid hemorrhage: a preliminary report of the Cooperative Aneurysm Study. *Neurology* 1983;33:981–988.

25. Hauerberg J, Eskesen V, Rosenorn J. The prognostic significance of intracerebral haematoma as shown on CT scanning after aneurysmal subarachnoid haemorrhage. *Br J Neurosurg* 1994;8:333–339.

26. Su CC, Saito K, Nakagawa A, Endo T, Suzuki Y, Shirane R. Clinical outcome following ultra-early operation for patients with intracerebral hematoma from aneurysm rupture—focusing on the massive intra-sylvian type of subarachnoid hemorrhage. *Acta Neurochir Suppl* 2002;82:65–69.

27. O'Sullivan MG, Whyman M, Steers JW, Whittle IR, Miller JD. Acute subdural haematoma secondary to ruptured intracranial aneurysm: diagnosis and management. *Br J Neurosurg* 1994;8:439–445.

28. McIver JI, Friedman JA, Wijdicks EFM, et al. Preoperative vetriculostomy and rebleeding after aneurysmal subarachnoid hemorrhage. *J Neurosurg* 2002;97:1042–1044.

29. Fujii Y, Takeuchi S, Sasaki O. Ultra-early rebleeding in spontaneous subarachnoid hemorrhage. *Neurosurgery* 1996;84:35–42.

30. Torner JC, Kassell NF, Wallace RB. Preoperative prognostic factors for rebleeding and survival in aneurysm patients receiving fibrinolytic therapy: report of the Cooperative Aneurysm Study. *Neurosurgery* 1981;9:506–513.

31. Brilstra EH, Rinkel GJE, Algra A, van Gijn J. Rebleeding, secondary ischemia, and timing of operation in patients with subarachnoid hemorrhage. *Neurology* 2000;55:1656–1660.

32. Broderick J, Brott T, Tomsick T. Management of intracerebral hemorrhage in a large metropolitan population. *Neurosurgery* 1994;34:882–887.

33. Vermuelen M, van Gijn J, Hijdra A. Causes of acute deterioration inpatients with a ruptured intracranial aneurysm. *J Neurosurg* 1984;60:935–939.

34. Van Crevel H. Pitfalls in the diagnosis of rebleeding from intracranial aneurysm. *Clin Neurol Neurosurg* 1984;660: 935–939.

35. Adams HP, Jr., Kassel NF, Torner JC. Early management of aneurysmal subarachnoid hemorrhage: a report of the Cooperative Aneurysm Study. *J Neurosurg* 1981;54:141.

36. Vermuelen M, Lindsay KW, Murray GD. Antifibrinolytic treatment in subarachnoid hemorrhage. *N Engl J Med* 1984;311:432–437.

37. Kassell NF, Torner JC, Adams HP, Jr. Antifibrinolytic therapy in the acute period following aneurysmal subarachnoid hemorrhage. Preliminary observations form the Cooperative Aneurysm Study. *J Neurosurg* 1984;61:225–230.

38. Leipzig TJ, Redelman K, Horner TG. Reducing the risk of rebleeding before early aneurysm surgery: a possible role for antifibrinolytic therapy. *J Neurosurg* 1997;86:220–225.

39. Roos Y, for the STAR Study Group. Antifibrinolytic treatment in subarachnoid hemorrhage. A randomized placebo-controlled trial. *Neurology* 2000;54:77–82.

40. Roos YB, Vermeulen M, Rinkel GJ, Algra A, van Gijn J. Systematic review of antifibrinolytic treatment in aneurysmal subarachnoid haemorrhage. *J Neurol Neurosurg Psychiatry* 1998;65:942–943.

41. Roos YB, Rinkel GJ, Vermeulen M, Algra A, van Gijn J. Antifibrinolytic therapy for aneurysmal subarachnoid haemorrhage. *Cochrane Database Syst Rev* 2000.

42. Hillman J, Fridriksson S, Nilsson O, Yu Z, Saveland H, Jakobsson K-E. Immediate administration of tranexamic acid and reduced incidence of early rebleeding after aneurysmal subarchnoid hemorrhage: a prospective randomized study. *J Neurosurg* 2002;97:771–778.

43. Mayberg MR, Batjer HH, Dacey R, et al. Guidelines for the management of aneurysmal subarachnoid hemorrhage. A statement for healthcare professionals from a special writing group of the Stroke Council, American Heart Association. *Stroke* 1994;25:2315–2328.

44. Schievink WI. Intracranial aneurysms. *N Engl J Med* 1997;336:25–40.

45. Miyaoka M, Sato K, Ishii S. A clinical study of the relationship of timing to outcome of surgery for ruptured

cerebral aneurysms: a retrospective analysis of 1,622 cases. *J Neurosurg* 1993;79:373–378.

46. Roos YB, Beenen LF, Groen RJ, Albrecht KW, Vermeulen M. Timing of surgery in patients with aneurysmal subarachnoid haemorrhage: rebleeding is still the major cause of poor outcome in neurosurgical units that aim at early surgery. *J Neurol Neurosurg Psychiatry* 1997;63:490–493.

47. Kassell NF, Torner JC, Haley EC, Jr., Jane JA, Adams HP, Jr., Kongable GL. The International Cooperative Study on the timing of aneurysm surgery. Part 1: overall management results. *J Neurosurg* 1990;73:18–36.

48. Kassell NF, Torner JC, Jane JA, Haley EC, Jr., Adams HP, Jr. The International Cooperative Study on the timing of aneurysm surgery. Part 2: surgical results. *J Neurosurg* 1990;73:37–47.

49. Ohman J, Heiskanen O. Timing of operation for ruptured supratentorial aneurysms: a prospective randomized study. *J Neurosurg* 1989;70:55.

50. Ross N, Hutchinson PJ, Seeley H, Kirkpatrick PJ. Timing of surgery for supratentorial aneurysmal subarachnoid haemorrhage: report of a prospective study. *J Neurol Neurosurg Psychiatry* 2002;72:480–484.

51. De Gans K, Nieuwkamp DJ, Rinkel GJ, Algra A. Timing of aneurysm surgery in subarachnoid hemorrhage: a systematic review of the literature. *Neurosurgery* 2002;50:336–340.

52. Nussbaum ES, Mendez A, Camarata P, Sebring L. Surgical management of fusiform aneurysms of the peripheral posteroinferior cerebellar artery. *Neurosurgery* 2003;53:831–834.

53. Leibowitz R, Do HM, Marcellus ML, Chang SD, Steinberg GK, Marks MP. Parent vessel occlusion for vertebrobasilar fusiform and dissecting aneurysms. *AJNR Am J Neuroradiol* 2003;24:902–907.

54. Jafar JJ, Russell SM, Woo HH. Treatment of giant intracranial aneurysms with saphenous vein extracranial-to-intracranial bypass grafting: indications, operative technique, and results in 29 patients. *Neurology* 2002;51:138–144.

55. CARAT Investigators. Rates of delayed rebleeding from intracranial aneurysms are low after surgical and endovascular treatment. *Stroke.* 2006;37:1437–1442.

56. Hope J, Byrne JV, Molyneux A. Factors influencing successful angiographic occlusion of aneurysms treated by coil embolization. *AJNR Am J Neuroradiol* 1999;20:391–399.

57. Cognard C, Weill A, Castaings L, Rey A, Moret J. Intracranial berry aneurysms: angiographic and clinical results after endovascular treatment. *Radiology* 1998;206:499–510.

58. Graves VB, Strother CM, Duff TA. Early treatment of ruptured aneurysms with Guglielmi detachable coils: effect on subsequent bleeding. *Neurosurgery* 1995;37:640–648.

59. Qureshi AI. Endovascular treatment of cerebrovascular diseases and intracranial neoplasms. *Lancet* 2004;363:804–813.

60. Eskridge J, Song J. Endovascular embolization of 150 basilar tip aneurysms with Guglielmi detachable coils: results of the Food and Drug Administration multicenter clinical trial. *J Neurosurg* 1998;89:81–86.

61. Konan AV, Raymond J, Roy D. Transarterial embolization of aneurysms associated with spinal cord arteriovenous

malformations—report of four cases. *J Neurosurg* 1999; 90:148–154.

62. Bavinzski G, Killer M, Gruber A, Reinprecht A, Gross CE, Richling B. Treatment of basilar artery bifurcation aneurysms by using Guglielmi detachable coils: a 6-year experience. *J Neurosurg* 1999;90:843–852.

63. Lefkowitz MA, Gobin YP, Akiba Y, et al. Balloon-assisted Guglielmi detachable coiling of wide-necked aneurysm: part II—clinical results. *Neurosurgery* 1999;45:531–537.

64. van den Berg R, Rinkel GJ, Vandertop WP. Treatment of unruptured intracranial aneurysms: implications of the ISAT on clipping versus coiling. *Eur J Radiol* 2003;46:172–177.

65. Mukonoweshuro W, Laitt RD, Hughes DG. Endovascular treatment of PICA aneurysms. *Neuroradiology* 2003;45:188–192.

66. Park HK, Horowitz M, Jungreis C, et al. Endovascular treatment of paraclinoid aneurysms: experience with 73 patients. *Neurosurgery* 2003;53:14–23.

67. Groden C, Eckert B, Ries T, Probst EN, Kucinski T, Zeumer H. Angiographic follow-up of vertebrobasilar artery aneurysms treated with detachable coils. *Neuroradiology* 2003;45:435–440.

68. Kremer C, Groden C, Lammers G, Weineck G, Zeumer H, Hansen HC. Outcome after endovascular therapy of ruptured intracranial aneurysms: morbidity and impact of rebleeding. *Neuroradiology* 2002;44:942–945.

69. Murayama Y, Nien YL, Duckwiler G, et al. Guglielmi detachable coil embolization of cerebral aneurysms: 11 years' experience. *J Neurosurg* 2003;98:959–966.

70. Weir RU, Marcellus ML, Do HM, Steinberg GK, Marks MP. Aneurysmal subarachnoid hemorrhage in patients with Hunt and Hess grade 4 or 5: treatment using the Guglielmi detachable coil system. *AJNR Am J Neuroradiol* 2003;42:585–590.

71. Wanke I, Doerfler A, Schoch B, Stolke D, Forsting M. Treatment of wide-necked intracranial aneurysms with a self-expanding stent system: initial clinical experience. *AJNR Am J Neuroradiol* 2003;24:1192–1199.

72. Han PP, Albuquerque FC, Ponce FA, et al. Percutaneous intracranial stent placement for aneurysms. *J Neurosurg* 2003;23:30.

73. Rabinstein AA, Pichelmann MA, Friedman JA, et al. Symptomatic vasospasm and outcomes following aneurysmal subarachnoid hemorrhage: a comparison between surgical repair and endovascular coil occlusion. *J Neurosurg* 2003;98:319–325.

74. Manabe H, Fujita S, Hatayama T, Suzuki S, Yagihashi S. Rerupture of a coil-embolized aneurysm during long-term observation. *J Neurosurg* 1998;88:1096–1098.

75. Horowitz MB, Jungreis CA, Genevro J. Delayed rupture of a previously coiled unruptured anterior communicating artery aneurysm: case report. *Neurosurgery* 2002;51:804–806.

76. Turner CL, Higgins JN, Kirkpatrick PJ. Assessment of transcranial color-coded duplex sonography for the surveillance of intracranial aneurysms treated with Guglielmi detachable coils. *Neurosurgery* 2003;53:866–871.

77. Friedman JA, Nichols DA, Meyer FB, et al. Guglielmi detachable coil treatment of ruptured saccular cerebral

aneurysms: retrospective review of a 10-year single-center experience. *AJNR Am J Neuroradiol* 2003;24:526–533.

78. Deinsberger W, Mewes H, Traupe H, Boeker DK. Surgical management of previously coiled intracranial aneurysms. *Br J Neurosurg* 2003;17:149–154.

79. Brilstra EH, Rinkel GJE, Van Der Graaf Y, van Rooij WJJ, Algra A. Treatment of intracranial aneurysms by embolization with coils—a systematic review. *Stroke* 1999;30:470–476.

80. Johnston SC, Dudley RA, Gress DR, Ono L. Surgical and endovascular treatment of unrupted cerebral aneurysms. *Neurology* 1999;52:1799–1805.

81. Lozier A, Connolly S, Lavine SD, Solomon RA. Guglielmi detachable coil embolization of posterior circulation aneurysms: a systematic review of the literature. *Stroke* 2002;33:2509–2518.

82. Arita K, Kurisu K, Ohba S, et al. Endovascular treatment of basilar tip aneurysms associated with moyamoya disease. *Neuroradiology* 2003;45:441–444.

83. Rabinov JD, Hellinger FR, Morris PP, Ogilvy CS, Putman CM. Endovascular management of vertebrobasilar dissecting aneurysms. *AJNR Am J Neuroradiol* 2003;24:1421–1428.

84. Anxionnat R, de Melo Neto JF, Bracard S, et al. Treatment of hemorrhagic intracranial dissections. *Neurosurgery* 2003;53:289–300.

85. Willing SJ, Skidmore F, Donaldson J, Nobo UL, Chernukha K. Treatment of acute intracranial vertebrobasilar dissection with angioplasty and stent placement: report of two cases. *AJNR Am J Neuroradiol* 2003;24:985–989.

86. Koivisto T, Vanninen R, Hurskainen H, Saari T, Hernesniemi J, Vapalahti M. Outcomes of early endovascular versus surgical treatment of ruptured cerebral aneurysms—a prospective randomized study. *Stroke* 2000;31:2369–2377.

87. Molyneux A, Kerr R, Stratton I, et al. International Subarachnoid Aneurysm Trial (ISAT) of neurosurgical clipping versus endovascular coiling in 2143 patients with ruptured intracranial aneurysms: a randomised trial. *Lancet* 2002;360:1267–1274.

88. International Subarachnoid Aneurysm Trial (ISAT) Collaborative Group. International Subarachnoid Aneurysm Trial (ISAT) of neurosurgical clipping versus endovascular coiling in 2143 patients with ruptured intracranial aneurysms: a randomised trial. *Lancet* 2002;360:1267–1274.

89. Rasmussen PA. Endovascular coiling: the end of conventional neurosurgery? *Cleve Clin J Med* 2004;71(suppl 1):S18.

90. Lawton MT, Guinones-Hinojosa A, Sanai N, Malek JY, Dowd CF. Combined microsurgical and endovascular management of complex intracranial aneurysms. *Neurosurgery* 2003;52:263–275.

91. Hop JW, Rinkel GJE. Secondary ischemia after subarachnoid hemorrhage. *Cerebrovasc Dis* 1996;6:264–265.

92. Mayberg MR. Cerebral vasospasm. *Neurosurg Clin N Am* 1998;9:615–627.

93. Roos YB, de Haan RJ, Beenen LF, Groen RJ, Albrecht KW, Vermeulen M. Complications and outcome in patients with aneurysmal subarachnoid haemorrhage: a prospective hospital based cohort study in the Netherlands. *J Neurol Neurosurg Psychiatry* 2000;68:337–341.

94. Kassell NF, Sasaki T, Colohan ART. Cerebral vasospasm following aneurysmal subarachnoid hemorrhage. *Stroke* 1985;16:562–572.

95. Findlay JM, Macdonald RL, Weir BKA. Current concepts of pathophysiology and management of cerebral vasospasm following aneurysmal subarachnoid hemorrhage. *Cerebrovasc Brain Metab Rev* 1991;3:336–361.

96. Weir B, Macdonald RL, Stoodley M. Etiology of cerebral vasospasm. *Acta Neurochir Suppl* 1999;72:27–46.

97. Dietrich HH, Dacey RG, Jr. Molecular keys to the problems of cerebral vasospasm. *Neurosurgery* 2000;46:517–530.

98. Rinkel GJE, Wijdicks EF, Vermeulen M, Hasan D, Brouwers PJAM, van Gijn J. The clinical course of perimesencephalic non-aneurysmal subarachnoid haemorrhage. *Ann Neurol* 1991;29:463–468.

99. Qureshi AI, Sung GY, Suri MA, et al. Prognostic value and determinants of ultraearly angiographic vasospasm after aneurysmal subarachnoid hemorrhage. *Neurosurgery* 1999;44:967–974.

100. Weir B, Grace M, Hansen J. Time course of vasospasm in man. *J Neurosurg* 1978;48:173–178.

101. Pasqualin A. Epidemiology and pathophysiology of cerebral vasospasm following subarachnoid hemorrhage. *J Neurosurg Sci* 1998;42:15–21.

102. Janjua N, Mayer SA. Cerebral vasospasm after subarachnoid hemorrhage. *Curr Opin Crit Care* 2003;9:113–119.

103. Dumont AS, Dumont RJ, Chow MM, et al. Cerebral vasospasm after subarachnoid hemorrhage: putative role of inflammation. *Neurosurgery* 2003;53:123–133.

104. Charpentier C, Audibert G, Guillemin F, et al. Multivariate analysis of predictors of cerebral vasospasm occurrence after aneurysmal subarachnoid hemorrhage. *Stroke* 1999;30:1402–1408.

105. Qureshi AI, Sung GY, Razumovsky AY, Lane K, Straw RN, Ulatowski JA. Early identification of patients at risk for symptomatic vasospasm after aneurysmal subarachnoid hemorrhage. *Crit Care Med* 2000;28:984–990.

106. Fisher CM, Kistler JP, Davis JM. Relation of cerebral vasospasm to subarachnoid hemorrhage visualized by computerized tomographic scanning. *Neurosurgery* 1980;6:1–9.

107. Adams HP, Jr., Kassell NF, Torner JC. Usefulness of computed tomography in predicting outcome after aneurysmal subarachnoid hemorrhage. *Neurology* 1985;35:1263–1267.

108. Hosoda K, Fujita S, Kawaguchi T, Shose Y, Hamano S, Iwakura M. Effect of clot removal and surgical manipulation on regional cerebral blood flow and delayed vasospasm in early aneurysm surgery for subarachnoid hemorrhage. *Surg Neurol* 1999;51:81–88.

109. Sasaki T, Ohta T, Kikuchi H. A phase II clinical trial of recombinant human tissue-type plasminogen activator against cerebral vasospasm after aneurysmal subarachnoid hemorrhage. *Neurosurgery* 1994;35:597–605.

110. Findlay JM, Kassell NF, Weir BKA. A randomized trial of intraoperative intracisternal tissue plasminogen activator for the prevention of vasospasm. *Neurosurgery* 1995;37:168–178.

111. Vora YY, Suarez-Almazor M, Steinke DE, Martin ML, Findlay JM. Role of transcranial Doppler monitoring in the diagnosis of cerebral vasospasm after subarachnoid hemorrhage. *Neurosurgery* 1999;44:1237–1248.

112. Grosset DG, Straiton J, McDonald I. Angiographic and Doppler diagnosis or cerebral artery vasospasm following subarachnoid hemorrhage. *Br J Neurosurg* 1993;7:291–298.

113. Laumer R, Steinmeier R, Gonner F. Cerebral hemodynamics in subarachnoid hemorrhage evaluated by transcranial Doppler sonography. *Neurosurgery* 1993;33:11–18.

114. Boecher-Schwarz HG, Ungersboeck K, Ulrich P, Fries G, Wild A, Perneczky A. Transcranial Doppler diagnosis of cerebral vasospasm following subarachnoid haemorrhage. Correlation and analysis of results in relation to the age of patients. *Acta Neurochir (Wien)* 1994;127:32–36.

115. Hasan D, Wijdicks EFM, Vermeulen M. Hyponatremia is associated with cerebral ischemia in patients with aneurysmal subarachnoid hemorrhage. *Ann Neurol* 1990; 27:106–108.

116. Vermeij FH, Hasan D, Bijvoet HW, Avezaat CJJ. Impact of medical treatment on the outcome of patients after aneurysmal subarachnoid hemorrhage. *Stroke* 1998;29: 924–930.

117. Feigin VL, Rinkel GJ, Algra A, van Gijn J. Circulatory volume expansion for aneurysmal subarachnoid hemorrhage. *Cochrane Database Syst Rev* 2000.

118. Egge A, Waterloo K, Sjoholm H, Solberg T, Ingebrigtsen T, Romner B. Prophylactic hyperdynamic postoperative fluid therapy after aneurysmal subarachnoid hemorrhage: a clinical, prospective, randomized, controlled study. *Neurosurgery* 2001;49:593–606.

119. Tseng M-Y, Al-Rawi PG, Pickard JD, Rasulo FA, Kirkpatrick PJ. Effect of hypertonic saline on cerebral blood flow in poor-grade patients with subarachnoid hemorrhage. *Stroke* 2003;34:1389–1397.

120. Pickard JD, Murray GD, Illingworth R, et al. Effect of oral nimodipine on cerebral infarction and outcome after subarachnoid haemorrhage: British aneurysm nimodipine trial. *Br Med J* 1989;298:636–642.

121. Barker FGI, Ogilvy CS. Efficacy of prophylactic nimodipine for delayed ischemic deficit after subarachnoid hemorrhage: a meta-analysis. *J Neurosurg* 1996;84:405–414.

122. Findlay JM. Current management of aneurysmal subarachnoid hemorrhage guidelines from the Canadian Neurosurgical Society. *Can J Neurol Sci* 1997;24:161–170.

123. Feigin VL, Rinkel GJ, Algra A, Vermeulen M, van Gijn J. Calcium antagonists for aneurysmal subarachnoid haemorrhage. *Cochrane Database Syst Rev* 2000.

124. Kasuya H, Onda H, Takeshita M, Okada Y, Hori T. Efficacy and safety of nicardipine prolonged-release implants for preventing vasospasm in humans. *Stroke* 2002;33:1011–1015.

125. Haley EC, Jr., Kassell NF, Torner JC, and the participants. A randomized trial of two doses of nicardipine in aneurysmal subarachnoid hemorrhage. A report of the Cooperative Aneurysm Study. *J Neurosurg* 1994;80:788.

126. Mori T, Katayama Y, Kawamata T, Hirayama T. Improved efficiency of hypervolemic therapy with inhibition of natriuresis by fludrocortisone in patients with aneurysmal subarachnoid hemorrhage. *J Neurosurg* 1999;91:947–952.

127. Mori K, Arai H, Nakajima K. Hemorheological and hemodynamic analysis of hypervolemic hemodilution therapy for cerebral vasospasm after aneurysmal subarachnoid hemorrhage. *Stroke* 1995;26:1620–1626.

128. Miller JA, Dacey RG, Jr., Diringer MN. Safety of hypertensive hypervolemic therapy with phenylephrine in the treatment of delayed ischemic deficits after subarachnoid hemorrhage. *Stroke* 1995;26:2260–2266.

129. Sen J, Belli A, Albon H, Morgan L, Petzold A, Kitchen N. Triple-H therapy in the management of aneurysmal subarachnoid haemorrhage. *Lancet Neurol* 2003;2:614–621.

130. Amin-Hanjani S, Schwartz RB, Sathi S, Stieg PE. Hypertensive encephalopathy as a complication of hyperdynamic therapy for vasospasm: report of two cases. *Neurosurgery* 1999;44:1113–1116.

131. Kassell NF, Peerless SJ, Durward QJ, Beck DW, Drake CG, Adams HP, Jr. Treatment of ischemic deficits from vasospasm with intravascular volume expansion and induced arterial hypertension. *Neurosurgery* 1982;11: 337–343.

132. European CGRP in Subarachnoid Hemorrhage Study Group. Effect of calcitonin-gene-related peptide in patients with delayed postoperative cerebral ischaemia after aneurysmal subarachnoid haemorrhage. *Lancet* 1992;339: 831–834.

133. Kassell NF, Haley EC, Jr., Apperson-Hansen C, et al. Randomized, double-blind, vehicle-controlled, trial of tirilazad mesylate in patients with aneurysmal subarachnoid hemorrhage: a cooperative study in Europe, Austarlia, and New Zealand. *J Neurosurg* 1996;84:221–228.

134. Lanzino G, Kassell NF, Dorsch NW, et al. Double-blind, randomized, vehicle-controlled study of high-dose tirilazad mesylate in women with aneurysmal subarachnoid hemorrhage. Part I. A cooperative study in Europe, Australia, New Zealand, and South Africa. *J Neurosurg* 1999;90:1011–1017.

135. Lanzino G, Kassell NF. Double-blind, randomized, vehicle-controlled study of high-dose tirilazad mesylate in women with aneurysmal subarachnoid hemorrhage. Part II. A cooperative study in North America. *J Neurosurg* 1999;90:1018–1024.

136. Haley ECJ, Kassell NF, Apperson-Hansen C, Maile MH, Alves WM. A randomized, double-blind, vehicle-controlled trial of tirilazad mesylate in patients with aneurysmal subarachnoid hemorrhage: a cooperative study in North America. *J Neurosurg* 1997;86:467–474.

137. Handa Y, Hayashi M, Takeuchi H. Effect of cyclosporine on the development of cerebral vasospasm in a primate model. *Neurosurgery* 1991;28:380.

138. Firlik KS, Kaufmann AM, Firlik AD, Jungreis CA, Yonas H. Intra-arterial papaverine for the treatment of cerebral vasospasm following aneurysmal subarachnoid hemorrhage. *Surg Neurol* 1999;51:66–74.

139. Saito I, Asano T, Sano K, et al. Neuroprotective effect of an antioxidant, ebselen, in patients with delayed neurological deficits after aneurysmal subarachnoid hemorrhage. *Neurosurgery* 1998;42:269–277.

140. Asano T, Takakura K, Sano K, et al. Effects of hydroxyl radical scavenger on delayed ischemic neurological deficits following aneurysmal subarachnoid hemorrhage: results of a multicenter, placebo-controlled double-blind trial. *J Neurosurg* 1996;84:792–803.

141. Andaluz N, Tomsick TA, Tew JM, Jr., van Loveren HR, Yeh HS, Zuccarello M. Indications for endovascular therapy

for refractory vasospasm after aneurysmal subarachnoid hemorrhage: experience at the University of Cincinnati. *Surg Neurol* 2002;58:131–138.

142. Kaku Y, Yonekawa Y, Tsukahara T, Kazekawa K. Superselective intra-arterial infusion of papaverine for the treatment of cerebral vasospasm after subarachnoid hemorrhage. *J Neurosurg* 1992;77:842.

143. Elliott JP, Newell DW, Lam DJ, et al. Comparison of balloon angioplasty and papaverine infusion for the treatment of vasospasm following aneurysmal subarachnoid hemorrhage. *J Neurosurg* 1998;88:277–284.

144. Fandino J, Kaku Y, Schuknect B, Valavanis A, Yonekawa Y. Improvement of cerebral oxygenation patterns and metabolic validation of superselective intraarterial infusion of papaverine for the treatment of cerebral vasospasm. *J Neurosurg* 1998;89:93–100.

145. Polin RS, Hansen CA, German P, Chadduck JB, Kassell NF. Intra-arterially administered papaverine for the treatment of symptomatic cerebral vasospasm. *Neurosurgery* 1998;42:1256–1264.

146. Chia RY, Hughes RS, Morgan MK. Magnesium: a useful adjunct in the prevention of cerebral vasospasm following aneurysmal subarachnoid haemorrhage. *J Clin Neurosci* 2002;9:279–281.

147. Schmid-Elsaesser R, Kunz M, Zausinger S, et al. Intravenous magnesium versus nimodipine in the treatment of patients with aneurysmal subarachnoid hemorrhage. A randomized study. *Neurosurgery*, 2006;58:1054–1065.

148. Pathak A, Mathuriya SN, Khandelwal N, Verma K. Intermittent low dose intrathecal sodium nitroprusside therapy for treatment of symptomatic aneurysmal SAH-induced vasospasm. *Br J Neurosurg* 2003;17:306–310.

149. Lesley WS, Lazo A, Chaloupka JC, Weigele JB. Successful treatment of cerebral vasospasm by use of transdermal nitroglycerin ointment (nitropaste). *AJNR Am J Neuroradiol* 2003;24:1234–1236.

150. Treggiari MM, Romand JA, Martin JB, Reverdin A, Rufenacht DA, De Tribolet N. Cervical sympathetic block to reverse delayed ischemic neurological deficits after aneurysmal subarachnoid hemorrhage. *Stroke* 2003;34:967–967.

151. Juvela S. Aspirin and delayed cerebral ischemia after aneurysmal subarachnoid hemorrhage. *J Neurosurg* 1995;82:945.

152. Hop JW, Rinkel GJ, Algra A, Berkelbach van der Sprenkel JW, van Gijn J. Randomized pilot trial of postoperative aspirin in subarachnoid hemorrhage. *Neurology* 2000;54:872–878.

153. Bejjani GK, Bank WO, Olan WJ, Sekhar LN. The efficacy and safety of angioplasty for cerebral vasospasm after subarachnoid hemorrhage. *Neurosurgery* 1998;42:979–986.

154. Nichols DA, Meyer FB, Piepgras DG, Smith PL. Endovascular treatment of intracranial aneurysms. *Mayo Clin Proc* 1994;69:272.

155. Firlik AD, Kaufmann AM, Jungreis CA, Yonas H. Effect of transluminal angioplasty on cerebral blood flow in the management of symptomatic vasospasm following aneurysmal subarachnoid hemorrhage. *J Neurosurg* 1997;86:830–839.

156. Eskridge JM, McAuliffe W, Song JK, et al. Balloon angioplasty for the treatment of vasospasm: results of first 50 cases. *Neurosurgery* 1998;42:510–516.

157. Murayama Y, Song JK, Uda K, et al. Combined endovascular treatment for both intracranial aneurysm and symptomatic vasospasm. *AJNR Am J Neuroradiol* 2003;24:133–139.

158. Hoelper BM, Hofmann E, Sporleder R, Soldner F, Behr R. Transluminal balloon angioplasty improves brain tissue oxygenation and metabolism in severe vasospasm after aneurysmal subarachnoid hemorrhage: case report. *Neurosurgery* 2003;52:970–974.

159. Muizelaar JP, Zwienenberg M, Rudisill NA, Hecht ST. The prophylactic use of transluminal balloon angioplasty in patients with Fisher Grade 3 subarachnoid hemorrhage: a pilot study. *J Neurosurg* 1999;91:51–57.

160. Linskey ME, Horton JA, Rao GR, Yonas H. Fatal rupture of the intracranial carotid artery during transluminal angioplasty for vasospasm induced by subarachnoid hemorrhage. *J Neurosurg* 1991;74:985–990.

161. Schoser BG, Heesen C, Eckert B, Thie A. Cerebral hyperperfusion injury after percutaneous transluminal angioplasty of extracranial arteries. *J Neurol* 1997;244:101–104.

162. Kreitschmann-Andermahr I, Hoff C, Niggemeier S, et al. Pituitary deficiency following aneurysmal subarachnoid haemorrhage. *J Neurol Neurosurg Psychiatry* 2003;74:1133–1135.

163. Bohmfalk GL, Story JL, Wissinger JP, et al. Bacterial intracranial aneurysm. *J Neurosurg* 1978;49:369–382.

164. Morawetz RB, Acker JD, Harsh GR, III. Management of mycotic (bacterial) intracranial aneurysms. *Contemp Neurosurgery* 1981;3:1–6.

165. Hartmann A, Mast H, Mohr JP, et al. Morbidity of intracranial hemorrhage in patients with cerebral arteriovenous malformation. *Stroke* 1998;29:931–934.

166. Brown RD, Jr., Wiebers DO, Torner JC, O'Fallon WM. Frequency of intracranial hemorrhage as a presenting symptom and subtype analysis: a population-based study of intracranial vascular malformation in Olmsted County, Minnesota. *J Neurosurg* 1996;85:29–32.

167. Kondziolka D, Lunsford LD, Kestle JRW. The natural history of cerebral cavernous malformations. *J Neurosurg* 1995;83:820–824.

168. Mast H, Young WL, Koennecke HC, et al. Risk of spontaneous haemorrhage after diagnosis of cerebral arteriovenous malformation. *Lancet* 1997;350:1065–1068.

169. Fleetwood IG, Marcellus ML, Levy RP, Marks MP, Steinberg GK. Deep arteriovenous malformations of the basal ganglia and thalamus: natural history. *J Neurosurg* 2003;98:747–750.

170. Langer DJ, Lasner TM, Hurst RW, Flamm ES, Zager EL, King JT, Jr. Hypertension, small size, and deep venous drainage are associated with risk of hemorrhagic presentation of cerebral arteriovenous malformations. *Neurosurgery* 1998;42:481–486.

171. Stefani MA, Porter PJ, TerBrugge KG, Montanera W, Willinsky RA, Wallace MC. Angioarchitectural factors present in brain arteriovenous malformations associated with hemorrhagic presentation. *Stroke* 2002;33:920–924.

172. Stapf C, Mohr JP, Sciacca RR, et al. Incident hemorrhage risk of brain arteriovenous malformations located in the arterial borderzones. *Stroke* 2000;31:2365–2368.

173. Apsimon H, Reef H, Phadke R, Popovic E. A population-based study of brain arteriovenous malformation: long-term treatment outcomes. *Stroke* 2002;33:2794–2800.

174. Hillman J. Population-based analysis of arteriovenous malformation treatment. *J Neurosurg* 2001;95:633–637.

175. Ondra SL, Troupp H, George ED, Schwab K. The natural history of symptomatic arteriovenous malformations of the brain: a 24-year follow-up assessment. *J Neurosurg* 1990;73:387–391.

176. Cunha e Sa MJ, Stein BM, Solomon RA, McCormick PC. The treatment of associated intracranial aneurysms and arteriovenous malformations. *J Neurosurg* 1992;77:853–859.

177. Stapf C, Mohr JP, Pile-Spellman J, et al. Concurrent arterial aneurysms in brain arteriovenous malformations with haemorrhagic presentation. *J Neurol Neurosurg Psychiatry* 2002;73:294–298.

178. Ogilvy CS, Stieg PE, Awad I, et al. Recommendations for the management of intracranial arteriovenous malformations. A statement for healthcare professionals from a special writing group of the Stroke Council, American Stroke Association. *Stroke* 2001;32:1458–1471.

179. Berman MF, Hartmann A, Mast H, et al. Determinants of resource utilization in the treatment of brain arteriovenous malformations. *AJNR Am J Neuroradiol* 1999;20:2004–2008.

180. Jafar JJ, Rezai AR. Acute surgical management of intracranial arteriovenous malformations. *Neurosurgery* 1994;34:8–13.

181. Ali MJ, Bendok BR, Rosenblatt S, Rose JE, Getch CC, Batjer HH. Recurrence of pediatric cerebral arteriovenous malformations after angiographically documented resection. *Pediatr Neurosurg* 2003;39:32–38.

182. Spetzler RF, Martin NA. A proposed grading system for arteriovenous malformations. *J Neurosurg* 1986;65:476–483.

183. Soderman M, Andersson T, Karlsson B, Wallace MC, Edner G. Management of patients with brain arteriovenous malformations. *Eur J Radiol* 2003;46:195–205.

184. Heros RC, Korosue K, Dibiold PM. Surgical excision of cerebral arteriovenous malformations: late results. *Neurosurgery* 1990;26:570–578.

185. Lawton MT. Spetzler–Martin Grade III arteriovenous malformations: surgical results and a modification of the grading scale. *Neurosurgery* 2003;52:740–748.

186. Steinberg GK, Chang SD, Gewirtz RJ, Lopez JR. Microsurgical resection of brainstem, thalamic, and basal ganglia angiographically occult vascular malformations. *Neurosurgery* 2000;46:260–270.

187. Huh SK, Lee KC, Lee KS, Kim DI, Park YG, Chung SS. Selection of treatment modalities for cerebral arteriovenous malformations: a retrospective analysis of 348 consecutive cases. *J Clin Neurosci* 2000;7:429–433.

188. Ferch RD, Morgan MK. High-grade arteriovenous malformations and their management. *J Clin Neurosci* 2002;9:37–40.

189. Han PP, Ponce FA, Spetzler RF. Intention-to-treat analysis of Spetzler–Martin Grades IV and V arteriovenous malformations: natural history and treatment paradigm. *J Neurosurg* 2003;98:3–7.

190. Pik JH, Morgan MK. Microsurgery for small arteriovenous malformations of the brain: results in 110 consecutive patients. *Neurosurgery* 2000;47:571–575.

191. Hartmann A, Stapf C, Hofmeister C, et al. Determinants of neurological outcome after surgery for brain arteriovenous malformation. *Stroke* 2000;31:2361–2364.

192. Zimmerman RS, Spetzler RF, Lee KS, Zabramski JM, Hargraves RW. Cavernous malformations of the brain stem. *J Neurosurg* 1991;75:32–39.

193. Schaller C, Urbach H, Schramm J, Meyer B. Role of venous drainage in cerebral arteriovenous malformation surgery, as related to the development of postoperative hyperperfusion injury. *Neurosurgery* 2002;51:921–927.

194. Morgan M, Sekhon L, Finfer S, Grinnell V. Delayed neurological deterioration following resection of arteriovenous malformations of the brain. *J Neurosurg* 1999;90:695–701.

195. Purdy PD, Batjer HH, Samson D. Management of hemorrhagic complications from preoperative embolization of arteriovenous malformations. *J Neurosurg* 1991;74:205–211.

196. Purdy PD, Samson D, Batjer HH, Risser RC. Preoperative embolization of cerebral arteriovenous malformations with polyvinyl alcohol particles: experience in 51 adults. *AJNR Am J Neuroradiol* 1990;11:501–510.

197. Cromwell LD, Harris AB. Treatment of cerebral arteriovenous malformations: combined neurosurgical and neuroradiologic approach. *AJNR Am J Neuroradiol* 1983;4:366–368.

198. Kinouchi H, Mizoi K, Takahashi A, Ezura M, Yoshimoto T. Combined embolization and microsurgery for cerebral arteriovenous malformation. *Neurol Med Chir* 2002;42:372–378.

199. Jafar JJ, Davis AJ, Berenstein A, Choi IS, Kupersmith MJ. The effect of embolization with *n*-butyl cyanoacrylate prior to surgical resection of cerebral arteriovenous malformations. *J Neurosurg* 1993;78:60–69.

200. Chang SD, Steinberg GK, Rosario M, Crowley RS, Hevner RF. Mixed arteriovenous malformation and capillary telangiectasia: a rare subset of mixed vascular malformations. *J Neurosurg* 1997;86:699–703.

201. Friedman JA, Pollock BE, Nichols DA, Gorman DA, Foote RL, Stafford SL. Results of combined stereotactic radiosurgery and transarterial embolization for dural arteriovenous fistulas of the transverse and sigmoid sinuses. *J Neurosurg* 2001;94:886–891.

202. Vinuela F, Dion JE, Duckwiler G, et al. Combined endovascular embolization and surgery in the management of cerebral arteriovenous malformations: experience with 101 cases. *J Neurosurg* 1991;75:856–864.

203. Gobin YP, Laurent A, Merienne L, et al. Treatment of brain arteriovenous malformations by embolization and radiosurgery. *J Neurosurg* 1996;85:19–28.

204. Liu HM, Wang YH, Chen YF, Tu YK, Huang KM. Endovascular treatment of brain-stem arteriovenous malformations: safety and efficacy. *Neuroradiology* 2003;45:644–649.

205. Hurst RW, Berenstein A, Kupersmith MJ, Madrid M, Flamm ES. Deep central arteriovenous malformations of the brain: the role of endovascular treatment. *J Neurosurg* 1995;82:190–195.

206. Spetzler RF, Martin NA, Carter LP, Flom RA, Raudzens PA, Wilkinson E. Surgical management of large AVM's by staged embolization and operative excision. *J Neurosurg* 1987;67:17–28.

207. Hartmann A, Pile-Spellman J, Stapf C, et al. Risk of endovascular treatment of brain arteriovenous malformations. *Stroke* 2002;33:1816–1820.

208. Deruty R, Pelissou-Guyotat I, Morel C, Bascoulergue Y, Turjman F. Reflections on the management of cerebral arteriovenous malformations. *Surg Neurol* 1998;50:245–255.

209. Keller E, Yonekawa Y, Imhof HG, Tanaka M, Valavanis A. Intensive care management of patients with severe intracerebral haemorrhage after endovascular treatment of brain arteriovenous malformations. *Neuroradiology* 2002;44:513–521.

210. Stein BM, Wolpert SM. Surgical and embolic treatment of cerebral arteriovenous malformations. *Surg Neurol* 1977; 7:359–369.

211. Greitz T, Lax I, Bergstrom M, et al. Stereotactic radiation therapy of intracranial lesions. Methodologic aspects. *Acta Radiol Oncol* 1986;25:81–89.

212. Steinberg GK, Fabrikant JI, Marks MP, et al. Stereotactic helium ion Bragg peak radiosurgery for intracranial arteriovenous malformations. Detailed clinical and neuroradiologic outcome. *Stereotact Funct Neurosurg* 1991;57:36–49.

213. Kurita H, Kawamoto S, Sasaki T, et al. Results of radiosurgery for brain stem arteriovenous malformations. *J Neurol Neurosurg Psychiatry* 2000;68:563–570.

214. Lunsford LD, Kondziolka D, Flickinger JC, et al. Stereotactic radiosurgery for arteriovenous malformations of the brain. *J Neurosurg* 1991;75:512–524.

215. Steiner L, Lindquist C, Torner JC, Alves W, Steiner M. Clinical outcome of radiosurgery for cerebral arteriovenous malformations. *J Neurosurg* 1992;77:1–8.

216. Colombo F, Pozza F, Chierego G, Casentini L, De Luca G, Francescon P. Linear accelerator radiosurgery of cerebral arteriovenous malformations: an update. *Neurosurgery* 1994;34:14–20.

217. Firlik AD, Levy EI, Kondziolka D, Yonas H. Staged volume radiosurgery followed by microsurgical resection: a novel treatment for giant cerebral arteriovenous malformations: technical case report. *Neurosurgery* 1998;43:1223–1228.

218. Flickinger JC, Pollock BE, Kondziolka D, Lunsford LD. A dose-response analysis of arteriovenous malformation obliteration after radiosurgery. *Int J Radiat Oncol Biol Phys* 1996;36:873–879.

219. Pollock BE, Flickinger JC. A proposed radiosurgery-based grading system for arteriovenous malformations. *J Neurosurg* 2002;96:79–85.

220. Karlsson B, Lindquist C, Steiner L. Prediction of obliteration after gamma knife surgery for cerebral arteriovenous malformations. *Neurosurgery* 1997;40:425–430.

221. Pollock BE, Garces YI, Stafford SL, Foote RL, Schomberg PJ, Link MJ. Stereotactic radiosurgery for cavernous malformations. *J Neurosurg* 2000;93:987–991.

222. Friedman WA, Bova FJ, Bollampally S, Bradshaw P. Analysis of factors predictive of success or complications in arteriovenous malformation radiosurgery. *Neurosurgery* 2003;52:296–307.

223. Pollock BE, Gorman DA, Coffey RJ. Patient outcomes after arteriovenous malformation radiosurgical management: results based on a 5- to 14-year follow-up study. *Neurosurgery* 2003;52:1291–1296.

224. Hasegawa T, McInerney J, Kondziolka D, Lee JY, Flickinger JC, Lunsford LD. Long-term results after stereotactic radiosurgery for patients with cavernous malformations. *Neurosurgery* 2002;50:1190–1197.

225. Smyth MD, Sneed PK, Ciricillo SF, et al. Stereotactic radiosurgery for pediatric intracranial arteriovenous malformations: the University of California at San Francisco experience. *J Neurosurg* 2002;97:48–55.

226. Karlsson B, Lax I, Soderman M. Risk for hemorrhage during the 2-year latency period following gamma knife radiosurgery for arteriovenous malformations. *Int J Radiat Oncol Biol Phys* 2001;49:1045–1051.

227. Kim DG, Choe WJ, Paek SH, Chung HT, Kim IH, Han DH. Radiosurgery of intracranial cavernous malformations. *Acta Neurochir (Wien)* 2002;144:869–878.

228. Inoue HK, Ohye C. Hemorrhage risks and obliteration rates of arteriovenous malformations after gamma knife radiosurgery. *J Neurosurg* 2002;97:474–476.

229. Pollock BE, Flickinger JC, Lunsford LD, Bissonette DJ, Kondziolka D. Hemorrhage risk after stereotactic radiosurgery of cerebral arteriovenous malformations. *Neurosurgery* 1996;38:652–659.

230. Flickinger JC, Kondziolka D, Maitz AH, Lunsford LD. Analysis of neurological sequelae from radiosurgery of arteriovenous malformations: how location affects outcome. *Int J Radiat Oncol Biol Phys* 1998;40:273–278.

231. van Rossum J, Wintzen AR, Endtz LJ, Schoen JH, de Jonge H. Effect of tranexamic acid on rebleeding after subarachnoid hemorrhage. A double-blind controlled clinical trial. *Ann Neurol,* 1977;2:238–242.

232. Chandra B. Treatment of subarachnoid hemorrhage from ruptured intracranial aneurysm with tranexamic acid. A double-blind clinical trial. *Ann Neurol,* 1978;3: 502–504.

233. Maurice-Williams RS. Prolonged antifibrinolysis. An effective non-surgical treatment for ruptured intracranial aneurysms? *Br Med J,* 1978;1(6118):945–947.

234. Kaste M, Ramsay M. Tranexamic acid in subarachnoid hemorrhage. A double-blind study. *Stroke,* 1979;10:519–522.

235. Fodstad H, Forsell A, Liliequist B, Schannong M. Antifibrinolysis with tranexamic acid in aneurysmal subarachnoid hemorrhage. A consecutive controlled clinical trial. *Neurosurgery,* 1981;8:158–165.

236. Tsementzis SA, Hitchcock ER, Meyer, CH Benefits and risks of antifibrinolytic therapy in the management of ruptured intracranial aneurysms. A double-blind placebo-controlled study. *Acta Neurochir (Wien).* 1990; 102:1–10.

CHAPTER 24

Management of Patients with Recent Stroke

► ADMISSION TO THE HOSPITAL

Decisions about admission to the hospital are made on a case-by-case basis. In general, most persons with recent stroke should be hospitalized in order to (1) observe for neurological worsening, (2) continue therapies initiated in the emergency department, (3) administer interventions that prevent or control complications, (4) promptly evaluate for the cause of stroke, (5) initiate rehabilitation and patient education, and (6) start medical or surgical therapies to treat the underlying vascular disease and prevent recurrent stroke (Table 24-1). Serious comorbid diseases also should be treated. The first 24 h following stroke are the most crucial.[1] There have been discussions about the need to hospitalize patients with recent stroke. Presumably, treatment at home setting would avoid the expense of hospitalization. This strategy appears to be unwise. No evidence exists to support a change in approach to early treatment of patients with stroke; it should remain hospital-based.[2]

Admission to the hospital should involve a smooth transition from the emergency department (see Chapter 21). In many instances, the physicians who treated the patient in the emergency department will continue management. In some circumstances, admission will follow treatment in an interventional radiology suite or an operating room, or additional physicians, such as intensive care specialists, are involved in care. Close communication among the physicians is crucial for success. Some patients may be transferred from a community hospital after acute treatment of the stroke to a larger medical center for subsequent management.

The length of stays for acute treatment of the stroke varies considerably among patients. During the last decade, a concerted effort by health care professionals stimulated by the demands of the government and insurance companies has resulted in considerable reductions in the duration of hospitalization in the United States. The pressure to shorten the hospitalization means that all components of management are implemented in parallel. Still, despite the thrust to reduce health care costs, the primary goal should be to assure that the patient receives excellent care. The period of acute hospitalization depends upon the severity of the patient's stroke and need for specific medical or surgical interventions. For a patient with relatively mild neurological impairments, the period of inpatient care could be limited to 1 or 2 days. On the other hand, patients with severe strokes, especially those with hemorrhages, often require a prolonged period of hospitalization.

Some exceptions to the rule for hospitalization do exist. Patients who do not seek medical attention until several days after the vascular event, particularly those with mild ischemic strokes, probably do not need admission. Their risk for complications is relatively low. Their evaluation can be performed on an outpatient basis. Medications to prevent recurrent stroke, such as antiplatelet agents, can be started and if surgery is needed, the patient can be admitted prior to the operation. Some patients with severe strokes are admitted to the hospital for palliative care. Other patients, especially those who already are residents of long-term care facilities and for whom no specific treatment is indicated, might be returned to their original institution.

With the development of regional stroke programs, patients will likely be treated at an emergency department in a community hospital. Following emergency management, possibly including the administration of

▶ **TABLE 24-1.** COMPONENTS OF ACUTE TREATMENT FOLLOWING ADMISSION TO THE HOSPITAL

Continue therapies to treat stroke started in the emergency department
Close observation of the patient's clinical status
   Neurological assessments
   Cardiovascular monitoring
Prevention or treatment of medical or neurological complications
Initiation of rehabilitation
Education of the patient and family
Evaluation for the cause of stroke
Initiation of therapies to prevent recurrent stroke
   Medications
      Antiplatelet agents
      Anticoagulants
   Surgical procedures
Discharge planning

recombinant tissue plasminogen activator (rtPA), the patient could be transferred to a tertiary hospital that has the expertise and special resources to treat stroke. The components of a specialized stroke center, both personnel and resources, are included in Chapter 3.

▶ STROKE UNITS AND SPECIALIZED STROKE CARE

The structure of a stroke unit is described in Chapter 3. It basically consists of physicians and other health care professionals who provide state-of-the-art treatment[1,3–7] The development of units that specialize in treatment of patients with life-threatening neurological illnesses, including recent stroke, is a major advance. Such an organized approach facilitates monitoring of the patient's neurological and medical status. An organized unit expedites the institution of therapies to prevent or control complications and speeds up the initiation of rehabilitative efforts (see Table 24-1). In a randomized trial that enrolled 267 patients with moderately severe stroke, Evans et al.[8] compared the usefulness of care in a stroke unit or treatment on a general medical ward with specialist stroke team support. At both 3 months and 1 year, mortality or need for institutionalized care was greater among the patients who were treated on the general medical wards. Several other reports have demonstrated similar benefits.[9–14] A systemic review found that stroke units reduce length of stay, rates of complications, and costs.[15] In addition, care in a stroke unit was associated with increased referral to rehabilitation centers and

▶ **TABLE 24-2.** COMPONENTS OF CARE MAPS IN THE TREATMENT OF PATIENTS WITH RECENT STROKE

Activity
  Usually require bed rest for the first 24 h
  Thereafter, encourage the patient to be out of bed
  Increase activity as tolerated by the patient
    Include measures to avoid falls
  Some patients require prolonged bed rest
    Implement measures to prevent pressure sores
      Mattress
      Moving patient
    Implement measures to prevent orthopedic problems
      Range-of-motion exercises
Observation performed at regular intervals
  Initially performed every 4 h
    Adjusted as the patient improves
    May be more frequent when patient treated with rtPA
Components of examination
    Neurological assessments
    Blood pressure
    Cardiac rate and rhythm
    Respiratory rate
    Temperature
Management of hydration and nutrition
  Initially not given food and water by mouth
  Assess swallowing—bedside or speech pathologist
  Adjust consistency of food and liquids to ability to swallow
  Modify diet to reflect needs of patient
    Diabetes
    Low fat, low cholesterol
    Low sodium
  Supplement diet with stool softeners to avoid constipation

General medical treatment
  Treat comorbid diseases
    (i.e., hypertension, diabetes mellitus, lung disease, heart disease, Parkinson disease, etc.)
  Symptomatic treatment
    (i.e., analgesics, antipyretics, antibiotics, sleeping aids, etc.)
  Management of urinary incontinence
    Short-term use of indwelling bladder catheter
    Remove catheter as patient's condition permits
  Prophylaxis of deep vein thrombosis for bedridden patients
    Subcutaneous anticoagulants
    Alternating pressure devices and support stockings
Consultation of rehabilitation and discharge services
  Social services
  Discharge planner
  Physical therapy
  Occupational therapy
  Speech therapy
Consultation of other physician services
Evaluation the cause of stroke
    Arterial imaging
    Cardiac imaging
    Special coagulation tests
    Tests for autoimmune disorders
Initiation of therapy to prevent recurrent stroke
    Antiplatelet agents
    Anticoagulants
    Surgical procedures

reduced discharges to long-term care facilities. Another systemic review found that persons admitted to a stroke unit are more likely to survive and to be independently living at home than those who do not receive such care.[16] The benefits are the most apparent in discrete units.

Care maps and stroke care protocols also reduce the length of hospitalization and improve care[17,18] (Table 24-2). Such protocols involve the collaboration of physicians, nurses, and rehabilitation specialists. While care maps include orders for general care, diet, activities, evaluation, general medical therapies, consultations, and discharge planning, these orders are revised so as to meet the requirements of the patient. A preprinted set of orders is helpful. Care maps are most useful for management of patients who are not hospitalized in an intensive care unit, where additional interventions, such as ventilatory assistance, add complexity to care. The care map in Table 24-2 does not list the special orders required for management of patients who require neurosurgical interventions. The use of protocols can shorten hospitalization. Besides improving coordination of treatment, such an approach is cost-effective because unnecessary tests and procedures might be avoided.

The role of specialized neurological treatment facilities for critically ill patients likely will increase during the years ahead. These units are becoming the standard for inpatient care. New technologies to examine brain function can complement current methods to monitor patients. For example, multimodal monitoring including assessments of cerebral blood flow, brain tissue oxygenation, and sampling of brain tissue fluid molecules might become an important future way to follow critically ill patients with acute neurological injuries, including stroke.[19]

▶ NEUROLOGICAL WORSENING AFTER ADMISSION TO THE HOSPITAL

Approximately 40 percent of patients have neurological worsening during the first week following stroke.[20,21] The causes of worsening and the timing of these events vary. Neurological deterioration secondary to the acute stroke itself usually develops during the first 24-48 h following stroke (Fig. 24-1). The leading causes are brain edema, hydrocephalus, and increased intracranial pressure (Table 24-3). These complications usually are found among patients with major vascular events or multilobar infarctions, especially those located in the posterior fossa. Patients with diabetes mellitus, hyperglycemia, or hypertension have the highest risk of neurological progression.[20] Recurrent stroke, seizures, or hemorrhagic transformation of an infarction also can lead to an increase in neurological impairments. In general, the neurological causes for deterioration reach a peak within the first week after the stroke. The time course for the neurological

▶ **TABLE 24-3.** CAUSES OF NEUROLOGICAL DETERIORATION FOLLOWING STROKE

Neurological events
  Early recurrent stroke
    Recurrent hemorrhage
    Recurrent embolization or infarction
Progression of the stroke
    Hemodynamic failure
    Biochemical mechanisms—neurotoxic agents
Symptomatic hemorrhagic transformation of infarction
Increased intracranial pressure
    Mass effects
    Brain edema
    Hydrocephalus
Medical events
  Cardiovascular
  Pulmonary embolism
  Infection
    Pneumonia
    Urinary tract infection
Complications of medications

complications following intracranial hemorrhage usually is shorter than that found in infarctions. However, the neurological causes of worsening are similar to hemorrhages or infarctions.

The most common medical complications that lead to increased neurological impairments, disability, or death

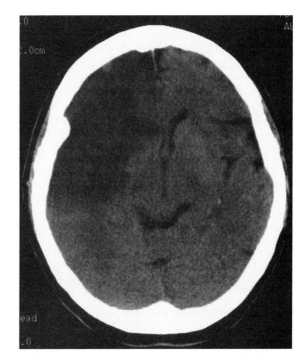

Figure 24-1. Large infarction of the right hemisphere is found in the right hemisphere. The infarction involves most of the deep and superficial branches of the middle cerebral artery and the anterior cerebral artery. The findings would be consistent with an occlusion of the internal carotid artery.

are infections and cardiovascular events, including deep vein thrombosis (DVT) and pulmonary embolism. The events, which generally occur for more than a week following stroke, complicate either hemorrhages or infarctions. These adverse events along with recurrent stroke are the leading causes of neurological worsening following stroke. In addition, serious comorbid diseases, such as diabetes, also can lead to a decline in neurological status. Thus, management of hospitalized patients involves treatment of the neurological and medical diseases.[22]

Brain Edema and Increased Intracranial Pressure

Management of brain edema is a critical component of treatment of patients with recent cerebral infarction or hemorrhage. Much of management is initiated in the emergency department (see Chapter 21). Most cases requiring urgent treatment of increased intracranial pressure in the emergency department are those with intracranial bleeding. In particular, decisions about emergency management of hydrocephalus or treatment of a mass-producing hematoma are made prior to admission to the hospital.

Brain edema is the most common neurological etiology for worsening among critically ill patients hospitalized with either hemorrhagic or ischemic stroke (Figs. 24-2 and 24-3). Malignant brain edema usually appears within

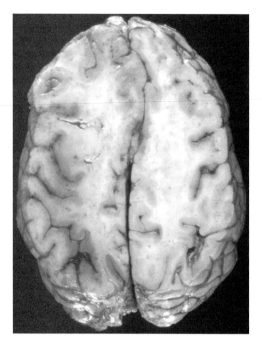

Figure 24-3. Axial autopsy specimen of the brain obtained from a patient dying of a major left hemisphere infarction. The infarction is in the territory of the middle cerebral artery. The hemisphere is swollen and the medial portion of the frontal lobe is shifted across the midline. (*Courtesy of S.S. Schochet, M.D., Department of Pathology, University of West Virginia, Morgantown, WV*)

24-48 h among patients with hemorrhages and 2-5 days among patients with infarctions.[3] Approximately 1–5 percent of patients with cerebral infarctions develop signs of malignant brain edema and increased intracranial pressure.[23] Malignant brain edema accounts for approximately three-fourths of the deaths that happen within 1 week of stroke.[22] Most deaths among patients with malignant brain edema are the consequence of herniation and secondary brain stem injury.[24,25] Secondary global brain ischemia also can complicate the increases in intracranial pressure. Mortality among patients with malignant brain edema following stroke is approximately 75 percent.[23] Patients surviving malignant brain edema often have major neurological sequelae.

The severity of the patient's stroke, as defined by the neurological impairments, predicts development of this complication. Malignant brain edema occurs with large hematomas or multilobar infarctions secondary to occlusions of major arteries (Fig. 24-4). These patients have declines in the level of consciousness, a high score on the National Institute of Health Stroke Scale (NIHSS), or a low score on the Glasgow Coma Scale.[26] Among patients with infarctions, those with hypertension, cardiac failure, and early nausea and vomiting have the highest risk for malignant brain edema.[26,27] Brain imaging findings of an infarction involving more than one-third

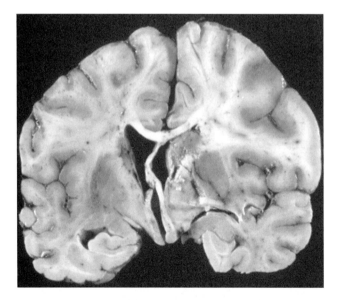

Figure 24-2. Coronal autopsy specimen obtained from a patient dying of a massive infarction of the left hemisphere. The left hemisphere is swollen with obliteration of the sulci and compression of the ipsilateral lateral ventricle. In addition, there is evidence of shift of the cingulate gyrus and the rostral brain stem and uncus across the midline. The findings are compatible with uncal herniation. (*Courtesy of S.S. Schochet, M.D., Department of Pathology, University of West Virginia, Morgantown, WV*)

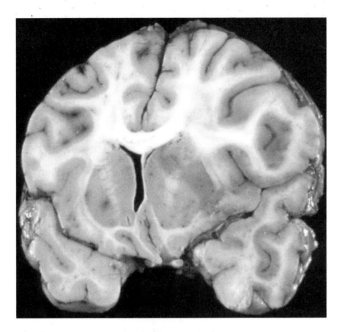

Figure 24-4. Coronal autopsy specimen of the brain demonstrates a malignant infarction of the left cerebral hemisphere secondary to embolic occlusion of the middle cerebral artery. The left hemisphere is swollen. The left lateral ventricle is obliterated and the third ventricle and left cingulate gyrus have been displaced across the midline. (*Courtesy of S.S. Schochet, M.D., Department of Pathology, University of West Virginia, Morgantown, WV*)

cephalus, is secondary to diffusion of cerebrospinal fluid through the ependymal lining of the ventricles and into periventricular white matter.[29] Thus, interstitial edema is usually seen among patients with intracranial hemorrhage or major infarctions in the posterior fossa that lead to obstruction of cerebrospinal fluid drainage pathways.[30,31]

No clinical treatment is established as effective in limiting development of brain edema following stroke.[28] Prophylaxis includes elevation of the head of the bed, avoidance of hypoosmolar fluids, and treating hypoxia, hypercarbia, and fever.[22,23,32,33] These measures have not been tested in clinical trials but their use seems reasonable. Corticosteroids are not effective (see Chapter 21). Patients with malignant brain edema usually need ventilatory assistance.[25] Most of these patients need airway support because of decreased levels of consciousness. Intubation also is helpful in preventing both hypoxia and hypercarbia, and hyperventilation is used to lower intracranial pressure (see Chapter 21). Still, hyperventilation is of limited utility and it should be considered as an adjunct to other measures to lower intracranial pressure. Data are limited about the utility of hyperosmolar therapy but the use of these agents, most commonly mannitol, is recommended[32,33] (see Chapter 21). There is considerable recent interest in the use of hypertonic saline. Hypertonic saline can lead to dehydration of the brain by creating an osmotic gradient, reducing viscosity, speeding reabsorption of cerebrospinal fluid, increasing

of a cerebral hemisphere, early sulcal effacement, early loss of the difference between the cortex and the adjacent white matter, or the presence of the dense artery sign (surrogate for a proximal middle cerebral artery occlusion) also forecast malignant brain edema among patients with infarctions (Fig. 24-5).

Most of the changes are secondary to an increase in brain volume due to the accumulation of water. Vascular engorgement probably has a minor contribution. Vasogenic edema is defined as fluid originating in blood vessels and accumulating around cells.[28] Cytotoxic edema involves the increase of water within the cells secondary to the cell injury; this is the edema that most commonly follows cerebral infarction.[28] Cytotoxic edema probably is in part due to transmembrane fluxes of sodium and water at the time of metabolic failure. Other factors including release of neurotransmitters and mitochondrial failure lead to changes in ionic gradients. Neurotoxic edema, which is a subtype of cytotoxic edema, is secondary to high concentrations of excitatory amino acids in the affected tissue. All three forms of edema coexist in stroke. Overall, the basic mechanism of brain edema involves the movement of cations (particularly, sodium and calcium) from extracellular spaces into cells. This movement is followed by chloride ions to maintain electrical balance, and water follows.[28] Interstitial edema, seen with hydro-

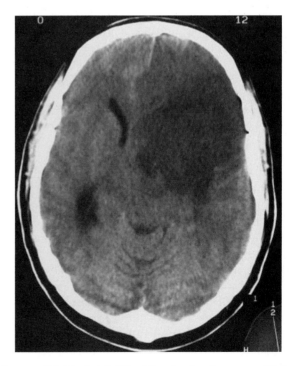

Figure 24-5. Axial CT of the brain shows multilobar left hemisphere infarction with secondary brain edema. Midline structures, including the hypothalamus and the rostral brain stem, have been displaced to the right. The right lateral ventricle is dilated.

▶ **TABLE 24-4.** SURGICAL TREATMENT OF MALIGNANT BRAIN EDEMA AND MASS EFFECTS OF PATIENTS WITH CEREBRAL INFARCTION

	Patients Treated	Survivors	Good Outcomes	
Study (Author)	N	N	N	%
Kondziolka and Fazl	5	5	5	100
Delashaw et al.	9	8	3	33
Steiger	8	6	4	50
Kalia and Yonas	4	4	4	100
Rieke et al.	32	21	15	46
Carver et al.	14	11	8	57
Sakai et al.	24	16	0	0
Schwab et al.	63	46	46	73
Mori et al.	13	11	3	23

Information obtained from.[40,176–182]

cardiac output, increasing blood pressure, improving oxygenation, and diminishing inflammatory reactions.[29] While hypothermia has been used to control intracranial pressure and brain edema, controlled trials of the intervention have not been done.[34,35]

Decompressive craniectomy is recommended for treatment of patients with rapid neurological worsening, deteriorating consciousness, massive cerebral ischemia, and edema[36] (Table 24-4). Considerable uncertainty exists about the role of decompressive operations, including hemicraniectomy for treatment of patients with malignant hemispheric infarctions.[37–40] The selection of patients and the timing of surgery have not been determined. Dohmen et al.[41] used positron emission tomographic (PET) imaging to select those patients who could be treated best with early surgical interventions. While this tactic is interesting, the use of PET or other ancillary tests to select patients for emergency surgery does not seem to be practical.

In a nonrandomized study involving 52 patients, Cho et al.[42] looked at the impact of the interval from onset of stroke until the timing of surgery. Patients who had very early decompressive surgery had lower mortality and better outcomes than those who had operation at latter time periods. They concluded that surgery before the patient becomes profoundly ill might improve outcomes. Pranesh et al.[43] performed hemicraniectomy for treatment of 19 patients with large middle cerebral artery infarctions; 10 had lesions of the dominant hemisphere. They concluded that speech function, especially comprehension, was improved following operation. However, the range of disabilities among survivors ranged from profound to mild. In a comparison of decompressive hemicraniectomy or moderate hypothermia to treat malignant brain edema following stroke, the surgical procedure seemed to be associated with lower rates of complications or death.[44] A systemic review concluded that evidence from clinical trials are lacking, and thus there is no solid evidence about the utility of decompressive surgery for treating patients with neurological deteriora-

tion secondary to brain edema following stroke.[45] A subsequent review of the potential utility of hemicraniectomy for treatment of malignant infarction in the territory of the middle cerebral artery looked at the results of 12 trials.[46] At follow-up, only 7 percent of 129 treated patients were independent, while 58 percent were dead or severely disabled. They found that patients older than 50 had extremely poor outcomes. They could not find a relationship to the timing of surgery, the side of infarction, or the presence of early signs of uncal herniation. Based on another review of available data, Hofmeijer et al.[47] concluded that no treatment modality had been shown as effective in treatment of space-occupying cerebral infarctions. They concluded that decompressive surgery is the most promising intervention.

A multicenter trial testing decompressive craniotomy for treatment of malignant cerebral infarctions showed benefit and another is underway.[48,49] These trials' results likely will influence future recommendations about surgical treatment of patients with malignant brain edema following cerebral infarction.

Hydrocephalus

Hydrocephalus may lead to neurological worsening in the first 7-10 days following intracranial bleeding, especially following aneurysmal subarachnoid hemorrhage. In addition, delayed (normal pressure) hydrocephalus is a potential cause of neurological symptoms, including gait disturbances, incontinence, and cognitive decline in the months or years after a ruptured aneurysm.[50,51] While some element of ipsilateral ventricular dilation can follow a major hemispheric infarction or ventricular enlargement can occur following multiple strokes, most patients with ischemic or hemorrhagic cerebrovascular disease do not develop symptoms secondary to the hydrocephalus.

Hemorrhagic Transformation of the Infarction

Postmortem examination of the brain of patients dying of recent cerebral infarction often demonstrates small areas of hemorrhagic transformation in the ischemic lesion[52] (Fig. 24-6). Some microscopic or petechial bleeding probably occurs in almost all infarctions. Still, these areas of hemorrhage do not produce neurological worsening and are probably of uncertain significance.[53] Sequential brain imaging studies detect these, usually asymptomatic, hemorrhagic changes with magnetic resonance imaging (MRI), including gradient-echo sequences, having a higher yield than computed tomography (CT)[54] (Fig. 24-7). The range of hemorrhagic changes spans from a small petechia, a confluent area of petechiae, a small homogenous area of bleeding, to a frank hematoma. The latter two patterns are most commonly associated with neurological worsening (Fig. 24-8). Symptomatic hemorrhagic transformation occurs most frequently among patients with large

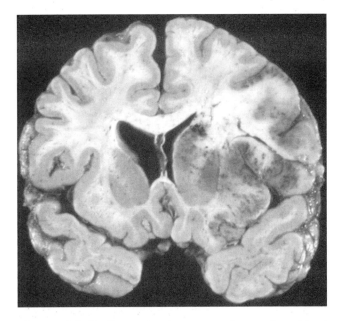

Figure 24-6. Coronal autopsy specimen of a patient dying of a large embolic infarction of the left hemisphere shows involvement of both superficial and deep structures. In addition, multiple areas of petechial hemorrhage are found primarily in gray matter structures. (*Courtesy of S.S. Schochet, M.D., Department of Pathology, University of West Virginia, Morgantown, WV*)

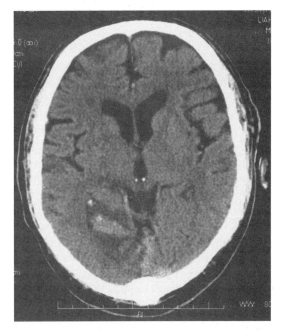

Figure 24-7. Unenhanced CT scan of the brain shows a hemorrhagic infarction in the distribution of the right posterior cerebral artery.

hemispheric infarctions. Patients with cardioembolic stroke also appear to have a higher risk of symptomatic hemorrhagic transformation. The administration of thrombolytic agents and anticoagulants has the potential to increase the severity of intracranial bleeding.[32,55–59] Because of the potential for bleeding complications, current guidelines recommend caution in administration of rtPA to patients with ischemic stroke who have severe neurological impairments (NIHSS score >20) or a large infarction on CT.[32] These recommendations are aimed at lowering the risk of symptomatic intracranial bleeding. The potential for symptomatic hemorrhagic transformation also is the reason for delaying the administration of antiplatelet agents or anticoagulants within the first 24 h after the use of rtPA.[32] Hemorrhagic transformation should be included in the differential diagnosis of any neurological worsening, especially when a patient has been treated with thrombolytic agents or anticoagulants. Emergency brain imaging (CT or MRI) should be performed and if bleeding is found, measures to treat any underlying coagulopathy should be instituted (see Chapter 21).

Early Recurrent Ischemic or Hemorrhagic Stroke

In the mid-1980s, the risk of early recurrent cardioembolic stroke was estimated to be approximately 10 percent.[60]

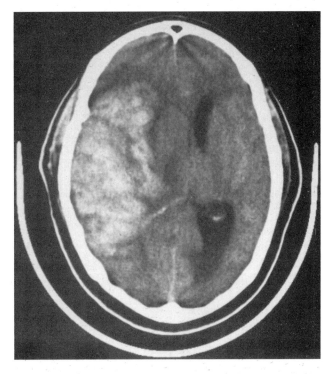

Figure 24-8. CT scan demonstrates massive hemorrhagic transformation of an infarction of the right hemisphere. Midline structures are shifted to the left, findings that are compatible with herniation. The ipsilateral lateral ventricle is obliterated, while the left lateral ventricle is dilated secondary to compression of the third ventricle.

This approximation is too high; the results of recent trials provide evidence that the risk of early recurrent stroke (within 1 week) is approximately 2 percent.[61–63] Some patients might have a higher risk. For example, the probability of recurrent embolism among patients with cardiac lesions is in the range of 2–8 percent.[63,64] Patients with evidence of a thrombus within a parent artery or heart might have an especially high risk. Patients with stroke secondary to large-artery atherosclerosis also have a high risk for early recurrent embolization. Unfortunately, data are limited about the potential likelihood of early recurrent embolization among such patients. Because early recurrent embolization would be considered as an important potential indication for urgent administration of anticoagulants, accurate knowledge is needed about the subgroups of patients who might benefit from treatment. At present, data do not demonstrate the utility of early anticoagulation to forestall recurrent stroke.[59,63,64]

Recurrent hemorrhage is an uncommon complication among patients hospitalized for treatment of intracranial bleeding. The highest risk persons are those who have bleeding diatheses or aneurysmal subarachnoid hemorrhage. Continued observation and monitoring for neurological worsening due to recurrent hemorrhage is important component of care in the hospital. The measures to treat the bleeding disorder are described in Chapter 21. The interventions used to prevent recurrent aneurysmal rupture, including surgical procedures, are described in Chapter 23.

Seizures

Seizures are reported in approximately 5 percent of hospitalized patients.[65–67] While most seizures develop at the time of the vascular event or within the subsequent few hours, convulsions also occur at later intervals (see Chapter 21). While patients with subarachnoid hemorrhage often receive prophylactic treatment with anticonvulsants, other patients do not receive these medications as part of management because of the relatively low risk of seizures.[32] Seizures happening more than 1 year following stroke usually occur among persons with large cortical lesions.[68] Patients with very delayed onset of seizures likely will have recurrent convulsions and they often require long-term treatment with anticonvulsants.

▶ OTHER NEUROLOGICAL COMPLICATIONS

Dementia

Approximately one-fourth of patients have confusion following stroke. Confusion is most common among elderly patients and those with preexisting cognitive impairments.[69] Patients with subarachnoid hemorrhage also can have a delirium. An acute confusion or delirium also results from concomitant medical conditions or complications including infections. Nonconvulsive status epilepticus also explains confusion or an acute delirium. In general, an acute delirium usually resolves with treatment of the stroke and severe comorbid diseases. Avoiding medications that potentiate confusion is another important component of management.

Although dementia is a potential consequence of a single vascular event, recurrent stroke is a potent risk factor or marker of dementia. Vascular dementia results from recurrent lacunar infarctions (multi-infarction dementia), amyloid angiopathy, Binswanger disease (presumably, microvascular disease), or multiple embolic events, which are the result of cardiac lesions, diseases of larger arteries, or prothrombotic disorders. Besides the development of cognitive or intellectual impairments directly related to the stroke, the vascular disease worsens the effects of degenerative diseases such as Alzheimer disease. Overall, a history of stroke increases likelihood of subsequent of dementia by a factor of approximately 9.[70] Tatemichi et al.[71] reported that approximately one-fourth of the patients older than 60 with stroke also had evidence of dementia. Besides age, other risk factors for dementia following stroke include diabetes mellitus, hyperglycemia, and lower educational background.[71,72] Patients with major vascular injuries to the dominant hemisphere also have a high risk. Memory disorders, which have a negative impact on recovery following stroke, are more common among patients with severe stroke.[73,74] The criteria for differentiating vascular dementia from degenerative dementia are described in Chapter 1.

Movement Disorders

Hemiballism and hemichorea are potential complications of either hemorrhagic or ischemic lesions of the basal ganglia, most commonly in the subthalamic nucleus.[75] Ballistic movements can be violent and lead to exhaustion. Usually, the hemiballism abates over several weeks following the stroke. Because of the severity of the movement disorder, patients are usually treated with medications such as phenothiazines or haloperidol.[76] Unilateral Parkinsonism is a rare complication of a stroke located in the putamen or globus pallidus.[77] More commonly, patients with multiple subcortical lacunar infarctions (lacunar state) can develop signs that mimic Parkinsonism. Focal tremors, dyskinesia, or dystonia are uncommon complications of vascular injuries to the basal ganglia or diencephalon.[78–80]

Autonomic Dysfunction

Besides cardiac arrhythmias and blood pressure instability (see Chapter 21), other evidence of autonomic nervous system dysfunction may be detected among persons with stroke. Patients develop swelling, temperature changes, or discoloration of the hand that is paralyzed. Presumably, these findings are secondary to an autonomic failure that occurs in conjunction with dysfunction of the corticospinal system.[81] Patients should be advised to protect the affected limb in cold weather. Shoulder–hand syndrome can complicate hemiplegia.[82] In this situation, the patient has pain and tenderness of the hand and arm. In some unusual cases, intense pain and the vasomotor changes of reflex sympathetic dystrophy develop.[83] Rare autonomic symptoms include hypohidrosis and gustatory disturbances.[84,85]

Pain

Hypersensitivity and pain (allodynia) secondary to minimal cutaneous stimuli most commonly complicate strokes in the dorsolateral medulla or the ventroposterolateral nucleus of the thalamus.[86–88] The abnormal pain, sometimes labeled the *thalamic pain syndrome*, is found in the same areas of the body in which the patient has a decreased perception to pain and temperature. Brain stem infarctions may produce symptoms that mimic trigeminal neuralgia.[89] Treatment of pain following stroke includes administration of tricyclic antidepressants, selective serotonin reuptake inhibitors (SSRI), anticonvulsants, and analgesics.

Hiccups

Persistent and severe hiccups, which can be uncomfortable, occur most commonly with infarctions involving the dorsolateral medulla or pons. The hiccups, which can happen in bouts of recurrent spasms, persist for several days and can be incapacitating. Affected patients also have dysphagia and dysarthria, reflecting dysfunction of the bulbar musculature. Patients with hiccups also have an increased chance of aspiration pneumonia and respiratory problems. In addition, nutrition is an issue because of the concomitant dysphagia. Treatment options include haloperidol, baclofen, chlorpromazine, and carbamazepine.[90]

Sleep Disorders

Disorders of sleep are both acute and long-term complications of stroke. Most affected patients have disturbances in the stages of sleep and complain of being fatigued or sleepy during the day. Obstructive sleep apnea and hypoventilation occur.[91,92] Sleep apnea following stroke is most commonly found among older persons, especially those with diabetes and obesity. In addition, patients with severe neurological impairments, including those with brain stem involvement or bulbar dysfunction, have a high rate of sleep disturbances. Palomaki et al.[93] reported that insomnia also is a common complaint following stroke. Hypersomnia is a potential complication of an infarction in the paramedian thalamus.[94]

Peripheral Nerve Injuries

Trauma to peripheral nerves, including repetitive compressive injuries, can complicate stroke. Among the possible causes of injury to the brachial plexus are pulling the patient up in the bed by the arms and compression with crutches. Increased use of the hand contralateral to a paralysis can induce carpal tunnel syndrome.[95]

▶ MEDICAL COMPLICATIONS

Heart Disease

A majority of patients with stroke have heart disease and in many instances, the cardiac disease is preexisting. The presence of cardiovascular disease adversely affects prognosis. Myocardial infarction and other cardiovascular complications of stroke are among the leading long-term causes of death. Because of the strong interactions between cardiovascular and cerebrovascular disease, management during the days following stroke includes measures to treat heart disease. Monitoring of the cardiovascular status is often continued for the first days after the event. Cardiac monitoring might be required for a longer period in critically ill patients. Many interventions started in the emergency department are continued throughout hospitalization (see Chapter 21). Treatment should also include long-term plans to prevent myocardial ischemia. Such measures include therapies to treat risk factors and antiplatelet aggregating agents (see Chapters 4 and 19).

Deep Vein Thrombosis and Pulmonary Embolism

DVT is an important complication among hospitalized patients.[96] Still, the incidence of symptomatic DVT is relatively low (Table 24-5). For example, a retrospective statewide review of the frequency of DVT among patients hospitalized with stroke noted that 74 of 15,599 patients hospitalized with ischemic stroke developed this complication.[97] The same group found that 37 of 1926 patients with hemorrhagic strokes had DVT. However, because these events were diagnosed by clinical findings, these numbers might be too low. Aggressive noninvasive evaluation for the presence of pelvic or lower extremity DVT would probably find a higher incidence of this complication. Such studies are not done routinely. DVT is most likely to develop among severely ill patients who are bedridden and have a paralyzed lower extremity. The thrombus commonly

► **TABLE 24-5.** PREVENTION OR TREATMENT OF DEEP VEIN THROMBOSIS—PULMONARY EMBOLISM

Acute prevention
  Mobilization
  Subcutaneous administration of anticoagulants
    Heparin
    LMW heparins
    Danaparoid
  Aspirin
  Compression stockings and pneumatic compression
    devices
Long-term prevention
  Oral anticoagulants
Treatment of acute deep vein thrombosis or pulmonary
  embolism
  Intravenous administration of anticoagulants
  Local administration of thrombolytic agents
  Placement of filter in inferior vena cava
  Plication of inferior vena cava

develops in the paralyzed limb. The presence of a painful, swollen limb secondary to the DVT hampers efforts for recovery. More importantly, DVT can be complicated by pulmonary embolism.

Because DVT can be prevented by several different methods and because of the potential relationship to pulmonary embolism, the frequency of DVT is an indicator of the quality of care. Mobilization is an effective form of prophylaxis. While the patient's activity is often restricted during the first hours after admission, the treatment plan should include efforts to encourage use of a chair, standing, or walking. Any increase in mobility is tailored to the patient's responses. Patients with more severe strokes, including many patients with hemorrhages, cannot be readily mobilized. In these circumstances, choices include physical methods (alternating pressure devices and compression stockings), antiplatelet agents, and anticoagulants. A systemic review of physical methods following stroke found a nonsignificant trend toward a reduction in DVT.[98] A reduction in mortality was not found. Some compressive methods are uncomfortable and they limit mobilization efforts. Clinical research is under way to test the utility of these physical methods. At present, physical efforts are a therapeutic option for treatment of bedridden patients who should not receive anticoagulants or antiplatelet agents.[99,100]

The data about the utility of anticoagulants following stroke are strongest for their ability to prevent DVT.[96] Current guidelines include a recommendation for the use of heparin or low-molecular-weight (LMW) heparin for management of patients at high risk for DVT, following stroke.[32] Several trials tested these medications.[101,102] In a randomized, double-blind trial, Hillbom et al.[103] compared 40 units of enoxaparin administered subcutaneously once

a day to 5000 units of conventional heparin given three times a day. Patients had a paralysis of the lower extremity and were treated within 48 h of onset of stroke. Enoxaparin was accompanied by fewer ischemic or hemorrhagic events than was heparin. A systemic review comparing LMW heparin to traditional heparin concluded that LMW heparin was equally effective in preventing venous thromboembolism and it significantly reduces the risk of bleeding or death.[104] The authors concluded that LMW heparin could be considered as the standard therapy for preventing DVT. Administration of LMW heparin as the initial step in prophylaxis against DVT is associated with shortening of the length of stay.[105] The shorter length of stay in the hospital probably compensates for the higher cost of the LMW heparins. Oral anticoagulants can be used as part of long-term management.[106] While aspirin appears to lower the risk of DVT, it is not widely prescribed.

Pulmonary embolism is an important nonneurological cause of death, following stroke. Patients at high risk for DVT also have the greatest risk for pulmonary embolism. Pulmonary embolism usually occurs days or weeks after the cerebrovascular event.[107] Because pulmonary embolism can cause sudden death, prevention is the key. Pulmonary embolization should be suspected if the patient suddenly develops respiratory distress, hypoxia, chest pain, or hemoptysis. The diagnosis of pulmonary embolism is supported by the findings of an abnormal chest X-ray and a perfusion defect on nuclide pulmonary scanning. Patients with respiratory distress need supplemental oxygen. In addition, anticoagulants are prescribed. A meta-analysis of controlled clinical trials concluded that fixed-dose LMW heparin was as effective and safe as adjusted doses of unfractionated heparin in the initial treatment of nonmassive pulmonary embolism.[108] Part of the rationale for the anticoagulants is to prevent recurrent embolization. A local infusion of a thrombolytic agent into the pulmonary artery can be used to speed lysis of the clot. Surgical plication of or placement of a filter within the inferior vena cava can be used to prevent recurrent embolization among patients who should not receive antithrombotic agents.

Respiratory Failure or Pneumonia

Within the first few days following stroke, pulmonary infections are diagnosed in approximately 10–30 percent of patients[109] (Tables 24-6 and 24-7). Pneumonia is an important cause of death; most deaths occur more than a week following the vascular event. Pneumonia also is a leading cause of death among patients requiring long-term institutionalized care. Pneumonia usually is secondary to atelectasis, hypoventilation, or aspiration.[110] Hilker et al.[111] found that pneumonia following stroke

► **TABLE 24-6.** CAUSES OF HYPOXIA OR RESPIRATORY FAILURE FOLLOWING STROKE

Airway compromise
Atelectasis
Aspiration pneumonia
Pneumonia
Pulmonary embolism
Pulmonary edema—congestive heart failure

was found among patients requiring mechanical ventilation or those with multiple strokes, brain stem stroke, dysphagia, or an abnormal chest X-ray. Dziewas et al.[110] found that approximately half of the cases of pneumonia occur among patients receiving nasogastric tube feedings. Important steps to lessen the risk of pneumonia include careful assessment and management of swallowing, early mobilization, and pulmonary care.

Pneumonia can lead to hypoxia; thus, it is included in the differential diagnosis as the cause of neurological worsening after stroke, especially if the decline happens more than a week following the vascular event. Other symptoms of pneumonia include fever and respiratory distress. In particular, the development of fever following stroke should prompt assessment for pneumonia. Besides a chest X-ray, cultures should be obtained. While prophylactic administration of antibiotics is not advised, clinical findings suggestive of pneumonia should prompt use of broad-spectrum antibiotics. Because many cases of pneumonia are hospital acquired, organisms resistant to conventional antibiotics often are encountered. The selection of antibiotics is influenced by the potential for antibiotic resistance.

Respiratory failure in the days following stroke can be secondary to aspiration, pneumonia, atelectasis, or pulmonary embolism. The existence of chronic lung disease also exacerbates the effects of any new pulmonary events. Respiratory failure also is a terminal component of severe neurological injuries, including cases of patients dying of brain edema and increased intracranial pressure. The steps to protect the airway and to give ventilatory assistance, as described in Chapter 21, might be needed to help these critically ill patients. Patients with respiratory failure usually require treatment in an intensive care unit. Their prognosis is poor.

Urinary Incontinence and Urinary Tract Infections

Urinary incontinence is a relatively common problem.[112] While approximately one-third to three-fourths of patients have one or more episodes of urinary incontinence within 1 week of stroke, this number declines by the time of discharge.[23] In general, the highest risk patients are those who have major brain injuries that cause them to be bedridden. Problems with bladder control should not be surprising. Hemorrhages or infarctions of the brain or spinal cord directly affect neural mechanisms that control the bladder, in particular a loss of voluntary control of the reflex arc between the bladder and the sacral spinal cord. Patients with parasagittal frontal lobe lesions also lose voluntary control of the bladder. Complications of stroke, such as hydrocephalus, also can impair bladder control. Detrusor hyperreflexia and urge incontinence happen. Some patients have cognitive impairments that impair judgment or recognition of a full bladder. Language impairments might not allow a patient to communicate the need to void. Other patients have motor impairments that limit mobility. A patient might not be able to use a commode or urinal. Patients are treated with diuretics that increase urinary volumes or medications that affect autonomic control of the bladder; these medications probably will increase the likelihood of incontinence. Diabetic patients may have an autonomic neuropathy that impairs bladder function.

Persistent incontinence is a marker of poor outcomes after stroke, probably because bladder dysfunction is secondary to severe neurological injury. Patients with incontinence have poor outcomes—often related to malnutrition and infections.[113] Repeated urinary incontinence can lead to skin breakdown. Incontinent patients can be treated with a chronic indwelling bladder catheter or intermittent catheterization. Male patients can be treated with a condom catheter but these devices are not very effective. In general, placement of an indwelling catheter is used for a limited period of time. However, critically ill patients usually require an indwelling catheter for long-term drainage of the bladder. Unfortunately, the use of an indwelling catheter is often complicated by urinary tract infections. As an alternative, regularly scheduled insertions of a catheter can be used to drain the bladder and help regain normal bladder regulatory responses. Nursing personnel or the patient can perform the intermittent catheterizations. Patients with persistent urinary incontinence following a stroke should be evaluated by studies of bladder function. Those with persistent bladder hyperreflexia can be treated with anticholingeric and antispasmodic medications.[23] Patients with overflow incontinence are often treated with cholinergic medications.[23]

► **TABLE 24-7.** CAUSES OF FEVER FOLLOWING STROKE

Pneumonia
Urinary tract infection
Sepsis
Thrombophlebitis
Drug-induced fever
Seizures
Central fever

Urinary tract infections occur in approximately 15 percent of patients and are a leading cause of fever following stroke[114–116] (see Table 24-7). Urinary tract infections most commonly occur among incontinent patients requiring catheterization. However, diabetic patients and others with an impaired immune status also have a high risk. Secondary bacteremia, pyelonephritis, or sepsis could cause a marked decline in the patient's status, including neurological worsening. Patients can die as the result of the septic complications.

Acidification of the urine by adding fluids, such as cranberry juice, which are high in vitamin C or adding 500 mg of vitamin C to the diet can be a prophylactic measure. Avoiding the use of bladder catheter is another prophylactic tactic. The development of a fever following stroke should prompt an examination of the urine, including a culture. While prophylactic administration of antibiotics is not recommended, these medications should be started if the evaluation suggests a urinary tract infection.

Fecal Incontinence and Constipation

Constipation is a relatively common problem. Patients are immobile and often dehydrated. Analgesics, including opiates, might impair bowel mobility. Abdominal pain, bloating, ileus, and fecal impaction are potential complications. Bowel care, including measures to avoid constipation, is an important component of ancillary management.[112] Maintaining adequate hydration and nutrition (sometimes via a feeding tube) and mobilization are ways to avoid severe constipation. Stool softeners or laxatives are useful adjunctive medications. Occasionally, enemas are needed.

Fecal incontinence is a very distressing complication for the patient, family, and medical personnel. Feces irritate the skin and are a potential source for infections, including urinary tract infections. Fecal incontinence is often associated with diarrhea. Severe diarrhea can lead to loss of proteins or electrolytes. The diarrhea may be the result of medical therapies, including antibiotics. Serious bowel secondary infections, including clostridium difficile colitis, can occur. In addition, hyperosmolar nasogastric feedings lead to diarrhea. In general, medications to control diarrhea are avoided because of their potential to induce constipation and impair bowel motility but if the diarrhea is severe, they can be given. Rarely, a rectal tube is necessary.

Gastrointestinal Bleeding

Upper gastrointestinal hemorrhage is an uncommon complication. It occurs primarily among patients with intracranial bleeding. Life-threatening hemorrhages develop more commonly among elderly persons and those with severe neurological injuries.[117] Recurrent vomiting among patients with infarctions in the posterior fossa or intracranial hemorrhages also is associated with bleeding, possibly due to esophageal tears.[118] Medications, most commonly aspirin, and other nonsteroid anti-inflammatory agents also lead to gastritis. The bleeding can be from erosive gastritis or stress or peptic ulcers. It can be aggravated by the administration of anticoagulants or thrombolytic agents. Severe bleeding can lead to hypotension or anemia.[118] Occasionally, the bleeding is sufficiently severe to require transfusions. Prophylactic interventions including antacids or histamine blocking agents can be given. However, some histamine blocking agents depress the central nervous system.

Electrolyte Disorders and Dehydration

Dehydration occurs especially among the elderly and those with severe vomiting. Patients with subarachnoid hemorrhage are at especially high risk, in part due to an inappropriate release of antidiuretic hormone (SIADH) or cerebral salt wasting. In the latter situation, reduced fluid volume occurs in addition to hyponatremia. Dehydration can result from lack of intake of fluids. Restriction of fluids to treat brain edema or SIADH also causes dehydration. Patients with fever or located in a warm environment can have insensible loss of fluids, which promotes dehydration. The use of diuretics to treat hypertension before or after the stroke also causes dehydration. Dehydration can induce a contraction in vascular volume and hemoconcentration, which reduces cerebral blood flow and promotes intravenous thrombosis or renal dysfunction.

Most patients receive at least 1.8–2.4 L of fluid daily. If the patient can take fluids by oral consumption or via a nasogastric tube, intravenous therapy is avoided. Otherwise patients should take intravenous fluids, most commonly normal saline. Hypoosmolar fluids, such as 5 percent dextrose and water, are avoided because they can aggravate hyponatremia.

Hyponatremia is the most frequent electrolyte disturbance; it is most commonly detected among patients with subarachnoid hemorrhage (see Chapter 23). Hyponatremia is the result of SIADH or cerebral salt wasting. It also is secondary to the use of medications. Hyponatremia can cause neurological worsening or seizures. Rapid correction of hyponatremia is avoided in order to lessen the risk of central pontine myelinolysis. Hypokalemia can be a complication of the use of diuretics. Management of the electrolyte disturbances, including the use of potassium supplementation, is part of general ancillary management.

Swallowing and Nutrition

Disturbances in swallowing are secondary to disturbances of supranuclear or bulbar innervation of the tongue, mouth, lips, or pharynx.[119–121] Dysphagia is found more commonly among patients with hemorrhagic stroke than among those with cerebral infarction.[121] Temporary dysphagia occurs in approximately 50 percent of patients with stroke.[122] Besides difficulty in swallowing food and fluids, patients with severe dysphagia can have problems handling their secretions. Patients often have more difficulty in swallowing clear liquids than handling soft or solid foods. Both dehydration and malnutrition are consequences. Patients with dysphagia also have a risk for aspiration pneumonia. Sudden death from airway compromise is a potential scenario.[123]

Patients with minor cortical or subcortical infarctions or hemorrhages of the cerebral hemisphere usually do not have major problems with swallowing. Still, dysphagia is found in approximately 30 percent of patients with hemispheric lesions and is most commonly found among persons with facial weakness, aphasia, or a weak voice.[124,125] Patients with larger hemispheric hemorrhages or infarctions and those with strokes in the brain stem or cerebellum have a much higher risk.[121] Dysphagia is found in approximately 90 percent of patients with bilateral hemispheric stroke.[126] Abnormal swallowing is prominent among persons with pontine or medullary strokes that cause bulbar dysfunction.[127]

Assessment of swallowing is part of the early evaluation of neurologically stable patients.[128–129] The goal is to rapidly determine if the patient will be able to eat and drink. Examination of the cough reflex provides an estimate on the risk of aspiration and pneumonia.[130] An intact reflex suggests that the airway is protected, while an abnormal response implies a high risk for pulmonary complications. Frequent coughing or a fall in pulse oximetry values following swallowing provides indirect evidence of aspiration.[131] Clinical and videofluoroscopic studies can identify the severity of the swallowing disturbance.[115,132] Sequential assessments can be used to guide advancement of the diet and drinking of liquids.

If the swallowing is impaired, oral exercises and positioning of the head can help improve swallowing. Changing the consistency of the diet, for example thickening of liquids or pureeing of solid food, expedites swallowing. Decreasing the volume of food with each meal and the use of frequent small meals can also be effective. Administering food via a syringe is another way to initiate swallowing.

Nutrition and hydration should be given via a nasogastric tube if the patient cannot swallow. A nasogastric tube should be inserted as soon as the patient is stable neurologically.[133] However, it should be considered as a temporary measure. Patients often do not tolerate the this tube. In addition, the use of this tube offers only limited protection against aspiration pneumonia.[110] Secondary lower esophageal sphincter or peristaltic dysfunction following the insertion of the nasogastric tube means that the patient is at risk for reflux and aspiration.[134] Sinusitis

is another potential complication. Patients often intentionally or inadvertently remove the tube, and repeated reinsertion of the tube often is necessary.

Percutaneous endoscopic gastrostomy (PEG) is recommended when a patient requires a prolonged course of enteral feeding. As a rule of thumb, a PEG should be inserted if the patient is likely to need tube feedings for more than 14 days.[135] In addition, many long-term care facilities require PEG for those patients who will need tube feedings. The chances of aspiration are lower with PEG than with a nasogastric tube. On the other hand, PEG is an invasive procedure. Potential complications include local skin breakdown and peritonitis.[135,136] Still, PEG is generally well tolerated. If the patient recovers the ability to swallow, the PEG or nasogastric tube can be removed.

Diabetes Mellitus

Management of diabetes mellitus is an important part of ancillary management. The goals are to avoid both hypoglycemia and profound hyperglycemia. The negative impact of hyperglycemia and the treatment of elevated blood glucose concentrations following stroke are described in Chapter 21. Measures to avoid excessively low blood glucose levels also are important.

Pressure Sores

Pressure sores (decubitus ulcers) develop in up to 15 percent of patients.[22,114] Skin breakdown at signs of bony prominences is most likely among elderly patients. Patients with diarrhea, fecal or urinary incontinence, or urinary catheters are at the highest risk. Thin or malnourished patients also are prone to pressure sores. Prophylaxis is key. Practice guidelines outline the steps to maintain the integrity of the skin.[137] Mobilization is the most effective measure. Bedridden patients should be turned and positioned properly. Special beds or mattresses can help relieve pressure against dependent areas. The skin is cleaned regularly and gently. Keeping the skin dry also helps.

Falls

Falls are a leading cause of trauma following stroke; they are relatively common as patients with moderate-to-severe impairments begin to be mobilized. Falls can occur during transfer from a bed, sitting, or ambulation.[138] Falls are an especially important problem during rehabilitation. A fracture of the hip, usually on the paralyzed side, is the most serious complication.[137] Serious bleeding also can complicate falls that happen among patients taking oral anticoagulants. The frequency of serious falls is estimated as approximately 9 per 1000 patient-days.[139] Overall, approximately 20 percent of patients with stroke will have one or more falls during the days following their vascular event.[114] Elderly persons, those with other neurological diseases, and patients with visual, sensory, hearing, or cognitive impairments are at the greatest risk. Nyberg and Gustafson[140] found that falls were most likely to occur among persons with poor postural stability, bilateral motor impairments, bilateral strokes, or neglect. Patients taking diuretics, anticonvulsants, and antidepressants also have a heightened fall risk.[140]

Prior to initiation of ambulation, the patient's environment should be assessed. Issues such as the lighting, floor surfaces, and trip hazards should be evaluated. Because many falls occur when the patient is trying to walk to the bathroom, the location and access of the toilet and bathing facilities should be examined. High-risk patients should be supervised and assisted in ambulation and transfer from the bed to the chair. Taking the patient to the toilet at regular intervals may help. Devices, such as canes or walkers, also assist in mobilization. In general, physical restraints should be avoided, whenever possible.[141]

Shoulder Pain and Adhesive Capsulitis

The shoulder is the joint most vulnerable to complications following stroke. Pain in the shoulder is a relatively common complaint.[142] Subluxation of the joint is among the causes of the pain. Changes in strength and tone of muscles about the shoulder predispose to subluxation.[143] In addition, moving the patient up in bed by pulling the shoulder aggravates this complication. Rather than using the arms of the patient to pull him/her toward the head of the bed, medical personnel should use a blanket or other device to reposition the patient. Linn et al.[144] suggest that electrical stimulation of the shoulder musculature can help maintain tone and lessen the risk of subluxation.

Immobility of the shoulder leads to adhesive capsulitis—a very painful complication, which appears within a few days following stroke. In order to avoid pain, patients often hold their arm next to their trunk and then try to limit movement. The use of slings can aggravate the process. Further restriction of motion and increase in pain result in worsening of the shoulder. Passive range of motion exercises, including external rotation, is an important part of ancillary care of a patient with a plegic arm. Both physical therapy and nursing service personnel perform the exercises. Anti-inflammatory agents, local injections of corticosteroids, or surgical interventions sometimes are needed to help control this complication.

Contractures

Contractures in the muscles of the paretic side appear relatively soon after stroke.[112] Painful contractures limit the patient's recovery from the stroke by restricting movement of the affected joints. Management focuses on splinting or casting of the joints to achieve anatomically correct postures.

Osteoporosis

Osteoporosis is a delayed complication. Bony changes are most prominent on the hemiparetic side.[145,146] The osteoporosis appears to be secondary to progressive reabsorption of bone and loss of bone mineral density.[147,148] Presumably, the osteoporosis is secondary to disuse of the affected limbs. In addition, changes might be secondary to changes in vascular flow or neural innervation. The use of oral anticoagulants that antagonize the effects of vitamin K, which is a key requirement for bone health, might accelerate development of osteoporosis.[149] Pathological fracture is a potential consequence. Supplementing the diet with calcium and vitamin D might help prevent the osteoporosis. In addition, administration of calcitriol or ipriflavone might help slow the loss of bone.[150,151]

Depression

Depression is a common acute and long-term complication.[152–155] Surveys show that depression can be diagnosed in approximately 20–25 percent of patients, and approximately 10 percent of patients have major depression.[156,157] It can persist for several years after the cerebrovascular event. An emotional reaction to the illness is not surprising. In addition, depression appears to be a direct consequence of the neurological injury.

Poststroke depression is more common among women, younger persons, highly educated persons, and those with large infarctions of the dominant hemisphere.[158,159] The data about the association of depression with left hemisphere lesions are controversial.[160] Additional research on this relationship is needed. Depression is also found among persons living alone or who have little social contact. The diagnosis is based on traditional findings, including a mood disorder and physical symptoms. Major depression slows recovery and can lead to decreased physical and cognitive functioning.[152] The presence of depression can prolong hospitalization and slow the process of rehabilitation.[161,162] Major depression also is associated with increased mortality and disability.[153,154,163]

Because of the high potential for adverse outcomes following stroke, interventions to control the mood disorder should be a component of management. The use of either tricyclic or SSRI antidepressants can improve outcome and lower mortality.[164] Among the effective medications are citralopam, fluoxetine, sertraline, and nortriptyline.[156,165,166]

Hypomania, Anxiety, and Disorders of Anger and Emotionality

Hypomania is an infrequent complication. It is most commonly associated with strokes of the nondominant hemisphere or thalamus.[167] Apathy or a catastrophic reaction also happens. Anxiety develops within the first few days after stroke and in some cases, the anxiety can persist for several years.[168] The frequency of generalized anxiety disorder following stroke is as high as 20 percent.[169] Some patients have a real fear of having another stroke. Some patients might need medications or counseling to treat these symptoms. Disinhibition, exaggerated responses to stimuli, and disorders of anger control are potential complications of strokes, especially with hemorrhages or infarctions of the frontal lobes.[170,171]

Pathological emotionality also can occur. The pseudobulbar syndrome occurs with severe bilateral lesions of the cerebral hemispheres. Affected patients have brief swings of physical behavior, with pathological crying or laughing that mimic depression or elation.[172] Sertraline, paroxetine, or citalopram have been used to treat these symptoms.[172,173]

▶ PALLIATIVE CARE

Patients with prolonged coma or other serious neurological impairments following stroke have a poor long-term prognosis. While some of these patients could survive with continued long-term care including efforts to prevent medical or neurological complications of the stroke and measures to treat concomitant diseases, the likelihood of good or functional recovery is often low. In such circumstances, the most likely disposition for the patient is long-term care in a nursing home—an outcome that most patients and their families do not want. Some patients have written advanced directives to guide decisions about their treatment if they cannot participate in such decision making themselves. However, these statements often do not provide specific comments about issues such as the use of measures to prevent or treat complications of stroke or the use of devices, such as feeding tubes, which can prolong their life. If the patient's prognosis is very poor, the physician should discuss treatment options with him/her. Because of the neurological impairments, the patient often cannot participate in this discussion. In this situation, the physician should have a frank and thoughtful conversation with family members about the situation. The physician should provide information about the prognosis and the most likelihood outcome of the stroke. The physician should review options in management, including resuscitation if a cardiopulmonary arrest occurs, the use of assistive devices including intubation and ventilators,

administration of medications that could prevent or treat complications such as pneumonia, and the maintenance of hydration and nutrition via tube feedings. In some cases, the most loving approach is not to implement interventions that would only prolong the patient's dying. In such circumstances, the patient and family should be advised that palliative care does include measures to treat pain and make the patient comfortable. Palliative care would permit the patient to die with dignity. The physician should give ample time so that the family can discuss these issues and ask questions. The physician should respect the family's decision and support them during the very difficult time. Some institutions have palliative care units that can be utilized. Some families will elect for palliative care after a prolonged course. Another solution is a referral to hospice.

▶ DISCHARGE PLANNING

While the priorities of treatment in the hospital should include prevention of acute or subacute complications, initiation of medical or surgical therapies to forestall recurrent strokes, and rehabilitation, management should also include education of the patient and family. In addition, management should include plans for discharge. Such planning should involve the collaboration of physicians, nursing personnel, rehabilitation specialists, social workers, and discharge specialists. The goal should be to arrange for the patient to be transferred to the appropriate setting for continued recovery from stroke (see Chapter 25). Early supported discharge can help speed referral to rehabilitation and reduce the length of acute hospitalization for management of stroke.[174] Fjaertoft et al.[175] recently demonstrated that stroke service based in a stroke unit with early supported discharge improves long-term clinical outcomes. Thus, this process can reduce costs of hospitalization and at the same time optimize the patient's continued treatment.

REFERENCES

1. Mitsias P. Ischemic stroke management in the critical care unit: the first 24 hours. *J Stroke Cerebrovasc Dis* 1999;8:151–159.
2. Langhorne P, Dennis MS, Kalra L, Shepperd S, Wade DT, Wolfe CDA. Services for helping acute stroke patients avoid hospital admission. *Cochrane Database Syst Rev* 2000;CD000444.
3. Norris JW, Hachinski VC. Intensive care management of stroke patients. *Stroke* 1976;7:573–577.
4. Dayno JM, Mansbach HH. Acute stroke units. *J Stroke Cerebrovasc Dis* 1999;8:160–170.
5. Bertram M, Schwarz S, Hacke W. Acute and critical care in neurology. *Eur Neurol* 1997;38:155–166.

6. Alberts MJ, Hademenos G, Latchaw RE, et al. Recommendations for the establishment of primary stroke centers. *JAMA* 2001;283:3102–3109.

7. Kennedy J, Ma C, Buchan AM. Organization of regional and local stroke resources: methods to expedite acute management of stroke. *Curr Neurol Neurosci Rep* 2004;4:13–18.

8. Evans A, Harraf F, Donaldson N, Kalra L. Randomized controlled study of stroke unit care versus stroke team care in different stroke subtypes. *Stroke* 2002;33:449–455.

9. Ronning OM, Guldvog B. Stroke unit versus general medical wards, II: neurological deficits and activities of daily living: a quasi-randomized controlled trial. *Stroke* 1998;29:586–590.

10. Ronning OM, Guldvog B. Stroke units versus general medical wards, I: twelve- and eighteen-month survival: a randomized, controlled trial. *Stroke* 1998;29:58–62.

11. Indredavik B, Bakke F, Slordahl SA, Rokseth R, Haheim LL. Treatment in a combined acute and rehabilitation stroke unit. *Stroke* 1999;30:917–923.

12. Indredavik B, Bakke F, Slordahl SA, Rokseth R, Haheim LL. Stroke unit treatment. 10-year follow-up. *Stroke* 1999;30:1524–1527.

13. Indredavik B. Stroke units—the Norwegian experience. *Cerebrovasc Dis* 2003;48:21–22.

14. Stegmayr B, Asplund K, Hulter-Asberg K, et al. Stroke units in their natural habitat: can results of randomized trials be reproduced in routine clinical practice? Risk–Stroke Collaboration. *Stroke* 1999;30:709–714.

15. Diez-Tejedor E, Fuentes B. Acute care in stroke: do stroke units make the difference? *Cerebrovasc Dis* 2001;11:31–39.

16. Stroke Unit Trialists' Collaboration. Organised inpatient (stroke unit) care for stroke. *Cochrane Database Syst Rev* 2002;CD000197.

17. Birbeck GL, Zingmond DS, Cui X, Vickrey BG. Multispecialty stroke services in California hospitals are associated with reduced mortality. *Neurology* 2006;66:1527–1532.

18. Awad IA, Fayad P, Abdulrauf SI. Protocols and critical pathways for stroke care. *Clin Neurosurg* 1999;45:86–100.

19. De Georgia MA. Multimodal monitoring in neurocritical care. *Cleve Clin J Med* 2004;71(suppl 1):S16–S17.

20. Toni D, Fiorelli M, Gentile M, et al. Progressing neurological deficit secondary to acute ischemic stroke. A study on predictability, pathogenesis, and prognosis. *Arch Neurol* 1995;52:670–675.

21. Davalos A, Cendra E, Teruel J, Martinez M, Genis D. Deteriorating ischemic stroke: risk factors and prognosis. *Neurology* 1990;40:1865–1869.

22. van der Worp HB, Kappelle LJ. Complications of acute ischaemic stroke. *Cerebrovasc Dis* 1998;8:124–132.

23. Kappelle LJ, van der Worp HB. Treatment or prevention of complications of acute ischemic stroke. *Curr Neurol Neurosci Rep* 2004;4:36–41.

24. Wijdicks EF, Diringer MN. Middle cerebral artery territory infarction and early brain swelling: progression and effect of age on outcome. *Mayo Clin Proc* 1998;73:829–836.

25. Hacke W, Schwab S, Horn M, Spranger M, De Georgia M, von Kummer R. "Malignant" middle cerebral artery territory infarction: clinical course and prognostic signs. *Arch Neurol* 1996;53:309–315.

26. Krieger DW, Demchuk AW, Kasner SE, Jauss M, Hantson L. Early clinical and radiological predictors of fatal brain swelling in ischemic stroke. *Stroke* 1999;30:287–292.

27. Kasner SE, Demchuk AM, Berrouschot J, et al. Predictors of fatal brain edema in massive hemispheric ischemic stroke. *Stroke* 2001;32:2117–2123.

28. Mamarou A. The pathophysiology of brain edema and elevated intracranial pressure. *Cleve Clin J Med* 2004;71(suppl 1):S6–S8.

29. Suarez JI. Hypertonic saline for cerebral edema and elevated intracranial pressure. *Cleve Clin J Med* 2004;71(suppl 1):S9–S13.

30. Horwitz NH, Ludolph C. Acute obstructive hydrocephalus caused by cerebellar infarction. Treatment alternatives. *Surg Neurol* 1983;20:13–19.

31. Greenberg J, Skubick D, Shenkin H. Acute hydrocephalus in cerebellar infarct and hemorrhage. *Neurology* 1979;29:409–413.

32. Adams HP, Adams RJ, Brott T, et al. Guidelines for the early management of patients with ischemic stroke. A scientific statement from the stroke council of the American Stroke Association. *Stroke* 2003;34:1056–1083.

33. Broderick JP, Adams HP, Jr., Barsan W, et al. Guidelines for the management of spontaneous intracerebral hemorrhage: a statement for healthcare professionals from a special writing group of the Stroke Council, American Heart Association. *Stroke* 1999;30:905–915.

34. Steiner T, Friede T, Aschoff A, Schellinger PD, Schwab S, Hacke W. Effect and feasibility of controlled rewarming after moderate hypothermia in stroke patients with malignant infarction of the middle cerebral artery. *Stroke* 2001;32:2833–2835.

35. Schwab S, Georgiadis D, Berrouschot J, Schellinger PD, Graffagnino C, Mayer SA. Feasibility and safety of moderate hypothermia after massive hemispheric infarction. *Stroke* 2001;32:2033–2035.

36. Koh MS, Goh KY, Tung MY, Chan C. Is decompressive craniectomy for acute cerebral infarction of any benefit? *Surg Neurol* 2000;53:225–230.

37. Sandalcioglu IE, Schoch B, Rauhut F. Hemicraniectomy for large middle cerebral artery territory infarction: do these patients really benefit from this procedure? *J Neurol Neurosurg Psychiatry* 2003;74:1600.

38. Attia M, Bakon M, Blatt I, Tanne D, Feldman Z. Decompressive hemicraniectomy as a lifesaving procedure in severe acute ischemic stroke. *Isr Med Assoc J* 2003;5:677–678.

39. Donnan GA, Davis SM. Surgical decompression for malignant middle cerebral artery infarction: a challenge to conventional thinking. *Stroke* 2003;34:2307–2307.

40. Schwab S, Hacke W. Surgical decompression of patients with large middle cerebral artery infarcts is effective. *Stroke* 2003;34:2304–2305.

41. Dohmen C, Bosche B, Graf R, et al. Predication of malignant course in MCA infarction by PET and microdialysis. *Stroke* 2003;34:2152–2158.

42. Cho DY, Chen TC, Lee HC. Ultra-early decompressive craniectomy for malignant middle cerebral artery infarction. *Surg Neurol* 2003;60:227–232.

43. Pranesh MB, Dinesh Nayak S, Mathew V, et al. Hemicraniectomy for large middle cerebral artery territory infarction: outcome in 19 patients. *J Neurol Neurosurg Psychiatry* 2003;74:800–802.

44. Georgiadis D, Schwarz S, Aschoff A, Schwab S. Hemicraniectomy and moderate hypothermia in patients with severe ischemic stoke. *Stroke* 2002;33:1568–1573.

45. Morley NCD, Berge E, Cruz-Flores S, Whittle IR. Surgical decompression for cerebral oedema in acute ischaemic stroke. *Cochrane Database Syst Rev* 2002;CD003435.

46. Gupta R, Connolly ES, Mayer S, Elkind MSV. Hemicraniectomy for massive middle cerebral artery territory infarction. A systematic review. *Stroke* 2004;35: 539–543.

47. Malm J, Bergenheim AT, Enblad P, et al. The Swedish Malignant Middle Cerebral Artery Infarction Study. Long-term results from a prospective study of hemicraniectomy combined with standardized neurointensive care. *Acta Neurol Scand* 2006;113:25–30

48. Frank JL, Krieger D, Chyatte D, Cancian S. Hemicraniectomy and durotomy upon deterioration from massive hemispheric infarction. A proposed multicenter, prospective, randomized study. *Stroke* 1999;30:243.

49. Hofmeijer J, van der Worp HB, Amelink GJ, Algra A, Kappelle LJ. Decompressive surgery in space occupying cerebral infarction. A randomized controlled trial. *Cerebrovasc Dis* 2001;11:34.

50. Boon AJ, Tans JT, Delwel EJ, et al. Dutch Normal-Pressure Hydrocephalus Study: the role of cerebrovascular disease. *J Neurosurg* 1999;90:221–226.

51. Graff-Radford NR, Torner J, Adams HP, Jr. Factors associated with hydrocephalus after subarachnoid hemorrhage: a report of the Cooperative Aneurysm Study. *Arch Neurol* 1989;46:744–752.

52. Hart RG. Hemorrhagic infarcts. *Stroke* 1986;17:586–589.

53. Hornig CR, Bauer T, Simon C, Trittmacher S, Dorndorf W. Hemorrhagic transformation in cardioembolic cerebral infarction. *Stroke* 1993;24:465–468.

54. Toni D, Fiorelli M, Bastianello S, et al. Hemorrhagic transformation of brain infarct: predictability in the first 5 hours from stroke onset and influence on clinical outcome. *Neurology* 1996;46:341–345.

55. Jaillard A, Cornu C, Durieux A, et al. Hemorrhagic transformation in acute ischemic stroke. The MAST-E study. MAST-E Group. *Stroke* 1999;30:1326–1332.

56. Hacke W, Kaste M, Fieschi C, et al. Intravenous thrombolysis with recombinant tissue plasminogen activator for acute hemispheric stroke. The European Cooperative Acute Stroke Study (ECASS). *JAMA* 1995;274:1017–1025.

57. Multicentre Acute Stroke Trial–Italy (MAST-I) Group. Randomised controlled trial of streptokinase, aspirin, and combination of both in treatment of acute ischaemic stroke. *Lancet* 1995;346:1509–1514.

58. The National Institute of Neurological Disorders and Stroke rt-PA Stroke Study Group. Tissue plasminogen activator for acute ischemic stroke. *N Engl J Med* 1995;333: 1581–1587.

59. Adams HP, Jr. Emergent use of anticoagulation for treatment of patients with ischemic stroke. *Stroke* 2002;33: 856–861.

60. Cerebral Embolism Task Force. Cardiogenic brain embolism. *Arch Neurol* 1986;43:71–84.

61. CAST (Chinese Acute Stroke Trial) Collaborative Group. CAST: randomised placebo-controlled trial of early aspirin use in 20,000 patients with acute ischaemic stroke. *Lancet* 1997;349:1641–1649.

62. International Stroke Trial Collaborative Group. The International Stroke Trial (IST): a randomised trial of aspirin, subcutaneous heparin, both, or neither among 19435 patients with acute ischaemic stroke. *Lancet* 1997; 349:1569–1581.

63. The Publications Committee for the Trial of ORG 10172 in Acute Stroke Treatment (TOAST) Investigators. Low molecular weight heparinoid, ORG 10172 (danaparoid), and outcome after acute ischemic stroke: a randomized controlled trial. *JAMA* 1998;279:1265–1272.

64. Berge E, Abdelnoor M, Nakstad PH, Sandset PM, on behalf of the HAEST Study Group. Low molecular-weight heparin versus aspirin in patients with acute ischaemic stroke and atrial fibrillation: a double-blind randomised study. *Lancet* 2000;355:1205–1210.

65. Giroud M, Gras P, Fayolle H, Andre N, Soichot P, Dumas R. Early seizures after acute stroke: a study of 1,640 cases. *Epilepsia* 1994;35:959–964.

66. So EL, Annegers JF, Hauser WA, O'Brien PC, Whisnant JP. Population-based study of seizure disorders after cerebral infarction. *Neurology* 1996;46:350–355.

67. Camilo O, Goldstein LB. Seizures and epilepsy after ischemic stroke. *Stroke* 2004;35:1769–1775.

68. Awada A, Omojola MF, Obeid T. Late epileptic seizures after cerebral infarction. *Acta Neurol Scand* 1999;99: 265–268.

69. Henon H, Lebert F, Durieu I, et al. Confusional state in stroke: relation to preexisting dementia, patient characteristics, and outcome. *Stroke* 1999;30:773–779.

70. Kokmen E, Whisnant JP, O'Fallon WM, Chu CP, Beard CM. Dementia after ischemic stroke: a population-based study in Rochester, Minnesota (1960-1984). *Neurology* 1996;46:154–159.

71. Tatemichi TK, Desmond DW, Mayeux R, et al. Dementia after stroke: baseline frequency, risks, and clinical features in a hospitalized cohort. *Neurology* 1992;42:1185–1193.

72. Tatemichi TK, Desmond DW, Paik M, et al. Clinical determinants of dementia related to stroke. *Ann Neurol* 1993;33:568–575.

73. Bowler JV, Eliasziw M, Steenhuis R, et al. Comparative evolution of Alzheimer disease, vascular dementia, and mixed dementia. *Arch Neurol* 1997;54: 697–703.

74. Bowler JV. Vascular cognitive impairment. *Stroke* 2004; 35:386–388.

75. Kase CS, Maulsby GO, deJuan E, Mohr JP. Hemichorea-hemiballism and lacunar infarction in the basal ganglia. *Neurology* 1981;31:452–455.

76. Johnson WG, Fahn S. Treatment of vascular hemiballism and hemichorea. *Neurology* 1977;27:634–636.

77. Fenelon G, Houeto JL. Unilateral Parkinsonism following a large infarct in the territory of the lenticulostriate arteries. *Mov Disord* 1997;12:1086–1090.

78. Kostic VS, Stojanovic-Svetel M, Kacar A. Symptomatic dystonias associated with structural brain lesions: report of 16 cases. *Can J Neurol Sci* 1996;23:53–56.

79. Wali GM. Shoulder girdle dyskinesia associated with a thalamic infarct. *Mov Disord* 1999;14:375–377.

80. Brannan T, Yahr MD. Focal tremor following striatal infarct—a case report. *Mov Disord* 1999;14:368–370.

81. Korpelainen JT, Sotaniemi KA, Myllyla VV. Asymmetrical skin temperature in ischemic stroke. *Stroke* 1995;26:1543–1547.

82. Braus DF, Krauss JK, Strobel J. The shoulder-hand syndrome after stroke: a prospective clinical trial. *Ann Neurol* 1994;36:728–733.

83. Wanklyn P, Forster A, Young J, Mulley G. Prevalence and associated features of the cold hemiplegic arm. *Stroke* 1995;26:1867–1870.

84. Korpelainen JT, Sotaniemi KA, Myllyla VV. Ipsilateral hypohidrosis in brain stem infarction. *Stroke* 1993;24:100–104.

85. Rousseaux M, Muller P, Gahide I, Mottin Y, Romon M. Disorders of smell, taste, and food intake in a patient with a dorsomedial thalamic infarct. *Stroke* 1996;27:2328–2330.

86. Peyron R, Garcia-Larrea L, Gregoire MC, et al. Allodynia after lateral-medullary (Wallenberg) infarct. A PET study. *Brain* 1998;121:345–356.

87. Bowsher D, Leijon G, Thuomas KA. Central poststroke pain: correlation of MRI with pain characteristics and sensory abnormalities. *Neurology* 1998;51:1352–1358.

88. MacGowan DJ, Janal MN, Clark WC, et al. Central poststroke pain and Wallenberg's lateral medullary infarction: frequency, character, and determinants in 63 patients. *Neurology* 1997;49:120–125.

89. Kim JS, Kang JH, Lee MC. Trigeminal neuralgia after pontine infarction. *Neurology* 1998;51:1511–1512.

90. Kumar A, Dromerick AW. Intractable hiccups during stroke rehabilitation. *Arch Phys Med Rehabil* 1998;79:697–699.

91. Dyken ME, Somers VK, Yamada T, Ren ZY, Zimmerman MB. Investigating the relationship between stroke and obstructive sleep apnea. *Stroke* 1996;27:401–407.

92. Bassetti C, Aldrich MS. Sleep apnea in acute cerebrovascular diseases: final report on 128 patients. *Sleep* 1999;22:217–223.

93. Palomaki H, Bery A, Meririnne E, et al. Complaints of poststroke insomnia and its treatment with mianserin. *Cerebrovasc Dis* 2003;15:56–62.

94. Bassetti C, Mathis J, Gugger M, Lovblad KO, Hess CW. Hypersomnia following paramedian thalamic stroke: a report of 12 patients. *Ann Neurol* 1996;39:471–480.

95. Sato Y, Kaji M, Tsuru T, Oizumi K. Carpal tunnel syndrome involving unaffected limbs of stroke patients. *Stroke* 1999;30:414–418.

96. Sandercock PA, van den Belt AG, Lindley RI, Slattery J. Antithrombotic therapy in acute ischaemic stroke: an overview of the completed randomised trials. *J Neurol Neurosurg Psychiatry* 1993;56:17–25.

97. Gregory PC, Kuhlemeier KV. Prevalence of venous thromboembolism in acute hemorrhagic and thromboembolic stroke. *Am J Phys Med Rehabil* 2003;82:364–369.

98. Mazzone C, Chiodo Grandi F, Sandercock P, Miccio M, Salvi R. Physical methods for preventing deep vein thrombosis in stroke. *Cochrane Database Syst Rev* 2002;CD001922.

99. Black PM, Crowell RM, Abbott WM. External pneumatic calf compression reduces deep venous thrombosis in patients with ruptured intracranial aneurysms. *Neurosurgery* 1986;18:25–28.

100. Kamran SI, Downey D, Ruff RL. Pneumatic sequential compression reduces the risk of deep vein thrombosis in stroke patients. *Neurology* 1998;50:1683–1688.

101. Gould MK, Dembitzer AD, Sanders GD, Garber AM. Low-molecular-weight heparins compared with unfractionated heparin for treatment of acute deep venous thrombosis. A cost-effectiveness analysis. *Ann Intern Med* 1999;130:789–799.

102. Koopman MM, Buller HR. Low-molecular-weight heparins in the treatment of venous thromboembolism. *Ann Intern Med* 1998;128:1037–1039.

103. Hillbom M, Erila T, Sotaniemi K, Tatlisumak T, Sarna S, Kaste M. Enoxaparin vs heparin for prevention of deep-vein thrombosis in acute ischaemic stroke: a randomized, double-blind study. *Acta Neurol Scand* 2002;106:84–92.

104. van den Belt AG, Prins MH, Lensing AWA, et al. Fixed dose subcutaneous low molecular weight heparins versus adjusted dose unfractionated heparin for venous thromboembolism. *Cochrane Database Syst Rev* 2000;CD001100.

105. Dunn A, Bioh D, Beran M, Capasso M, Siu A. Effect of intravenous heparin administration on duration of hospitalization. *Mayo Clin Proc* 2004;79:159–163.

106. Hyers TM, Agnelli G, Hull RD, et al. Antithrombotic therapy for venous thromboembolic disease. *Chest* 1998;114:561S–578S.

107. Wijdicks EF, Scott JP. Pulmonary embolism associated with acute stroke. *Mayo Clin Proc* 1997;72:297–300.

108. Quinlan DJ, McQuillan A, Eikelboom JW. Low-molecular-weight heparin compared with intravenous unfractionated heparin for treatment of pulmonary embolism. A meta-analysis of randomized, controlled trials. *Ann Intern Med* 2004;140:175–183.

109. Bounds JV, Wiebers DO, Whisnant JP, Okazaki H. Mechanisms and timing of deaths from cerebral infarction. *Stroke* 1981;12:474–477.

110. Dziewas R, Ritter M, Schilling M, et al. Pneumonia in acute stroke patients fed by nasogastric tube. *J Neurol Neurosurg Psychiatry* 2004;75:852–856.

111. Hilker R, Poetter C, Findeisen N, et al. Nosocomial pneumonia after acute stroke: implications for neurological intensive care medicine. *Stroke* 2003;34:975–981.

112. Zorowitz RD, Tietjen GE. Medical complications after stroke. *J Stroke Cerebrovasc Dis* 1999;8:192–196.

113. Gariballa SE. Potentially treatable causes of poor outcome in acute stroke patients with urinary incontinence. *Acta Neurol Scand* 2003;107:336–340.

114. Davenport RJ, Dennis MS, Wellwood I, Warlow CP. Complications after acute stroke. *Stroke* 1996;27:415–420.

115. Dromerick A, Reding M. Medical and neurological complications during inpatient stroke rehabilitation. *Stroke* 1994;25:358–361.

116. Langhorne P, Stott DJ, Robertson L, et al. Medical complications after stroke. A multicenter study. *Stroke* 2000; 31:1223–1229.

117. Davenport RJ, Dennis MS, Warlow CP. Gastrointestinal hemorrhage after acute stroke. *Stroke* 1996;27:421–424.

118. Wijdicks EF, Fulgham JR, Batts KP. Gastrointestinal bleeding in stroke. *Stroke* 1994;25:2146–2148.

119. Daniels SK, Ballo LA, Mahoney MC, Foundas AL. Clinical predictors of dysphagia and aspiration risk: outcome measures in acute stroke patients. *Arch Phys Med Rehabil* 2000;81:1030–1033.

120. Vigderman AM, Chavin JM, Kososky C, Tahmoush AJ. Aphagia due to pharyngeal constrictor paresis from acute lateral medullary infarction. *J Neurol Sci* 1998;155:208–210.

121. Paciaroni M, Mazzotta G, Corea F, et al. Dysphagia following stroke. *Eur Neurol* 2004;51:162–167.

122. Dziewas R, Schilling M, Konrad C, Stogbauer F, Ludemann P. Placing nasogastric tubes in stroke patients with dysphagia: efficiency and tolerability of the reflex placement. *J Neurol Neurosurg Psychiatry* 2003;74:1429–1431.

123. Finestone HM, Fisher J, Greene-Finestone LS, Teasell RW, Craig ID. Sudden death in the dysphagic stroke patient— a case of airway obstruction caused by a food bolus: a brief report. *Am J Phys Med Rehabil* 1998;77:550–552.

124. Horner J, Massey EW. Silent aspiration following stroke. *Neurology* 1988;38:317–319.

125. Mann G, Hankey GJ. Initial clinical and demographic predictors of swallowing impairment following acute stroke. *Dysphagia* 2001;16:208–215.

126. Horner J, Brazer SR, Massey EW. Aspiration in bilateral stroke patients: a validation study. *Neurology* 1993;43:430–433.

127. Horner J, Buoyer FG, Alberts MJ, Helms MJ. Dysphagia following brain-stem stroke. Clinical correlates and outcome. *Arch Neurol* 1991;48:1170–1173.

128. Finestone HM, Woodbury MG, Foley NC, Teasell RW, Greene-Finestone LS. Tracking clinical improvement of swallowing disorders after stroke. *J Stroke Cerebrovasc Dis* 2002;11:23–27.

129. Smithard DG. Swallowing and stroke. Neurological effects and recovery. *Cerebrovasc Dis* 2002;14:1–8.

130. Addington WR, Stephens RE, Gilliland K, Rodriguez M. Assessing the laryngeal cough reflex and the risk of developing pneumonia after stroke. *Arch Phys Med Rehabil* 1999;80:150–154.

131. Collins MJ, Bakheit AM. Does pulse oximetry reliably detect aspiration in dysphagic stroke patients? *Stroke* 1997;28:1773–1775.

132. Mann G, Hankey GJ, Cameron D. Swallowing function after stroke: prognosis and prognostic factors at 6 months. *Stroke* 1999;30:744–748.

133. Dennis MS, Lewis SC, Warlow C, FOOD Trial collaboration. Effect of timing and method of enteral tube feeding for dysphagic stroke patients (FOOD). A multicentre randomised controlled trial. *Lancet* 2005;365:764–772.

134. Lucas CE, Yu P, Vlahos A, Ledgerwood AM. Lower esophageal sphincter dysfunction often precludes safe gastric feeding in stroke patients. *Arch Surg* 1999;134:55–58.

135. O'Mahony D, McIntyre AS. Artificial feeding for elderly patients after stroke. *Age Ageing* 1995;24:533–535.

136. Klor BM, Milianti FJ. Rehabilitation of neurogenic dysphagia with percutaneous endoscopic gastrostomy. *Dysphagia* 1999;14:162–164.

137. Gresham GE, Duncan PW, Stason WB, et al. Post-stroke rehabilitation. *Clinical Practice Guideline, No. 16.* Rockville, MD: U.S. Department of Health and Human Services, 1995.

138. Nyberg L, Gustafson Y. Patient falls in stroke rehabilitation. A challenge to rehabilitation strategies. *Stroke* 1995; 26:838–842.

139. Tutuarima JA, van der Meulen JH, de Haan RJ, van Straten A, Limburg M. Risk factors for falls of hospitalized stroke patients. *Stroke* 1997;28:297–301.

140. Nyberg L, Gustafson Y. Fall prediction index for patients in stroke rehabilitation. *Stroke* 1997;28:716–721.

141. Schleenbaker RE, McDowell SM, Moore RW, Costich JF, Prater G. Restraint use in inpatient rehabilitation: incidence, predictors, and implications. *Arch Phys Med Rehabil* 1994; 75:427–430.

142. Gamble GE, Jones AK, Tyrrell PJ. Shoulder pain after stroke: case report and review. *Ann Rheum Dis* 1999;58:451.

143. Arsenault AB, Bilodeau M, Dutil E, Riley E. Clinical significance of the V-shaped space in the subluxed shoulder of hemiplegics. *Stroke* 1991;22:867–871.

144. Linn SL, Granat MH, Lees KR. Prevention of shoulder subluxation after stroke with electrical stimulation. *Stroke* 1999;30:963–968.

145. Sato Y, Kaji M, Saruwatari N, Oizumi K. Hemiosteoporosis following stroke: importance of pathophysiologic understanding and histologic evidence. *Stroke* 1999;30:1978–1979.

146. Ramnemark A, Nyberg L, Lorentzon R, Englund U, Gustafson Y. Progressive hemiosteoporosis on the paretic side and increased bone mineral density in the nonparetic arm the first year after severe stroke. *Osteoporos Int* 1999;9:269–275.

147. Beaupre GS, Lew HL. Bone-density changes after stroke. *Am J Phys Med Rehabil* 2006;85:464–472.

148. Ramnemark A, Nyberg L, Lorentzon R, Olsson T, Gustafson Y. Hemiosteoporosis after severe stroke, independent of changes in body composition and weight. *Stroke* 1999; 30:755–760.

149. Sato Y, Honda Y, Kunoh H, Oizumi K. Long-term oral anticoagulation reduces bone mass in patients with previous hemispheric infarction and nonrheumatic atrial fibrillation. *Stroke* 1997;28:2390–2394.

150. Sato Y, Maruoka H, Oizumi K. Amelioration of hemiplegia-associated osteopenia more than 4 years after stroke by 1 alpha-hydroxyvitamin D3 and calcium supplementation. *Stroke* 1997;28:736–739.

151. Sato Y, Metoki N, Iwamoto J, Satoh K. Amelioration of osteoporosis and hypovitaminosis D by sunlight exposure in stroke patients. *Neurology* 2003;61:338–342.

152. Sharpe M, Hawton K, Seagroatt V, et al. Depressive disorders in long-term survivors of stroke. Associations with demographic and social factors, functional status, and brain lesion volume. *Br J Psychiatry* 1994;164:380–386.

153. Pohjasvaara T, Leppavuori A, Siira I, Vataja R, Kaste M, Erkinjuntti T. Frequency and clinical determinants of poststroke depression. *Stroke* 1998;29:2311–2317.

154. Pohjasvaara T, Leskela M, Vataja R, et al. Post-stroke depression, executive dysfunction and functional outcome. *Eur J Neurol* 2002;9:269–275.

155. Eriksson M, Asplund K, Glader E-L, et al. Self-reported depression and use of antidepressants after stroke: a national survey. *Stroke* 2004;35:936–941.

156. Robinson RG. Poststroke depression: prevalence, diagnosis, treatment, and disease progression. *Biol Psychiatry* 2003;54:376–387.

157. Kauhanen M-L, Korpelainen JT, Hiltunen P, et al. Poststroke depression correlates with cognitive impairment and neurological deficits. *Stroke* 1999;30:1875–1880.

158. Paradiso S, Robinson RG. Minor depression after stroke: an initial validation of the DSM-IV construct. *Am J Geriatr Psychiatry* 1999;7:244–251.

159. Shimoda K, Robinson RG. The relationship between poststroke depression and lesion location in long-term follow-up. *Biol Psychiatry* 1999;45:187–192.

160. Bhogal SK, Teasell R, Foley N, Speechley M. Lesion location and poststroke depression. Systematic review of the methodological limitations in the literature. *Stroke* 2004;35:794–802.

161. Galynker I, Prikhojan A, Phillips E, Focseneanu M, Ieronimo C, Rosenthal R. Negative symptoms in stroke patients and length of hospital stay. *J Nerv Ment Dis* 1997;185:616–621.

162. van de Weg FB, Kuik DJ, Lankhorst GJ. Post-stroke depression and functional outcome: a cohort study investigating the influence of depression on functional recovery from stroke. *Clin Rehabil* 1999;13:268–272.

163. Everson SA, Roberts RE, Goldberg DE, Kaplan GA. Depressive symptoms and increased risk of stroke mortality over a 29-year period. *Arch Intern Med* 1998;158:1133–1138.

164. Teasell RW, Merskey H, Deshpande S. Antidepressants in rehabilitation. *Phys Med Rehabil Clin N Am* 1999;10:237–253.

165. Jorge RE, Robinson RG, Arndt S, Starkstein S. Morality and poststroke depression: a placebo-controlled trial of antidepressants. *Am J Psychiatry* 2003;160:1823–1829.

166. Rasmussen A, Lunde M, Poulsen DL, Sorensen K, Qvitzau S, Bech P. A double-blind, placebo-controlled study of sertraline in the prevention of depression in stroke patients. *Psychosomatics* 2003;44:216–221.

167. Vuilleumier P, Ghika-Schmid F, Bogousslavsky J, Assal G, Regli F. Persistent recurrence of hypomania and prosopoaffective agnosia in a patient with right thalamic infarct. *Neuropsychiatry Neuropsychol Behav Neurol* 1998;11:40–44.

168. Bruggimann L, Annoni JM, Staub F, et al. Chronic post-traumatic stress symptoms after nonsevere stroke. *Neurology* 2006;66:513–516.

169. Leppavuori A, Pohjasvaara T, Vataja R, Kaste M, Erkinjuntti T. Generalized anxiety disorders three to four months after ischemic stroke. *Cerebrovasc Dis* 2003;16:257–264.

170. Everson SA, Kaplan GA, Goldberg DE, Lakka TA, Sivenius J, Salonen JT. Anger expression and incident stroke. *Stroke* 1999;30:523–528.

171. Eslinger PJ, Warner GC, Grattan LM, Easton JD. "Frontal lobe" utilization behavior associated with paramedian thalamic infarction. *Neurology* 1991;41:450–452.

172. Mukand J, Kaplan M, Senno RG, Bishop DS. Pathological crying and laughing: treatment with sertraline. *Arch Phys Med Rehabil* 1996;77:1309–1311.

173. Derex L, Ostrowsky K, Nighoghossian N, Trouillas P. Severe pathological crying after left anterior choroidal artery infarct. Reversibility with paroxetine treatment. *Stroke* 1997;28:1464–1466.

174. Early Supported Discharge Trialists. Services for reducing duration of hospital care for acute stroke patients. *Cochrane Database Syst Rev* 2002;CD000443.

175. Fjaertoft H, Indredavik B, Lydersen S. Stroke unit care combined with early supported discharge: long-term follow-up of a randomized controlled trial. *Stroke* 2003;34:2687–2691.

176. Kalia KK, Yonas H. An aggressive approach to massive middle cerebral artery infarction. *Arch Neurol* 1993;50:1293–1297.

177. Sakai K, Iwahashi K, Terada K, et al. Outcome after external decompression for massive cerebral infarction. *Neurologia Medico Chirurgica* 1998;38:131–135.

178. Delashaw JB, Broaddus WC, Kassell NF, et al. Treamtne of right hemispheric cerebral infarction by hemicraniectomy. *Stroke* 1990;21:874–881.

179. Kondziolka D, Fazl M. Functional recovery after decompressive craniectomy for cerebral infarction. *Neurosurgery* 1988;23:143–147.

180. Mori K, Ishimaru S, Maeda M. Unco-parahippocampectomy for direct surgical treatment of downward transtentorial herniation. *Acta Neurochir* 1998;140:1239–1244.

181. Rieke K, Schwab D, Krieger R, et al. Decompressive surgery in space-occupying hemispheric infarction. Results of an open, prospective trial. *Crit Care Med* 1995;23:1576–1587.

182. Steiger HJ. Outcome of acute supratentorial cerebral infarction in patients under 60. *Acta Neurochir* 199;111:73–79.

CHAPTER 25

Rehabilitation and Return to Society

► GENERAL PRINCIPLES FOR REHABILITATION

Some survivors of stroke have such minimal neurological impairments that interventions to help recover from any residual deficits are not necessary. Such individuals are able to return to their prestroke activities without any restrictions. The goal of modern stroke management is to increase the number of such patients. Unfortunately, many survivors require extensive rehabilitation. The aim is to compensate for the residual impairments from stroke through aggressive efforts to maximize recovery. Physicians treating patients with stroke should know the goals and aims of rehabilitation.[1,2] Measures to help the patient to compensate for the neurological impairments and thereby maximize recovery are the foundation of rehabilitation. Rehabilitation is as important as treatment of the acute stroke itself and the prevention of recurrent neurological events (Fig. 25-1). Rehabilitation is a part of comprehensive management and involves the collaboration of multiple disciplines.[3] It should be started in the acute care setting and followed by measures that are prescribed through inpatient and outpatient rehabilitation programs.[3,4]

A stroke rehabilitation team assesses and treats patients and it may be part of the acute stroke care team in a hospital.[5] A stroke team now is the standard to which other types of rehabilitation are compared. Members of the stroke rehabilitation team include physicians, nurses, discharge planners, social service specialists, physical therapists, occupational therapists, speech pathologists, and neuropsychologists (Table 25-1). Each member of the team has his/her own expertise that complements the efforts of the other professionals. The physicians and nurses are responsible for the patient's overall care. A physician usually directs the other members of the rehabilitation team. Physical therapists focus on improving ambulation and major limb movements. Speech pathologists treat language and speech impairments and help in the assessment and treatment of swallowing. Occupational therapists specialize in improving function of the affected hand and provide assistance devices to improve independence and the performance of activities of daily living. Neuropsychologists assess the severity and types of cognitive impairments and assist in cognitive rehabilitation. Social workers aid the patient in obtaining proper insurance coverage and other assistance as the patient returns to society. The team develops recommendations about subsequent rehabilitation, including the setting. Depending upon the patient's progress, transition from one type of rehabilitation setting to another is implemented (Tables 25-2 and 25-3). For example, the patient might be discharged from an acute hospital directly to an inpatient rehabilitation unit. Subsequently, the patient might be discharged home with continued outpatient rehabilitation either in a clinic or in his/her home.

During the course of rehabilitation, priorities and components of rehabilitation often change. For example, assessment of swallowing and initiation of efforts to improve maintenance of nutrition and hydration by an oral route is often the first step in rehabilitation. Thereafter, other activities including initiation of mobilization begin within the first few days following stroke.

The goal of rehabilitation is to allow the patient to return home and in as independent a state as possible. While helping a patient return to all his/her prestroke

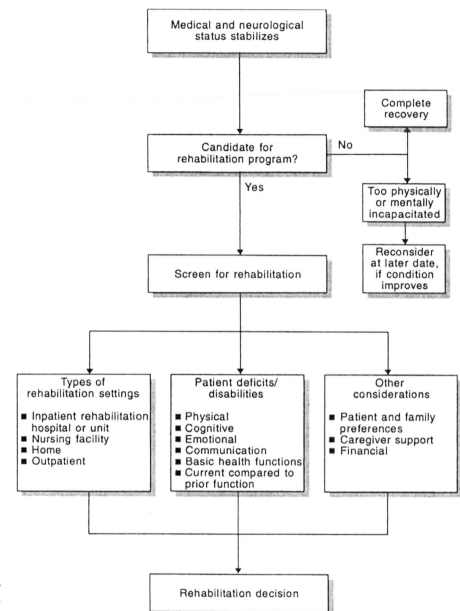

Figure 25-1. Outline of decisions in regard to rehabilitation. (*Reprinted from Ref. 1*)

▶ **TABLE 25-1.** PROFESSIONALS INVOLVED IN REHABILITATION

Physician
    Physical medicine and rehabilitation
    Neurology
    Other specialty
Nurse
    Care manager
Physical therapist
Occupational therapist
Speech pathologist
Neuropsychologist
Recreation therapist
Social worker
Vocational counselor

activities is laudable, many patients cannot achieve this aim. Although those patients with minimal or no neurological impairments can reach this goal, others with severe strokes likely will not. The aims should reflect the patient's potential for recovery. Setting a goal that cannot be realistically achieved during rehabilitation does not help the patient, the family, or society. The target should be to reduce disability and handicap as much as possible and should therefore reflect the nature of the patient's neurological impairments and other factors. The goals should be clearly explained to the patient and family (Fig. 25-2). They must be involved in all stages of the rehabilitation decision-making process. The patient and family should also be educated about the type of rehabilitation

▶ **TABLE 25-2.** SITES FOR REHABILITATION

Inpatient rehabilitation
   Part of another hospital
   Independent rehabilitation hospital
Skilled nursing facility
Nursing home with rehabilitation capacities
Outpatient rehabilitation
   Home based
   Day hospital programs
   Outpatient clinics

measures and the frequency, intensity, and duration of these interventions, as well as the planned stages and settings of rehabilitation. In addition, rehabilitation personnel should outline the long-term management plan at the beginning of rehabilitation.

During rehabilitation, physicians, therapists, and other medical personnel regularly evaluate the patient's progress (see Fig. 25-2). The frequency of these assessments depends upon the nature and location of the rehabilitation. Guidelines recommend that these evaluations be done at least weekly when patients are treated in an inpatient unit.[1] In other situations, follow-up assessments may be done every 2-4 weeks. The goals of these evaluations are to monitor the patient's progress with all components of rehabilitation, to adjust the treatment plan in response to the patient's performance, and to readjust the goals or markers of success. An increase or decrease in rehabilitation activities is developed in response to the contents of the evaluation. For example, a decrease in intensity of therapy may relate to the patient no longer needing the intervention. Conversely, a therapy may also be eliminated if the patient does not appear benefited.

▶ **TABLE 25-3.** STEPS IN REHABILITATION

Baseline assessment
   Severity of neurological impairments
   Medical conditions
      Comorbid diseases
      Overall health and stamina
   Personal status
      Age
      Family support or caregivers
      Ability to cooperate with rehabilitation
Periodic assessments for responses to treatment
Goal planning
   Living environment
   Occupation
   Family support and caregiver
Needed individual interventions
Organization of rehabilitation efforts
Plans for long-term care

▶ **TABLE 25-4.** SCREENING FOR REHABILITATION

Demographic
   Age
   Gender
   Race, ethnicity, or cultural beliefs
   Primary language
Social
   Level of education
   Financial resources
   Health insurance
   Size of community and availability of resources
      Health care
      Rehabilitation
      Transportation
      Home care
   Membership in religious groups
   Membership in special interest groups
   Members in household—relationships
   Other potential caregivers
   Structure of family
   Prior activities including work
   Prior socialization, leisure activities, and hobbies
   Willingness to seek assistance
   Expectations
   Living environment
Medical
   History of mental illness
   History of alcohol or drug abuse

Because rehabilitation is expensive, time-consuming, and involves the use of limited resources, only carefully selected patients should have treatment (Fig. 25-3). Yet, most patients with mild-to-severe neurological impairments should have rehabilitation. Several factors predict poor responses to rehabilitation, including severe neurological impairments, cognitive impairments, advanced age, or absence of supportive family members[6–11] (Tables 25-4 to 25-6). Serious comorbid diseases including diabetes, arthritis, heart disease, lung disease, or other neurological diseases also hamper responses to treatment[12–15] (Tables 25-7 and 25-8). Factors such as the patient's stamina can affect plans for rehabilitation. The interval from stroke to rehabilitation is not as crucial as other factors.[16] In addition, the wishes and goals of the patient and family are important factors in selecting the type and location of rehabilitation.

The initial site for rehabilitation depends upon the factors outlined in Table 25-2. If the deficits are isolated or mild, rehabilitation might be on an outpatient basis. Patients with moderate-to-severe impairments usually require the gamut of rehabilitative services. Inpatient rehabilitation is often recommended for those patients with mild-to-severe neurological impairments that require at least two rehabilitation interventions (speech therapy, physical therapy, and occupational therapy)

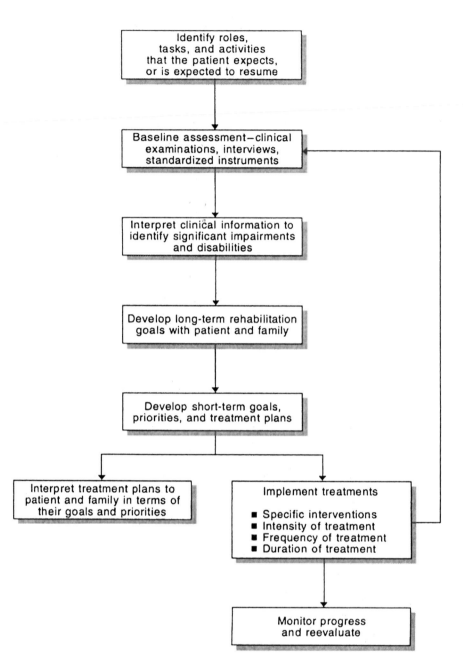

Figure 25-2. Outline of assessments and timing of monitoring of responses to rehabilitation. (*Reprinted from Ref. 1*)

and can tolerate at least 3 h of therapy per day (Fig. 25-4; Table 25-9). More intensive daily physical therapy and other rehabilitation procedures might shorten the length of stay for rehabilitation.[17] In general, inpatient rehabilitation immediately follows acute hospitalization and it continues for several weeks. Inpatient rehabilitation is the most expensive option and involves the collaboration of physicians and several other rehabilitation specialists. Medical therapies started in the acute care hospital usually are continued. In addition, patients transferred to inpatient rehabilitation need interventions to prevent or treat subacute or new medical complications.[18,19] Among the complications that require surveil-

lance and attention are incontinence, urinary tract infections, pneumonia, deep vein thrombosis, orthopedic problems, and pressure sores. Many patients demonstrate dramatic gains during this period.

Other options for rehabilitation include admission to a skilled nursing facility (see Table 25-2). Patients who cannot be discharged to an outpatient program and who are not candidates for inpatient rehabilitation are often referred to such institutions. The intensity of rehabilitation is less than that found with inpatient programs, but improvement often does occur.[20] Elderly patients and patients with very severe strokes or serious comorbid diseases are admitted to long-term care treatment

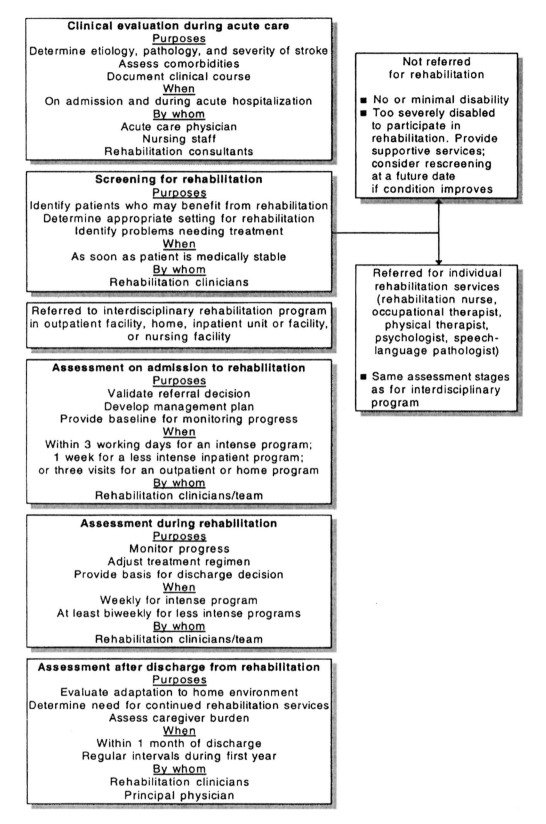

Figure 25-3. Screening, selecting, and monitoring of patients undergoing rehabilitation after stroke. (*Reprinted from Ref. 1*)

▶ **TABLE 25-5.** NEUROLOGICAL SCREENING OF PATIENTS WITH STROKE—REHABILITATION

Altered consciousness or coma precludes most rehabilitation
Cognitive and mental status, including language
    Severe deficits preclude rehabilitation
    Moderate deficits impede rehabilitation
        Severe aphasia impedes rehabilitation
        Severe neglect impedes rehabilitation
    Mild-to-moderate deficits should receive aggressive rehabilitation
    Focal deficits should receive aggressive rehabilitation
    Mild-to-severe aphasia should receive aggressive rehabilitation
Vision
    Severe visual loss impedes rehabilitation
Articulation
    Mild-to-severe dysarthria should receive aggressive rehabilitation
Swallowing
    Severe dysphagia often does not respond to rehabilitation
    Mild-to-moderate dysphagia should receive aggressive rehabilitation
Pain
    Generally impedes rehabilitation—usually requires treatment
Sensory loss
    Generally impedes rehabilitation
    Usually a focus of rehabilitation
Motor loss
    Severe deficits (paralysis) usually respond poorly to rehabilitation
    Mild-to-moderate deficits should receive aggressive rehabilitation
Impairments of balance or coordination
    Severe deficits usually impede rehabilitation
    Mild-to-moderate deficits should receive aggressive rehabilitation

▶ **TABLE 25-6.** NEUROLOGICAL OR MEDICAL DISEASES THAT AFFECT REHABILITATION

Presence of other neurological diseases
    Peripheral neuropathy
    Movement disorders
    Dementia
    Epilepsy
Presence of medical diseases
    Heart disease—heart failure, coronary artery disease
    Lung disease—emphysema
    Diabetes mellitus
    Poor vision
    Poor hearing
    Psychiatric disease
    Arthritis
Functional health patterns
    Nutrition
    Hydration
    Ability to swallow
    Urinary incontinence
    Fecal incontinence
    Skin integrity
    Activity tolerance—stamina
    Sleep patterns

facilities (nursing homes).[21] In these institutions, limited rehabilitation generally is offered.

Outpatient rehabilitation can be centered in the patient's home, in which case rehabilitation specialists visit the patient (Tables 25-7, 25-8, and 25-10). Outpatient rehabilitation may also involve the patient participating in programs in a clinic. It could also be the setting for initial rehabilitation of mildly affected patients, such as those who might need only one intervention. It also follows rehabilitation done in an inpatient unit or skilled nursing facility.[22] Since outpatient therapy is usually less intensive with less-frequent sessions and shorter periods of treatment than inpatient care, it is less expensive than treatment in these other locations.

Each type of outpatient rehabilitation has advantages. For example, coming to the outpatient clinic helps the patient to practice traveling, it provides an opportunity for socialization with others, and it is usually more comprehensive than visits to a patient's home.[23] Some types of rehabilitation cannot be performed easily in a patient's home. In-home rehabilitation can include the traditional rehabilitation modalities in combination with home health care and nursing personnel. It also allows for the implementation of rehabilitation strategies in the actual living situation of the patient. Rehabilitation in the patient's home is shown to be effective in improving outcomes.[24,25] Follow-up outpatient rehabilitation services are associated with continued improvements in outcomes.[26] Depending upon the patient's wishes and other characteristics, additional measures may include follow-up house calls, instructions and treatment by therapists, and usual follow-up by nursing and home health personnel. Therapy-based rehabilitation services for stroke patients living at home reduce the odds of deterioration in the performance of activities of daily living and increase the ability of personal activities.[27] These data support the

▶ **TABLE 25-7.** FACTORS THAT PREDICT A FAVORABLE RESPONSE TO REHABILITATION

Relatively discrete neurological impairments
Early initiation of rehabilitation
A comprehensive rehabilitation program
Absence of severe comorbid diseases
Strong family support
Strong financial support
High level of education
Upper socioeconomic class

▶ **TABLE 25-8.** PREDICTORS THAT PREDICT A POOR RESPONSE TO REHABILITATION

Strongly negative predictors
  Coma or prolonged period or unresponsiveness
  Poor cognition—including preexisting dementia
    Neglect
    Severe apraxia
    Visual-spatial deficits
    Aphasia with poor comprehension
  Urinary or fecal incontinence (>2 weeks after stroke)
  Severe motor impairments
    Little motor recovery >1 month after stroke
    Poor sitting balance
  Severe comorbid diseases (especially heart disease)
Negative predictors
  Advanced intellect
  Low intellect
  Language impairments
  Sensory loss—especially nondominant hemisphere
  Homonymous hemianopia
  Absence of spouse or close family members

▶ **TABLE 25-9.** CRITERIA FOR ADMISSION INPATIENT REHABILITATION PROGRAM

Moderate-to-severe neurological impairments
Normal consciousness
Limited cognitive impairments
Requirement for at least two of the following interventions
  Physical therapy
  Occupational therapy
  Speech therapy
  Ability to perform at least 3 h of therapy per day
Younger age
Absence of severe comorbid medical diseases
Absence of severe comorbid neurological diseases
Relatively good functional status before stroke
Well-motivated patient
Strong support from family

rehabilitation is relatively expensive, and it may not eliminate the need for treatment in other environments.

utility of outpatient-based rehabilitation for patients who have been able to return home. Such services often follow hospitalization in an acute care setting or are used after a period of more intensive inpatient rehabilitation. In-home

▶ **REHABILITATION PROCEDURES**

Experimental research is providing the scientific underpinnings for a better understanding of how rehabilitation

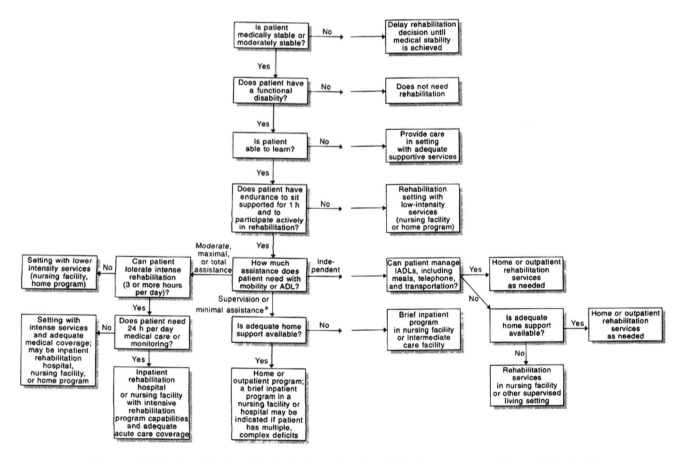

Figure 25-4. Decision tree including important variables in recommending rehabilitation after stroke. (*Reprinted from Ref. 1*)

▶ **TABLE 25-10.** COMPONENTS OF HOME
HEALTH CARE

Nurses
   Prepare, supervise, or administer medications
   Administer other medical therapies
   Assess patient's status
   Arrange clinic visits
   Interact with patient's physician
Rehabilitation personnel
   Continue specific rehabilitation activities
Home health care aides
   Prepare meals and assist in dining
   Assist in dressing
   Assist in bathing and other activities of daily living
   Assist in toilet
   Household cleaning
   Laundry

can speed recovery from a brain injury, such as stroke.[9] This field is likely to receive considerable attention in the future. Because the number of patients who might benefit from such interventions is considerably higher than the group that can be treated with acute therapies, the potential impact is huge. Virtually, all patients with stroke (and possibly other brain diseases) could be treated with various rehabilitation or restorative modalities.

Functional magnetic resonance imaging (MRI) and transcortical magnetic stimulation allow demonstration of the reorganization of the brain in patients who suffered a stroke.[9] Important concepts including plasticity therefore are being studied. Plasticity may result from dendritic arborization, synaptogenesis, and modification of synapses via horizontal connections in the cerebral cortex.[9]

Medications

Medications are being evaluated for their ability to speed or help recovery by modulating relearning of cognitive or other skills. Neurotrophic growth factors and tissue transplantation are among the interventions that might be used[28–30] (see Chapter 22). While such interventions hold considerable promise, evidence about their utility in improving outcomes is currently lacking.[31,32]

Pharmacological interventions might assist other rehabilitation measures to maximize improvements. Amphetamines, antidepressants, and gamma-aminobutyric acid (GABA) agonists are among the medications that are under evaluation. For example, Crisostomo et al.[33] reported that adjunctive administration of amphetamines could speed motor recovery during physical therapy. This observation was supported by the results of another small study.[34] In a series of 45 patients treated within 72 h of stroke, Martinsson and Wahlgren[35] found that dexamphetamine increased blood pressure and

heart rate. While no differences in temperature or consciousness were noted with the medication, they had the impression that the dexamphetamine improved outcomes. In a small clinical trial, Treig et al.[36] could not find any benefit from the concomitant administration of D-amphetamine and physical therapy for treatment of patients with stroke. Patients had improvements in arm function whether or not they received D-amphetamine. Knecht et al.[37] found that D-amphetamine did not improve somatosensory training in healthy patients with stroke. However, based upon a systemic review, Martinsson et al.[38] concluded that there were no definitive data about the utility or lack of efficacy of amphetamines. They concluded that there was no evidence that these medications reduced death and disability. Dam et al.[39] reported that adjunctive use of fluoxetine could help improve recovery of hemiparetic patients undergoing physical therapy. In another study, nimodipine was shown to improve recovery of memory following stroke.[40] Additional experimental and clinical research is needed to determine if any pharmacological intervention could speed the recovery after stroke.[41]

Conversely, some medications might actually hamper recovery. For example, major tranquilizers appear to have negative effects.[9] Clonidine, prazosin, most neuroleptic agents, some anticonvulsants, and dopamine antagonists are among the agents that may slow the motor responses.[42,43] Some of the negative effects may be secondary to a global depression of consciousness. In addition, the effects of dopamine antagonists and neuroleptic agents raise the possibility of specific negative influences on dopaminergic systems within the brain. While the current data are not sufficiently strong to advise against the use of these medications, the possible negative influence of these agents may prompt physicians to recommend other therapies as substitutes.

Cognitive Rehabilitation

Impairments in higher executive function, judgment, attention, and memory are frequent sequelae that affect the patient's ability to return home, and hamper other efforts to maximize recovery.[44] The types of neuropsychological impairments correlate closely with the individual's ability to recover independence.[45] For example, patients with infarctions in the nondominant (right) hemisphere often have anosognosia, asomatognosia, or neglect that affects their ability to understand the pragmatic and social nuances, which hampers efforts to recover from stroke.[46] Unfortunately, measures to counteract these impairments are not particularly successful. The effects of cognitive rehabilitation were evaluated in systemic reviews.[47–49] These reviews found limited data and the authors concluded that there were insufficient data to support or refute the use of measures to improve memory or other aspects of higher brain function. Measures to improve attention help sustain alertness.[49] Bowen et al.[47] found some effect of rehabilitative strategies addressing spatial neglect, but the impact on reducing disability is not clear. Considerable research is needed in the cognitive component of rehabilitation and this should be made a high priority.

Other behavioral impairments also follow stroke. Spontaneous recovery of visual loss is uncommon. Most affected patients have some residual deficits that hamper activities such as driving. To date, little rehabilitation is available other than training the individual to consciously look into the affected field. Computer-assisted training may help diminish residual visual field defects.[50] Such strategies require additional research.

Persisting depression hinders efforts in all spheres of rehabilitation; thus, its treatment is an important component of management. Mild depression may often be alleviated by the attention and encouragement of rehabilitation personnel, family, and friends. More severe or unrelenting depression requires pharmacological interventions (see Chapter 24).

Speech Therapy

Speech pathologists generally are the first rehabilitation specialists contacted (Table 25-11). Their initial task is to help evaluate the patient's ability to swallow and handle oral secretions. Some of the issues related to swallowing are described in Chapter 24. Some patients need aggressive therapy to regain swallowing. Strategies include using cool substances to stimulate normal pharyngeal swallowing reflexes. As the patient improves, the content of the diet is advanced. Fortunately, most patients

recover swallowing in the first 6 months after stroke. Only 5 percent of patients have moderate-to-severe eating impairments.[51] The number of patients requiring prolonged enteral nutrition is relatively small.

A second component of speech therapy involves treatment of disorders of articulation, including disturbances of respiration, phonation, resonation, articulation, or prosody.[1] The goal is to restore clarity of speech. Possible interventions include sensory stimulation; strengthening of the muscles of pharynx, mouth, lips, and tongue; positioning; and methods to improve respiratory capacity. In some cases, communication devices are used, including communication boards, pacing boards, or electronic communication devices.

Aphasia leads to severe incapacity following stroke (Fig. 25-5). Most patients cannot return to their usual activities or work. The inability to understand another person's language or to convey one's thoughts greatly impairs the quality of life. While many patients salvage part of language function, several factors including the patient's age, sex, handedness, and level of education significantly influence recovery.[52] The severity and type of aphasia also affect responses to rehabilitation.[53] Selnes et al.[54] found that recovery of language was correlated with the location of the stroke. These investigators proposed that plasticity might be helpful in reorganizing language function in the nondominant hemisphere. In some patients, differences between the language and the

► **TABLE 25-11.** ACTIVITIES OF SPEECH THERAPY

Swallowing
  Assess severity of impairments
  Monitor improvements
  Advise on consistency of foods to be swallowed
  Assist in efforts to improve swallowing
Articulation
  Assess severity of impairments
  Assist in efforts to improve articulation
  Use of communication assistance devices
    Communication board
    Electronic communication devices
Language
  Assess severity of impairments
    Aural comprehension
    Reading
    Oral production
    Writing
  Assist in efforts to improve language

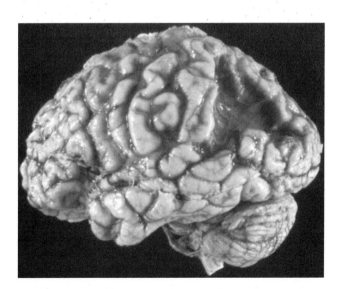

Figure 25-5. Lateral view of the left hemisphere shows a large infarction involving the parietal lobe. A stroke of this size and location likely would produce focal cognitive or language impairments that would necessitate a prolonged course of rehabilitation. (*Courtesy of S.S. Schochet, M.D., Department of Pathology, University of West Virginia, Morgantown, WV*)

melody (prosody) of speech might help modulate recovery.[55] Greener et al.[56] proposed that adjunctive administration of piracetam may be effective in improving aphasia following stroke. Several studies evaluated the utility of speech therapy in speeding recovery from stroke but the data are mixed.[57–61] A systemic review found that there were insufficient data to determine if the interventions were effective or ineffective in improving outcomes.[62] Thus, additional research is needed. Despite such limited data supporting the utility of speech therapy, patients and families expect this intervention. It should be prescribed to patients with language impairments. The regular support and encouragement by speech pathologists and other family members probably do help speed the recovery of language.[57]

Physical Therapy

Physical therapy is often the primary focus of rehabilitation following stroke (Table 25-12). Physical therapists aid the patient in regaining mobility through the use of exercises, compensatory techniques, and devices.[1] There is evidence that aggressive physical therapy helps reduce mortality and speed recovery.[63,64] In a randomized trial, Duncan et al.[65] found that therapeutic exercises improve endurance, balance, and mobility. There is evidence that physical therapy speeds recovery of

▶ **TABLE 25-12.** ACTIVITIES—PHYSICAL THERAPY

Mobility and balance
   Improve sitting, standing, transferring, and walking
   Improve reaching, turning, and changing directions
   Ability to care objects
   Going up and down stairs or ramps
Range of motion
   Passive or active exercises of motion
   In particular, proximal joints—shoulder and hip
Motor activity
   Assist contraction of weak muscles
   Assist in isokinetic, isometric, eccentric, or concentric
     exercises
   Exercise agonist and antagonist muscle groups
   Increase complexity of motor movements
Sensory function
   Assist in compensation for sensory loss, in particular
     Proprioception and position sense
Pain
   Help in reducing pain
     Use of slings and supports
     Elevation of limb
     Nonpharmacological interventions
     Teach patient to avoid exercises that increase pain
   Advise in selection of orthotic devices
   Advise in selection of therapies to treat spasticity

important brain circuitry. For example, Miyai et al.[66] showed that locomotor recovery was associated with activation of both the premotor cortex and the medial aspects of the primary sensorimotor cortex. This finding implies that rehabilitation probably involves physiological changes as well as reeducation. Unfortunately, some patients have little recovery of limb function despite extensive physical therapy.[67]

Motor recovery, including mobility, is important for independence and performing activities of daily living. Approximately 70 percent of persons surviving stroke have residual motor impairments at 1 month; by 6 months, the number declines to approximately 60 percent.[68] Patients with moderate motor impairments achieve the greatest recovery.[69] Motor recovery is most rapid and dramatic during the first few days after stroke.[70] Patients generally achieve sitting balance on the day of stroke, standing balance within 3 days, and 10-step walking by 6 days.[71,72] The rate of recovery is very slow after the first 3 months following stroke.[73,74] Still, patients have improved motor function with interventions prescribed months or even years following a stroke.[75] Thus, a program of physical therapy that involves long-term interventions can help patients.

The types and patterns of motor and sensory deficits in the upper and lower extremities affect decisions about physical therapy (see Table 25-12). Because many infarctions are in the territory of the middle cerebral artery, more severe impairments are found in the upper extremity. The amount of functional recovery of the arm and hand is often less than that in the lower extremity. The hand, in particular fine motor movements, has the least opportunity for recovery. Recovery of limb function involves the activation of areas of the brain that are often remote from the stroke, including the contralateral hemisphere.[76–78] Measures that address sensory function are an important aspect of rehabilitation.[73] Very severe sensory loss, in particular loss of vibratory or position sense, decreases mobility and hampers recovery. Impairments of visuospatial function, which may be accompanied by distortions of perceived space or neglect, also affect motor recovery.[79–81] Strategies, such as the use of mirrors, may help lessen the effects of neglect.[82]

In general, physical therapy is started as soon as the patient's medical status is stable. Emphasizing strength and coordination of the hemiplegic side appears to be an important goal in maximizing recovery.[83] Attention to balance also is critical as the patient's mobilization begins. Activities that involve synchronous activation of axial trunk muscles on both sides of the body appear to be critical in recovering mobility and motor function.[84] Several physical therapy models are used when treating stroke survivors (Table 25-13). Research on these strategies is considerable. Traditional remediation involves sensory stimulation modalities, exercises, and resistance

▶ **TABLE 25-13.** TYPES OF PHYSICAL THERAPY TECHNIQUES

Remediation
Compensation
Constraint-induced movement
Treadmill
Intermittent pneumatic compression devices
Acupuncture
Sensory stimulation
Electrical stimulation
Robot training
Biofeedback

training to enhance motor recovery.[1] Compensatory techniques involve methods to achieve independence by improving motor function rather than stimulating motor behavior. In addition, physical therapists have used specific interventions that involve task-specific motor control. At present, no strategy is established as superior. A systemic review could not find evidence that one type of physiotherapy was better than the others.[72]

Submaximal aerobic training helps improve the patient's overall health and increases functional levels following stroke.[85] Low-intensity treadmill exercises are used to improve the gait of hemiparetic patients, including those with heart disease.[86] Methods to use treadmill training for walking in wheelchair-bound patients are available.[9] Supported treadmill training involves the placement of a patient in a sling while he is receiving treatment to improve walking. Such a tactic appears to be safe and feasible.[87] Other systems include a parachute harness and body-weight-supported devices. In a small, randomized trial, Ada et al.[88] demonstrated that a program involving treadmill and overground walking improved gait among persons with chronic motor impairments following stroke. The intervention involved 30 min of structured walking three times per week.

One approach that has received considerable recent attention is constraint-induced movement therapy.[89,90] In this situation, the unaffected limb is constrained so that the patient must use the paralyzed arm. With constraint-induced therapy, expansion of the areas of representation of the extremity in the damaged area can be found.[9] This intervention focuses on recovery of the function of the upper extremity and it may be prescribed several months after the stroke. The intervention is intensive and involves several hours with a therapist every day. A randomized trial of constraint-induced movement therapy revealed improved upper extremity function.[91] Page et al.[92] tested a modified version of constraint-induced physical therapy. Patients were given regular therapy in association with constraint of the unaffected arm for 5 h, 5 days a week. They also noted

improved function of the paralyzed arm using this approach. Additional studies testing the utility of constraint-induced therapy are currently under way.

Another approach to physical therapy involves active neuromuscular stimulation and repetitive practice. Cauragh and Kim[93] reported that this strategy could be used to help patients with chronic upper extremity motor impairments. However, in another study, Moreland et al.[94] found no benefit from progressive resistance strengthening exercises. Orthopedic complications, such as adhesive capsulitis and contracture of muscle groups, can hamper physical therapy.[73] Interventions to treat these complications of stroke need to be prescribed on a case-by-case basis.

Adjunctive Interventions to Treat Motor Impairments

A loss of autonomic innervation of the fine arteries of the paralyzed limb may lead to trophic changes including edema of the hand or foot. The swelling can be considerable and it can cause pain or limit rehabilitation efforts. Intermittent pneumatic compression is sometimes used to lessen limb edema. Roper et al.[95] found that this intervention was effective. However, it is not used widely. At present, the best tactic to reduce swelling of the hand probably is elevation of the limb.

Compression devices are also used to help recovery from sensory impairments. Cambier et al.[96] administered this intervention in addition to standard physical therapy. Some patients reported improvement in sensation.

Muellbacher et al.[97] recently looked at whether deafferentation of an affected body part, through the use of local anesthesia, would enhance cortical representations of adjacent body parts and thus improve recovery. They tested this approach in combination with transcranial magnetic stimulation evoked output to the hand. Some improvement in hand function was apparent. Pain, dysesthesias, and paresthesias can limit recovery or affect efforts for rehabilitation. Acupuncture or biofeedback is also reported to supplement conventional physical therapy but evidence for efficacy is inconclusive.[98,99] Sensory stimulation also has been found to improve recovery and posture.[100] Yu et al.[101] reported that intramuscular neuromuscular electric stimulation can reduce shoulder pain among those patients with secondary shoulder subluxation. Price and Pandyan[102] reviewed the results of several small studies that tested electrical stimulation to prevent or treat shoulder pain following stroke. The intervention seemed to improve the pain-free range of motion of the shoulder and reduced the severity of glenohumeral subluxation. However, no net improvement in functional recovery was noted.

Robotic training is also used to enhance motor recovery following stroke.[103] Fasoli et al.[104] tested the utility of robotic therapy to increase goal-directed exercises of the upper extremity. They found that the intervention reduced residual deficits among patients with moderate-to-severe chronic motor impairments. This strategy holds promise and requires testing in additional clinical trials. Neuromuscular electrical stimulation (EMG-triggered NMES) can facilitate patterned, repetitive exercise while supplying cutaneous feedback immediately locked to each movement.[9] It can cause contraction of paralyzed hand muscles and has been employed to improve function of the extensors of the wrist.[105,106] However, one study found that electrical stimulation did not help either biomechanical or functional movements of the hand.[107]

Orthotic or adaptive devices are adjuncts to conventional physical therapy (Table 25-14). These devices are recommended when a patient cannot otherwise achieve independence. Devices are used to help sensorimotor function, improve independence, or increase mobility. A wheelchair is recommended if the patient does not recover sufficient function to walk either independently or with the use of other devices. Both poor stamina and major neurological impairments also are indications for the use of a wheelchair. The wheelchair should be adapted to the individual patient's needs and, in some cases, should be a motorized unit. Some patients with gait instability or moderately severe residual motor impairments need walkers. Canes, including quad canes, are used to help improve spatial variables among patients with hemiparesis.[108] Orthotic devices are most commonly used to stabilize the ankle. Because of the potential for spasticity, spring-loaded ankle braces are not administered. Less commonly, devices are used to support the knee or wrist. Other specific devices may assist in activities of daily living. The patient, family, and other caregivers need to be trained in the proper use of these devices. Because many devices are expensive, issues such as insurance coverage should be addressed before they are ordered.

▶ **TABLE 25-14.** DEVICES TO IMPROVE MOBILITY

Manual or electrically powered wheelchair
Pickup or rolling walker (often with brakes)
Single or quad cane
Transfer board
Hydraulic or electric lift
Elevator
Gait/transfer belt
Braces—in particular at ankle
Seats to heighten toilet and chairs
Rails or bars on toilet seat
Bedside commode, urinal, or bedpan
Shower chair with rails or bars
Nonskid mats in shower

▶ **TABLE 25-15.** MEDICAL MANAGEMENT OF SEVERE SPASTICITY

Injections of botulinum toxin
Baclofen
   Oral
   Intrathecal
Dantrolene
Alcohol nerve block
Phenol nerve block
Resection of nerve

Treatment of Spasticity

Spasticity impedes recovery of motor function by limiting joint movement.[12] It also causes muscular or orthopedic pain. In some patients, the spasticity can be more disabling than the weakness. The signs of spasticity usually evolve over several months following stroke. Physical therapy strategies involve range of motion exercises and placement of limbs in positions that antagonize the effects of spasticity. In addition, medications including tizanidine, baclofen, diazepam, dantrolene, clonidine, and gabapentin are prescribed to lessen spasticity[109] (Table 25-15). Each medication has side effects, most commonly sedation and increased weakness. Still, these therapies are an option for treatment. Baclofen can be given orally or intrathecally. Its primary effects are via the GABA transmission in the spinal cord. Oral doses are gradually increased as the patient tolerates the medication. Large doses of baclofen may cause sedation or confusion, and sudden termination of the medication can produce seizures, hallucinations, or a psychosis.[110] Intrathecal infusions of baclofen also are used to treat patients with multiple sclerosis, spinal cord injury, and cerebral palsy.[111] This intervention is used to treat spasticity following stroke.[112] A small study found that intrathecal baclofen combined with physical therapy might improve walking speed and functional mobility in patients with poststroke spastic hemiplegia.[113] Diazepam also can lessen spasticity but its sedating effects and the potential for abuse limit its administration. Dantrolene reduces intracellular transport of calcium within the muscle cells, and as a result muscle contractility is lessened.[114] While dantrolene can cause hepatotoxicity, it can be prescribed as an alternative to baclofen or other therapies to treat severe spasticity. Evidence that it relieves spasticity following stroke is meager.[115]

The most widely used and promising treatment is injections of botulinum toxin into severely affected muscle groups. It is very effective at improving mobility and relieving pain in areas affected by severe spasticity. Randomized trials demonstrate the utility of the medication in treating spasticity in either the upper or lower extremity.[116–120] Pittock et al.[121] tested 500, 1000, or 1500 units of botulinum toxin in treatment of spastic calf muscles and found that the medication improved mobility. In a randomized trial, Brashear et al.[122] administered intramuscular injections of botulinum toxin to reduce spasticity of wrist and finger muscles. The medication was successful in improving mobility and reducing hand impairments. Johnson et al.[123] reported that the combination of localized injections of botulinum toxin and electric stimulation could lessen spastic foot drop and increase mobility. The effects of botulinum usually last for a few months, which means that the patient requires repeated injections. Some patients eventually develop antibodies to the agent, which limits the efficacy of repeated injections. The doses are not sufficiently large as to cause clinical botulism. The success of botulinum toxin has resulted in it being the first intervention used to treat patients with severe spasticity.

Patients with profound spasticity that does not respond to other interventions may require surgical procedures. These interventions result in irreversible changes and their use should be restricted to treating only those patients who are bed-bound and in a great deal of pain. Choices include nerve blocks with alcohol or phenol, chronic stimulation of the spinal cord, surgical rhizotomy, and myelotomy.[124]

Occupational Therapy

Occupational therapy uses interventions that augment functional independence, including therapies aimed at improving hand and finger function (Table 25-16). The occupational therapist assesses the patient's ability to perform activities of daily living and also recommends the use of adaptive devices that can improve independence (Table 25-17). Therapy started in an inpatient setting is often extended to continued interactions following the patient's return to home. Inpatient occupational therapy improves recovery on standard disability scales and improves activities of daily living.[125] However, in another trial, the combination of the intensive use of physical therapy and occupational therapy did not improve outcomes of upper limb function.[126] Despite the results of this recent trial, occupational therapy remains a key component of initial, inpatient rehabilitation as well as chronic long-term efforts to maximize recovery and functional independence following stroke.

▶ **TABLE 25-16.** ACTIVITIES OF OCCUPATIONAL THERAPY

Assess the ability of patient to be independent
Assess the ability of the patient to use devices
Assess the hand function of the patient
Assist in recovery of activities of daily living
Advise on the use of devices to improve independence

▶ **TABLE 25-17.** DEVICES TO AUGMENT INDEPENDENCE ACTIVITIES OF DAILY LIVING

Motor or hand devices
  Large handles on eating utensils
  Rocker knife
  Nonskid place mat on table
  Plate guards or scoop dishes
  Modified cups with large handles
  Long-handled sponge
  Adapted razor, toothbrush, and combing
  Self-adhesive (Velcro®) closures
    Shoes
    Clothes
  One-handed buttoning devices
  Elastic shoestrings
  Long-handled shoehorn
Communication
  Communication board
  Electronic communication devices

▶DISCHARGE FROM REHABILITATION AND A RETURN TO SOCIETY

Discharge from the hospital or an inpatient rehabilitation unit is often stressful for the patient and family. Adjustments to the realities of the consequences of the stroke are critical. The family and patient should be aware of the transitions back into society or the usual living environment.

Unfortunately, some patients will never return home. Instead, they are admitted to a long-term care facility (nursing home) (Table 25-18). Approximately one-sixth of patients surviving stroke need such institutionalized care.[1] Persons most likely to go to a nursing home are the elderly and those with very severe neurological deficits. Since elderly women more often live alone, they also are more likely to go to a nursing home than are elderly men.[127] Some patients require general nursing care that is

▶ **TABLE 25-18.** FACTORS THAT LEAD TO LONG-TERM INSTITUTIONALIZED CARE FOLLOWING STROKE

Severe neurological impairments
  Coma or prolonged unresponsiveness
  Major cognitive impairments or dementia
  Major sensorimotor impairments
Severe preexisting, comorbid neurological diseases
Severe preexisting, comorbid medical diseases
Advanced age
Living alone
No close family members to provide care
Close family members cannot provide care
  Poor health
  Other reasons

beyond the scope of family members to provide. Because long-term nursing home care is expensive, this option presents concerns to the family and patient. Issues such as insurance or governmental programs must be addressed. In some instances, family members feel guilty if they do not assume the caregiver role. Some cultures and religions emphasize the importance of family support and caring for relatives, particularly parents.

Patient and Family Issues

Both the patient and the family should be informed about the warning symptoms of stroke and the proper response to such events. They should also be informed about the importance of medical therapies to prevent recurrent stroke and rehabilitation. Family-specific plans for continued management after discharge need to be reviewed. Several factors influence the decision about the patient returning home. The health of the spouse and other members of the household require evaluation (Table 25-19). An elderly, frail spouse might not be able to give the necessary support. The presence of small children or another person with a disability might also affect decisions about a severely disabled person returning home. Family members with alcohol or drug abuse or mental illness may not be able to cope with or provide the care needed for a stroke survivor.[128–130] In addition, social, occupational, and leisure activities of the spouse should be addressed because the patient's return to home can greatly affect the partner's quality of life.[131,132]

Family members should be encouraged to collaborate in the patient's efforts to recover. The presence of strong support from family members helps improve recovery from stroke.[133] If a patient lives in a household, another family member, most commonly a spouse or adult child, often assumes the role of a primary caregiver. Attention to the psychological well-being of the caregiver is important. For example, a day care program, respite

care, or home services should be included in the management program.[134,135] In addition, these programs may be necessary if the primary caregiver must also work outside the home.

Home Environment

The patient's living environment should be assessed (Table 25-20). Persons who live alone are much less likely to return home than those patients who live with a spouse, other family members, or other caregivers.[136,137] Some patients may need community services including nursing care, home health aides, day care centers, and delivery of meals.[137] The living quarters should be evaluated. Issues such as stairs or the number of stories of the house or apartment building are considered. For example, a patient may not be able to return to an apartment in a building that does not have an elevator. A two-story house also could present problems, particularly if the bathroom and bedroom are located on different floors. A narrow hallway might preclude the use of a wheelchair or walker. The hallway might need to be modified with the addition of a handrail to permit mobility. The patient may require a hospital bed or a lift to help transfer from the bed to a chair. The patient might need to have a bedside commode, bedpan, urinal, or modifications of the toilet or bathing facility. Lightening and floor surfaces should be assessed. For example, trip hazards should be removed. Devices that can improve the patient's independence should be purchased.

Returning to Work

Returning to work following stroke is not important for those patients who are elderly or who have retired (Table 25-21). However, returning to work is a central issue for younger patients. Several factors affect the individual's ability to return to work. Those patients with the mildest strokes, in particular those who are without language impairments, have the best opportunity to return to their usual occupation.[138] Patients with severe neurological impairments usually are not able to work again. While some causes of disability such as motor deficits are obvious, other impairments such as disturbances in attention,

▶ **TABLE 25-19.** DISCHARGE TO HOME—ISSUES THAT NEED TO BE ADDRESSED

Severity of neurological impairments
Severity of comorbid diseases
Required medical interventions
Living situation in patient's home
    Family member or other caregiver
    Physical situation at home
Community or neighborhood support
    Home health care resources
        Nursing care
        Rehabilitation services
        General home care (meals, etc.)
    Transportation
        Medical care
        Rehabilitation
        Recreation and socialization

▶ **TABLE 25-20.** LIVING ENVIRONMENT ISSUES TO BE ADDRESSED BEFORE RETURNING HOME

Stairs and floors
    Availability of elevator
Location of rooms on single floor
Arrangement of kitchen, bedroom, toilet, and bath
Toilet and bath/shower modifications
Chairs and bed transfer
Lighting
Trip hazards including rugs
Railings in hallways

▶ **TABLE 25-21.** FACTORS THAT AFFECT THE PATIENT'S ABILITY TO RETURN TO WORK FOLLOWING STROKE

Age
Previous occupation and level of income
Level of education
Workers compensation
Social welfare system and disability programs
Personal motivation to return to work
Family support
Transportation
   Requirement to drive to work—ability
   Public or other transportation
Severity and types of neurological impairments
   Ability to return to previous occupation
   Ability to learn a new occupation
Severity and types of comorbid diseases
Required continued medical therapies or rehabilitation

judgment, or thinking can preclude the person's return to prestroke work activities. Professional persons with higher incomes and those with mild deficits also have a higher likelihood of returning to work than do other patients.[139] Some patients may not be able to return to potentially dangerous operations or require additional training for another job. Vocational rehabilitation can be an important step in returning to work.[1,140] Since most patients have some recovery in the first weeks following stroke, insurance companies and governmental bodies often do not determine disability immediately following stroke. The loss of income can be an important cause of emotional distress to the patient and family.

Driving

Most persons consider driving a motor vehicle as a key component of independence and the inability to return to driving limits returning to prestroke activities. The inability to return to driving might hamper the ability of the patient to regain employment. It also affects the patient's emotional status. Patients with minimal neurological impairments following stroke usually are able to return to driving. However, most patients with moderate-to-severe impairments cannot safely operate a motor vehicle.[141] Among the impairments are visual field deficits or sensory loss, including neglect, which hamper the ability to recognize hazards while driving. Motor or sensory loss, disorders of judgment or attention, and the potential for seizures are additional reasons for not allowing the person to drive. The patient and family should be advised strongly about the limitations in driving.

Sexuality

Dissatisfaction with sexual function is a relatively common complaint among patients and their partners.[142–144]

Issues include decreased libido, sexual arousal, and sexual satisfaction; impaired erection and ejaculation; or decreased vaginal lubrication. Social and psychological factors are key. These issues should be addressed during rehabilitation. On occasion, sexual dysfunction is secondary to other medical problems, such as diabetes mellitus or neuropathy, or secondary to medications. If appropriate, medications to help sexual function can be administered but these agents should be prescribed with caution especially if the patient has hypertension or heart disease.

Quality of Life Issues

Most patients consider their health worse following stroke.[145] This finding should not be surprising. Patients lose independence and their status in the family and society declines. All aspects of life, including work and social activities, are altered.[146,147] In addition to the obvious neurological deficits and changes in life, many patients develop emotional problems including anxiety, decreased self-esteem, decreased energy, irritability, or depression, which lessen the quality of life.[148–151] Some patients have severe psychological or social problems such as social withdrawal, apathy, emotionality, apathy, or self-neglect.[152–154] These consequences should be addressed as the person returns to society. Planning for long-term measures to improve the patient's psychological symptoms by providing adequate support is important.[155] Medications or counseling may be needed. Psychological and social interventions and education also can help the transition. Close communication with the patient and family by health care professionals is particularly important.

REFERENCES

1. Gresham GE, Duncan PW, Stason WB, et al. Post-stroke rehabilitation. *Clinical Practice Guideline, No. 16.* Rockville, MD: U.S. Department of Health and Human Services, 1995.
2. Wade DT. Stroke: rehabilitation and long-term care. *Lancet* 1992;339:791–793.
3. Cifu DX, Stewart DG. Factors affecting functional outcome after stroke: a critical review of rehabilitation interventions. *Arch Phys Med Rehabil* 1999;80:S35–S39.
4. Jorgensen HS, Kammersgaard LP, Houth J, et al. Who benefits from treatment and rehabilitation in a stroke unit? A community-based study. *Stroke* 2000;31:434–439.
5. Wood-Dauphinee S, Shapiro S, Bass E, et al. A randomized trial of team care following stroke. *Stroke* 1984;15:864–872.
6. Alexander MP. Stroke rehabilitation outcome. A potential use of predictive variables to establish levels of care. *Stroke* 1994;25:128–134.

7. Wade DT, Hewer RL, Wood VA. Stroke: influence of patient's sex and side of weakness on outcome. *Arch Phys Med Rehabil* 1984;65:513–516.

8. Paolucci S, Antonucci G, Gialloreti LE, et al. Predicting stroke inpatient rehabilitation outcome: the prominent role of neuropsychological disorders. *Eur Neurol* 1996; 36:385–390.

9. Dombovy ML. Understanding stroke recovery and rehabilitation: current and emerging approaches. *Curr Neurol Neurosci Rep* 2004;4:31–35.

10. Kwakkel G, Wagenaar RC, Kollen BJ, Lankhorst GJ. Predicting disability in stroke—a critical review of the literature. *Age Ageing* 1996;25:479–489.

11. Deutsch A, Granger CV, Heinemann AW, et al. Poststroke rehabilitation. Outcomes and reimbursement of inpatient rehabilitation facilities and subacute rehabilitationprograms. *Stroke* 2006;37:1477–1482.

12. Black-Schaffer RM, Kirsteins AE, Harvey RL. Stroke rehabilitation. 2. Co-morbidities and complications. *Arch Phys Med Rehabil* 1999;80:S8–16.

13. Roth EJ, Mueller K, Green D. Stroke rehabilitation outcome: impact of coronary artery disease. *Stroke* 1988;19: 42–47.

14. Roth EJ. Heart disease in patients with stroke. Part II: impact and implications for rehabilitation. *Arch Phys Med Rehabil* 1994;75:94–101.

15. Tirschwell DL, Kukull WA, Longstreth WT, Jr. Medical complications of ischemic stroke and length of hospital stay: experience in Seattle, Washington. *J Stroke Cerebrovasc Dis* 1999;8:336–343.

16. Novack TA, Satterfield WT, Lyons K, Kolski G, Hackmeyer L, Connor M. Stroke onset and rehabilitation: time lag as a factor in treatment outcome. *Arch Phys Med Rehabil* 1984;65:316–319.

17. Slade A, Tennant A, Chamberlain MA. A randomised controlled trial to determine the effect of intensity of therapy upon length of stay in a neurological rehabilitation setting. *J Rehabil Med* 2002;34:260–266.

18. Kalra L, Yu G, Wilson K, Roots P. Medical complications during stroke rehabilitation. *Stroke* 1995;26:990–994.

19. Dromerick A, Reding M. Medical and neurological complications during inpatient stroke rehabilitation. *Stroke* 1994;25:358–361.

20. Gladman JR, Lincoln NB, Barer DH. A randomised controlled trial of domiciliary and hospital-based rehabilitation for stroke patients after discharge from hospital. *J Neurol Neurosurg Psychiatry* 1993;56:960–966.

21. Brown RD, Jr., Ransom J, Hass S, et al. Use of nursing home after stroke and dependence on stroke severity: a population-based analysis. *Stroke* 1999;30:924–929.

22. Werner RA, Kessler S. Effectiveness of an intensive outpatient rehabilitation program for postacute stroke patients. *Am J Phys Med Rehabil* 1996;75:114–120.

23. Marsh M. A day rehabilitation stroke program. *Arch Phys Med Rehabil* 1984;65:320–323.

24. Baskett JJ, Broad JB, Reekie G, Hocking C, Green G. Shared responsibility for ongoing rehabilitation: a new approach to home-based therapy after stroke. *Clin Rehabil* 1999;13: 23–33.

25. Young A. Assessment for rehabilitation after stroke. *Ann Acad Med Singapore* 1988;17:267–274.

26. Andersen HE, Eriksen K, Brown A, Schultz-Larsen K, Forchhammer BH. Follow-up services for stroke survivors after hospital discharge—a randomized control study. *Clin Rehabil* 2002;16:593–603.

27. Outpatient Service Trialists. Rehabilitation therapy services for stroke patients living at home: systematic review of randomised trials. *Lancet* 2004;363:352–356.

28. Wechsler LR, Kondziolka D. Cell therapy: replacement. *Stroke* 2003;34:2081–2082.

29. Wechsler LR. Stem cell transplantation for stroke. *Cleve Clin J Med* 2004;71(suppl 1):S40–S41.

30. Yenari MA, Zhao H, Giffard RG, Sobel RA, Sapolsky RM, Steinberg GK. Gene therapy and hypothermia for stroke treatment. *Ann N Y Acad Sci* 2003;993:54–68.

31. Bogousslavsky J, Victor SJ, Salinas EO, et al. Fiblast (trafermin) in acute stroke: results of the European–Australian phase II/III safety and efficacy trial. *Cerebrovasc Dis* 2002;14:239–251.

32. Wahlgren NG, Ahmed N. Neuroprotection in cerebral ischaemia: facts and fancies—the need for new approaches. *Cerebrovasc Dis* 2004;17(suppl 1):153–166.

33. Crisostomo EA, Duncan PW, Propst M, Dawson DV, Davis JN. Evidence that amphetamine with physical therapy promotes recovery of motor function in stroke patients. *Ann Neurol* 1988;23:94–97.

34. Walker-Batson D, Smith P, Curtis S, Unwin H, Greenlee R. Amphetamine paired with physical therapy accelerates motor recovery after stroke. Further evidence. *Stroke* 1995;26:2254–2259.

35. Martinsson L, Wahlgren NG. Safety of dexamphetamine in acute ischemic stroke: a randomized, double-blind, controlled dose-escalation trial. *Stroke* 2003;34: 475–481.

36. Treig T, Werner C, Sachse M, Hesse S. No benefit from D-amphetamine when added to physiotherapy after stroke: a randomized, placebo-controlled study. *Clin Rehabil* 2003;17:590–599.

37. Knecht S, Imai T, Kamping S, et al. D-amphetamine does not improve outcome of somatosensory training. *Neurology* 2001;57:2248–2252.

38. Martinsson L, Hardemark HG, Wahlgren NG. Amphetamines for improving stroke recovery. A systematic Cochrane review. *Stroke* 2003;34:2766.

39. Dam M, Tonin P, De Boni A, et al. Effects of fluoxetine and maprotiline on functional recovery in poststroke hemiplegic patients undergoing rehabilitation therapy. *Stroke* 1996;27:1211–1214.

40. Sze KH, Sim TC, Wong E, Cheng S, Woo J. Effect of nimodipine on memory after cerebral infarction. *Acta Neurol Scand* 1998;97:386–392.

41. Zorowitz RD, Smout RJ, Gassaway JA, Horn SD. Neurostimulant medication usage during stroke rehabilitation. The Post-Stroke Rehabilitation Outcomes Project (PSROP). *Top Stroke Rehabil* 2005;12:28–36.

42. Goldstein LB. Common drugs may influence motor recovery after stroke. The Sygen in Acute Stroke Study Investigators. *Neurology* 1995;45:865–871.

43. Goldstein LB. Potential effects of common drugs on stroke recovery. *Arch Neurol* 1998;55:454–456.

44. Clark MS, Smith DS. Psychological correlates of outcome following rehabilitation from stroke. *Clin Rehabil* 1999; 13:129–140.

45. Bourestom NC, Howard MT. Behavioral correlates of recovery of self-care in hemiplegic patients. *Arch Phys Med Rehabil* 1968;49:449–454.

46. Happe F, Brownell H, Winner E. Acquired "theory of mind" impairments following stroke. *Cognition* 1999; 70: 211–240.

47. Bowen A, Lincoln NB, Dewey M. Cognitive rehabilitation for spatial neglect following stroke. *Cochrane Database Syst Rev* 2002;CD003586.

48. Majid MJ, Lincoln NB, Weyman N. Cognitive rehabilitation for memory deficits following stroke. *Cochrane Database Syst Rev* 2000;CD002293.

49. Lincoln NB, Majid MJ, Weyman N. Cognitive rehabilitation for attention deficits following stroke. *Cochrane Database Syst Rev* 2000;CD002842.

50. Julkunen L, Tenovuo O, Jaaskelainen S, Hamalainen H. Rehabilitation of chronic post-stroke visual field defect with computer-assisted training: a clinical and neurophysiological study. *Restor Neurol Neurosci* 2003;21:19–28.

51. Perry L, McLaren S. Eating difficulties after stroke. *J Adv Nurs* 2003;43:360–369.

52. Ferro JM, Mariano G, Madureira S. Recovery from aphasia and neglect. *Cerebrovasc Dis* 1999;9(suppl 5):6–22.

53. Basso A, Capitani E, Vignolo LA. Influence of rehabilitation on language skills in aphasic patients. A controlled study. *Arch Neurol* 1979;36:190–196.

54. Selnes OA. Recovery from aphasia: activating the "right" hemisphere. *Ann Neurol* 1999;45:419–420.

55. Barrett AM, Crucian GP, Raymer AM, Heilman KM. Spared comprehension of emotional prosody in a patient with global aphasia. *Neuropsychiatry Neuropsychol Behav Neurol* 1999;12:117–120.

56. Greener J, Enderby P, Whurr R. Pharmacological treatment for aphasia following stroke. *Cochrane Database Syst Rev* 2001;CD000424.

57. David R, Enderby P, Bainton D. Treatment of acquired aphasia: speech therapists and volunteers compared. *J Neurol Neurosurg Psychiatry* 1982;45:957–961.

58. Greener J, Grant A. Beliefs about effectiveness of treatment for aphasia after stroke. *Int J Lang Commun Disord* 1998;33(suppl):162–163.

59. Greener J, Enderby P, Whurr R, Grant A. Treatment for aphasia following stroke: evidence for effectiveness. *Int J Lang Commun Disord* 1998;33(suppl):158–161.

60. Lincoln NB, Parry RH, Vass CD. Randomized, controlled trial to evaluate increased intensity of physiotherapy treatment of arm function after stroke. *Stroke* 1999; 30:573–579.

61. Lincoln NB, McGuirk E, Mulley GP, Lendrem W, Jones AC, Mitchell JR. Effectiveness of speech therapy for aphasic stroke patients. A randomised controlled trial. *Lancet* 1984;1197–1200.

62. Greener J, Enderby P, Whurr R. Speech and language therapy for aphasia following stroke. *Cochrane Database Syst Rev* 2001;CD000424.

63. Langhorne P, Wagenaar R, Partridge C. Physiotherapy after stroke: more is better? *Physiother Res Int* 1996;1:75–88.

64. Langhorne P. Intensity of rehabilitation: some answers and more questions? *J Neurol Neurosurg Psychiatry* 2002; 72:430–431.

65. Duncan P, Studenski S, Richards L, et al. Randomized clinical trial of therapeutic exercise in subacute stroke. *Stroke* 2003;34:2173–2180.

66. Miyai I, Yagura H, Hatakenaka M, Oda I, Konishi I, Kubota K. Longitudinal optical imaging study for locomotor recovery after stroke. *Stroke* 2003;34:2866–2870.

67. Parry RH, Lincoln NB, Vass CD. Effect of severity of arm impairment on response to additional physiotherapy early after stroke. *Clin Rehabil* 1999;13:187–198.

68. Bonita R, Beaglehole R. Recovery of motor function after stroke. *Stroke* 1988;19:1497–1500.

69. Chiu L, Shyu WC, Chen TR. A cost-effectiveness analysis of home care and community-based nursing homes for stroke patients and their families. *J Adv Nurs* 1997;26:872–878.

70. Duncan PW, Goldstein LB, Horner RD, et al. Similar motor recovery of upper and lower extremities after stroke. *Stroke* 1994;25:1181–1188.

71. Smith MT, Baer GD. Achievement of simple mobility milestones after stroke. *Arch Phys Med Rehabil* 1999;80:442–447.

72. Pollock A, Baer G, Pomeroy V, Langhorne P. Physiotherapy treatment approaches for the recovery of postural control and lower limb function following stroke. *Cochrane Database Syst Rev* 2003;CD001920.

73. Broeks JG, Lankhorst GJ, Rumping K, Prevo AJ. The long-term outcome of arm function after stroke: results of a follow-up study. *Disabil Rehabil* 1999;21:357–364.

74. Skilbeck CE, Wade DT, Hewer RL, Wood VA. Recovery after stroke. *J Neurol Neurosurg Psychiatry* 1983;46:5–8.

75. Wade DT, Collen FM, Robb GF, Warlow CP. Physiotherapy intervention late after stroke and mobility. *BMJ* 1992;304: 609–613.

76. Silvestrini M, Cupini LM, Placidi F, Diomedi M, Bernardi G. Bilateral hemispheric activation in the early recovery of motor function after stroke. *Stroke* 1998;29:1305–1310.

77. Seitz RJ, Azari NP, Knorr U, Binkofski F, Herzog H, Freund HJ. The role of diaschisis in stroke recovery. *Stroke* 1999;30:1844–1850.

78. Muellbacher W, Artner C, Mamoli B. The role of the intact hemisphere in recovery of midline muscles after recent monohemispheric stroke. *J Neurol* 1999;246:250–256.

79. Sveen U, Bautz-Holter E, Sodring KM, Wyller TB, Laake K. Association between impairments, self-care ability and social activities 1 year after stroke. *Disabil Rehabil* 1999; 21:372–377.

80. Harvey M, Milner AD. Residual perceptual distortion in "recovered" hemispatial neglect. *Neuropsychologia* 1999; 37:745–750.

81. Paolucci S, Antonucci G, Guariglia C, Magnotti L, Pizzamiglio L, Zoccolotti P. Facilitatory effect of neglect rehabilitation on the recovery of left hemiplegic stroke patients: a cross-over study. *J Neurol* 1996;243:308–314.

82. Ramachandran VS, Altschuler EL, Stone L, Al-Aboudi M, Schwartz E, Siva N. Can mirrors alleviate visual hemineglect? *Med Hypotheses* 1999;52:303–305.

83. De Q, I, Simon SR, Leurgans S, Pease WS, McAllister D. Gait pattern in the early recovery period after stroke. *J Bone Joint Surg Am* 1996;78:1506–1514.

84. Dickstein R, Heffes Y, Laufer Y, Ben-Haim Z. Activation of selected trunk muscles during symmetric functional activities in poststroke hemiparetic and hemiplegic patients. *J Neurol Neurosurg Psychiatry* 1999;66:218–221.

85. Katz-Leurer M, Shochina M, Carmeli E, Friedlander Y. The influence of early aerobic training on the functional capacity in patients with cerebrovascular accident at the subacute stage. *Arch Phys Med Rehabil* 2003;84:1609–1614.

86. Macko RF, DeSouza CA, Tretter LD, et al. Treadmill aerobic exercise training reduces the energy expenditure and cardiovascular demands of hemiparetic gait in chronic stroke patients. A preliminary report. *Stroke* 1997;28:326–330.

87. da Cunha IT, Jr., Lim PA, Qureshy H, Henson H, Monga T, Protas EJ. Gait outcomes after acute stroke rehabilitation with supported treadmill ambulation training: a randomized controlled pilot study. *Arch Phys Med Rehabil* 2002;83:1258–1265.

88. Ada L, Dean CM, Hall JM, Bampton J, Crompton S. A treadmill and overground walking program improves walking in persons residing in the community after stroke: a placebo-controlled, randomized trial. *Arch Phys Med Rehabil* 2003;84:1486–1491.

89. Pohl PS, Winstein CJ. Practice effects on the less-affected upper extremity after stroke. *Arch Phys Med Rehabil* 1999;80:668–675.

90. Miltner WH, Bauder H, Sommer M, Dettmers C, Taub E. Effects of constraint-induced movement therapy on patients with chronic motor deficits after stroke: a replication. *Stroke* 1999;30:586–592.

91. Winstein CJ, Miller JP, Blanton S, et al. Methods for a multisite randomized trial to investigate the effect of constraint-induced movement therapy in improving upper extremity function among adults recovering from a cerebrovascular stroke. *Neurorehabil Neural Repair* 2003;17:137–152.

92. Page SJ, Sisto S, Johnston MV, Levine P. Modified constraint-induced therapy after subacute stroke: a preliminary study. *Neurorehabil Neural Repair* 2002;16:290–295.

93. Cauraugh JH, Kim SB. Stroke motor recovery: active neuromuscular stimulation and repetitive practice schedules. *J Neurol Neurosurg Psychiatry* 2003;74:1562–1566.

94. Moreland JD, Goldsmith CH, Huijbregts MP, et al. Progressive resistance strengthening exercises after stroke: a single-blind randomized controlled trial. *Arch Phys Med Rehabil* 2003;84:1433–1440.

95. Roper TA, Redford S, Tallis RC. Intermittent compression for the treatment of the oedematous hand in hemiplegic stroke: a randomized controlled trial. *Age Ageing* 1999;28:9–13.

96. Cambier DC, De Corte E, Danneels LA, Witvrouw EE. Treating sensory impairments in the post-stroke upper limb with intermittent pneumatic compression. Results of a preliminary trial. *Clin Rehabil* 2003;17:14–20.

97. Muellbacher W, Richards C, Ziemann U, et al. Improving hand function in chronic stroke. *Arch Neurol* 2002;59:1278–1282.

98. Wolf SL. Use of biofeedback in the treatment of stroke patients. *Stroke* 1990;21:II22–II23

99. Glanz M, Klawansky S, Stason W, et al. Biofeedback therapy in poststroke rehabilitation: a meta-analysis of the randomized controlled trials. *Arch Phys Med Rehabil* 1995;76:508–515.

100. Magnusson M, Johansson K, Johansson BB. Sensory stimulation promotes normalization of postural control after stroke. *Stroke* 1994;25:1176–1180.

101. Yu DT, Chae J, Walker ME, et al. Intramuscular neuromuscular electric stimulation for poststroke shoulder pain: a multicenter randomized clinical trial. *Arch Phys Med Rehabil* 2004;85:695–704.

102. Price CIM, Pandyan AD. Electrical stimulation for preventing and treating post-stroke shoulder pain. *Cochrane Database Syst Rev* 2000;CD001698.

103. Volpe BT, Krebs HI, Hogan N, Edelsteinn L, Diels CM, Aisen ML. Robot training enhanced motor outcome in patients with stroke maintained over 3 years. *Neurology* 1999;53:1874–1876.

104. Fasoli SE, Krebs HI, Stein J, Frontera WR, Hogan N. Effects of robotic therapy on motor impairment and recovery in chronic stroke. *Arch Phys Med Rehabil* 2003;84:477–482.

105. Powell J, Pandyan AD, Granat M, Cameron M, Stott DJ. Electrical stimulation of wrist extensors in poststroke hemiplegia. *Stroke* 1999;30:1384–1389.

106. Kraft GH, Fitts SS, Hammond MC. Techniques to improve function of the arm and hand in chronic hemiplegia. *Arch Phys Med Rehabil* 1992;73:220–227.

107. Hummelsheim H, Maier-Loth ML, Eickhof C. The functional value of electrical muscle stimulation for the rehabilitation of the hand in stroke patients. *Scand J Rehabil Med* 1997;29:3–10.

108. Kuan TS, Tsou JY, Su FC. Hemiplegic gait of stroke patients: the effect of using a cane. *Arch Phys Med Rehabil* 1999;80:777–784.

109. Al-Shahrani AM. Anti-spasticity medications. *Saudi Med J* 2003;24:19–22.

110. Rivas DA, Chancellor MB, Hill K, Freedman MK. Neurological manifestations of baclofen withdrawal. *J Urol* 1993;150:1903–1905.

111. Ochs GA. Intrathecal baclofen. *Baillieres Clin Neurol* 1993;2:73–86.

112. Albright AL, Barron WB, Fasick MP, Polinko P, Janosky J. Continuous intrathecal baclofen infusion for spasticity of cerebral origin. *JAMA* 1993;270:2475–2477.

113. Francisco GE, Boake C. Improvement in walking speed in poststroke spastic hemiplegia after intrathecal baclofen therapy: a preliminary study. *Arch Phys Med Rehabil* 2003;84:1194–1199.

114. Ward A, Chaffman MO, Sorkin EM. Dantrolene. A review of its pharmacodynamic and pharmacokinetic properties and therapeutic use in malignant hyperthermia, the neuroleptic malignant syndrome and an update of its use in muscle spasticity. *Drugs* 1986;32:130–168.

115. Katrak PH, Cole AM, Paulos CJ, McCauley JC. Objective assessment of spasticity, strength, and function with early exhibition of dantrolene sodium after cerebrovascular

accident: a randomized double-blind study. *Arch Phys Med Rehabil* 1992;73:4–9.

116. Simpson DM, Alexander DN, O'Brien CF, et al. Botulinum toxin type A in the treatment of upper extremity spasticity: a randomized, double-blind, placebo-controlled trial. *Neurology* 1996;46:1306–1310.

117. Burbaud P, Wiart L, Dubos JL, et al. A randomised, double blind, placebo controlled trial of botulinum toxin in the treatment of spastic foot in hemiparetic patients. *Neurol Neurosurg Psychiatry* 1996;61:265–269.

118. Hesse S, Krajnik J, Luecke D, Jahnke MT, Gregoric M, Mauritz KH. Ankle muscle activity before and after botulinum toxin therapy for lower limb extensor spasticity in chronic hemiparetic patients. *Stroke* 1996;27:455–460.

119. Bhakta BB, Cozens JA, Bamford JM, Chamberlain MA. Use of botulinum toxin in stroke patients with severe upper limb spasticity. *J Neurol Neurosurg Psychiatry* 1996;61: 30–35.

120. Brashear A, McAfee AL, Kuhn ER, Fyffe J. Botulinum toxin type B in upper-limb poststroke spasticity: a double-blind, placebo-controlled trial. *Arch Phys Med Rehabil* 2004;85:705–709.

121. Pittock SJ, Morre AP, Hardiman O, et al. A double-blind randomised placebo-controlled evaluation of three doses of botulinum toxin type A (Dysport®) in the treatment of spastic equinovarus deformity after stroke. *Cerebrovasc Dis* 2003;15:289–300.

122. Brashear A, Gordon MF, Elovic E, et al. Intramuscular injection of botulinum toxin for the treat of wrist and finger spasticity after a stroke. *N Engl J Med* 2002;347: 395–400.

123. Johnson CA, Burridge JH, Strike PW, Wood DE, Swain ID. The effect of combined use of botulinum toxin type A and functional electric stimulation in the treatment of spastic drop foot after stroke: a preliminary investigation. *Arch Phys Med Rehabil* 2004;85:902–909.

124. Dimitrijevic MR, Sherwood AM. Spasticity: medical and surgical treatment. *Neurology* 1980;30:19–27.

125. Walker MF, Gladman JR, Lincoln NB, Siemonsma P, Whiteley T. Occupational therapy for stroke patients not admitted to hospital: a randomised controlled trial. *Lancet* 1999;354:278–280.

126. Rodgers H, Mackintosh J, Price C, et al. Does an early increased-intensity interdisciplinary upper limb therapy programme following acute stroke improve outcome? *Clin Rehabil* 2003;17:579–589.

127. Smurawska LT, Alexandrov AV, Bladin CF, Norris JW. Cost of acute stroke care in Toronto, Canada. *Stroke* 1994;25: 1628–1631.

128. Bishop DS, Evans RL. Family functioning assessment techniques in stroke. *Stroke* 1990;21:II50–II51.

129. Han B, Haley WE. Family caregiving for patients with stroke. *Stroke* 1999;30:1478–1485.

130. Noonan WC, Evans RL, Hendricks R. Using personal and family variates to predict patients' adjustment after stroke. *Psychol Rep* 1988;63:247–251.

131. Van Heutgen C, Visser-Meily A, Post M, Lindeman E. Care for cares of stroke patients. Evidence-based clinical practice guidelines. *J Rehabil Med* 2006;38:153–158.

132. Forsberg-Warleby G, Moller A, Blomstrand C. Life satisfaction in spouses of patients with stroke during the first year of stroke. *J Rehabil Med* 2004;36:4–11.

133. Basmajian JV, Gowland CA, Finlayson MA, et al. Stroke treatment: comparison of integrated behavioral-physical therapy vs traditional physical therapy programs. *Arch Phys Med Rehabil* 1987;68:267–272.

134. Forster A, Smith J, Young J, Knapp P, House A, Wright J. Information provision for stroke patients and their caregivers. *Cochrane Database Syst Rev* 2001;CD001919.

135. Dennis M, O'Rourke S, Lewis S, Sharpe M, Warlow C. A quantitative study of the emotional outcome of people caring for stroke survivors. *Stroke* 1998;29: 1867–1872.

136. Wilson DB, Houle DM, Keith RA. Stroke rehabilitation: a model predicting return home. *West J Med* 1991;154: 587–590.

137. Legh-Smith J, Wade DT, Langton-Hewer R. Services for stroke patients one year after stroke. *J Epidemiol Community Health* 1986;40:161–165.

138. Black-Schaffer RM, Osberg JS. Return to work after stroke: development of a predictive model. *Arch Phys Med Rehabil* 1990;71:285–290.

139. Wozniak M, Kittner SJ. Return to work after ischemic stroke: a methodological review. *Neuroepidemiology* 2002; 21:159–166.

140. Flick CL. Stroke rehabilitation. 4. Stroke outcome and psychosocial consequences. *Arch Phys Med Rehabil* 1999;80: S21–S26.

141. Legh-Smith J, Wade DT, Hewer RL. Driving after a stroke. *J R Soc Med* 1986;79:200–203.

142. Korpelainen JT, Kauhanen M-L, Kemola H, Malinen U, Myllya VV. Sexual dysfunction in stroke patients. *Acta Neurol Scand* 1998;98:400–405.

143. Korpelainen JT, Nieminen P, Myllya VV. Sexual functioning among stroke patients and their spouses. *Stroke* 1999; 30:715–719.

144. Monga TN, Lawson JS, Inglis J. Sexual dysfunction in stroke patients. *Arch Phys Med Rehabil* 1986;67:19–22.

145. Duncan PW, Samsa GP, Weinberger M, et al. Health status of individuals with mild stroke. *Stroke* 1997;28: 740–745.

146. Gresham GE, Kelly-Hayes M, Wolf PA, et al. Survival and functional status 20 or more years after first stroke: the Framingham Study. *Stroke* 1998;29:793–797.

147. Naess H, Waje-Andreassen U, Thomassen L, Nyland H, Myhr KM. Health-related quality of life among young adults with ischemic stroke on long-term follow-up. *Stroke* 2006;37:1232–1236.

148. Williams LS, Weinberger M, Harris LE, Biller J. Measuring quality of life in a way that is meaningful to stroke patients. *Neurology* 1999;53:1839–1843.

149. Chang AM, Mackenzie AE. State self-esteem following stroke. *Stroke* 1998;29:2325–2328.

150. Astrom M, Adolfsson R, Asplund K. Major depression in stroke patients. *Stroke* 1993;24:976–982.

151. Ahlsio B, Britton M, Murray V, Theorell T. Disablement and quality of life after stroke. *Stroke* 1984;15: 886–890.

152. Angeleri F, Angeleri VA, Foschi N, Giaquinto S, Nolfe G. The influence of depression, social activity, and family stress on functional outcome after stroke. *Stroke* 1993; 24:1478–1483.

153. Neau JP, Ingrand P, Mouille-Brachet C, et al. Functional recovery and social outcome after cerebral infarction in young adults. *Cerebrovasc Dis* 1998;8: 296–302.

154. Jonkman EJ, de Weerd AW, Vrijens NL. Quality of life after a first ischemic stroke. Long-term developments and correlations with changes in neurological deficit, mood and cognitive impairment. *Acta Neurol Scand* 1998;98:169–75.

155. Evans RL, Bishop DS. Psychosocial outcomes in stroke survivors. Implications for research. *Stroke* 1990; II48–II49.

INDEX